THE COMPLETE LEARNING DISABILITIES RESOURCE GUIDE

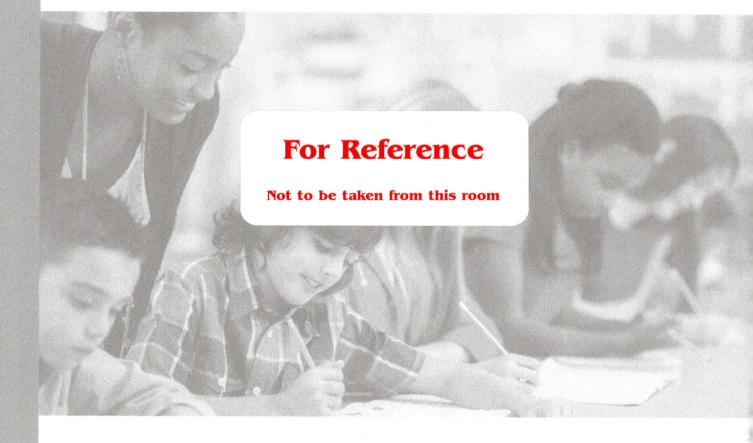

2019
TWENTY-FIRST EDITION

THE COMPLETE LEARNING DISABILITIES RESOURCE GUIDE

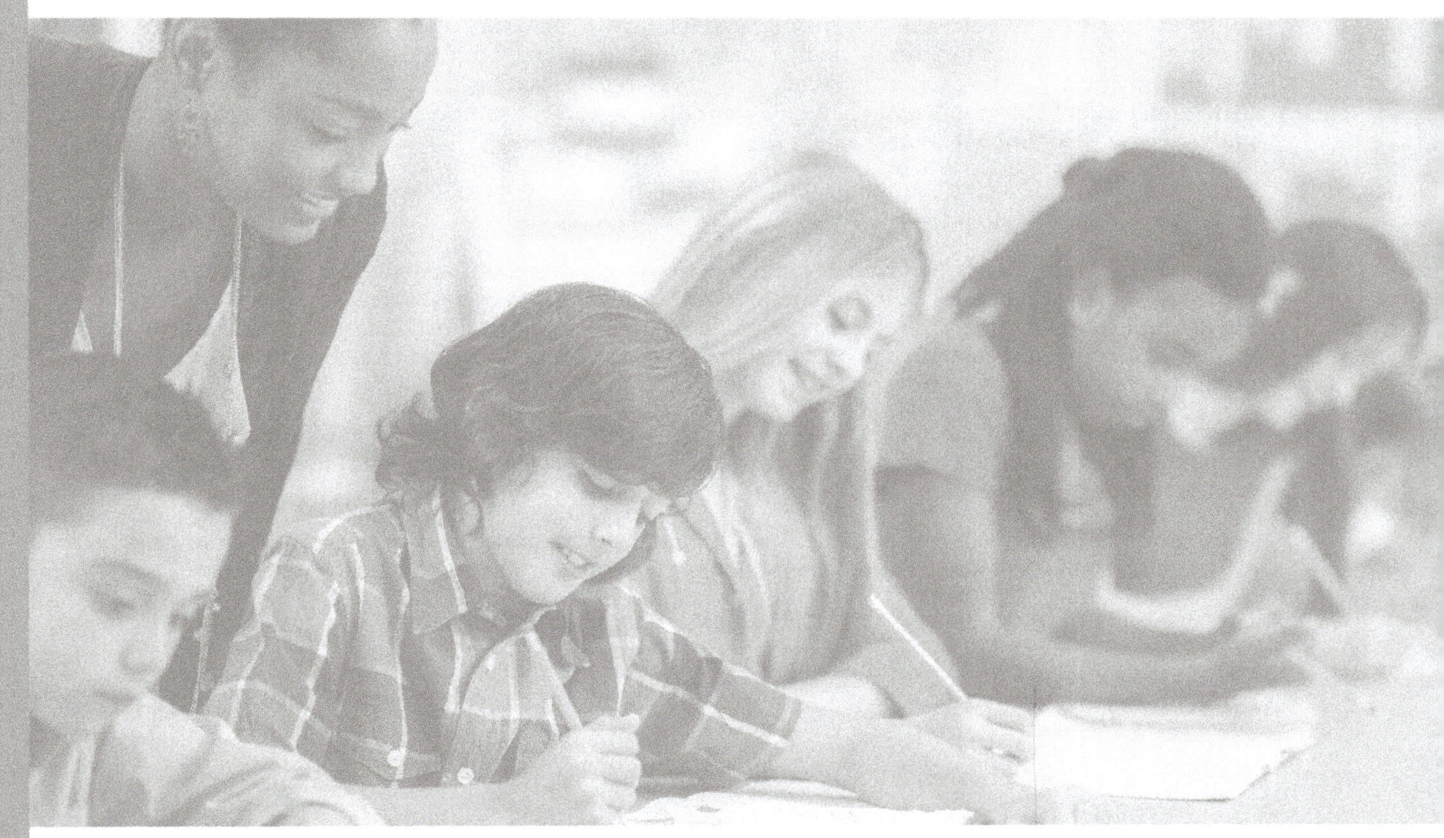

A SEDGWICK PRESS BOOK
GREY HOUSE PUBLISHING

PRESIDENT: Richard Gottlieb
PUBLISHER: Leslie Mackenzie
EDITORIAL DIRECTOR: Laura Mars
PRODUCTION MANAGER & COMPOSITION: Kristen Hayes
ASSOCIATE EDITORS: Melanie Benard, Olivia Parsonson
MARKETING DIRECTOR: Jessica Moody

A Sedgewick Press Book
Grey House Publishing, Inc.
4919 Route 22
Amenia, NY 12501
518.789.8700
FAX 845.373.6390
www.greyhouse.com
e-mail: books@greyhouse.com

While every effort has been made to ensure the reliability of the information presented in this publication, Grey House Publishing neither guarantees the accuracy of the data contained herein nor assumes any responsibility for errors, omissions or discrepancies. Grey House accepts no payment for listing; inclusion in the publication of any organization, agency, institution, publication, service or individual does not imply endorsement of the editors or publisher.

Errors brought to the attention of the publisher and verified to the satisfaction of the publisher will be corrected in future editions.

First edition published 1993
Twenty-first edition published 2018

Publisher's Cataloging-In-Publication Data
(Prepared by The Donohue Group, Inc.)

Names: Grey House Publishing, Inc., publisher.
Title: The complete learning disabilities resource guide : associations, products, resources, conferences, services, web sites.
Description: Amenia, NY : Grey House Publishing, 2018- | "A Sedgewick Press book." | Includes indexes.
Subjects: LCSH: Learning disabled--Services for--Directories. | Developmentally disabled--Services for--Directories. | Special education--Directories. | LCGFT: Directories.
Classification: LCC LC4704.6 .C65 | DDC 371.9025--dc23

Table of Contents

Introduction

The Complete Learning Disabilities Resource Guide (formerly *The Complete Learning Disabilities Directory*) has been a comprehensive and sought-after resource for professionals, families and individuals with learning disabilities since 1992. This twenty-first edition is the most comprehensive and current source of resources for the LD community available today, and a continual National Health Information Awards Winner for providing "...the Nation's Best Consumer Health Information Programs and Materials in the category of Health Promotion/ Disease and Injury Prevention Information."

The Complete Learning Disabilities Resource Guide supports the LD population, from those with a learning disability to their support network, in a number of ways. This edition starts with valuable front matter—both statistics about children and adults with learning disabilities—and a summary report from the National Center for Learning Disabilities (NCLSD). The report includes information about:

1. Understanding Learning and Attention Issues
2. Identifying Struggling Students
3. Supporting Academic Success
4. Social, Emotional and Behaviorial Challenges
5. Transitioning to Life After High School
6. Recommended Policy Changes

This twenty-first edition, with 4,614 listings, provides a comprehensive look at the variety of resources available for the many different types of learning disabilities, from those that occur in spoken language, to those that affect organizational skills. It includes a wide array of testing resources, crucial for early diagnosis, and is arranged in subject-specific chapters for quick, effective research.

The Table of Contents is your guide to this database in print form. *The Complete Learning Disabilities Resource Guide* is arranged into 21 major chapters and 100 subchapters, making it easy to pinpoint the exact type of desired reference, including Associations, National/State Programs, Publications, Audio/Video, Web Sites, Products, Conferences, Schools, Learning/Testing Centers, and Summer Programs. Listings provide thousands of valuable contact points, including 4,339 key executives, web sites, fax numbers, descriptions, founding year, designed-for age products, and size of LD population for schools.

With valuable information for not only those individuals with LD, but also for parents, teachers and professionals, this edition offers answers to legal and advocacy questions, as well as specially designed computer software and a full range of assistive devices. *The Complete Learning Disabilities Resource Guide* gives you the confidence that this one resource is all you need. It assures those in the LD community that this crucial information is readily available at every school and library across the country, not just at state or district level special education resource centers. Now, every special education teacher, student, and parent can have, right at their fingertips, a wealth of information on the critical resources that are available to help individuals achieve in school and in their community.

This valuable resource includes three indexes: Entry Name & Publisher, Geographic, and Subject.

Praise for previous editions:

> *"This is a must-have resource for individuals who work with people with different types of learning disabilities. . . . any professional, parent, or student wanting to learn more. This is by far the best of all the resources available for learning disabled individuals. No need to search the Internet to find this information; this book provides it all at your fingertips!"*
>
> —Doody's Review Service

> *"This title would be a tremendous asset to any professional, parent, or student who seeks to deepen their knowledge about challenges and rewards of recognizing different learning styles and behaviours which may one day not be seen as a 'disability.'"*
>
> —Pinnacle Health System

> *"By virtue of its size, comprehensiveness, and frequency of updates, this directory stands out as a singularly important resource for academic and public libraries. It is highly recommended."*
>
> —ARBA

Data in *The Complete Learning Disabilities Resource Guide* is also available for subscription on G.O.L.D.—Grey House OnLine Databases. Subscribers to G.O.L.D. can access their subscription via the Internet and do customized searches that make finding information quicker and easier. Visit http://gold.greyhouse.com for more information.

Learning Disabilities: Condition Information

What are learning disabilities?

Learning disabilities are conditions that affect how a person learns to read, write, speak, and calculate numbers. They are caused by differences in brain structure and affect the way a person's brain processes information.[1]

Learning disabilities are usually discovered after a child begins attending school and has difficulties in one or more subjects that do not improve over time. A person can have more than one learning disability.[2] Learning disabilities can last a person's entire life, but they may be alleviated with the right educational supports.[3]

A learning disability is not an indication of a person's intelligence. Also, learning disabilities are not the same as learning problems due to intellectual and developmental disabilities, or emotional, vision, hearing, or motor skills problems.[4]

Some of the most common learning disabilities include the following:

- **Dyslexia.** This condition causes problems with language skills, particularly reading. People with dyslexia may have difficulty spelling, understanding sentences, and recognizing words they already know.[5]
- **Dysgraphia.** People with dysgraphia have problems with their handwriting. They may have problems forming letters, writing within a defined space, and writing down their thoughts.[6,7]
- **Dyscalculia.** People with this math learning disability may have difficulty understanding arithmetic concepts and doing such tasks as addition, multiplication, and measuring.[8]
- **Dyspraxia.** This condition, also termed sensory integration disorder, involves problems with motor coordination that lead to poor balance and clumsiness. Poor hand-eye coordination also causes difficulty with fine motor tasks such as putting puzzles together and coloring within the lines.[9]
- **Apraxia of speech.** Sometimes called verbal apraxia, this disorder involves problems with speaking. People with this disorder have trouble saying what they want to say correctly and consistently.[10]
- **Central auditory processing disorder.** People with this condition have trouble understanding and remembering language-related tasks. They have difficulty explaining things, understanding jokes, and following directions. They confuse words and are easily distracted.[11]
- **Nonverbal learning disorders.** People with these conditions have strong verbal skills but great difficulty understanding facial expression and body language. In addition, they are physically clumsy and have trouble generalizing and following multistep directions.[12]
- **Visual perceptual/visual motor deficit.** People with this condition mix up letters; they might confuse "m" and "w" or "d" and "b," for example. They may also lose their place while reading, copy inaccurately, write messily, and cut paper clumsily.[13]
- **Aphasia.** Aphasia (pronounced *uh-FEY-zhuh*), also called dysphasia (pronounced *dis-FEY-zhuh*), is a language disorder. A person with this disorder has difficulty understanding spoken language, poor reading comprehension, trouble with writing, and great difficulty finding words to express thoughts and feelings.[14]Aphasia occurs when the language areas of the brain are damaged. In

adults, it often is caused by stroke, but children may get aphasia from a brain tumor, head injury, or brain infection.[15]

What are the indicators of learning disabilities?

Many children have difficulty with reading, writing, or other learning-related tasks at some point, but this does not mean they have learning disabilities. A child with a learning disability often has several related signs, and these persist over time. The signs of learning disabilities vary from person to person. Common signs that a person may have learning disabilities include the following:

- Difficulty with reading and/or writing
- Problems with math skills
- Difficulty remembering
- Problems paying attention
- Trouble following directions
- Poor coordination
- Difficulty with concepts related to time
- Problems staying organized[1]

A child with a learning disability also may exhibit one or more of the following[2]:

- Impetuous behavior
- Inappropriate responses in school or social situations
- Difficulty staying on task (easily distracted)
- Difficulty finding the right way to say something
- Inconsistent school performance
- Immature way of speaking
- Difficulty listening well
- Problems dealing with new things in life
- Problems understanding words or concepts

These signs alone are not enough to determine that a person has a learning disability. A professional assessment is necessary to diagnose a learning disability.

Each learning disability has its own signs. Also, not every person with a particular disability will have all of the signs of that disability.

Children being taught in a second language that they are learning sometimes act in ways that are similar to the behaviors of someone with a learning disability. For this reason, learning disability assessment must take into account whether a student is bilingual or a second language learner.

Below are some common learning disabilities and the signs associated with them:

Dyslexia

People with dyslexia usually have trouble making the connections between letters and sounds and with spelling and recognizing words.[3]

People with dyslexia often show other signs of the condition. These may include[4,5]:

- Failure to fully understand what others are saying
- Difficulty organizing written and spoken language
- Delayed ability to speak
- Poor self-expression (for example, saying "thing" or "stuff" for words not recalled)
- Difficulty learning new vocabulary, either through reading or hearing
- Trouble learning foreign languages
- Slowness in learning songs and rhymes
- Slow reading as well as giving up on longer reading tasks
- Difficulty understanding questions and following directions
- Poor spelling
- Difficulty recalling numbers in sequence (for example, telephone numbers and addresses)
- Trouble distinguishing left from right

Dysgraphia

Dysgraphia is characterized by problems with writing. This disorder may cause a child to be tense and awkward when holding a pen or pencil, even to the extent of contorting his or her body. A child with very poor handwriting that he or she does not outgrow may have dysgraphia.[6]

Other signs of this condition may include [6]:

- A strong dislike of writing and/or drawing
- Problems with grammar
- Trouble writing down ideas
- A quick loss of energy and interest while writing
- Trouble writing down thoughts in a logical sequence
- Saying words out loud while writing
- Leaving words unfinished or omitting them when writing sentences

Dyscalculia

Signs of this disability include problems understanding basic arithmetic concepts, such as fractions, number lines, and positive and negative numbers.

Other symptoms may include[7]:

- Difficulty with math-related word problems
- Trouble making change in cash transactions
- Messiness in putting math problems on paper
- Trouble recognizing logical information sequences (for example, steps in math problems)
- Trouble with understanding the time sequence of events
- Difficulty with verbally describing math processes

Dyspraxia

A person with dyspraxia has problems with motor tasks, such as hand-eye coordination, that can interfere with learning.

Some other symptoms of this condition include[7]:

- Problems organizing oneself and one's things
- Breaking things
- Trouble with tasks that require hand-eye coordination, such as coloring within the lines, assembling puzzles, and cutting precisely
- Poor balance
- Sensitivity to loud and/or repetitive noises, such as the ticking of a clock
- Sensitivity to touch, including irritation over bothersome-feeling clothing

How many people are affected/at risk for learning disabilities?

There is a wide range in estimates of the number of people affected by learning disabilities and disorders. Some of the variation results from differences in requirements for diagnosis in different states.

Some reports estimate that as many as 15% to 20% of Americans are affected by learning disabilities and disorders.[1] In contrast, a major national study found that approximately 5% of children in the United States had learning disabilities. It also found that approximately 4% had both a learning disability and attention deficit/hyperactivity disorder (ADHD). Other research, conducted in 2006, estimated that 4.6 million school-age children in the United States have been diagnosed with learning disabilities.[2]

What causes it?

Researchers do not know exactly what causes learning disabilities, but they appear to be related to differences in brain structure. These differences are present from birth and often are inherited. To improve understanding of learning disabilities, researchers at the NICHD and elsewhere are studying areas of the brain and how they function. Scientists have found that learning disabilities are related to areas of the brain that deal with language[1] and have used imaging studies to show that the brain of a dyslexic person develops and functions differently from a typical brain.[2]

Sometimes, factors that affect a developing fetus, such as alcohol or drug use, can lead to a learning disability. Other factors in an infant's environment may play a role as well. These can include poor nutrition and exposure to toxins such as lead in water or paint. In addition, children who do not receive the support necessary to promote their intellectual development early on may show signs of learning disabilities once they start school.[3]

Sometimes a person may develop a learning disability later in life. Possible causes in such a case include dementia or a traumatic brain injury (TBI).[4]

How is it diagnosed?

Learning disabilities are often identified when a child begins to attend school. Educators may use a process called "response to intervention" (RTI) to help identify children with learning disabilities. Specialized testing is required to make a clear diagnosis, however.

RTI

RTI usually involves the following[1]:

- Monitoring all students' progress closely to identify possible learning problems
- Providing a child identified as having problems with help on different levels, or tiers
- Moving this youngster through the tiers as appropriate, increasing educational assistance if the child does not show progress

Students who are struggling in school can also have individual evaluations. An evaluation can[2]:

- Identify whether a child has a learning disability
- Determine a child's eligibility under federal law for special education services
- Help construct an individualized education plan (IEP) that outlines supports for a youngster who qualifies for special education services
- Establish a benchmark for measuring the child's educational progress

A full evaluation for a learning disability includes the following[3]:

- A medical examination, including a neurological exam, to identify or rule out other possible causes of the child's difficulties, including emotional disorders, intellectual and developmental disabilities, and brain diseases
- Exploration of the youngster's developmental, social, and school performance
- A discussion of family history
- Academic achievement testing and psychological assessment

Usually, several specialists work as a team to perform an evaluation. The team may include a psychologist, special education expert, and speech-language pathologist (SLP). Many schools also have reading specialists on staff who can help diagnosis a reading disability.[4]

Role of School Psychologists

School psychologists are trained in both education and psychology. They can help to identify students with learning disabilities and can diagnose the learning disability. They can also help the student with the disability, parents, and teachers come up with plans that improve learning.[5]

Role of SLPs

All SLPs are trained in diagnosing and treating speech- and language-related disorders. A SLP can provide a complete language evaluation as well as an assessment of the child's ability to organize his or her thoughts and possessions. The SLP may evaluate various age-appropriate learning-related skills in the child, such as understanding directions, manipulating sounds, and reading and writing.[6]

Is there a cure for learning disabilities?

Learning disabilities have no cure, but early intervention can provide tools and strategies to lessen their effects. People with learning disabilities can be successful in school and work and in their personal lives. More information is available about interventions for learning disabilities.

What are the treatments for learning disabilities?

People with learning disabilities and disorders can learn strategies for coping with their disabilities. Getting help earlier increases the likelihood for success in school and later in life. If learning disabilities remain untreated, a child may begin to feel frustrated with schoolwork, which can lead to low self-esteem, depression, and other problems.[1]

Usually, experts work to help a child learn skills by building on the child's strengths and developing ways to compensate for the child's weaknesses.[2] Interventions vary depending on the nature and extent of the disability.

Special Education Services

Children diagnosed with learning and other disabilities can qualify for special educational services. The Individuals with Disabilities Education Improvement Act(IDEA) requires that the public school system provide free special education supports to children with disabilities.[3]

In most states, each child is entitled to these services beginning when he or she is 3 years old and extending through high school or until age 21, whichever comes first. The specific rules of IDEA for each state are available from the National Early Childhood Technical Assistance Center.

IDEA states that children must be taught in the least restrictive environments appropriate for them. This means the teaching environment should be designed to meet a child's specific needs and skills and should minimize restrictions on the youngster's access to typical learning experiences.

IEPs

A child who qualifies for special education services should receive his or her own Individualized Education Program, or IEP. This personalized and written education plan[4]:

- Lists individualized goals for the child
- Specifies the plan for services the youngster will receive
- Lists the specialists who will work with the child

Qualifying for Special Education

To qualify for special education services, a child must be evaluated by the school system and meet specific criteria outlined in federal and state guidelines. To learn how to have a child assessed for special services, parents and caregivers can contact a local school principal or special education coordinator. Parents can also visit these Web resources:

- The Parent Technical Assistance Center Network website
- The Parent Guide to IDEA

Interventions for Specific Learning Disabilities

Below are just a few examples of ways educators help children with specific learning disabilities.

Dyslexia[5]

- **Special teaching techniques.** These can include helping a child learn through multisensory experiences and by providing immediate feedback to strengthen a child's ability to recognize words.
- **Classroom modifications.** For example, teachers can give students with dyslexia extra time to finish tasks and provide taped tests that allow the child to hear the questions instead of reading them.
- **Use of technology.** Children with dyslexia may benefit from listening to books on tape or using word-processing programs with spell-check features.

Dysgraphia[6]

- **Special tools.** Teachers can offer oral exams, provide a note-taker, and/or allow the child to videotape reports instead of writing them.
- **Use of technology.** A child with dysgraphia can be taught to use word-processing programs or an audio recorder instead of writing by hand.
- **Other ways of reducing the need for writing.** Teachers can provide notes, outlines, and preprinted study sheets.

Dyscalculia[6]

- **Visual techniques.** For example, teachers can draw pictures of word problems and show the student how to use colored pencils to differentiate parts of problems.
- **Use of memory aids.** Rhymes and music are among the techniques that can be used to help a child remember math concepts.
- **Use of computers.** A child with dyscalculia can use a computer for drills and practice.

Dyspraxia[6]

- **Quiet learning environment.** To help a child deal with sensitivity to noise and distractions, educators can provide the youngster with a quiet place for tests, silent reading, and other tasks that require concentration.
- **Alerting the child in advance.** For example, a child who is sensitive to noise may benefit from knowing in advance about such events as fire drills and assemblies.
- **Occupational therapy.** Exercises that focus on the tasks of daily living can help a child with poor coordination.

Other Treatments

A child with a learning disability may struggle with low self-esteem, frustration, and other problems. Mental health professionals can help the youngster understand these feelings, develop coping tools, and build healthy relationships.

Children with learning disabilities sometimes have other conditions such as ADHD. These conditions require their own treatments, which may include therapy and medications.

Courtesy: *Eunice Kennedy Shriver* National Institute of Child Health and Human Development

Footnotes

Learning Disabilities: Condition Information

1. National Dissemination Center for Children with Disabilities. (2011). *Learning disabilities*. Retrieved June 26, 2012, from http://nichcy.org/wp-content/uploads/docs/fs7.pdf
2. National Institute of Neurological Disorders and Stroke. (2011). *NINDS learning disabilities information page*. Retrieved June 26, 2012, from https://www.ninds.nih.gov/Disorders/All-Disorders/Learning-Disabilities-Information-Page
3. LD OnLine. (n.d.). *What is a learning disability?* Retrieved June 26, 2012, from http://www.ldonline.org/ldbasics/whatisld
4. LD OnLine. (n.d.). *What is a learning disability?* Retrieved June 26, 2012, from http://www.ldonline.org/ldbasics/whatisld
5. International Dyslexia Association. (2008). *Dyslexia basics*. Retrieved June 21, 2012, from http://www.interdys.org/ewebeditpro5/upload/BasicsFactSheet.pdf
6. National Institute of Neurological Disorders and Stroke. (2011). *What is dysgraphia?* Retrieved June 26, 2012, from https://www.ninds.nih.gov/Disorders/All-Disorders/Dysgraphia-Information-Page
7. National Center for Learning Disabilities. (2010). *What is dysgraphia?* Retrieved June 26, 2012, from https://www.understood.org/en/learning-attention-issues/child-learning-disabilities/dysgraphia/understanding-dysgraphia
8. National Center for Learning Disabilities. (2010). *What is dyscalculia?* Retrieved June 26, 2012, from https://www.understood.org/en/learning-attention-issues/child-learning-disabilities/dyscalculia/understanding-dyscalculia
9. Learning Disabilities Association of America. (n.d.). *Dyspraxia*. Retrieved June 15, 2012, from http://ldaamerica.org/types-of-learning-disabilities/dyspraxia/
10. National Institute on Deafness and Other Communication Disorders. (2010). *Apraxia of speech*. Retrieved August 30, 2012, from http://www.nidcd.nih.gov/health/voice/Pages/apraxia.aspx
11. Learning Disabilities Association of America. (n.d.). *Central auditory processing disorder*. Retrieved June 15, 2012, from http://ldaamerica.org/types-of-learning-disabilities/auditory-processing-disorder/
12. Learning Disabilities Association of America. (n.d.). *Non-verbal learning disorders*. Retrieved June 15, 2012, from http://ldaamerica.org/types-of-learning-disabilities/non-verbal-learning-disabilities/
13. Learning Disabilities Association of America. (n.d.). *Visual perceptual/visual motor deficit*. Retrieved June 15, 2012, from http://ldaamerica.org/types-of-learning-disabilities/visual-perceptual-visual-motor-deficit/
14. Learning Disabilities Association of America. (n.d.). *Language disorders: Aphasia, dysphasia, or global aphasia*. Retrieved June 15, 2012, from http://ldaamerica.org/types-of-learning-disabilities/language-processing-disorder/
15. National Institute on Deafness and Other Communication Disorders. (2008). *Aphasia*. Retrieved June 29, 2012, from http://www.nidcd.nih.gov/health/voice/Pages/aphasia.aspx

What are the indicators of learning disabilities?

1. American Academy of Child and Adolescent Psychiatry. (2011). *Children with learning disabilities*. Retrieved June 26, 2012, from http://www.aacap.org/AACAP/Families_and_Youth/Facts_for_Families/FFF-Guide/Children-With-Learning-Disorders-016.aspx
2. Learning Disabilities Association of America. (n.d.). *Symptoms of learning disabilities*. Retrieved June 15, 2012, from http://www.ldaamerica.us/aboutld/parents/ld_basics/symptoms.asp
3. National Institute of Neurological Disorders and Stroke. (2011). *What is dyslexia?* Retrieved June 26, 2012, from https://www.ninds.nih.gov/Disorders/All-Disorders/Dyslexia-Information-Page
4. International Dyslexia Association. (2008). *Dyslexia basics*. Retrieved June 21, 2012, fromhttp://www.interdys.org/ewebeditpro5/upload/BasicsFactSheet.pdf (PDF - 43 KB)

5. American Speech-Language-Hearing Association. (n.d.). *Language-based learning disabilities*. Retrieved June 15, 2012, from http://www.asha.org/public/speech/disorders/LBLD.htm
6. National Center for Learning Disabilities. (2010). *What is dysgraphia?* Retrieved June 21, 2012, from https://www.understood.org/en/learning-attention-issues/child-learning-disabilities/dysgraphia/understanding-dysgraphia
7. Learning Disabilities Association of America. (n.d.). *Dyscalculia*. Retrieved June 15, 2012, from http://ldaamerica.org/types-of-learning-disabilities/dyscalculia/

How many people are affected/at risk for learning disabilities?

1. Department of Education. (2010). *Twenty-ninth annual report to congress on the implementation of the Individuals with Disabilities Education Act, Parts B and C. 2007*. Retrieved June 12, 2012, from http://www2.ed.gov/about/reports/annual/osep/2007/parts-b-c/
2. Pastor, P. N., & Reuben, C. A. (2008). Diagnosed attention deficit hyperactivity disorder and learning disability: United States, 2004-2006. *Vital and Health Statistics, 10*. Retrieved June 26, 2012, from http://www.cdc.gov/nchs/data/series/sr_10/Sr10_237.pdf (PDF - 327 KB)

What causes it?

1. American Speech-Language-Hearing Association. (n.d.). *Language-based learning disabilities: Causes and number*. Retrieved June 26, 2012, from http://www.asha.org/public/speech/disorders/LBLD.htm
2. American Speech-Language-Hearing Association. (2008). *Brain activity in those with dyslexia pre and post treatment: A review*. Retrieved June 17, 2012, from http://www.asha.org/Events/convention/handouts/2008/1794_Kors_Alicia
3. National Center for Learning Disabilities. (2012). *What are learning disabilities?*Retrieved June 26, 2012, from https://www.understood.org/en/learning-attention-issues/child-learning-disabilities
4. National Institute of Neurological Disorders and Stroke. (2011). *What is dyslexia?*Retrieved June 26, 2012, from https://www.ninds.nih.gov/Disorders/All-Disorders/Dyslexia-Information-Page

How is it diagnosed?

1. National Dissemination Center for Children with Disabilities. (2010). *Response to intervention*. Retrieved June 26, 2012, from http://nichcy.org/schools-administrators/rti#elements
2. Learning Disabilities Association of America. (2001). *Evaluation: What does it mean for your child?* Retrieved June 17, 2012, from http://ldaamerica.org/category/assessment-evaluation/assessment-evaluation-for-parents/
3. National Library of Medicine. (2010). *Developmental reading disorder*. Retrieved June 15, 2012, from http://www.nlm.nih.gov/medlineplus/ency/article/001406.htm
4. International Reading Association. (2010) *Teaching all children to read: The roles of a reading specialist*. A position statement of the International Reading Association. Retrieved August 30, 2012, from https://www.literacyworldwide.org/docs/default-source/where-we-stand/reading-specialist-position-statement.pdf
5. National Association of School Psychologists. (n.d.) *What is a school psychologist?* Retrieved August 30, 2012, from http://www.nasponline.org/about-school-psychology/who-are-school-psychologists
6. American Speech-Language-Hearing Association. (n.d.). *Language-based learning disabilities*. Retrieved June 15, 2012, from http://www.asha.org/public/speech/disorders/LBLD.htm

What are the treatments for learning disabilities?

1. American Speech-Language-Hearing Association. (n.d.). *Language-based learning disabilities: Benefits of speech-language pathology services*. Retrieved June 15, 2012, from http://www.asha.org/public/speech/disorders/LBLDslpBenefits.htm
2. National Institute of Neurological Disorders and Stroke. (2011). *NINDS learning disabilities information page*. Retrieved June 26, 2012, from https://www.ninds.nih.gov/Disorders/All-Disorders/Learning-Disabilities-Information-Page
3. Department of Education. (2010). *Building the legacy: IDEA 2004*. Retrieved January 28, 2011, from http://idea.ed.gov/
4. National Dissemination Center for Children with Disabilities. (n.d.). *10 basic steps in special education*. Retrieved January 28, 2011, from http://nichcy.org/schoolage/steps
5. International Dyslexia Association. (2008). *Dyslexia basics*. Retrieved June 21, 2012, from http://www.interdys.org/ewebeditpro5/upload/BasicsFactSheet.pdf
6. Learning Disabilities Association of America. (n.d.). *Dysgraphia*. Retrieved June 16, 2012, from http://www.ldanatl.org/aboutld/parents/ld_basics/dysgraphia.asp

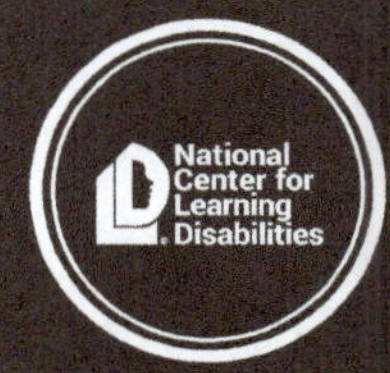

The State of Learning Disabilities: Understanding the 1 in 5

Executive Summary

Chapter 1: Understanding Learning and Attention Issues

Learning and attention issues are more common than many people think, affecting 1 in 5 children. With supportive policies and increased awareness among parents, educators and communities, these students can thrive academically, socially and emotionally.

SNAPSHOT

Children with learning and attention issues are as smart as their peers and, with the right support, can achieve at high levels. This chapter features a snapshot of learning and attention issues that includes:

- Risk factors
- Barriers to success
- Ways to help

Download the "1 in 5" Snapshot

NEUROSCIENCE

New research is deepening our understanding of the differences in brain structure and function in children with learning and attention issues. Brain scans and other tools are also helping researchers measure the biological impact that instructional interventions have on children who learn differently, including those with dyslexia, ADHD and other issues.

STIGMA

Recent surveys indicate widespread confusion and stigma:

- 33% of educators say that sometimes what people call a learning or attention issue is really just laziness.
- 43% of parents say that they wouldn't want others to know if their child had a learning disability.
- Doctors who recommend evaluating a child for learning and attention issues say parents follow their recommendation only 54% of the time.

FEDERAL LAWS AND FUNDING

Several laws, including some that were recently enacted, protect the rights of children and adults with disabilities and guarantee supports and services that can help improve outcomes for the 1 in 5. But these laws have never been adequately funded. In 2016, the federal government covered 16% of the extra cost of special education—far below the 40% that Congress promised to fund—leaving states to grapple with this multibillion-dollar shortfall.

DEFINITION

Learning and attention issues are brain-based difficulties in reading, writing, math, organization, focus, listening comprehension, social skills, motor skills or a combination of these. Learning and attention issues are not the result of low intelligence, poor vision or hearing, or lack of access to quality instruction.

Examples include:

- ADHD
- Dyscalculia
- Dysgraphia
- Dyslexia
- Dyspraxia
- Executive function deficits
- Nonverbal learning disabilities

PREVALENCE

1 in 5

children in the U.S. have learning and attention issues, but only a small subset are formally identified with a disability in school

1 in 16

public school students have Individualized Education Programs (IEPs) for specific learning disabilities (SLD) such as dyslexia and for other health impairments (OHI), the disability category that covers ADHD and dyspraxia

1 in 50

public school students receive accommodations for disabilities through a civil rights statute called Section 504

Chapter 2: Identifying Struggling Students

Early and accurate identification of learning disabilities and ADHD in schools can set struggling students on a path for success. But identification can be influenced by many factors—and too often is not happening early enough.

DISPARITIES IN SPECIAL EDUCATION IDENTIFICATION

Learning and attention issues affect children from all income levels and across all races and ethnicities. Yet low-income children, students of color and English language learners are more likely to be identified as having specific learning disabilities (SLD). Bias plays a key role in over- and underrepresentation.

SLD Identification by Income Level

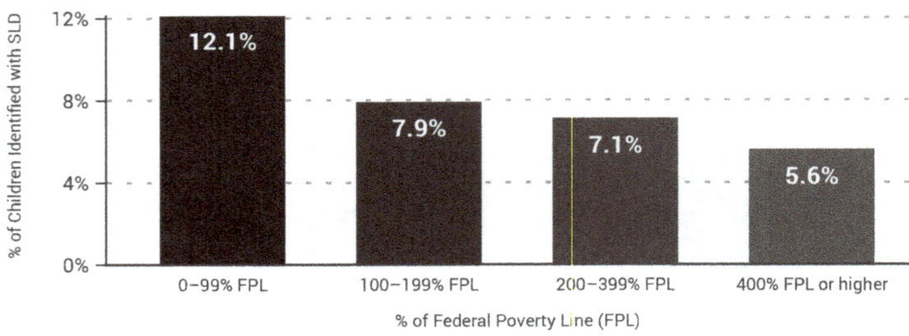

DELAYS IN SLD IDENTIFICATION

Learning disabilities don't suddenly appear in third grade. Researchers have noted that the achievement gap between typical readers and those with dyslexia is evident as early as first grade. But many students struggle for years before they are identified with SLD and receive needed support.

IDENTIFYING ADHD IN SCHOOLS

Though many children have ADHD, it's hard to tell how many have been identified in school as having a disability under the Individuals with Disabilities Education Act (IDEA). Federal guidance has made clear to states that when ADHD is the main reason students qualify for special education, they should be classified under Other Health Impairments (OHI). That category accounted for 15% of students receiving special education in 2015–2016, up from 11% in 2008–2009. (SLD remains the largest disability category, accounting for nearly 39% of students receiving special education in 2015–2016.)

Some students with ADHD may be receiving accommodations under Section 504 rather than IDEA, but Section 504 doesn't require schools to classify students by disability type. The percentage of students with 504 plans has nearly doubled since 2009.

OPPORTUNITIES

A multi-tier system of supports (MTSS) can help schools with early intervention and accurate identification. The Every Student Succeeds Act (ESSA) offers funding to develop this type of decision-making framework, which uses data from frequent progress monitoring to help educators quickly respond to students' needs and provide targeted instruction and support. One key component of MTSS—universal screening—aids teachers' observations by assessing all students, not just the ones showing outward signs of struggle.

Signed into law in 2016, the **Research Excellence and Advancements for Dyslexia (READ) Act** directs funding for research that may lead to:

- Identifying dyslexia earlier
- Training educators to better understand and instruct students with SLD or dyslexia
- Developing curriculum and tools for students with SLD and dyslexia
- Implementing and scaling successful models of dyslexia intervention

A majority of states have passed laws that focus on **third-grade reading proficiency** and/or early identification of dyslexia. These laws are expanding the use of early intervention in many states.

Many states are using **kindergarten entry assessments** to identify students who may need further testing. A few states have started identifying students with SLD before age 6.

Chapter 3: Supporting Academic Success

Lack of effective instruction can limit opportunities and lead to poor outcomes for students with learning and attention issues, who are often misunderstood as not trying hard or not being capable of more. With the right support, these students can achieve at high levels. But schools that lower expectations or standards can make it harder for students with learning disabilities and ADHD to graduate with the skills needed to succeed in college or the workforce.

ACHIEVEMENT GAP

Children with specific learning disabilities (SLD) have average or above-average intelligence, but the National Assessment of Educational Progress (NAEP) points to a wide achievement gap between students with SLD and without disabilities.

2013 NAEP Reading Scores

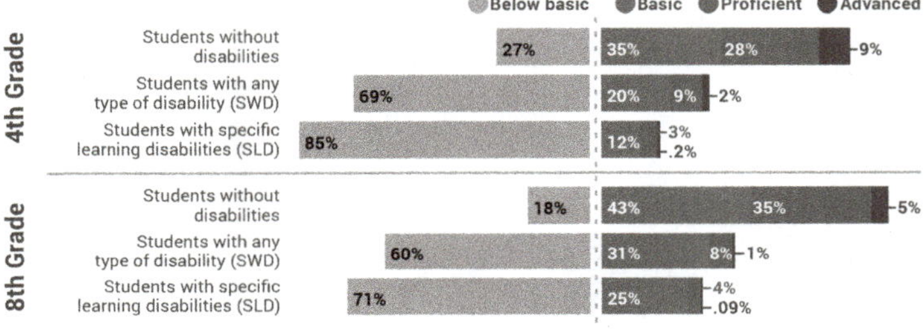

INCLUSION

7 out of 10 students with SLD and other health impairments (OHI) spent 80% or more of their day in general education classrooms in 2015–2016. Inclusion can improve outcomes—but only if teachers can meet the needs of diverse learners.

RETENTION

Students with IEPs were 85% more likely—and students with 504 plans were 110% more likely—to repeat a grade than their peers without disabilities in 2013–2014. Retention increases the risk of dropping out.

GRADUATION

70.8% of students with SLD—and 72.1% of students with OHI—left school in 2013–2014 with a regular diploma, lagging behind the national average by about 10 percentage points. The graduation gap for students with disabilities is even worse among some racial and ethnic groups. Approximately 35% of African American, Hispanic and Native American students with disabilities left high school without a regular diploma in 2014–2015, compared to less than 25% of Asian and white students.

OPPORTUNITIES

The Every Student Succeeds Act (ESSA) includes **accountability requirements** that disaggregate outcome data by subgroups including disability status and provides funding to increase the use of evidence-based interventions at schools with large learning gaps. The law also includes new initiatives that focus on struggling readers, including a **Comprehensive Literacy Center** to help educators and parents recognize early signs of dyslexia and to offer training on effective instructional strategies.

Recent guidance from the U.S. Department of Education **clarifies how to use IEPs to set high standards and provide appropriate supports**:

- IEPs can include terms like dyslexia, dysgraphia and dyscalculia
- IEP goals must be tied to grade-level standards

Amid the growing movement to embrace neurodiversity, **Universal Design for Learning (UDL)** and other best practices can help educators design curricula that meet the needs of all students. **Personalized learning** builds on UDL in ways that enable students to master a standard set of rigorous competencies while working at their own pace, with choices in how they access information and demonstrate their learning—with support in areas of need such as executive function and self-advocacy.

Chapter 4: Social, Emotional and Behavioral Challenges

When schools fail to provide enough support for students, the social, emotional and behavioral challenges that often come along with learning and attention issues can lead to serious consequences. These include social isolation, disproportionate disciplinary rates and an increased likelihood of skipping school, dropping out and becoming involved with the criminal justice system.

CHRONIC ABSENTEEISM

Nearly 1 in 5 students (19%) with IEPs miss three or more weeks of school each year, compared to about 1 in 8 students (13%) without IEPs. School aversion and chronic absenteeism can be a sign of unidentified or inadequately addressed learning and attention issues.

DISCIPLINE

Students with disabilities are more than twice as likely to be suspended as students without disabilities, and the loss of instructional time increases the risk of repeating a grade and dropping out. In 2013–2014, 65% of all special education disciplinary removals involved students with SLD or OHI. Many removals are made at the discretion of school officials.

% of Students Who Received One or More Out-of-School Suspensions

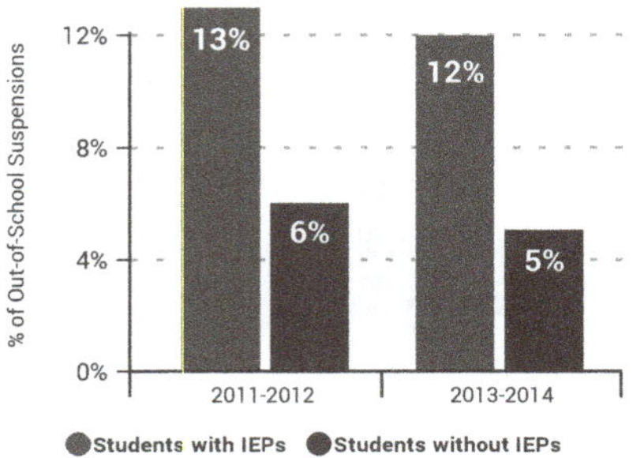

DROPPING OUT

In 2013–2014, 18.1% of students with SLD and 17.6% of students with OHI dropped out, nearly three times the rate of all students (6.5%). In a national longitudinal survey, the most common reason students with SLD gave for dropping out was that they disliked school.

JUSTICE INVOLVEMENT

Failure to address learning and attention issues too often leads to students being incarcerated, which further disrupts their education and contributes to high dropout and recidivism rates. Some studies indicate a third or more of incarcerated youth have learning disabilities, and an even greater proportion may show signs of ADHD. Inadequate instruction while incarcerated or inadequate support upon reentering school helps explain why more than a quarter of reentering students drop out within six months, and nearly half return to confinement within three years.

OPPORTUNITIES

More schools and mentoring programs are incorporating **social and emotional learning (SEL)** into their curricula. SEL may be especially beneficial for students with learning and attention issues because it helps them understand their strengths and needs. But schools should be prepared to provide targeted SEL supports to help students who struggle with self-reflection and self-regulation.

Equity in IDEA regulations issued in 2016 aim to reduce disproportionate identification and disciplinary rates among students of color with disabilities by requiring states to use a standard approach to compare racial and ethnic groups. The regulations also provide funding that districts can use to address disproportionality.

Early warning systems use data on attendance, disciplinary incidents, and coursework to identify students at risk of dropping out, provide more effective interventions and keep students on track to graduate.

Collaboration among schools, healthcare professionals, and judges is critical to preventing juvenile justice involvement and addressing the factors that may lead to delinquency. **Diversion programs**—which offer screening, services, and family supports—may be particularly helpful to students with learning and attention issues who are already struggling academically, socially and emotionally.

Chapter 5: Transitioning to Life After High School

After 12th grade, individuals with learning and attention issues will only receive accommodations in college or the workplace if they disclose their disabilities. But many students leave high school without the self-awareness, self-advocacy skills or self-confidence to successfully navigate their new independence and seek out support when needed.

COLLEGE ENROLLMENT AND COMPLETION

Success in college and the workplace is heavily influenced by internal resilience factors such as temperament and self-perception. Low self-esteem and stigma help explain why young adults with learning disabilities—who are as smart as their peers—enroll in four-year colleges at half the rate of all young adults. Lack of self-advocacy and self-regulation skills may explain why students with learning disabilities who attend any type of postsecondary school are less likely to graduate than students without disabilities.

LACK OF DISCLOSURE

Stigma and other factors deter many undergraduates from accessing key resources in college, where only one-fourth of students with learning disabilities disclose that they have a disability. Reasons for low disclosure rates may include:

- Wanting to establish an identity independent of disability status
- Shame or fear of being perceived as lazy or unintelligent
- Underestimating how important accommodations are to their academic success
- Not knowing what kinds of disability services are available in college or not having the paperwork needed to access them

24% of students with learning disabilities informed their college they have a learning disability

7% did not inform their college even though they still considered themselves to have a learning disability

69% did not inform their college because they no longer considered themselves to have a learning disability (even though people don't "grow out" of learning disabilities)

EMPLOYMENT

Working-age adults with learning disabilities are twice as likely to be jobless as their peers who do not have disabilities. Stigma, low rates of college completion, and lack of awareness about workplace accommodations may all contribute to difficulty attaining employment and succeeding in the workplace. Research shows:

- 19% of young adults with learning disabilities reported that their employers were aware of their disability
- 5% of young adults with learning disabilities reported that they were receiving accommodations in the workplace

OPPORTUNITIES

Self-advocacy and other factors that help students stay in college can be taught, practiced and supported. To ask for and receive accommodations in college and the workplace, young adults must not only understand their needs but also be able to explain them to others. Developing K–12 and community-based programs that provide more opportunities to work on self-advocacy skills—and the confidence to use them—will contribute greatly to social and emotional well-being, academic success and career readiness.

Transition planning is critical to preparing students with disabilities for life after high school. New research shows that when transition plans specify the accommodations students will need in college, the odds of students seeking and using postsecondary supports increase significantly.

Recent changes in standardized testing like the SAT and legislative proposals like the RISE Act, which was introduced in December 2016, may **remove barriers to receiving accommodations** and increase college and workforce opportunities for students with disabilities.

The **Workforce Innovation and Opportunity Act (WIOA)**, which became law in 2014, provides pre-employment transition planning, job training and employment services for students with disabilities, including those with 504 plans.

Chapter 6: Recommended Policy Changes

To help the 1 in 5 thrive in school, in the workplace and in life, targeted policy change is needed in several areas to create a more open, supportive and inclusive society that recognizes the potential of all individuals.

MAJOR POLICY AREA	KEY ASPECTS
Expand Early Screening	• Invest in early screening • Build expertise of educators and healthcare providers to recognize early signs
Empower Students and Families	• Prepare students for a successful transition to postsecondary education and employment • Focus on social and emotional learning (SEL) • Increase access and build capacity of institutions of higher education to meet student needs • Invest in research on outcomes after young adulthood
Cultivate Creative, Informed Educators	• Create more supportive classrooms by rethinking educator preparation programs and professional development • Partner to erase discipline disparities • Expand research on ways to prevent youth involvement in the justice system
Drive Innovation for Effective Teaching and Learning	• Transform teaching by investing in research on the science of learning • Expand evidence-based literacy and math instruction • Promote personalized learning • Use Universal Design for Learning (UDL) and a multi-tier system of supports (MTSS) to reach every student • Invest in integrated student supports
Strengthen and Enforce Civil Rights Laws and Invest in Public Schools	• Strengthen and enforce civil rights laws • Invest in public schools (including programs funded through IDEA and ESSA as well as related programs like Head Start and Medicaid) and reject private school voucher proposals

STATE SNAPSHOTS

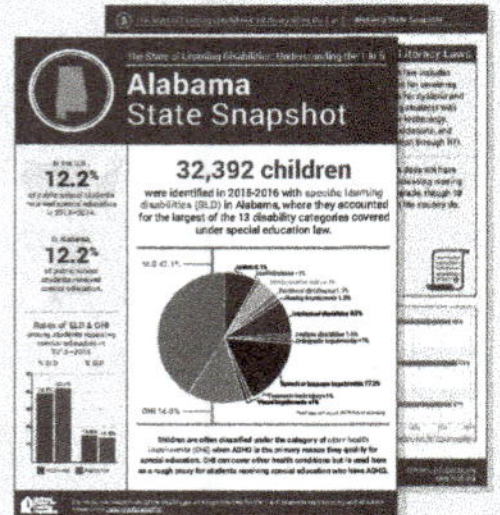

The State of Learning Disabilities includes two-page snapshots for each state and for the District of Columbia, highlighting key data points and comparisons to national averages in several areas:

- Identification rates for specific learning disabilities (SLD) and other health impairments (OHI)
- Inclusion in general education classrooms
- Discipline
- Graduation and dropout rates
- State literacy laws

Go to State Snapshots

HOW TO CITE THIS REPORT

Horowitz, S. H., Rawe, J., & Whittaker, M. C. (2017). ***The State of Learning Disabilities: Understanding the 1 in 5.*** New York: National Center for Learning Disabilities.

MEDIA INQUIRIES

Contact NCLD at (646) 616-1210 or media-inquiries@ncld.org.

Children and Youth With Disabilities

In 2015–16, the number of students ages 3–21 receiving special education services was 6.7 million, or 13 percent of all public school students. Among students receiving special education services, 34 percent had specific learning disabilities.

Enacted in 1975, the Individuals with Disabilities Education Act (IDEA), formerly known as the Education for All Handicapped Children Act, mandates the provision of a free and appropriate public school education for eligible students ages 3–21. Eligible students are those identified by a team of professionals as having a disability that adversely affects academic performance and as being in need of special education and related services. Data collection activities to monitor compliance with IDEA began in 1976.

From school year 2000–01 through 2004–05, the number of students ages 3–21 who received special education services increased from 6.3 million, or 13 percent of total public school enrollment, to 6.7 million, or 14 percent of total public school enrollment.[1] Both the number and percentage of students served under IDEA declined from 2004–05 through 2011–12. Between 2011–12 and 2015–16, the number of students served increased from 6.4 million to 6.7 million, while the percentage served remained at 13 percent of total public school enrollment.

Figure 1. Percentage distribution of students ages 3–21 served under the Individuals with Disabilities Education Act (IDEA), Part B, by disability type: School year 2015–16

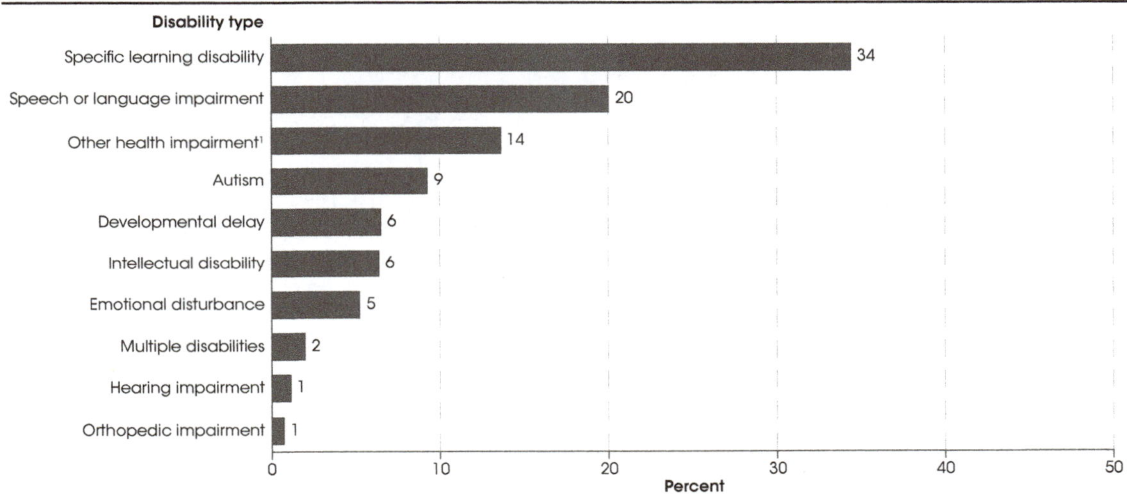

[1] Other health impairments include having limited strength, vitality, or alertness due to chronic or acute health problems such as a heart condition, tuberculosis, rheumatic fever, nephritis, asthma, sickle cell anemia, hemophilia, epilepsy, lead poisoning, leukemia, or diabetes.
NOTE: Deaf-blindness, traumatic brain injury, and visual impairment are not shown because they each account for less than 0.5 percent of students served under IDEA. Due to categories not shown, detail does not sum to 100 percent. Although rounded numbers are displayed, the figures are based on unrounded estimates.
SOURCE: U.S. Department of Education, Office of Special Education Programs, Individuals with Disabilities Education Act (IDEA) database, retrieved July 10, 2017, from https://www2.ed.gov/programs/osepidea/618-data/state-level-data-files/index.html#bcc. See *Digest of Education Statistics 2017*, table 204.30.

In school year 2015–16, a higher percentage of students ages 3–21 received special education services under IDEA for specific learning disabilities than for any other type of disability. A specific learning disability is a disorder in one or more of the basic psychological processes involved in understanding or using language, spoken or written, that may manifest itself in an imperfect ability to listen, think, speak, read, write, spell, or do mathematical calculations. In 2015–16, some 34 percent of all students receiving special education services had specific learning disabilities, 20 percent had speech or language impairments, and 14 percent had other health impairments (including having limited strength, vitality, or alertness due to chronic or acute health problems such as a heart condition, tuberculosis, rheumatic fever, nephritis, asthma, sickle cell anemia, hemophilia, epilepsy, lead poisoning, leukemia, or diabetes). Students with autism, intellectual disabilities, developmental delays, and emotional disturbances each accounted for between 5 and 9 percent of students served under IDEA. Students with multiple disabilities, hearing impairments, orthopedic impairments, visual impairments, traumatic brain injuries, and deaf-blindness each accounted for 2 percent or less of those served under IDEA.

Figure 2. Percentage of students ages 3–21 served under the Individuals with Disabilities Education Act (IDEA), Part B, by race/ethnicity: School year 2015–16

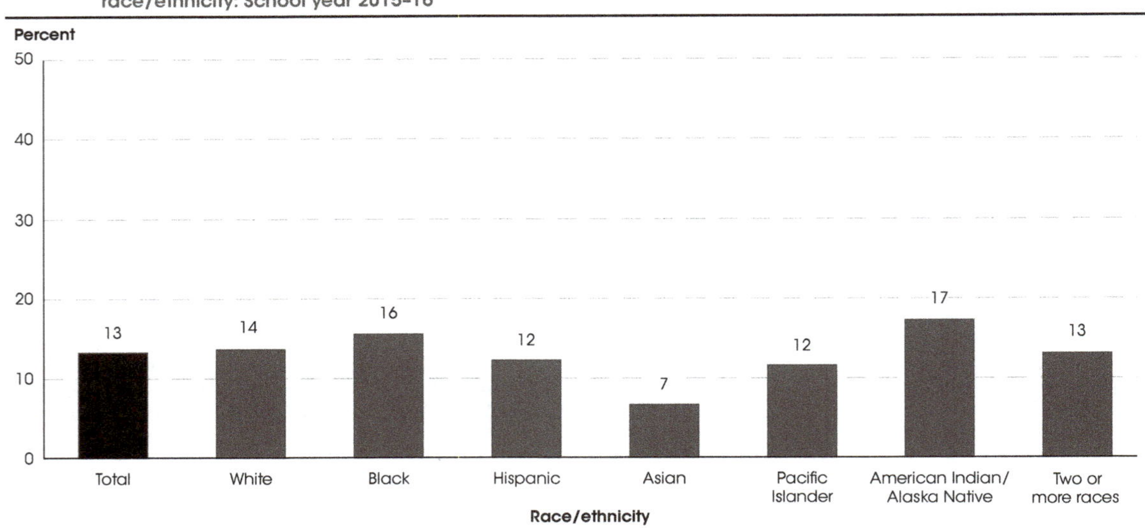

NOTE: Based on the total enrollment in public schools, prekindergarten through 12th grade. Race categories exclude persons of Hispanic ethnicity. Although rounded numbers are displayed, the figures are based on unrounded estimates.
SOURCE: U.S. Department of Education, Office of Special Education Programs, Individuals with Disabilities Education Act (IDEA) database, retrieved July 10, 2017, from http://www2.ed.gov/programs/osepidea/618-data/state-level-data-files/index.html#bcc; and National Center for Education Statistics, Common Core of Data (CCD), "State Nonfiscal Survey of Public Elementary/Secondary Education," 2015–16. See *Digest of Education Statistics 2017*, table 204.50.

In school year 2015–16, the percentage (out of total public school enrollment) of students ages 3–21 served under IDEA differed by race/ethnicity. The percentage of students served under IDEA was highest for those who were American Indian/Alaska Native (17 percent), followed by those who were Black (16 percent), White (14 percent), of Two or more races (13 percent), Hispanic and Pacific Islander (both at 12 percent), and Asian (7 percent).

In each racial/ethnic group except for Asian, the percentage of students receiving services for specific learning disabilities combined with the percentage receiving services for speech or language impairments accounted for over 50 percent of students served under IDEA. The percentage distribution of various types of special education services received by students ages 3–21 in 2015–16 differed by race/ethnicity. For example, the percentage of students with disabilities receiving services under IDEA for specific learning disabilities was lower among Asian students (21 percent), students of Two or more races (30 percent), and White students (31 percent) than among students overall (34 percent). However, the percentage of students with disabilities receiving services under IDEA for autism was higher among Asian students (21 percent), students of Two or more races (10 percent), and White students (10 percent) than among students overall (9 percent). Additionally, among students who were served under IDEA, 7 percent of Black students and 7 percent of students of Two or more races received services for emotional disturbances. In comparison, 5 percent of all students served under IDEA received services for emotional disturbances. Among students who received services under IDEA, each racial/ethnic group other than Hispanic (5 percent) had a higher percentage of students receiving services for developmental delays than the overall percentage of students receiving services for developmental delays (6 percent).

Separate data on special education services for males and females are available only for students ages 6–21, rather than ages 3–21. Among those 6- to 21-year-old students enrolled in public schools in 2015–16, a higher percentage of males (17 percent) than of females (9 percent) received special education services under IDEA. The percentage distribution of students who received various types of special education services in 2015–16 differed by sex. For example, the percentage of students served under IDEA who received services for specific learning disabilities was higher among female students (44 percent) than among male students (35 percent), while the percentage served under IDEA who received services for autism was higher among male students (12 percent) than among female students (4 percent).

Figure 3. Percentage of students ages 6–21 served under the Individuals with Disabilities Education Act (IDEA), Part B, by amount of time spent inside general classes: Selected school years, 2000–01 through 2015–16

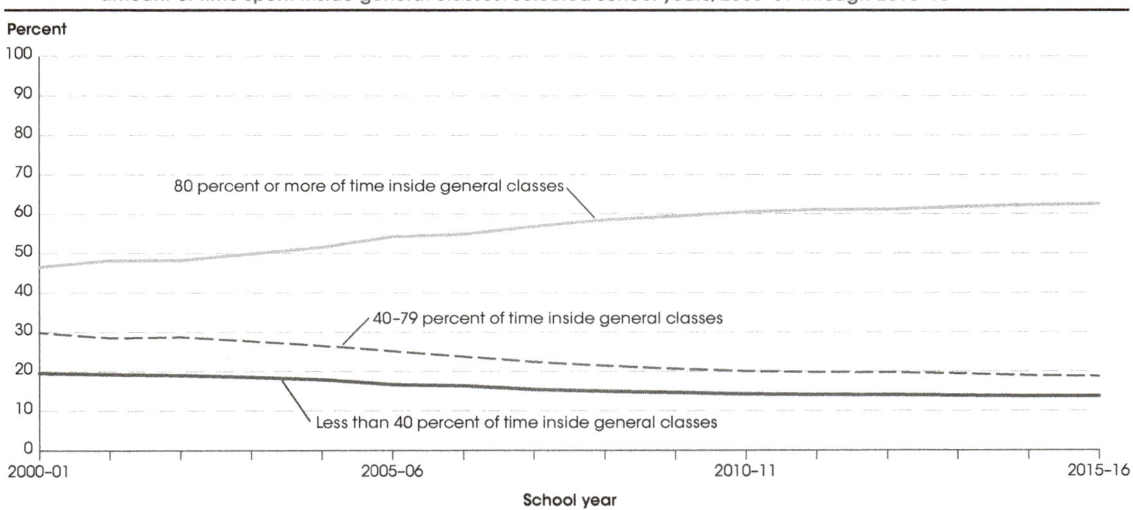

SOURCE: U.S. Department of Education, Office of Special Education Programs, Individuals with Disabilities Education Act (IDEA) database, retrieved July 15, 2017, from http://www2.ed.gov/programs/osepidea/618-data/state-level-data-files/index.html#bcc. See *Digest of Education Statistics 2017*, table 204.60.

Educational environment data are also available for students ages 6–21 served under IDEA. About 95 percent of students ages 6–21 served under IDEA in fall 2015 were enrolled in regular schools. Some 3 percent of students served under IDEA were enrolled in separate schools (public or private) for students with disabilities; 1 percent were placed by their parents in regular private schools; and less than 1 percent each were homebound or in hospitals, in separate residential facilities (public or private), or in correctional facilities. Among all students ages 6–21 served under IDEA, the percentage who spent most of the school day (i.e., 80 percent or more of their time) in general classes in regular schools increased from 47 percent in fall 2000 to 63 percent in fall 2015. In contrast, during the same period, the percentage of those who spent 40 to 79 percent of the school day in general classes declined from 30 to 19 percent, and the percentage of those who spent less than 40 percent of their time inside general classes also declined, from 20 to 14 percent. In fall 2015, the percentage of students served under IDEA who spent most of the school day in general classes was highest for students with speech or language impairments (87 percent). Approximately two-thirds of students with specific learning disabilities (70 percent), visual impairments (67 percent), other health impairments (65 percent), and developmental delays (64 percent) spent most of the school day in general classes. In contrast, 16 percent of students with intellectual disabilities and 13 percent of students with multiple disabilities spent most of the school day in general classes.

Data are also available for students ages 14–21 served under IDEA who exited school during school year 2014–15, including exit reason.[2] Approximately 395,000 students ages 14–21 who received special education services under IDEA exited school in 2014–15: about two-thirds (69 percent) graduated with a regular high school diploma, 18 percent dropped out, 11 percent received an alternative certificate,[3] 1 percent reached maximum age, and less than one-half of 1 percent died.

Figure 4. Percentage of students ages 14–21 served under the Individuals with Disabilities Education Act (IDEA), Part B, who exited school, by selected exit reason and race/ethnicity: School year 2014–15

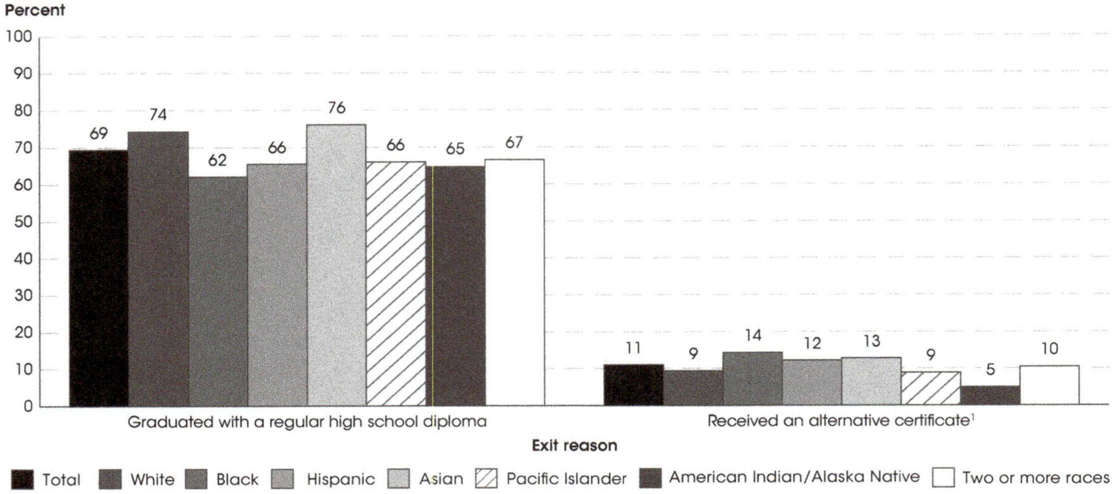

Exit reason	Total	White	Black	Hispanic	Asian	Pacific Islander	American Indian/Alaska Native	Two or more races
Graduated with a regular high school diploma	69	74	62	66	76	66	65	67
Received an alternative certificate[1]	11	9	14	12	13	9	5	10

[1] Received a certificate of completion, modified diploma, or some similar document, but did not meet the same standards for graduation as those for students without disabilities.

NOTE: Data in this figure are for the 50 states, the District of Columbia, the Bureau of Indian Education, American Samoa, the Federated States of Micronesia, Guam, the Northern Marianas, Puerto Rico, the Republic of Palau, the Republic of the Marshall Islands, and the U.S. Virgin Islands. Data for all other figures in this indicator are for the 50 states and the District of Columbia only. Race categories exclude persons of Hispanic ethnicity.

SOURCE: U.S. Department of Education, Office of Special Education Programs, Individuals with Disabilities Education Act (IDEA) Section 618 Data Products: State Level Data Files. Retrieved July 14, 2017, from http://www2.ed.gov/programs/osepidea/618-data/state-level-data-files/index.html. See *Digest of Education Statistics 2017*, table 219.90.

Of the students ages 14–21 served under IDEA who exited school in 2014–15, the percentages who graduated with a regular high school diploma, received an alternative certificate, and dropped out differed by race/ethnicity. The percentage of exiting students who graduated with a regular high school diploma was highest among Asian students (76 percent) and lowest among Black students (62 percent). The percentage of exiting students who received an alternative certificate was highest among Black students (14 percent) and lowest among American Indian/Alaska Native students (5 percent). The percentage of exiting students who dropped out in 2014–15 was highest among American Indian/Alaska Native students (29 percent) and lowest among Asian students (7 percent).

Of the students ages 14–21 served under IDEA who exited school in 2014–15, the percentages who graduated with a regular high school diploma, received an alternative certificate, and dropped out also differed by type of disability. The percentage of exiting students who graduated with a regular high school diploma was highest among students with visual impairments (82 percent) and lowest among those with intellectual disabilities (42 percent). The percentage of exiting students who received an alternative certificate was highest among students with intellectual disabilities (34 percent) and lowest among students with speech or language impairments (5 percent). The percentage of exiting students who dropped out in 2014–15 was highest among students with emotional disturbances (35 percent) and lowest among those with autism and visual impairments (both at 7 percent).

Endnotes:

[1] Data for students ages 3–21 and 6–21 served under IDEA are for the 50 states and the District of Columbia only.

[2] Data for students ages 14–21 served under IDEA who exited school are for the 50 states, the District of Columbia, the Bureau of Indian Education, American Samoa, the Federated States of Micronesia, Guam, the Northern Marianas, Puerto Rico, the Republic of Palau, the Republic of the Marshall Islands, and the U.S. Virgin Islands.

[3] Received a certificate of completion, modified diploma, or some similar document, but did not meet the same standards for graduation as those for students without disabilities.

Reference tables: *Digest of Education Statistics 2017*, tables 204.30, 204.50, 204.60, and 219.90; *Digest of Education Statistics 2015*, table 204.30

Related indicators and resources: Disability Rates and Employment Status by Educational Attainment [*The Condition of Education 2017 Spotlight*]; English Language Learners in Public Schools; Students with Disabilities [*Status and Trends in the Education of Racial and Ethnic Groups*]

Glossary: Disabilities, children with; Enrollment; High school completer; High school diploma; Individuals with Disabilities Education Act (IDEA); Private school; Public school or institution; Racial/ethnic group; Regular school

McFarland, J., Hussar, B., Wang, X., Zhang, J., Wang, K., Rathbun, A., Barmer, A., Forrest Cataldi, E., and Bullock Mann, F. (2018). The Condition of Education 2018 (NCES 2018-144). U.S. Department of Education. Washington, DC: National Center for

User Guide

Descriptive listings in *The Complete Learning Disabilities Resource Guide* are organized into 21 chapters and 100 subchapters. You will find the following types of listings throughout the book:

- National Agencies & Associations
- State Agencies & Associations
- Camps & Summer Programs
- Exchange Programs
- Classroom & Computer Resources
- Print & Electronic Media
- Schools & Learning Centers
- Testing & Training Resources
- Conferences & Workshops

Below is a sample listing illustrating the kind of information that is or might be included in an entry. Each numbered item of information is described in the paragraphs on the following page.

1→ 1234

2 → **Association for Children and Youth with Disabilities**

3 → **1704 L Street NW**

Washington, DC 20036

4 → **075-785-0000**

5 → **FAX: 075-785-0001**

6 → **800-075-0002**

7 → **TDY: 075-785-0002**

8 → **info@AGC.com**

9 → **www.AGC.com**

10→ Peter Rancho, Director
Nancy Williams, Information Specialist
Tanya Fitzgerald, Marketing Director
William Alexander, Editor

11→ Advocacy organization that ensures children and youth with learning disabilities receive the best possible education. Services include speaking with an informed specialist, free publications, database searches, and referrals to other organizations.

12→ *$6.99*

13→ *204 pages*

14→ *Paperback*

User Key

1 → **Record Number**: Entries are listed alphabetically within each category and numbered sequentially. The entry numbers, rather than page numbers, are used in the indexes to refer to listings.

2 → **Organization Name**: Formal name of organization. Where organization names are completely capitalized, the listing will appear at the beginning of the alphabetized section. In the case of publications, the title of the publication will appear first, followed by the publisher.

3 → **Address**: Location or permanent address of the organization.

4 → **Phone Number**: The listed phone number is usually for the main office of the organization, but may also be for sales, marketing, or public relations as provided by the organization.

5 → **Fax Number**: This is listed when provided by the organization.

6 → **Toll-Free Number**: This is listed when provided by the organization.

7 → **TDY**: This is listed when provided by the organization. It refers to Telephone Device for the Deaf.

8 → **E-Mail**: This is listed when provided by the organization and is generally the main office e-mail.

9 → **Web Site**: This is listed when provided by the organization and is also referred to as an URL address. These web sites are accessed through the Internet by typing http:// before the URL address.

10 → **Key Personnel**: Name and title of key executives within the organization.

11 → **Organization Description**: This paragraph contains a brief description of the organization and their services.

The following apply if the listing is a publication:

12 → **Price:** The cost of each issue or subscription, often with frequency information. If the listing is a school or program, you will see information on age group served and enrollment size.

13 → **Number of Pages**: Total number of pages for publication.

14 → **Paperback:** The available format of the publication: paperback; hardcover; spiral bound.

National

1 **AVKO Educational Research Foundation**
3084 Willard Rd.
Birch Run, MI 48415-9404 810-686-9283
866-285-6612
http://www.avko.org
AVKO is a non-profit membership organization that focuses on the development and production of materials and techniques to help students with learning disabilities achieve literacy. Resource subjects focus on reading and spelling, handwriting (manuscript and cursive), and key boarding.

2 **America's Health Insurance Plans**
601 Pennsylvania Ave. NW
South Building, Suite 500
Washington, DC 20004 202-778-3200
Fax: 202-331-7487
http://www.ahip.org
info@ahip.org
Matt Eyles, President/CEO
Dawn Banda, Chief Financial Officer
Richard Bankowitz, Chief Medical Officer
Purpose is to represent the interests of members on legislative and regulatory issues at the federal and state levels, and with the media, consumers, and employers. Provides information and services such as newsletters, publications, a magazine, and online services. Conducts education, research, and quality assurance programs and engages in a host of other activities to assist members.

3 **American Association of Collegiate Registrars and Admissions Officers**
One Dupont Circle NW
Suite 520
Washington, DC 20036 202-293-9161
Fax: 202-872-8857
http://www.aacrao.org
corporateinfo@aacrao.org
Tina Falkner, President
Luisa Havens, President Elect
Jack Miner, Vice President, Operations
Provides professional development, guidelines, and voluntary standards to be used by higher education officials regarding the best practices in records management, admissions, enrollment management, administrative information technology, and student services.

4 **American Association of People with Disabilities (AAPD)**
2013 H St NW
5th Fl
Washington, DC 20006 202-521-4316
800-840-8844
http://www.aapd.com
Helena Berger, President & CEO
Amy Naoum, Chief Financial Officer
Jason Mida, Director of Development
Advocacy group dedicated to improving the lives of persons with disabilities and their families by eliminating barriers and allowing them to exercise their civil, legal, and human rights.

5 **American Bar Association Center on Children and the Law**
1050 Conneticut Ave.
Suite 400
Washington, DC 20036 202-662-1720
http://www.americanbar.org/groups
ctrchildlaw@americanbar.org
Prudence Beidler Carr, Director
Claire Chiamulera, Legal Editor
Anne Maries Lancour, Associate Director
Aims to improve children's lives through advances in law, justice, knowledge, practice, and public policy.
1978

6 **American Camp Association**
5000 State Rd. 67 N
Martinsville, IN 46151-7902 765-342-8456
800-428-2267
Fax: 765-342-2065
http://www.acacamps.org
contactus@acacamps.org
Tom Rosenberg, President/CEO
Ross Turner, Chair
Tony Oyenarte, Vice Chair
The American Camp Association brings together camping professionalsdedicated to ensuring the quality of camp programs, and providing children with the unique enjoyment of camp experiences.
11,000+ members

7 **American College Testing**
P.O. Box 414
Iowa City, IA 52243-0414 319-337-1270
http://www.act.org
Marten Roorda, Chief Executive Officer
Suzana Delanghe, Chief Commercial Officer
Lucas Kuhlmann, Chief Technology Officer
An independent, not-for-profit organization that provides more than a hundred assessment, research, information, and program management services in the broad areas of education and workforce development.

8 **American Counseling Association**
6101 Stevenson Ave.
Alexandria, VA 22304 703-823-9800
800-347-6647
Fax: 703-823-0252
http://www.counseling.org
membership@counseling.org
Richard Yep, CEO
Simone Lambert, President
Heather Trepal, Presient Elect
The ACA is a non-profit organization working towards the growth and enhancement of the counseling profession.
1952

9 **American Dance Therapy Association (ADTA)**
10632 Little Patuxent Pkwy.
Suite 108
Columbia, MD 21044 410-997-4040
Fax: 410-997-4048
http://www.adta.org
info@adta.org
Margaret Migliorati, Board President
Leslie Armeniox, Secretary
Vicky Wilder, Treasurer
Works to establish and maintain high standards of professional education and competence in the field of dance/movement therapy. ADTA stimulates communication among dance/movement therapists and members of allied professions through publication of the ADTA Newsletter, the American Journal of Dance Therapy, monographs, bibliographies, and conference proceedings.

10 **American Dyslexia Association**
442 S. Tamiami Trail
Osprey, FL 34229
http://www.american-dyslexia-association.com
office@american-dyslexia-association.com
The American Dyselxia Association Inc. is a non-profit organization, providing information and teaching aids for dyslexic and dyscalculic people with free information and teaching aids.

11 **American Occupational Therapy Association**
4720 Montgomery Ln.
Suite 200
Bethesda, MD 20814 301-652-6611
800-729-2682
http://www.aota.org

Amy J. Lamb, President
Wendy C. Hildenbrand, President Elect
Debra Young, Vice President
Founded to represent the interests and concerns of occupational therapy practitioners and students of occupational therapy and to improve the quality of occupational therapy services. Advances the quality, availability, use, and support of occupational therapy through standard-setting, advocacy, education, and research on behalf of its members and the public.
60,000 members 1917

12 **American Psychological Association**
750 First St. NE
Washington, DC 20002-4242 202-336-5500
800-374-2721
TTY: 202-336-6123
http://www.apa.org
Jessica Henderson Daniel, President
Jennifer F. Kelly, Secretary
Arthur C. Evans, Jr., CEO/Executive Vice President
Its objectives are to advance psychology as a science and profession and as a means of promoting health, education, and human welfare.
115,700 members

13 **American Public Human Services Association (APHSA)**
1133 19th St. NW
Suite 400
Washington, DC 20036 202-682-0100
Fax: 202-289-6555
http://www.aphsa.org
memberservice@aphsa.org
Tracy Wareing Evans, President/CEO
Nicole York, Human Resources Director
Jessica Garon, Communications Manager
A non-profit, bipartisan organization of state and local human service agencies and individuals who work in or are interested in public human service programs. Mission is to develop and promote policies and practices that improve the health and well-being of families, children, and adults

14 **American Red Cross (National Headquarters)**
431 18th St., NW
Washington, DC 20006 202-303-4498
800-733-2767
http://www.redcross.org
info@usa.redcross.org
Gail J. McGovern, President/CEO
Bonnie McElveen-Hunter, Chairman of the Board
Brian J. Rhoa, Chief Financial Officer
A humanitarian organization led by volunteers, guided by its Congressional Charter and the fundamental principles of the International Red Cross Movement to provide relief to victims of disasters and help people prevent, prepare for, and respond to emergencies.

15 **American Rehabilitation Counseling Association (ARCA)**
5999 Stevenson Ave
Alexandria, VA 22304-3304 703-823-9800
800-347-6647
Fax: 703-461-9260
TDD: 937-775-3153
http://www.arcaweb.org
Noel Ysasi, President
Michael Hartley, President-Elect
Cecilia Guyton, Treasurer
An organization of rehabilitation counseling practitioners, educators, and students who are concerned with improving the lives of people with disabilities. The mission is to enhance the lives of people with disabilities and to promote excellence in the rehabilitation counseling profession.

16 **American Speech-Language-Hearing Association (ASHA)**
2200 Research Blvd.
Rockville, MD 20850-3289 301-296-5700
800-498-2071
Fax: 301-296-8580
TTY: 301-296-5650
http://www.asha.org
nsslha@asha.org
Elise Davis-McFarland, President
Shari B. Robertson, President Elect
Arlene A. Pietranton, Chief Executive Officer
Promotes the interests of and provides the highest quality services for professionals in audiology, speech-language pathology, and speech and hearing science. ASHA advocates for people with communication disabilities.
198,000 members 1958

17 **Association of Educational Therapists**
7044 S. 13th St.
Oak Creek, WI 53154 414-908-4949
http://www.aetonline.org
customercare@AETOnline.org
Judith Brennan, President
Polly Brophy, Treasurer
Kaye Ragland, Secretary
A national professional organization dedicated to establishing ethical professional standards, defining the roles and responsibilities of the educational therapist, providing opportunities for professional growth, and to studying techniques and technologies, philosophies, and research related to the practice of educational therapy.
1979

18 **Association on Higher Education and Disability (AHEAD)**
8015 West Kenton Circle
Suite 230
Huntersville, NC 28078 704-947-7779
Fax: 704-948-7779
http://www.ahead.org
Jamie Axelrod, President
Gaeir Dietrich, Treasurer
Stephan Smith, Executive Director
Membership for professionals invloved in the development of policy and the provision of quality services to meet the needs of persons with disabiities in all aspects of higher education.
3,000 members 1977

19 **Attention Deficit Disorder Association**
800-939-1019
http://www.add.org
Duane Gordon, President
Michelle Frank, Vice President
Melissa Reskof, Secretary
The Attention Deficit Disorder Association is an organization focused on the needs of adults and young adults with ADD/ADHD, offering resources and research to help children, families, and professionals.

20 **Autism Research Institute**
4182 Adams Ave.
San Diego, CA 92116 833-281-7165
http://www.autism.com
Stephen Edelson, Ph.D., Executive Director
Marvin Natowicz, Chairman
Founded to conduct and foster scientific research designed to improve methods of diagnosing, treating, and preventing autism. ARI also disseminates research findings to parents and others worldwide seeking help.
1967

21 **Autism Risk & Safety Management**
2338 SE Holland St
Port St. Lucie, FL 34953 772-398-9756
http://www.autismriskmanagement.com
ddpi@flash.net

Dennis Debbaubt, Founder & Director
Develops current and relevant autism and law enforcement cirriculum and content. Materials include training, course outlines, learning outcomes, and more information pertinent to autism.

22 **Autism Society**
4340 East-West Hwy.
Suite 350
Bethesda, MD 20814 800-328-8476
http://www.autism-society.org
info@autism-society.org
Scott Badesch, President/CEO
John Dabrowski, CFO/COO
Kim Musheno, Vice President, Public Policy
Works to increase public awareness about the day-to-day issues faced by those on the autism spectrum. Offers a national contact center, local chapters throughout the country, a quarterly magazine, and an annual conference.
1965

23 **Autism Speaks**
1 E 33rd St
4th Fl
New York, NY 10016 646-385-8500
888-288-4762
Fax: 212-252-8676
http://www.autismspeaks.org
familyservices@autismspeaks.org
Philip H. Geier, Jr., Director Emeritus
Angela Geiger, President & CEO
Kevin Roy, EVP, Advocacy
Austism Speaks is a nonprofit organization dedicated to finding solutions to the needs of individuals with autism and their families and improving quality of life. Austism Speaks is an vessel for advocacy and support.
1905

24 **Autism Treatment Center of America**
2080 S. Undermountain Rd.
Sheffield, MA 01257 413-229-2100
877-766-7473
http://www.autismtreatmentcenter.org
Barry Neil Kaufman, Co-Founder/CEO
Samahria Lyte Kaufman, Co-Founder
Raun K. Kaufman, Group Facilitator
Provides innovative training programs for parents and professionals caring for children challenged by Autism, Autism Spectrum Disorders, Pervasive Developmental Disorder (PDD) and other developmental difficulties. The Son-Rise Program teaches a specific yet comprehensive system of treatment and education designed to help families and caregivers enable their children to dramatically improve in all areas of learning.

25 **Best Buddies International**
100 Southeast Second St.
Suite 2200
Miami, FL 33131 305-374-2233
Fax: 305-789-5577
http://www.bestbuddies.org
info@bestbuddies.org
Anthony K. Shriver, Founder/Chairman
Maria Valle, Chief of Staff
Jen Miller, SVP, Finance/Operations
A non-profit organization dedicated to enhancing the lives of people with intellectual disabilities by providing opportunities for one-to-one friendships and integrated employment. Best Buddies is an international community that reaches students in middle schools, high schools, and college campuses across the country and abroad.

26 **Birth Defect Research for Children (BDRC)**
976 Lake Baldwin Ln.
Suite 104
Orlando, FL 32814 407-895-0802
http://www.birthdefects.org
staff@birthdefects.org
Betty Mekdeci, Co-Founder
Mike Mekdeci, Co-Founder
A non-profit organization that provides parents and expectant parents with information about birth defects and support services for children. BDRC also has a parent-matching program that links families who have children with similar birth defects.

27 **Boy Scouts of America**
1325 West Walnut Hill Ln.
Irving, TX 75038 972-580-2000
http://www.scouting.org
myscouting@scouting.org
Mike Surbaugh, Chief Scout Officer
Provides an educational program for boys and young adults to build character, to train in responsible citizenship, and to develop personal fitness.
1910

28 **Brain Injury Association of America**
1608 Spring Hill Rd.
Suite 110
Vienna, VA 22182 703-761-0750
800-444-6443
Fax: 703-761-0755
http://www.biausa.org
info@biausa.org
Douglas L. Brewer, Chairman
Harold Ginsburg, Vice Chairman
Susan H. Connors, President/CEO
A national organization serving and representing individuals, families, and professionals who are touched by a life-altering traumatic brain injury.

29 **CASANA**
1501 Reedsale St.
Suite 202
Pittsburgh, PA 15233 412-785-7072
http://www.apraxia-kids.org
Angela Grimm, Executive Director
David Hammer, Vice President, Programs
Brandice Wilburn, Program Manager
The Childhood Apraxia of Speech Association is a non-profit publicly funded charity whose mission is to strengthen the support systems in the lives of children with apraxia so that each child is afforded their best opportunity to develop speech and communication.

30 **Career Education Colleges and Universities (CECU)**
1530 Wilson Blvd.
Suite 1050
Arlington, VA 22209 571-970-3941
Fax: 571-970-6753
http://www.career.org
David Vice, Chairman
Nick Mansour, Vice Chairman
Lynelle Lynch, Treasurer
Formerly APSCU, CECU provides education, advocacy, and training for professionals in postsecondary and higher education.

31 **Center for Applied Linguistics**
4646 40th St., NW
Washington, DC 20016-1859 202-362-0700
Fax: 202-362-3740
http://www.cal.org
info@cal.org
Joel Gomez, President/CEO
Ruben Rodriguez, COO/CFO
Sophia Birdas, Director, Marketing & Outreach
The Center for Applied Linguistics is a non-profit organization promoting access, equity, and mutual understanding for linguistically and culturally diverse people around the world.

32 **Center for Applied Special Technology (CAST)**
40 Harvard Mills Square
Suite 3
Wakefield, MA 01880 781-245-2212
http://www.cast.org
cast@cast.org
Anne Meyer, Co-Founder
David H. Rose, Co-Founder
Sheldon H. Berman, Chair
CAST has earned international recognition for innovative, technology-based educational resources and strategies based on the principals of Universal Design for Learning (UDL). The mission is to expand opportunities for all individuals, especially those with disabilities, through the research and development of innovative, technology-based educational resources and strategies.

33 **Center for Parent Information & Resources**
c/o Statewide Parent Advocacy Ntwk
35 Halsey St., 4th Fl.
Newark, NJ 07102 973-642-8100
http://www.parentcenterhub.org
malizo@spanadvocacy.org
Myriam Alizo, Project Assistant
Formerly housing the National Dissemination Center for Children with Disabilities, CPIR is a website that now houses NICHCY's legacy resources, in addition to resources of their own, continuing to offer informational assistance to parents of children with disabilities.

34 **Closing the Gap**
P.O. Box 68
Henderson, MN 56044 507-248-3294
Fax: 507-248-3810
http://www.closingthegap.com
info@closingthegap.com
Dolores Hagen, Co-Founder
Budd Hagan, Co-Founder
Megan Turek, Director
An organization that focuses on computer technology for people with special needs through its bi-monthly newsletter, annual international conference, and other professional development resources.

35 **Commission on the Accreditation of Rehabilitation Facilities (CARF)**
6951 East Southpoint Rd.
Tucson, AZ 85756-9407 520-325-1044
888-281-6531
Fax: 520-318-1129
TTY: 520-495-7077
http://www.carf.org
Brian J. Boon, President/CEO
Cindy L. Johnson, Strategic Development Officer
Leslie Ellis-Lang, Managing Director
An independent, non-profit accreditor of human service providers in the areas of aging services, behavioral health, child and youth services, DMEPOS, employment, and medical rehabilitation.

36 **Council for Accreditation of Counseling & Related Educational Programs**
1001 North Fairfax St.
Suite 510
Alexandria, VA 22314 703-535-5990
Fax: 703-739-6209
http://www.cacrep.org
Chris Hull, Chair
Vilia Tarvydas, Vice Chair
Charles McAdams, Treasurer
An accreditation organiztion for professional preparation programs in the areas of education and counseling. CACREP promotes excellence in the development and practice of preparation standards. CACREP is working to incorporate disability concepts into their practices with the merger of the Council on Rehabilitation Education (CORE).

37 **Council for Exceptional Children (CEC)**
2900 Crystal Dr.
Suite 100
Arlington, VA 22202-3557 888-232-7733
TTY: 866-915-5000
http://www.cec.sped.org
service@cec.sped.org
Laurie VanderPloeg, President
Mary Lynn Boscardin, President Elect
Jim McCormick, Treasurer
An international professional organization dedicated to improving educational outcomes for individuals with exceptionalities, students with disabilities, and/or the gifted. Advocates for appropriate governmental policies, sets professional standards, provides continual professional development, advocates for underserved individuals with exceptionalities, and helps professionals obtain resources necessary for effective professional practice.

38 **Council for Learning Disabilities**
11184 Antioch Rd.
Box 405
Overland Park, KS 66210 913-491-1011
Fax: 913-491-1011
http://council-for-learning-disabilities.org
CLDInfo@cldinternational.org
Deborah Reed, President
Lindy Crawford, Vice President
Linda Nease, Executive Director
An international organization concerned about issues related to students with learning disabilities. Working to build a better future for students with LD has been the primary goal of CLD for more than 20 years. Involvement in CLD helps members stay abreast of current issues that are shaping the field, affecting the lives of students, and influencing professional careers.

39 **Council of Administrators of Special Education (CASE)**
101 Katelyn Circle
Suite E
Warner Robins, GA 31088 478-333-6892
Fax: 478-333-2453
http://www.casecec.org/
Dr. Luann Purcell, Executive Director
CASE is an international professional organization that provides leadership and support to its members by working to affect policies and practices relation to special education.

40 **Department of VSA and Accessibility**
Kennedy Center for the Performing Arts
2700 F St., NW
Washington, DC 20566 202-467-4600
800-444-1324
http://www.kennedy-center.org
David M. Rubenstein, Chairman
Deborah F. Rutter, President
Gianandrea Noseda, Music Director, NSO
An international, non-profit organization founded to create a society where all people with disabilities learn through, participate in, and enjoy the arts.

41 **Disability Resource Center**
170 Scoggins Dr
Demorest, GA 30535 706-778-5355
888-534-7144
http://disabilityresourcecenter.org
Judy Presley, President
Nancy Peeples, Executive Director
Angie Lance, Operations Director
A nonprofit organization dedicated to enhancing independence, access and equal rights for people with disabilities.
1999

42 **Disability Rights Education & Defense Fund (DREDF)**
3075 Adeline St.
Suite 210
Berkeley, CA 94703
510-644-2555
Fax: 510-841-8645
TTY: 510-841-8645
http://www.dredf.org
info@dredf.org
Susan Henderson, Executive Director
Arlene B. Mayerson, Directing Attorney
Mary Lou Breslin, Senior Policy Advisor
A national civil rights law and policy center directed by individuals with disabilities and parents who have children with disabilities. Advances the civil and human rights of people with disabilities through legal advocacy, training, education, and public policy and legislative development.
1979

43 **Distance Education Accrediting Commission (DEAC)**
1101 17th St., NW
Suite 808
Washington, DC 20036
202-234-5100
Fax: 202-332-1386
http://www.deac.org
info@deac.org
Leah K. Matthews, Executive Director
Nan Ridgeway, Director, Accreditation
Robert Chalifoux, Director, Media and Events
A non-profit educational association founded to promote sound educational standards and ethical business practices within the correspondence and distance education fields.

44 **Division for Communicative Disabilities and Deafness (DCDD)**
Council for Exceptional Children
2900 Crystal Dr.
Suite 100
Arlington, VA 22202-3557
888-232-7733
TTY: 866-915-5000
http://community.cec.sped.org/dcdd/home
dcdd.us@gmail.com
Suzanne Raschke, President
Caron Mellblom-Nishioka, President Elect
The DCDD is concerned with the well-being, development, and education of infants, toddlers, children, and youth with communication and learning disorders, and/or who are deaf or hard of hearing.

45 **Division for Culturally & Linguistically Diverse Exceptional Learners**
Council for Exceptional Children
2900 Crystal Dr.
Suite 100
Arlington, VA 22202-3557
888-232-7733
TTY: 866-915-5000
http://community.cec.sped.org/ddel
Mildred Boveda, President
Charmion Rush, Secretary
Evette Simmons-Reed, President Elect
The official division of the Council for Exceptional Children that promotes the advancement and improvement of educational opportunities for culturally and linguistically diverse learners with disabilities and/or gifts and talents, their families, and the professionals who serve them.

46 **Division for Early Childhood of CEC**
Council for Exceptional Children
2900 Crystal Dr.
Suite 100
Arlington, VA 22202-3557
310-428-7209
Fax: 855-678-1989
http://www.dec-sped.org/
dec@dec-sped.org
Peggy Kemp, Executive Director
Ben Rogers, Assistant Director
Sharon Walsh, Government Relations
An international membership association that aims to assist those those who work with or on behalf of children with disabilities from birth through age eight and their families. The Division promotes and advocates for policies that hope to ensure the best outcomes for child development.
1973

47 **Division of Research**
Council for Exceptional Children
2900 Crystal Dr.
Suite 100
Arlington, VA 22202-3557
888-232-7733
TTY: 866-915-5000
http://www.cecdr.org
info@cec.sped.org
Kristen McMaster, President
David Lee, President Elect
Tom Farmer, Vice President
Devoted to the advancement of research related to the education of individuals with disabilities and/or who are gifted. CEC-DR aims to promote equal partnership with practitioners in designing, conducting, and interpreting research in special education.

48 **Division on Career Development & Transition (DCDT)**
Council for Exceptional Children
2900 Crystal Dr.
Suite 100
Arlington, VA 22202-3557
888-232-7733
TTY: 866-915-5000
http://community.cec.sped.org/dcdt/home
jrazeghi@gmu.edu
Jusy Shanley, President
Karrie Shogren, Vice President
Jane Razeghi, Executive Director
Promotes national and international efforts to improve the quality of and access to career, vocational, and transition services. Works to influence policies affecting career development and transition services for persons with disabilities.

49 **Division on Visual Impairments and Deafblindness**
Council for Exceptional Children
2900 Crystal Dr.
Suite 100
Arlington, VA 22202-3557
888-232-7733
TTY: 866-915-5000
http://community.cec.sped.org/dvi/home
service@cec.sped.org
Amy Parker, President
Tessa McCarthy, Secretary
Karen Vay Walker, Director
Division offering support and resources to further the education of visually impaired individuals, and assist the CEC in its efforts to improve educational accessibility for persons who are gifted and exceptional.

50 **Dyscalculia International Consortium (DIC)**
7420 Calhoun St.
Dearborn, MI 48126
313-300-1901
http://www.dyscalculia.org
help@dyscalculia.org
Renee M. Newman, President/Founder
Samira Guyot, Chief Attorney, Education Law
Rodrick Coffee, Director, Communications
A non-profit educational organization dedicated to advancing understanding and treatment of dyscalculia. This organization aims to provide free information to the public about dyscalculia and the best practices for diagnosis and treatment.

51 **Easterseals**
141 W. Jackson Blvd.
Suite 1400A
Chicago, IL 60604
312-726-6200
800-221-6827
Fax: 312-726-1494
http://www.easterseals.com
info@easterseals.com

Angela F. Williams, President/CEO
Julie Hubbard, SVP, Finance
Jed Johnson, VP, National Programs
Easter Seals' mission is to create solutions that change lives for children and adults with disabilities, their families, and their communities, by identifying the needs of people with disabilities and providing appropriate developmental and rehabilitation services. Easter Seals operates 550 websites that provide services to children and adults with disabilities and their families.

52 **Eden Autism Services**
2 Merwick Rd.
Princeton, NJ 08540
609-987-0099
Fax: 609-987-0243
http://edenautism.org
info@edenservices.org
Michaek K. Decker, President/CEO
Jennifer Bizub, Chief Operating Officer
David Napoleon, Chief Financial Officer
A non-profit ogranization that provides year round educational services, early intervention, parent training, respite care, outreach services, community based residential services, and employment opportunities for individuals with autism.
1975

53 **Federation for Children with Special Needs**
529 Main St.
Suite 1M3
Boston, MA 02129
617-236-7210
800-331-0688
Fax: 617-241-0330
http://www.fcsn.org
fcsninfo@fcsn.org
Richard Robison, Executive Director
Tom Hamel, Director, Business/Finance
Jennetta Hyatt, Director, Human Resources
The mission of the Federation is to provide information, support and assistance to parents of children with disabilities, their professional partners and their communities. Major services include information and referral and parent and professional training.

54 **Higher Education for Learning Problems (HELP)**
Marshall University
Myers Hall
520 18th St.
Huntington, WV 25755
304-696-6252
Fax: 304-696-3231
http://www.marshall.edu/help
help@marshall.edu
Debbie Painter, Director
Missi Fisher, Assistant Director
Renna Moore, Administrative Assistant
Provides educational support, remediation, and mentoring to individuals diagnosed with a learning disability and/or ADD/ADHD. Comprised of Community H.E.L.P., College H.E.L.P., Medical/Law H.E.L.P., and Diagnostic H.E.L.P.

55 **Independent Living Research Utilization Program**
TIRR Memorial Hermann Research Center
1333 Moursund
Houston, TX 77030
713-520-0232
Fax: 713-520-5785
TTY: 713-520-0232
http://www.ilru.org
ilru@ilru.org
Lex Frieden, Director
Richard Petty, Co-Director
Darrell Jones, Program Director
A national center for information, training, research, and technical assistance in independent living. ILRU collects and disseminates information relating to the field of independent living.

56 **Institute for Educational Leadership**
4301 Connecticut Ave., NW
Suite 100
Washington, DC 20008
202-822-8405
Fax: 202-872-4050
http://www.iel.org
iel@iel.org
Johan Uvin, President
Karen Mapp, Chair
Sara A. Sneed, Vice Chair
The Institute aims to improve education and the lives of children and their families through positive and visionary change.

57 **Institute for Human Centered Design (IHCD)**
200 Portland St.
Suite 1
Boston, MA 02114
617-695-1225
800-949-4232
Fax: 617-482-8099
TTY: 617-695-1225
http://humancentereddesign.org
info@HumanCenteredDesign.org
Ralph Jackson, President
Valerie Fletcher, Executive Director
Gabriela Bonome-Sims, Director, Administration
The IHCD seeks to improve accessibility standards for disabled people through improvement and innovation in design. The institute offers information on both legal standards and best practices for universal design.
1978

58 **Institutes for the Achievement of Human Potential (IAHP)**
8801 Stenton Ave.
Wyndmoor, PA 19038
215-233-2050
800-207-2948
Fax: 215-233-9646
http://www.iahp.org
institutes@iahp.org
Janet Doman, Director
Dr. Denise Malkowicz, Medical Director
Non-profit educational organization that serves children by introducing parents to the field of child brain development. Parents learn how to enhance significantly the development of their children physically, intellectually, and socially.
1955

59 **International Dyslexia Association**
40 York Rd.
4th Fl.
Baltimore, MD 21204
410-296-0232
Fax: 410-321-5069
http://www.dyslexiaida.org
info@ydslexiaida.org
Rick Smith, Chief Executive Officer
Newton Guerin, Chief Operating Officer
David Holste, Chief Financial Officer
The International Dyslexia Association is an international organization that concerns itself with the complex issues of dyslexia. The IDA membership consists of a variety of professionals in partnership with people with dyslexia and their families and all others interested in The Association's mission.

60 **International Literacy Association (ILA)**
800 Barksdale Rd.
Newark, DE 19711-3204
302-731-1600
800-336-7323
Fax: 302-731-1057
http://www.literacyworldwide.org
customerservice@reading.org
Bernadette Dwyer, President
Marcie Craig Post, Executive Director
Stephen Sye, Associate Executive Director
The mission of the International Literacy Association is to promote reading by continuously advancing the quality of literacy instruction and research worldwide.

61 **LD OnLine**
2775 South Quincy St.
Arlington, VA 22206 *Fax:* 703-998-2060
http://www.ldonline.org
Noel Gunther, Executive Director
Christian Lindstrom, Director, Learning Media
Kelly Deckert, Associate Manager, Online Media
A national educational service that provides information and referrals to both parents and educators dealing with children that are diagnosed with learning disabilities.

62 **Landmark School Outreach Program**
Landmark School
429 Hale St.
P.O. Box 227
Prides Crossing, MA 01965 978-236-3216
Fax: 978-927-7268
http://www.landmarkoutreach.org
outreach@landmarkschool.org
Dan Ahearn, Director of Outreach
Keryn Kwedor, Associate Director, Outreach
Jenna Lanoue, Operations Manager
Offers strategies, research, and professional development to help educators improve learning for children with language-based learning disabilities.
1971

63 **Learning Ally: National Headquarters**
20 Roszel Rd.
Princeton, NJ 08540 800-221-4792
http://www.learningally.org
Andrew Friedman, President/CEO
Connie Murphy, Executive Vice President
Cynthia Hamburger, Chief Operating Officer/CIO
National, non-profit organization working to provide better access to learning aids that can assist children with reading-related disabilities. Offers informational resources for educators, parents, and professionals intended to help connect them with access to these learning aids and guides on implementing them at home or in the classroom.

64 **Learning Disabilities Association of America (LDAA)**
4156 Library Rd.
Pittsburgh, PA 15234-1349 412-341-1515
Fax: 412-344-0224
http://www.ldaamerica.org
info@ldaamerica.org
Mary-Clare Reynolds, Executive Director
Stephanie Fedro-Byrom, Operations Manager
Myrna Mandlawitz, Policy Director
LDA is a grassroots, membership organization seeking to improve policy and accessibility for individuals with learning disabilities.

65 **Learning Resource Network**
P.O. Box 9
River Falls, WI 54022 800-678-5376
Fax: 888-234-8633
http://www.lern.org
info@lern.org
William A. Draves, President
Julie Coates, SVP, Information Services
Greg Marsello, SVP, Organizational Development
An organization dedicated to offering informational resources and consultative expertise on continuing education and lifelong learning. Disseminates publications, newsletters, webinars, and conferences that provide strategies and methodologies for professionals in educational institutions.
1974

66 **Matrix Parent Network & Resource Center**
94 Galli Dr.
Suite C
Novato, CA 94949 415-884-3535
800-578-2592
Fax: 415-884-3555
http://www.matrixparents.org
info@matrixparents.org
Alexis Lynch, Board President
Nora Thompson, Executive Director
Alyssa DiFilippo, Director, Parent Services
Providing families who have children with disabilities and other special needs with the tools they need to effectively advocate for themselves.
1983

67 **McRel International**
4601 DTC Blvd.
Suite 500
Denver, CO 80237-2596 303-337-0990
800-858-6830
http://www.mcrel.org
info@mcrel.org
Sue Desch, Chief Financial Officer
Bryan Goodwin, President/CEO
Melissa Gray, Chief People Officer
Organization offering educational services through evaluation, analysis, and research in order to assist schools with providing optimal learning outcomes.

68 **Menninger Clinic**
12301 Main St.
Houston, TX 77035 713-275-5000
Fax: 713-275-5107
http://www.menningerclinic.com
Tony Gaglio, Interim President/CEO
Bella Schanzer, Interim Chief of Staff
Avni Cirpili, SVP/Chief Nursing Officer
The mission of Menninger is to be a national resource providing psychiatric care and treatment of the highest standard, searching for better understanding of mental illness and human behavior, disseminating their findings, and applying this knowledge in useful ways to promote individual growth and better mental health.

69 **NASDSE**
225 Reinekers Ln.
Suite 420
Alexandria, VA 22314 703-519-3800
Fax: 703-519-3808
http://www.nasdse.org
Santina Thibedeau, President
Bill East, Executive Director
Nancy Reder, Deputy Executive Director
The National Association of State Directors of Special Education provides leadership focused on the improvement of educational services and positive outcomes for children and youth with disabilities throughout the United States.

70 **NASP**
4340 East West Hwy.
Suite 402
Bethesda, MD 20814 301-657-0270
866-331-6277
Fax: 301-657-0275
http://nasponline.org
Kathleen Minke, Executive Director
Laura Benson, Chief Operating Officer
Lisa Kelly-Vance, President
The National Association of School Psychologists empowers school psychologists by advancing effective practices to improve students' learning, behavior, and mental health.

71 **National ARD/IEP Advocates**
4510 Redstart
Houston, TX 77035 281-265-1506
http://www.narda.org
nationalardadvocates@gmail.com
Louis H. Geigerman, Founder/President
National ARD Advocates is dedicated to obtaining the appropriate educational services for children with special needs.

72 **National Adult Education Professional Development Consortium (NAEPDC)**
444 North Capitol St., NW
Suite 422
Washington, DC 20001
202-624-5250
Fax: 202-624-1497
http://www.naepdc.org
ptyler@naepdc.org

Patricia H. Tyler, Executive Director
Reecie Stagnolia, Chair
Gene Sofer, Director, Government Relations
An organization dedicated to enhancing adult education through professional development and dissemination of information and assistive resources.

73 **National Association for Adults with Special Learning Needs (NAASLN)**
P.O. Box 716
Bryn Mawr, PA 19010
http://www.naasln.org

Richard Cooper, President
Joan Hudson-Miller, Co-President
Frances A. Holthaus, Vice President
An association for those who serve adults with special learning needs. Members include educators, trainers, employers, and human service providers

74 **National Association for Child Development (NACD)**
5492 S. 500 E.
Washington Terrace, UT 84405
801-621-8606
http://www.nacd.org

Robert J. Doman, Jr., Founder/Director
Laird Doman, COO/Family Liason
Ellen R. Doman, Educational Director
Provides neurodevelopmental evaluations and individualized programs for children and adults, updated on a quarterly basis. Stresses parent training and parent implementation of the program.

75 **National Association for Community Mediation (NAFCM)**
P.O. Box 5246
Louisville, KY 40255
602-633-4213
http://www.nafcm.org
info@nafcm.org

D.G. Mawn, President
Brennan Frazier, Membership Coordinator
Renata Valree, Chair
Supports the maintenance and growth of community-based mediation programs and processes; acts as a resource for mediation information; and locates a center to help individuals and groups resolve disputes.

76 **National Association for Gifted Children (NAGC)**
1331 H St., NW
Suite 1001
Washington, DC 20005
202-785-4268
Fax: 202-785-4248
http://www.nagc.org
nagc@nagc.org

Sally Krisel, President
M. René Islas, Executive Director
Adriane Wiles, Manager, Member Services
An organization of parents, teachers, educators, other professionals, and community leaders who unite to address the unique needs of children and youth with demonstrated gifts and talents as well as those children who may be able to develop their talent potential with appropriate educational experiences.

77 **National Association for the Education of Young Children (NAEYC)**
1313 L St., NW
Suite 500
Washington, DC 20005-4101
202-232-8777
800-424-2460
Fax: 202-328-1846
http://www.naeyc.org
naeyc@naeyc.org

Rhian Evans Allvin, Chief Executive Officer
Nancy Griswold, General Counsel
Cindy Chesnut, Senior Director, Human Resources
Dedicated to improving the well-being of all children, with particular focus on the quality of educational and developmental services for children from birth through age 8. Also the largest organization working on behalf of young adults with nearly 60,000 members; a national network of over 50 local, state, and regional affiliates; and a growing global alliance of like-minded organizations.

78 **National Association of Councils on Developmental Disabilities (NACDD)**
1825 K. St., NW
Suite 600
Washington, DC 20006
202-506-5813
http://www.nacdd.org
info@nacdd.org

Shannon Buller, President
Steve Gieber, Vice President
Charles Hughes, Secretary
A national member-driven organization consisting of 56 State and Territorial Councils. Places high value on meaningful participation and contribution by Council members and staff of all Member Councils, and continually works towards positive system change on behalf of individuals with developmental disabilities and their families.

79 **National Association of Parents with Children in Special Education (NAPCSE)**
3642 E Sunnydale Dr.
Chandler Heights, AZ 85142
800-754-4421
Fax: 800-424-0371
http://www.napcse.org
contact@napcse.org

Dr. George Giuliani, President
A national membership organization dedicated to supporting and assisting parents whose children receive special education services, both in and outside of school. NAPCSE was founded to promote a sense of community and provide a national forum for ideas.

80 **National Association of Private Special Education Centers (NAPSEC)**
601 Pennsylvania Ave., NW
Suite 900 - South Building
Washington, DC 20004
202-434-8225
http://www.napsec.org
napsec@napsec.org

Tom Dempsey, President
Dr. Tom McCool, Vice President
Tom Celli, Treasurer
A non-profit association whose mission is to ensure access for individuals to private special education as a vital component of the continuum of appropriate placement and services in American education. The association consists solely of private special education programs that serve both both privately and publicly placed individuals of all ages with disabilities.

81 **National Association of Special Education Teachers (NASET)**
1250 Connecticut Ave., NW
Suite 200
Washington, DC 20036
800-754-4221
Fax: 800-754-4421
http://www.naset.org
contactus@naset.org

Dr. Roger Pierangelo, Executive Director
Dr. George Giuliani, Executive Director
A national membership organization dedicated to providing support and assistance to those preparing for or teaching in the field of special education.

82 **National Autism Association**
One Park Ave.
Suite 1
Portsmouth, RI 02871
401-293-5551
877-622-2884
Fax: 401-293-5342
http://nationalautismassociation.org
naa@nationalautism.org
Claire Bothwell, Board Chair
Wendy Fournier, President/Founding Board Member
Krystal Higgins, Executive Director
The National Autism Association deals with and provides help for the most urget needs of the autism community.

83 **National Business and Disability Council at The Viscardi Center**
201 I.U. Willets Rd.
Albertson, NY 11507
516-465-1400
Fax: 516-465-1591
http://www.viscardicenter.org/nbdc/
info@viscardicenter.org
Scott Wright, Manager
Michael J. McGowan, Corporate Services Specialist
A leading resource for employers seeking to integrate people with disabilities into the workplace and companies seeking to reach them in the consumer marketplace. The NBDC has played a major role in helping businesses create accessible work conditions for employees and accessible products and services for consumers.

84 **National Center for Families Learning (NCFL)**
325 West Main St.
Suite 300
Louisville, KY 40202
502-584-1133
http://www.familieslearning.org
Sharon Darling, President/Founder
Mission is to create a literate nation by leveraging the power of family. Family literacy is an intergenerational approach based on the indisputable evidence that low literacy is an unfortunate and debilitating family tradition.

85 **National Center for Learning Disabilities (NCLD)**
32 Laight St.
2nd Fl.
New York, NY 10013
888-575-7373
http://www.ncld.org
Frederic M. Poses, Chairman of the Board
Mimi Corcoran, President/CEO
Rashonda Ambrose, Director, Strategic Partnerships
Works to ensure that the nation's 15 million children, adolescents, and adults with learning disabilities have every opportunity for succees in school, work, and life. NCLD also provides essential information to parents, professionals, and individuals with learning disabilities; promotes research and programs to foster effective learning; and advocates for policies to protect and strengthen educational rights and opportunities.

86 **National Center for Youth Law**
405 14th St.
15th Fl.
Oakland, CA 94612
510-835-8098
Fax: 510-835-8099
http://www.youthlaw.org
info@youthlaw.org
Peter B. Edelman, President
Jesse Hahnel, Executive Director
Christopher Wu, Vice President
Uses the law to improve the lives of low-income children. Also works to ensure that low-income children have the resources, support, and opportunities they need for a healthy and productive future. Much of NCYL's work is focused on poor children who are additionally challenged by abuse and neglect, disability, or other disadvantage.

87 **National Council of Juvenile and Family Court Judges (NCJFCJ)**
P.O. Box 8970
Reno, NV 89507
775-507-4777
Fax: 775-507-4848
http://www.ncjfcj.org
contactus@ncjfcj.org
Anthony Capizzi, President
Joey Orduna Hastings, Chief Executive Officer
Cheryl Dailey, Chief Financial Officer
The vision of the NCJFCJ is that every child and young person be reared in a safe, permanent, and nuturing family, where love, self-control, concern for others, and responsibility for the consequences of one's actions are experienced and taught as fundamental values for a successful life. Also advocates that every family in need of judicial oversight has access to fair, effective, and timely justice.

88 **National Council on Rehabilitation Education (NCRE)**
1099 E. Champlain Dr.
Suite A, #137
Fresno, CA 93720
559-906-0787
http://www.ncre.org
info@ncre.org
Denise Catalano, President
Matt Bruinekool, 1st Vice President
David A. Rosenthal, 2nd Vice President
A professional organization of educators that provide quality services for persons with disabilities. NCRE advocates for maintaining professional standards in the rehabilitation field.
1955

89 **National Disabilities Rights Network (NDRN)**
820 1st St. NE
Suite 740
Washington, DC 20002
202-408-9514
Fax: 202-408-9520
TTY: 202-408-9521
http://www.ndrn.org
info@ndrn.org
Michael Kirkman, President
Curtis L. Decker, Executive Director
Zachary Martin, Director, Operations
Non-profit membership organization for the federally mandated Protection and Advocacy Systems and Client Assistance Programs for individuals with disabilities. Serves a wide range of individuals with disabilities including those with cognitive, mental, sensory, and physical disabilities. Services include guarding against abuse; advocating for basic rights; and ensuring accountability in health care, education, employment, housing, and transportation.

90 **National Education Association (NEA)**
1201 16th St., NW
Washington, DC 20036-3290
202-833-4000
Fax: 202-822-7974
http://www.nea.org
Lily Eskelsen Garc¡a, President
Becky Pringle, Vice President
John C. Stocks, Executive Director
The National Education Association, along with it's state-wide affiliates, seeks to advance public education, working with professionals and members at every educational level—from pre-school to university.

91 **National Federation of the Blind**
200 E. Wells St.
at Jernigan Place
Baltimore, MD 21230
410-659-9314
Fax: 410-685-5653
http://www.nfb.org
pmaurer@nfb.org
Mark A. Riccobono, President
Pam Allen, First VP/Board Chair
Ron Brown, Second Vice President

The largest and most influential membership organization of blind people in the United States. The NFB improves the lives of the blind through advocacy, education, research, technology, and programs encouraging independence and self-confidence. It is also the leading force in the blindness field today and the voice of the nation's blind.

92 **National Institute for Learning Development**

1540 Breezeport Way
Suite 500
Suffolk, VA 23435
757-423-8646
Fax: 757-451-0970
http://nild.org

Kristin Barbour, Executive Director
Allison Jenson, Program Development Manager
Susie Hartung, Program Coordinator

NILD is a global institute offering services to parents, students, and educators in areas of accreditation, professional development, and educational therapy.

93 **National Institute of Art and Disabilities Art Center**

551 23rd St.
Richmond, CA 94804
510-620-0290
http://www.niadart.org

Deborah Dyer, Executive Director
Tim Buckwalter, Director, Exhibitions
Arden Fredman, Director of Client Services

An innovative visual arts center assisting adults with developmental and other physical disabilities. Provides an art program that promotes creativity, independence, dignity, and community integration for people with developmental and other disabilities.

94 **National Joint Committee on Learning Disabilities**

http://www.ldonline.org/njcld
Elsa.Hagan@times.uh.edu

Elsa Cardenas-Hagan, NJCLD Chair
Stan Dublinske, NJCLD Secretary/Treasurer

A partner of LD OnLine, the NJCLD's mission is to provide multi-organizational leadership and resources to optimize outcomes for individuals with learning disabilities. LD OnLine serves as the official website for the NJCLD.
1975

95 **National Organization for Rare Disorders (NORD)**

55 Kenosia Ave.
Danbury, CT 06810
203-744-0100
800-999-6673
Fax: 203-263-9938
http://www.rarediseases.org

Marshall Summar, Board Chairman
Peter Saltonstall, President/CEO
Pamela Gavin, Chief Strategy Officer

A unique federation of voluntary health organizations dedicated to helping people with rare diseases and assisting the organizations that serve them. Committed to the identification, treatment, and cure of rare disorders through programs of education, advocacy, research, and service.

96 **National Organization on Disability (NOD)**

77 Water St.
Suite 204
New York, NY 10005
646-505-1191
Fax: 646-505-1184
http://www.nod.org
info@nod.org

Gov. Tom Ridge, Board Chairman
Carol Glazer, President
Miranda Pax, Director, External Affairs

The mission of the National Organization on Disability is to expand the participataion and contribution of America's 57 million men, women, and children with disabilities in all aspects of life.

97 **National Rehabilitation Association**

P.O. Box 150235
Alexandria, VA 22315
703-836-0850
888-258-4295
Fax: 703-836-0848
http://www.nationalrehab.org
membership@nationalrehab.org

Greg Mason, President
Dr. Fredric Schroeder, Executive Director
James Liin, Membership Coordinator

A membership organization that promotes ethical and state of the art practice in rehabilitation with the goal of the personal and economic independence of persons with disabilities. Members include rehabilitation counselors, physical, speech and occupational therapists, job trainers, consultants, independent living instructors, students in rehabilitation programs, and other professionals involved in the advocacy of programs and services for people with disabilities.

98 **National Rehabilitation Information Center (NARIC)**

8400 Corporate Dr.
Suite 500
Landover, MD 20785
800-346-2742
Fax: 301-459-4263
TTY: 301-459-5984
http://www.naric.com
naricinfo@heitechservices.com

Mark X. Odum, Project Director
Jessica H. Chaiken, Media & Info Services Manager
Natalie J. Collier, Library and Acquisitions Manager

The mission of the Center is to collect and disseminate the results of research funded by the National Institute on Disability, Independent Living and Rehabilitation Research (NIDLRR); and provide information and referral on disability and rehabilitation from the layperson to the professional.

99 **Nonverbal Learning Disorders Association (NLDA)**

507 Hopmeadow St.
Simsbury, CT 06070
860-658-5522
Fax: 860-658-6688
http://www.nlda.org
info@nlda.org

Patricia Carrin, Founder/President
Marcia Rubinstein, Founder/Executive Liaison

A non-profit organization dedicated to research, education, and advocacy for nonverbal learning disorders.

100 **Parent Advocacy Coalition for Educational Rights (PACER)**

8161 Normandale Blvd.
Bloomington, MN 55437
952-838-9000
800-537-2237
Fax: 952-838-0199
http://www.pacer.org
pacer@pacer.org

Matthew Woods, Board President
Tammy Pust, Board Vice President
Paula F. Goldberg, Executive Director

The mission of PACER is to expand opportunities and enhance the quality of life of children and young adults with disabilities and their families, based on the concept of parents helping parents.

101 **Parent Educational Advocacy Training Center (PEATC)**

8003 Forbes Place
Suite 310
Springfield, VA 22151
703-923-0010
800-869-6782
Fax: 800-693-3514
TTY: 703-923-0010
http://www.peatc.org
partners@peatc.org

Suzanne Bowers, Executive Director
Nichole Drummond, Deputy Director
Vanessa Rakestraw, President

A non-profit that believes children with disabilities reach their full potential when families and professionals enjoy an equal, respectful partnership. PEATC also provides support education, and training to families, schools, and other professionals committed to helping children with disabilities.

102 **Parents Helping Parents**
Sobrato Center for Nonprofits-San Jose
1400 Parkmoor Ave.
Suite 100
San Jose, CA 95126
408-727-5775
855-727-5775
Fax: 408-286-1116
http://www.php.com
info@php.com
Maria Daane, Executive Director
Jane Floethe Ford, Director, Education Services
Mark Fishler, Development Director
Helping children with special needs receive the resources, love, hope, respect, health care, education, and other services they need to achieve their full potential by helping to create strong families and dedicated professionals.

103 **Rehabilitation Engineering and Assistive Technology Society of North America (RESNA)**
1560 Wilson Blvd.
Suite 850
Arlington, VA 22209
703-524-6686
Fax: 703-524-6630
http://www.resna.org
info@resna.org
Roger O. Smith, President
Michael J. Brogioli, Executive Director
An interdisciplinary association of people with a common interest in technology and disability. The purpose is to use technology to improve the potential of people with disabilities and enable them to achieve their goals.

104 **Rehabilitation International (RI Global)**
866 United Nations Plaza
Office 422
New York, NY 10017
212-420-1500
Fax: 212-505-0871
http://www.riglobal.org
info@riglobal.org
Zhang Haidi, President
Venus Ilagan, Secretary General
Susan Parker, Treasurer
A global network of people with disabilities, service providers, researchers, government agencies, and advocates promoting and implementing the rights and inclusion of people with disabilities.

105 **Sertoma Inc.**
1912 East Meyer Blvd.
Kansas City, MO 64132
816-333-8300
Fax: 816-333-4320
http://www.sertoma.org
infosertoma@sertomahq.org
Edwin Dlugopolski, President
John Kelly, President Elect
Joy Newman, Senior Vice President
Activities focus on helping people with speech and hearing problems, but also have programs in the areas of youth, national heritage, drug awareness, and community services.

106 **Smart Kids with Learning Disabilities**
38 Kings Hwy. North
Westport, CT 06880
203-226-6831
Fax: 203-226-6708
http://smartkidswithld.org
Smart Kids with Learning Disabilities is a non-profit organization dedicated to empowering the parents of children with learning disabilites (LD) and attention-deficit disorder (ADHD) by providing resources to help understand and evaluate their child's capabilities.

107 **Son-Rise Program**
Autism Treatment Center of America
2080 S. Undermountain Rd.
Sheffield, MA 01257
413-229-2100
877-766-7473
http://www.autismtreatmentcenter.org
Barry Neil Kaufman, Co-Founder
Raun K. Kaufman, Group Facilitator
Samahria Lyte Kaufman, Co-Founder
Since 1983, the Autism Treatment Center of America has provided innovative training programs and workshops for parents and professionals caring for children challenged by Autism, Autism Spectrum Disorders, Pervasive Developmental Disorder (PDD), and other developmental difficulties.
1983

108 **Stuttering Foundation of America**
P.O. Box 11749
Memphis, TN 38111-0749
901-761-0343
800-992-9392
Fax: 901-761-0484
http://www.stutteringhelp.org
info@stutteringhelp.org
Jane H. Fraser, President
Founded with the goal to provide the best and most up-to-date information and help available for the prevention of stuttering in young children and the most effective treatment available for teenagers and adults.

109 **Team of Advocates for Special Kids (TASK)**
100 West Cerritos Ave.
Anaheim, CA 92805
714-533-8275
Fax: 714-533-2533
http://www.taskca.org
Mario Haug, Executive Director
Dr. John Hess, President
Katherine Patel, Vice President
TASK's mission is to enable children with disabilities to reach their maximum potential by providing them, their families, and the professionals who serve them, with training, support information resources and referrals, and by providing community awareness programs. TASK's TECH Center is a place for children, parents, adult consumers, and professionals to learn about assistive technology by providing hands-on access to computer hardware, software, and adaptive equipment.

110 **Technology and Media Division**
Council for Exceptional Children
2900 Crystal Dr.
Suite 1000
Arlington, VA 22202-3557
888-232-7733
TTY: 866-915-5000
http://www.tamcec.org
aevmenov@gmu.edu
Sean Smith, President
Marci Kinas Jerome, Treasurer
Sara Heintzelman, Secretary
TAM works to promote the availability and effective use of technology and media for children, birth to 21, with disabilities and/or who are gifted.

111 **The American Printing House for the Blind, Inc.**
1839 Frankfort Ave.
Louisville, KY 40206-0085
502-895-2405
800-223-1839
Fax: 502-899-2284
http://www.aph.org
info@aph.org
Jane Hardy, Board Chair
A non-profit organization providing educational, work place, and independent living products and services for people who are visually impaired.

112 **The College Board**
250 Vesey St.
New York, NY 10281
212-713-8000
866-630-9305
http://www.collegeboard.org
David Coleman, President/CEO
Jeremy Singer, Chief Operating Officer
John McGrath, Senior VP, Communications
Founded in 1900, The College Board offers testing accommodations that minimize the effect of disabilities on test performance. The SAT Program tests eligible students with documented visual, physical, hearing, or learning disabilities who require testing accommodations for SAT.

113 **US Autism & Asperger Association**
12180 S. 300 E.
Suite 532
Draper, UT 84020-0532-0532
888-928-8476
http://usautism.org
Lawrence Kaplan, Chairman/CEO
Phillip C. DeMio, Chief Medical Officer
Richard Dunie, Secretary/Treasurer
US Autism & Asperger Association (USAAA) is a non-profit organization for Autism and Asperger education, support, and solutions.

114 **US Department of Education: Office for Civil Rights**
400 Maryland Ave., SW
Washington, DC 20202-1100
800-421-3481
Fax: 202-453-6012
TTY: 800-877-8339
http://www.ed.gov
ocr@ed.gov
Kenneth L. Marcus, Assistant Secretary
William E. Trachman, Dep. Assistant Secretary, Policy
The mission of the Office for Civil Rights is to ensure equal access to education and to promote educational excellence throughout the nation.

115 **Washington PAVE: Specialized Training of Military Parents (STOMP)**
6316 South 12th St.
Tacoma, WA 98465
253-565-2266
800-572-7368
Fax: 253-566-8052
TTY: 800-573-7368
http://www.wapave.org
pave@wapave.org
Tracy Kahlo, Executive Director
Nicol Walsh, Communications Specialist
Elma Rounds, CFO/Office Manager
STOMP is a parent-directed project that exists to empower military parents, individuals with disabilities, and service providers with knowledge, skills, and resources so that they might access services to create a collaborative environment for a family and professional partnerships without regard to geographic location.

116 **World Institute on Disability (WID)**
3075 Adeline St.
Suite 155
Berkeley, CA 94703
510-225-6400
Fax: 510-225-0477
TTY: 510-225-0478
http://www.wid.org
wid@wid.org
Loretta Herrington, Manager, Special Projects
Anita Shafer Aaron, Executive Director
Thomas Foley, Managing Director
A non-profit public policy center dedicated to promoting independence and full societal inclusion of people with disabilities.

117 **YACHAD/National Jewish Council for Disabilities**
11 Broadway
13th Fl.
New York, NY 10004
212-613-8229
Fax: 212-613-0796
http://www.yachad.org
njcd@ou.org
Dr. Jeffrey Lichtman, International Director
Ken Saibel, Associate Director
Becca Zebovitz, Acting Director, Operations
Yachad/NJCD is dedicated to addressing the needs of all individuals with disabilities and including them in the Jewish community. Summer Programs include a variety of summer experiences for youth and adults with developmental disabilities.

118 **YAI Network**
460 West 34th St.
11th Fl.
New York, NY 10001-2382
212-273-6100
http://www.yai.org
staff@yai.org
George Contos, Chief Executive Officer
Jeffrey A. Mordos, Chairman
Lewis A. Lindenberg, Vice Chairman
A national leader in the provision of services, education, and training in the field of developmental and learning disabilities.

Alabama

119 **Easter Seals - Alabama**
5960 E Shirley Ln
Montgomery, AL 36117
334-395-4489
Fax: 334-395-4492
http://www.easterseals.com/alabama
info@al.easterseals.com
John Ives, Chairman
Randy Thomas, Chairman Elect
Lynne Stokley, Chief Executive Officer
Easter Seals provides services to children and adults with disabilities and other special needs, and support to their families.
1926

120 **Easter Seals - Birmingham Area**
2717 3rd Avenue S
Birmingham, AL 35233
205-942-6277
Fax: 205-945-5568
http://www.eastersealsbham.org
info@eastersealsbham.org
Paul Ebert, Chair
Jennifer Shaw, Vice Chair
David Higgins, Executive Director
From child development centers to physical rehabilitation and job training for people with disabilities, Easter Seals offers a variety of services to help people with disabilities address life's challenges and achieve personal goals.

121 **Easter Seals - Central Alabama**
2185 Normandie Dr
Montgomery, AL 36111
334-288-0240
Fax: 334-288-7171
http://eastersealscentralalabama.org
info@eastersealsca.org
Debbie Lynn, Executive Director
Ed Collier, Director, Programs
Frankie Thomas, Senopr Employment Program
Provides quality life enhancing programs and services to meet the needs of children and adults with disabilities.

122 **Easter Seals - West Alabama**
1140 James I Harrison, Jr. Pkwy E
Tuscaloosa, AL 35405 205-759-1211
800-726-1216
Fax: 205-349-1162
http://www.eswaweb.org
eswa@eswaweb.org
Kenneth Gaddy, Chair
Sandra Ray, Vice Chair
Ronny Johnston, Executive Director
Serves children and adults with disabilities through programs such as job training and skill development, speech therapy, and family nursing.

123 **International Dyslexia Association of Alabama**
2925 Chantry Place SE
Gurley, AL 35748 256-337-1889
http://al.dyslexiaida.org
tcrowecrnp@msn.com
Denise Gibbs, President
Gladys Shaefer, Vice President
Townley Crowe, Secretary
ALIDA provides dyslexic individuals in Alabama with a unified voice to represent their interests to the public, to the educational community, to the legislature, and to others. ALIDA also serves as a vehicle to increase awareness and understanding of dyslexia in Alabama.
1903

124 **Learning Disabilities Association of Alabama**
PO Box 244023
Montgomery, AL 36124 334-277-9151
http://ldaalabama.org
Tamara Massey-Garrett, President
A non-profit grassroots organization whose members are individuals with learning disabilities, their families, and the professionals who work with them. LDAA is dedicated to identifying causes and promoting prevention of learning disabilities and to enhance the quality of life for all individuals with learning disabilities and their families by encouraging effective identification and intervention, fostering research, and protecting their rights under the law.

125 **The Arc of Alabama**
557 S Lawrence St
Montgomery, AL 36104 334-262-7688
http://www.thearcofal.org
advocacy@thearcofalabama.com
Bruce Koppenhoefer, President
Johnna Breland, Treasurer
Terrie Platt, Secretary
A non-profit organization dedicated to improving the quality of life for people with learning disabilities and developmental disabilities.

Alaska

126 **Adam's Camp - Alaska**
PO Box 242003
Anchorage, AK 99524 907-885-1758
http://adamscampalaska.org
alaska@adamscamp.org
Kellie Newland, President
Cindy Wells, Vice President
Clay Waller, Treasurer
Designed to give children and teens with physical and developmental disabilities the opportunity to development life skills, make friends, and foster self esteem.
1986

127 **Center for Human Development (CHD)**
University of Alaska Anchorage
2702 Gambell St
Ste 103
Anchorage, AK 99503 907-272-8270
800-243-2199
Fax: 907-274-4802
http://www.alaskachd.org
info@alaskachd.org
Karen Ward, Director
Jenny Miller, LEND Training Director
Ken Hamrick, AWP Program Director
One of 67 University Centers located in every state and territory, which attempts to bring together the resources of the university and the community in support of individuals with developmental disabilities.

128 **Community Connections**
721 Stedman St
Ketchikan, AK 99901 907-225-7825
Fax: 907-225-1541
http://comconnections.org
Bess Clark, Executive Director
Brynn Bolling, Program Dir., Early Learning
Shawn Shotwell, Program Dir., Senior/Disability
Operates three specialized programs: Children's Mental Health, Early Learning, and Senior & Disability Services. Community Connections serves individuals with developmental disabilities in Ketchikan, Metlakatla, and Prince of Wales Island, Alaska.
1985

129 **Easter Seals - Alaska**
670 W Fireweed Ln
Ste 105
Anchorage, AK 99503 907-277-7325
Fax: 907-272-7325
http://www.easterseals.com/alaska
Vilma Gutierrez-Osborne, Chief Executive Officer
Easter Seals assists more than one million children and adults with disabilities and their families annually through a nationwide network of more than 450 service sites.

Arizona

130 **Arizona Center for Disability Law**
5025 E Washington St
Ste 202
Phoenix, AZ 85034 602-274-6287
800-927-2260
Fax: 602-274-6779
http://www.azdisabilitylaw.org
center@azdisabilitylaw.org
Sami Hamed, President
Sherri Collins, Secretary
Floyd Galloway, Treasurer
Advocates for the legal rights of persons with disabilities to be free from abuse, neglect and discrimination; and to have access to education, healthcare, housing and jobs, and other services in order to maximize independence and achieve equality.

131 **Institute for Human Development: Northern Arizona University**
912 Riordan Rd, Bldg 27A
PO Box 5630
Flagstaff, AZ 86011-5630 *Fax:* 928-523-9127
TTY: 928-523-1695
http://www.nau.edu
ihd@nau.edu
Emily McRobbie, Program Coordinator
Aimee Barerra, Administrative Assistant
The Institute values and supports the independence, productivity and inclusion of Arizona's citizens with disabilities. Based on the values and beliefs, the Institute conducts training, research and services that further these goal.

132 **International Dyslexia Association of Arizona**
PO Box 13116
Phoenix, AZ 85002-3116
http://az.dyslexiaida.org
arizona.ida@gmail.com
Rebekah Dyer, President
Courtney Gilstrap LeVinus, Vice President
Tina Wildoner, Secretary
The Arizona Branch of The International Dyslexia Association (AIDA) non-profit, scientific organization dedicated to educating the public about the learning disability, dyslexia. The Arizona Branch has four objectives: to increase awareness in the dyslexic and general community; to network with other learning disability groups and legislators in education; to increase membership; to raise funds for future projects that will make a difference in the community.

133 **Parent Information Network**
Arizona Department of Education
1535 W. Jeffer St.
Phoenix, AZ 85007
602-542-5393
800-352-4558
http://www.azed.gov
adeinbox@azed.gov
Alissa Trollinger, Deputy Associate Superintendent
Provides free training and information to parents on federal and state laws and regulations for special education, parental rights and responsibilities, parent involvement, advocacy, behavior, standards and disability related resources. Provides a clearinghouse of information targeted to parents of children with disabilities. Also assists schools in promoting positive parent/professional/regional partnerships.

Arkansas

134 **Easter Seals - Arkansas**
3920 Woodland Heights Rd
Little Rock, AR 72212-2495
501-227-3600
Fax: 501-227-3658
http://www.easterseals.com/arkansas
Jay Heflin, Chair
Dr. James Hunt, Vice Chair
Elaine Eubank, President & CEO
Easter Seals' mission is to provide exceptional services to ensure that all people with disabilities or special needs have equal opportunities to live, learn, work and play in their communities.

135 **Learning Disabilities Association of Arkansas (LDAA)**
PO Box 23514
Little Rock, AR 72221
501-666-8777
http://www.ldarkansas.org
Kaci Smith, President
Kimberly Newton, Vice President
Doris Pierce, Treasurer
A nonprofit, volunteer organization of parents and professionals. LDAA is devoted to defining and finding solutions to the broad spectrum of learning disabilities.

California

136 **California Association of Private Special Education Schools (CAPSES)**
921 11th St
Ste 501
Sacramento, CA 95814
916-447-7061
Fax: 916-447-1320
http://www.capses.com
director@capses.com
Teresa Malekzadeh, President
Rebecca Foo, Secretary
Susan Lane, Executive Director
Dedicated to preserving and enhancing the leadership role of the private sector in offering quality alternative services to students with disabilities.
191 members 1973

137 **Community Alliance for Special Education (CASE)**
1550 Bryant St
Ste 735
San Francisco, CA 94103
415-431-2285
Fax: 415-431-2289
http://www.caseadvocacy.org
info@caseadvocacy.org
Heather Selick, Parent/Child Advocate
Provides special education advocacy, representation at individual education program (IEP) meetings and due process proceedings, free technical assistance consultations and training throughout the San Francisco Bay area.
1979

138 **Easter Seals - Bay Area, Lakeport**
1950 Parallel Dr
Lakeport, CA 95453
707-263-3949
http://www.eastersealsbayarea.org
customerservice@esba.org
Susan Armiger, President & CEO
Jeff Bruner, Chief Financial Officer
Sheldon Orloff, Chair
Easter Seals provides services to children and adults with autism and other disabilities needs and support to their families.

139 **Easter Seals - Camp Heron**
16403 Hwy 9
Boulder Creek, CA 95006
831-338-3383
http://www.campharmon.org
campharmon@es-cc.org
Devin Laming, Coordinator
Camp Harmon offers camping opportunities to people with disabilities. Offers sessions designed for a specific age group and specific to developmental and/or physical disabilities.
1963

140 **Easter Seals - Central California, Aptos**
9010 Soquel Dr
Ste 1
Aptos, CA 95003-4002
831-684-2166
Fax: 831-684-1018
http://www.easterseals.com/centralcal
Scott Webb, Executive Director
Twila Chaffee, Finance Manager
Jeff Terpstra, Chair
Create solutions that change lives of children and adults with disabilities or other special needs and their families.

141 **Easter Seals - Central California, Fresno**
2505 W Shaw Ave
Ste 2
Fresno, CA 93711
559-241-7233
Fax: 559-492-1409
http://www.easterseals.com/centralcal
Scott Webb, Executive Director
Twila Chaffee, Finance Manager
Jeff Terpstra, Chair
Create solutions that change lives of children and adults with disabilities or other special needs and their families.

142 **Easter Seals - Southern California**
1063 McGaw Ave
Irvine, CA 92614
714-834-1111
http://www.easterseals.com/southerncal
Mark Whitley, Chief Executive Officer
Molly Pyott, Chair
Andre Bertrand, First Vice Chair
Provides exceptional services to ensure that all people with disabilities or other special needs and their families have equal opportunities to live, learn, work and play in their communities.

143 **International Dyslexia Association of Los Angeles**
PO Box 66662
Los Angeles, CA 90066
http://dyslexiala.org
info@dyslexiala.org

Barb Langeloh, President
Stephanie Funk, Treasurer
Megan Jensen, Secretary
The Los Angeles County Branch of The International Dyslexia Association believes that all individuals have the right to realize their potential, that individual learning abilities can be strengthened, and that language and reading skills can be achieved.

144 **International Dyslexia Association of Northern California (NCBIDA)**
PO Box 5010
San Mateo, CA 94402-0010 650-328-7667
http://norcal.dyslexiaida.org
info.norcal@dyslexiaida.org
Cawley Carr, President
John Santonastaso, Vice President
David Futterman, Treasurer
Formed to increase public awareness of dyslexia in Northern California and Northern Nevada. Have been serving individuals with dyslexia, their families and professionals in the field in this community for 30 years.

145 **International Dyslexia Association of San Diego**
12285 Oak Knoll Rd.
Poway, CA 92064 619-295-3722
800-657-0381
http://sdcal.dyslexiaida.org
sdidainfo@gmail.com
Steve Mayo, President
Julie Seki Sulzmaier, Vice President
Dana Gordon, Secretary
A nonprofit scientific and educational organization dedicated to the study and treatment of the learning disability. This branch was informed to increase public awareness of dyslexia.

146 **Legal Services for Children**
1254 Market St
3rd Fl
San Francisco, CA 94102 415-863-3762
Fax: 415-863-7708
http://www.lsc-sf.org
Reyna Burgos, DICP Coordinator
Ron Gutierrez, Clinical Director
Abigail Trillin, Executive Director
Nonprofit law firm for children and youth. Legal Services for Children provides free legal and social services to children and youth under 18 years old in the San Francisco Bay area.
1975

147 **Los Angeles Learning Disabilities Association**
PO Box 1067
Sierra Madre, CA 91025 626-355-0240
http://lalda.org
lalda@lalda.org
A nonprofit volunteer organization of parents, professionals and adults with learning disabilities. Its purpose is to promote and support the education and general welfare of children and adults of potentially normal intelligence who manifest learning, perceptual, and/or behavioral handicaps.

148 **Lutheran Braille Workers**
13471 California St.
P.O. Box 5000
Yucaipa, CA 92399 909-795-8977
800-925-6092
Fax: 909-795-8970
http://www.lbwinc.org
lbw@lbwinc.org
Loyd Coppenger, Executive Director
The mission of Lutheran Braille Workers is to provide the message of salvation, through faith in Jesus Christ, to individuals who are blind or visually impaired throughout the world.
1943

Colorado

149 **Colorado Council for Learning Disabilities**
CO http://cocld.org
contactus@cocld.org
Sabrina Raugutt, President
Cassie Harrelson, Treasurer/MOP Coordinator
Annemarie Dempsey, Secretary
Provides resources to educators, families, and other educating professionals who are impacted by learning disabilities.

150 **Easter Seals - Colorado Camp Rocky Mountain Village**
PO Box 115
Empire, CO 80438 303-569-2333
Fax: 303-569-3857
http://www.easterseals.com/co
Lynn Robinson, Chief Executive Officer
Nancy Hanson, VP, Human Resources
Krasimir Koev, Primary Contact
Provides services to children and adults with disabilities and other special needs, and support to their families.

151 **International Dyslexia Association Rocky Mountain Branch**
740 Yale Rd.
Boulder, CO 80305 303-721-9425
855-543-2762
http://idarmb.org
ida_rmb@yahoo.com
Lynn Kuhn, President
Tammy Curran, Vice President
Diane Mayer, Vice President
dedicated to ensuring that every student with the learning difference of Dyslexia will recieve scientifically based instruction and services consistent with his/her needs. Serves communities in Colorado, Utah, and Wyoming.

152 **PEAK Parent Center**
917 E Moreno Ave
Ste 140
Colorado Springs, CO 80903 719-531-9400
http://www.peakparent.org
info@peakparent.org
Barbara Buswell, Executive Director
David Meeks, President
Sid Inamdar, Vice President
A federally-designated Parent Traning and Information Center (PTI). As a PTI, PEAK supports and empowers parents, providing them with information and strategies to use when advocating for their children with disabilities by expanding knowledge of special education and offering new strategies for success.

153 **Rocky Mountain ADA Center**
3630 Sinton Rd
Ste 103
Colorado Springs, CO 80907 719-444-0268
800-949-4232
TTY: 719-444-0268
http://www.rockymountainada.org
email@rockymountainada.org
Dana Barton, Director
Emily Shuman, Media Coordinator
Provides information on the Americans with Disabilities Act to Colorado, Utah, Montana, Wyoming, North Dakota and South Dakota.

154 **Rocky Mountain International Dyslexia Association**
740 Yale Rd
Boulder, CO 80305 303-721-9425
855-5-IDA-RM
http://idarmb.org
ida_rmb@yahoo.com
Lynn Kuhn, President
Tammy Curran, Vice President
Karen Leopold, Treasurer

The mission of the International Dyslexia Association of Colorado is to pursue and provide the most comprehensive range of evidence-based information, education, and services that address the full scope of dyslexia and other associated learning disabilities and to have a meaningful impact on the lives of individuals and families affected by dyslexia so they may advocate for themselves and achieve their highest potential.
300+ members 1949

Connecticut

155 **Capitol Region Education Council**
111 Charter Oak Ave
Hartford, CT 06106 860-247-CREC
http://www.crec.org
Greg J. Florio, Executive Director
Mason Thrall, Director, Operations
Regina Burgess-Terrell, Director, Human Resources
Will promote cooperation and collaboration with local school districts and other organizations committed to the improved quality of public education; provide cost-effective services to member districts and other clients; listen and respond to client needs for the improved quality of public education; and provide leadership in the region through the quality of its services and its ability to identify and share quality services of its member districts and other organizations to public education.
1966

156 **Connecticut Association of Private Special Education Facilities (CAPSEF)**
701 Hebron Ave
3rd Floor
Glastonbury, CT 06033 860-525-1318
Fax: 860-541-6484
http://www.capsef.org
info@capsef.org
A voluntary association of provate schools which provides quality, cost effective, special education and related services to the special needs of children and adolescents (birth to 21 years) of Connecticut. The focus of these education services is social and vocation programs designed to enable students to succeed in the least restrictive environment.
2,500 members 1974

157 **Easter Seals - Capital Region & Eastern Connecticut**
100 Deerfield Rd
Windsor, CT 06095 860-270-0600
http://www.easterseals.com/hartford/
Tracey May, Chair
V. Vanessa Williams, Vice Chair
Allen Gouse, PhD, President & CEO
Easter Seals Connecticut creates solutions that change the lives of children and adults with disabilities or special needs, their families and communities.
1966

158 **Nonverbal Learning Disorders Association**
507 Hopmeadow St.
Simsbury, CT 06070 860-658-5522
Fax: 860-658-6688
http://www.nlda.org
info@nlda.org
Patricia Carrin, Founder/President
Marcia Rubinstein, Founder/Executive Liaison
A non-profit corporation dedicated to research, education, and advocacy for nonverbal learning disorders.

159 **SpEd Connecticut**
75 Charter Oak Ave
Ste 105
Hartford, CT 06106-1903 860-560-1711
http://www.spedconnecticut.com
info@spedconnecticut.org
SpEd Connecticut is a non-profit organization of parents, professionals, and persons with learning disabilities. Formerly known as the Learning Disabilities Association of Connecticut, SpEd is dedicated to promoting a better understanding of learning disabilities, securing appropriate educational and employment opportunities for children and adults with learning disabilities.

160 **State Education Resources Center of Connecticut (SERC)**
100 Roscommon Dr
Middletown, CT 06457-1520 860-632-1485
Fax: 860-632-8870
http://www.ctserc.org
info@ctserc.org
Ingrid Canady, Executive Director
Matthew Dugan, Director, Program Services
Alice Henley, Director, Program Development
Non-profit educational organization. Provides high-quality Profession Development to teachers, educators, parents and families throughout the state of CT.
1969

Delaware

161 **Easter Seals - Delaware & Maryland's Easten Shore, New Castle**
61 Corporate Cir
New Castle, DE 19720 302-324-4444
Fax: 302-324-4441
TDD: 302-324-4442
http://www.easterseals.com/de
Kenan Sklenar, Chief Executive Officer
Jeffrey Gosnear, Chair
Gary W Spitzer, Vice Chair
Provides exceptional services to ensure that all people with disabilities or special needs and their families have equal opportunities to live, learn, work and play in their communities.

162 **Easter Seals - Georgetown**
22317 DuPont Blvd
Georgetown, DE 19947-2153 302-253-1100
Fax: 302-856-7296
http://www.easterseals.com/de/
Pam Reuther, Primary Contact
Kenan Sklenar, Chief Executive Officer
Jeffrey Gosnear, Chair
Provides exceptional services to ensure that all people with disabilities or special needs and their families have equal opportunities to live, learn, work and play in their communities.

163 **Parent Information Center of Delaware**
404 Larch Cir
Wilmington, DE 19804 302-999-7394
888-547-4412
Fax: 302-999-7637
http://www.picofdel.org
Tika Hartsock, Chair
Meedra Surratte, Special Programs Manager
Jazmone Taylor, Executive Director
A statewide non-profit organization dedicated to providing information, education and support, to families and caregivers of children with disabilites or special needs.

District of Columbia

164 **Association for Childhood Education International (ACEI)**
1875 Connecticut Ave NW
10 Fl
Washington, DC 20009 202-372-9986
800-423-3563
http://www.acei.org

Pilar Fort, President
Diane Whitehead, Executive Director
Michelle Allen, Director, Operations
Mission is to promote and support in global community the optimal education and development of children, from birth through early adolescence, and to influence the professional growth of educators and the efforts of others who are committed to the needs of children in a changing society.

165 **Center for Child and Human Development**
Georgetown University
PO Box 571485
Washington, DC 20057-1485 202-687-5000
Fax: 202-687-1954
http://gucchd.georgetown.edu
gucchd@georgetown.edu
Phyllis Magrab, PhD, Executive Director
Established over four decades ago to improve the quality of life for all children and youth, especially those with, or at risk for, special needs and their families. Brings together policy, research and clincal practice for the betterment of individuals and families, especially childre, youth and those with special needs including: developmental disabilities and special health care needs, mental health needs, young children and those in the child welfare system.

Florida

166 **International Dyslexia Association of Florida**
6088 Sabal Hammock Cir
Port Orange, FL 32128 http://fl.dyslexiaida.org
info.fl@dyslexiaida.org
Pat Sekel, President
Charlotte Chase, Treasurer
Frank McKeown, Secretary
A non-profit, scientific and educational organization, which was formed to increase public awareness of dyslexia in Florida.
1949

167 **Learning Disabilities Association of Florida**
7100 W Camino Real
Boca Raton, FL 33433 http://lda-florida.org
A nonprofit volunteer organization of parents, professionals, and LD adults. It is devoted to defining and finding solutions to the broad spectrum of learning issues.

168 **Miami Lighthouse for the Blind and Visually Impaired**
601 SW 8th Ave
Miami, FL 33130 305-856-2288
Fax: 305-285-6967
http://www.miamilighthouse.com
info@miamilighthouse.com
Virginia A. Jacko, President & CEO
Richard Fernandez, Chief Financial Officer
Carol Brady-Simmons, Chief Program Officer
The oldest and largest private agency in Florida to serve people of all ages who are blind or the visually impaired.

169 **The Arc of Florida**
2898 Mahan Dr
Ste 1
Tallahassee, FL 32308 800-226-1155
http://www.arcflorida.org
Dick Bradley, President
Greg Roe, Vice President of Administration
Bobbie Lake, Secretary
A nonprofit organization dedicated to improving the quality of life for people with learning disabilities and developmental disabilities. The Arc of Florida partners with local, state and national associations to advocate for and support people with autism, spina bifida, cerebral palsy, and other developmental disabilities.

Georgia

170 **Easter Seals - North Georgia**
53 Perimeter Center E
Ste 550
Atlanta, GA 30346 404-943-1070
http://www.easterseals.com/northgeorgia
Donna Davidson, President & CEO
Robert Gwaltney, VP of Early Education and Care
Bipin Nagar, Chief Financial Officer
Provides information and referral, physical, occupational, and speech therapy, child care, Head Start and teacher training.

171 **Easter Seals - Southern Georgia**
1906 Palmyra Rd
Albany, GA 31701 229-439-7061
Fax: 229-435-6278
http://www.easterseals.com/southerngeorgia
Kyle Nichols, Chairman
Matt Hatcher, Chief Operating Officer
Beth English, Executive Director
Creates solutions that change the lives of children, adults and families with disabilities or special needs by offering a variety of programs and services that enable individuals to lead lives of equality, dignity and independence.

172 **International Dyslexia Association of Georgia**
7778 McGinnis Ferry Rd
Ste 291
Suwanee, GA 30024 404-256-1232
http://ga.dyslexiaida.org
info@idaga.org
Karen Huppertz, President
Renee Bernhardt, Vice President
Meredith Chase, Treasurer
Formed to increase public awareness about dyslexia in the State of Georgia. The Branch encourages teachers to train in multisensory language instruction. Provides a network for individuals with dyslexia, their families and professionals in the educational and medical fields.
300 members

173 **Learning Ally: Athens Recording Studio**
320 S Hull St
Athens, GA 30605 800-221-4792
http://www.learningally.org
Andrew Friendman, President & CEO
Harold J Logan, Chair
Therese Llorente, Vice Chair
To create opportunities for students who cannot read standard print because of a visual impairment, learning disability or other physical disability, to succeed in school by providing accessible educational materials.

174 **Learning Disabilities Association of Georgia**
4105 Briarcliff Rd NE
Ste 3
Atlanta, GA 30345 404-502-5358
http://www.ldag.org
ldaofgeorgia@gmail.com
For over 30 years, LDAG has been enhancing the quality of life for individuals of all ages with Learning Disabilities and/or Attention Deficit and Hyperactivity Disorders.

Hawaii

175 **Assistive Technology Resource Centers of Hawaii (ATRC)**
200 N Vineyard Blvd
Ste 430
Honolulu, HI 96817-5362 808-532-7110
800-645-3007
Fax: 808-532-7120
http://www.atrc.org
atrc-info@atrc.org

Barbara Fischlowitz-Leong, MEd, Executive Director & CEO
Monty Anderson-Nitahara, JD, Program Manager
Edna Kaahaaina, Office Manager
A statewide, nonprofit organization committed to ensuring access to assistive technology for persons with disabilities. ATRC links individuals with technology so all people can participate in every aspect of community life. Also empowers individuals to maintain dignity and control their lives by promoting technology thorough, advocacy, training, information, and education.

176 **Easter Seals - Hawaii**
710 Green St
Honolulu, HI 96813 808-536-1015
http://www.eastersealshawaii.org
info@eastersealshawaii.org
Ron Brandvold, President & CEO
Harvey Henderson, Jr., Chair
Josh Stinson, Vice Chair
Provide exceptional services to ensure that all people with disabilities of special needs and their families have equal opportunities to live, learn, work and play in their communities.

177 **International Dyslexia Association of Hawaii**
913 Alewa Dr
Honolulu, HI 96817 808-538-7007
http://hi.dyslexiaida.org
info.hi@dyslexiaida.org
Natalie Haggerty, MEd, President
M'Liss Moore, Secretary
Mark Murakami, Treasurer
HIDA's mission is to increase awareness of dyslexia in the community, provide support for parents and teachers, and promote teacher training. HIDA also offers tutoring and testing referrals and information about other resources in Hawaii.
1986

178 **Learning Disabilities Association of Hawaii (LDAH)**
245 N Kukui St
Ste 205
Honolulu, HI 96817 808-536-9684
Fax: 808-537-6780
http://www.ldahawaii.org
Sam Yee, President
Tayne Sekimura, Vice President
Rosie Rowe, Executive Director
A non-profit organization founded by parents of children with learning disabilities.
1968

179 **The Arc in Hawaii**
3989 Diamond Head Rd
Honolulu, HI 96816 800-737-7995
Fax: 808-732-9531
http://www.thearcinhawaii.org
info@thearcinhawaii.org
Lei Fountain, Executive Director
A nonprofit organization dedicated to improving the quality of life for people with learning disabilities and developmental disabilities.
1954

Idaho

180 **Disability Rights - Idaho**
4477 Emerald St
Ste B-100
Boise, ID 83706-2066 208-336-5353
800-632-5125
Fax: 208-336-5396
TDD: 208-336-5353
http://www.disabilityrightsidaho.org
info@disabilityrightsidaho.org
Rick Huber, President
The designated Protection and Advocacy System for Idaho provides advocacy for people with disabilities who have been abused/neglected; denied services or benefits; have experienced rights violations or discrimination because of their disability; or have voting accessibility problems. Also provides information & referral; negotiation & mediation; short term & technical assistance; legal advice and representation.
1977

Illinois

181 **Child Care Association of Illinois**
413 W Monroe
1st Fl
Springfield, IL 62704 217-528-4409
Fax: 217-528-6498
http://ilchildcare.net
ilccamb@aol.com
Margaret M. Berglind, ACSW-LCSW, President & CEO
A voluntary, not-for-profit organization dedicated to improving the delivery of social services to the abused, neglected, and troubled children, youth and families of Illinois.
1964

182 **Easter Seals - Metropolitan Chicago**
1939 W 13th St
Ste 300
Chicago, IL 60608-1226 312-491-4110
Fax: 312-733-0247
http://www.easterseals.com/chicago
F. Timothy Muri, President & CEO
Gary Kaatz, Chair
Mark T. O'Toole, Vice Chair
Provides comprehensive services for individuals with disabilities or other special needs and their families to improve quality of life and maximize independence.

183 **Illinois Protection & Advocacy Agency: Equip for Equality**
20 N Michigan Ave
Ste 300
Chicago, IL 60602 312-341-0022
800-537-2632
TTY: 800-610-2779
http://www.equipforequality.org
Zena Naiditch, President & CEO
John K. Holton, PhD, Chair
Sue Suter, Vice Chair
Advances the human and civil rights of children and adults with physical and mental disabilities in Illinois. The only statewide, cross-disability, comprehensive advocacy organization providing self-advocacy assistance, legal services, and disability rights education while also engaging in public policy and legislative advocacy and conducting abuse investigations and other oversight activities.
1985

184 **International Dyslexia Association of Illinois**
751 Roosevelt Rd
Ste 116
Glen Ellyn, IL 60137 630-469-6900
Fax: 630-469-6810
http://www.readibida.org
info@readibida.org
Dedicated to the study and remediation of dyslexia and to the support and encouragement of individuals with dyslexia and their families.
1949

185 **Jewish Child & Family Services Downtown Chicago - Central Office**
216 W Jackson Blvd
Ste 800
Chicago, IL 60606
312-357-4800
855-275-5237
http://www.jcfs.org
ask@jcfs.org
Howard Sitron, President & CEO
Wendy Platt Newberger, VP & COO
Vincent Everson, VP & CFO
Provides a range of comprehensive programs designed to enable individuals and families to grow and develop positively throughout their lives.

186 **Learning Disabilities Association of Illinois**
10101 S Roberts Rd
Ste 205
Palos Hills, IL 60465
708-430-7532
Fax: 708-430-7592
http://www.ldail.com
A resource office with information for parents, professionals and adults with learning disabilities.

187 **National Council of Teachers of English**
1111 W Kenyon Rd
Urbana, IL 61801-1096
217-328-3870
877-369-6283
Fax: 217-328-9645
http://www.ncte.org
Jocelyn A. Chadwick, President
Leah Zuidema, Vice President
Emily Kirkpatrick, Executive Director
The National Council of Teachers of English, with over 30,000 members and subscribers worldwide, is dedicated to improving the teaching and learning of English and the language arts at all levels of education.

188 **Second Sense**
65 E Wacker Pl
Ste 1010
Chicago, IL 60601
312-236-8569
http://www.second-sense.org
info@second-sense.org
Brett Christenson, President
Laura Rounce, Secretary
Steven Zelner, Executive Director
Support and information for families and individuals with visual disabilities. Formerly Guild for the Blind.

Indiana

189 **Dyslexia Institute of Indiana**
8395 Keystone Crossing
Ste 110
Indianapolis, IN 46240
317-222-6635
http://www.diin.org
Bill Herman, Chief Executive Officer
Lynn Leonard, Director of Programs
Travis Cox, Chair
DII is dedicated to helping students, parents, and educators impacted by dyslexia and other language learning dificulties.
1989

190 **Easter Seals - Arc of Northeast Indiana**
4919 Coldwater Rd
Fort Wayne, IN 46825
260-456-4534
http://www.easterseals.com/neindiana
Donna K. Elbrecht, President & CEO
Sheri Ward, Director, Development
Misty Woltman, CFO/Controller
Provides services to children and adults with disabilities and other special needs, and support to their families.

191 **Easter Seals - Southwestern Idiana**
Easter Seals Rehabilitation Center
3701 Bellemeade Ave
Evansville, IN 47714
812-479-1411
http://www.easterseals.com/in-sw
Kelly Schneider, President
Guy Davis, VP, Administration
Laura Terhune, VP, Development
The Easter Seals Rehabilitation Center in Evansville, IN provides services to children and adults with disabilities and other special needs and support to their families.

192 **International Dyslexia Association of Indiana**
2511 E 46th St
Indianapolis, IN 46205
317-926-1450
http://in.dyslexiaida.org
info.in@dyslexiaida.org
Sara Silvey, President
Tracy Powell, Vice President & Treasurer
Laura Williams, Secretary
A non-profit organization dedicated to helping individuals with dyslexia, their families and the communities that support them. Promotes and disseminates researched-based knowledge for early identification, effective teaching approaches and intervention strategies for dyslexics.
1971

193 **Learning Disabilities Association of Indiana**
176 W Logan St
Ste 158
Noblesville, IN 46060
http://www.ldaofindiana.net
Patty Useem, President
Dr. Tammy Mahon, Vice President
Mary Tremmel Koenig, Secretary
A non-profit, volunteer organization of parents, educators, and other individuals who are committed to promoting awareness, knowledge and acceptance of individuals with learning disabilities and associated disorders such as attention deficit/hyperactivity disorders.
1972

Iowa

194 **Center for Disabilities and Development**
University of Iowa Children's Hospital
100 Hawkins Dr
213 CDD
Iowa City, IA 52242
319-356-1346
855-543-2884
http://www.uichildrens.org/cdd
Dianne McBrien, MD, Medical Director
Ellen Eulberg, RN, Nurse Manager
Jennifer Fitzpatrick, BS, MPT, Rehab Therapies Manager
Improve the health and independence of people with disabilities and advance the community systems on which they rely.
1947

195 **Easter Seals Iowa Assistive Technology Program**
401 NE 66th Ave
Des Moines, IA 50313
http://www.iowaat.org
atinfo@eastersealsia.org
Tracy Keninger, Director
Kim Karwal, Coordinator
Miranda Cantrell, Program & Support Specialist
The Easter Seals Iowa Assistive Technology Program educates the public about and provide access assistive technology.
1989

196 **International Dyslexia Association of Iowa**
PO Box 11188
Cedar Rapids, IA 52410-1188
765-507-9432
http://ia.dyslexiaida.org
info@iowaida.org

Denise Little, President
Tricia Krsek, Vice President
Genevieve Monthie, Secretary
Provides workshops, hands-on simulations, and resources to incease public awareness of dyslexia.

197 **Learning Disabilities Association of Iowa**
5665 Greendale Rd
Ste D
Johnston, IA 50131
888-690-5324
Fax: 515-243-1902
http://www.lda-ia.org
info@ldaiowa.org
Paula Hamp, President
Dedicated to identifying causes and promoting prevention of learning disabilities and to enhancing the quality of life for all individuals with learning disabilities and their families by: encouraging effective identification and intervention, fostering research, and protecting the rights of individuals with learning disabilities under the law.

Kansas

198 **Disability Rights Center of Kansas (DRC)**
214 SW 6th Ave
Ste 100
Topeka, KS 66603
785-273-9661
877-776-1541
Fax: 785-273-9414
TDD: 877-335-3725
http://www.drckansas.org
Rocky Nichols, MPA, Executive Director
Nick Cobos, Office Assistant
Bev Masters, Administrative Assistant
Formerly Kansas Advocacy & Protection Services, a public interest legal advocacy agency empowered by federal law to advocate for the civil and legal rights of Kansans with disabilities.

199 **Easter Seals - Capper Foundation**
3500 SW 10th Ave
Topeka, KS 66604-1904
785-272-4060
http://capper.easterseals.com
Bruce Meyers, Chair
Emily McGee, Vice Chair
Jim Leiker, President & CEO
A community resource providing services to enhance the independence of people with disabilities, primarily children.

200 **Goodwill Industries of Kansas**
3351 N Webb Rd
Wichita, KS 67226
316-744-9291
Fax: 316-744-1428
http://goodwillks.org
Emily Compton, President & CEO
Greg Sandlin, VP, Administration & CFO
Curtis Tatum, VP, Workforce Development
Education, training and employment for people with disabilities and other barriers to employment.

201 **Learning Disabilities Association of Kansas**
Olathe, KS 66603
http://www.ldakansas.org
LDAK is a nonprofit, volunteer organization whose purpose is to advance the education and general well-being of children and adults with learning disabilities.

Kentucky

202 **Learning Disabilities Association of Kentucky**
2210 Goldsmith Ln
Ste 118
Louisville, KY 40218
502-473-1256
http://www.ldaofky.org
LDAofKY@yahoo.com
Tim Woods, Executive Director
A non-profit organization of individuals with learning differences and attention difficulties, their parents, educators, and other service providers.
1966

Louisiana

203 **Advocacy Center of Louisiana: Lafayette**
600 Jefferson St
Ste 812
Lafayette, LA 70501
337-237-7380
TTY: 855-861-3577
http://www.advocacyla.org
advocacycenter@advocacyla.org
Bob Whitney, Interim Executive Director
Jason Kehoe, Chief Financial Officer
Sarah Voigt, Legal Director
Protects and advocates for the human and legal rights of persons living in Louisiana who are elderly or disabled.

204 **Advocacy Center of Louisiana: New Orleans**
8325 Oak Street
New Orleans, LA 70118
800-960-7705
http://www.advocacyla.org
advocacycenter@advocacyla.org
Bob Whitney, Interim Executive Director
Jason Kehoe, Chief Financial Officer
Sarah Voigt, Legal Director
Protects and advocates for the human and legal rights of persons living in Louisiana who are elderly or disabled.

205 **Advocacy Center of Louisiana: Shreveport**
2620 Centenary Blvd
Shreveport, LA 71104
318-227-6186
800-960-7705
http://www.advocacyla.org
advocacycenter@advocacyla.org
Bob Whitney, Interim Executive Director
Jason Kehoe, Chief Financial Officer
Sarah Voigt, Legal Director
Protects and advocates for the human and legal rights of persons living in Louisiana who are elderly or disabled.

206 **Autism Society Louisiana**
PO Box 14587
Baton Rouge, LA 70898
225-221-7873
800-328-8476
http://www.lastateautism.org
autismsociety_lastatechapter@yahoo.com
Provides resources and services for people with austim and their families. The Society has chapters in Baton Rouge, New Orleans, Bayou, Acadiana, and Southwest Louisiana.
1975

207 **The Arc of Louisiana**
606 Colonial Dr
Ste G
Baton Rouge, LA 70714
225-383-1033
866-966-6260
http://www.thearcla.org
info@thearcla.org
Kelly Monroe, Executive Director
Linda Wilson, Project Manager
Stephanie Bell, Support Coordinator
A nonprofit organization dedicated to improving the quality of life for people with learning disabilities and developmental disabilities.

Maine

208 **Easter Seals - Maine**
125 Presumpscot St
Portland, ME 04103
207-828-0754
Fax: 207-828-5355
http://maine.easterseals.com

Joseph Reagan, Director of Development
Kaili Irvin, Director of Clinical Services
Creates solutions that change lives of children and adults with disabilities or other special needs and their families.

209 **Learning Disabilities Association of Maine (LDA)**
Windham, ME 04062
http://www.ldame.org
info@ldame.org
Dedicated to assisting individuals with learning and attention disabilities through support, education and advocacy.

210 **Maine Parent Federation**
484 Maine Ave
Ste 2D
Farmingdale, ME 04344
207-588-1933
800-870-7746
Fax: 207-588-1938
TTY: 207-588-1933
http://mpf.org
parentconnect@mpf.org
Carrie Woodcock, Executive Director
Jane K. Morse, Chair
Anne Osolinski, Vice Chair
The Maine Parent Federation is a statewide organiztion that provides information, advocacy, education, and training to benefit all children. We promote individual aspirations and community inclusion for people with disabilities.
1984

Maryland

211 **Accessibility & Disability Service**
University of Maryland
4281 Chapel Ln
College Park, MD 20742
301-314-7682
Fax: 301-405-0813
http://www.counseling.umd.edu/ads/
Jo Ann Hutchinson, RhD, Director
Julia Barlis, Counselor
Tessa DiPerri, MA, Disability Specialist
Coordinates services that ensure individuals with disabilities equal access to University of Maryland College Park programs.
800 members

212 **Division of Rehabilitation Services**
Maryland State Department of Education
200 W Baltimore St
Baltimore, MD 21201-2595
410-767-0100
888-246-0016
TTY: 443-798-2840
http://marylandpublicschools.org
dors@maryland.gov
Scott Dennis, Asst. State Superintendent
Enables persons with disabilities to achieve employment, economic self-sufficiency and independence.

213 **Easter Seals - DC, MD, VA**
1420 Spring St
Silver Spring, MD 20910
301-588-8700
http://www.easterseals.com/DCMDVA
Jonathan Horowitch, President & CEO
Cindy Hallberlin, JD, Chief Operating Officer
Michael Piemonte, Chief Financial Officer
Provides exceptional services to ensure that all people with disabilities or special needs and their families have equal opportunities to live, learn, work and play in their communities. Proudly servinf Washington-Baltimore Region and the surrounding communities in Maryland, Northern Virginia and West Virginia.

214 **International Dyslexia Association of Maryland**
PO Box 233
Brooklandville, MD 21022-0233
800-509-4980
http://md.dyslexiaida.org
info@idamd.org
Annette Fallon, President
Karen Fallon, Vice President
Timothy Yearick, Secretary
Believes that all individuals have the right to achieve their full potential and that individual learning abilities can be strengthen. MBIDA will promote and organize classes and workshops to provide informtion and training for dyslexic individuals, educators, parents and others.

215 **International Dyslexia Association of DC Capital Area**
5715 Brewer House Cir
T2
Rockville, MD 20852
301-906-1630
http://dc.dyslexiaida.org
Laurie Moloney, President
Amy Vandent Boogart, Secretary
Allan Freedman, Treasurer
The DC Capital Area Branch of the International Dyslexia Association is a non-profit, scientific and educational organization dedicated to the study and treatment of dyslexia.

216 **Learning Disabilities Association of Maryland**
Dunkirk, MD 20754
888-265-6459
http://www.ldamd.org
ldamd@ldamd.org
Dedicated to enhancing the quality of life for all individuals with learning disabilities and their families through awareness, advocacy, education, service and collaborative efforts.

217 **Maryland Association of University Centers on Disabilities**
1100 Wayne Ave
Ste 1000
Silver Spring, MD 20910
301-588-8252
Fax: 301-588-2842
http://www.aucd.org
aucdinfo@aucd.org
Bruce Keisling, PhD, President
Sachin Pavithran, PhD, Secretary
Andrew J. Imparato, JD, Executive Director
The mission of AUCD is to advance policy and practice for and with people living with developmental and other disabilities, their families, and communities by supporting members to engage in research, education, and service activities.

218 **National Federation of Families for Children's Mental Health**
12320 Parklawn Dr
Rockville, MD 20852-6390
240-403-1901
http://www.ffcmh.org
ffcmh@ffcmh.org
Lynda Gargan, PhD, Executive Director
Barbara Huff, Social Marketing TA Provider
Michelle Covington, Project Manager
Dedicated exclusively to helping children with mental health needs and their families achieve a better quality of life.

Massachusetts

219 **Adaptive Environments**
Institute for Human Centered Design
200 Portland St
Ste 1
Boston, MA 02114
617-695-1225
Fax: 617-482-8099
TTY: 617-695-1225
http://humancentereddesign.org
info@humancentereddesign.org
Valerie Fletcher, Executive Director
Ralph Jackson, President
Gabriela Bonome-Sims, Director of Administration
Committed to advancing the role of design in expanding opportunity and enhancing experience for people of all ages and abiliites.
1978

220 **Easter Seals - Massachusetts**
484 Main St
Worcester, MA 01608-1817 800-244-2756
http://www.easterseals.com/ma
Paul Nedeiros, President & CEO
Kathy Kittle, Chair
David Hoffman, Vice Chair
Statewide, community based organization that has been helping people with disabilities to live full and independent lives for over 60 years.

221 **International Dyslexia Association of Massachusetts**
PO Box 562
Lincoln, MA 01773 617-650-0011
http://ma.dyslexiaida.org
massbranchida@gmail.com
Nathan Doty, President
Caroline Legor, Vice President
Charlotte Lunde, Secretary
The Massachusetts Branch of The International Dyslexia Association (MABIDA) is a non-profit, scientific and educational organization dedicated to the study and treatment of dyslexia. This Branch was formed to increase public awareness of dyslexia in Massachusetts.

222 **Learning Disabilities Worldwide (LDW)**
179 Bear Hill Rd
Ste 104
Waltham, MA 02451 http://www.ldworldwide.org
help@ldworldwide.org
Emmanuel Chinweoke Aja, MD, Chair
Nicholas D. Young, PhD, EdD, Vice Chair
Teresa Allissa Citro, Chief Executive Officer
Formerly the Learning Disabilities Association of Massachusetts, works to enhance the lives of individuals with learning disabilities, with a specail emphasis on the underserved. The purpose is to identify and support the unrecognized strengths and capabilities of a person with learning disabilities.
15,000 members 1965

223 **Massachusetts Association of Approved Private Schools (MAAPS)**
607 North Ave
15 Lakeside Office Park
Wakefield, MA 01880 781-245-1220
http://www.maaps.org
info@maaps.org
Mark P. de Chabert, Chief Operating Officer
James V. Major IOM, CAE, Executive Director
Kristen Brown, Business Manager
Nonprofit association dedicated to providing educational programs and services to students with special needs throughout Massachusetts. Concerned that children with special needs have appropriate, quality education and that they and their families know the rights, policies, procedures and options that make the education process a productive reality for special needs children.

Michigan

224 **Easter Seals - Michigan**
2399 E Walton Blvd
Auburn Hills, MI 48326 248-475-6400
http://www.easterseals.com/michigan
Brent Wirth, President & CEO
Juliana Harper, Chief Program Officer/SVP
Ron Hocking, Chief Financial Officer/SVP
Offers programs and services for children and adults with disabilities and special needs.

225 **International Dyslexia Association of Michigan**
5735 Big Pine Dr
Ypsilanti, MI 48197-7184 888-432-6424
http://mi.dyslexiaida.org
info@idamich.org
Heidi Turchan, MEd, President
Nancy Williams, Vice President
Randy Meyer, Treasurer
The purpose of the Michigan Branch of the International Dyslexia Association is to develop awareness and provide information about Dyslexia.

Minnesota

226 **International Dyslexia Association Upper Midwest Branch**
5021 Vernon Ave
Ste 159
Minneapolis, MN 55436 612-486-4242
http://umw.dyslexiaida.org
info.umw@dyslexiaida.org
Brian Pittenger, President
Jennifer Bennett, Secretary
Informs and educates people about dyslexia and related difficulties in learning to read and write, in a way that supports and encourages, promotes effective change, and gives individuals the opportunity to lead productive and fulfilling lives, which benefits society with the resource that is liberated. this branch serves Minnesota, North Dakota, and South Dakota.

227 **Learning Disabilities Association of Minnesota**
6100 Golden Valley Rd
Golden Valley, MN 55422 952-582-6000
Fax: 952-582-6031
http://www.ldaminnesota.org
info@ldaminnesota.org
Jeff Fox, President
Sherry Holtz, Vice President
Jerry Golden, Treasurer
Nonprofit educational agency helping children, youth, and adults at risk for learning disabilities and other learning difficulties.

228 **PACER Center, Inc.**
8161 Normandale Blvd.
Bloomington, MN 55437 952-838-9000
800-537-2237
Fax: 952-838-0199
http://www.pacer.org
Paula F. Goldberg, Executie Director
Matthew Woods, President
Tammy Pust, Vice President
The PACER Center provides assistance, workshops, and materials for parents of children with disabilities and professionals whose work is focused on children with disabilities.

229 **Technical Assistance Alliance for Parent Centers: PACER Center**
8161 Normandale Blvd
Minneapolis, MN 55437 952-838-9000
http://www.pacer.org
Matthew Woods, President
Tammy Pust, Vice President
Paula Goldberg, Executive Director
An innovative project that supports a unified technical assistance system for the purpose of developing, assisting and coordinating Parent Training Information Projects and Community Parent Resource Centers.

Mississippi

230 **Learning Disabilities Association of Mississippi**
Jackson, MS 888-300-6710
http://ldaamerica.org/lda-chapters/mississippi
info@ldaamerica.org
A nonprofit, volunteer organization that is an informational Support Center for parents of children with learning disabilities, adults with learning disabilities, and professionals providing services related to learning disabilities.

Missouri

231 **Easter Seals - Heartland**
13975 Manchester Rd
Ste 2
Manchester, MO 63011 636-227-6030
Fax: 636-779-2270
http://www.ucpheartland.org
Brenda Wrench, President & CEO
Judy Grainger, Vice President Programs
Lori Burch, Chief Financial Officer
Provides exceptional services to ensure all people with disabilities have equal opportunities to live, learn, work and play in their communities.

232 **Missouri Protection & Advocacy Services**
925 S Country Club Dr
Jefferson City, MO 65109 573-659-0678
800-392-8667
Fax: 573-659-0677
TDD: 800-735-2966
http://www.moadvocacy.org
app.unit@mo-pa.org
Sharon Williams, Chair
Jason Mize, Vice Chair
Katharine Kinder, Secretary/Treasurer
A federally mandated system in the state which provides protection of the rights of persons with disabilities through leagally-based advocacy. The mission is to protect the rights of individuals with disabilities by providing advocacy and legal services.
1977

233 **St Louis Learning Disabilities Association**
13537 Barrett Pkwy Dr
Ste 100
Ballwin, MO 63021 314-966-3088
Pam Kortum, Chief Executive Officer
Sheryl Silvey, Chair
James Hartman, Vice Chair
Provides information and support to parents, individuals with learning disabilities and professionals.

Montana

234 **Montana Parents, Let's Unite for Kids (PLUK)**
2345 King Ave W
Ste B
Billings, MT 59102 406-255-0540
800-222-7585
Fax: 406-255-0523
http://www.mtpluk.org
info@mtpluk.org
Roger Holt, Executive Director
PLUK is a private, nonprofit organization formed by parents of children with disabilities and chronic illnesses. Its purpose is to provide information, support, training and assistance to aid parents with their children at home, in school and as adults.
1984

Nebraska

235 **Autism Society of Nebraska**
P.O. Box 83559
Lincoln, NE 68501-3559 800-580-9279
http://autismnebraska.org
autismsociety@autismnebraska.org
Megan Misegadis, President
Julie Czepa, Vice President
Robyn Roberts, Treasurer
An affiliate of the Autism Society of America, the Autism Society of Nebraska aims to improve the lives of individuals with autism spectrum disorders and their families.

236 **Disability Rights Nebraska**
134 South 12th St.
Suite 600
Lincoln, NE 68508 402-474-3183
800-422-6691
http://www.disabilityrightsnebraska.org
info@disabilityrightsnebraska.org
Eric Evans, Chief Executive Officer
Tania Diaz, Legal Services Director
Judy Sinner, Director, Fiscal/Human Resources
A protection and advocacy organization that utilizes various forms of advocacy, such as legal advocacy, self-advocacy, advocacy education, and more in order to protect people with disabilities.

237 **Easter Seals - Nebraska**
12565 W Center Rd
Ste 100
Omaha, NE 68144 800-650-9880
Fax: 855-376-1234
http://www.easterseals.com/ne
James C. Summerfelt, President & CEO
Angela Howell, Vice President
Lily Sughroue, Director of Camp, Respite, Rec.
Provides exceptional services to help ensure all people with disabilities have an equal opportunity to live, learn, work and play.

238 **Learning Disabilities Association of Nebraska**
11118 N 62nd St
Omaha, NE 68152 402-571-7771
http://ldaamerica.org/lda-chapters/nebraska/
ldaofneb@yahoo.com
Support groups for parents and teachers, information for school and the community about ADHD and LD children/adults. Offers book and video library, educational seminars and conferences, parent panels. Quarterly newsletter.
1984

239 **Nebraska Association of Service Providers**
1200 Libra Dr.
Suite 100
Lincoln, NE 68513 402-802-8312
http://neserviceproviders.org
bolznasp@gmail.com
Kate Bolz, Executive Director
Brian Kanter, President
A membership organization made up of community organizations who provide supports to people with disabilities.

240 **The Arc of Nebraska**
215 Centennial Mall S.
Suite 508
Lincoln, NE 68508-1825 402-475-4407
http://www.arc-nebraska.org
info@arc-nebraska.org
Julie Stahla, President
Lynn Redding, Vice President
Melissa Mazzula, Treasurer
A non-profit organization dedicated to improving the quality of life for people with learning disabilities and developmental disabilities.

Nevada

241 **Children's Cabinet**
1090 S Rock Blvd
Reno, NV 89502 775-856-6200
Fax: 775-856-6208
http://www.childrenscabinet.org
mail@childrenscabinet.org
Michael Russell, Chair
Rob Gaedtke, Co-Chair
Lauren Sankovich, Treasurer

The Children's Cabinet strives to ensure every child and family in our community has the services and resources to meet fundamental development, care, and learning needs.
1985

242 **Easter Seals - Nevada**
7281 W Charleston Blvd
Las Vegas, NV 89117 702-870-7050
http://www.easterseals.com/nevada
Kimberly Trueba, Chair
Karl Armstrong, Esq., Vice Chair
Brian Patchett, Chief Executive Officer
Provides services to children and adults with disabilities and other special needs, and support to their families.

243 **Learning Disabilities Association of Nevada**
Reno, NV 888-300-6710
http://www.ldaamerica.org/ida-chapters/nevada
info@ldaamerica.org
To create opportunities for success for all individuals affected by learning disabilities and to reduce the incidence of learning disabilities in future generations.

New Hampshire

244 **Crotched Mountain**
1 Verney Dr
Greenfield, NH 03047 603-547-3311
http://www.crotchedmountain.org
info@crotchedmountain.org
Michael Coughlin, President & CEO
Scott Graff, CFO/COO
Melissa White, Chief Program Officer
Serves individuals with disabilities and their families, embracing personal choice and development, and building communities of mutual support.

245 **Easter Seals - New Hampshire**
555 Auburn St
Manchester, NH 03103 603-623-8863
800-870-8728
http://www.easterseals.com/nh/
Larry Gammon, President & CEO
Elin Treanor, Chief Financial Officer
Nancy Rollins, Chief Operating Officer
Easter Seals New Hampshire is one of the most comprehensive affiliates in the nation, assisting more than 18,000 children and adults with disabilities through a network of more than a dozen service sites around the state and in Vermont. Each center provides top-quality, family-focused and innovative services tailored to meet the specific needs of the particular community it serves.
1936

246 **NH Family Ties**
70 Pembroke Rd
Concord, NH 03301 800-499-4153
A network of families with special needs children sharing resources and experiences.
1989

247 **New Hampshire Disabilities Rights Center (DRC)**
64 N Main St
Ste 2, 3 Fl
Concord, NH 03301-4913 603-228-0432
800-834-1721
Fax: 603-225-2077
TTY: 800-834-1721
http://www.drcnh.org
advocacy@drcnh.org
Lisa DiMartino, President
John Tobin, Vice President
Cynthia Trottier, Treasurer
A statewide organization that is independent from state government or service providers and is dedicated to the full and equal enjoyment of civil and other legal rights by people with disabilities. The DRC is New Hampshire's designated Protection and Advocacy agency and authorized by federal statute to pursue legal, administrative and other appropriate remedies on behalf of individuals with disabilities.
1978

New Jersey

248 **ASPEN Autism Spectrum Education Network**
9 Aspen Cir
Edison, NJ 08820 732-321-0880
http://www.aspennj.org
info@aspennj.org
Lori Shery, President
Rich Meleo, Vice President
Elizabeth Yamashita, Vice President
Provides families and individuals whose lives are affected by Autism Spectrum Disorders (Asperger Syndrome, Pervasive Developmental Disorder-NOS, High Functioning Autism), and Nonverbal Learning Disabilities with education, support and advocacy.

249 **Disability Rights New Jersey**
210 S Broad S
3rd Fl
Trenton, NJ 08608 609-292-9742
800-922-7233
Fax: 609-777-0187
TTY: 609-633-7106
http://www.drnj.org
advocate@drnj.org
Mitch Friedman, Chair
Tasha Jones, Vice Chair
Joseph Young, Executive Director
A consumer-directed, nonprofit organization that serves as New Jersey's designated protection and advocacy system for people with disabilities in the state.

250 **Easter Seals - New Jersey**
25 Kennedy Blvd
Ste 600
East Brunswick, NJ 08816 732-257-6662
http://www.easterseals.com/nj
Brian Fitzgerald, President & CEO
Aleisha Hart, CFO & Assistant Treasurer
Shelley Samuels, Chief Program Officer
To enable individuals with disabilities or special needs and their families to live, learn, work and play in their communities with equality, dignity and independence.

251 **Family Resource Associates, Inc.**
35 Haddon Ave
Shrewsbury, NJ 07702 732-747-5310
Fax: 732-747-1896
http://www.frainc.org
info@frainc.org
Christopher Curcia, President
Allan Proske, Vice President
Nancy Phalanukorn, Executive Director
A nonprofit agency with the mission of helping children, adolescents and people of all ages with disabilities to reach their fullest potenttial. Provides home-based early intervention for infants, therapeutic recreation programs and assistive technology services, along with family and sibling support groups.
1979

252 **Family Support Center of New Jersey**
1 AAA Dr
Ste 203
Trenton, NJ 08691 800-336-5843
Fax: 609-392-5621
http://www.fscnj.org
ejoice@familyresourcenetwork.org

Eric M. Joice, Executive Director
Liza Gundell, Deputy Director
Jessica Goldsmith Barzilay, Assistant Director
The Family Support Center of New Jersey (FSCNJ) is a clearing house of up-to-date information on national, state and local family support programs, services and disabilities. FSCNJ offers a one stop shopping approach to individuals seeking information on disabilities and services by providing them with easy acces to a comprehensive array of services.

253 **International Dyslexia Association of New Jersey**
PO Box 32
Long Valley, NJ 07853 *Fax:* 908-876-0092
http://nj.dyslexiaida.org
njida@msn.com
Patricia Barden, President
An international nonprofit, scientific and educational organization dedicated to the study of dyslexia. Offers tutoring and testing referrals, as well as support teacher education and hold outreach programs.
700 members

254 **Learning Disabilities Association of New Jersey**
P.O. Box 6268
East Brunswick, NJ 08816 732-645-2738
http://www.ldanj.org
info@ldanj.org
To create opportunities for success in all individuals affected by learning disabilities and to reduce the incidence of learning disabilities in future generations.

255 **New Jersey Self-Help Group Clearinghouse**
673 Morris Ave
Ste 100
Springfield, NJ 07801 973-571-4100
800-367-6274
Fax: 973-218-0636
TTY: 877-294-4356
http://www.njgroups.org
njgroups@mhanj.org
Puts callers in touch with any of several hundred national and international self-help groups covering a wide range of illnesses, disabilities, addictions, bereavement and stressful life situations.
1981

256 **Special Child Health and Early Intervention Services**
NJ Department of Health
PO Box 360
Trenton, NJ 08625 http://www.nj.gov/health/fhs/sch
Assists families caring for children with long-term medical and developmental disabilities. Programs include Early Intervention Services, Case Management, Special Child Health Services, Registry, Autism Registry, Early Hearing Detection & Intervention, and Newborn Screening and Genetics Services and Hemophilia Program.

New Mexico

257 **Easter Seals - Santa Maria El Mirador**
10 A-Van-Nu-Po
Santa Fe, NM 87508 505-424-7700
Fax: 505-424-7707
http://www.easterseals.com/elmirador
Patsy Romero, Chief Executive Officer
Jamie Coleman, Primary Contact
Provides an array of quality supports for individuals with developmental disabilities in community integrated environments centered on personl choice, self value, and dignity.
1971

258 **International Dyslexia Association Southwest Branch**
3915 Carlisle Blvd NE
Albuquerque, NM 87107 505-255-8234
http://sw.dyslexiaida.org
swida@southwestida.org
Claudia Gutierrez, President
Erin Brown, Vice President
Cammie Archuleta, Treasurer
Deeply committed to the training of teachers, speech pathologists, parents, literacy volunteers, and other professionals in appropriate instructional methods for individuals with dyslexia. IDA's Southwest Branch encourages the use of Orton-Gilligham multisensory structured language based (MSL-based) methodology, which has proven to be the most effective way to teach individuals with dyslexia and related learning disabilities.
1985

259 **The Arc of New Mexico**
3655 Carlisle NE
Albuquerque, NM 87110 505-883-4630
800-358-6493
Fax: 505-883-5564
http://www.arcnm.org
Veronica Chavez Neuman, Chief Executive Officer
Elaine Palma, President
Ling Faith-Heuertz, Secretary
The Arc of New Mexico helps aid in the inclusion and participation of individuals with intellectual and developmental disabilities in their communities.

New York

260 **Advocates for Children of New York**
151 W. 30th St.
5th Fl.
New York, NY 10001 212-947-9779
Fax: 212-947-9790
http://www.advocatesforchildren.org
info@advocatesforchildren.org
Kim Sweet, Executive Director
Matthew Lenaghan, Deputy Director
Rebecca Shore, Director of Litigation
Works on behalf of children from infancy to age 21 who are at greatest risk for school-based discrimination and/or academic failure. AFC provides a full range of services: free individual case advocacy, technical assistance, and training for parents, students, and professionals about children's educational entitlements and due process rights in New York City.

261 **American Autism Association**
P.O. Box 1703
New York, NY 10156 877-654-4483
http://myautism.org
info@myautism.org
Caitlin Bendersky, President
Chris Gurciullo, Vice President
Luba Dulman, Treasurer
The American Autism Association offers educational services, financial aid, and informational resources to assist families of children with autism.

262 **Easterseals New York**
633 Third Ave.
6th Fl.
New York, NY 10017 212-220-2290
Fax: 212-695-4807
http://www.easterseals.com/newyork/
Craig Stenning, Executive Director
Aris Pavlides, Senior VP, Development
Kevin Carey, Director of Finance

Provides programs and services to children and adults with disabilities and other special needs, and their families. The goal is to help individuals with special needs gain dignity, equality, and independence. Also provides the highest quality services in the most caring and cost-effective manner.
1922

263 **Everyone Reading, Inc.**
11 Broadway
Ste 868
New York, NY 10004 917-903-2648
http://everyonereading.org
info@everyonereading.org
Candace Carponter, President
Lavinia Mancuso, Executive Director
Laura Guerrero, Administrative Assistant
Everyone Reading, formerly the New York Branch of the International Dyslexia Association, provides a variety of resources to enable children and adults with dyslexia to succeed in school and in life.

264 **INCLUDEnyc**
116 E. 16th St.
5th Fl.
New York, NY 10003 212-677-4650
Fax: 212-254-4070
http://www.includenyc.org
info@includenyc.org
Ellen Miller-Wachtel, Chair
Barbara A. Glassman, Executive Director
Jane Heaphy, Deputy Exec. Director, Programs
An information, referral, advocacy, tranining, and support center for NYC parents and professionals looking for services for children, ages birth to 26, with learning, developmental, emotional or physical disabilities.

265 **International Dyslexia Association Long Island**
1550 Deer Park Ave.
Suite C
Deer Park, NY 11729 631-261-7441
Fax: 631-261-7834
http://www.lidyslexia.org
info@lidyslexia.org
Concetta Russo, EdD, President
Caryl Deiches, Vice President
Randi Burns, 2nd Vice President
Objectives are to increase awareness of dyslexia in the community; provide support for parents and teachers; and promote teacher training. They offer a telephone message system for information requests, sponsor an annual conference and four topic workshops, as well as a summer Orton-Gillingham course. They have a network of local school officials, parents, attorneys, and other professionals to help parents navigate the channels of the school system.

266 **LAUNCH**
212 East Manlius St.
East Syracuse, NY 13057 315-432-0665
Fax: 315-431-0606
http://www.launchcny.org
info@launchcny.org
Rebecca Grossman, President
Amy Zwecker, Manager, Marketing/Development
Paulette Purdy, Executive Director
LAUNCH, formerly the Learning Disabilities Association of Central New York, partners children with adults to provide individualzed learning.

267 **Learning Ally: New York Recording Studio**
545 Fifth Ave
Ste 1005
New York, NY 10017 800-221-4792
http://www.learningally.org
Andrew Friendman, President & CEO
Harold J. Logan, Chair
Therese Llorente, Vice Chair
To create opportunities for students who cannot read standard print because of a visual impairment, learning disability or other physical disability, to succeed in school by providing accessible educational materials.

268 **Learning Disabilities Association of New York State (LDANYS)**
2555 Elmwood Ave.
Kenmore, NY 14217 518-608-8992
Fax: 518-608-8993
http://ldanys.org
info@ldaamerica.org
Jeffrey Baker, President
Charles Giglio, Vice President
Helene Fallon, Treasurer
LDANYS works with the Governor's office, members of the state legislature, Board of Regents, and key state agencies that oversee programs and services that touch the lives of individuals who have learning disabilities and their families to ensure policies are fair and provide equal access to programs and services for individuals who have learning disabilities.

269 **Learning Disabilities Association of Western New York**
2555 Elmwood Ave.
Kenmore, NY 14217 716-874-7200
Fax: 716-874-7205
http://www.ldaofwny.org
information@ldaofwny.org
Jane Bedore, President
Valerie Franczyk, Executive Vice President
Pauli Chameli, Vice President
To create conditions under which persons with learning disabilities, neurological impairments, and developmental disabilities are given opportunities to make choices and develop and achieve independence. The association also addresses each individual's health, future, participation in the community, and personal relationships. LDA Southern Fredonia Tier branch can be reached at 716-679-1601.

270 **Northeast ADA Center**
201 Dolgen Hall
Ithaca, NY 14853 800-949-4232
Fax: 607-255-2763
TTY: 607-255-6686
http://northeastada.org
northeastada@cornell.edu
Wendy Strobel-Gower, Director
Joe Zesski, Assistant Director
The Northeast ADA Center provides information and training on the Americans with Disabilities Act (ADA) in New York, New Jersey, Puerto Rico, and the U.S. Virgin Islands.

271 **Starbridge**
1650 South Ave.
Suite 200
Rochester, NY 14620 585-546-1700
Fax: 585-224-7100
http://www.starbridgeinc.org
info@starbridgeinc.org
Colin Garwood, President/CEO
Jason Blackwell, VP, Programs & Services
Terry O'Hare, VP, Finance/Operations
A non-profit agency that partners with individuals who seek help in learning, so that they can succeed in school, work, and community life. The primaty constituents include people who are working to overcome cognitive or developmental barriers to learning. Also serves as a resource to people who are involved in the lives of these individuals, such as family members, employers, teachers, and health care professionals.

272 **Strong Center for Developmental Disabilities**
Golisano Children's Hospital at Strong
601 Elmwood Ave.
P.O. Box 671
Rochester, NY 14642 585-275-0355
http://www.urmc.rochester.edu/
Stephen B. Sulkes, Co-Director
Susan A. Hetherington, Co-Director

A University Center of Excellence for Developmental Disabilities, Education, Research and Service. Provides services, advocacy, education, technical assistance, and research to ensure full inclusion of persons with developmental disabilities in their communities and to maximize their potentional for leading independent and productive lives.

273 **Westchester Institute for Human Development**
Westchester Medical Center
Cedarwood Hall
Valhalla, NY 10595 914-493-8150
http://www.wihd.org
info@WIHD.org
Susan Fox, President/CEO
David O'Hara, Vice President, Programs
Marianne Ventrice, VP, Finance/Administration
WIHD advances policies and practices that foster the healthy development and ensure the safety of all children, strenghten families and communities, and promote health and well-being among people of all ages with disabilities and special health care needs.
1950

274 **Yellin Center for Mind, Brain, and Education**
104 W. 29th St.
12th Fl.
New York, NY 10001 646-775-6646
Fax: 646-775-6602
http://www.yellincenter.com
info@yellincenter.com
Dr. Paul B. Yellin, MD, FAAP, Director
Susan Yellin, Director, Advocacy/Transition
Rishara Maharaj, Director, Operations
Comprehensive Neurodevelopmental and Psychoeducational Evaluation for students in Pre-K, K-12, College, Graduate and Professional Schools, and for adults. Ongoing support including Academic Coaching, Medication Management, Progress Monitoring and College Transition Support. Outreach to School, Teachers, and other providers where indicated. Professional development presentations for schools and parent organizations. Sliding scale available.

North Carolina

275 **Autism Society of North Carolina**
5121 Kingdom Way
Suite 100
Raleigh, NC 27607 800-442-2762
http://www.autismsociety-nc.org
Tracey Sheriff, Chief Executive Officer
Paul Wendler, Chief Financial Officer
Kristy White, Chief Development Officer
Provides support and opportunities to succeed to people with autism and their families.

276 **Disability Rights North Carolina**
3724 National Dr.
Suite 100
Raleigh, NC 27612 919-856-2195
877-235-4210
Fax: 919-856-2244
http://www.disabilityrightsnc.org
info@disabilityrightsnc.org
Denise Jones, Chair
Rachel Fuerst, Vice Chair
Itnuit Janovitz Freireich, Treasurer
Protects and advocates for the rights of people with disabilities in North Carolina. Legal services and advocacy are provided at no cost.

277 **Easter Seals - UCP North Carolina & Virginia**
5171 Glenwood Ave.
Suite 211
Raleigh, NC 27612 800-662-7119
Fax: 919-782-5486
http://eastersealsucp.com
info@nc.eastersealsucp.com
Luanna Welch, President/CEO
A lifeling partner for people managing disabilities and mental health challenges. Services are centered around each person's individual needs to live, learn, and participate fully in his or her community.

278 **First In Families of North Carolina**
3109 University Dr.
Suite 100
Durham, NC 27707 919-251-8368
http://fifnc.org
info@fifnc.org
Betsy MacMichael, Executive Director
Karen Luken, President
Mark Bullock, Vice President
A non-profit corporation that helps people with disabilities and their families achieve their goals. First In Families is supported in part by funding from the North Carolina Division of Mental Health.

279 **Mind Matters**
Southeast Psych
6060 Piedmont Row Dr. S.
Suite 120
Charlotte, NC 28287 704-552-0116
Fax: 704-552-7550
http://www.southeastpsych.com
Karen Amrhein, Director, Finance
Marti Flowers, Office Manager
Elle Neese, Operations Coordinator
Mind Matters at Southeast Psych believes in describing learners, identifying strengths, explaining findings clearly, collaborating to support struggling learners, and improving the self-insight of all learners.

280 **Success in Mind**
324 Blackwell St.
Suite 1240
Durham, NC 27701 919-680-8921
http://www.success-in-mind.org
info@success-in-mind.org
Beth Briere, MD, Executive Director
Craig Pohlman, PhD, Learning Specialist
Marianne Zura, MD, Neurodevelopmentalist
Provides students, families, teachers and others involved in a student's education with a deep understanding and a common language that demystifies learning, values individual learning differences, and promotes success for each learner.

281 **The Arc North Carolina**
343 E. Six Forks Rd.
Suite 320
Raleigh, NC 27609 919-782-4632
800-662-8706
http://www.arcnc.org
info@arcnc.org
John Nash, Executive Director
A state chapter of the Arc of the United States, the Arc North Carolina aims to advocate for and provide services to people with intellectual and developmental disabilities.

North Dakota

282 **Easter Seals Goodwill North Dakota: Bismarck**
1031 Interstate Ave.
Suite 1
Bismarck, ND 58503 701-751-0863
800-247-0698
http://www.esgwnd.org
Gordon Hauge, CEO

Easter Seals provides services to children and adults with disabilities and other special needs, and support to their families.

283 **Easter Seals Goodwill North Dakota: Dickson**
2125 Sims St.
P.O. Box 361
Dickson, ND 58602-0361
701-264-1060
866-895-1587
Fax: 701-264-1099
http://www.esgwnd.org
Gordon Hauge, CEO
Easter Seals provides services to children and adults with disabilities and other special needs, and support to their families.

284 **Easter Seals Goodwill North Dakota: Fargo**
3333 7th Ave. N
Fargo, ND 58102
701-893-3456
866-895-1588
Fax: 701-234-9390
http://www.esgwnd.org
Gordon Hauge, CEO
Easter Seals provides services to children and adults with disabilities and other special needs, and support to their families.

285 **Easter Seals Goodwill North Dakota: Jamestown**
402 14th Ave. N.E.
Suite 1
Jamestown, ND 58401
701-251-1446
866-897-6004
Fax: 701-252-9527
http://www.esgwnd.org
Gordon Hauge, CEO
Easter Seals provides services to children and adults with disabilities and other special needs, and support to their families.

286 **Easter Seals Goodwill North Dakota: Minot**
800 12th Ave. S.W.
Minot, ND 58701-9114
701-839-4121
866-895-1589
Fax: 701-838-5998
http://www.esgwnd.org
Gordon Hauge, CEO
Easter Seals provides services to children and adults with disabilities and other special needs, and support to their families.

287 **Easter Seals Goodwill: Headquarters**
211 Collins Ave.
Mandan, ND 58554-3106
701-663-6828
Fax: 701-663-6859
http://www.esgwnd.org
Gordon Hauge, CEO
Easter Seals provides services to children and adults with disabilities and other special needs, and support to their families.

288 **North Dakota Association For The Disabled (NDAD)**
2660 S. Columbia Rd.
Grand Forks, ND 58201
701-775-5577
800-532-6323
http://www.ndad.org
grandforks@ndad.org
Ronald Gibbens, President
Don Sater, Chief Executive Officer
Traci LaDouceur, Chief Financial Officer
NDAD is a non-profit organization that assists people with disabilities who are not eligable for services from other agencies.
1975

289 **North Dakota Association for Lifelong Learning (NDALL)**
1605 E. Capitol Ave.
Bismarck, ND 58501
701-355-4458
Fax: 701-227-8847
http://sites.google.com/site/northdakotaall/
jgreuel@clearwatercommunications.net
Penny Veit-Hetletved, President
Beth Hurt, Vice President
Joe Kalvoda, Secretary/Treasurer
The North Dakota Association for Lifelong Learning (NDALL) supports educators, adult students, and partners in alternative education. Formerly it was known as the North Dakota Association of Adult Basic & Secondary Education (NDABSE).

290 **North Dakota Autism Center**
647 13th Ave. E.
West Fargo, ND 58078
701-277-8844
Fax: 701-227-8847
http://www.ndautismcenter.org
Eric Mauch, Board Chair
Amy Beito, Board Member
Lane Huseby, Board Member
The Autism Center supports families and individuals affected by autism spectrum disorders through care, therapy, advocacy, and more. Is also the home of the AuSome Kids Day Program which focuses on the needs of preschool and school age children with Autism Spectrum Disorders or related disabilities and behaviours.

291 **North Dakota Center for Persons with Disabllities (NDCPD)**
Minot State University
500 University Ave. W.
Memorial Hall 203
Minot, ND 58707
701-858-3580
800-233-1737
Fax: 701-858-3483
TTY: 701-858-3580
http://www.ndcpd.org
ndcpd@minotstateu.edu
Dr. Brent Askvig, Executive Director
Dr. Lori Garnes, Associate Director, Development
Susie Mack, Coordinator for Operations
The NDCPD provides services, education, and research designed to encourage communities to welcome, value, and ensure the well-being of the differently abled. It is part of the University Center of Excellence on Developmental Disabilities, Education, Research and Services.

292 **North Dakota Protection & Advocacy Project**
400 E. Broadway
Suite 409, Wells Fargo Bank Bldg.
Bismarck, ND 58501-4071
701-328-2950
800-472-2670
Fax: 701-328-3934
http://www.ndpanda.org
panda@nd.gov
Teresa Larsen, Executive Director
David Boeck, Director, Legal Services
Dotty Simes, Fiscal Manager
The Protection & Advocacy Project advocates for the rights of North Dakotans with disabilities.

293 **Pathfinder Services**
1015 S. Broadway
Suite 42
Minot, ND 58701
701-837-7500
http://www.psnd.co/index.php
info@pathfinder-nd.org
David King, Board President
Jodi Webb, Executive Director
Jacki Harasym, Director, Family/Finance Support
Pathfinder seeks to support North Dakota families of children and youth with learning difficulties. Programs include webinars, workshops, and parent advising.
1987

Ohio

294 Easterseals Youngstown
299 Edwards St.
Youngstown, OH 44502-1599 330-743-1168
Fax: 330-743-1616
http://www.easterseals.com/mtc/
Kenan J. Sklenar, President/CEO
Easterseals of Mahoning, Trumbull, and Columbiana Counties pledges to help persons with disabilities or special needs live with equality, dignity, and independence.

295 International Dyslexia Association of Central Ohio
P.O. Box 1601
Westerville, OH 43086 614-899-5711
http://coh.dyslexiaida.org
info@cobida.org
Mike McGovern, President
Blythe Wood, Vice President
Diana McGovern, Treasurer
Increases awareness of dyslexia and related learning disabilities; assists professionals, dyslexics, and their families; promotes use of effective teaching methods; and disseminates research-based knowledge. Serves Central Ohio and parts of West Virginia.

296 International Dyslexia Association of Northern Ohio
P.O. Box 172
Richfield, OH 44286 216-556-0883
http://noh.dyslexiaida.org
nobidainfo@gmail.com
Jennifer LaHaie, President
Theresa Kaska, 1st Vice President
Nicole Smyk, 2nd Vice President
A non-profit, scientific and educational organization dedicated to the study and treatment of the language-based reading disability, dyselxia.

297 International Dyslexia Association: Ohio Valley Branch
6682 Hitching Post Ln.
Cincinnati, OH 45230 513-651-4747
http://ohv.dyslexiaida.org
tutor@cincinnatidyslexia.org
Kennetha Schmits, President
A non-profit, scientific and educational organization dedicated to the study and treatment of the learning disability, dyslexia. This Branch was formed to increase public awareness of dyslexia on the Southern Ohio, Southeast Indiana, Kentucky and Huntington, West Virginia areas.

298 Learning Disabilities Association of Ohio
P.O. Box 784
Springfield, OH 45501 http://ldaamerica.org/lda-chapters/ohio/
DaveSaunders1111@gmail.com
Dave Saunders
Empowers those with specific learning disabilities to realize their potential and achieve their goals.

Oklahoma

299 Learning Disabilities Association of Oklahoma
P.O. Box 1134
Jenks, OK 74037 405-269-6279
http://oklahoma.ldaamerica.net/
hrice@cameron.edu
Holly Rice
A non-profit organization committed to enhancing the lives of individuals with learning disabilities and their families through education, advocacy, research, and service.

300 Oklahoma Parents Center, Inc.
223 North Broadway
P.O. Box 512
Holdenville, OK 74848 405-379-6015
877-553-4332
Fax: 405-379-2106
http://oklahomaparentscenter.org
info@oklahomaparentscenter.org
Sharon Coppedge Long, Executive Director
Ellen Kimbrell, Associate Director
Deidra Edwards, Training Specialist
The Oklahoma Parents Center (OPC) is a federally funded Parent and Training Information Center that provides services to families of children with disabilities, teachers, and other professionals.

301 WovenLife, Inc.
701 N.E. 13th St.
Oklahoma City, OK 73104 405-239-2525
Fax: 405-239-2278
http://wovenlifeok.org
Paula Porter, President/CEO
Debbie Rucker, Chief Operating Officer
Samantha Pascoe, Vice President, Programs
Formerly the Oklahoma branch of Easter Seal Society, WovenLife became an independent organization in 2017. WovenLife focuses on their local community, offering services such as medical rehabilitation and caregiver support groups. There are programs for children and adults, including the Intergenerational Program, which offers therapeutic activities designed to develop communication skills, problem solving, and promoting self-esteem.
1925

Oregon

302 Easterseals Oregon
7300 SW Huntziker St.
Portland, OR 97223 503-228-5108
Fax: 503-228-1352
http://www.easterseals.com/oregon/
David Cheveallier, CEO
Provides services to children and adults with disabilities and other special needs, helping them to live with equality, dignity, and independence.

303 International Dyslexia Association of Oregon
P.O. Box 2609
Portland, OR 97208-2609 503-228-4455
http://or.dyslexiaida.org/
info@orbida.org
Jane Cooper, President
Danielle Thompson, Vice President
Anne Mauboussin, Treasurer
The Oregon Branch of the International Dyslexia Association (ORBIDA) focuses on increasing public awareness of how dyslexia affects both children and adults.

304 Learning Disabilities Association of Oregon
10175 S.W. Barbur Blvd.
Suite 214B
Portland, OR 97219 503-997-3181
http://www.ldaor.org
rosal24@comcast.net
Laura Rosal
Works to promote the welfare of children and adults with learning disabilities. A non-profit organization that serves as a resource, referral, and information center for adults with learning disabilities, parents of children with learning disabilities, and profesionals working in the field of learning disabilities.

305 **Oregon's Deaf and Hard of Hearing Services**
500 Summer St. NE
Suite E-15
Salem, OR 97301
503-454-6100
Fax: 503-947-4245
TTY: 503-945-6214
http://www.odc.state.or.us
odhhs.info@state.or.us
Clark Anderson, Co-Chair
Mark Hill, Co-Chair
Provides information and referral sources on deafness and hearing loss issues, training on deaf awareness and sensitivity, and how to communicate with those with hearing loss.

306 **University of Oregon Center for Excellence in Developmental Disabilities**
Center on Human Development College of Education
5252 University of Oregon
Eugene, OR 97403-5252
541-346-3591
http://www.uoucedd.org/
uocedd@uoregon.edu
Jane Squires, PhD, Co-Director
Christopher Murray, PhD, Co-Director
Annette Tognazzini, Business Manager
UCEDD provides assistance in the quality of life for individuals with disabilities and their familes.

Pennsylvania

307 **AAC Institute**
1100 Washington Ave.
Suite 317
Carnegie, PA 51506
412-489-5527
Fax: 412-489-5726
http://www.aacinstitute.org
khill@aacinstitute.org
Katya Hill, PhD, Clinic Director
Established in 2000, a resource for all who are interested in enhancing the communication of people who rely on augmentative and alternative communication (AAC). A not-for-profit charitable organization, offers information and provides services worldwide.

308 **Easterseals Eastern Pennsylvania**
1501 Lehigh St.
Suite 201
Allentown, PA 18103
610-289-0114
http://www.easterseals.com/esep/
Dolores Bertoti, Chair
Nancy Knoebel, President/CEO
Deborah F. Hill, Chief Financial Officer
An organization that offers services such as child development centers, physical rehabilitation, and job training for people with disabilities.

309 **Easterseals Southeastern Pennsylvania**
3975 Conshohocken Ave.
Philadelphia, PA 19131
215-879-1000
Fax: 215-879-8424
http://www.easterseals.com/sepa/
Roy Yaffe, President
Don Maxfield, Vice President
Cummins Catherwood, Jr., Secretary
An organization that offers services such as child development centers, physical rehabilitation, and job training for people with disabilities.

310 **Easterseals Western & Central Pennsylvania**
875 Greentree Rd., 6 Pkwy Center
Suite 150
Pittsburgh, PA 15220
412-281-7244
http://www.easterseals.com/wcpenna/
development@eastersealswcpenna.org
Ronald Palmer, Chairman
Pete Licastro, 1st Vice Chairman
Bill Warfel, Treasurer
An organization that offers services such as child development centers, physical rehabilitation, and job training for people with disabilities.

311 **Huntingdon County PRIDE**
1301 Mount Vernon Ave.
Huntingdon, PA 16652
814-643-5724
Fax: 814-643-6085
http://www.huntingdonpride.org
apfingstl@huntingdonpride.org
Adam Pfingstl, Executive Director
Kathleen Renninger, Service Coordinator
Jody McCartney, PRIDE Cares Coordinator
Provides programs which enable people who are developmentally and/or physically disabled to function at their optimal level of performance.

312 **International Dyslexia Association of Pennsylvania**
1062 E. Lancaster Ave.
Suite 15H
Rosemont, PA 19010
610-527-1548
855-220-8885
http://www.pbida.org
Monica McHale-Small, President
The Pennsylvania Branch of the International Dyslexia Association (PBIDA), serving Pennsylvania and Delaware provides support and information for individuals, families, and educational professionals concerned with the issues of dyslexia and learning differences.

313 **Learning Disabilities Association of Pennsylvania**
4156 Library Rd.
Suite 1
Pittsburg, PA 15234
412-341-1515
888-300-6710
http://ldaamerica.org
A non-profit organization dedicated to serving Pennsylvania residents by providing accurate, up-to-date information regarding learning disabilities as well as support.

314 **Pennsylvania Client Assistance Program**
Center for Disability Law and Policy
1515 Market St.
Suite 1300
Philadelphia, PA 19102
215-557-7112
888-745-2357
Fax: 215-557-7602
TTY: 215-557-7112
http://www.equalemployment.org
Stephen S. Pennington, Executive Director
Francella Porter, Office Manager
Margaret Passio-McKenna, Senior Advocate
An advocacy program for people with disabilities administered by the Center for Disability Law & Policy. CAP helps people, free of charge, who are seeking services from the Office of Vocational Rehabilitation, Blindness and Visual Services, Centers for Independent Living, and other progrmas funded under federal law.

Rhode Island

315 **International Dyslexia Association of Rhode Island**
P.O. Box 603144
Providence, RI 02906
401-521-0020
Fax: 401-847-6720
http://idarhodeisland.weebly.com
ida.Rhodeisland@gmail.com
A non-profit, scientific and educational organization dedicated to the study and treatment of dyslexia.

316 **Looking Upwards**
438 E Main Rd
PO Box 4289
Middletown, RI 02842
401-847-0960
http://www.lookingupwards.org

Michele Banks, Program Admin., Day Enrichment
Tanya Howard, Admin., Supported Living
Jenn Szcesniak, Employment Team Coordinator
A nonprofit agency serving adults with developmental disabilities through a variety of programs. Services include supported living, employment assistance, day activities and classes.
1978

317 **The Arc of Blackstone Valley**
500 Prospect St.
Wing A
Pawtucket, RI 02860
401-727-0150
800-257-6092
Fax: 401-727-1545
http://www.bvcriarc.org
John J. Padien III, Chief Executive Officer
Katherine S. Hunt, Chief Operating Officer
Catherine Gilligan, Chief Financial Officer
Serving approximately 300 adults with disabilities, The Arc of Blackstone Valley advocates for and protects the rights of individuals with intellectual and developmental disabilities.

South Carolina

318 **Easterseals South Carolina**
P.O. Box 5715
Columbia, SC 29250
803-466-4089
Fax: 803-356-6902
http://www.easterseals.com/southcarolina
Drew Royall, Chair
Deanna Lewis, President & CEO
Paul Guinn, Director, Finance
Provides services to children and adults with disabilities and other special needs, and support to their families.

319 **International Dyslexia Association of South Carolina**
30 Southampton Dr.
Charleston, SC 29407
http://sc.dyslexiaida.org
southcarolinabranchida@gmail.com
Ann Whitten, President
Robert Whetsell, Vice President
Jessica Overstreet, Treasurer
The South Carolina Branch provides general information about dyslexia and makes referrals to various professionals and schools serving individuals with learning disabilities.
130 members

320 **The Arc South Carolina**
1202 12th St.
Cayce, SC 29033
803-748-5020
Fax: 803-445-1026
http://www.arcsc.org
Margie Williamson, Executive Director
Carly Fieldhouse, Director, Operations
Breanna Neely, Project Director
A state chapter of The Arc of the United States, The Arc of South Carolina supports the inclusion and participation of individuals with intellectual and developmental disabilities in their communities.

South Dakota

321 **South Dakota Center for Disabilities**
Health Science Center
1400 W. 22nd St.
Sioux Falls, SD 57105
800-658-3080
Fax: 605-357-1438
http://www.usd.edu/cd
cd@usd.edu
Wendy Parent-Johnson, Executive Director
John R. Johnson, Research & Development Director
Kristin Berg, Assistant Director
A division of the Department of Pediatrics at the Sanford School of Medicine at the University of South Dakota. The Center for Disabilities is South Dakota's University Center for Excellence in Developmental Disabilities Education, Research and Service sometimes referred to as University Centers for Excellence in Developmental Disabilities.

Tennessee

322 **Easterseals Tennessee**
750 Old Hickory Blvd.
Suite 2-260
Brentwood, TN 37027
615-292-6640
Fax: 615-251-0994
http://www.easterseals.com/tennessee/
Tim Ryerson, President/CEO
Susan Brown, Chief Financial Officer
Jennifer Wang, Director, Programs & Services
Creates solutions that change the lives of children and adults with disabilities or other special needs and their families.

323 **International Dyslexia Association of Tennessee**
6731 Ridgerock Ln.
Knoxville, TN 37909
877-836-6432
Fax: 931-528-3916
http://www.tnida.org
Emily Dempster, President
Erin Alexander, Senior Vice President
Michele Richter, Secretary
The Tennessee Branch of the International Dyslexia Association was formed to increase awareness about Dyslexia in the state of Tennessee. TN-IDA supports efforts to provide information regarding appropriate language arts instruction to those involved with language-based learning differences and to encourage the identity of these individuals at-risk for such disorders as soon as possible. This branch also serves individuals in the state of Kentucky.

324 **Learning Disabilities Association of Tennessee**
P.O. Box 40237
Memphis, TN 38174-0237
901-788-5328
http://www.learningdisabilitiesoftennessee.org
info@learningdisabilitiesoftennessee.org
The Learning Disabilities Association of Tennessee has a mission to provide information concerning awareness, advocacy, parent information, and community education to maximize the quality of life for individuals and families affected by Learning Disabilities and related disorders in the state of Tennessee.

325 **LifeLine, Inc.**
1400 McCallie Ave.
Suite 112
Chattanooga, TN 37404
423-622-4007
http://lifelinefamilies.org
info@lifelinefamilies.org
Becky Cunningham, Chair
Emily Calloway, Vice Chair
Lisa Mattheiss, Executive Director
A non-profit church organization that aims to help meet the unique needs of families of those with special needs.

326 **STAR Center, Inc.**
1119 Old Humboldt Rd.
Jackson, TN 38305
731-668-3888
Fax: 731-668-1666
http://www.star-center.org
info@star-center.org
Dave Bratcher, President
The STAR Center aims to help any person with any type of disability realize their potential by providing services for education, employment, and quality of life.

327 **The Arc Tennessee**
545 Mainstream Dr.
Suite 100
Nashville, TN 37228-1213
615-248-5878
800-835-7077
Fax: 615-248-5879
http://www.thearctn.org
info@thearctn.org
Carrie Hobbs Guiden, Executive Director
Loria Hubbard, Director, Programs
Nicole Ramsey, Business Manager
A non-profit, statewide advocacy agency that empowers people with intellectual and developmental disabilities to participate in the community.

Texas

328 **Easterseals Central Texas**
8505 Cross Park Dr.
Suite 120
Austin, TX 78754
512-478-2581
http://www.easterseals.com/centraltx/
Tod Marvin, President/CEO
Mia Martin, Chief Financial Officer
Lucas Wells, Chief Program Officer
Easterseals Central Texas provides exceptional services so people with disabilities and their families can fully participate in their communities.

329 **Easterseals North Texas**
1424 Hemphill St.
Fort Worth, TX 76104
888-617-7171
http://www.easterseals.com/northtexas/
Donna Dempsey, President/CEO
Nancy Q. Quimby, Executive VP/CFO
Denise Wilkerson, Vice President, Development
Created by the merger of Easter Seals of Greater Dallas and Easter Seals Greater Northwest Texas. Creates opportunities that advance the independence of individuals with disabilities and other special needs.

330 **International Dyslexia Association of Austin**
P.O. Box 92604
Austin, TX 78709
512-666-8190
http://aus.dyslexiaida.org
Mary Bach, President
Karen Monteith, Vice President
Herman H. Klare, Treasurer
The Austin Area Branch of the International Dyslexia Association is a non-profit organization dedicated to promoting reading excellence for all children through early identification of dyslexia, effective literacy education for adults and children with dyslexia, and teacher training.

331 **International Dyslexia Association of Dallas**
14070 Proton Dr.
Suite 100
Dallas, TX 75244
972-233-9107
Fax: 972-490-4219
http://dal.dyslexiaida.org
admin.dal@dyslexiaida.org
Emily Visinsky, President
Shanara Hawkins, Vice President
Paul Niemyski, Treasurer
The Dallas Branch of The International Dyslexia Association is committed to leadership and advocacy for people with dyslexia by providing support for individuals and group interactions; programs to inform and educate; and information for professionals and the general public.

332 **International Dyslexia Association of Houston**
P.O. Box 540504
Houston, TX 77254-0504
832-282-7154
http://www.houstonida.org
HoustonBIDA@gmail.com
Mary Yarus, President
Anson J. Koshy, Vice President
Karen Priputen, Treasurer
A non-profit organization dedicated to helping individuals with dyslexia and related learning disorders, their families, and the communities that support them.

333 **Learning Ally: Austin Recording Studio**
1314 W 45th St
Austin, TX 78756
800-221-4792
http://www.learningally.org
Andrew Friendman, President & CEO
Harold J Logan, Chair
Therese Llorente, Vice Chair
To create opportunities for students who cannot read standard print because of a visual impairment, learning disability or other physical disability, to succeed in school by providing accessible educational materials.

334 **Learning Disabilities Association of Texas**
P.O. Box 831392
Richardson, TX 75083
800-604-7500
http://www.ldatx.org
contact@ldatx.org
Promotes the educational and general welfare of individuals with learning disabilities.
1963

335 **North Texas Rehabilitation Center**
1005 Midwestern Pkwy.
Wichita Falls, TX 76302
940-322-0771
http://www.ntrehab.org
sthompson@ntrehab.org
Mike Castles, President/CEO
Lesa Enlow, Program Director
Sheila Moeller, Financial Officer
A not-for-profit organization providing nationally accredited outpatient medical, academic, and developmental rehabilitation to North Texas and Southern Oklahoma. From the Early Childhood Intervention program to the Aquatics programs, these services are designed to help patients acheive their highest level of independence.
1948

Utah

336 **International Dyslexia Association Rocky Mountain Branch**
740 Yale Rd.
Boulder, CO 80305
303-721-9425
855-543-2762
http://idarmb.org
ida_rmb@yahoo.com
Lynn Kuhn, President
Tammy Curran, Vice President
Diane Mayer, Vice President
Dedicated to ensuring that every student with the learning difference of Dyslexia will receive scientifically based instruction and services consistent with his/her needs. Serves communities in Colorado, Utah, and Wyoming.

337 **Learning Disabilities Association of Utah**
P.O. Box 900726
Sandy, UT 84090-0726
801-553-9156
http://www.ldau.org
contact@ldau.org
A non-profit volunteer organization supporting people with learning disabilities and their families. Their mission is to create opportunities for individuals with learning disabilities to succeed and for their families to participate in their success.

338 **Utah Parent Center**
230 West 200 South
Suite 1101
Salt Lake City, UT 84101
801-272-1051
800-468-1160
Fax: 801-272-8907
http://utahparentcenter.org
info@utahparentcenter.org
Helen Post, Executive Director
Gina Money, Associate Director
Jennie Dopp, Development Coordinator
UPC aims to help parents help their children with disabilities life the bet life possible by offering free training, information, referral, and assistance. UPC also aids professionals in their efforts to help children with disabilities through professional development workshops, webinars, and more.

Vermont

339 **Vermont Family Network**
600 Blair Park Rd.
Suite 240
Williston, VT 05495
800-800-4005
Fax: 802-876-6291
http://www.vermontfamilynetwork.org
info@vtfn.org
Pam McCarthy, President/CEO
Holly Brooks, Vice President, Operations
Charles Teske, Finance Manager
An organization that supports and empowers the families of children with special needs. Vermont Family network provides information, connections, and support about the development, education, and heath of children with disabilities.

340 **Vermont Protection & Advocacy**
Disability Rights Vermont
141 Main St.
Suite 7
Montpelier, VT 05602
802-229-1355
800-834-7890
Fax: 802-229-1359
http://www.disabilityrightsvt.org/programs.html
info@disabilityrightsvt.org
Ed Paquin, Executive Director
Sarah Wendell-Launderville, President
David LaCroix, Vice President
Dedicated to addressing problems, questions, and complaints brought to it by Vermonters with disabilities. VP&A's mission is to promote the equality, dignity, and self-determination of people with disabilities. VP&A provides infomration, referral, and advocacy services, including legal representation when appropriate, to individuals with disabilities throughout Vermont.

Virginia

341 **Easter Seals - UCP North Carolina & Virginia**
5171 Glenwood Ave.
Suite 211
Raleigh, NC 27612
800-662-7119
Fax: 919-782-5486
http://eastersealsucp.com
info@nc.eastersealsucp.com
Luanne Welch, President/CEO
A lifelong partner for people managing disabilities and mental health challenges. Services are centered around each person's individual needs to live, learn, and participate fully in his or her community.

342 **International Dyslexia Association of Virginia**
3126 West Cary St.
Suite 102
Richmond, VA 23221
866-893-0583
http://va.dyslexiaida.org/
info@vbida.org
Lisa Snider, President
Lisa Harrah, Vice President
Robin Hegner, Secretary
Formed to increase public awareness of dyslexia in the State of Virginia. They serve the entire state, with the exception of Northern Virginia, which is part of the DC-Capital Branch in Washington, DC. They serve individuals with dyslexia, their families, and professionals in the field.

343 **The Arc of Virginia**
2147 Staples Mill Rd.
Richmond, VA 23230
804-649-8481
888-604-2677
Fax: 804-649-3585
http://thearcofva.org
info@thearcofva.org
Tonya Milling, Executive Director
Kim Goodloe, President
Burt Hudson, Vice President
Promotes and protects the rights of individuals with intellectual and developmental disabilities.

344 **The READ Center**
4915 Radford Ave.
Suite 204
Richmond, VA 23230
804-288-9930
http://readcenter.org
frontdesk@readcenter.org
Karen La Forge, Executive Director
Samuel Baronian, Jr., President
Nora Crouch, Vice President
A non-profit organization that aims to help adults with low-level literacy skills achieve basic reading/communication skills.

Washington

345 **Disability Rights Washington**
315 5th Ave. S.
Suite 850
Seattle, WA 98104
206-324-1521
800-562-2702
Fax: 206-957-0729
TTY: 206-957-0728
http://www.disabilityrightswa.org
info@dr-wa.org
Mark Stroh, Executive Director
David Carlson, Director, Advocacy
David Lord, Director, Public Policy
Disability Rights Washington is a private, non-profit organization that has been protecting the rights of people with disabilities.
1974

346 **Easterseals Washington**
220 W. Mercer St.
Suite 210E
Seattle, WA 98119-3954
206-281-5700
Fax: 206-284-0938
http://wa.easterseals.com
Jeff Pavey, Board Chair
Cathy Bisaillon, President/CEO
Carol Basile, Vice Chair
Provides exceptional services to ensure that people living with autism and other disabilities have equal opportunities to live, learn, work, and play.

347 **International Dyslexia Association of Washington State**
P.O. Box 27435
Seattle, WA 98165
206-382-1020
http://www.wabida.org
info@wabida.org
Jessica Ruger, President
Jamie Geddis, Vice President
Dana Mott, Managing Director

The Washington State Branch of the International Dyslexia Association is a non-profit, scientific and educational organization dedicated to the study and treatment of dyslexia. They seek to increase public awareness of dyslexia in their branch's area which includes Washington, Idaho, and Western Montana.

348 **Learning Disabilities Association of Washington**
16315 NE., 87th St.
Suite B-10
Redmond, WA 98052 425-882-0820
http://www.ldawa.org
nsobich@ldawa.org
Nancy Sobich, Program Manager, Info./Referral
Promotes and provides services and support to improve the quality of life for individuals and families affected by learning and attentional disabilities.
1964

349 **Washington Assistive Technology Act Program**
University of Washington
UW Box 354237
Seattle, WA 98195-4237 800-214-8731
Fax: 206-543-4779
TTY: 866-866-0162
http://watap.org
watap@uw.edu
Alan Knue, Director
Scott Canaan, Program Coordinator
Offers services and advocacy pertaining to assistive technology for persons with disabilities.

350 **Washington Parent Training Project: PAVE**
6316 S. 12th St.
Tacoma, WA 98465 253-565-2266
800-572-7368
Fax: 253-566-8052
http://www.wapave.org
pave@wapave.org
Tracy Kahlo, Executive Director
Nicol Walsh, Communications Specialist
Elma Rounds, CFO/Office Manager
A parent directed organization that exists to increase independence, empowerment, future opportunities and choices for consumers with special needs, their families and communities through training, information, referral, and support.
1979

West Virginia

351 **Disability Rights West Virginia**
1207 Quarrier St.
Suite 400
Charlston, WV 25301 304-346-0847
800-950-5250
Fax: 304-346-0867
http://www.drofwv.org
Susan Given, Executive Director
Jeremiah Underhill, Legal Director
Taniua Hardy, Program Director
Disability Rights West Virginia is a protection and advocacy organization for people with disabilities in West Virginia. They provide information, training, education, and assistance to people with disabilities, their families, and agencies or professionals who serve disabled persons.

352 **Easter Seals West Virginia**
1305 National Rd.
Wheeling, WV 26003 304-242-1390
Fax: 304-243-5880
http://www.easterseals.com/wv/
Tom Tuttle, President
J. David Diosi, Vice President
Deborah Joseph, Secretary
Easter Seals helps children and adults with Autism Spectrum Disorder and other disabilities.

353 **The Disability Action Center**
102 Benoni Ave.
Fairmont, WV 26554 304-366-3213
http://disabilityactioncenter.com
jsole@disabilityactioncenter.com
Julie Sole, Executive Director
Since 1958 the Disability Action Center has been providing programs and services to individuals with disabilities and their families. Current programs include a Career Readiness Center, Experience IT Co-Op, education and training, health and wellness, life skills and independent living, reading and literacy, self-advocacy, and more.

Wisconsin

354 **Disability Rights Wisconsin**
6737 W. Washington St.
Suite 3230
Milwaukee, WI 53214 414-733-4646
800-928-8778
http://www.disabilityrightswi.org
Barbara Beckert, Office Director
Laura Hanson, Director, Operations/Quality
Lea Kitz, Program Manager
A non-profit organization protecting the rights of people with disabilities in the state of Wisconsin.

355 **Easterseals Southeast Wisconsin**
2222 S. 114th St.
West Allis, WI 53227 414-449-4444
Fax: 414-571-5568
http://www.easterseals.com/wi-se/
Roger Schaus, Jr., Chair
Peter Engel, Chief Executive Officer
Michelle Schaefer, Chief Operating Officer
Provides services across the lifespan to individuals with autism and other disabilities. Services include: autism therapies, early intervention, day services, and work service training.

356 **International Dyslexia Association of Wisconsin**
1616 Graham Ave.
Eau Claire, WI 54701 608-355-0911
http://wi.dyslexiaida.org
wibida@gmail.com
Dr. Tammy Tillotson, President
Kimberly Chan, Treasurer
Mary Brod, Secretary
A membership organization of parents, teachers, tutors, and diagnosticians interested in learning about reading disabilities and learning the skills needed to help deal with dyslexia.

357 **Learning Disabilities Association of Wisconsin**
7625 Lechler Ln.
Kiel, WI 53042 http://www.ldawisconsin.com
info@LDAwisconsin.com
Diane Sixel, President
Lisa Olig, Vice President
Jan Anderson, Secretary
Affiliated with the national organization the Learning Disabilities Association of America, LDA Wisconsin provides support to children and adults with learning disabilities through advocacy, education, information, and research.

358 **Wisconsin FACETS**
600 W. Virginia St.
Suite 501
Milwaukee, WI 53204 414-374-4645
877-374-0511
Fax: 414-374-4655
http://wifacets.org
Courtney Salzer, Executive Director
Cheryl Peterson, Accounting Director

Wisconsin Family Assistance Center for Education, Training & Support, known as WI FACETS, is a non-profit organization that aims to help children and youth with special needs and their families by being an information center that connects them to much needed resources.

359 **Wisconsin Institute for Learning Disabilities/Dyslexia Inc. (WILDD)**
6525 Grand Teton Plaza
Suite B
Madison, WI 53719 608-824-8980
Fax: 608-831-3840
http://wildd.org
madison@wildd.org
Ervin Carpenter, Co-Founder/Executive Director
Kim Campbell-Carpenter, Co-Founder/Director, Operations
Tim Mueller, Chairman
Through identification, remediation, therapy, support, community education, and advocacy the Wisconsin Institute for Learning Disabilities/Dyslexia helps children with learning disabilities achieve success in school and in their community.

Wyoming

360 **Cheyenne Habilitation & Theraputic Center (CHAT)**
1100 Storey Blvd.
Cheyenne, WY 82009 307-433-1110
Fax: 307-433-1114
http://www.chatcenterinc.com
Kim Elfering, Director
CHAT Center finds employment and volunteer opportunities for disabled participants in their programs to be involved in the community.
1972

361 **Children's Learning Center**
P.O. Box 4100
Jackson, WY 83001 307-733-1616
Fax: 307-733-0478
http://www.childrenlearn.org
info@learningcenterwy.org
Audrey Cohen-Davis, Chair
Karen Horstmann, Vice Chair
Lance Windey, Treasurer
Provides quality child development services to the Counties of Teton and Sublette, for children age six weeks to three years. CLC has more than 80 staff, 14 classrooms, 3 therapy facilities, and 6 campuses.
1972

362 **Easter Seals Wyoming**
991 Joe St.
Sheridan, WY 82801-1363 307-672-2816
http://www.easterseals.com/wyoming/
Scott L. Wilson, Board Chair
Michelle Belknap, President/CEO
Dawn Mellinger, Secretary
Provides life improving programs and services to benefit children and adults with disabilities.

363 **International Dyslexia Association Rocky Mountain Branch**
740 Yale Rd.
Boulder, CO 80305 303-721-9425
855-543-2762
http://idarmb.org
ida_rmb@yahoo.com
Lynn Kuhn, President
Tammy Curran, Vice President
Diane Mayer, Vice President
Dedicated to ensuring that every student with the learning differene of Dyslexia will receives scientifically based instruction and services consistent with his/her needs. Serves communities in Colorado, Utah, and Wyoming.

364 **Northwest Community Action Programs - Casper (NOWCAP)**
345 North Walsh Dr.
P.O. Box 51248
Casper, WY 82609 307-237-9146
Fax: 307-234-1029
http://www.nowcapservices.org
rpullen@nowcapservices.org
Renate Pullen, Executive Director
Kari Cornella, Operations Director
E. Joe Stolns, CEO
NOWCAP Services is a provider of services for people with disabilities in Natrona County.

365 **Northwest Community Action Programs - Rock Springs (NOWCAP)**
649 North Front St., Building B
P.O. Box 1666
Rock Springs, WY 82901 307-382-2683
Fax: 307-362-3035
http://www.nowcapservices.org
rlloyd@nowcapservices.org
Roy Lloyd, Community Services Director
NOWCAP Services is a provider of services for people with disabilities in Natrona County.

366 **The Arc of Natrona County**
355 N. Lincoln St.
Casper, WY 82601 307-577-4913
Fax: 307-577-4014
http://arcofnatronacounty.org
Dr. Nathan Edwards, President
Aaron Yeigh, Vice President
Bethany Young, Executive Director
The Arc provides education, research, advocacy, and support to individuals with cognitive, intellectual, and developmental disabilities, as well as for their families and friends in the Natrona County.

National Programs

367 **Attention Deficit Disorder Association**

800-939-1019
http://www.add.org

Duane Gordon, President
Michelle Frank, Vice President
Melissa Reskof, Secretary

The Attention Deficit Disorder Association is an organization focused on the needs of adults and young adults with ADD/ADHD, offering resources and research to help children, families, and professionals.

368 **Children and Adults with Attention Deficit Hyperactivity Disorder (CHADD)**

4601 Presidents Drive
Suite 300
Lanham, MD 20706
301-306-7070
800-233-4050
Fax: 301-306-7090
http://www.chadd.org
help@chadd.org

Michael MacKay, President
M. Jeffry Spahr, MBA, JD, Secretary
Patricia Michel, CPA, MBA, Treasurer

Children and Adults with Attention-Deficit/Hyperactivity Disorder (CHADD), is a national non-profit, tax-exempt (Section 501) organization providing education, advocacy and support for individuals with AD/HD. In addition to an informative Web site, CHADD also publishes a variety of printed materials to keep members and professionals current on research advances, medications and treatments affecting individuals with AD/HD.

16,000 members

369 **Council for Exceptional Children (CEC)**

2900 Crystal Dr.
Suite 100
Arlington, VA 22202-3557
888-232-7733
TTY: 866-915-5000
http://www.cec.sped.org
service@cec.sped.org

Laurie VanderPloeg, President
Mary Lynn Boscardin, President Elect
Jim McCormick, Treasurer

The Council for Exceptional Children (CEC) is an international organization dedicated to improving educational outcomes for individuals with exceptionalities, students with disabilities, and/or the gifted. CEC advocates for appropriate governmental policies, sets professional standards, provides continual professional development, advocates for newly and historically underserved individuals with exceptionalities, and helps professionals obtain resources necessary for professional practice.

370 **Council for Learning Disabilities (CLD)**

11184 Antioch Rd.
Box 405
Overland Park, KS 66210-2420
913-491-1011
Fax: 913-491-1011
http://council-for-learning-disabilities.org
CLDInfo@cldinternational.org

Deborah Reed, President
Lindy Crawford, Vice President
Linda Nease, Executive Director

The mission of the Council for Learning Disabilities/CLD is to enhance the education and life span development of individuals with learning disabilities. CLD establishes standards of excellence and promotes innovative strategies on research and practice through interdisciplinary education, collaboration, and advocacy. CLD's publication, Learning Disability Quarterly, focuses on the latest research in the field of learning disabilities with an applied focus.

371 **Dyslexia Research Institute**

5746 Centerville Rd
Tallahassee, FL 32309
850-893-2216
Fax: 850-893-2440
http://www.dyslexia-add.org
dri@dyslexia-add.org

Patricia K. Hardman, PhD, Founder, CEO
Robyn Rennick, Program Director

Addresses academic, social and self-concept issues for dyslexic and ADD children and adults. College prep courses, study skills, advocacy, diagnostic testing, seminars, teacher training, day school, tutoring and an adult literacy and life skills program is available using an accredited MSLE approach.

372 **Learning Disabilities Association of America (LDAA)**

4156 Library Rd.
Pittsburgh, PA 15234-1349
412-341-1515
Fax: 412-344-0224
http://www.ldaamerica.org
info@ldaamerica.org

Mary-Clare Reynolds, Executive Director
Stephanie Fedro-Byrom, Operations Manager
Myrna Mandlawitz, Policy Director

An information and referral center for parents and professionals dealing with Attention Deficit Disorders, and other learning disabilities. Free materials and referral service to nearest chapter.

373 **National Alliance on Mental Illness (NAMI)**

3803 N. Fairfax Drive
Suite 100
Arlington, VA 22203
703-524-7600
888-999-6264
Fax: 703-524-9094
http://www.nami.org
info@nami.org

David Levy, Chief Financial Officer
Lynn Borton, Chief Operating Officer
Jean-Michel Texier, Chief Information Officer

NAMI/National Alliance on Mental Illness is a mental health organization dedicated to improving the lives of persons living with serious mental illness and their families. NAMI members, leaders, and friends work across all levels to meet a shared NAMI mission of support, education, advocacy, and research for people living with mental illness.

374 **National Center for Learning Disabilities (NCLD)**

32 Laight St.
2nd Fl.
New York, NY 10013
888-575-7373
http://www.ncld.com

Frederic M. Poses, Chairman of the Board
Mimi Corcoran, President/CEO
Rashonda Ambrose, Director, Strategic Partnerships

NCLD develops and delivers programs and promotes research to improve instruction, assessment, and support services for individuals with learning disabilities. They create and disseminate essential information for parents and educators, providing help and hope.

375 **National Clearinghouse of Rehabilitation Training Materials (NCRTM)**

Utah State University
6524 Old Main Hill
Logan, UT 84322-6524
866-821-5355
Fax: 435-797-7537
http://www.nchrtm.okstate.edu
ncrtm@cc.us.edu

Chenyong Zhu, M.S., Instructional Designer
Jared Schultz, Principal Investigator
Sylvia Sims, Office Assistant

The mission of the NCRTM is to advocate for the advancement of best practice in rehabilitation counseling through the development, collection, dissemination, and utilization of professional information, knowledge and skill.

376 **National Dissemination Center for Children with Disabilities**
1825 Connecticut Ave NW
Suite 700
Washington, DC 20009
202-884-8200
800-695-0285
Fax: 202-884-8441
http://www.nichcy.org
emulligan@fhi360.org
Suzanne Ripley, Director
National Dissemination Center for Children with Disabilities is a central source of information on: disabilities in infants, toddlers, children, and youth; IDEA, which is the law authorizing special education; No Child Left Behind (as it relates to children with disabilities); and research-based information on effective educational practices.

377 **National Institute of Mental Health (NIMH) Nat'l Institute of Neurological Disorders and Stroke**
NIMH Neurological Institute
P.O. Box 5801
Bethesda, MD 20824-0001
800-352-9424
Fax: 301-496-5751
TTY: 301-408-5981
http://www.ninds.nih.gov
nimhinfo@nih.gov
Story C Landis Ph.D, Director NINDS
Thomas Inseo, Director NIMH
NINDS is part of the National Institutes of Health which support research on developmental disorders such as ADHD. Research programs of the NINDS, the National Institute of Mental Health (NIMH), and the National Institute of Child Health and Human Development (NICHD) seek to address unanswered questions about the causes of ADHD, as well as to improve diagnosis and treatment.

378 **National Resource Center on AD/HD**
4601 Presidents Drive
Suite 300
Lanham, MD 20706
301-306-7070
800-233-4050
Fax: 301-306-7090
http://www.help4adhd.org/
Timothy J MacGeorge MSW, Director
The National Resource Center on AD/HD (NRC): A Program of CHADD (Children and Adults with Attention-Deficit/Hyperactivity Disorder), was established in 2002 to be the national clearinghouse for the latest evidence-based information on AD/HD. The NRC provides comprehensive information and support to individuals with AD/HD, their families and friends, and the professionals involved in their lives.

379 **U.S. Department of Health & Human Services Administration on Developmental Disabilities**
370 L'Enfant Promenade SW
Mailstop HHH 405-D
Washington, DC 20447-0001
202-690-6590
Fax: 202-690-6904
http://www.acf.hhs.gov/programs/add
fmccormick@acf.hhs.gov
Faith McCormick, Director
The Administration on Developmental Disabilities ensures that individuals with developmental disabilities and their families participate in the design of and have access to culturally competent services, supports, and other assistance and opportunities that promotes independence, productivity, and integration and inclusion into the community.

Publications/Videos

380 **A New Look at ADHD: Inhibition, Time, and Self-Control**
Guilford Publications
72 Spring St
New York, NY 10012-4019
212-431-9800
800-365-7006
Fax: 212-966-6708
http://www.guilford.com
info@guilford.com
Russell A. Barkley PhD, Author
This video provides an accessible introduction to Russell A. Barkley's influential theory of the nature and origins of ADHD. The companion manual reviews and amplifies key ideas and contains helpful suggestions for further reading. The package also includes a leader's guide, providing tips on the optimal use of the video with a variety of audiences.
$99.00
Video & Manual
ISBN 1-593854-21-8

381 **AD/HD For Dummies**
American Psychiatric Publishing, Inc (APPI)
1000 Wilson Boulevard
Suite 1825
Arlington, VA 22209-3924
703-907-7322
800-368-5777
Fax: 703-907-1091
http://www.appi.org
appi@psych.org
John McDuffie, Associate Publisher
Jeff Strong, Author
Michael O Flanagan, Author
This book provides answers for parents of children who may have either condition, as well as for adult sufferers. Written in a friendly, easy-to-understand style, it helps people recognize and understand ADD and ADHD symptoms and offers an authoritative, balanced overview of both drug and non-drug therapies. *$29.95*
Paperback
ISBN 0-764537-12-7

382 **ADD and Creativity: Tapping Your Inner Muse**
Taylor Publishing
7211 Circle S Road
Austin, TX 78745
512-444-0571
800-225-3687
Fax: 512-440-2160
http://www.taylorpublishing.com
Yearbooks@balfour.com
Lynn Weiss PhD, Author
Raises and answers questions about the dynamic between the two components and shows how they can be a wonderful gift but also a painful liability if not properly handled. Real-life stories and inspirational affirmations throughout.
216 pages Paperback
ISBN 0-878339-60-4

383 **ADD and Romance: Finding Fulfillment in Love, Sex and Relationships**
Taylor Publishing
7212 Circle S Road
Austin, TX 78745
512-444-0571
800-225-3687
Fax: 512-440-2160
http://www.taylorpublishing.com
Yearbooks@balfour.com
Jonathan Halverstadt, Author
A look at how attention deficit disorder can damage romantic relationships when partners do not take time, or do not know how to address this problem. This book provides the tools needed to build and sustain a more satisfying relationship.
240 pages Paperback
ISBN 0-878332-09-X

384 **ADD and Success**
Taylor Publishing
7213 Circle S Road
Austin, TX 78745
512-444-0571
800-225-3687
Fax: 512-440-2160
http://www.taylorpublishing.com
Yearbooks@balfour.com

Lynn Weiss PhD, Author
Presents the stories of 13 individuals and their experiences and challenges of living with adult attention disorder and achieving success.
224 pages Paperback
ISBN 0-878339-94-9

385 **ADD in Adults**
Taylor Publishing
7214 Circle S Road
Austin, TX 78745
512-444-0571
800-225-3687
Fax: 512-440-2160
http://www.taylorpublishing.com
Yearbooks@balfour.com

Lynn Weiss PhD, Author
Updated version of this best-selling book on the topic of ADD helps others to understand and live with the issues related to ADD. *$17.95*
192 pages Paperback
ISBN 0-878338-50-0

386 **ADD/ADHD Behavior-Change Resource Kit: Ready-to-Use Strategies & Activities for Helping Children**
With Attention Deficit Disorder
1000 Wilson Boulevard
Suite 1825
Arlington, VA 22209-3924
703-907-7322
800-368-5777
Fax: 703-907-1091
http://www.appi.org
appi@psych.org

John McDuffie, Associate Publisher
Grad L Flick Ph.D, Author
Rebecca D. Rinehart, Publisher
For teachers, counselors and parents, this comprehensive new resource is filled with up-to-date information and practical strategies to help kids with attention deficits learn to control and change their own behaviors and build the academic, social, and personal skills necessary for success in school and in life. The Kit first explains ADD/ADHD behavior, its biological bases and basic characteristics and describes procedures used for diagnosis and various treatment options. *$29.95*
Paperback
ISBN 0-876281-44-4

387 **ADHD - What Can We Do?**
Guilford Publications
72 Spring St
New York, NY 10012-4019
212-431-9800
800-365-7006
Fax: 212-966-6708
http://www.guilford.com
info@guilford.com

Seymour Weingarten, Editor-in-Chief
Russell A. Barkley PhD, Author
Bob Matloff, President
This program introduces viewers to a variety of the most effective techniques for managing ADHD in the classroom, at home, and on family outings. Illustrated are ways that parents, teachers, and other professionals can work together to implement specific strategies that help children with the disorder improve their school performance and behavior. Informative interviews, demonstrations of techniques, and commentary from Dr. Barkley illuminate the significant difference that treatment can make. *$99.00*
Manual-DVD/VHS
ISBN 1-593854-25-0

388 **ADHD - What Do We Know?**
Guilford Publications
72 Spring St
New York, NY 10012-4019
212-431-9800
800-365-7006
Fax: 212-966-6708
http://www.guilford.com
info@guilford.com

Seymour Weingarten, Editor-in-Chief
Bob Matloff, President
Russell A. Barkley PhD, Author
Covering all the basic issues surrounding ADHD, this program is highly instructive. Through commentary from Dr. Barkley and interviews with parents, teachers, and children, viewers gain an understanding of: the causes and prevalence of ADHD; effects on children's learning and behavior; other conditions that may accompany ADHD, and, long-term prospects for children with the disorder. *$99.00*
Manual-DVD/VHS
ISBN 1-593854-17-X

389 **ADHD Challenge Newsletter**
PO Box 2277
Peabody, MA 01960-7277
800-233-2322
Fax: 978-535-3276
http://www.dyslexiacenter.org/ar/000039.shtml
info@dyslexiacenter.org

Joan T Esposito, Founder and Program Director
Leslie V. Esposito, C.F.R.E, Development Director
Valerie Allen, Center Coordinator
National newsletter on ADD/ADHD that presents interviews with nationally-known scientists, as well as physicians, psychologists, social workers, educators, and other practitioners in the field of ADHD. *$35.00*
Bimonthly

390 **ADHD Report**
Guilford Publications
72 Spring St
New York, NY 10012-4019
212-431-9800
800-365-7006
Fax: 212-966-6708
http://www.guilford.com
info@guilford.com

Seymour Weingarten, Editor-in-Chief
Russell A. Barkley PhD, Author
Bob Matloff, President
Presents the most up-to-date information on the evaluation, diagnosis and management of ADHD in children, adolescents and adults. This important newsletter is an invaluable resource for all professionals interested in ADHD. *$79.00*
16 pages Bimonthly
ISSN 1065-8025

391 **ADHD and the Nature of Self-Control**
Guilford Publications
72 Spring St
New York, NY 10012-4019
212-431-9800
800-365-7006
Fax: 212-966-6708
http://www.guilford.com
info@guilford.com

Seymour Weingarten, Editor-in-Chief
Russell A. Barkley PhD, Author
Bob Matloff, President
This instructive program integrates information about ADHD with the experiences of adults from different walks of life who suffer from the disorder. Including interviews with these individuals, their family members, and the clinicians who treat them, the program addresses such important topics as the symptoms and behaviors that are characteristic of the disorder, how adult ADHD differs from the childhood form, the effects of ADHD on the family, and successful coping strategies. *$55.00*
Hardcover
ISBN 1-593853-89-0

392 **ADHD in Adolescents: Diagnosis and Treatment**
Guilford Publications
72 Spring St
New York, NY 10012-4019
212-431-9800
800-365-7006
Fax: 212-966-6708
http://www.guilford.com
info@guilford.com

Seymour Weingarten, Editor-in-Chief
Arthur L Robin, Author
Russell A Barkley PhD, Co-Author
This highly practical guide presents an empirically based approach to understanding, diagnosing, and treating ADHD in adolescents. Practitioners learn to conduct effective assessments and formulate goals that teenagers can comprehend, accept, and achieve. Educational, medical, and family components of treatment are described in depth, illustrated with detailed case material. Included are numerous reproducible handouts and forms. *$32.00*
Paperback
ISBN 1-572305-45-2

393 **ADHD in Adults: What the Science Says**
Guilford Publications
72 Spring St
New York, NY 10012-4019
212-431-9800
800-365-7006
Fax: 212-966-6708
http://www.guilford.com
info@guilford.com

Seymour Weigarten, Editor-in-Chief
Russell Barkley PhD, Author
Kevin R. Murphy, Author
Providing a new perspective on ADHD in adults, this book analyzes findings from two major studies directed by leading authority Russell A. Barkley. Information is presented on the significant impairments produced by the disorder across major functional domains and life activities, including educational outcomes, work, relationships, health behaviors, and mental health. Accessible tables, figures, and sidebars encapsulate the study results and offer detailed descriptions of the methods. *$50.00*
Hardcover
ISBN 1-593855-86-9

394 **ADHD in the Schools: Assessment and Intervention Strategies**
Guilford Publications
72 Spring St
New York, NY 10012-4019
212-431-9800
800-365-7006
Fax: 212-966-6708
http://www.guilford.com
info@guilford.com

Seymour Weigarten, Editor-in-Chief
George J DupPaul, Author
Gary Stoner, Author
This popular reference and text provides essential guidance for school-based professionals meeting the challenges of ADHD at any grade level. Comprehensive and practical, the book includes several reproducible assessment tools and handouts. A team-based approach to intervention is emphasized in chapters offering research-based guidelines for identifying and assessing children with ADHD and those at risk. *$29.00*
Paperback
ISBN 1-593850-89-1

395 **ADHD/Hyperactivity: A Consumer's Guide For Parents and Teachers**
P.O.Box 746
DeWitt, NY 13214-0746
315-446-4849
800-550-2343
Fax: 315-446-2012
http://www.gsi-add.com
info@gsi-add.com

The publication is designed to assist parents and teachers in understanding ADHD/Hyperactivity, providing guidance in the selection of educational programs, effective evaluations, and offers suggestions for choosing medications. Dr. Gordon discusses 30 easy-to-understand principles that will help parents, teachers, and clinicians avoid the many pitfalls along the path to effective diagnosis and treatment. *$14.95*

396 **ADHD: Attention Deficit Hyperactivity Disorder in Children, Adolescents, and Adults**
Oxford University Press
198 Madison Ave
New York, NY 10016-4308
212-726-6000
800-445-9714
Fax: 919-677-1303
http://www.oup.com/us
custserv.us@oup.com

Paul H. Wender, Author
ADHD provides parents and adults whose lives have been touched by this disorder an indispensable source of help, hope, and understanding. Explains the vital importance of drug therapy in treating ADHD; provides practical and extensive instructions for parents of ADHD sufferers; includes personal accounts of ADHD children, adolescents, and adults; and, offers valuable advice on where to find help. *$13.95*
ISBN 0-195113-49-7

397 **Assessing ADHD in the Schools**
Guilford Publications
72 Spring St
New York, NY 10012-4019
212-431-9800
800-365-7006
Fax: 212-966-6708
http://www.guilford.com
info@guilford.com

Seymour Weingarten, Editor-in-Chief
George J DuPaul, Author
Gary Stoner, Author
This dynamic program demonstrates an innovative model for assessing ADHD in the schools. In a departure from other approaches, DuPaul and Stoner depict assessment as a collaborative, problem-solving process that is inextricably linked to the planning of individualized interventions. A range of crucial assessment techniques are considered, including parent interviews, behavior and academic performance rating scales, and direct observation. *$99.00*
Manual-DVD/VHS
ISBN 1-572304-14-6

398 **Attention Deficit Disorder Warehouse**
300 Northwest 70th Avenue
Suite 102
Plantation, FL 33317-2360
954-792-8100
800-233-9273
Fax: 954-792-8545
http://www.addwarehouse.com
websales@addwarehouse.com

Roberta Parker, Co-Founder/Owner/Manager
Harvey Parker PhD, Co-Founder/Owner/Manager
A comprehensive resource for the understanding and treatment of all developmental disorders, including ADHD and related problems, the ADD Warehouse provides a vast collection of ADHD-related books, videos, training programs, games, professional texts and assessment products.

399 **Attention Deficit Disorder in Adults Workbook**
Taylor Publishing
7214 Circle S Road
Austin, TX 78745
512-444-0571
800-225-3687
Fax: 512-440-2160
http://www.taylorpublishing.com
Yearbooks@balfour.com

Lynn Weiss, Author

Dr. Lynn Weiss's best-selling Attention Deficit Disorder In Adults has sold over 125,000 copies since its publication in 1991. This updated volume still contains all the original information — how to tell if you have ADD, ways to master distraction, ADD's impact on the family, and more—plus the newest treatments available. *$17.99*
192 pages Paperback
ISBN 0-878338-50-0

400 **Attention Deficit Disorder: A Concise Source of Information for Parents**
Temeron Books
6531-111 Street
Edmonton, AB T6H 4R5
780-989-0910
855-283-0900
Fax: 780-989-0930
http://www.brusheducation.ca
contact@brusheducation.ca
Hossein Moghadam MD, Author
Lauri Seidlitz, Managing Editor
Fraser Seely, Partner
The authors travel from a brief historical review of ADD, through a description of symptoms and consequences, to a discussion of treatment. *$12.95*
128 pages Paperback
ISBN 1-550590-82-0

401 **Attention Deficit Hyperactivity Disorder: Handbook for Diagnosis & Treatment**
Guilford Publications
72 Spring St
New York, NY 10012-4019
212-431-9800
800-365-7006
Fax: 212-966-6708
http://www.guilford.com
info@guilford.com
Bob Matloff, President
Russell Barkley PhD, Author
Seymour Weingarten, Editor-in-Chief
This second edition helps clinicians diagnose and treat Attention Deficit Hyperactivity Disorder. Written by an internationally recognized authority in the field, it covers the history of ADHD, its primary symptoms, associated conditions, developmental course and outcome, and family context. A workbook companion manual is also available.
700 pages Hardcover

402 **Attention Deficit/Hyperactivity Disorder Fact Sheet**
National Dissemination Center for Children
1825 Connecticut Ave NW
Suite 700
Washington, DC 20009
202-884-8200
800-695-0285
Fax: 202-884-8441
http://www.nichcy.org
emulligan@fhi360.org
Stephen F Moseley, President
An 8 page informational fact sheet, a publication of the National Dissemination Center for Children with Disabilities, that provides information on attention deficit/hyperactivity disorder in infants, toddlers, children, and youth. The brochure provides suggestions and tips for parents and teachers in addition to providing links to organizations where individuals can obtain further details on ADHD.

403 **Attention-Deficit Disorders and Comorbidities in Children, Adolescents, and Adults**
American Psychiatric Publishing, Inc (APPI)
1000 Wilson Boulevard
Suite 1825
Arlington, VA 22209-3924
703-907-7322
800-368-5777
Fax: 703-907-1091
http://www.appi.org
appi@psych.org
John McDuffie, Associate Publisher
Thomas E. Brown, Editor
Rebecca D. Rinehart, Publisher
Book provides in-depth discussion of both ADD/Attention Deficit Disorders and that of ADHD/Attention Deficit-Hyperactivity Disorders, providing readers with information that focuses on several perspectives including learning disorders in children and adolescents; cognitive therapy for adults with ADHD; educational interventions for students with ADDs; tailoring treatments for individuals with ADHD; clinical and research perspectives, etc. *$82.00*
Hardcover
ISBN 0-880487-11-9

404 **Attention-Deficit Hyperactivity Disorder: A Clinical Workbook**
Guilford Publications
72 Spring St
New York, NY 10012-4019
212-431-9800
800-365-7006
Fax: 212-966-6708
http://www.guilford.com
info@guilford.com
Seymour Weingarten, Editor-in-Chief
Russell A Barkley PhD, Author
Kevin R. Murphy, Co-Author
The revised and expanded third edition of this user-friendly workbook provides a master set of the assessment and treatment forms, questionnaires, and handouts recommended by Barkley in the third edition of the Handbook. Formatted for easy photocopying, many of these materials are available from no other source. Includes interview forms and rating scales for use with parents, teachers, and adult clients; checklists and fact sheets; daily school report cards for monitoring academic progress. *$34.00*
Paperback
ISBN 1-593852-27-4

405 **Attention-Deficit/Hyperactivity Disorder: A Clinical Guide To Diagnosis and Treatment**
American Psychiatric Publishing, Inc (APPI)
1000 Wilson Boulevard
Suite 1825
Arlington, VA 22209
703-907-7322
800-368-5777
Fax: 703-907-1091
http://www.appi.org
appi@psych.org
Robert E Hales, M.D., M.B.A., Editor-in-Chief
Larry B Silver, Author
Rebecca D. Rinehart, Publisher
This new edition of Dr. Larry Silver's groundbreaking clinical book incorporates recent research findings on attention-deficit/hyperactivity disorder (ADHD), covering the latest information on diagnosis, associated disorders, and treatment, as well as ADHD in adults. The publication thoroughly reviews disorders often found to be comorbid with ADHD, including specific learning disorders, anxiety disorders, depression, anger regulation problems, obsessive-compulsive disorder, and tic disorders. *$52.00*
Paperback
ISBN 1-585621-31-6

406 **CHADD Educators Manual**
CHADD
4601 Presidents Drive
Suite 300
Lanham, MD 20706
301-306-7070
800-233-4050
Fax: 301-306-7090
http://www.chadd.org
help@chadd.org
Michael F. MacKay, JD, CPA, MSIA, President
Christine Hoch, Director of Development
Susan Buningh, MRE, Executive Editor
An in-depth look at Attention Deficit Disorders from an educational perspective. *$10.00*

407 **Children with ADD: A Shared Responsibility**
Council for Exceptional Children
2900 Crystal Drive
Suite 1000
Arlington, VA 22202-3557
703-620-3660
888-232-7733
Fax: 703-264-9494
TDD: 866-915-5000
TTY: 703-264-9446
http://www.cec.sped.org
service@cec.sped.org

George J DuPaul, Author
Gary Stoner, Co-Author
Robin D. Brewer, President
This book represents a consensus of what professionals and parents believe ADD is all about and how children with ADD may best be served. Reviews the evaluation process under IDEA and 504 and presents effective classroom strategies.
35 pages
ISBN 0-865862-33-8

408 **Classroom Interventions for ADHD**
Guilford Publications
72 Spring St
New York, NY 10012-4019
212-431-9800
800-365-7006
Fax: 212-966-6708
http://www.guilford.com
info@guilford.com

Seymour Weingarten, Editor-in-Chief
George J DupPaul, Author
Gary Stoner, Co-Author
This informative video provides an overview of intervention approaches that can be used to help students with ADHD enhance their school performance while keeping the classroom functioning smoothly. The video features an illuminating discussion among DuPaul, Stoner, and Russell A. Barkley, addressing provocative questions on the benefits of proactive, preventive measures, on the one hand, and reactive techniques, on the other. *$99.00*
Manual-DVD/VHS
ISBN 1-572304-15-4

409 **Coping: Attention Deficit Disorder: A Guide for Parents and Teachers**
Temeron Books
6531-111 Street
Edmonton, AB T6H 4R5
780-989-0910
855-283-0900
Fax: 780-989-0930
http://www.brusheducation.ca
contact@brusheducation.ca

Mary Ellen Beugin, Author
Lauri Seidlitz, Managing Editor
Fraser Seely, Partner
The author investigates medical and behavioral interventions that can be tried with ADD children and gives suggestions on coping with these children at home and at school.
$15.95
173 pages Paperback
ISBN 1-550590-13-8

410 **Driven to Distraction: Attention Deficit Disorder from Childhood Through Adulthood**
Hallowell Center
144 North Rd
Suite 2450
Sudbury, MA 01776-1142
978-287-0810
Fax: 978-287-5566
http://www.drhallowell.com
HallowellReferralsNYC@gmail.com

Edward M Hallowell, Author
John J. Ratey MD, Co-Author
Through vivid stories of the experience of their patients, Drs. Hallowell and Ratey show the varied forms ADD takes — from the hyperactive search for high stimulation to the floating inattention of daydreaming — and the transforming impact of precise diagnosis and treatment. *$10.40*
336 pages
ISBN 0-684801-28-0

411 **E-ssential Guide: A Parent's Guide to AD/HD Basics**
Schwab Learning
160 Spear Street
Suite 1020
San Francisco, CA 94105
650-655-2410
Fax: 650-655-2411
http://www.schwablearning.org

Bill Jackson, Founder, President, and CEO
Matthew Nelson, Chief Operating Officer
Gretchen Anderson, Vice President, Product
This guide covers the fundamental facts about Attention-Deficit/Hyperactivity Disorder (AD/HD) that will provide a better understanding of AD/HD. Included is: A general overview of AD/HD and helpful strategies for managing your child's AD/HD at home and at school.

412 **Fact Sheet-Attention Deficit Hyperactivity Disorder**
Attention Deficit Disorder Association
PO Box 7557
Wilmington, DE 19803-9997
856-439-9099
800-939-1019
Fax: 800-939-1019
http://www.add.org
info@add.org

Evelyn Polk Green, MS.Ed, President
Linda Roggli, PCC, Vice President
Duane Gordon, Communications Committee Chair
A pamphlet offering factual information on ADHD. *$10.00*

413 **Family Therapy for ADHD - Treating Children, Adolescents, and Adults**
Guilford Publications
72 Spring St
New York, NY 10012-4019
212-431-9800
800-365-7006
Fax: 212-966-6708
http://www.guilford.com
info@guilford.com

Seymour Weingarten, Editor-in-Chief
Craig A. Everett, Author
Sandra Volgy Everett, Co-Author
Presents an innovative approach to assessing and treating ADHD in the family context. Readers learn strategies for diagnosing the disorder and evaluating its impact not only on affected young persons but also on their parents and siblings. From expert family therapists, the volume outlines how professionals can help families mobilize their resources to manage ADHD symptoms; improve functioning in school and work settings; and develop more effective coping strategies.
$ 29.00
Paperback
ISBN 1-572307-08-0

414 **Focus Magazine**
Attention Deficit Disorder Association
PO Box 7557
Wilmington, DE 19803-9997
856-439-9099
800-939-1019
Fax: 800-939-1019
http://www.add.org
info@add.org

Evelyn Polk Green, MS.Ed, President
Linda Roggli, PCC, Vice President
Duane Gordon, Communications Committee Chair
Comprehensive magazine of the National Attention Deficit Disorder Association. It focuses on the needs of adults and young adults with ADD/ADHD, their children and families, teachers and friends. Free with membership.
Quarterly

415 **Getting a Grip on ADD: A Kid's Guide to Understanding & Coping with ADD**
Educational Media Corporation
1443 Old York Road
Warminster, PA 18974
763-781-0088
800-448-2197
Fax: 215-956-9041
http://www.educationalmedia.com
help@marcoproducts.com
Kim T. Frank, Author
Susan Smith, Co-Author
Help your elementary and middle school students cope more effectively with Attention Deficit Disorders. *$9.95*
64 pages Paperback
ISBN 0-932796-60-5

416 **How to Reach & Teach Teenagers With ADHD**
John Wiley & Sons Inc
111 River Street
Hoboken, NJ 07030-5774
201-748-6000
800-225-5945
Fax: 201-748-6088
http://http://as.wiley.com
info@wiley.com
Grad L Flick PhD, Author
Stephen M. Smith, President/CEO
Ellis E. Cousens, EVP, COO
This comprehensive resource is pack with tested, up-to-date information and techniques to help teachers, counselors and parents understand and manage adolescents with attention deficit disorder, including step-by-step procedures for behavioral intervention at school and home and reproducible handouts, checklists and record-keeping forms. *$29.00*
ISBN 0-130320-21-6

417 **Hyperactive Child Book**
St. Martin's Press
175 5th Ave
New York, NY 10010-7703
646-307-5151
888-330-8477
Fax: 212-677-7456
http://us.macmillan.com
permissions@stmartins.com
Patricia Kennedy, Author
Lief G Terdal, Co-Author
The Hyperactive Child Book contains a comprehensive review of information about raising, treating, and educating a child with Attention Deficit-Hyperactivity Disorder. The book will be useful to parents, teachers, and health care professionals in their efforts to provide for the ADHD child. *$12.95*
288 pages
ISBN 0-312112-86-6

418 **Hyperactive Child, Adolescent and Adult**
Oxford University Press
198 Madison Ave
New York, NY 10016-4308
212-726-6000
800-445-9714
Fax: 919-677-1303
http://www.oup.com/us
custserv.us@oup.com
Paul H Wender, Author
How does one know if a youngster is hyperactive? How do you know if you are hyperactive yourself? The answers may lie in this easy-to-read and comprehensive volume written by one of the leading researchers in the field. *$27.00*
172 pages Hardcover
ISBN 0-195042-91-3

419 **Hyperactive Children Grown Up: ADHD in Children, Adolescents, and Adults**
Guilford Publications
72 Spring St
New York, NY 10012-4019
212-431-9800
800-365-7006
Fax: 212-966-6708
http://www.guilford.com
info@guilford.com
Seymour Weingarten, Editor-in-Chief
Gabrielle Weiss, Author
Lily Trokenberg Hechtman, Co-Author
Based on the McGill prospective studies, research that now spans more than 30 years, the volume reports findings on the etiology, treatment, and outcome of attention deficits and hyperactivity at all stages of development. This second edition includes entirely new chapters that describes new developments in Attention Deficit Hyperactivity Disorder (ADHD) in addition to the assessment, diagnosis, and treatment of ADHD adults. *$35.00*
Paperback
ISBN 0-898625-96-3

420 **I Would if I Could: A Teenager's Guide To ADHD/Hyperactivity**
PO Box 746
DeWitt, NY 13214
315-446-4849
800-550-2343
Fax: 315-446-2012
http://www.gsi-add.com
info@gsi-add.com
Michael Gordon Ph.D, Author
Janet H. Junco, Illustration
Arthur L. Robin, PhD., Co-Author
Provides youngsters with straightforward information about the disorder in addition to exploring its impact on family relationships, self-esteem, and friendships. Dr. Gordon uses humor and candor to educate and encourage teenagers who too often find themselves confused and frustrated, providing youngsters with straightforward information about the disorder and exploring its impact on family relationships, self-esteem, and friendships. *$12.50*

421 **I'd Rather Be With a Real Mom Who Loves Me: A Story for Foster Children**
PO Box 746
DeWitt, NY 13214
315-446-4849
800-550-2343
Fax: 315-446-2012
http://www.gsi-add.com
info@gsi-add.com
Michael Gordon Ph.D, Author
Janet H. Junco, Illustration
This book tells the story of a young boy who's lived most of his life away from his birth parents. It's an honest, realistic account of the frustrations and heartache he endures. This fully illustrated book sensitively but forthrightly deals with the entire range of concerns that confront foster children with ADHD/Hyperactivity disorder. *$12.00*

422 **Identifying and Treating Attention Deficit Hyperactivity Disorder: A Resource for School and Home**
U S Department of Education/Special Ed-Rehab Srvcs
PO Box 1398
Jessup, MD 20794-1398
877-433-7827
Fax: 301-470-1244
TDD: 877-576-7734
http://www.ed.gov/rschstat/research/pubs/adhd
edpubs@inet.ed.gov
Alexa Posny, Editor
Danny Harris, Chief Information Officer
Arne Duncan, Secretary of Education
Publication from the U S Department of Education that provides comprehensive information on attention deficit hyperactivity disorders, including causes, medical evaluation and treatment options in addition to helpful hints and tips for both the home and school environments. *$6.00*

423 **International Reading Association Newspaper: Reading Today**
International Reading Association
PO Box 8139
800 Barksdale Rd.
Newark, DE 19714-8139
302-731-1600
800-336-7323
Fax: 302-731-1057
http://www.reading.org
customerservice@reading.org

Alan Farstrup, Editor
Jill Lewis-Spector, President
Diane Barone, Vice-President
Reading Today, the Association's bimonthly newspaper, is the first choice of IRA members for news and information on all these topics and more. It is available in print exclusively as an IRA membership benefit.
Bimonthly

424 **Jumpin' Johnny**
Gordon Systems, Inc.
PO Box 746
DeWitt, NY 13214 315-446-4849
800-550-2343
Fax: 315-446-2012
http://www.gsi-add.com
info@gsi-add.com
Michael Gordon Ph.D, Author
Janet H. Junco, Illustration and Design
Harvey C. Parker, PhD., Co-Author
This entertaining and informative book will help children understand the basic ideas about the evaluation of ADHD/Hyperactivity. Jumpin' Johnny tells what it is like to be inattentive and impulsive, and how his family and school work with him to make life easier. Children find this book amusing, educational, and accurate in its depiction of the challenges that confront them daily. *$11.00*

425 **LD Child and the ADHD Child**
1406 Plaza Dr
Winston Salem, NC 27103-1470 336-768-1374
800-222-9796
Fax: 336-768-9194
http://www.blairpub.com
sakowski@blairpub.com
Steve Kirk, Editor
Suzanne H Stevens, Author
Carolyn Sakowski, President
It is a brief, upbeat, always realistic look at what learning disabilities are and what problems LD children and parents face at home and at school. It contains a wealth of valuable suggestions, and its tempered optimism may dimish one's sense of futility and helplessness. *$12.95*
261 pages Paperback
ISBN 0-895871-42-4

426 **Learning Times**
Learning Disabilities Association of Georgia
2566 Shallowford Road
Suite 104 PMB 353
Atlanta, GA 30345-1200 404-303-7774
Fax: 404-467-0190
http://www.ldag.org
ldaga@bellsouth.net
Tia Powell, Editor
Information and helpful articles on learning disabilities. *$40.00*
Bimonthly

427 **Making the System Work for Your Child with ADHD**
Guilford Publications
72 Spring St
New York, NY 10012-4019 212-431-9800
800-365-7006
Fax: 212-966-6708
http://www.guilford.com
info@guilford.com
Seymour Weingarten, Editor-in-Chief
Perter S Jensen, Co-Author
Bob Matloff, President
Child psychiatrist Dr. Peter Jensen guides parents over the rough patches and around the hairpin curves in this empowering, highly informative book. Readers learn the whats, whys, and how-tos of making the system work and in getting their money's worth from the healthcare system, cutting through red tape at school, and making the most of fleeting time with doctors and therapists. *$17.95*
Paperback
ISBN 1-572308-70-2

428 **Managing Attention Deficit Hyperactivity Disorder: A Guide for Practitioners**
John Wiley & Sons Inc
111 River Street
Hoboken, NJ 07030-5774 201-748-6000
800-225-5945
Fax: 201-748-6088
http://http://as.wiley.com
info@wiley.com
Sam Goldstein, Author
Michael Goldstein, Co-Author
Stephen M. Smith, President/CEO
A valuable working resource for practitioners who manage children with ADHD, Managing Attention Deficit Hyperactivity in Children, Second Edition features: in-depth reviews of the latest research into the etiology and development of ADHD; Step-by-step guidelines on evaluating ADHD-medically, at home, and in school; a multidisciplinary approach to treating ADHD that combines medical, family, cognitive, behavioral, and school interventions; and critical discussions of controversial new treatments. *$130.00*
Hardcover
ISBN 0-471121-58-9

429 **Mastering Your Adult ADHD A Cognitive-Behavioral Treatment Program**
Oxford University Press
198 Madison Ave
New York, NY 10016-4308 212-726-6000
800-445-9714
Fax: 919-677-1303
http://www.oup.com/us
custserv.us@oup.com
Steven A Safren, Author
Used in conjunction with the corresponding client workbook, this therapist guide offers effective treatment strategies that follow an empirically-supported treatment approach. It provides clinicians with effective means of teaching clients skills that have been scientifically tested and shown to help adults cope with ADHD. *$35.00*
ISBN 0-195188-18-7

430 **Maybe You Know My Kid: A Parent's Guide to Identifying ADHD**
119 West 40th Street
New York, NY 10018 212-407-1500
800-221-2647
Fax: 212-935-0699
http://www.kensingtonbooks.com/
SZacharius@kensingtonbooks.com
Mary Cahill Fowler, Author
Steven Zacharius, Chairman, President & CEO
A guide for parents of children diagnosed with ADD discusses the recent changes in the education of these children and offers practical guidelines for improving educational performance.

431 **Meeting the ADD Challenge: A Practical Guide for Teachers**
Research Press
P.O. Box 7886
Champaign, IL 61826-9177 217-352-3273
800-519-2707
Fax: 217-352-1221
http://www.researchpress.com
orders@researchpress.com
Steve B Gordon, Author
Michael J Asher, Co-Author
Provides educators with practical information about the needs and treatment of children and adolescents with ADD. The book addresses the defining characteristics of ADD, common treatment approaches, myths about ADD, matching intervention to student, use of behavior-rating scales and checklists evaluating interventions, regular verses, special class placement, helps students regulate their own behavior and more. Case examples are used throughout. *$17.95*
196 pages
ISBN 0-878223-45-2

432 **My Brother is a World Class Pain A Sibling's Guide To ADHD/Hyperactivity**
Gordon Systems, Inc.
P.O.Box 746
DeWitt, NY 13214-0746
315-446-4849
800-550-ADHD
Fax: 315-446-2012
http://www.gsi-add.com
info@gsi-add.com
Michael Gordon Ph.D, Author
A book for the often forgotten group of those affected by ADHD, the brothers and sisters of ADHD children, this story about an older sister's efforts to deal with her active and impulsive brother sends the clear message to siblings of the ADHD child that they can play an important role in a family's quest for change. *$11.00*

433 **NIMH-Attention Deficit-Hyperactivity Disorder Information Fact Sheet**
National Institute of Mental Health
6001 Executive Blvd.
Room 6200, MSC 9663
Bethesda, MD 20892-9663
301-443-4536
866-615-6464
Fax: 301-443-4279
TTY: 301-443-8431
http://www.nimh.nih.gov
nimhinfo@nih.gov
Thomas Insel MD, Director
Marlene Guzman, Senior Advisor to the Director
William Potter, Senior Advisor to the Director
NINDS (National Institute of Neurological Disorders and Stroke) is part of the National Institutes of Health several components of which support research on developmental disorders such as ADHD. Informational fact sheet provides data relative to research, symptons and diagnosis, in addition to links for organizational resources relative to the disorder.

434 **National Alliance on Mental Illness (NAMI) Attention-Deficit/Hyperactivity Disorder Fact Sheet**
3803 N. Fairfax Drive
Suite 100
Arlington, VA 22203
703-524-7600
888-999-6264
Fax: 703-524-9094
TDD: 703-516-7227
http://www.nami.org
info@nami.org
Jim Payne, J.D., Interim President, First VP
Linda E. Jensen, Second Vice President
Mary Giliberti, J.D., Executive Director
NAMI/National Alliance on Mental Illness is a mental health organization dedicated to improving the lives of persons living with serious mental illness and their families. ADHD fact sheet provides information on attention-deficit/hyperactivity disorder through NAMI's mission of support, education, advocacy, and research for people living with mental illness.

435 **Natural Therapies for Attention Deficit Hyperactivity Disorder**
Comprehensive Psychiatric Resources, Inc.
203 Crescent Street
Suite 110
Waltham, MA 02453-2741
781-647-0066
Fax: 781-899-4905
http://www.integrativepsychmd.com
office@integrativepsychmd.com
James M Greenblatt MD, Director
A full day workshop professionally recorded on six audiotapes featuring Dr. James M. Greenblatt, M.D., neuropsychiatrist. Dr. Greenblatt explores updated research on nutrition and ADD, food additives, food allergies, fatty acids and more, provides practical treatment strategies and helps you make informed choices between effective and worthless therapies. *$59.95*

436 **Nutritional Treatment for Attention Deficit Hyperactivity Disorder**
Comprehensive Psychiatric Resources, Inc.
203 Crescent Street
Suite 110
Waltham, MA 02453
781-647-0066
Fax: 781-899-4905
http://www.integrativepsychmd.com
office@integrativepsychmd.com
James M Greenblatt MD, Director
A full day workshop professionally recorded on six audiotapes featuring Dr. James M. Greenblatt, M.D., neuropsychiatrist. Dr. Greenblatt explores updated research on nutrition and ADD, food additives, food allergies, fatty acids and more, provides practical treatment strategies and helps you make informed choices between effective and worthless therapies.

437 **Power Parenting for Children with ADD/ADHD A Parent's Guide for Managing Difficult Behaviors**
111 River Street
Hoboken, NJ 07030-5774
201-748-6000
Fax: 201-748-6088
http://www.wiley.com
info@wiley.com
Grad L Flick, Author
A Practical Parent's Guide for Managing Difficult Behaviors. Written in clear, non-technical language, this much-needed guide provides practical, real-life techniques and activities to help parents. *$19.95*
ISBN 0-876288-77-1

438 **Putting on the Brakes: Young People's Guide to Understanding ADHD**
American Psychological Association
750 First Street Northeast
Washington, DC 20002-4242
202-336-5500
800-374-2721
TDD: 202-336-6123
TTY: 202-336-6123
http://www.maginationpress.com/4414576.html
executiveoffice@apa.org
Patricia O Quinn, Author
Judith Stern, Co-Author
This book allows children to put their understanding of ADHD into action. Using pictures, puzzles, and other techniques to assist in the learning of a range of skills, this book helps teach problem solving, organizing, setting priorities, planning, maintaining control — all of those hard-to-learn skills that make everyday life just a little more manageable.
$14.95
ISBN 0-945354-57-6

439 **Rethinking Attention Deficit Disorders**
Brookline Books
8 Trumbull Rd
Suite B-001
Northampton, MA 01060
413-584-0184
800-666-2665
Fax: 413-584-6184
http://www.brooklinebooks.com
brbooks@yahoo.com
Susan Sharp, Author
Jonathan Stolzenberg, Author
This ground-breaking work argues that the two behavioral manifestations of attention deficit disorder—hyperactivity and impulsivity—represent a person's attempts at self-regulation. The authors view Attention Deficit Disorder as a problem with control and fluency of attention; people with ADD have sustaining focus when faced with novel and/or intense stimulae. *$27.95*
272 pages
ISBN 1-571290-37-0

440 **Ritalin Is Not The Answer: A Drug-Free Practical Program for Children Diagnosed With ADD or ADHD**
John Wiley & Sons Inc
111 River Street
Hoboken, NJ 07030-5774 201-748-6000
Fax: 201-748-6088
http://www.wiley.com
info@wiley.com
David P Stein, Author
Ritalin Is Not the Answer confronts and challenges what has become common practice and teaches parents and educators a healthy, comprehensive behavioral program that really works as an alternative to the epidemic use of medication-without teaching children to use drugs in order to handle their behavioral and emotional problems. *$15.00*
Paperback
ISBN 0-787945-14-5

441 **Shelley, the Hyperactive Turtle**
Woodbine House
6510 Bells Mill Rd
Bethesda, MD 20817-1636 301-897-3570
800-843-7323
Fax: 301-897-5838
http://www.woodbinehouse.com
info@woodbinehouse.com
Deborah M Moss, Author
Shelley the turtle has a very hard time sitting still, even for short periods of time. During a visit to the doctor, Shelley learns that he is hyperactive, and that he can take medicine every day to control his wiggly feeling. *$ 14.95*
20 pages Hardcover
ISBN 1-890627-75-5

442 **Stimulant Drugs and ADHD Basic and Clinical Neuroscience**
Oxford University Press
198 Madison Ave
New York, NY 10016-4308 212-726-6000
800-445-9714
Fax: 919-677-1303
http://www.oup.com/us
custserv.us@oup.com
Mary Solanto, Editor
This volume is the first to integrate advances in the basic and clinical neurosciences in order to shed new light on this important question. The chapter topics span basic research into the neuroanatomy, neurophysiology and neuropsychology of catecholamines, animal models of ADHD, and clinical studies of neuroimaging, genetics, pharmacokinetics and pharmacodynamics, and the cognitive pharmacology of stimulants. *$81.50*
ISBN 0-195133-71-4

443 **The ADD/ADHD Checklist**
American Psychiatric Publishing, Inc (APPI)
1000 Wilson Boulevard
Suite 1825
Arlington, VA 22209 703-907-7322
800-368-5777
Fax: 703-907-1091
http://www.appi.org
appi@psych.org
Robert E Hales, M.D., M.B.A., Editor-in-Chief
Sandra F Rief MA, Author
Rebecca D. Rinehart, Publisher
Written by a nationally known educator with two decades of experience in working with ADD/ADHD students. This unique resource is packed with up-to-date facts, findings, and proven strategies and techniques for understanding and helping children and adolescents with attention deficit problems and hyperactivity- all in a handy list format. *$12.95*
Paperback
ISBN 0-137623-95-2

444 **The ADHD Book of Lists: A Practical Guide for Helping Children and Teens With ADD**
American Psychiatric Publishing, Inc (APPI)
1000 Wilson Boulevard
Suite 1825
Arlington, VA 22209 703-907-7322
800-368-5777
Fax: 703-907-1091
http://www.appi.org
appi@psych.org
Robert E Hales, M.D., M.B.A., Editor-in-Chief
Sandra F Rief MA, Author
Rebecca D. Rinehart, Publisher
The ADHD Book of Lists is a comprehensive, reliable source of answers, practical strategies, and tools written in a convenient list format. Created for teachers (K-12), parents, school psychologists, medical and mental health professionals, counselors, and other school personnel, this important resource contains the most current information about Attention Deficit/Hyperactivity Disorder (ADHD). *$29.95*
Paperback
ISBN 0-787965-91-4

445 **The Down & Dirty Guide to Adult ADD**
Gordon Systems, Inc.
P.O.Box 746
DeWitt, NY 13214-0746 315-446-4849
800-550-ADHD
Fax: 315-446-2012
http://www.gsi-add.com
info@gsi-add.com
Michael Gordon Ph.D, Author
A book about Adult ADD that is informative, and uncomplicated. Drs. Gordon and McClure spare no effort or humor in clearly describing concepts essential to understanding how this disorder is best identified and treated. You'll find a refreshing absence of jargon and an abundance of common sense, practical advice, and healthy skepticism. This fine brew of scientific evidence and clinical wisdom is so cleverly presented that even the most inattentive reader will breeze through its pages. *$16.95*

446 **The Hidden Disorder: A Clinician's Guide to Attention Deficit Hyperactivity Disorder in Adults**
American Psychological Association
750 First Street Northeast
Washington, DC 20002-4242 202-336-5500
800-374-2721
Fax: 202-336-5500
TTY: 202-336-6123
http://www.apa.org/publications
nkaslow@emory.edu
Robert J Resnick PhD, Author
Through accessible writing and engaging case studies, Robert J. Resnick, PhD, provides expert clinical guidance on etiology, differential diagnosis, assessment, and treatment. Adults with ADHD often require intermittent treatment at different points in their lives. This book provides various treatment interventions over the livespan. Also covered are the various co-morbid and look alike disorders that can confound diagnosis and lead to unsuccessful treatment. *$34.95*
Hardcover
ISBN 1-557987-24-2

447 **Treating Huckleberry Finn: A New Narrative Approach to Working With Kids Diagnosed ADD/ADHD**
John Wiley & Sons Inc
111 River Street
Hoboken, NJ 07030-5774 201-748-6000
Fax: 201-748-6088
http://www.wiley.com
info@wiley.com
David Nylund, Author

Ritalin Is Not the Answer confronts and challenges what has become common practice and teaches parents and educators a healthy, comprehensive behavioral program that really works as an alternative to the epidemic use of medication-without teaching children to use drugs in order to handle their behavioral and emotional problems. *$32.00*
Paperback
ISBN 0-787961-20-6

448 **Understanding and Teaching Children With Autism**
John Wiley & Sons Inc
111 River Street
Hoboken, NJ 07030-5774
201-748-6000
Fax: 201-748-6088
http://www.wiley.com
info@wiley.com
Rita Jordan, Author
Stuart Powell, Co-Author
The triad of impairment: social, language and communication and thought behavior aspects of development discussed. Difficulties in interacting, transfer of learning and bizarre behaviors are part of syndrome. Many LD are associated with autism. *$65.00*
188 pages Paperback
ISBN 0-471957-14-3

449 **Understanding and Treating Adults With Attention Deficit Hyperactivity Disorder**
American Psychiatric Publishing, Inc (APPI)
1000 Wilson Boulevard
Suite 1825
Arlington, VA 22209
703-907-7322
800-368-5777
Fax: 703-907-1091
http://www.appi.org
appi@psych.org
Robert E Hales, M.D., M.B.A., Editor-in-Chief
Brian B Doyle MD, Author
Rebecca D. Rinehart, Publisher
Understanding the evolution of the concept and treatment of ADHD in children illuminates current thinking about the disorder in adults. Dr. Doyle presents guidelines for establishing a valid diagnosis, including clinical interviews and standardized rating scales. He covers genetic and biochemical bases of the disorder. He also addresses the special challenges of forming a therapeutic alliance-working with coach caregivers; cultural, ethnic, and racial issues; and legal considerations. *$52.00*
Paperback
ISBN 1-585622-21-4

450 **What Causes ADHD?: Understanding What Goes Wrong and Why**
Guilford Press
72 Spring St
New York, NY 10012-4019
800-365-7006
Fax: 212-966-6708
http://www.guilford.com
info@guilford.com
Seymour Weingarten, Editor
Joel T Nigg, Author
This book focuses on the multiple pathways by which attention-deficit/ hyperactivity disorder (ADHD) develops. Joel T. Nigg discusses the processes taking place within the symptomatic child's brain and the reasoning for such activity, tracing intersecting causal influences of genetic, neural, and environmental factors. Specific suggestions are provided for studies that might further refine the conceptualization of the disorder, with significant potential benefits for treatment and prevention. *$44.00*
Hardcover
ISBN 1-593852-67-3

451 **Why Can't My Child Behave?**
Feingold Association of the United States
11849 Suncatcher Drive
Fishers, IN 46037
631-369-9340
800-321-3287
Fax: 631-369-2988
http://www.feingold.org/book.html
janeFAUS@aol.com
Jane Hersey, Author & Director
This book shows how foods and food additives can trigger learning and behavior problems in sensitive people. It provides practical guidance on using a simple diet to uncover the causes of ADD and ADHD. *$22.00*
473 pages Paperback
ISBN 0-965110-50-8

452 **You Mean I'm Not Lazy, Stupid or Crazy?**
Simon & Schuster, Inc.
1230 Avenue of the Americas
New York, NY 10020-1513
212-698-7000
800-622-6611
Fax: 212-698-7007
http://www.simonsays.com
Peggy Ramundo, Author
Kate Kelly, Co-Author
This book is written by ADD adults for other ADD adults. A comprehensive guide, it provides accurate information, practical how-to's, and moral support. Among other issues, readers will get information on: unique differences in ADD adults; the impact on their lives; up-to-date research findings; treatment options available for adults; and much more. *$16.00*
464 pages
ISBN 0-743264-48-7

Web Sites

453 **www.add.org**
Attention Deficit Disorder Association
The National Attention Deficit Disorder Association is an organization focused on the needs of adults and young adults with ADD/ADHD, and their children and families. We seek to serve individuals with ADD, as well as those who love, live with, teach, counsel and treat them.

454 **www.addhelpline.org**
ADD Helpline for Help with ADD
A site dedicated to providing information and support to all parents, regardless of their choice of treatment, belief or approach toward ADD/ADHD.

455 **www.additudemag.com**
Attitude Magazine
Information and inspiration for adults and children with attention deficit disorder.

456 **www.addvance.com**
ADDvance Online Newsletter
A resource for individuals with ADD and ADHD.

457 **www.addwarehouse.com**
ADD Warehouse
The world's largest collection of ADHD-related books, videos, training programs, games, professional texts and assessment products.

458 **www.adhdnews.com/ssi.htm**
Guidance in applying for Social Security disability benefits on behalf of a child who has ADHD.

459 **www.cec.sped.org**
Council for Exceptional Children
Dedicated to improving educational outcomes for individuals with exceptionalities, students with disabilities, and/or the gifted.

460 **www.chadd.org**
National Resource Center on AD/HD
CHADD works to improve the lives of people affected by AD/HD.

461 **www.childdevelopmentinfo.com**
Child Development Institute
Online information on child development, child psychology, parenting, learning, health and safety as well as childhood disorders such as attention deficit disorder, dyslexia and autism. Provides comprehensive resources and practical suggestions for parents.

462 **www.dyslexia.com**
Davis Dyslexia Association International
Links to internet resources for learning. Includes dyslexia, Autism and Asperger's Syndrome, ADD/ADHD and other learning disabilities.

463 **www.ldonline.org**
LD Online
LD OnLine seeks to help children and adults reach their full potential by providing accurate and up-to-date information and advice about learning disabilities and ADHD. The site features hundreds of helpful articles, monthly columns by noted experts, first person essays, children's writing and artwork, a comprehensive resource guide, very active forums, and a Yellow Pages referral directory of professionals, schools, and products.

464 **www.ncgiadd.org**
National Center for Gender Issues and AD/HD
Offers knowledge and understanding of girls and women with ADHD to improve their lives.

465 **www.nichcy.org**
Nat'l Dissemination Center for Children Disabiliti
Provides information on disabilties in children and youth and programs and services.

466 **www.oneaddplace.com**
One A D D Place
A virtual neighborhood of information and resources relating to ADD, ADHD and learning disorders.

467 **www.therapistfinder.net**
Locate psychologists, psychiatrists, social workers, family counselors, and more specializing in all disorders.

468 **www.webmd.com**
Web MD Health
Medical website with information which includes learning disabilities, ADD/ADHD, etc.

Alabama

469 **Camp ASCCA**
Easter Seals of Alabama
PO Box 21
5278 Camp ASCCA Dr
Jacksons Gap, AL 36861 256-825-9226
Fax: 256-269-0714
http://www.campascca.org
info@campascca.org
Matt Rickman, Camp Director
Abbey Murray, Director of Health Services
John Stephenson, Administrator
Helps children and adults with disabilities achieve equality, dignity and maximum independence. This is to be accomplished through a safe and quality program of camping, recreation and education in a year-round barrier-free environment.
1976

470 **Good Will Easter Seals Golf Coast**
2440 Gordon Smith Dr
Mobile, AL 36617 251-471-1581
http://www.gesgc.org
Frank Harkins, President & CEO
Cindy Larry, Chief Financial Officer
Jane Gardner, VP, Operations
Easter Seals camping and recreation programs serve children, adults and families of all abilities. Various programs are available with the united purpose of giving disabled individuals a fun and safe camping or recreational experience. Camperships are available.

471 **Happy Camp**
Merrimack Hall Performing Arts Center
3320 Triana Blvd SW
Huntsville, AL 35805 256-534-6455
http://www.merrimackhall.com
jsap@merrimackhall.com
Performing arts education camp for children with Autism, Down Syndrome, Cerebral Palsy and cancer.
1909Grade Range: Ages 3-12

Arizona

472 **Camp Civitan**
Civitan Foundation
5008 N Civitan Rd
PO Box 457
Williams, AZ 86046 928-635-2944
Fax: 928-635-2730
http://www.civitanfoundationaz.com
info@campcivitan.org
Dawn Trapp, Chief Executive Officer
Lizzy Adams, Camp Program Director
Rob Adams, Camp Civitan Director
Week-long camp sessions for developmentally disabled children and adults. The camp offers a variety of recreational programs that promote self-esteem, teamwork and socialization.

Arkansas

473 **A-Camp**
Camp Aldersgate
2000 Aldersgate Rd
Little Rock, AR 72205-7018 http://www.acamp4kids.com
info@a-camp4kids.com
Amanda Laboy, President
Amy Morris, Treasurer
Caitlin Vestal, Secretary
A 6 week therapeutic day camp that serves children with Autism Spectrum Disorders. Activities include canoeing, finishing, hiking, swimming, and arts and crafts. With a 1:3 counselor to camper ratio, A-Camp is dedicated to helping children thrive.

474 **Leaping Beyond**
1500 Wilson
Ward, AR 72176 501-941-5630
http://leapingbeyond.goddysites.com
A nonprofit organization offering a variety of summer sport camps and swimming programs for individuals with disabilities, ages ranging from 5 to 20+. Programs include adaptive basketball, baseball, soccer, kickball, volleyball, tennis, dance, and aquatics. Leaping Beyond is focused on improving the health and fitness of individuals with disabilities.

California

475 **Camp Krem: Camping Unlimited**
102 Brook Lane
Boulder Creek, CA 95006 831-338-3210
http://www.campingunlimited.com
campkrem@campingunlimited.org
Katie Giampa, Program Director
Christina Krem, Program Director
Layla Sharief, Administrative Director
Provides year-round, recreation programs for children and adults with disabilities, Down Syndrome, Cerebral Palsy, Autism, wide range of physical/emotional disabilities.

476 **Camp ReCreation**
9272 Madison Ave
Orangevale, CA 95662 916-988-6835
http://www.camprecreation.org
camprecreation@outlook.com
Camp ReCreation is a residential summer camp program for persons with developmental disabilities, offering participants opportunities for fun, social interaction, and spiritual growth while providing valuable respite for parents and care givers. Camp ReCreation is held at Camp Ronald McDonald at Eagle Lake, owned and operated by Ronald McDonald House Charities Northern California and is sponsored by the Catholic Diocese of Sacramento.
1983

477 **Camp Ronald McDonald at Eagle Lake**
2555 49th St
Sacramento, CA 95817 916-734-4230
Fax: 916-734-4238
http://www.campronald.org
mdamos@RMHCNC.org
Maria Damos, Camp Director
Camp Ronald McDonald at Eagle Lake is a fully accessible residential summer camp for children who are at-risk with a variety of special medical needs, economic hardship and/or emotional, developmental or physical disabilities. Traditional camping activities include arts & crafts, hikes, fishing, canoeing, sports, swimming, talent show and campfires.

478 **Easter Seals - Bay Area, San Jose**
Easter Seals - Bay Area
180 Grand Ave
Ste 225
Oakland, CA 94612 510-451-5800
http://www.eastersealsbayarea.org
customerservice@esba.org
Susan Armiger, President & CEO
Jeff Bruner, Chief Financial Officer
Sheldon Orloff, Chair
Easter Seals provides services to children and adults with autism and other disabilities needs and support to their families.

479 **Easter Seals - Superior California, Stockton**
7273 Murray Dr
Ste 1
Stockton, CA 95210
916-485-6711
Fax: 916-485-2653
http://www.easterseals.com
Gary Kasai, Chief Executive Officer
Easter Seals camping and recreation programs serve children, adults and families of all abilities. Various programs are available with the united purpose of giving disabled individuals a fun and safe camping or recreational experience. Camping and recreational services offered are: Swim programs.

480 **Easterseals Camp Harmon**
Easter Seals of Central California
16403 Hwy 9
Boulder Creek, CA 95006
831-338-3383
http://www.campharmon.org
campharmon@es-cc.org
Devin Laming, Coordinator
Camp Harmon offers camping opportunities to people with disabilities. Offers sessions designed for a specific age group and specific to developmental and/or physical disabilities.
1963

481 **Kaleidoscope After School Program**
Easter Seals - Bay Area
7425 Larkdale Ave
Dublin, CA 94568-1500
925-849-8999
http://www.easterseals.com
Susan Armiger, Chief Executive Officer
Easter Seals camping and recreation programs serve children, adults and families of all abilities. Various programs are available with the united purpose of giving disabled individuals a fun and safe camping or recreational experience.

482 **Via West**
2851 Park Ave
Santa Clara, CA 95050
408-867-1115
Fax: 408-867-4817
http://www.viaservices.org
Leslie Davis, Chief Executive Officer
Leslie Leger, Vice President, Administration
Shannon McDaniel, Vice President, Advancement
Camp Costanoan is a residential, respite and recreational camp for children and adults with physical and/or developmental disabilities. Camp Costanoan enhances camper self-esteem, improves socialization skills and provide hands-on learning and therapeutic recreation opportunities. Additionally, Camp provides respite for families of individuals with disabilities.

Colorado

483 **Adam's Camp - Colorado**
6767 S Spruce St
Ste 102
Centennial, CO 80112
303-563-8290
Fax: 303-563-8291
http://adamscampcolorado.org
contact@adamscamp.org
Kellie Newland, President
Cindy Wells, Vice President
Clay Waller, Treasurer
Designed to give children and teens with physical and developmental disabilities the opportunity to development life skills, make friends, and foster self esteem.
1986

484 **Rocky Mountain Village Camp**
Easter Seals of Colorado
393 S Harlan St
Ste 250
Lakewood, CO 80226
303-233-1666
http://www.easterseals.com
Lynn Robinson, President & CEO
Nancy Hanson, VP, Human Resources
Camping and recreational services are: Adventure, camp respite for adults, camp respite for children, camperships, conference rental, family retreats, recreational services for adults, recreational services for children, residential camping programs, swim programs and therapeutic horseback riding.

485 **The Learning Camp**
Gypsum, CO
970-524-2706
http://www.learningcamp.com
ann@learningcamp.com
Ann Cathcart, Director & CEO
Tom Macht, Director & CFO
Summer camp that focuses on helping children with learning disabilities, such as dyslexia, ADD, ADHD and other learning challenges. The Learning Camp provides adventurous summer camp fun for boys and girls ages 7 - 14 combined with carefully designed academic programs. Camp activities include swimming, horseback riding, backpacking, archery, arts and crafts, fishing, canoeing, board games, and Colorado River rafting.
1996

Connecticut

486 **Cyber Launch Pad Camp**
Ben Bronz Foundation, Inc.
11 Wampanoag Dr
West Hartford, CT 06117
860-236-5807
http://www.benbronzacademy.org
Kim Holley, Executive Director & CEO
Jason Devin, Chief Operating Officer
Christina Lamphere, Education Director
Summer program where children and their parents learn to use CyberSlate which is learning keyboarding, word processing, programming and remedial sessions in reading, writing and arithmetic for learning disabled children.

487 **Eagle Hill Summer Program**
Eagle Hill School
45 Glenville Rd
Greenwich, CT 06831-5331
203-622-9240
http://www.eaglehillschool.org
Deane Flood, Summer Academic Program Director
Brian Dayton, Summer Activities Director
Emma Lipman, Summer Academic Program Advisor
Designed for children experiencing academic difficulty. Some of the programs offered are mathematics, spelling, reading tutorials, writing workshops, oral language, handwriting, and study skills. Students attending the morning classes may also sign up for the Summer Activities Extended Program which is held in the afternoon.

488 **Easter Seals - Camp Hemlocks**
Easter Seals - Connecticut
85 Jones St
Hebron, CT 06248
860-228-0393
TTY: 860-228-2091
http://www.easterseals.com/cfc
Jillian.McCarthy@oakhillct.org
Jillian McCarthy, Camp Director
Offers an environment that allows campers with disabilities optimal independence. Camping and recreational services are: Aquatics, Family Camp, Recreational Services for Adults and Children, Residential Camping Programs, Adventure/Traveling Program.

489 **Horizons, Inc.**
127 Babcock Hill Rd
PO Box 323
South Windham, CT 06266
860-456-1032
Fax: 860-456-4721
http://www.horizonsct.org
Adam Milne, Chair
Chris Mcnaboe, President
Kathleen Mcnaboe, Vice President

The mission of Horizons is to provide high quality residential, recreational support and work programs for people who have developmental disabilties or who have other challenging social and emotional needs.
1979

490 **Our Victory Day Camp**
46 Vineyard Ln
Stamford, CT 06902 203-329-3394
http://www.ourvictory.com
ourvictory@aol.com
Fred Tunick, Executive Director
Our Victory Day Camp is a 7-week day camping program for children from 5 to 12 years of age. It is oriented toward children with learning disabilities and/or attention deficit disorder. The program is designed to expose each camper to a wide variety of activities. The goal is to create an opportunity for each camper to achieve success, whatever the camper's ability. Activities include arts and crafts, drama, music, nature, dancing, hiking, jewelry making, swimming, and sports.

491 **Summer Day Programs**
Middletown Recreation Services Division
61 Durant Terrace
Middletown, CT 06457 860-638-4500
Fax: 860-344-3319
http://www.cityofmiddletown.com
rec@middletownct.gov
Catherine Lechowicz, Director
Debbie Stanley, Manager
Karen Nocera, Inclusion Specialist
These camps offer a variety of recreational and social activities. Each camp will be integrated with at least 12% population of children with disabilities. Campers must be Middletown residents.

492 **Valley-Shore YMCA**
201 Spencer Plains Rd
Westbrook, CT 06498 860-399-9622
http://www.vsymca.org
vsymca@vsymca.org
Mike Storiale, 1st Vice President
Melissa Ozols, Secretary
Chris Pallatto, CEO/Executive Director
Family Play Dates, an adaptive recreation program designed for special language need children (Pervasive Developmental Disorder and high functioning Autism, Asperger's, Down Syndrome). Daycamp with swimming, hiking, sports, games, nature study, archery and low ropes course.

493 **Wheeler Regional Family YMCA**
149 Farmington Ave
Plainville, CT 06062 860-793-9631
Fax: 860-793-2092
http://www.ghymca.org
wheeler.membership@ghymca.org
Harold Sparrow, President & CEO
Joseph Weist, VP & Chief Financial Officer
Howard Goodrow, Cheif Development Officer
The Wheeler Regional Family YMCA is a non-profit charitable community organization. The YMCA provides a wide variety of programs for all ages. The YMCA's main programs include Child Care, Aquatic Programs, Day Camp, Teen programs, Wellness and Fitness Programs. The Wheeler Regional Family YMCA serves Plainville, Bristol, Farmington, Burlington and Plymouth.

494 **Winston Prep School Summer Program**
57 West Rocks Road
Norwalk, CT 06851 646-638-2705
http://www.winstonprep.edu
summer@winstonprep.edu
Peter Hill, Summer Program Director
For 6th through 12th grade students with learning differences such as dyslexia, nonverbal learning disabilities, expressive or receptive language disorders and attention deficit problems. The Summer Enrichment Program at their New York City branch school is designed to enhance academic skills. Students from area parochial, public and private schools attend the program every year. They receive daily one-on-one instruction in addition to attending class in the courses they have selected.

Delaware

495 **Brandywine Center for Autism**
210 Bellefonte Ave
Wilmington, DE 19809 302-762-2636
http://brandywinecenterforautism.com
bcainfo@brandywinecenterforautism.com
Marcus A. Henry, Owner & CEO
Valpresious Ham, Director, Operations
Kate Prukalski, Lead Therapist
Offers week long camp programs from 9 am to 2 pm during school breaks. Activities range from field trips, outdoor games, and arts and crafts designed to improve social skills and academia.

Florida

496 **3D Learner Program**
3D Learner, Inc.
7100 W Camino Real
Ste 215
Boca Raton, FL 33433 561-361-7495
http://www.3dlearner.com
Mira Stulberg-Halpert MEd, Educational Director
Eva Schmeichler, Operations Manager
Julie Halpert, Director
3D Learner Program, a one-week program for struggling students who learn best when they see and experience information.

497 **Camp Challenge**
Easter Seals Florida
31600 Camp Challenge Rd
Sorrento, FL 32776 352-383-4711
Fax: 352-383-0744
http://www.easterseals.com/florida
Susan Ventura, CEO
Suzanne Caporina, Primary Contact
At Easter Seals Camp Challenge, campers participate in arts & crafts, nature activities, a universal high and low ropes course, music and dancing, outside entertainers, farm animals and other camp activities.

498 **Camp Kavod**
Adolph & Rose Levis Jewish Community Center
9801 Donna Klein Blvd
Boca Raton, FL 33428-1755 561-852-3269
http://www.levisjcc.org/special-needs/camp-kavo
alil@levisjcc.org
Ali Landman, Camp Director
An 8-week summer camp program for children and teens with special needs in the Jewish community. Activities are specially designed to improve social, motor and language skills in order to achieve greater independence.

499 **Camp Thunderbird**
Quest, Inc.
500 E Colonial Dr
Orlando, FL 32803 407-218-4300
http://www.questinc.org
rcage@questinc.org
John Gill, President & CEO
Brooke Eakins, Chief Operating Officer
Todd Thrasher, Chief Financial Officer

Dedicated to providing a real summer camp experience for people with special needs. Camp Thunderbird is designed for children and adults with Down syndrome, autism, Cerebral Palsy and other developmental disabilities.
1969

500 **Easter Seals - Florida**
520 N Semoran Blvd
Ste 280
Orlando, FL 32807
407-306-9766
Fax: 407-306-9767
http://www.easterseals.com/florida
Susan Ventura, President & CEO
Gladys Epps, Chief Financial Officer
Rob Porcaro, Chief Operating Officer
Easter Seals camping and recreation programs serve children, adults and families of all abilities. Various programs are available with the united purpose of giving disabled individuals a fun and safe camping or recreational experience. Camping and recreational services are: Day camping for children.

Georgia

501 **Camp Hollywood**
FOCUS
3825 Presidential Pkwy
Ste 103
Atlanta, GA 30340
770-234-9111
Fax: 770-234-9131
http://www.focus-ga.org
inquiry@focus-ga.org
Keith Mauriello, President
Lucy Cusick, Executive Director
Joy Trotti, Associate Director
Unique camp for children with developmental delays, neurological involvement, cerebral palsy, heart problems and immune deficiencies. FOCUS also hosts Camp TEAM and Camp Infinity.

502 **United Cerebral Palsy Of Georgia**
3300 Northeast Expy NE
Bldg 9
Atlanta, GA 30341
770-676-2000
888-827-9455
Fax: 770-455-8040
http://ucpga.org
info@ucpga.org
Diane Wilush, President & CEO
Kevin Walton, Chief Program Director
Jonessa Alexander, Chief Operating Officer
UCP offers afterschool programs that help to develop cognitive, motors, language and communication skills, while fostering self-image and independence.

Hawaii

503 **Healing Horses, Kauai**
PO Box 2082
Kapaa, HI 96746
808-634-3896
http://healinghorseskauai.com
hhkauai@gmail.com
A nonprofit equine therapy services designed to improve physical, cognitive, social and/or emotional well-being. Program is offered to people of all ages.

Illinois

504 **Camp Little Giant: Touch of Nature Environmental Center**
Southern Illinois University
1206 Touch of Nature Rd
Makanda, IL 62958
618-453-1121
http://ton.siu.edu
tonec@siu.edu
JD Tanner, Director
Erik Oberg, Program Coordinator
Vicki Lang-Mendenhall, Program Coordinator
A residential camp program designed to meet the recreational needs of adults and children with disabilities. The programs are designed for individuals with physical/developmental disabilities, visual & hearing impairements, muscular dystrophy, cerebral palsy, autism, ADD/ADHD, traumatic brain injury and special needs.
1952

505 **Camp Timber Pointe**
Easter Seals Central Illinois
20 Timber Pointe Ln
Hudson, IL 61748
309-365-8021
Fax: 309-365-8934
http://www.easterseals.com/ci
Steven Thompson, President & CEO
Don Young, Chair
Wes Blumenshine, Vice Chair
Camping and respite program for children and adults with disabilities or special needs and their families. Campers can participate in recreational activities susch as fishing, boating, swimming, music, sports, horseback riding and arts and crafts.

506 **Easter Seals - Central Illinois**
507 E Armstrong Ave
Peoria, IL 61603-3197
309-686-1177
http://www.easterseals.com/ci
Steven Thompson, CEO
Don Young, Chair
Wes Blumenshine, Vice Chair
Easter Seals camping and recreation programs serve children, adults and families of all abilities. Various programs are available with the united purpose of giving disabled individuals a fun and safe camping or recreational experience. The following are Camping and Recreational services offered: Recreational services for adults and recreational services for children.

507 **Easter Seals - Joliet**
212 Barney Dr
Regional Pediatric Center and Corporate
Joliet, IL 60435-2830
815-725-2194
http://www.easterseals.com/joliet
Debbie Condotti, CEO
Edna Brass, Chair
Ralph Schultz, Vice Chair
Easter Seals camping and recreation programs serve children, adults and families of all abilities. Various programs are available with the united purpose of giving disabled individuals a fun and safe camping or recreational experience. The following are camping and recreational services offered: Camperships.

508 **Jayne Shover Center**
Easter Seals DuPage and the Fox Valley Region
799 S McLean Blvd
Elgin, IL 60123
847-742-3264
Fax: 847-742-9436
http://www.easterseals.com/dfv
Theresa Forthofer, President & CEO
Kimberly Garcia, Primary Contact
John Jostrand, Chair

Easter Seals camping and recreation programs serve children, adults and families of all abilities. Various programs are available with the united purpose of giving disabled individuals a fun and safe camping or recreational experience. The following are Camping and Recreational services offered: Recreational services for adult and recreational services for children.

Indiana

509 **Easter Seals - Arc of Northeast Indiana**
4919 Coldwater Rd
Fort Wayne, IN 46825 260-456-4534
http://www.easterseals.com/neindiana
Donna K. Elbrecht, President & CEO
Sheri Ward, Director, Development
Misty Woltman, CFO/Controller
Easter Seals camping and recreation programs serve children, adults and families of all abilities. Various programs are available with the united purpose of giving disabled individuals a fun and safe camping or recreational experience. The following are camping and recreational services offered: Recreational services for adults and camp respite for adults and children.

510 **Easter Seals - Crossroads**
4740 Kingsway Dr
Indianapolis, IN 46205 317-466-1000
Fax: 317-466-2000
http://www.eastersealscrossroads.org
Patrick Sandy, President & CEO
Susan Saunders, Chief Financial Officer
Angela Danner, Director, Human Resources
Easter Seals camping and recreation programs serve children, adults and families of all abilities. Various programs are available with the united purpose of giving disabled individuals a fun and safe camping or recreational experience. The following are camping and recreational services offered: Camperships and recreational services for children.

Iowa

511 **Camp Albrecht Acres**
14837 Sherrill Road
PO Box 50
Sherrill, IA 52073 563-552-1771
Fax: 563-552-2732
http://www.albrechtacres.org
office@albrechtacres.org
Eric Veltstra, Executive Director
Barb Kurt, President
Joe Kane, Vice President
For children with special needs. Activities include cookouts, swimming, fishing, hay wagon rides, volleyball, dances and arts and crafts.

512 **Camp Sunnyside**
Easter Seals Of Iowa
401 NE 66th Ave
Des Moines, IA 50313 515-289-1933
http://www.easterseals.com/ia
Sherri Nielsen, President & CEO
Krable Mentzer, Chief Administrative Officer
Kevin Small, Chief Financial Officer
Easter Seals camping and recreation programs serve children, adults and families of all abilities. Various programs are available with the united purpose of giving disabled individuals a fun and safe camping or recreational experience. The following are Camping and Recreational services offered: Adventure, camp respite for children, day camping for children, easter seals own and operated camps and residential camping programs.

Kentucky

513 **Easter Seals Cardinal Hill**
2050 Versailles Rd
Lexington, KY 40504 859-246-8816
http://cardinalhill.org
cindy.jacobelli@cardinalhill.org
Jenny Wurzback, Executive Director
Cindy Jacobelli, Dir., Adaptive Recreation
The Adaptive Recreation program offers adults with disabilities a full range of adaptive sports, including downhill skiing, kayaking, sled hockey, wheelchair basketball, hand cycling, golf, bowling, rock climing, fishing, wheelchair tennis, and baseball.

Louisiana

514 **Camp ABLE**
Easter Seals Of Louisiana
1010 Common Street
Ste 2440
New Orleans, LA 70112 504-523-7325
http://www.easterseals.com/louisiana
Tracy Garner, President & CEO
Joseph Oliveri, COO & CFO
Dawn Huber, Vice President
A nonprofit, community-based health agency whose mission is to help children and adults with disabilities achieve independence through a variety of programs and services. Campers enjoy boating, nature walks, swimming, arts & crafts and campfire sing-a-longs.
1951

515 **Easter Seals - Louisiana**
New Orleans Corporate Office
1010 Common St
Ste 2440
New Orleans, LA 70112 504-523-7325
http://www.easterseals.com/louisiana
Tracy Garner, President & CEO
Joseph Oliveri, COO & CFO
Dawn Huber, Vice President
Easter Seals camping and recreation programs serve children, adults and families of all abilities. Various programs are available with the united purpose of giving disabled individuals a fun and safe camping or recreational experience. The following are camping and recreational services offered: Camperships.

Maine

516 **Camp Alsing**
81 Brighton Ave
Portland, ME 04102 207-805-4155
http://campalsing.com
Emily Chaleff, Founder & Camp Director
Andy Lilienthal, Founder
Matthew Siegel, Clinical Advisor
A sleep-away camp for boys and girls with social communication disorders, Asperger's Syndrome and/or high-functioning Autism. Includes all traditional camp activities, such as canoeing, campfires, swimming, and nature trails.

517 **Camp Ketcha**
336 Black Point Rd
Scarborough, ME 04074 207-883-8977
http://campketcha.org
Thomas Doherty, Executive Director
Liz Tully, Director, Operations
Kate Connolly, Montessori Director
Camp Ketcha accepts all children for its day camp summer program. Activities include equestrian clinics, drama and musi, arts and crafts, swimming, archery, gardening, and a variety of sports.
1964

Maryland

518 **Camp Accomplish**
5606 Dower House Rd
Upper Marlboro, MD 20772
301-599-8000
Fax: 301-599-0180
http://www.melwood.org
Carol Ann Desantis, President & CEO
Myron Thomas, Chief Operating Officer
Larysa Kautz, Chief of Staff & General Counsel
A sleep-away camp for children and teens with disabilities, such as developmental, physical, and emotional. However, the camp is unable to support children with extreme behavioral issues or intense medical needs. Located on 108 acres of land and equipped with air-conditioned cabins, Activities include fishing, boating and hiking.

519 **Camp Fairlee**
Easter Seals of Delaware-Maryland
22242 Bay Shore Rd
Chestertown, MD 21620
410-778-0566
Fax: 410-778-0567
http://www.easterseals.com/de
Jeffrey Gosnear, Chair
Gary W. Spitzer, Vice Chair
Kenan J. Sklenar, President & CEO
For children with physical disabilities and/or cognitive impairements. Activities include arts & crafts, sports, games, nature walks, fishing, swimming and much more.

Massachusetts

520 **Camp Connect**
The Bridge Center
470 Pine St
Bridgewater, MA 02324
508-697-7557
http://www.thebridgectr.org
info@TheBridgeCtr.org
Jackie Ross, Executive Director
Tom Walsh, President
Stephen Abisso, 1st Vice President
Camp for children and teens with high functioning Autism and Asperger's Syndrome. The programs offers to help support social skills and thinking development and practice.

521 **Camp Discovery**
The Bridge Center
470 Pine St
Bridgewater, MA 02324
508-697-7557
http://www.thebridgectr.org
info@TheBridgeCtr.org
Jackie Ross, Executive Director
Tom Walsh, President
Stephen Abisso, 1st Vice President
For campers with intellectual and developmental disabilities who benefit from extensive or pervasive support. Campers have access to all activities and also have staff support with daily living activities.

522 **Camp Endeavor**
The Bridge Center
470 Pine St
Bridgewater, MA 02324
508-697-7557
http://www.thebridgectr.org
info@TheBridgeCtr.org
Jackie Ross, Executive Director
Tom Walsh, President
Stephen Abisso, 1st Vice President
For children and adolescents with learning, intellectual and developmental disabilities. The program offers campers the chance to meet new people, try new activities and feel successfull.

523 **Camp Joy**
Boston Centers for Youth & Families
1483 Tremont St
Boston, MA 02120-2908
617-635-4920
TTY: 617-635-5041
http://www.cityofboston.gov/bcyf
Roberta.Smalls@boston.gov
Roberta Smalls, Program Manager
A therapeutic recreational program for special needs children and adults. Serves the physically and cognitively challenged, multi-handicapped, behaviorally involved, legally blind/visually impaired, deaf/hearing impaired, learning disabled, and pre-school special needs children. The camp also welcomes their siblings between the ages 3 and 7.

524 **Camp Lapham**
119 Myrtle St
Duxbury, MA 02332
617-765-7556
Fax: 781-765-2701
http://crossroadsma.org
info@crossroadsma.org
Kevin Phelan, Chair
Simon Hess, President
Caroline Warren, Governance Co-Chair
Designed to meet the needs of children who thrive in a small, structured environment. The program emphasis includes anger and behavior management, along with strong self-image building all in a fun, noncompetitive camp atmosphere. With a maximum of 50 children enrolled per session and a low camper to counselor ratio of 1 to 4, the campers experience success in a more family-like atmosphere which enables each child to focus on personal goals and nonviolent methods of interaction.

525 **Camp Ramah**
1206 Boston Providence Hwy
Ste 201
Norwood, MA 02062
781-702-5290
Fax: 781-702-5239
http://www.campramahne.org
info@campramahne.org
Rabbi Ed Gelb, Director
Josh Edelglass, Assistant Director
Marggi Shechanah, Registrar/Office Manager
Young people have fun while developing skills, strong friendships and a Jewish conciousness that lasts a lifetime through a variety of experiences such as sports, nature, music, arts and crafts, boating, study, Shabbat and Judaica. Campers have developmental disabilities. Some campers with LD are included in typical divisions.

526 **Camp Starfish**
636 Great Rd
Ste 2
Stow, MA 01775
978-637-2617
Fax: 603-899-9590
http://www.campstarfish.org
info@campstarfish.org
Beth McCollum, Camp Director
Year-round camp for children and young adults with ADHD, Aspergers, behavioral issues and learning disabilities. The focus is on teaching the children how to interact appropriately in a soocial group, and work on individual goals, while developing self-esteem and self-confidence.

527 **Camp Sunshine**
The Bridge Center
470 Pine St
Bridgewater, MA 02324
508-697-7557
http://www.thebridgectr.org
info@TheBridgeCtr.org
Tom Walsh, President
Stephen Abisso, 1st Vice President
Jackie Ross, Executive Director
For children between ages 4-14 with or without disabilities. A 22 acre campus. Activities include fishing, hiking, soccer and baseball, and swimming.

528 **Create & Collaborate Program**
The Bridge Center
470 Pine St
Bridgewater, MA 02324 508-697-7557
http://www.thebridgectr.org
info@TheBridgeCtr.org
Jackie Ross, Executive Director
Visual and performing arts, music, drama and dance. Children learn how to express themselves with art specific skills.

529 **Horse Camp**
The Bridge Center
470 Pine St
Bridgewater, MA 02324 508-697-7557
http://www.thebridgectr.org
info@TheBridgeCtr.org
Tom Walsh, President
Stephen Abisso, 1st Vice President
Jackie Ross, Executive Director
For ages 8 and up who love to ride horses. The camp offers riding center activities and mounted riding lessons.

530 **Landmark School Summer Boarding Program**
Landmark School
429 Hale St
PO Box 227
Prides Crossing, MA 01965 978-236-3216
Fax: 978-921-7268
http://www.landmarkoutreach.org
outreach@landmarkschool.org
Meg Arnio, Director, Summer Institute
Jenna Lanoue, Operations Manager
Our Summer Program accepts boys and girls age 7-20, in grades 1-12, who possess average to superior intelligence, a history of healthy emotional development, and have been diagnosed with a language-based learning disability. Landmark's Summer Boarding Program excels at providing a safe, fun, and exciting summer experience.
1971

531 **Moose Hill Nature Day Camp**
208 S Great Rd
Lincoln, MA 01773 781-259-9500
800-283-8266
http://www.massaudubon.org
Gary Clayton, President
Bancroft Poor, Vice President, Operations
Nature Day Camp is a welcoming environment with fewer than one hundred campers in each weekly session. The goal is to educate children and enrich their lives through outdoor exploration, focused activities, games, hikes, and crafts. Most weeks include special visitors and camp-wide theme days. The camp day runs from 9 a.m. to 3 p.m. with before and after camp programs available. The camp uses the Nature Center of Moose Hill Wildlife Sanctuary as its base.

532 **Summer@Carroll**
The Carroll School
25 Baker Bridge Rd
Lincoln, MA 01773 781-314-9731
http://www.carrollschool.org
gsummers@carrollschool.org
Greely Summers, Director
Donna Brown, Assistant Director
Summer at Carroll is designed to offer academic intervention and remediation to children diagnosed with primary language learning difficulties, such as dyslexia. Small group teaching, individualized instruction and attention to the needs of goals of the students are what Carroll prides themselves on.

533 **The Bridge Center Summer Camp Program**
470 Pine St
Bridgewater, MA 02324 508-697-7557
http://www.thebridgectr.org
info@TheBridgeCtr.org
Jackie Ross, Executive Director
Tom Walsh, President
Stephen Abisso, 1st Vice President
Program offers teens and young adults the skills necessary for independent living and vocational success, as well as structured social and recreational opportunities.

534 **The Drama Play Connection, Inc.**
6 Abbott Rd
Wellesley Hills, MA 02481 781-237-3200
http://www.dramaplayconnection.com
info@dramaplayconnection.com
Liana P Morgens, PhD, President
Sean Hyde O'Brien, PsyD, Board Member
Carol Singer, EdD, Board Member
The Summer Pragmatic Language Drama Program serves primarily children and adolescents with Asperger's Disorder, Nonverbal Learning Disabilities, and those with related social pragmatic difficulties. The pragmatic program is designed to help children acquire the skills necessary to function more competently with their peers. The program includes drama curriculum that focuses on teaching nonverbal language skills through the use of improvisation and other drama techniques.

Michigan

535 **Camp Barefoot**
The Fowler Center For Outdoor Learning
2315 Harmon Lake Rd
Mayville, MI 48744 989-673-2050
Fax: 989-673-6355
http://www.thefowlercenter.org
Kyle L. Middleton, CTRS, Executive Director
Lynn M. Seeloff, CTRS, Assistant Director
Specifically designed for teens and young adults age 18 and older with traumatic brain injuries or closed head injuries. Campers can request their daily activities.

536 **Children's Therapy Programs**
Easter Seals - Michgan
2399 E Walton Blvd
Auburn Hills, MI 48326 248-475-6400
http://www.easterseals.com/michigan/
Brent Wirth, President & CEO
Juliana Harper, Chief Program Officer/SVP
Ron Hocking, Chief Financial Officer/SVP
Various programs designed for children with autism, speech and language delays, amotional, motor and social skill issues.

537 **Eagle Village Retreats**
5044 175th Ave
Hersey, MI 49639 231-832-2234
http://www.eaglevillage.org
Cathey Prudhomme, President & CEO
Marjie Wirth, VP, Operations
Chad Saxton, Director, Camps
Eagle Village offers a variety of fun camp experiences for any child, including those with emotional and/or behavioral impairments. Challenging activities make the camps rewarding experiences.

538 **Easter Seals - Genesee County Greater Flint Therapy Center**
1420 University Ave
Flint, MI 48504-6208 810-238-0475
Fax: 810-238-9270
http://mi.easterseals.com
Diane Austin, Program Manager
Children and adults with mental and physical disabilities and other special needs have access to services designed to meet their individual needs. Health professionals from a variety of disciplines work with each person to overcome obstacles to independence, and to reach his/her personal goals through person centered planning. The following are camping and recreational services offered: Recreational services for adults and children, residential camping programs, therapeutic horseback riding.

539 **Easter Seals - Michigan**
2399 E Walton Blvd
Auburn Hills, MI 48326 248-475-6400
http://www.easterseals.com/michigan/
Brent Wirth, President & CEO
Juliana Harper, Chief Program Officer/SVP
Ron Hocking, Chief Financial Officer/SVP
Offers a variety of programs to individuals with disabilities and special needs.

540 **The Fowler Center For Outdoor Learning**
2315 Harmon Lake Rd
Mayville, MI 48744-9737 989-673-2050
Fax: 989-673-6355
http://www.thefowlercenter.org
info@thefowlercenter.org
Lynn Sealoff, Director
The Fowler Center is an outdoor recreation and education facility that provides programs for children, teens and adults with disabilities. Along with day camp programs, the camp also offers autism weekend camps and respite camps.

541 **The JCC Center**
Jewish Community Center of Metropolitan Detroit
D. Dan & Betty Kahn Building
6600 West Maple
West Bloomfield, MI 48322-3022 248-661-1000
Fax: 248-661-3680
http://www.jccdet.org
dstone@jccdet.org
Brian D. Siegel, Chair
Florine Mark, President
Ilana Glazier, Vice President
Programs that support Jewish unity, ensure Jewish continuity and enrich Jewish life while conveying the importance of well-being within the Jewish and general community and the people of Israel.

542 **The Play Project**
3031 Miller Rd
Ann Arbor, MI 48103 734-585-5333
http://www.playproject.org
info@playproject.org
Kate Bernhardt, Program Director
Shana Wirth, Training Director
Kristen Suzio, Communications Coordinator
An early intervention program for children with autism and their parents. Designed to engage children, develop a strong bond between parent and child, and improve their overall social and functional skills.

Minnesota

543 **Camp Buckskin**
4124 Quebec Avenue North
Suite 300
Minneapolis, MN 55427 763-208-4805
Fax: 763-208-8668
http://www.campbuckskin.com
info@campbuckskin.com
Tom Bauer, Director
Mary Bauer, Director
Jared Griffin, Program Director
Overnight summer camp program that specializes in serving boys and girls ages 6 - 18 who are experiencing social skill and academic difficulties. While not an entrance requirement, the majority of our campers have a primary diagnosis of AD/HD, Learning Disabilities, or Aspergers while others may have a secondary or related diagnosis.

544 **Camp Confidence**
1620 Mary Fawcett Memorial Dr
East Gull Lake, MN 56401-7538 218-828-2344
Fax: 218-828-2618
http://www.campconfidence.com
info@campconfidence.com
Jeff Olson, Executive Director
Bob Slaybaugh, Program Director
Kelly Brooking, Director of Finance
A year-round center for persons with developmental disabilities specializing in recreation and outdoor education. Aimed at promoting self confidence and self esteem and the necessary skills to become full, contributing members of society.

545 **Camp Friendship**
Friendship Ventures
10509 108th St NW
Annandale, MN 55302-2912 952-852-0101
800-450-8376
Fax: 952-852-0123
http://truefriends.org
fv@friendshipventures.org
Floyd Adelman, Chairman
Jeff Bangsberg, Board Member
Jerry Caruso, Board Member
A summer resident camp that is open to anyone five or older who has developmental and/or physical disabilities.

546 **Camp New Hope**
Friendship Ventures
10509 108th Street NW
Annandale, MN 55302-4598 952-852-0101
800-450-8376
Fax: 952-852-0123
http://truefriends.org
fv@friendshipventures.org
Floyd Adelman, Chairman
Jeff Bangsberg, Board Member
Jerry Caruso, Board Member
A summer resident camp that is open to anyone five or older who has developmental and/or physical disabilities.

547 **Camp Winnebago**
19708 Camp Winnebago Rd
Caledonia, MN 55921-5738 507-724-2351
Fax: 507-724-3786
http://www.campwinnebago.org
director@campwinnebago.org
Terry Chiglo, President
Eileen Loken, Vice President
Jane Palen, Secretary
Individuals with developmental disabilities, six years of age and older, are eligable to attend Camp Winnebago. A variety of traditional summer camp activities abound: swimming, cooking over a fire, games, arts and crafts, hay-wagon rides, dancing and more. Activities are adapted to the age and ability of each camper to ensure maximum participation.

Missouri

548 **Camp Encourage**
208 West Linwood Boulevard
Kansas City, MO 64111 816-830-7171
http://www.campencourage.org
info@campencourage.org
Jenny Hines, Board President/Parent Liason
Kelly Lee, M.S.Ed., Executive Director
Marita Burrow, Ph.D., Secretary
For children and young adults with Autism Spectrum disorders. The camp offers activities such as horseback riding, archery, fishing, swimming, hayrides, horseback riding, and art activities.

549 **H.O.R.S.E.**
C/O BJ Wright
19021 Long Grove Road
Higginsville, MO 64037 660-909-5381
http://www.horsehelpspeople.org
Brenda@HORSEhelpspeople.org
Brenda Wright, Executive Director
Athena Sharp, Director
Colleen White, Director

Combines the healing power of horses to deliver alternative therapeutic services to children with autism spectrum disorders and emotionally troubled individuals. The programs help to develop emotional awareness & expression, social skills and relationship building, as well as to help them build more self-esteem and self confidence.

Montana

550 **Christikon**
1108 24th St W
Billings, MT 59102-3810 406-656-1969
http://www.christikon.org
director@christikon.org
Mark Donald, Pastor & Director
Christikon offers camp sessions for adults 18 and over with developmental disabilities. Activities include hiking, arts & crafts, and music.

Nebraska

551 **Camp Kitaki**
YMCA Of Lincoln Nebraska
570 Fallbrook Blvd.
Suite 210
Lincoln, NE 68521-3110 402-434-9200
Fax: 402-434-9226
http://www.ymcalincoln.org
CampKitaki@ymcalincoln.org
Barb Bettin, President/CEO
J.P. Lauterbach, Chief Operations Officer
Misty Muff, Chief Administrative Officer
A Christian camp for children with ADD and other disabilities. Archery, climbing, horseback riding, fishing and aquatic activities are some of the activities.

552 **Easter Seals - Nebraska**
12565 W Center Rd
Ste 100
Omaha, NE 68144 800-650-9880
Fax: 855-376-1234
http://www.easterseals.com/ne
James C. Summerfelt, President & CEO
Andela Howell, Vice President
Lily Sughroue, Director of Camp, Respite, Rec.
Camp respite for adults and children, camperships, recreational services for children and residential camping programs.

Nevada

553 **Camp Lotsafun**
Amplify Life
480 Galletti Way
Bldg 2
Sparks, NV 89436 775-827-3866
Fax: 775-560-6211
http://www.amplifylife.org
info@amplifylife.org
Cyndy Gustafson, Chair
Gayla , Executive Director
A nonprofit 1 week sleep-away camp designed to be recreational and therapeutic for children, teens and adults with disabilities.
1978Grade Range: Ages 7-70+

New Hampshire

554 **Calumet Camp**
Calumet Lutheran Ministries
1090 Ossipee Lake Road
P.O. Box 236
West Ossipee, NH 03890-0236 603-539-4773
Fax: 603-539-5343
http://www.calumet.org
karl@Calumet.org
Brian Eckblom, Chair
Jim Nye, Treasurer
Karl Ogren, Executive Director of Calumet Lu
Camp Calumet is for kids, adults, seniors, singles, church groups, families and the developmentally disabled.

555 **Easter Seals - New Hempshire**
555 Auburn St
Manchester, NH 03103 603-623-8863
800-870-8728
http://www.easterseals.com/nh/
Larry Gammon, President & CEO
Elin Treanor, Chief Financial Officer
Nancy Rollins, Chief Operating Officer
Easter Seals camping and recreation programs serve children, adults and families of all abilities. Various programs are available with the united purpose of giving disabled individuals a fun and safe camping or recreational experience.

New Jersey

556 **Camp Merry Heart**
Easter Seals Of New Jersey
21 O Brien Rd
Hackettstown, NJ 07840-4839 908-852-3896
Fax: 908-852-9263
http://www.easterseals.com/nj
msimpson@nj.easterseals.org
Richard W. Davidson, Chairman
Sandra L. Bouwman, 1st Vice Chairman
Joseph G. Kern, 2nd Vice Chairman
Camp Merry Heart provides a safe, supervised and beautiful setting for iindividuals with disabilities and special needs. Activities include swimming, boating, fishing, arts and crafts, singing, dance and nature studies.

557 **Camp Moore**
New Jersey State Elks Association
P.O. Box 1596
Woodbridge, NJ 07095 732-326-1300
Fax: 732-326-1319
TDD: 609-271-0138
http://www.njelks.org
elkscampmoore@njelks.org
Todd Garmer, Camp Director
Elks Camp Moore offers a fun filled vacation away from home for children with special needs. A week at Elks Camp Moore is a remarkable experience not soon to be fogotten. The primary goal of the camp is to further develop the recreational and social skills of each child. In a relaxed and accepting atmosphere, each camper experiences new adventures, lasting friendships, and opportunities that promote independence and greater self-confidence.

558 **Round Lake Camp**
21 Plymouth St
Fairfield, NJ 07004-1615 973-575-3333
Fax: 973-575-4188
http://www.roundlakecamp.org
rlc@njycamps.org
David Friedman, Camp Director
A camp for children with learning differences and social communication disorders. The camp is designed so that all the educational, recreational and social activities are planned to meet the capabilities of each child.

559 **Summit Camp**
Summit Camp & Travel Programs
322 Route 46 West
Suite 210
Parsippany, NJ 07054-6266 973-732-3230
Fax: 973-732-3226
http://www.summitcamp.com
info@summitcamp.com
Mayer Stiskin, Executive Director
Eugene Bell, Senior Director
Leah Love, Assistant Director
Summit offers co-ed 4 week and 8 week programs, along with a 10 day Mini-Camp, providing many camp activities that feature a heated swimming pool, complete lake activities, climbing wall, go-karts, computer labs, adventure programs, field trips, etc. The programs and staffing are tailored to the needs of the children dealing with social/emotional challenges, Aspergers, Tourette's, Non-verbal LD, Bipolar Disorder. The camp serves 300 children and provides a staff of 270.

New Mexico

560 **Camp Without Barriers**
Easter Seals Of New Mexico - Santa Fe
2041 S. Pacheco Street
Suite 100
Santa Fe, NM 87505 505-424-7700
Fax: 505-424-7707
http://www.smem.easterseals.com
Jane Carr, Camp Director
Camp Easter Seals New Mexico provides fun for children and adults with disabilities. Its unique combination of comfortable accessible facilities and energetic, outgoing staff offers a fun, exciting, summer experience with memories to last a lifetime. Camp Easter Seals is held at Kamp Kiwanis' site, located in Vanderwagen, New Mexico.

New York

561 **Adirondack Leadership Expeditions**
82 Church St
Saranac Lake, NY 12983-1858 518-897-5011
Fax: 518-897-5017
http://www.adirondackleadership.com
rtheisen@adkle.com
Robert Theisen, Ph.D, Executive Director
Specializes in helping young adults age 13 to 17 who are experiencing / exhibiting any of the following: entitlement, manipulation, family conflict, isolation, low self-esteem, substance use, defiant behavior, attention deficit, learning differences, school failure, and negative peer relationships.

562 **Camp Akeela**
3 New King Street
White Plains, NY 10604 866-680-4744
Fax: 866-462-2828
http://www.campakeela.com
info@campakeela.com
Eric Sasson, Director
Debbie Sasson, Director
Kevin Trimble, Assistant Director
Akeela campers thrive in a world in which they are surrounded by peers with similar experiences and a staff who understands and embraces them. Not only do they have the time of their lives at camp, but they return home with skills and a newfound self-confidence that they carry with them throughout the year.

563 **Camp Bari Tov**
92ny Street Y
1395 Lexington Ave
New York, NY 10128-1612 212-415-5500
Fax: 212-415-5788
http://www.92y.org
Stuart J. Ellman, President
Laurence D. Belfer, Vice President
Marc S. Lipschultz, Vice President
Summer recreational program for children and young adults ages 5-13 with severe developmental disabilities. Campers participate in a variety of camp activities which include adaptive sports, music, art, nature and more.

564 **Camp Colonie**
Easter Seals New York
292 Washington Avenue Ext.
Suite 112
Albany, NY 12203-6385 212-220-2290
800-727-8785
Fax: 518-456-5094
http://www.ny.easterseals.com
info@ny.easter-seals.org
John McGrath, MPA, Chief Executive Director
Aris Pavlides, SVP, Development
Thomas Renart, M.A., M.S., SVP Program Services
Week long sessions for children and young adults age 5-21 years of age with developmental, emotional or physical disabilities.

565 **Camp Dunnabeck at Kildonan School**
425 Morse Hill Rd
Amenia, NY 12501-5240 845-373-8111
Fax: 845-373-9793
http://www.kildonan.org
admissions@kildonan.org
Kevin Pendergast, Head Master
Specializes in helping intelligent children with specific reading, writing and spelling disabilities. Provides Orton-Gillingham tutoring with camp activities, including swimming, sailing, waterskiing, horseback riding, ceramics, tennis and woodworking.

566 **Camp Huntington**
Registration & Billing Office
P.O. Box 37
High Falls, NY 12440-0037 866-514-5281
Fax: 845-853-1172
http://www.camphuntington.com
dfalk@camphuntington.com
Michael Bednarz, Executive Director
Alex Mellor, Program Director
Cathy Crowley, Program Supervisor
Coed camp for children and young adults ages 6-21 who have learning and developmental disabililties, Autism Spectrum Disorders, Apsperger's, and ADD/ADHD. Programs emphasize development of social skills and independent living, vocational orientation, speech and language.

567 **Camp Kehilla**
Sid Jacobson JCC
300 Forest Dr
East Hills, NY 11548-1231 516-484-1545
Fax: 516-484-7354
http://www.campkehilla.org
pzimmer@sjjcc.org
Pam Zimmer, MS Ed., Camp Director
Karen Kiernan, LMSW., Director
Marissa Gonta, Assistant Director
A summer day camp for children and teens with special needs.

568 **Camp Northwood**
132 State Route 365
Remsen, NY 13438-5700 315-831-3621
Fax: 315-831-5867
http://www.nwood.com
northwoodprograms@hotmail.com
Gordon Felt, Camp Director
Coed camp providing structured programs and activities to children and young adults ages 8-18 with Asperger's Syndrome, HFA, and Attention Deficit Disorders.

569 **Camp Sunshine-Camp Elan**
Mosholu Montefiore Community Center
3450 Dekalb Ave
Bronx, NY 10467-2302
718-882-4000
Fax: 718-882-6369
http://www.mmcc.org
info@mmcc.org
Natly Esnard, Co-Chair
Jon Lefkowitz, Co-Chair
Helen Kornblau, Vice-President
Provides programs, services and seasonal camping for children and adults. The camp serves children who are intellectually limited, emotionally impaired, and/or those who demonstrate special learniing disabilities.

570 **Camp Tova**
1395 Lexington Avenue
New York, NY 10128
212-415-5500
Fax: 212-415-5788
http://www.92y.org
Stuart J. Ellman, President
Laurence D. Belfer, Vice President
Marc S. Lipschultz, Vice President
Camp Tova is for children and young adults ages 6-13 with learning and other developmental disabilities. Campers develop a wide variety of social and creative skills while enjoying a variety of camp activites.

571 **Clover Patch Camp**
55 Helping Hand Ln
Glenville, NY 12302-5801
518-384-3081
Fax: 518-384-3001
http://www.cloverpatchcamp.org
cloverpatchcamp@cfdsny.org
Laura Taylor, Camp Director
Clover Patch is a summer camp for individuals with disabilities where each camper is encouraged to reach his or her fullest potential. Campers enjoy a wide variety of programs and are able to make new friends and create everlasting memories.

572 **EBL Coaching Summer Programs**
17 E 89th St
Ste 1D
New York, NY 10128-0615
212-249-0147
Fax: 212-937-2305
http://www.eblcoaching.com
info@eblcoaching.com
Emily Levy, Director
Lauren Hosking, Education Coordinator
Provides one-on-one tutoring and small group summer programs for students with learning disabilities and ADHD. They use all research-based, multi-sensory strategies, including the Orton Gillingham technique.

573 **Easter Seals - Albany**
292 Washington Avenue Ext
Ste 112
Albany, NY 12203-6385
518-456-0828
800-727-8785
Fax: 518-456-5094
http://ny.easterseals.com
info@ny.easter-seals.org
John McGrath, MPA, Chief Executive Director
Aris Pavlides, SVP Development
Thomas Renart, M.A., M.S., SVP Program Services
Easter Seals camping and recreation programs serve children, adults and families of all abilities. Various programs are available with the united purpose of giving disabled individuals a fun and safe camping or recreational experience. The following are camping and recreational services offered: Camp respite for children, camperships, day camping for children and recreational services for children.

574 **Gow School Summer Programs**
PO Box 85
South Wales, NY 14139-0085
716-652-3450
Fax: 716-652-3457
http://www.gow.org
summer@gow.org
David Mendlewski, Director
Doug Cotter, Admissions Director
M. Bradley Rogers, Jr., Headmaster
For boys and girls who have experienced past academic difficulties and have learning differences but possess the potential for success. The five week co-educational Gow School Summer Program (GSSP) serves students ages 8-16. Academic classes are combined with traditional camp activities and weekend trips.

575 **Kamp Kiwanis**
NY District Kiwanis Foundation
9020 Kiwanis Rd
Taberg, NY 13471-2727
315-336-4568
Fax: 315-336-3845
http://www.kiwanis.org
kamp@kiwanis-ny.org
Rebecca Lopez, Executive Director
Jessica Dymond, Chief Development Officer
Jerry Huncosky, CEO
Coed camp for children aged 8-14 who have special needs, are austistic, or physically/mentally challenged.

576 **Mainstreaming at Camp**
Frost Valley YMCA
2000 Frost Valley Rd
Claryville, NY 12725-5221
845-985-2291
Fax: 845-985-0056
http://www.frostvalley.org
nfo@frostvalley.org
Joe Medler, Camp Director
Serves children with developmental disabilities. The YMCA's 'Mainstreaming at Camp' allows campers to integrate with other campers throughout the day and reside in their own village with specially trained staff in the evenings.

577 **Rockland County Association for the Learning Disabled (YAI/RCALD)**
2 Crosfield Avenue
Suite 411
West Nyack, NY 10994-2212
845-358-2032
Fax: 845-358-6119
http://www.yai.org
link@yai.org
Melissa Yu, MD, CEO
YAI/RCALD conducts a wide variety of programs, supervised by experienced and professional staff, designed to build life skills, promote self-esteem, provide information exchange and offer other support services for individuals with learning and other developmental disabilities. The programs include, vocational evaluation and placements, recreational, residential, camping, service coordination and support groups.

578 **Samuel Field Y**
58-20 Little Neck Pkwy
Little Neck, NY 11362-2595
718-225-6750
Fax: 718-255-3910
http://sfysummercamps.org
sfy@sfy.org
Danielle Hersch, Program Director
Andy Gavora, Assistant Director
Robin Topol, Director of Special Services
Day camps specialize in serving children who have developmental disabilities 5-21 years old. Younger campers enjoy the center-based Childhood Program where they swim, play in the gym, cook, dance, as well as share arts and crafts activities and music. Activities for older campers include swimming, nature fun, an overnight at the Little Neck Site, community field trips, as well as a wide variety of specialty activities, such as drama, music, sports and arts and crafts.

579 **School Vacation Camps: Youth with Developmental Disabilities**
YWCA of White Plains-Central Westchester
515 North St
White Plains, NY 10605-3002 914-949-6227
Fax: 914-949-8903
http://ywcawpcw.org
frontdesk@ywcawpcw.org
Maria L. Imperial, CEO
L. Danielle Cylich, Chief Operating Officer
Mary Lee, Director Information Technology
Camp for people with developmental disabilities.

580 **Shield Summer Play Program**
144-61 Roosevelt Avenue
Flushing, NY 11354-6252 718-939-8700
Fax: 718-961-7669
http://www.shield.org
sprovenzano@shield.org
Dr. Susan Provenzano, Ed.D, Executive Director
Beth Anisman, B&Co., LLC, President
Michael E. Katz, Treasurer
The School Program provides a school for children, adolescents, and young adults, ages 6 to 21, who have been diagnosed with either mental retardation or other developmental disabilities. The program provides special education and related services based on each student's skills and potential for independence. Instruction focuses on developing and enhancing skills in community, recreational, and vocational settings. Year-round services are available.

North Carolina

581 **Camp Sky Ranch**
634 Sky Ranch Rd
Blowing Rock, NC 28605 828-264-8600
lori@campskyranchevents.com
Serves developmentally and mentally disabled individuals of all ages, from all over the world. Children and adults with Down Syndrome, Prader-Willie Syndrome, ADD/HD, Fragile X Syndrome, and Autism attend our camp each year.

582 **Discovery Camp**
Talisman Camps & Programs
64 Gap Creek Rd
Zirconia, NC 28790 828-697-6313
http://talismancamps.com
info@talismancamps.com
Linda Tatsapaugh, Operations Director & Owner
Douglas Smathers, Camp Director & Owner
Robiyn Mims, Admissions Director
Discovery Camp is a 2-week program designed for children who may have ADD, learning disabilities, or experiencing some social anxiety. The activity packed schedule and 1:2.5 staff-camper ratio allows campers to have a positive experience at camp. In a nurturing yet structured environment, campers are challenged to become more independent and outgoing within the emotionally and physically safe setting that small group living provides. A good introduction to camp for younger kids.

583 **Millstone 4-H Camp**
1296 Mallard Dr
Ellerbe, NC 28338 910-652-5905
http://www.millstone4hcamp.com
hkrussel@ncsu.edu
Keith Russell, Director
Erehn Moss, Program Director
The type of 4-H Camp program operating in North Carolina offers campers a greater chance to learn, develop life skills and form attitudes that will help them to become self-directing and productive members of society. At camp, youth focus on subjects that might be difficult to handle at home due to need for special equipment. Camp then becomes a learning laboratory that allows youth to apply their new knowledge to real-life situations.

584 **SOAR Adventure Camps - Balsam**
SOAR, Inc.
226 SOAR Ln
PO Box 388
Balsam, NC 28707 828-456-3435
Fax: 801-820-3050
http://www.soarnc.org
admissions@soarnc.org
John Willson, MS, Executive Director
Laura Pate, Director of Operations
Catey Terry, CFO/Controller
Emphasis is placed on developing self-confidence, social skills, problem-solving techniques, a willingness to attempt new challenges and the motivation which comes through successful goal orientation. Full semester and summer programs are available.

585 **SUWS Wilderness Program**
363 Graphite Rd
Old Fort, NC 28762 844-334-2878
http://www.suwscarolinas.com
Bryan Delaney, Program Director
Daniel Fishburn, Executive Director & CEO
Camille Edmonds, Operations Director
Programs specialize in helping troubled teens and defiant teens with behavioral and emotional problems. SUWS wilderness programs have assisted young people to identify and work through internal conflicts and emotional obstacles that have kept them from responding to parental efforts, schools, and treatment.

586 **Talisman Camps & Programs**
64 Gap Creek Rd
Zirconia, NC 28790 828-697-6313
http://talismancamps.com
info@talismancamps.com
Linda Tatsapaugh, Operations Director & Owner
Douglas Smathers, Camp Director & Owner
Robiyn Mims, Admissions Director
Programs are co-educational, for children ages 9-13 who have been diagnosed with LD, ADD, ADHD, and mild behavior issues. Participants live on campus in rustic cabins participating in a variety of activities designed to promote better communication and cooperation skills. Limited enrollment helps to facilitate an extended-family environment. The 2.5 to 1 camper-to-staff ratio ensures that no child is lost in the crowd.

587 **Victory Junction Gang Camp**
4500 Adam's Way
Randleman, NC 27317 336-498-9055
http://victoryjunction.org
info@victoryjunction.org
Chad Coltrane, President & CEO
Lisa Weber, Chief Financial Officer
Jonathan Lemmon, Executive Program Director
Enriches the lives of children with chronic medical conditions or serious illnesses by providing life-changing camping experiences that are exciting, fun, and empowering, in a safe and medically sound environment.

Ohio

588 **Academic Fun & Fitness Camp**
Creative Education Institute
31300 Solon Rd
Ste 1
Solon, OH 44139 440-914-0200
http://www.cei4learning.org
info@cei4learning.org
Carole Richards, President & CEO
John Kusik, Chair
Sharon Miles, Manager of Field Projects
For children with special needs and learning differences such as ADD/ADHD, Asperger's Syndrome, and Dyslexia. 6 weeks in June & July; 5:1 camper/counselor ratio.

589 **Akron Rotary Camp**
4460 Rex Lake Dr
Akron, OH 44319
330-644-4512
877-GOT-CAMP
Fax: 330-644-1013
http://www.akronymca.org/RotaryCamp
rotarycamp@akronymca.org
Dan Reynolds, Camp Director
Amanda Warner, Dir. Volunteering/Special Events
Rotary Camp offers children with special needs a place to spend their summers. Children with physical or developmental disabilities are eligible to participate in this fun-filled camping experience.
1924Grade Range: Ages 6-17

590 **Camp Courageous**
12701 Waterville-Swanton Rd
Whitehouse, OH 43571
419-875-6828
http://www.campcourageous.com
camping@campcourageous.com
Mark Frey, President
Jim Cady, Treasurer
Joe Stanford, Secretary
Camp Courageous is a year-round recreational and respite facility for individuals with disabilities. The camp provides the opportunity to campers for social and personal growth within a supportive environment while helping them to develop enhanced self-esteem. Some of the recreational activities include bocce ball, canoeing, games, hikes, scavenger hunts and arts & crafts.

591 **Camp Echoing Hills**
36272 County Road 79
Warsaw, OH 43844
740-327-2311
http://www.ehvi.org
info@ehvi.org
Emily Smith, Camp Program Director
Lauren Unger, Camp Administrator
Doreen Peterson, Camp Secretary
Camp Echoing Hills is a nonprofit Christian camp for adults and children with physical and developmental disabilities. The 7 week camp is designed to build strong communities and provide an opportunities for individuals to develop friendships, skills and life-long memories.
1967

592 **Camp Happiness**
Catholic Charities Disability Services
7911 Detroit Ave
Cleveland, OH 44102
216-334-2963
http://ccdocle.org/disability
mjscott@ccdocle.org
Dennis C. McNulty, Director
Marilyn Scott, Program Director
A summer camp program for persons with developmental disabilities, Camp Happiness is a six-week day camp offered at several sites throughout the Diocese of Cleveland that provides educational, social and recreational services to children and adults with developmental disabilities during the summer months.
1996Grade Range: Ages 5-21

593 **Camp Nuhop**
Township Road 2916
Perrsville, OH 44864
419-938-7151
http://nuhop.org/camp-nuhop
Trevor Dunlap, Executive Director
Chris Clyde, Associate Director
A residential camp for all children with learning disabilities, attention deficit disorders and behavior disorders.

594 **Easter Seals - Broadview Heights**
Easter Seals North East Ohio
1929 A East Royalton Rd
Broadview Heights, OH 44147
440-838-0990
Fax: 440-838-8440
TTY: 440-838-0990
http://www.easterseals.com/noh
Sheila Dunn, CEO
Amy Kullik, Esq., Chair
Susan Vasu, Vice Chair
Camperships and day camping for children and adults with disabilities.

595 **Easter Seals - Central & Southeast Ohio**
3830 Trueman Ct
Hilliard, OH 43026
614-228-5523
http://www.easterseals.com/centralohio
Jim Kelley, President
Tony Kickeisen, Vice President
Trisha Krejci, Treasurer
Aquatics Summer Day Camp is open to toddlers, ages 18 months to 2 years, and preschoolers and young school-aged children from 3-8 years of age with and without disabilities.

596 **Easter Seals - Cincinnati**
2901 Gilbert Ave
Cincinnati, OH 45206
513-281-2316
http://www.easterseals.com/gc
Pamela Green, President and CEO
David Dreith, Chief Operating Officer
Jenn Zugelder, Chief Financial Officer
Easter Seals camping and recreation programs serve children, adults and families of all abilities. Various programs are available with the united purpose of giving disabled individuals a fun and safe camping or recreational experience.

597 **Easter Seals - Northeast Ohio**
2173 N Ridge Rd
Ste G
Lorain, OH 44055
888-325-8532
http://www.easterseals.com/noh
Amy Kullik, Esq., Chair
Sheila Dunn, President & CEO
Suzanne Meehan, Secretary
Easter Seals camping and recreation programs serve children, adults and families of all abilities. Various programs are available with the united purpose of giving disabled individuals a fun and safe camping or recreational experience.

598 **Easter Seals - Youngstown**
299 Edwards St
Youngstown, OH 44502-1599
330-743-1168
TTY: 330-743-1616
http://www.easterseals.com/mtc
Tim Nelson, President & CEO
Easter Seals camping and recreation programs serve children, adults and families of all abilities. Various programs are available with the united purpose of giving disabled individuals a fun and safe camping or recreational experience.

599 **Marburn Academy Summer Programs**
9555 Johnstown Rd
New Albany, OH 43054
614-433-0822
Fax: 614-433-0812
http://www.marburnacademy.org
Jamie Williamson, Headmaster
Scott Burton, Associate Head of School
Beth Weakley, Chief Financial Officer
A four program academic day camp for children with LD and dyslexia, offering remediation in reading, math, phonemic awareness, or writing.

600 **Recreation Unlimited Camps & Retreat Center**
Recreation Unlimited Foundation
7700 Piper Rd
Ashley, OH 43003
740-548-7006
Fax: 740-747-2640
http://www.recreationunlimited.org
info@recreationunlimited.org
Paul L. Huttlin, Executive Director & CEO
Provides year round programs in recreation, sports and education for individuals with developmental or physical disabilities. Campers build self-confidence and self-esteem while gaining positive relationships, attitudes and behaviors.

Oklahoma

601 **Camp Loughridge**
4900 W 71st St
Tulsa, OK 74131 918-446-4194
http://www.camploughridge.org
mstaires@camploughridge.org
Michael Staires, Camp Program Director
A Christian summer day camp offering all the traditional camp activities such as archery, arts and crafts, canoeing, challenge and ropes courses, sports, hikes, swimming, and chapel sessions. Offers a Autism Inclusion program.

602 **TMA Camp**
Therapy & Beyond
308 Aspen Ave
Broken Arrow, OK 74012 972-295-9322
844-422-2669
http://www.therapyandbeyond.com/tmacamp
info@therapyandbeyond.com
Regiona M. Crone, Founder & Director
Teach Me Academy is an academic summer day camp designed to encourage children with Autism Spectrum Disorders and other developmental disabilities to achieve their highest potential while participating in summer outdoor activities.

Oregon

603 **Easter Seals - Medford**
119 N Oakdale Ave
Salem, OR 97501 541-776-6060
Fax: 888-710-6157
http://www.easterseals.com/oregon
J. David Cheveallier, CEO
Programs offered in Medford include summer day camp, Recreation & Respite, and the popular First Saturday dance and social event. Programs are held at various community centers in Medford.

604 **Easter Seals - Oregon**
7300 SW Hunziker Rd
Ste 103
Portland, OR 97223 503-228-5108
http://www.easterseals.com/oregon
J. David Cheveallier, CEO
Easter Seals camping and recreation programs serve children, adults and families of all abilities. Various programs are available with the united purpose of giving disabled individuals a fun and safe camping or recreational experience. In addition, the Portland program center hosts a warm water aquatic facility.

Pennsylvania

605 **Amica**
1272 Knox Dr
Yardley, PA 19067 267-258-3974
http://www.amica4autism.com
amica4autism@gmail.com
Stephanie DeSouza, Owner
Meghann Hernandez, Director
Amy Ellison, Senior Counselor
Offers year-round camps for children and teens with high-functioning autism, Asperger's Syndrom, PDD-NOS, and nonverbal learning disabilities. Amica's mission is to foster social skills and provide an opportunity for campers to develop friendships with their peers.

606 **Autism Drama Program**
Theatre Horizon
401 DeKalb St
Norristown, PA 19401 610-283-2230
http://www.theatrehorizon.org
info@theatrehorizon.org
Jennifer Pratt Johnson, Executive Director
Molly Braverman, Managing Director
The Theatre Horizon Autism Drama Program fosters imagination, communication and personal relationships through the techniques of performing arts. Classes help students develop social and verbal skills.

607 **Camp Hope**
12300 Perry Hwy
Ste 100
Wexford, PA 15090 724-933-4673
Fax: 724-799-8365
http://www.thehopelearningcenter.org
info@thehopelearningcenter.org
Asha Persaud, Executive Director
Meaghan Nescot, Center Director
Audrey Mackie, Officer Manager
A 6 week day camp focused on the Pennsylvania Academic Standards and ABA Standards for teaching Verbal Behavior. Camp Hope's goal is to develop new learning skills through group activities.

608 **Camp Lee Mar**
805 Redgate Road
Dresher, PA 19025 215-658-1708
Fax: 215-658-1710
http://www.leemar.com
Lynsey@leemar.com
Ari Segal, MSW, Director
Lynsey Trohoske, BA, Assistant Director
Laura Leibowitz, BA, M.Ed, Assistant Director
Private residential special needs camp for children and young adults with mild to moderate learning and developmental challenges, including but not limited to the following: mental retardation, developmental disabilities, down syndrome, autism, learning disabilities, Williams Syndrome, Asperger Syndrome, ADD, Prader Willi, and ADHD. A structured environment, individual attention and guidance are emphasized at all times.
1953Grade Range: Ages 7-21

609 **Creative Arts Program**
Wesley Family Services
100 Emerson Ln
Ste 1525
Bridgeville, PA 15017 412-342-2270
http://wfspa.org/service/creative-arts-program
Doug Muetzel, Chief Executive Officer
Marc Cosentino, VP, Facilities
Tiffany Jimenez, Director, Development
Music therapy for children and teens with behavioral, social, psychological, communication, physical, and congnitive functioning disabilities. Designed for children and their families to use performance art as a therapeutic and rehabilitation tool.

Rhode Island

610 **Camp Wannagoagain!**
The Autism Project
1516 Atwood Ave
Johnston, RI 02919 401-785-2666
Fax: 401-785-2272
http://www.theautismproject.org
jmoran1@lifespan.org
Jennie Moran, Office Manager
Caren Skurka, Program Manager
Joanne G. Quinn, Executive Director
A 2 week summer camp for children with Austim, Asperger Syndrom or other communication disorders. Designed to foster communication skills and provide an opportunity for campers to develop new friendships.

South Carolina

611 **Camp Spearhead**
Greenville County Rec
4806 Old Spartangburg Dr
Taylors, SC 29687
864-288-6470
Fax: 864-288-6499
http://greenvillerec.org
An 8 week residential summer camp for children and adults with developmental disabilities and communication disorders. Activities include canoeing, kayaking, zip lining, high ropes course, nature trails, archery, wimming, gem mining, yoga, basketball, and group games.
1968Grade Range: Ages 8+

Tennessee

612 **Camp Conquest**
Arlington, TN
901-490-7164
http://www.campconquest.com
markp@campconquest.com
Mark Price, Co-Founder
Amanda Price, Co-Founder
A Christ-centered, weeklong, overnight camp for children and adults with special needs, chronic illnesses and disabilities. Camp Conquest encourages campers to try new things and gain self-confidence. Activities include a 3 story water slide, rope swing, rock climbing wall, horseback riding, zip lines, and more.

Texas

613 **Charis Hills**
498 Faulkner Rd.
Sunset, TX 76270
940-964-2145
Fax: 940-964-2147
http://www.charishills.org
info@charishills.org
Rand Southard, President
Colleen Southard, Director
Molly Southard, Assistant Program Director
Those with special learning needs have an opportunity to meet others, both children and their counselors, who share similar experiences who are on the road to success. They have the opportunity to learn new activities in an environment that is safe, physically and socially.

Utah

614 **Summer Reading Camp at Reid Ranch**
2965 E Evergreen Ave
Salt Lake City, UT 84109
801-486-5083
800-468-3274
Fax: 801-485-0561
http://www.reidranch.com
Dr. Mervin R Reid, President
Dr. Ethna R. Reid, Director
The camp offers daily reading and language arts programs for children and young adults. Recreational activities include horseback riding, swimming, paddle boats and canoes, mountain climbing, volleyball and other other sports.
1987

Vermont

615 **Camp Akeela**
314 Bryn Mawr Ave
Bala Cynwyd, PA 19004
802-866-0380
Fax: 866-462-2828
http://www.campakeela.com
Greg Walker, Program Director
Eric Sasson, Executive Director
Debbie Sasson, Executive Director
Camp Akeela is a sleepaway camp in Vermont. The camp is small in order to help campers with communication disorders feel comfortable. Camp Akeela is designed to foster self-confidence and improve social skills.

616 **Camp Kaleidoscope**
Common Ground Center
473 Tatro Rd.
Starksboro, VT 05487
802-453-2592
800-430-2667
http://www.cgcvt.org
info@cgcvt.org
Carole Blane, Camp Director
Connor Timmons, Executive Director
Camp Kaleidoscope is a summer camp retreat for families experiencing autism. A place for families to relax and spend time together in a stress-free environment.

Virginia

617 **Summer PLUS Program**
Blue Ridge Autism and Achievement Center
312 Whitwell Dr
Roanoke, VA 24019
540-366-7399
http://braacroanoke.org
braac.roanoke@svhservices.org
Christina Giuliano, Executive Director
Lisa Hensley, Business Manager
Jeanne Lawrence, Development Coordinator
Summer camp program for children with learning disabilities and Autism. Programs put emphasis on social play and social skill development, communication and social skills all while targeting learning goals.

Washington

618 **Aspiring Youth**
2400 NE 95th St
Seattle, WA 98115
206-517-0241
http://www.aspiringyouth.net
info@aspiringyouth.net
Benjamin Wahl, Program Coordinator
Offering a variety of summer camps for children and teens with behavioral disabilities across Washington state.
1904Grade Range: Ages 8-18

619 **Blue Compass Camps**
1725 SW Roxbury St
Seattle, WA 98106
206-486-4893
http://www.bluecompasscamps.com
Joel , Executive Director
Debi , Non-Profit President
Summer camps for children and teens with high-functioning Autism, Aspergers and ADHD. Programs place emphasis on the outdoors experience within a small and intimate environment for campers.

Wisconsin

620 **YMCA Camp Glacier Hollow**
Stevens Point Area YMCA
1000 Division St
Stevens Point, WI 54481
715-342-2980
Fax: 715-342-2987
http://www.glacierhollow.com
pmatthai@spymca.org
Pete Matthai, Camp Director
Tiffany Praeger, Camp Program Director
Offers day camps and adventure trips for children with physical and developmental disabilities.

Wyoming

621 **SOAR Adventure Camps - Dubois**
SOAR, Inc.
Eagle View Ranch
184 Uphill Rd
Dubois, WY 82513
307-455-3084
Fax: 801-820-3050
http://www.soarnc.org
evr@soarnc.org

John Willson, MS, Executive Director
Laura Pate, Director of Operations
Catey Terry, CFO/Controller

Emphasis is placed on developing self-confidence, social skills, problem-solving techniques, a willingness to attempt new challenges and the motivation which comes through successful goal orientation. Full semester and summer programs are available.

Language Arts

622 **Analogies 1, 2 & 3**
Educators Publishing Service
PO Box 9031
Cambridge, MA 02139-9031
617-547-6706
800-225-5750
Fax: 617-547-3805
http://www.epsbooks.com
CustomerService.EPS@schoolspecialty.com
Arthur Liebman, Author
Rick Holden, President
Jeff Belanger, Regional Sales Manager
Studying analogies helps students to sharpen reasoning ability, develop critical thinking, understand relationships between words and ideas, learn new vocabulary, and prepare for the SAT's and for standardized tests.

623 **AtoZap!**
Sunburst Technology
1550 Executive Dr
Elgin, IL 60123-9311
800-321-7511
Fax: 888-608-0344
http://store.sunburst.com
service@sunburst.com
Michael Guillory, Channel Sales/Marketing Manager
A whimsical world of magical talking alphabet blocks and energetic playful characters this program provides young children with exciting opportunities to explore new concepts through open-ended activities and games. Mac/Win CD-ROM

624 **Basic Signing Vocabulary Cards**
Harris Communications
15155 Technology Dr
Eden Prairie, MN 55344-2273
952-906-1180
800-825-6758
Fax: 952-906-1099
TTY: 800-825-9187
http://www.harriscomm.com
info@harriscomm.com
Dr. Robert Harris, President
Darla Hudson, Customer Service
Lori Foss, Marketing Director
Harris Communications is the sign language superstore and sells a full line of sign language materials for children, students, teachers and interpreters. Please visit us on-line to view all of our sign language products. Catalog is also available to view on-line or sent via USPS. *$7.95*
100 cards/set

625 **Bubbleland Word Discovery**
Sunburst Technology
1550 Executive Dr
Elgin, IL 60123-9311
800-321-7511
Fax: 888-608-0344
http://store.sunburst.com
service@sunburst.com
Michael Guillory, Channel Sales/Marketing Manager
Build and sharpen language arts skills with this multimedia dictionary. Students explore ten familiar locations that include a pet shop, zoo, toy store, hospital, playground, beach and airport where they engage in 40 activities that build word recognition, pronunciation and spelling skills.

626 **Carolina Picture Vocabulary Test (CPVT): For Deaf and Hearing Impaired Children**
Pro-Ed
8700 Shoal Creek Blvd
Austin, TX 78757-6897
512-451-3246
800-897-3202
Fax: 800-397-7633
http://www.proedinc.com
info@proedinc.com
Cheri Richardson, Permissions Editor
Thomas Layton, Author
David Holmes, Co-Author
A norm-referenced, validated, receptive sign vocabulary test for deaf and hearing-impaired children. *$147.00*

627 **Curious George Pre-K ABCs**
Sunburst Technology
1550 Executive Dr
Elgin, IL 60123-9311
800-321-7511
Fax: 888-608-0344
http://store.sunburst.com
service@sunburst.com
Michael Guillory, Channel Sales/Marketing Manager
Children go on a lively adventure with Curious George visiting six multi level activities that provide an animated introduction to letters and their sounds. Students discover letter names and shapes, initial letter sounds, letter pronunciations, the order of the alphabet and new vocabulary words during the fun exursions with Curious George. Mac/Win CD-ROM

628 **Early Communication Skills for Children with Down Syndrome**
Therapro
225 Arlington St
Framingham, MA 01702-8773
508-872-9494
800-257-5376
Fax: 508-875-2062
http://www.therapro.com
info@therapro.com
Libby Kumin PhD, Author
Karen Conrad, President
Provides professional expertise in understandable terms. Parents and professionals learn how their skills are evaulated by professionals, and what activities they can practice with a child immediately to encouarge a childs's communication skill development. *$19.95*
368 pages

629 **Early Listening Skills**
Therapro
225 Arlington St
Framingham, MA 01702-8773
508-872-9494
800-257-5376
Fax: 508-875-2062
http://www.therapro.com
info@therapro.com
Diana Williams, Author
Karen Conrad, President
Two hundred activities designed to be photocopied for classroom or home. Includes materials on auditory detection, discrimination, recognition, sequencing and memory. Describes listening projects and topics for the curriculum. Activity sheets for parents are included. A practical, comprehensive and effective manual for professionals working with preschool children or the older child with special needs. *$63.50*

630 **Earobics Step 2: Home Version**
Abilitations Speech Bin
PO Box 1579
Appleton, WI 54912-1579
419-589-1600
888-388-3224
Fax: 888-388-6344
http://www.schoolspecialty.com
orders@schoolspecialty.com
Joseph M. Yorio, President, CEO
Rick Holden, Executive Vice President
Kevin Baehler, Vice President, Acting CFO
Step 2 teaches critical language comprehension skills and trains the critical auditory skills children need for success in learning. It offers hundreds of levels of play, appealing graphics, and entertaining music to train the critical auditory skills young children need for success in learning. Item number C483. *$58.99*

631 **Earobics Step 2: Specialist/Clinician Version**
Abilitations Speech Bin
PO Box 1579
Appleton, WI 54912-1579
419-589-1600
888-388-3224
Fax: 888-388-6344
http://www.schoolspecialty.com
orders@schoolspecialty.com
Joseph M. Yorio, President, CEO
Rick Holden, Executive Vice President
Kevin Baehler, Vice President, Acting CFO
Earobics features: tasks and level counter with real time display; adaptive training technology for individualized programs; and reporting to track and evaluate each individual's progress. Step 2 teaches critical language comprehension skills and trains the critical auditory skills children need for success in learning. Item number C484. *$298.99*

632 **Every Child a Reader**
Sunburst Technology
1550 Executive Dr
Elgin, IL 60123-9311
800-321-7511
Fax: 888-608-0344
http://store.sunburst.com
service@sunburst.com
Michael Guillory, Channel Sales/Marketing Manager
Traditional reading strategies in a rich literary context. Designed to promote independent reading and develop oral and written language expression.

633 **Explode the Code: Wall Chart**
Educators Publishing Service
PO Box 9031
Cambridge, MA 02139-9031
617-547-6706
800-225-5750
Fax: 617-547-3805
http://www.epsbooks.com
CustomerService.EPS@schoolspecialty.com
Nancy M Hall, Author
Rick Holden, President
Jeff Belanger, Regional Sales Manager
Learning sounds is exciting with the new Explode The Code alphabet chart! Each letter is represented by a colorful character from the series and is stored inside a felt pocket embroidered with the letter's name.

634 **First Phonics**
Sunburst Technology
1550 Executive Dr
Elgin, IL 60123-9311
800-321-7511
Fax: 888-608-0344
http://store.sunburst.com
service@sunburst.com
Michael Guillory, Channel Sales/Marketing Manager
Targets the phonics skills that all children need to develop, sounding out the first letter of a word. This program offers four different engaging activities that you can customize to match each child's specific need.

635 **Fun with Language: Book 1**
Therapro
225 Arlington St
Framingham, MA 01702-8773
508-872-9494
800-257-5376
Fax: 508-875-2062
http://www.therapro.com
info@therapro.com
Kathleen Yardley, Author
Karen Conrad, President
A wonderful reproducible workbook of thinking and language skill exercises for children ages 4-8. Perfect when you need something on a moment's notice. Over 100 beautifully illustrated exercises in the following categories: Spatial Relationships; Opposites; Categorizing; Following Directions; Temporal Concepts; Syntax & Morphology; Same and Different; Plurals; Memory; Reasoning; Storytelling; and Describing. Targets both receptive and expressive language as well as problem- solving skills. *$59.50*

636 **Goldman-Fristoe Test of Articulation: 2nd Edition**
Abilitations Speech Bin
PO Box 1579
Appleton, WI 54912-1579
419-589-1600
888-388-3224
Fax: 888-388-6344
http://www.schoolspecialty.com
orders@schoolspecialty.com
Joseph M. Yorio, President, CEO
Ronald Goldman, Author
Macalyne Fristoe, Co-Author
It systematically measures a child's production of 39 consonant sounds and blends. Its age range is 2-21 years, and age based standard scores have separate gender norms. In this revised edition, inappropriate stimulus words have been replaced based on multicultural review, and all new artwork is featured. Item number 190915116. *$229.99*

637 **HearFones**
Abilitations Speech Bin
PO Box 1579
Appleton, WI 54912-1579
419-589-1600
888-388-3224
Fax: 888-388-6344
http://www.schoolspecialty.com
orders@schoolspecialty.com
Joseph M. Yorio, President, CEO
Rick Holden, Executive Vice President
Kevin Baehler, Vice President, Acting CFO
This unique nonelectronic self-contained headset is made of composite and plastic materials, and it's easy to clean. It lets users hear themselves more directly and clearly so they can analyze their own speech sound production and voice quality. Item number N261. *$28.99*

638 **I Can Say R**
Abilitations Speech Bin
PO Box 1579
Appleton, WI 54912-1579
419-589-1600
888-388-3224
Fax: 888-388-6344
http://www.schoolspecialty.com
orders@schoolspecialty.com
Joseph M. Yorio, President, CEO
Rick Holden, Executive Vice President
Kevin Baehler, Vice President, Acting CFO
Helping children overcome problems saying R sounds is one of the most perplexing dilemmas speech and language pathologists face in their caseloads. Here's a terrific book packed with innovative practice materials to make that task easier. Item number 190728116. *$26.99*

639 **Idiom's Delight**
Academic Therapy Publications
20 Leveroni Court
Novato, CA 94949-5746
415-883-3314
800-422-7249
Fax: 888-287-9975
http://www.academictherapy.com
sales@academictherapy.com
Jim Arena, President
Joanne Urban, Manager
Cynthia Coverston
Offers 75 idioms and accompanying reproducible activities. Delightful illustrations portraying humorous literal interpretations of idioms are sprinkled throughout the book to enhance enjoyment. *$14.00*
64 pages
ISBN 0-878798-89-7

640 **Island Reading Journey**
Sunburst Technology
1550 Executive Dr
Elgin, IL 60123-9311
800-321-7511
Fax: 888-608-0344
http://store.sunburst.com
service@sunburst.com
Michael Guillory, Channel Sales/Marketing Manager

Enhance your reading program with meaningful summary and extension activities for 100 intermediate level books. Students read for meaning while they engage in activities that test for comprehension, build writing skills with reader response and essay questions, develop usage skills with cloze activities and improve vocabulary/word attack skills.

641 **Kaufman Speech Praxis Test**
Abilitations Speech Bin
PO Box 1579
Appleton, WI 54912-1579 419-589-1600
888-388-3224
Fax: 888-388-6344
http://www.schoolspecialty.com
orders@schoolspecialty.com
Nancy R. Kaufman, Author
Joseph M. Yorio, President, CEO
Rick Holden, Executive Vice President
This standardized test utilizes a hierarchy of simple to complex motor-speech movements, from oral movement and simple phonemic/syllable to complex phonemic/syllable level. The complete kit contains manual, guide, and 25 test booklets. Item number 192126116. *$185.00*

642 **LILAC**
Abilitations Speech Bin
PO Box 1579
Appleton, WI 54912-1579 419-589-1600
888-388-3224
Fax: 888-388-6344
http://www.schoolspecialty.com
orders@schoolspecialty.com
Joseph M. Yorio, President, CEO
Rick Holden, Executive Vice President
Kevin Baehler, Vice President, Acting CFO
LILAC uses direct and naturalistic teaching in a creative approach that links spoken language learning to reading and writing. Activities to develop semantic, syntactic, expressive, and receptive language skills are presented sequentially from three-to five-year-old developmental levels. Item number 190825116. *$27.99*

643 **Language Activity Resource Kit: LARK**
Abilitations Speech Bin
PO Box 1579
Appleton, WI 54912-1579 419-589-1600
888-388-3224
Fax: 888-388-6344
http://www.schoolspecialty.com
orders@schoolspecialty.com
Joseph M. Yorio, President, CEO
Richard A Dressler, Author
Kevin Baehler, Vice President, Acting CFO
The LARK: Language Activity Resource Kit has been revised! This perennially popular language kit is now more portable and versatile for use with persons who have moderate to severe language disorders. Item number 190613116. *$ 217.99*

644 **Max's Attic: Long & Short Vowels**
Sunburst Technology
1550 Executive Dr
Elgin, IL 60123-9311 800-321-7511
Fax: 888-608-0344
http://store.sunburst.com
service@sunburst.com
Michael Guillory, Channel Sales/Marketing Manager
Filled to the rafters with phonics fun, this animated program builds your students' vowel recognition skills.

645 **Pair-It Books: Early Emergent Stage 2**
Houghton Mifflin Harcourt
222 Berkeley Street
Boston, MA 02116 617-351-5000
855-969-4642
Fax: 800-269-5232
http://www.hmhco.com
school.permissions@hmhco.com
Michael Opitz, Author
Linda K. Zecher, President, CEO & Director
Eric Shuman, Chief Financial Officer
John K. Dragoon, EVP and Chief Marketing Officer
A series of 20 books, each containing 16 pages, that gradually become more difficult and reflect more complex text structures such as dialogue, content vocabulary and question and answer formats. All stories are available on audio cassette, and four are available in big book format.

646 **PhonicsMart CD-ROM**
HMH Supplemental Publishers
222 Berkeley Street
Boston, MA 02116 617-351-5000
855-969-4642
Fax: 800-269-5232
http://www.hmhco.com
school.permissions@hmhco.com
Linda K. Zecher, President, CEO & Director
Eric Shuman, Chief Financial Officer
John K. Dragoon, EVP and Chief Marketing Officer
Five interactive games offer practice and reinforcement in 19 phonics skills at a variety of learning levels! Over 700 key words are vocalized, and each is accompanied by sound effects, colorful illustrations, animation, or video clips!

647 **Polar Express**
Sunburst Technology
1550 Executive Dr
Elgin, IL 60123-9311 800-321-7511
Fax: 888-608-0344
http://store.sunburst.com
service@sunburst.com
Michael Guillory, Channel Sales/Marketing Manager
Share the magic and enchantment of the holiday season with this CD-ROM version of Chris Van Allsburg's Caldecott-winning picture book.

648 **Python Path Phonics Word Families**
Sunburst Technology
1550 Executive Dr
Elgin, IL 60123-9311 800-321-7511
Fax: 888-608-0344
http://store.sunburst.com
service@sunburst.com
Michael Guillory, Channel Sales/Marketing Manager
Your students improve their word-building skills by playing three fun strategy games that involve linking one-or two-letter consonant beginnings to basic word endings.

649 **Ridgewood Grammar**
Educators Publishing Service
PO Box 9031
Cambridge, MA 02139-9031 617-547-6706
800-225-5750
Fax: 617-547-3805
http://www.epsbooks.com
CustomerService.EPS@schoolspecialty.com
Terri Wiss, Author
Nancy Bison, Co-Author
Rick Holden, President
Grammar is an important part of any student's education. This new series, from the school district that developed the popular Ridgewood Analogies books, teaches 3rd, 4th, and 5th graders about the parts of speech and their use in sentences.

650 **Sequential Spelling 1-7 with Student Respose Book**
AVKO Educational Research Foundation
3084 Willard Rd
Birch Run, MI 48415-9404 810-686-9283
866-285-6612
Fax: 810-686-1101
http://www.avko.org
webmaster@avko.org
Don McCabe, President/Research Director
Linda Heck, Vice-President
Michael Lane, Treasurer

Sequential Spelling uses immediate student self-correction. It builds from easier words of a word family such as all and then builds on them to teach; all, tall, stall, install, call, fall, ball, and their inflected forms such as: stalls, stalled, stalling, installing, installment. *$89.95*
72 pages
ISBN 1-664003-00-0

651 **Soaring Scores CTB: TerraNova Reading and Language Arts**
HMH Supplemental Publishers
222 Berkeley Street
Boston, MA 02116 617-351-5000
855-969-4642
Fax: 800-269-5232
http://www.hmhco.com
school.permissions@hmhco.com
Linda K. Zecher, President, CEO & Director
Eric Shuman, Chief Financial Officer
John K. Dragoon, EVP and Chief Marketing Officer
Through a combination of targeted instructional practice and test-taking tips, these workbooks help students build better skills and improve CTB-TerraNova test scores. Initial lessons address reading comprehension and language arts. The authentic practice test mirrors the CTB's format and content.

652 **Soaring Scores in Integrated Language Arts**
HMH Supplemental Publishers
222 Berkeley Street
Boston, MA 02116 617-351-5000
855-969-4642
Fax: 800-269-5232
http://www.hmhco.com
school.permissions@hmhco.com
Linda K. Zecher, President, CEO & Director
Eric Shuman, Chief Financial Officer
John K. Dragoon, EVP and Chief Marketing Officer
Help your students develop the right skills and strategies for success on integrated arts assessments. Soaring Scores presents three sets of two lengthy, thematically linked literature selections. Students develop higher-order thinking skills as they respond to open-ended questions about the selections.

653 **Soaring Scores on the CMT in Language Arts& on the CAPT in Reading and Writing Across Disciplines**
HMH Supplemental Publishers
222 Berkeley Street
Boston, MA 02116 617-351-5000
855-969-4642
Fax: 800-269-5232
http://www.hmhco.com
school.permissions@hmhco.com
Linda K. Zecher, President, CEO & Director
Eric Shuman, Chief Financial Officer
John K. Dragoon, EVP and Chief Marketing Officer
Make every minute count when you are preparing for the CMT or CAPT. Fine tune your language arts test preparation with the program developed specifically for the Connecticut's assessments. Questions are correlated to Connecticut's content standards for reading and responding, producing text, applying English language conventions, and exploring and responding to texts.

654 **Soaring Scores on the NYS English Language Arts Assessment**
HMH Supplemental Publishers
222 Berkeley Street
Boston, MA 02116 617-351-5000
855-969-4642
Fax: 800-269-5232
http://www.hmhco.com
school.permissions@hmhco.com
Linda K. Zecher, President, CEO & Director
Eric Shuman, Chief Financial Officer
John K. Dragoon, EVP and Chief Marketing Officer
With these workbooks, students receive instructional practice for approaching the assessment's reading, listening and writing questions.

655 **Soaring on the MCAS in English Language Arts**
HMH Supplemental Publishers
222 Berkeley Street
Boston, MA 02116 617-351-5000
855-969-4642
Fax: 800-269-5232
http://www.hmhco.com
school.permissions@hmhco.com
Linda K. Zecher, President, CEO & Director
Eric Shuman, Chief Financial Officer
John K. Dragoon, EVP and Chief Marketing Officer
Instructional practice in the first section builds skills for the MCAS language, literacy, and composition questions. A practice test models the MCAS precisely in design and length.

656 **Spelling: A Thematic Content-Area Approach**
HMH Supplemental Publishers
222 Berkeley Street
Boston, MA 02116 617-351-5000
855-969-4642
Fax: 800-269-5232
http://www.hmhco.com
school.permissions@hmhco.com
Linda K. Zecher, President, CEO & Director
Eric Shuman, Chief Financial Officer
John K. Dragoon, EVP and Chief Marketing Officer
Help students master the words they will use most frequently in the classroom. Organized lessons incorporate word analysis of letter patterns, correlations to appropriate literature, writing exercises, and application and extension activities.

657 **Stories and More: Time and Place**
Riverdeep, Inc.
100 Pine Street
Suite 1900
San Francisco, CA 94111-5205 415-659-2000
Fax: 415-659-2020
http://web.riverdeep.net
info@riverdeep.net
Barry O'Callaghan, Executive Chairman/CEO
Jim Rudy, Chief Revenue Officer
Tom Mulderry, Executive Vice President
Combines three well-loved stories - The House on Maple Street, Roxaboxen, and Galimoto with engaging activities that strengthen students' reading comprehension.

658 **Sunken Treasure Adventure: Beginning Blends**
Sunburst Technology
1550 Executive Dr
Elgin, IL 60123-9311 800-321-7511
Fax: 888-608-0344
http://store.sunburst.com
service@sunburst.com
Michael Guillory, Channel Sales/Marketing Manager
Focus on beginning blends sounds and concepts with three high-spirited games that invite students to use two letter consonant blends as they build words.

659 **Teaching Phonics: Staff Development Book**
HMH Supplemental Publishers
222 Berkeley Street
Boston, MA 02116 617-351-5000
855-969-4642
Fax: 800-269-5232
http://www.hmhco.com
school.permissions@hmhco.com
Linda K. Zecher, President, CEO & Director
Eric Shuman, Chief Financial Officer
John K. Dragoon, EVP and Chief Marketing Officer
Fine-tune your instructional approach with fresh insights from phonics experts. This resource offers informative articles and timely tips for teaching phonics in the integrated language arts classroom.

660 **Test of Early Language Development**
Pro-Ed, Inc.
8700 Shoal Creek Blvd
Austin, TX 78757-6897
512-451-3246
800-897-3202
Fax: 800-397-7633
http://www.proedinc.com
info@proedinc.com
Wayne Hresko, Author
D Kim Reid, Co-Author
Don Hammill, Co-Author
A normed test appropriate for children 0-2 through 7-11. It quickly and easily measures Receptive and Expressive language and yields an overall Spoken Language Score. *$295.00*

661 **Vocabulary Connections**
HMH Supplemental Publishers
222 Berkeley Street
Boston, MA 02116
617-351-5000
855-969-4642
Fax: 800-269-5232
http://www.hmhco.com
school.permissions@hmhco.com
Linda K. Zecher, President, CEO & Director
Eric Shuman, Chief Financial Officer
John K. Dragoon, EVP and Chief Marketing Officer
Keep students engaged in building vocabulary through crossword puzzles and cloze passages, and by using words in context and making analogies. Lessons build around thematically organized literature and nonfiction selections provide meaningful context for essential vocabulary words.

662 **Workbook for Aphasia**
Wayne State University Press
4809 Woodward Ave
Detroit, MI 48201-1309
313-577-6120
800-978-7323
Fax: 313-577-6131
http://www.wsupress.wayne.edu
bookorders@wayne.edu
Susan Howell Brubaker, Author
Jane Hoehner, Director
Gabe Gloden, Community Engagement Officer
This book gives you materials for adults who have recovered a significant degree of speaking, reading, writing, and comprehension skills. It includes 106 excercises divided into eight target areas. *$65.00*
500 pages

663 **Workbook for Language Skills**
Wayne State University Press
4809 Woodward Ave
Detroit, MI 48201-1309
313-577-6120
800-978-7323
Fax: 313-577-6131
http://wsupress.wayne.edu
bookorders@wayne.edu
Susan Howell Brubaker, Author
Jane Hoehner, Director
Gabe Gloden, Community Engagement Officer
This workbook features 68 real-world exercises designed for use with mildly to severely cognitive and language-impaired individuals. The workbook is divided in seven target areas: Sentence Completion; General Knowledge; Word Recall; Figurative Language; Sentence Comprehension; Sentence Construction and Spelling. *$50.00*
288 pages

Life Skills

664 **Activities for the Elementary Classroom**
Curriculum Associates
153 Rangeway Rd
North Billerica, MA 01862-2013
978-667-8000
800-225-0248
Fax: 800-366-1158
http://www.curriculumassociates.com
cainfo@curriculumassociates.com
Ernest L Kern, Editor
Robert Waldron, President and CEO
Dave Caron, Chief Financial Officer
Challenge your students to make a hole in a 3x5 index card large enough to poke their heads through. Or offer to pour them a glass of air. You'll have their attenion — the first step toward learning — when you use the high-interest, hands-on activities in these exciting teacher resource books.

665 **Activities of Daily Living: A Manual of Group Activities and Written Exercises**
Therapro
225 Arlington St
Framingham, MA 01702-8773
508-872-9494
800-257-5376
Fax: 508-875-2062
http://www.therapro.com
info@therapro.com
Karen McCarthy COTA, Author
Karen Conrad, President
Designed to provide group leaders easy access to structured plans for Activities of Daily Living (ADL) Groups. Organized into five modules: Personal Hygiene; Laundry Skills; Money Management; Leisure Skills and Nutrition. Each includes introduction, assessment guidelines, worksheets to copy, suggested board work, and wrap-up discussions. Appropriate for adult or adolescent programs, school systems and programs for the learning disabled. *$25.00*
136 pages

666 **Aids and Appliances for Independent Living**
Maxi-Aids
42 Executive Blvd
Farmingdale, NY 11735-4710
631-752-0521
800-522-6294
Fax: 631-752-0689
TTY: 631-752-0738
http://www.maxiaids.com
Elliot Zaretsky, President
Thousands of products to make life easier. Eating, dressing, communications, bed, bath, kitchen, writing aids and more.

667 **Changes Around Us CD-ROM**
222 Berkeley Street
Boston, MA 02116
617-351-5000
855-969-4642
Fax: 800-269-5232
http://www.hmhco.com
school.permissions@hmhco.com
Linda K. Zecher, President, CEO & Director
Eric Shuman, Chief Financial Officer
John K. Dragoon, EVP and Chief Marketing Officer
Nature is the natural choice for observing change. By observing and researching dramatic visual sequences such as the stages of development of a butterfly, children develop a broad understanding of the concept of change. As they search this multimedia database for images and information about plant and animal life cycles and seasonal change, students strengthen their abilities in research, analysis, problem-solving, critical thinking and communication.

668 **Classroom Visual Activities**
Therapro
225 Arlington St
Framingham, MA 01702-8773
508-872-9494
800-257-5376
Fax: 508-875-2062
http://www.therapro.com
info@therapro.com

Regina G Richards MA, Author
Karen Conrad, President
This work presents a wealth of activities for the development of visual skills in the areas of pursuit, scanning, aligning, and locating movements; eye hand coordination, and fixation activity. Each activity lists objectives and criteria for success and gives detailed instuctions. *$15.00*
80 pages

669 **Cognitive Strategy Instruction for Middleand High Schools**
Brookline Books
PO Box 1209
Brookline, MA 02446
617-734-6772
800-666-2665
Fax: 617-734-3952
http://www.brooklinebooks.com
brbooks@yahoo.com
Eileen Wood, Editor
Vera E Woloshyn, Editor
Teena Willoughby, Editor
Presents cognitive strategies empirically validated for middle and high school students, with an emphasis for teachers on how to teach and support the strategies. *$26.95*
286 pages
ISBN 1-571290-07-9

670 **Fine Motor Activities Guide and Easel Activities Guide**
Therapro
225 Arlington St
Framingham, MA 01702-8773
508-872-9494
800-257-5376
Fax: 508-875-2062
http://www.therapro.com
info@therapro.com
Jayne Berry OTR, Author
Carol Ann Meyers OTR, Co-Author
Karen Conrad, President
Useful for activity plans or teacher-educator-parent consultations. Perfect hand-outs as part of your inservice packet (no need to write out ideas, photocopy materials, etc). Package of 10 booklets. *$19.00*

671 **Finger Frolics: Fingerplays**
Therapro
225 Arlington St
Framingham, MA 01702-8773
508-872-9494
800-257-5376
Fax: 508-875-2062
http://www.therapro.com
info@therapro.com
Liz Cromwell, Author
Dixie Hibner, Co-Author
John Faitel, Editor
Invaluable for occupational therapists, speech/language pathologists and teachers. Over 350 light and humorous fingerplays help children with rhyming and performing actions which develop fine motor and language skills. *$13.25*

672 **Hands-On Activities for Exceptional Students**
Sage/Corwin Press
2455 Teller Rd
Thousand Oaks, CA 91320-2218
805-499-9734
800-233-9936
Fax: 805-499-5323
http://www.corwinpress.com
order@corwin.com
Mike Soules, President
Beverly Thorne, Author
Lisa Shaw, Executive Director Editorial
This exceptional new release is developed for educators of students who have cognitive delays who will eventually work in a sheltered employment environment. If you need new ideas at your fingertips, this practical book is for you. *$25.95*
112 pages Special Ed
ISBN 1-890455-31-8

673 **Health**
HMH Supplemental Publishers
222 Berkeley Street
Boston, MA 02116
617-351-5000
855-969-4642
Fax: 800-269-5232
http://www.hmhco.com
school.permissions@hmhco.com
Linda K. Zecher, President, CEO & Director
Eric Shuman, Chief Financial Officer
John K. Dragoon, EVP and Chief Marketing Officer
Lessons and projects focus on nutrition, outdoor safety, smart choices, and exercise. Designed to make children more health conscious. Activity formats include fill in the blank, word puzzles, multiple choice, crosswords, and more.

674 **Life-Centered Career Education Training**
Council for Exceptional Children
2900 Crystal Drive
Ste 1000
Arlington, VA 22202-3557
703-620-3660
888-232-7733
Fax: 703-264-9494
TDD: 866-915-5000
TTY: 866-915-5000
http://www.cec.sped.org
service@cec.sped.org
Robin D. Brewer, President
James P. Heiden, President Elect
Christy A. Chambers, Immediate Past President
LCCE teaches you to prepare students to function independently and productively as family members, citizens, and workers, and to enjoy fulfilling personal lives. LCCE is a motivating and effective classroom, home, and community-based curriculum.

675 **MORE: Integrating the Mouth with Sensory & Postural Functions**
Therapro
225 Arlington St
Framingham, MA 01702-8773
508-872-9494
800-257-5376
Fax: 508-875-2062
http://www.therapro.com
info@therapro.com
Patricia Oetter OTR, Author
Eileen Richter OTR, Co-Author
Karen Conrad, President
MORE is an acronym for Motor components, Oral organization, Respiratory demands and Eye contact and control; elements of toys and items that can be used to facilitate integration of the mouth with sensory and postural development, as well as self-regulation and attention. A theoretical framework for the treatment of both sensorimotor and speech/language problems is presented, methods for evaluating therapeutic potential of motor toys, and activities designed to improve functions. *$49.95*

676 **Memory Workbook**
Therapro
225 Arlington St
Framingham, MA 01702-8773
508-872-9494
800-257-5376
Fax: 508-875-2062
http://www.therapro.com
info@therapro.com
Karen Conrad, President
Kathleen Anderson, Author
Pamela Crow Miller, Co-Author
Recalling daily activities, seasons, months of the year, shapes, words and pictures. *$12.50*

677 **One-Handed in a Two-Handed World**
Therapro
225 Arlington St
Framingham, MA 01702-8773
508-872-9494
800-257-5376
Fax: 508-875-2062
http://www.therapro.com
info@therapro.com

Tommye K Mayer, Author
Karen Conrad, President
A personal guide to managing single handed. Written by a woman who has lived one-handed for many years, this book shares a methodology and mindset necessary for managing. It details a wide array of topics including personal care, daily chores, office work, traveling, sports, relationships and many more. A must for patients and therapists. *$19.95*
250 pages

678 **People at Work**
Pearson AGS Globe
PO Box 2500
Lebanon, IN 46052-3009
800-992-0244
Fax: 877-260-2530
http://www.pearsonschool.com
Marjorie Scardino, CEO
Victor Coira, Sales Representative
Victoria Ramos, Digital Sales Rep
With an interest level of High School through Adult, ABE and ESL and a reading level of Grades 3-4, this program is a simple, thorough teaching plan for every day of the school year. The program's 180 sessions are divided into eighteen study units that each survey an entire occupational cluster of eight jobs while focusing on one or two writing skills. *$26.95*

679 **Responding to Oral Directions**
Pro-Ed
8700 Shoal Creek Blvd
Austin, TX 78757-6897
512-451-3246
800-897-3202
Fax: 800-397-7633
http://www.proedinc.com
info@proedinc.com
Robert A Mancuso, Author
Help children of all ages who function at first through sixth-grade levels learn to identify unclear directions and ask for clarification. Nine units teach them how to handle: recognizing directions, carryover and generalization; unreasonable, distorted, vague, unfamiliar, lenngthy, unknown, and mixed directions. Item number 190575116. *$59.00*

680 **So What Can I Do?**
Therapro
225 Arlington St
Framingham, MA 01702-8773
508-872-9494
800-257-5376
Fax: 508-875-2062
http://www.therapro.com
info@therapro.com
Gail Kushnir, Author
Karen Conrad, President
A book to help children develop their own solutions to everyday problems. Cartoon illustrations feature common situations for children to analyze. The adult asks the child, so what can you do? The child is then encouraged to think of creative solutions, developing their emotional intelligence and improving coping skills. 58 problems to solve. *$10.95*

681 **Special Needs Program**
Dallas Metro Care
1380 River Bend Drive
Dallas, TX 75247
214-743-1200
877-283-2121
Fax: 214-630-3469
http://www.metrocareservices.org
metrocare@metrocareservices.org
Jill Martinez, Chairman
Judy N. Myers, Vice Chairman
Corey Golomb, Secretary
The special needs curriculum teaches students with disabilities the life skills they need to achieve self-sufficiency. The program focuses on and enhances coping skills.

682 **Stepwise Cookbooks**
Therapro
225 Arlington St
Framingham, MA 01702-8773
508-872-9494
800-257-5376
Fax: 508-875-2062
http://www.therapro.com
info@therapro.com
Beth Jackson, Author
Karen Conrad, President
A chance for children and adults at all developmental levels to participate in fun-filled hands-on cooking activities while developing independence. These cookbooks were developed by an OT working with children and teenagers with cognitive and physical challenges. Only one direction is presented on a page to reduce confusion. Recipes are represented by large Boardmaker symbols from Mayer Johnson. Large, easy-to-read text with dividing lines for visual clarity. *$52.50*

683 **Strategies for Problem-Solving**
Houghton Mifflin Harcourt
222 Berkeley Street
Boston, MA 02116
617-351-5000
855-969-4642
Fax: 800-269-5232
http://www.hmhco.com
school.permissions@hmhco.com
Arnold Yellin, Author
Linda K. Zecher, President, CEO & Director
Eric Shuman, Chief Financial Officer
Show students more than one way to approach a problem, and you hand them the key to effective problem solving. These reproducible activities build math reasoning and critical thinking skills, reinforce core concepts, and reduce math anxiety too. *$11.99*

684 **Survey of Teenage Readiness and Neurodevelopmental Status**
Educators Publishing Service
PO Box 9031
Cambridge, MA 02139-9031
617-547-6706
800-225-5750
Fax: 617-547-3805
http://www.epsbooks.com
CustomerService.EPS@schoolspecialty.com
Melvin D Levine MD FAAP, Author
Stephen R. Hooper, Ph.D., Co-Author
Rick Holden, President
Developed by Dr. Mel Livine and Dr.Stephen Hooper, The Survey of Teenage Readiness and Neurodevelopmental Status capitalizes on adolescents' evolving metacognitive abilities by directly asking them for their perceptions of how they are functioning in school and how they process information across a variety of neurocognitive and psychosocial domains.

685 **Swallow Right 2nd Edition**
Therapro
225 Arlington St
Framingham, MA 01702-8773
508-872-9494
800-257-5376
Fax: 508-875-2062
http://www.therapro.com
info@therapro.com
Roberta B Pierce, Author
Karen Conrad, President
This 12-session program evaluates and treats oral myofunctional disorders. 40 reproducible sequential exercises train individuals from five years to adult how to swallow correctly. Easy-to-use evaluation and tracking forms, checklist, and carryover strategies make this book a real time-saver! Item number Q858. *$55.00*

686 **Target Spelling**
Houghton Mifflin Harcourt
222 Berkeley Street
Boston, MA 02116
617-351-5000
855-969-4642
Fax: 800-269-5232
http://www.hmhco.com
school.permissions@hmhco.com
Linda K. Zecher, President, CEO & Director
Eric Shuman, Chief Financial Officer
John K. Dragoon, EVP and Chief Marketing Officer
You can differentiate instructions to address a variety of learning styles and profiles and meet the needs of special education students.

687 **Teaching Dressing Skills: Buttons, Bowsand More**
Therapro
225 Arlington St
Framingham, MA 01702-8773
508-872-9494
800-257-5376
Fax: 508-875-2062
http://www.therapro.com
info@therapro.com
Marcy Coppelman Goldsmith, Author
Karen Conrad, President
Consists of 5 fold-out pamphlets for teaching children and adults of varying abilities the basic dressing skills: shoe tying, buttoning, zippering, dressing and undressing. Each task is broken down with every step clearly illustrated and specific verbal directions given to avoid confusion and to eliminate excess verbiage that can distract the learner. The author, an experienced OT, has included the needed prerequisites for each task, many great teaching tips and more.
$10.50
5 Pamphlets

688 **ThemeWeavers: Animals Activity Kit**
Riverdeep
14046 Collections Center Drive
Chicago, IL 60693
855-969-4642
Fax: 800-269-5232
http://www.hmhinnovation.com
school.permissions@hmhco.com
Linda K. Zecher, President and CEO
Eric Shuman, Chief Financial Officer
John K. Dragoon, EVP
ThemeWeavers: Animals is the essential companion for theme-based teaching. Dozens of animal-themed, interactive activities immediately engage your students to practice fundamental skills in math, language arts, science, social studies and more. Easy-to-use tools allow you to modify these activities or create your own to meet specific classroom needs.

689 **ThemeWeavers: Nature Activity Kit**
Riverdeep
14046 Collections Center Drive
Chicago, IL 60693
855-969-4642
Fax: 800-269-5232
http://www.hmhinnovation.com
school.permissions@hmhco.com
Linda K. Zecher, President and CEO
Eric Shuman, Chief Financial Officer
John K. Dragoon, EVP
ThemeWeavers: Nature Activity Kit is an all-in-one solution for theme-based teaching. In just a few minutes, you can select from dozens of ready-to-use activities centering on the seasons and weather and be ready for the next day's lesson! Interactive and engaging activities cover multiple subject areas such as language arts, math, science, social studies and art.

690 **Thinkin' Science ZAP**
Riverdeep
14046 Collections Center Drive
Chicago, IL 60693
855-969-4642
Fax: 800-269-5232
http://www.hmhinnovation.com
school.permissions@hmhco.com
Linda K. Zecher, President and CEO
Eric Shuman, Chief Financial Officer
John K. Dragoon, EVP
It is a dark and stormy night as you step backstage to be guest director at the Wonder Dome, the world-famous auditorium of light, sound, and electricity. But great zotz! The Theater has been zapped by lightning, and the Laser Control System is on the fritz! Can you learn all about light, sound and electricity to rescue the show? *$69.95*

691 **Time: Concepts & Problem-Solving**
Houghton Mifflin Harcourt
222 Berkeley Street
Boston, MA 02116
617-351-5000
855-969-4642
Fax: 800-269-5232
http://www.hmhco.com
school.permissions@hmhco.com
Linda K. Zecher, President, CEO & Director
Eric Shuman, Chief Financial Officer
John K. Dragoon, EVP and Chief Marketing Officer
Develop concepts of telling time, identifying intervals, calculating elapsed time, and solving problems that deal with time changes, lapses, and changes over the AM/PM cusp.

692 **Travel the World with Timmy Deluxe**
Riverdeep
14046 Collections Center Drive
Chicago, IL 60693
855-969-4642
Fax: 800-269-5232
http://www.hmhinnovation.com
school.permissions@hmhco.com
Linda K. Zecher, President and CEO
Eric Shuman, Chief Financial Officer
John K. Dragoon, EVP
France and Russia are the newest destinations for Edmark's favorite world traveler, Timmy! In this delightful and improved program, students will enjoy expanding their understanding of the world around them. With wonderful stories, songs, games, and printable crafts, early learners discover how their international neighbors live, dress, sing, eat and play.

693 **Workbook for Reasoning Skills**
Wayne State University Press
4809 Woodward Ave
Detroit, MI 48201-1309
313-577-6120
800-978-7323
Fax: 313-577-6131
http://wsupress.wayne.edu
bookorders@wayne.edu
Susan Howell Brubaker, Author
Jane Hoehner, Director
Gabe Gloden, Community Engagement Officer
This workbook is designed for adults and children who need practice in reasoning, thinking, and organizing. Includes 67 exercises created for individuals with closed head injuries and mild to moderate cognitive deficits. Item number W332.
$60.00
328 pages

Math

694 **Algebra Stars**
Sunburst Technology
1550 Executive Dr
Elgin, IL 60123-9311
800-321-7511
Fax: 888-608-0344
http://store.sunburst.com
service@sunburst.com
Michael Guillory, Channel Sales/Marketing Manager
Students build their understanding of algebra by constructing, categorizing, and solving equations and classifying polynomial expressions using algebra tiles.

695 **Attack Math**
Educators Publishing Service
PO Box 9031
Cambridge, MA 02139-9031
617-547-6706
800-225-5750
Fax: 617-547-3805
http://www.epsbooks.com
CustomerService.EPS@schoolspecialty.com
Carole Greenes, Author
George Immerzeel, Co-Author
Linda Schulman, Co-Author
This series, for grades 1-6, teaches the four arithmetic operations: addition, subtraction, multiplication and division. Each operation is covered in three books, with book one teaching the basic facts and books two and three teaching multi-digit computation with whole numbers. A checkpoint and testpoint monitor progress at the middle and end of each book.

696 **Awesome Animated Monster Maker Math**
Sunburst Technology
1550 Executive Dr
Elgin, IL 60123-9311
800-321-7511
Fax: 888-608-0344
http://store.sunburst.com
service@sunburst.com
Michael Guillory, Channel Sales/Marketing Manager
With an emphasis on building core math skills, this humorous program incorporates the monstrous and the ridiculous into a structured learning environment. Students choose from six skill levels tailored to the 3rd to 8th grade.

697 **Basic Essentials of Math: Whole Numbers, Fractions, & Decimals Workbook**
Houghton Mifflin Harcourt
222 Berkeley Street
Boston, MA 02116
617-351-5000
855-969-4642
Fax: 800-269-5232
http://www.hmhco.com
school.permissions@hmhco.com
James T Shea, Author
Linda K. Zecher, President, CEO & Director
Eric Shuman, Chief Financial Officer
Ideal for basic math skill instruction, test practice, or any situation requiring a thorough, confidence-building review. It provides a complete lesson - instruction, examples, and computation exercises. *$19.00*

698 **Building Mathematical Thinking**
Educators Publishing Service
PO Box 9031
Cambridge, MA 02139-9031
617-547-6706
800-225-5750
Fax: 617-547-3805
http://www.epsbooks.com
CustomerService.EPS@schoolspecialty.com
Marsha Stanton, Author
Rick Holden, President
Jeff Belanger, Regional Sales Manager
In this new math program, the units covered are presented as a series of Skinny Concepts that serve as manageable building blocks that eventually become entire topics. The Students Journal provides exercises for each Skinny Concept, encourages students to seek their own conclusions for problem solving, and provides space for the students ideas.

699 **Building Perspective**
Sunburst Technology
1550 Executive Dr
Elgin, IL 60123-9311
800-321-7511
Fax: 888-608-0344
http://store.sunburst.com
service@sunburst.com
Michael Guillory, Channel Sales/Marketing Manager
Develop spatial perception and reasoning skills with this award-winning program that will sharpen your students' problem-solving abilities.

700 **Building Perspective Deluxe**
Sunburst Technology
1550 Executive Dr
Elgin, IL 60123-9311
800-321-7511
Fax: 888-608-0344
http://store.sunburst.com
service@sunburst.com
Michael Guillory, Channel Sales/Marketing Manager
New visual thinking challenges await your students as they engage in three spacial reasoning activities that develop their 3D thinking, deductive reasoning and problem solving skills

701 **Combining Shapes**
Sunburst Technology
1550 Executive Dr
Elgin, IL 60123-9311
800-321-7511
Fax: 888-608-0344
http://store.sunburst.com
service@sunburst.com
Michael Guillory, Channel Sales/Marketing Manager
Students discover the properties of simple geometric figures through concrete experience combining shapes. Measurements, estimating and operation skills are part of this fun program.

702 **Concert Tour Entrepreneur**
Sunburst Technology
1550 Executive Dr
Elgin, IL 60123-9311
800-321-7511
Fax: 888-608-0344
http://store.sunburst.com
service@sunburst.com
Michael Guillory, Channel Sales/Marketing Manager
Your students improve math, planning and problem solving skills as they manage a band in this music management business simulation.

703 **Creating Patterns from Shapes**
Sunburst Technology
1550 Executive Dr
Elgin, IL 60123-9311
800-321-7511
Fax: 888-608-0344
http://store.sunburst.com
service@sunburst.com
Michael Guillory, Channel Sales/Marketing Manager
Students discover patterns by exploring the properties of radiating and tiling patterns through Native American basket weaving and Japanese fish print themes.

704 **Data Explorer**
Sunburst Technology
1550 Executive Dr
Elgin, IL 60123-9311
800-321-7511
Fax: 888-608-0344
http://store.sunburst.com
service@sunburst.com
Michael Guillory, Channel Sales/Marketing Manager
This easy-to-use CD-ROM provides the flexibility needed for eleven different graph types including tools for long-term data analysis projects.

705 **Decimals: Concepts & Problem-Solving**
Houghton Mifflin Harcourt
222 Berkeley Street
Boston, MA 02116
617-351-5000
855-969-4642
Fax: 800-269-5232
http://www.hmhco.com
school.permissions@hmhco.com
Linda K. Zecher, President, CEO & Director
Eric Shuman, Chief Financial Officer
John K. Dragoon, EVP and Chief Marketing Officer
This easy to implement, flexible companion to the classroom mathematics curriculum emcompasses decimal concepts such as values and names, equivalent decimals, mixed decimals, patterns, comparing, ordering, estimating and more.

706 **Equation Tile Teaser**
Sunburst Technology
1550 Executive Dr
Elgin, IL 60123-9311
800-321-7511
Fax: 888-608-0344
http://store.sunburst.com
service@sunburst.com
Michael Guillory, Channel Sales/Marketing Manager
Students develop logic thinking and pre-algebra skills solving sets of numbers equations in three challenging problem-solving activities.

707 **Factory Deluxe**
Sunburst Technology
1550 Executive Dr
Elgin, IL 60123-9311
800-321-7511
Fax: 888-608-0344
http://store.sunburst.com
service@sunburst.com
Michael Guillory, Channel Sales/Marketing Manager
Five activities explore shapes, rotation, angles, geometric attributes, area formulas, and computation. Includes journal, record keeping, and on-screen help. This program helps sharpen geometry, visual thinking and problem solving skills.

708 **Focus on Math**
Houghton Mifflin Harcourt
222 Berkeley Street
Boston, MA 02116
617-351-5000
855-969-4642
Fax: 800-269-5232
http://www.hmhco.com
school.permissions@hmhco.com
Linda K. Zecher, President, CEO & Director
Eric Shuman, Chief Financial Officer
John K. Dragoon, EVP and Chief Marketing Officer
omnsists of four sections and in each you will learn more about addition and subtraction, multiplication and division, fractions, decimals, measurements, geometry and problem solving.

709 **Fraction Attraction**
Sunburst Technology
1550 Executive Dr
Elgin, IL 60123-9311
800-321-7511
Fax: 888-608-0344
http://store.sunburst.com
service@sunburst.com
Michael Guillory, Channel Sales/Marketing Manager
Build the fraction skills of ordering, equivalence, relative sizes and multiple representations with four, multi-level, carnival style games.

710 **Fractions: Concepts & Problem-Solving**
Houghton Mifflin Harcourt
222 Berkeley Street
Boston, MA 02116
617-351-5000
855-969-4642
Fax: 800-269-5232
http://www.hmhco.com
school.permissions@hmhco.com
Linda K. Zecher, President, CEO & Director
Eric Shuman, Chief Financial Officer
John K. Dragoon, EVP and Chief Marketing Officer
This companion to the classroom mathematics curriculum emcompasses many of the standards established at each grade level. Each activity page targets a specific skill to help bolster students who need additional work in a particular area of fractions.

711 **GEPA Success in Language Arts Literacy and Mathematics**
Houghton Mifflin Harcourt
222 Berkeley Street
Boston, MA 02116
617-351-5000
855-969-4642
Fax: 800-269-5232
http://www.hmhco.com
school.permissions@hmhco.com
Estell Kleinman, Author
Linda K. Zecher, President, CEO & Director
Eric Shuman, Chief Financial Officer
Build skills as you improve scores on the GEPA. Better test scores don't always mean better skills. With these workbooks, you can ensure that your students are becoming more proficient users of language and math as well as more skilled test-takers. Your students will gain valuable practice answering the types of questions found on the GEPA, such as open-ended and enhanced multiple-choice items. *$17.60*

712 **Geometry for Primary Grades**
Houghton Mifflin Harcourt
222 Berkeley Street
Boston, MA 02116
617-351-5000
855-969-4642
Fax: 800-269-5232
http://www.hmhco.com
school.permissions@hmhco.com
Linda K. Zecher, President, CEO & Director
Eric Shuman, Chief Financial Officer
John K. Dragoon, EVP and Chief Marketing Officer
Self-explanatory lessons ideal for independent work or as homework. Transitions from concrete to pictorial to abstract.

713 **Get Up and Go!**
Sunburst Technology
1550 Executive Dr
Elgin, IL 60123-9311
800-321-7511
Fax: 888-608-0344
http://store.sunburst.com
service@sunburst.com
Michael Guillory, Channel Sales/Marketing Manager
Students interpret and construct timelines through three descriptive activities in the animated program. Students are introduced to timelines as they participate in an interactive story.

714 **Grade Level Math**
Houghton Mifflin Harcourt
222 Berkeley Street
Boston, MA 02116
617-351-5000
855-969-4642
Fax: 800-269-5232
http://www.hmhco.com
school.permissions@hmhco.com
Linda K. Zecher, President, CEO & Director
Eric Shuman, Chief Financial Officer
John K. Dragoon, EVP and Chief Marketing Officer
Easy to understand practice exercises help students build conceptual knowledge and computation skills together. Each book addresses essential grade appropriate math areas.

715 **Graphers**
Sunburst Technology
1550 Executive Dr
Elgin, IL 60123-9311
800-321-7511
Fax: 888-608-0344
http://store.sunburst.com
service@sunburst.com
Michael Guillory, Channel Sales/Marketing Manager
Students develop data analysis skills with this easy to use graphing tool. With over 30 pictorial data sets and 16 lessons, students learn to construct and interpret six different graph types.

716 **Green Globs & Graphing Equations**
Sunburst Technology
1550 Executive Dr
Elgin, IL 60123-9311
800-321-7511
Fax: 888-608-0344
http://store.sunburst.com
service@sunburst.com
Michael Guillory, Channel Sales/Marketing Manager
As students explore parabolas, hyperbolas, and other graphs, they discover how altering an equation changes a graph's shape or position.

717 **Hidden Treasures of Al-Jabr**
Sunburst Technology
1550 Executive Dr
Elgin, IL 60123-9311
800-321-7511
Fax: 888-608-0344
http://store.sunburst.com
service@sunburst.com
Michael Guillory, Channel Sales/Marketing Manager
Beginning algebra students undertake three challenges that develop skills in the areas of solving linear equations, substituting variables, grouping like variables, using systems of equations and translating algebra word problems into equations.

718 **High School Math Bundle**
Sunburst Technology
1550 Executive Dr
Elgin, IL 60123-9311
800-321-7511
Fax: 888-608-0344
http://store.sunburst.com
service@sunburst.com
Michael Guillory, Channel Sales/Marketing Manager
Each program in this bundle focuses on a specific area to ensure that your students master the math skills they need. This bundle allows students to master basics of Algebra, explore equations and graphs, practice learning with algebra graphs, use trigonometric functions, apply math concepts to practical situations and improve problem solving and data analysis skills.

719 **Higher Scores on Math Standardized Tests**
Harcourt Achieve
222 Berkeley Street
Boston, MA 02116
617-351-5000
855-969-4642
Fax: 800-269-5232
http://www.hmhco.com
school.permissions@hmhco.com
Linda K. Zecher, President, CEO & Director
Eric Shuman, Chief Financial Officer
John K. Dragoon, EVP and Chief Marketing Officer
These grade level math test preparation series provide focused practice in areas where students have shown a weakness in previous standardized tests. Improves test scores by zeroing in on the skills requiring remediation.

720 **Hot Dog Stand: The Works**
Sunburst Technology
1550 Executive Dr
Elgin, IL 60123-9311
800-321-7511
Fax: 888-608-0344
http://store.sunburst.com
service@sunburst.com
Michael Guillory, Channel Sales/Marketing Manager
Students practice math, problem-solving, and communication skills in a multimedia business simulation that challenges students with unexpected events.

721 **How the West Was 1+3x4**
Sunburst Technology
1550 Executive Dr
Elgin, IL 60123-9311
800-321-7511
Fax: 888-608-0344
http://store.sunburst.com
service@sunburst.com
Michael Guillory, Channel Sales/Marketing Manager
Students use order of operations to construct equations and race along number line trails.

722 **Ice Cream Truck**
Sunburst Technology
1550 Executive Dr
Elgin, IL 60123-9311
800-321-7511
Fax: 888-608-0344
http://store.sunburst.com
service@sunburst.com
Michael Guillory, Channel Sales/Marketing Manager
Elementary students learn important problem solving, strategic planning and math operation skills, as they become owners of a busy ice cream truck.

723 **Intermediate Geometry**
Houghton Mifflin Harcourt
222 Berkeley Street
Boston, MA 02116
617-351-5000
855-969-4642
Fax: 800-269-5232
http://www.hmhco.com
school.permissions@hmhco.com
Linda K. Zecher, President, CEO & Director
Eric Shuman, Chief Financial Officer
John K. Dragoon, EVP and Chief Marketing Officer
Prepares intermediate and middle school students for a successful experience in high school geometry. Intermediate geometry provides a study of the concepts, computation, problem-solving, and enrichment of topics identified by NCTM standards. This three-book series links the informal explorations of geometry in primary grades to more formalized processes taught in high school.

724 **Introduction to Patterns**
Sunburst Technology
1550 Executive Dr
Elgin, IL 60123-9311
800-321-7511
Fax: 888-608-0344
http://store.sunburst.com
service@sunburst.com
Michael Guillory, Channel Sales/Marketing Manager
Students discover patterns found in art and nature, exploring linear and geometric designs, predicting outcomes and creating patterns of their own.

725 **Mastering Math**
Houghton Mifflin Harcourt
222 Berkeley Street
Boston, MA 02116
617-351-5000
855-969-4642
Fax: 800-269-5232
http://www.hmhco.com
school.permissions@hmhco.com
Linda K. Zecher, President, CEO & Director
Eric Shuman, Chief Financial Officer
John K. Dragoon, EVP and Chief Marketing Officer
Now low level readers can succeed at math with this easy to read presentation. Makes basic math concepts accessible to all students.

726 **Measurement: Practical Applications**
Houghton Mifflin Harcourt
222 Berkeley Street
Boston, MA 02116
617-351-5000
855-969-4642
Fax: 800-269-5232
http://www.hmhco.com
school.permissions@hmhco.com
Linda K. Zecher, President, CEO & Director
Eric Shuman, Chief Financial Officer
John K. Dragoon, EVP and Chief Marketing Officer
Concentrated practice on the measurement skills we use on a daily basis. This practical presentation of both customary and metric units helps the student to understand the importance of measurement skills in everyday life. Hands on activities and real life situations create logical applications so measurements make sense.

727 **Memory Fun!**
Sunburst Technology
1550 Executive Dr
Elgin, IL 60123-9311
800-321-7511
Fax: 888-608-0344
http://store.sunburst.com
service@sunburst.com
Michael Guillory, Channel Sales/Marketing Manager
Welcome to Tiny's attic where students build memory, matching, counting and money sense through a variety of fun matching activities.

728 **Middle School Math Bundle**
Sunburst Technology
1550 Executive Dr
Elgin, IL 60123-9311
800-321-7511
Fax: 888-608-0344
http://store.sunburst.com
service@sunburst.com
Michael Guillory, Channel Sales/Marketing Manager
This bundle helps improve student's logical thinking, number sense and operation skills. This product comes with Math Arena, Building Perspective Deluxe, Equation Tile Teasers and Easy Sheet.

729 **Middle School Math Collection Geometry Basic Concepts**
Houghton Mifflin Harcourt
222 Berkeley Street
Boston, MA 02116
617-351-5000
855-969-4642
Fax: 800-269-5232
http://www.hmhco.com
school.permissions@hmhco.com
Linda K. Zecher, President, CEO & Director
Eric Shuman, Chief Financial Officer
John K. Dragoon, EVP and Chief Marketing Officer
Provides students with enough comprehensive, skill specific practice in the key areas of geometry to ensure mastery. Ideal for junior high or high school students in need of remediation.

730 **MindTwister Math**
Riverdeep
14046 Collections Center Drive
Chicago, IL 60693
855-969-4642
Fax: 800-269-5232
http://www.hmhinnovation.com
school.permissions@hmhco.com
Linda K. Zecher, President and CEO
Eric Shuman, Chief Financial Officer
John K. Dragoon, EVP
MindTwister Math provides a challenging review of third grade math and problem-solving skills in a fast-paced, multi-player game show format. Thousands of action-packed challenges encourage students to practice essential math facts including addition, subtraction, mutiplication and division and develop more advanced mathematical problem-solving skills such as visualization, deduction, sequencing, estimating and pattern recognition.

731 **Mirror Symmetry**
Sunburst Technology
1550 Executive Dr
Elgin, IL 60123-9311
800-321-7511
Fax: 888-608-0344
http://store.sunburst.com
service@sunburst.com
Michael Guillory, Channel Sales/Marketing Manager
Students advance their understanding of geometric properties and spatial relationships by exploring lines of symmetry within a single geometric shape.

732 **Multiplication & Division**
Houghton Mifflin Harcourt
222 Berkeley Street
Boston, MA 02116
617-351-5000
855-969-4642
Fax: 800-269-5232
http://www.hmhco.com
school.permissions@hmhco.com
Linda K. Zecher, President, CEO & Director
Eric Shuman, Chief Financial Officer
John K. Dragoon, EVP and Chief Marketing Officer
Skill specific activities focus on the concepts and inverse relationships of multiplication and division. Explains in simplified terms how the process of multiplication undoes the process of division, and vice versa.

733 **My Mathematical Life**
Sunburst Technology
1550 Executive Dr
Elgin, IL 60123-9311
800-321-7511
Fax: 888-608-0344
http://store.sunburst.com
service@sunburst.com
Michael Guillory, Channel Sales/Marketing Manager
Students discover the math involved in everyday living as they take a character from high school graduation to retirement, advising on important health, education, career, and financial decisions.

734 **Nimble Numeracy: Fluency in Counting and Basic Arithmetic**
Oxton House Publishers
PO Box 209
Farmington, ME 04938
207-779-1923
800-539-7323
Fax: 207-779-0623
http://www.oxtonhouse.com
info@oxtonhouse.com
Dr. Phyllis E. Fischer, Author
William Berlinghoff PhD, Managing Editor
Bobby Brown, Marketing Director
Dr. Phyllis Fischer, Author
This is a richly detailed handbook for teachers, tutors, and parents who want to help children develop fluent arithmetric skills. It provides explicit techniques for teaching counting and basic arithmetic, with special emphasis on the language of our base-ten, place-value system for speaking about and writing numbers. *$19.95*
136 pages
ISBN 1-881929-19-1

735 **Number Meanings and Counting**
Sunburst Technology
1550 Executive Dr
Elgin, IL 60123-9311
800-321-7511
Fax: 888-608-0344
http://store.sunburst.com
service@sunburst.com
Michael Guillory, Channel Sales/Marketing Manager
Students develop their understanding of number meaning and uses with experiences practicing estimating, using number meanings, and making more-and-less comparisons.

736 **Number Sense & Problem Solving CD-ROM**
Sunburst Technology
1550 Executive Dr
Elgin, IL 60123-9311
800-321-7511
Fax: 888-608-0344
http://store.sunburst.com
service@sunburst.com
Michael Guillory, Channel Sales/Marketing Manager
Build number and operation skills with these three programs: How the West Was One + Three x Four, Divide and Conquer and Puzzle Tanks.

737 **Numbers Undercover**
Sunburst Technology
1550 Executive Dr
Elgin, IL 60123-9311
800-321-7511
Fax: 888-608-0344
http://store.sunburst.com
service@sunburst.com
Michael Guillory, Channel Sales/Marketing Manager
As children try to solve the case of missing numbers, they practice telling time, measuring and estimating, counting, and working with money.

738 **Penny Pot**
Sunburst Technology
1550 Executive Dr
Elgin, IL 60123-9311
800-321-7511
Fax: 888-608-0344
http://store.sunburst.com
service@sunburst.com
Michael Guillory, Channel Sales/Marketing Manager
Students learn about money as they count combinations of coins in this engaging program.

739 **Problemas y mas**
Houghton Mifflin Harcourt
222 Berkeley Street
Boston, MA 02116
617-351-5000
855-969-4642
Fax: 800-269-5232
http://www.hmhco.com
school.permissions@hmhco.com
Alan Handel, Author
Linda K. Zecher, President, CEO & Director
Eric Shuman, Chief Financial Officer
This ESL math practice and strategy tool is in three levels the same as Problems Plus, but expressly for your Spanish fluent ESL learners. *$13.40*
ISBN 0-811495-93-0

740 **Problems Plus Level H**
Houghton Mifflin Achieve
222 Berkeley Street
Boston, MA 02116
617-351-5000
855-969-4642
Fax: 800-269-5232
http://www.hmhco.com
school.permissions@hmhco.com
Francis J Gardella, Author
Linda K. Zecher, President, CEO & Director
Eric Shuman, Chief Financial Officer
A one-of-a-kind guide to solving open-ended math problems. Doesn't just give answers to test questions. With its innovative problem-solving plan, this series teaches math thinking and problem attack strategies, plus offers practice in higher order thinking skills students need to solve open-ended math problems successfully. *$15.10*

741 **Puzzle Tanks**
Sunburst Technology
1550 Executive Dr
Elgin, IL 60123-9311
800-321-7511
Fax: 888-608-0344
http://store.sunburst.com
service@sunburst.com
Michael Guillory, Channel Sales/Marketing Manager
A problem-solving program that uses logic puzzles involving liquid measurements.

742 **Representing Fractions**
Sunburst Technology
1550 Executive Dr
Elgin, IL 60123-9311
800-321-7511
Fax: 888-608-0344
http://store.sunburst.com
service@sunburst.com
Michael Guillory, Channel Sales/Marketing Manager
In this investigation students work with one interpretation of a fraction and the relationship between parts and wholes by working with symbolic and visual representations.

743 **Sequencing Fun!**
Sunburst Technology
1550 Executive Dr
Elgin, IL 60123-9311
800-321-7511
Fax: 888-608-0344
http://store.sunburst.com
service@sunburst.com
Michael Guillory, Channel Sales/Marketing Manager
Text, pictures, animation, and video clips provide a fun-filled program that encourages critical thinking skills.

744 **Shape Up!**
Sunburst Technology
1550 Executive Dr
Elgin, IL 60123-9311
800-321-7511
Fax: 888-608-0344
http://store.sunburst.com
service@sunburst.com
Michael Guillory, Channel Sales/Marketing Manager
Students actively create and manipulate shapes to discover important ideas about mathematics in an electronic playground of two and three dimensional shapes.

745 **Shapes Within Shapes**
Sunburst Technology
1550 Executive Dr
Elgin, IL 60123-9311
800-321-7511
Fax: 888-608-0344
http://store.sunburst.com
service@sunburst.com
Michael Guillory, Channel Sales/Marketing Manager
Students identify shapes within shapes, then rearrange them to develop spatial sense and deepen their understanding of the properties of shapes.

746 **Spatial Relationships**
Sunburst Technology
1550 Executive Dr
Elgin, IL 60123-9311
888-492-8817
Fax: 888-608-0344
http://store.sunburst.com
service@sunburst.com
Michael Guillory, Channel Sales/Marketing Manager
Students explore location by identifying the positions of objects and creating paths between places. Children develop spatial abilities and language needed to communicate about our world.

747 **Speed Drills for Arithmetic Facts**
Oxton House Publishers
PO Box 209
Farmington, ME 04938
207-779-1923
800-539-7323
Fax: 207-779-0623
http://www.oxtonhouse.com
info@oxtonhouse.com
William Berlinghoff PhD, Managing Editor
Bobby Brown, Marketing Director
Dr. Phyllis Fischer, Author
This looseleaf packet is a set of 48 pages of carefully constructed exercises to promote automaticity with basic arithmetic facts. The worksheets reinforce the interrelationship of three numbers in addition/subtraction and multiplication/division statements. Also included are six pages of detailed teaching advice and a chart template for tracking student progress. *$24.95*
54 pages
ISBN 1-881929-16-7

748 **Splish Splash Math**
Sunburst Technology
1550 Executive Dr
Elgin, IL 60123-9311
800-321-7511
Fax: 888-608-0344
http://store.sunburst.com
service@sunburst.com
Michael Guillory, Channel Sales/Marketing Manager

Students learn and practice basic operation skills as they engage in this high interest program that keeps them motivated. Great visual rewards and three levels of difficulty keep students challanged.

749 **Strategies for Problem-Solving**
Houghton Mifflin Harcourt
222 Berkeley Street
Boston, MA 02116
617-351-5000
855-969-4642
Fax: 800-269-5232
http://www.hmhco.com
school.permissions@hmhco.com
Arnold Yellin, Author
Linda K. Zecher, President, CEO & Director
Eric Shuman, Chief Financial Officer
Show students more than one way to approach a problem, and you hand them the key to effective problem solving. These reproducible activities build math reasoning and critical thinking skills, reinforce core concepts, and reduce math anxiety, too. *$11.99*
ISBN 0-817267-61-1

750 **Strategies for Success in Mathematics**
Houghton Mifflin Harcourt
222 Berkeley Street
Boston, MA 02116
617-351-5000
855-969-4642
Fax: 800-269-5232
http://www.hmhco.com
school.permissions@hmhco.com
June Coultas, Author
Linda K. Zecher, President, CEO & Director
Eric Shuman, Chief Financial Officer
Teach your students specific problem-solving skills and test taking strategies for success with math and math assessments. Practice thoroughly covers five math clusters: numerical operations, patterns and functions, algebraic concepts, measurement and geometry, and data analysis. *$16.60*

751 **Sunbuddy Math Playhouse**
Sunburst Technology
1550 Executive Dr
Elgin, IL 60123-9311
800-321-7511
Fax: 888-608-0344
http://store.sunburst.com
service@sunburst.com
Michael Guillory, Channel Sales/Marketing Manager
An entertaining play, hidden math-related animations, and four multi-level interactive activities encourage children to explore math and reading.

752 **Ten Tricky Tiles**
Sunburst Technology
1550 Executive Dr
Elgin, IL 60123-9311
800-321-7511
Fax: 888-608-0344
http://store.sunburst.com
service@sunburst.com
Michael Guillory, Channel Sales/Marketing Manager
Students develop their arithmetic and logic skills with three levels of activities that involve solving sets of numbers sentences.

753 **Tenth Planet: Combining and Breaking Apart Numbers**
Sunburst Technology
1550 Executive Dr
Elgin, IL 60123-9311
800-321-7511
Fax: 888-608-0344
http://store.sunburst.com
service@sunburst.com
Michael Guillory, Channel Sales/Marketing Manager
Students develop their number sense as they engage in real life dilemmas, which demonstrates the basic concepts of operations.

754 **Tenth Planet: Comparing with Ratios**
Sunburst Technology
1550 Executive Dr
Elgin, IL 60123-9311
800-321-7511
Fax: 888-608-0344
http://store.sunburst.com
service@sunburst.com
Michael Guillory, Channel Sales/Marketing Manager
Students learn that ratio is a way to compare amounts by using multiplication and division. Through five engaging activities, students recognize and describe ratios, develop proportional thinking skills, estimate ratios, determine equivalent ratios, and use ratios to analyze data.

755 **Tenth Planet: Equivalent Fractions**
Sunburst Technology
1550 Executive Dr
Elgin, IL 60123-9311
800-321-7511
Fax: 888-608-0344
http://store.sunburst.com
service@sunburst.com
Michael Guillory, Channel Sales/Marketing Manager
This exciting investigation develops students' conceptual understanding that every fraction can be named in many different but equivalent ways.

756 **Tenth Planet: Fraction Operations**
Sunburst Technology
1550 Executive Dr
Elgin, IL 60123-9311
800-321-7511
Fax: 888-608-0344
http://store.sunburst.com
service@sunburst.com
Michael Guillory, Channel Sales/Marketing Manager
Students build on their concepts of fraction meaning and equivalence as they learn how to perform operations with fractions.

757 **Tenth Planet: Grouping and Place Value**
Sunburst Technology
1550 Executive Dr
Elgin, IL 60123-9311
800-321-7511
Fax: 888-608-0344
http://store.sunburst.com
service@sunburst.com
Michael Guillory, Channel Sales/Marketing Manager
Students develop their understanding of our number system, learning to think about numbers in groups of ones, tens, and hundreds, and discovering the meaning of place value.

758 **Zap! Around Town**
Sunburst Technology
1550 Executive Dr
Elgin, IL 60123-9311
800-321-7511
Fax: 888-608-0344
http://store.sunburst.com
service@sunburst.com
Michael Guillory, Channel Sales/Marketing Manager
Students develop mapping and direction skills in this easy-to-use, animated program featuring Shelby, your friendly Sunbuddy guide.

Preschool

759 **2's Experience Fingerplays**
Building Blocks
38w567 Brindlewood Ln
Elgin, IL 60124-7976
800-233-2448
Fax: 847-742-1054
http://www.bblocksonline.com
sales@bblocksonline.com
Liz Wilmes, Author
Dick Wilmes, Co-Author

A wonderful collection of fingerplays, songs and rhymes for the very young child. Fingerplays are short, easy to learn, and full of simple movement. Chant or sing the fingerplays and then enjoy the accompanying games and activities. *$12.95*
144 pages

760 **Curious George Preschool Learning Games**
Sunburst Technology
1550 Executive Dr
Elgin, IL 60123-9311 800-321-7511
Fax: 888-608-0344
http://store.sunburst.com
service@sunburst.com
Michael Guillory, Channel Sales/Marketing Manager
Join Curious George in Fun Town and play five arcade-style games that promote the visual and auditory discrimination skills all students need before they begin to read. Mac/Win CD-ROM

761 **Devereux Early Childhood Assessment (DECA)**
Kaplan Early Learning Company
1310 Lewisville Clemmons Rd
Lewisville, NC 27023-9635 336-766-7374
800-334-2014
Fax: 800-452-7526
http://www.kaplanco.com
info@kaplanco.com
Paul A. LeBuffe, Author
Jack A Naglieri, Co-Author
Hal Kaplan, President & CEO
Strength-based standardized, norm-referenced behavior rating scale designed to promote resilience and measure protective factors in children ages 2-5. Through the program, early childhood professionals and families learn specific strategies to support young children's social and emotional development and to enhance the ovall quality of early childhood programs. *$125.95*

762 **Devereux Early Childhood Assessment: Clinical Version (DECA-C)**
Kaplan Early Learning Company
1310 Lewisville Clemmons Rd
Lewisville, NC 27023-9635 336-766-7374
800-334-2014
Fax: 800-452-7526
http://www.kaplanco.com
info@kaplanco.com
Paul A. LeBuffe, Author
Jack A Naglieri, Co-Author
Hal Kaplan, President & CEO
DECA-C is designed to support early intervention efforts to reduce or eliminate significant emotional and behavioral concerns in preschool children. This can be used for guide interventions, identify children needing special services, assess outcomes and help programs meet Head Start, IDEA, and similar requirements. Kit includes: 1 Manual, 30 Record Forms, and 1 Norms Reference Card. *$125.95*

763 **Early Movement Skills**
Therapro
225 Arlington St
Framingham, MA 01702-8773 508-872-9494
800-257-5376
Fax: 508-875-2062
http://www.therapro.com
info@therapro.com
Naomi Benari, Author
Karen Conrad, President
Easy to follow, reproducible gross motor activities are graded from very simple (even for the passive child) to more demanding (folk dancing). Each of the 150 pages offers an activity with its objective, a clear instruction of the activity, rationale, and alternative movements and games. Many activities involve music and rythm. A great source for early intervention and early childhood programs. *$58.00*

764 **Early Screening Inventory: Revised**
Pearson Assessments
5601 Green Valley Dr
Bloomington, MN 55437-1099 800-627-7271
Fax: 800-232-1223
http://www.pearsonassessments.com
clinicalcustomersupport@pearson.com
Samuel J Meisels, Author
Martha S Wiske, Co-Author
Laura W Henderson, Co-Author
A developmental screening instrument for 3-to-6-year olds. Provides a norm-referenced overview of visual-motor/adaptive, language and cognition, and gross motor development. Meets IDEA and Head Start requirements for early identification and parental involvement. Test in English or Spanish in 15-20 minutes. Training video and materials available.

765 **Early Sensory Skills**
Therapro
225 Arlington St
Framingham, MA 01702-8773 508-872-9494
800-257-5376
Fax: 508-875-2062
http://www.therapro.com
info@therapro.com
Jackie Cooke, Author
Karen Conrad, President
A wonderful book filled with practical and fun activities for stimulating vision, touch, taste and smell. Invaluable for anyone working with children 6 months to 5 years, this manual outlines basic principals followed by six sections containing activities, games and topics to excite the senses. Introductions are easy to follow, and materials for the sensory work are readily accessible in the everyday environment. *$57.75*

766 **Early Visual Skills**
Therapro
225 Arlington St
Framingham, MA 01702-8773 508-872-9494
800-257-5376
Fax: 508-875-2062
http://www.therapro.com
info@therapro.com
Diana Williams, Author
Karen Conrad, President
A beautifully designed, easy to follow reproducible book for working with young children on visual perceptual skills. Most of the activities are nonverbal and can be used with children who have limited language. Each section has both easy and challenging activities for school and for parents working with children at home. Activities include sorting, color and shape matching, a looking walk, games to develop visual memory and concentration and many more. *$62.50*
208 pages

767 **HELP for Preschoolers at Home**
Therapro
225 Arlington St
Framingham, MA 01702-8773 508-872-9494
800-257-5376
Fax: 508-875-2062
http://www.therapro.com
info@therapro.com
Karen Conrad, President
Three hundred pages of practical, home-based activities that can be easily administered by the parents or the child's home-care provider. Upon completion of their assessments, teachers and therapists provide parents with these handouts to help them work on skills at home in conjunction with the program. *$72.50*

768 **LAP-D Kindergarten Screen Kit**
Kaplan Early Learning Company
1310 Lewisville Clemmons Rd
Lewisville, NC 27023-9635 336-766-7374
800-334-2014
Fax: 800-452-7526
http://www.kaplanco.com
info@kaplanco.com

Hal Kaplan, President & CEO
Concise, standardized screening deice normed on 5 year old children. Tasks are in four domains: fine, motor, gross motor, cognititve, and language. The Kindergarten Kit includes the technical manual, examiners, manual, and materials to assist in determining pure outcomes. *$124.95*

769 **Learning Accomplishment Profile Diagnostic Normed Screens for Age 3-5**
Kaplan Early Learning Company
1310 Lewisville Clemmons Rd
Lewisville, NC 27023-9635
336-766-7374
800-334-2014
Fax: 800-452-7526
http://www.kaplanco.com
info@kaplanco.com
Hal Kaplan, President & CEO
For 3-5 years. Create reliable developmental snapshots in fine motor, gross motor, cognitive, language, personal/social, and self-help skill domains. *$349.95*

770 **Learning Accomplishment Profile (LAP-R) KIT**
Kaplan Early Learning Company
1310 Lewisville Clemmons Rd
Lewisville, NC 27023-9635
336-766-7374
800-334-2014
Fax: 800-452-7526
http://www.kaplanco.com
info@kaplanco.com
Hal Kaplan, President & CEO
Mike Mathers, Author
A criterion-referenced assessment instrument measuring development in six domains: gross motor, fine motor, cognitive, language, self-help and social/emotional. Kit includes all materials necessary for assessing 20 children. *$ 299.95*

771 **Learning Accomplishment Profile Diagnostic Normed Assessment (LAP-D)**
Kaplan Early Learning Company
1310 Lewisville Clemmons Rd
Lewisville, NC 27023-9635
336-766-7374
800-334-2014
Fax: 800-452-7526
http://www.kaplanco.com
info@kaplanco.com
Belinda J. Hardin, Ph.D., Author
Ellen S. Peisner-Feinberg, Ph.D, Co-Author
Stephanie W. Weeks, Ph.D., Co-Author
A comprehensive developemtal assessment tool for children between the ages of 30 and 72 months. LAP-D consists of a hierarchy of developmental skills arranged in four developmental domains: fine motor, gross motor, cognitive and language. *$624.95*

772 **Partners for Learning (PFL)**
Kaplan Early Learning Company
1310 Lewisville Clemmons Rd
Lewisville, NC 27023-9635
336-766-7374
800-334-2014
Fax: 800-452-7526
http://www.kaplanco.com
info@kaplanco.com
Hal Kaplan, President & CEO
This resource uses cards, books, posters, and support materials to supply teaching ideas and to support child development. PARTNERS for Learning encourages cognitive, social, motor, and language development. The kit provides materials for curriculum planning and self-assessment. *$199.95*

773 **Right from the Start: Behavioral Intervention for Young Children with Autism**
Therapro
225 Arlington St
Framingham, MA 01702-8773
508-872-9494
800-257-5376
Fax: 508-875-2062
http://www.therapro.com
info@therapro.com
Sandra Harris PhD, Author
Mary Jane Weiss PhD, Co-Author
Karen Conrad, President
This informative and user-friendly guide helps parents and service providers explore programs that use early intensive behavioral intervention for young children with autism and related disorders. Within these programs, many children improve in intellectual, social and adaptive functioning, enabling them to move on to regular elementary and preschools. Benefits all children, but primarily useful for children age five and younger. *$16.95*
138 pages

774 **Sensory Motor Activities for Early Development**
Therapro
225 Arlington St
Framingham, MA 01702-8773
508-872-9494
800-257-5376
Fax: 508-875-2062
http://www.therapro.com
info@therapro.com
Chia Swee Hong, Author
Helen Gabriel, Co-Author
Cathy St John, Co-Author
A complete package of tried and tested gross and fine motor activities. Many activities to stimulate sensory and body awareness, encourage basic movement, promote hand skills, and enhance spatial/early perceptual skills. Master handouts throughout to give to parents for home practice activities for working in small groups. *$51.50*
93 pages

Reading

775 **Animals of the Rainforest Classroom Library**
HMH Supplemental Publishers
222 Berkeley Street
Boston, MA 02116
617-351-5000
855-969-4642
Fax: 800-269-5232
http://www.hmhco.com
school.permissions@hmhco.com
Linda K. Zecher, President and CEO
Eric Shuman, Chief Financial Officer
John K. Dragoon, EVP and Chief Marketing Officer
When reading is a struggle, academic success is even harder to achieve. Now you can put social studies and science curriculum content within reach of every student with this series. Designed specifically for limited readers. *$ 46.50*
ISBN 0-739849-32-8

776 **Ants in His Pants: Absurdities and Realities of Special Education**
Sage Publications
2455 Teller Rd
Thousand Oaks, CA 91320-2218
805-499-9774
800-818-7243
Fax: 800-583-2665
http://www.sagepub.com
orders@sagepub.com
Michael Giangreco, Author
Kevin Ruelle, Co-Author
Blaise R. Simqu, President
With wit, humor and profound one liners, Michael Giangreco will transform your thinking as you take a lighter look at the sometimes comical and occasionally harsh truths in the ever changing field of special education. *$20.95*
128 pages
ISBN 1-890455-42-3

777 **AppleSeeds**
Cobblestone Publishing
Ste C
30 Grove St
Peterborough, NH 03458-1453 603-924-7209
800-821-0115
Fax: 603-924-7380
http://www.cobblestonepub.com
customerservice@caruspub.com
Susan Buckley, Editor
An award winning magazine of adventure and exploration for children ages 7 to 9. Provides kids with themed issues that explore a different topic with insightful articles, cool photographs, and a unique you-are-there perspective on culture and history. *$29.95*
36 pages 9 times a year

778 **Basic Level Workbook for Aphasia**
Wayne State University Press
4809 Woodward Ave
Detroit, MI 48201-1309 313-577-6120
800-978-7323
Fax: 313-577-6131
http://wsupress.wayne.edu
bookorders@wayne.edu
Susan Howell Brubaker MS, Author
Jane Hoehner, Director
Gabe Gloden, Community Engagement Officer
If you work with adolescents and adults with mild to moderate language deficits or limited, impaired, or emerging reading skills, this workbook is what you've been waiting for! The mMaterial is relevant to their lives, interests, experiences, and vocabulary. Item number W324. *$50.00*
360 pages
ISBN 0-814326-20-X

779 **Beyond the Code**
Educators Publishing Service
PO Box 9031
Cambridge, MA 02139-9031 617-547-6706
800-225-5750
Fax: 617-547-3805
http://www.epsbooks.com
CustomerService.EPS@schoolspecialty.com
Nancy M Hall, Author
Rick Holden, President
Jeff Belanger, Regional Sales Manager
Beyond the Code gives beginning readers experience reading original stories as well as thinking about what they have read. This companion series follows the same phonetic progression as the frist 4 books of the popular Explode the Code program.

780 **Chess with Butterflies**
Oxton House Publishers
PO Box 209
Farmington, ME 04938 207-779-1923
800-539-7323
Fax: 207-779-0623
http://www.oxtonhouse.com
info@oxtonhouse.com
William Berlinghoff PhD, Managing Editor
Bobby Brown, Marketing Director
Sandi Hawkins, Representative
This is a phoneticaly controlled sequel to 'Fishing with Balloons.' It continues the adventures of the main character as it develops more sophisticated word families. Lists for those word families and notes on using them for reading instruction are included in the back of the book. *$5.95*
66 pages
ISBN 1-881929-43-4

781 **Claims to Fame**
Educators Publishing Service
PO Box 9031
Cambridge, MA 02139-9031 617-547-6706
800-225-5750
Fax: 617-547-3805
http://www.epsbooks.com
CustomerService.EPS@schoolspecialty.com
Carol Einstein, Author
Rick Holden, President
Jeff Belanger, Regional Sales Manager
The three exercises after each reading are tailored to the content of each story. In Thinking About What You Have Read, students check and extend their understanding of the story. Working with Words asks students to think about and experiment with vaious word meanings.

782 **Clues to Meaning**
Educators Publishing Service
PO Box 9031
Cambridge, MA 02139-9031 617-547-6706
800-225-5750
Fax: 617-547-3805
http://www.epsbooks.com
CustomerService.EPS@schoolspecialty.com
Ann L Staman, Author
Rick Holden, President
Jeff Belanger, Regional Sales Manager
A versatile series which teaches beginning readers to use the sounds of letters as one strategy among many in learning to read.

783 **Concept Phonics**
Oxton House Publishers
PO Box 209
Farmington, ME 04938 207-779-1923
800-539-7323
Fax: 207-779-0623
http://www.oxtonhouse.com
info@oxtonhouse.com
William Berlinghoff PhD, Managing Editor
Bobby Brown, Marketing Director
Dr. Phyllis Fischer, Author
This is a remarkably effective, research-based, multisensory program for teaching reading-decoding and speech to students with learning disabilities at any age or grade level. Its 13 component pieces include a book on understanding phonics, detailed teacher's guides, and sets of contrast cards, speed drills, worksheets, visual teaching aids, and comprehensive word lists. *$315.00*
ISBN 1-881929-36-1

784 **Cosmic Reading Journey**
Sunburst Technology
1550 Executive Dr
Elgin, IL 60123-9311 800-321-7511
Fax: 888-608-0344
http://store.sunburst.com
service@sunburst.com
Michael Guillory, Channel Sales/Marketing Manager
This reading comprehension program provides meaningful summary and writing activities for the 100 books that early readers and their teachers love most.

785 **Creepy Cave Initial Consonants**
Sunburst Technology
1550 Executive Dr
Elgin, IL 60123-9311 800-321-7511
Fax: 888-608-0344
http://store.sunburst.com
service@sunburst.com
Michael Guillory, Channel Sales/Marketing Manager
Help your students develop letter recognition and phonemic awareness skills matching words with the same initial consonant letter in a Creepy Cave.

786 **Decoding Automaticity Materials for Reading Fluency**
Oxton House Publishers
PO Box 209
Farmington, ME 04938
207-779-1923
800-539-7323
Fax: 207-779-0623
http://www.oxtonhouse.com
info@oxtonhouse.com
William Berlinghoff PhD, Managing Editor
Bobby Brown, Marketing Director
Dr. Phyllis Fischer, Author
This six-part set is designed to bring students from decoding to automaticity in reading words. The two sets of worksheets train the brain's visual processor to recognize letter units in words; the contrast cards train the brain's speech processor to say the sounds for the letter units; and the speed drills put these two tasks together for reading whole words automatically. Also included are comprehensive sets of lists of one-and two syllable words for designing customized materials. *$150.00*
ISBN 1-881929-37-X

787 **Dyslexia Training Program**
Educators Publishing Service
PO Box 9031
Cambridge, MA 02139-9031
617-547-6706
800-225-5750
Fax: 617-547-3805
http://www.epsbooks.com
CustomerService.EPS@schoolspecialty.com
Kathryn Hansen, Key Accounts Coordinator
Ryan Todd, Sales Consultant
Jeff Belanger, Regional Sales Manager
Introduces reading and writing skills to dyslexic children through a two-year, cumulative series of daily one-hour videotaped lessons and accompanying student's books and teacher's guides.

788 **Earobics® Clinic Version Step 1**
Abilitations Speech Bin
PO Box 1579
Appleton, WI 54912-1579
419-589-1600
888-388-3224
Fax: 888-388-6344
http://www.schoolspecialty.com
orders@schoolspecialty.com
Joseph M. Yorio, President, CEO
Rick Holden, Executive Vice President
Kevin Baehler, Vice President, Acting CFO
Earobics is a dazzling software that teaches phonological awareness and auditory processing. It systematically — anf enjoyably — trains these critical skills for development ages four to seven years. Item number C482. *$298.99*

789 **EarobicsM® Step 1 Home Version**
Abilitations Speech Bin
PO Box 1579
Appleton, WI 54912-1579
419-589-1600
888-388-3224
Fax: 888-388-6344
http://www.schoolspecialty.com
orders@schoolspecialty.com
Joseph M. Yorio, President, CEO
Rick Holden, Executive Vice President
Kevin Baehler, Vice President, Acting CFO
Step 1 offers hundreds of levels of play, appealing graphics, and entertaining music to train the critical auditory skills young children need for success in learning. Item number C481. *$58.99*

790 **Emergent Reader**
Sunburst Technology
1550 Executive Dr
Elgin, IL 60123-9311
800-321-7511
Fax: 888-608-0344
http://store.sunburst.com
service@sunburst.com
Michael Guillory, Channel Sales/Marketing Manager
This story-reading program supports the efforts of beginning readers by developing their sight word vocabularies.

791 **Every Child a Reader**
Sunburst Technology
1550 Executive Dr
Elgin, IL 60123-9311
800-321-7511
Fax: 888-608-0344
http://store.sunburst.com
service@sunburst.com
Michael Guillory, Channel Sales/Marketing Manager
Traditional reading strategies in a rich literary context. Designed to promote independent reading and develop oral and written language expression.

792 **Explode the Code**
Educators Publishing Service
PO Box 9031
Cambridge, MA 02139-9031
617-547-6706
800-225-5750
Fax: 617-547-3805
http://www.epsbooks.com
CustomerService.EPS@schoolspecialty.com
Nancy M Hall, Author
Rick Holden, President
Jeff Belanger, Regional Sales Manager
Explode the Code provides a sequential, systematic approach to phonics in which students blend sounds to build vocabulary and read words, phrases, sentences, and stories.

793 **Fishing with Balloons**
Oxton House Publishers
PO Box 209
Farmington, ME 04938
207-779-1923
800-539-7323
Fax: 207-779-0623
http://www.oxtonhouse.com
info@oxtonhouse.com
William Burlinghoff PhD, Owner
Bobby Brown, Marketing Director
Dion , Author
This is a phonetically controlled chapter book about a 10 year old who learns how his physical disability need not be a barrier to his aspirations. As the story holds the reader's interest, it also emphasizes certain families of words. Lists for those word families and notes on using them for reading instruction are included in the back of the book. *$5.95*
68 pages
ISBN 1-881929-34-5

794 **Great Series Great Rescues**
HMH Supplemental Publishers
222 Berkeley Street
Boston, MA 02116
617-351-5000
855-969-4642
Fax: 800-269-5232
http://www.hmhco.com
school.permissions@hmhco.com
Henry Billings, Author
Linda K. Zecher, President, CEO & Director
Eric Shuman, Chief Financial Officer
Human drama makes beginning reading worth the effort. Eight exciting titles build confidence as they build skills. Short, easy-to-read selections enable limited readers to succeed with material that matters. *$15.00*
ISBN 0-811441-76-8

795 **Handprints**
Educators Publishing Service
PO Box 9031
Cambridge, MA 02139-9031
617-547-6706
800-225-5750
Fax: 617-547-3805
http://www.epsbooks.com
CustomerService.EPS@schoolspecialty.com
Ann L Staman, Author
Rick Holden, President
Jeff Belanger, Regional Sales Manager

Handprints is a set of 50 storybooks and 4 workbooks for beginning readers in kindergarten and first grade. The storybooks increase in difficulty very gradually and encourage the new readers to use meaning, language, and print cues as they read.

796 **High Noon Books**
Academic Therapy Publications
20 Leveroni Court
Novato, CA 94949-5746
415-883-3314
800-422-7249
Fax: 888-287-9975
http://www.academictherapy.com
sales@academictherapy.com
Jim Arena, President
Joanne Urban, Manager
Cynthia Coverston
Serving the field of learning disabilities for the past 25 years. High-interest books for reluctant readers. Reading solution programs, phonics, spelling, writing, visual tracking materials.

797 **I Can Read**
Teddy Bear Press
3703 S Edmunds St
Ste 67
Seattle, WA 98118
206-402-6947
Fax: 866-870-7323
http://www.teddybearpress.com
fparker@teddybearpress.net
Fran Parker, Author
A series of 7 reading books and 7 workbooks, a set of 52 flashcards and teacher manual which uses a sight word approach to teach beginning readers. These teacher created books and workbooks present an easy to use beginning reading program which provides repetition, visual motor, visual discrimination and word comprehension activities. It was created to teach young, learning disabled children and has been successfully employed to teach beginning readers of varying ages and abilities. *$90.00*

798 **I Can See the ABC's**
Teddy Bear Press
3703 S Edmunds St
Ste 67
Seattle, WA 98118
206-402-6947
Fax: 866-870-7323
http://www.teddybearpress.com
fparker@teddybearpress.net
Fran Parker, Author
A big 11x17 which contains the pre-primer words found in the I Can Read program while introducing the alphabet. *$25.00*

799 **Inclusion: Strategies for Working with Young Children**
Corwin Press
2455 Teller Road
Thousand Oaks, CA 91320-2218
805-499-9734
800-233-9936
Fax: 805-499-5323
http://www.corwinpress.com
webmaster@corwin.com
Lorraine O Moore PhD, Author
Mike Soules, President
Lisa Shaw, Executive Director
This exceptional resource is a gold mine of developmentally based ideas to help children between the ages of 3-7 or older students who may be developmentally delayed. This is a very practical and easy-to-use publication which is appropriate for early childhood teachers, K-2 general and special education teachers. *$28.95*
144 pages Educators
ISBN 1-890455-33-4

800 **Island Reading Journey**
Sunburst Technology
1550 Executive Dr
Elgin, IL 60123-9311
800-321-7511
Fax: 888-608-0344
http://store.sunburst.com
service@sunburst.com
Michael Guillory, Channel Sales/Marketing Manager
Enhance your reading program with meaningful summary and extension activities for 100 intermediate level books. Students read for meaning while they engage in activities that test for comprehension, build writing skills with reader response and essay questions, develop usage skills with cloze activities and improve vocabulary/word attack skills.

801 **Kids Media Magic 2.0**
Sunburst Technology
1550 Executive Dr
Elgin, IL 60123-9311
800-321-7511
Fax: 888-608-0344
http://store.sunburst.com
service@sunburst.com
Michael Guillory, Channel Sales/Marketing Manager
The first multimedia word processor designed for young children. Help your child become a fluent reader and writer. The Rebus Bar automatically scrolls over 45 vocabulary words as students type.

802 **Let's Go Read 1: An Island Adventure**
Riverdeep
14046 Collections Center Drive
Chicago, IL 60693
855-969-4642
Fax: 800-269-5232
http://www.hmhinnovation.com
school.permissions@hmhco.com
Linda K. Zecher, President, CEO & Director
Eric Shuman, Chief Financial Officer
John K. Dragoon, EVP and Chief Marketing Officer
Take off with Robby the Raccoon, Emily the Squirrel and the Reading Rover on an exciting adventure to an island inhabited by the alphabet. Motivated by the delight of mastering new challenges, your child will play through more than 35 fun activties that install and reinforce the essential skills for successful reading.

803 **Let's Go Read 2: An Ocean Adventure**
Riverdeep
14046 Collections Center Drive
Chicago, IL 60693
855-969-4642
Fax: 800-269-5232
http://www.hmhinnovation.com
school.permissions@hmhco.com
Linda K. Zecher, President, CEO & Director
Eric Shuman, Chief Financial Officer
John K. Dragoon, EVP and Chief Marketing Officer
Building upon your child's mastery of letters, Let's Go Read: 2 explores how letters combine to form words, and how words combine to express meaning. Dozens of captivating, skill-building activities teach your child the skills to sound out, recognize, build and comprehend hundreds of new words. It's an endlessly fun voyage toward reading fluency!

804 **Let's Read**
Educators Publishing Service
PO Box 9031
Cambridge, MA 02139-9031
617-547-6706
800-225-5750
Fax: 617-547-3805
http://www.epsbooks.com
CustomerService.EPS@schoolspecialty.com
Leonard Bloomfield, Author
Clarence L Barnhart, Co-Author
Robert K Barnhart, Co-Author
Using a linguistic approach to teaching reading skills, this series emphasizes relationship of spelling to sound, presenting the concepts together, and providing nine reading books and accompanying workbooks for practice. Provides classroom directions and suggestions for supplementary exercises.

805 **Lighthouse Low Vision Products**
Lighthouse International
111 E 59th St
New York, NY 10022-1202
212-821-9200
800-829-0500
Fax: 212-821-9707
TTY: 212-821-9713
http://www.lighthouse.org
info@lighthouse.com
Mark G. Ackermann, President, CEO
Maura J. Sweeney, SVP/COO
John Vlachos, SVP, Chief Financial Officer
Empowers people of all ages who are visually impaired to lead safe, active and independent lives

806 **Megawords**
Educators Publishing Service
PO Box 9031
Cambridge, MA 02139-9031
617-547-6706
800-225-5750
Fax: 617-547-3805
http://www.epsbooks.com
CustomerService.EPS@schoolspecialty.com
Kristin Johnson, Author
Polly Baird, Co-Author
Rick Holden, President
A series with a systematic, multisensory approach to learning the longer words encountered from fourth grade on. Students first work with syllables, then combine the syllables into words, use them in context, and work to increase their reading and spelling proficiency. Teacher's Guide and Answer Key available.

807 **Mike Mulligan & His Steam Shovel**
Houghton Mifflin
222 Berkeley Street
Boston, MA 02116
617-351-5000
855-969-4642
Fax: 800-269-5232
http://www.hmhco.com
school.permissions@hmhco.com
Virginia Lee Burton, Author
Linda K. Zecher, President, CEO & Director
Eric Shuman, Chief Financial Officer
This CD-ROM version of the Caldecott classic lets students experience interactive book reading and participate in four skills-based extension activities that promote memory, matching, sequencing, listening, pattern recognition and map reading skills.
ISBN 0-395664-99-3

808 **More Primary Phonics**
Educators Publishing Service
PO Box 9031
Cambridge, MA 02139-9031
617-547-6706
800-225-5750
Fax: 617-547-3805
http://www.epsbooks.com
CustomerService.EPS@schoolspecialty.com
Barbara W Makar, Author
Rick Holden, President
Jeff Belanger, Regional Sales Manager
Reinforces and expands skills developed in Primary Phonics. Workbooks and storybooks contain the same phonetic elements, sight words and phonetic sequences as workbooks 1 and 2.

809 **Multi-Sequenced Speed Drills for Fluency Multi-Sequenced Speed Drills for Fluency in Decoding**
Oxton House Publishers
PO Box 209
Farmington, ME 04938
207-779-1923
800-539-7323
Fax: 207-779-0623
http://www.oxtonhouse.com
info@oxtonhouse.com
William Burlinghoff PhD, Owner
Bobby Brown, Marketing Director
Dr. Phyllis Fischer, Author
This 179-page set of reading speed drills are carefully constructed to promote decoding automaticity and the fluent recognition of words. They follow the traditional Orton-Gillingham spelling and sound sequences. The set also includes eight pages of teaching advice and a master chart fro tracking student programs. *$29.95*
195 pages
ISBN 1-881929-14-0

810 **Next Stop**
Educators Publishing Service
PO Box 9031
Cambridge, MA 02139-9031
617-547-6706
800-225-5750
Fax: 617-547-3805
http://www.epsbooks.com
CustomerService.EPS@schoolspecialty.com
Tanya Auger, Author
Rick Holden, President
Jeff Belanger, Regional Sales Manager
Increase reading and language skills while exploring different literacy genres. This series is intended for students who are ready to move beyond phonetically controlled readers to the nest stop-real chapter books that will help prepare them for the more challenging literature they will encounter in later grades.

811 **Patterns of English Spelling**
AVKO Educational Research Foundation
3084 Willard Rd
Birch Run, MI 48415-9404
810-686-9283
866-285-6612
Fax: 810-686-1101
http://www.avko.org
webmaster@avko.org
Don Mc Cabe, President/Research Director
Linda Heck, Vice-President
Michael Lane, Treasurer
Use the index to locate the page upon which you can find all the words that share the same patterns. If you look up the word cat, you will find all the pages where all the at words are located. If you look up the word precious you will find all the words ending in cious. There are ten volumes which can be purchased all together or separately. *$119.95*
Whole set

812 **Phonemic Awareness: The Sounds of Reading**
Corwin Press
2455 Teller Rd
Thousand Oaks, CA 91320-2218
805-499-9734
800-233-9936
Fax: 805-499-5323
http://www.corwinpress.com
order@corwin.com
Victoria Groves Scott, Author
Mike Soules, President
Lisa Shaw, Executive Director Editorial
In this dynamic new video, Dr. Scott demonstrates the principal components of phonemic awareness: identification; comparison; segmentation; blending and rhyming. This video will help you to better understand phonemic awareness training and will show you how to apply these components not only to the reading curriculum but to all subjects through the school day. Filmed in actual classroom settings.
$69.95
25 minute video
ISBN 1-890455-29-6

813 **Polar Express**
Houghton Mifflin
222 Berkeley Street
Boston, MA 02116
617-351-5000
855-969-4642
Fax: 800-269-5232
http://www.hmhco.com
school.permissions@hmhco.com
Chris Van Allsburg, Author
Linda K. Zecher, President, CEO & Director
Eric Shuman, Chief Financial Officer

Share the magic and enchantment of the holiday season with this CD-ROM version of the Caldecott-winning picture book.

814 **Prehistoric Creaures Then & Now**
HMH Supplemental Publishers
222 Berkeley Street
Boston, MA 02116 617-351-5000
855-969-4642
Fax: 800-269-5232
http://www.hmhco.com
school.permissions@hmhco.com
K S Rodriguez, Author
Linda K. Zecher, President, CEO & Director
Eric Shuman, Chief Financial Officer
When reading is a struggle, academic success is even harder to achieve. Now you can put social studies and science curriculum content within reach of every students with Steadwell Books — the series designed specifically for limited readers. Attention-getting photos and informative illustrations, maps, and time lines communicate the social studies and science concepts found in the text.
ISBN 0-739821-47-4

815 **Primary Phonics**
Educators Publishing Service
PO Box 9031
Cambridge, MA 02139-9031 617-547-6706
800-225-5750
Fax: 617-547-3805
http://www.epsbooks.com
CustomerService.EPS@schoolspecialty.com
Barbara W Makar, Author
Rick Holden, President
Jeff Belanger, Regional Sales Manager
This revised program of storybooks and coordinated workbooks teaches reading for grades K-2. There is a set of ten storybooks to go with each of the first five workbooks. A Primary Phonics Picture Dictionary contains 2,500 commonly used words, including most of the words in the series. This series' individualized nature permits students to progress at their own speed. Teacher's manual available.

816 **Read On! Plus**
Sunburst Technology
1550 Executive Dr
Elgin, IL 60123-9311 800-321-7511
Fax: 888-608-0344
http://store.sunburst.com
service@sunburst.com
Michael Guillory, Channel Sales/Marketing Manager
Promote skills and strategies that improve reading comprehension, and build appreciation for literature and the written word.

817 **Reader's Quest I**
Sunburst Technology
1550 Executive Dr
Elgin, IL 60123-9311 800-321-7511
Fax: 888-608-0344
http://store.sunburst.com
service@sunburst.com
Michael Guillory, Channel Sales/Marketing Manager
These reading workshops provide students with direct reading instruction, interactive practice activities, and practical strategies to ensure reading success.

818 **Reader's Quest II**
Sunburst Technology
1550 Executive Dr
Elgin, IL 60123-9311 800-321-7511
Fax: 888-608-0344
http://store.sunburst.com
service@sunburst.com
Michael Guillory, Channel Sales/Marketing Manager
These reading workshops provide students with direct reading instruction, interactive practice activities, and practical strategies to ensure reading success.

819 **Reading Comprehension Bundle**
Sunburst Technology
1550 Executive Dr
Elgin, IL 60123-9311 800-321-7511
Fax: 888-608-0344
http://store.sunburst.com
service@sunburst.com
Michael Guillory, Channel Sales/Marketing Manager
This collection for the intermediate-level classroom develops the skills students need to read for meaning and understanding.

820 **Reading Comprehension in Varied Subject Matter**
Educators Publishing Service
PO Box 9031
Cambridge, MA 02139-9031 617-547-6706
800-225-5750
Fax: 617-547-3805
http://www.epsbooks.com
CustomerService.EPS@schoolspecialty.com
Jane Ervin, Author
Rick Holden, President
Jeff Belanger, Regional Sales Manager
Ten workbooks that present a wide range of people and situations with new reading selections, new vocabulary, and a new writing exercise. Each book contains 31 selections in the subject areas of social studies, science, literature, mathematics, philosophy, logic, language, and the arts.

821 **Reading Pen**
Wizcom Technologies
20 Haganan St.
Einav Industrial Park 073-290-6133
http://www.wizcomtech.com
customer_service@wizcomtech.com
Isaac Soibelman, President
Tiran Fartouk, CEO
Portable assitive reading device that reads words aloud and can be used anywhere. Scans a word from printed text, displays the word in large characters, reads the word aloud from built-in speaker or ear phones and defines the word with the press of a button. Displays syllables, keeps a history of scanned words, adjustable for left or right-handed use. Includes a tutorial video and audio cassette. Not recommended for persons with low vision or impaired fine motor control.
$279.00

822 **Reading Who? Reading You!**
Sunburst Technology
1550 Executive Dr
Elgin, IL 60123-9311 800-321-7511
Fax: 888-608-0344
http://store.sunburst.com
service@sunburst.com
Michael Guillory, Channel Sales/Marketing Manager
Teach beginning reading skills effectively with phonics instruction built into engaging games and puzzles that have children asking for more.

823 **Reading for Content**
Educators Publishing Service
PO Box 9031
Cambridge, MA 02139-9031 617-547-6706
800-225-5750
Fax: 617-547-3805
http://www.epsbooks.com
CustomerService.EPS@schoolspecialty.com
Carol Einstein, Author
Rick Holden, President
Jeff Belanger, Regional Sales Manager
Reading for Content is a series of 4 books designed to help students improve their reading comprehension skills. Each book contains 43 pasages followed by 4 questions. Two questions ask for a recall of main ideas, and two ask the student to draw conclusions from what they have just read.

824 **Reading for Job and Personal Use**
PO Box 2500
Lebanon, IN 46052-3009
800-848-9500
Fax: 877-260-2530
http://www.pearsonschool.com
k12cs@custhelp.com
Marjorie Scardino, CEO
Victor Coira, Sales Representative
Victoria Ramos, Digital Sales Rep
The practical, real-life exercises in these texts teach students how to read and comprehend catalogs, training manuals, letters and memos, signs, reports, charts, and more.

825 **Reasoning & Reading Series**
Educators Publishing Service
PO Box 9031
Cambridge, MA 02139-9031
617-547-6706
800-225-5750
Fax: 617-547-3805
http://www.epsbooks.com
CustomerService.EPS@schoolspecialty.com
Joanne Carlisle, Author
Rick Holden, President
Jeff Belanger, Regional Sales Manager
These workbooks develop basic language and thinking skills that build the foundation for reading comprehension. Exercises reinforce reading as a critical reasoning activity. Many exercises encourage students to come up with their own response in instances where there is no single correct answer. In other cases, exercises lend themselves to students working collaboratively to see how many different answers satisfy a question.

826 **Right into Reading: A Phonics-Based Reading and Comprehension Program**
Educators Publishing Service
PO Box 9031
Cambridge, MA 02139-9031
617-547-6706
800-225-5750
Fax: 617-547-3805
http://www.epsbooks.com
CustomerService.EPS@schoolspecialty.com
Jane Ervin, Author
Rick Holden, President
Jeff Belanger, Regional Sales Manager
Right into Reading introduces phonics skills in a carefully ordered sequence of bite-size lessons so that students can progress easily and successfully from one reading level to the next. The stories and selections are unusually diverse and interactive.

827 **See Me Add**
Teddy Bear Press
3703 S Edmunds St
Ste 67
Seattle, WA 98118
206-402-6947
Fax: 866-870-7323
http://www.teddybearpress.com
fparker@teddybearpress.net
Fran Parker, Author
Introduces the concept of addition using simple story problems and the basic sight word vocabulary found in the I Can Read and Reading Is Fun programs. *$25.00*

828 **See Me Subtract**
Teddy Bear Press
3703 S Edmunds St
Ste 67
Seattle, WA 98118
206-402-6947
Fax: 866-870-7323
http://www.teddybearpress.com
fparker@teddybearpress.net
Fran Parker, Author
Introduces the concept of subtraction using simple story problems. *$25.00*

829 **Sounds and Spelling Patterns for English**
Oxton House Publishers
PO Box 209
Farmington, ME 04938
207-779-1923
800-539-7323
Fax: 207-779-0623
http://www.oxtonhouse.com
info@oxtonhouse.com
William Burlinghoff PhD, Owner
Bobby Brown, Marketing Director
Dr. Phyllis Fischer, Author
This book is a clear, concise, practical, jargon-free overview of the sounds that make up the English languate and the symbols that we use to represent them in writing. It includes an explanatory chapter on phonological and phonemic awareness and a broad range of strategies for helping beginning readers develop fluent decoding skills. *$24.95*
140 pages
ISBN 1-881929-01-9

830 **Specialized Program Individualizing Reading Excellence (SPIRE)**
Educators Publishing Service
PO Box 9031
Cambridge, MA 02139-9031
617-547-6706
800-225-5750
Fax: 617-547-3805
http://www.epsbooks.com
CustomerService.EPS@schoolspecialty.com
Sheila Clark Edmands, Author
Rick Holden, President
Jeff Belanger, Regional Sales Manager
SPIRE is a comprehensive multisensory reading and language arts program for students with learning differences.

831 **Starting Comprehension**
Educators Publishing Service
PO Box 9031
Cambridge, MA 02139-9031
617-547-6706
800-225-5750
Fax: 617-547-3805
http://www.epsbooks.com
CustomerService.EPS@schoolspecialty.com
Ann L Staman, Author
Rick Holden, President
Jeff Belanger, Regional Sales Manager
A reading series of 12 workbooks that develops essential comprehension skills at the earliest reading level. It is divided into two different strands, one for students who have a strong visual sense, the other for those who learn sounds easily. Vocabulary introduced within context of exercises, using most of the words in the books. Student relates the details of the passage to the main idea.

832 **Stories and More: Animal Friends**
Riverdeep, Inc.
14046 Collections Center Drive
Chicago, IL 60693
855-969-4642
Fax: 800-269-5232
http://www.hmhinnovation.com
school.permissions@hmhco.com
Linda K. Zecher, President, CEO & Director
Eric Shuman, Chief Financial Officer
John K. Dragoon, EVP and Chief Marketing Officer
Stories and More: Animal Friends features three well-known stories — The Gunnywolf, The Trek, and Owl and the Moon — with engaging activities that strengthen students reading comprehension. A scaffolding of pre-reading, reading, and post-reading activities for each story helps kindergarten and 1st grade students practice prediction and sequencing skills; appreciate the importance of character and setting; and respond to literature through writing, drawing, and speaking. *$ 69.95*

833 **Stories and More: Time and Place**
Riverdeep, Inc.
14046 Collections Center Drive
Chicago, IL 60693
855-969-4642
Fax: 800-269-5232
http://www.hmhinnovation.com
school.permissions@hmhco.com
Linda K. Zecher, President, CEO & Director
Eric Shuman, Chief Financial Officer
John K. Dragoon, EVP and Chief Marketing Officer
Stories and More: Time and Place combines three well-loved stories — The House on Maple Street, Roxaboxen, and Galimoto — with — angaging activities that strengthen students' reading comprehension. In these books, the setting plays a primary role. Second and third grade students learn the importance of time, culture, and place in our lives.

834 **Stories from Somerville**
Oxton House Publishers
PO Box 209
Farmington, ME 04938
207-779-1923
800-539-7323
Fax: 207-779-0623
http://www.oxtonhouse.com
info@oxtonhouse.com
William Berlinghoff PhD, Managing Editor
Bobby Brown, Marketing Director
Kim Ramsey, Author
This set of two readers and three workbooks contains a total of 75 separate but interconnected, phonetically-controlled stories that follow a careful pattern of skill development. They are compatible with most phonics-based reading programs. The realistic personal interactions of the characters also provide opportunities for rich class discussion about various social skills that may be troublesome for many students, including those with learning disabilities. *$69.95*
ISBN 1-881929-40-4

835 **Take Me Home Pair-It Books**
Harcourt Achieve
222 Berkeley Street
Boston, MA 02116
617-351-5000
855-969-4642
Fax: 800-269-5232
http://www.hmhco.com
school.permissions@hmhco.com
Linda K. Zecher, President and CEO
Eric Shuman, Chief Financial Officer
John K. Dragoon, EVP and Chief Marketing Officer
Make reading time a family favorite. Our most popular Pair-It Book titles in convenient take-home packages make it easy to get parents involved in reinforcing reading. *$346.10*

836 **Taking Your Camera To...Steadwell**
Harcourt Achieve
222 Berkeley Street
Boston, MA 02116
617-351-5000
855-969-4642
Fax: 800-269-5232
http://www.hmhco.com
school.permissions@hmhco.com
Linda K. Zecher, President, CEO
Eric Shuman, Chief Financial Officer
John K. Dragoon, EVP and Chief Marketing Officer
Give limited readers unlimited access to major countries! Each title devotes a spread to the land, the people, major cities, lifestyles, places to visit, government and religion, earning a living, sports and school, food and holidays, quick facts, statistics and maps, and the future. *$7.80*

837 **Teaching Comprehension: Strategies for Stories**
Oxton House Publishers
PO Box 209
Farmington, ME 04938
207-779-1923
800-539-7323
Fax: 207-779-0623
http://www.oxtonhouse.com
info@oxtonhouse.com
William Burlinghoff PhD, Managing Editor
Bobby Brown, Marketing Director
Dr. Phyllis Fischer, Author
This handbook gives teachers a richly detailed roadmap for providing students with effective strategies for comprehending and remembering stories. It inlcudes story-line masters for helping students to organize their thinking about a story and to accurately depict characters and sequence events. *$24.95*
62 pages
ISBN 1-881929-27-2

838 **Tenth Planet: Roots, Suffixes, Prefixes**
Sunburst Technology
1550 Executive Dr
Elgin, IL 60123-9311
800-321-7511
Fax: 888-608-0344
http://store.sunburst.com
service@sunburst.com
Michael Guillory, Channel Sales/Marketing Manager
Students learn to decode difficult and more complex words as they engage in six activities where they construct and dissect words with roots, prefixes and suffixes.

839 **Transition Stage 2-3**
Harcourt Achieve
222 Berkeley Street
Boston, MA 02116
617-351-5000
855-969-4642
Fax: 800-269-5232
http://www.hmhco.com
school.permissions@hmhco.com
Linda K. Zecher, President and CEO
Eric Shuman, Chief Financial Officer
John K. Dragoon, EVP and Chief Marketing Officer
A series of 20 books, each containing 16 pages, that provide readers with a gradual transition into early fluency. All stories are available on audio cassette, and four are available in big book format. *$951.80*

840 **Vowels: Short & Long**
Sunburst Technology
1550 Executive Dr
Elgin, IL 60123-9311
800-321-7511
Fax: 888-608-0344
http://store.sunburst.com
service@sunburst.com
Michael Guillory, Channel Sales/Marketing Manager
Introduce students to vowels and the role they play in the structure of words. By engaging in word building activities, students learn to identify short and long vowels and regular spelling patterns.

841 **Wilson Language Training**
47 Old Webster Rd
Oxford, MA 01540-2705
508-368-2399
800-899-8454
Fax: 508-368-2300
http://www.wilsonlanguage.com
info@wilsonlanguage.com
Barbara A Wilson, Co-Founder/President
Ed Wilson, Co-Founder/Publisher
Dedicated to providing educators with the resources they need to help their students become fluent, independent readers. Provides professional development and research-based reading and spelling curricula for all ages.

842 **Wordly Wise 3000 ABC 1-9**
Educators Publishing Service
PO Box 9031
Cambridge, MA 02139-9031
617-547-6706
800-225-5750
Fax: 617-547-3805
http://www.epsbooks.com
CustomerService.EPS@schoolspecialty.com
Kenneth Hodkinson, Author
Sandra Adams, Co-Author
Rick Holden, President

Three thousand new and carefully selected words taken from literature, textbooks and SAT-prep books, are the basis of this new series that teaches vocabulary through reading, writing, and a variety of exercises for grades 4-12.

843 **Wordly Wise ABC 1-9**
Educators Publishing Service
PO Box 9031
Cambridge, MA 02139-9031 617-547-6706
800-225-5750
Fax: 617-547-3805
http://www.epsbooks.com
CustomerService.EPS@schoolspecialty.com
Kenneth Hodkinson, Author
Sandra Adams, Co-Author
Rick Holden, President
Vocabulary workbook series employs crossword puzzles, riddles, word games and a sense of humor to make the learning of new words an interesting experience.

Science

844 **Learn About Life Science: Animals**
Sunburst Technology
1550 Executive Dr
Elgin, IL 60123-9311 800-321-7511
Fax: 888-608-0344
http://store.sunburst.com
service@sunburst.com
Michael Guillory, Channel Sales/Marketing Manager
Learn about animal classification, adaptation to climate, domestication and special relationships between humans and animals.

845 **Learn About Life Science: Plants**
Sunburst Technology
1550 Executive Dr
Elgin, IL 60123-9311 800-321-7511
Fax: 888-608-0344
http://store.sunburst.com
service@sunburst.com
Michael Guillory, Channel Sales/Marketing Manager
Students explore the world of plants. From small seeds to tall trees students learn what plants are and what they need to grow.

846 **Learn About Physical Science: Simple Machines**
Sunburst Technology
1550 Executive Dr
Elgin, IL 60123-9311 800-321-7511
Fax: 888-608-0344
http://store.sunburst.com
service@sunburst.com
Michael Guillory, Channel Sales/Marketing Manager
Students delve into the mechanical world learning about the ways simple machines make our work easier.

847 **Life Cycles Beaver**
HMH Supplemental Publishers
222 Berkeley Street
Boston, MA 02116 617-351-5000
855-969-4642
Fax: 800-269-5232
http://www.hmhco.com
school.permissions@hmhco.com
Sabrina Crewe, Author
Linda K. Zecher, President, CEO & Director
Eric Shuman, Chief Financial Officer
Dramatic photos tell the story of animal growth and development. This softcover series enriches any classroom science curriculum. Animal development is a complex subject but this series makes it understandable for young readers with simple text and informative images that follow each animal from birth to maturity. *$8.80*

848 **Maps & Navigation**
Sunburst Technology
1550 Executive Dr
Elgin, IL 60123-9311 800-321-7511
Fax: 888-608-0344
http://store.sunburst.com
service@sunburst.com
Michael Guillory, Channel Sales/Marketing Manager
This exciting nautical simulation provides students with opportunities to use their math and science skills.

849 **Our Universe**
HMH Supplemental Publishers
222 Berkeley Street
Boston, MA 02116 617-351-5000
855-969-4642
Fax: 800-269-5232
http://www.hmhco.com
school.permissions@hmhco.com
Gregory Vogt, Author
Linda K. Zecher, President, CEO & Director
Eric Shuman, Chief Financial Officer
Unravel the mysteries of space! A complex universe becomes amazingly clear in these easy-to-read titles. *$96.00*
ISBN 0-739833-55-3

850 **Prehistoric Creaures Then & Now**
HMH Supplemental Publishers
222 Berkeley Street
Boston, MA 02116 617-351-5000
855-969-4642
Fax: 800-269-5232
http://www.hmhco.com
school.permissions@hmhco.com
K S Rodriguez, Author
Linda K. Zecher, President, CEO & Director
Eric Shuman, Chief Financial Officer
Now limited readers can dig into the details of dinosaurs! Each information-packed title includes a special spread with a project, a profile of a dinosaur expert, or a description of a recent dinosaur discovery.
ISBN 0-739821-47-4

851 **Space Academy GX-1**
Riverdeep
14046 Collections Center Drive
Chicago, IL 60693 855-969-4642
Fax: 800-269-5232
http://www.hmhinnovation.com
school.permissions@hmhco.com
Linda K. Zecher, President, CEO & Director
Eric Shuman, Chief Financial Officer
John K. Dragoon, EVP and Chief Marketing Officer
Explore the solar system with Space Academy GX-1! Fully aligned with national science standards and state curricula, Space Academy GX-1, students investigate the astronomical basis for seasons, phases of the moon, gravity, orbits, and more. As students succeed, Grow Slides adjust to offer more advanced topics and problems.

852 **Talking Walls**
Riverdeep
14046 Collections Center Drive
Chicago, IL 60693 855-969-4642
Fax: 800-269-5232
http://www.hmhinnovation.com
school.permissions@hmhco.com
Linda K. Zecher, President, CEO & Director
Eric Shuman, Chief Financial Officer
John K. Dragoon, EVP and Chief Marketing Officer
The Talking Walls Software Series is a wonderful springboard for a student's journey of exploration and discovery. This comprehensive collection of researched resources and materials enables students to focus on learning while conducting a guided search for information.

853 **Talking Walls: The Stories Continue**
Riverdeep
14046 Collections Center Drive
Chicago, IL 60693
855-969-4642
Fax: 800-269-5232
http://www.hmhinnovation.com
school.permissions@hmhco.com
Linda K. Zecher, President, CEO & Director
Eric Shuman, Chief Financial Officer
John K. Dragoon, EVP and Chief Marketing Officer
Using the Talking Walls Software Series, students discover the stories behind some of the world's most fascinating walls. The award-winning books, interactive software, carefully chosen Web sites, and suggested classroom activities build upon each other, providing a rich learning experience that includes text, video, and hands-on projects.

854 **ThemeWeavers: Nature Activity Kit**
Riverdeep
14046 Collections Center Drive
Chicago, IL 60693
855-969-4642
Fax: 800-269-5232
http://www.hmhinnovation.com
school.permissions@hmhco.com
Linda K. Zecher, President, CEO & Director
Eric Shuman, Chief Financial Officer
John K. Dragoon, EVP and Chief Marketing Officer
ThemeWeavers: Nature Activity Kit is an all-in-one solution for theme-based teaching. In just a few minutes, you can select from dozens of ready-to-use activities centering on the seasons and weather and be ready for the next day's lesson! Interactive and engaging activities cover multiple subject areas such as language arts, math, science, social studies and art.

855 **Thinkin' Science**
Sunburst Technology
1550 Executive Dr
Elgin, IL 60123-9311
800-321-7511
Fax: 888-608-0344
http://store.sunburst.com
service@sunburst.com
Michael Guillory, Channel Sales/Marketing Manager
Five environments introduce students to the scientific methods and concepts needed to understand basic earth, life and physical sciences. Students learn to think like scientists as they solve problems using hypothesis, experimentation, observation and deduction.

856 **Thinkin' Science ZAP!**
Sunburst Technology
1550 Executive Dr
Elgin, IL 60123-9311
800-321-7511
Fax: 888-608-0344
http://store.sunburst.com
service@sunburst.com
Michael Guillory, Channel Sales/Marketing Manager
Working with laser beams, electrical circuits, and visible sound waves, students practice valuable thinking skills, observation, prediction, dedutive reasoning, conceptual modeling, theory building and hypothesis testing while experimenting within scientifically accurate learning environment.

857 **True Tales**
HMH Supplemental Publishers
222 Berkeley Street
Boston, MA 02116
617-351-5000
855-969-4642
Fax: 800-269-5232
http://www.hmhco.com
school.permissions@hmhco.com
Henry Billings, Author
Linda K. Zecher, President, CEO & Director
Eric Shuman, Chief Financial Officer
If you have been looking for reading comprehension materials for limited readers, your search is over. True Tales presents powerful real-lfe events with direct connections to geography and science at reading level 3. Gripping accounts of personal triumph and tragedy put geography and science in a very real context. Accompanying activities develop reading and language arts, science, and geography skills students need to boost test scores. *$205.00*
ISBN 0-739834-49-5

858 **Virtual Labs: Electricity**
Riverdeep
14046 Collections Center Drive
Chicago, IL 60693
855-969-4642
Fax: 800-269-5232
http://www.hmhinnovation.com
school.permissions@hmhco.com
Linda K. Zecher, President, CEO & Director
Eric Shuman, Chief Financial Officer
John K. Dragoon, EVP and Chief Marketing Officer
Five environments introduce students to the scientific methods and conepts needed to understand basic Earth, life, and physical sciences. Students will learn to think like scientists as they solve problems using hypothesis, experimentation, observation, and deduction. *$69.95*

Social Skills

859 **Activities Unlimited**
Therapro
225 Arlington St
Framingham, MA 01702-8773
508-872-9494
800-257-5376
Fax: 508-875-2062
http://www.therapro.com
info@therapro.com
A Cleveland, Author
B Caton, Co-Author
L Adler, Co-Author
Helps young children develop fine and gross motor skills, increase their language, become self-reliant and play cooperatively. An innovative resource that immediately attracts and engages children. Short of time? Need a good idea? Count on Activites Unlimited. *$17.95*

860 **Activity Schedules for Children with Autism: Teaching Independent Behavior**
Therapro
225 Arlington St
Framingham, MA 01702-8773
508-872-9494
800-257-5376
Fax: 508-875-2062
http://www.therapro.com
info@therapro.com
Lynn McClannahan PhD, Author
Patricia Krantz PhD, Co-Author
Karen Conrad, President
An activity schedule is a set of pictures or words that cue a child to follow a sequence of activities. When mastered, the children are more self-directed and purposeful at home, school and leisure activites. In this book, parents and professionals can find detailed instructions and examples, assess a child's readiness to use activity schedules, and understand graduated guidance and progress monitoring. Great for promoting independence in children with autism. *$16.95*
117 pages

861 **Alert Program with Songs for Self-Regulation**
Therapro
225 Arlington St
Framingham, MA 01702-8773
508-872-9494
800-257-5376
Fax: 508-875-2062
http://www.therapro.com
info@therapro.com
Mary Sue Williams OTR, Author
Sherry Shellenberger OTR, Co-Author
Karen Conrad, President

This program compares the body to an engine, running either high, low, or just right. Side A is an overview, Side B has 15 songs for self-regulation. Extremely successful in helping kids recognize and change their own engine speeds. *$23.95*
Audio Tape

862 An Introduction to How Does Your Engine Run?
Therapro
225 Arlington St
Framingham, MA 01702-8773
508-872-9494
800-257-5376
Fax: 508-875-2062
http://www.therapro.com
info@therapro.com
Mary Sue Williams OTR, Author
Sherry Shellenberger OTR, Co-Author
Karen Conrad, President
Introduces the entire Alert Program, which explains how we regulate our arousal states. Describes the use of sensorimotor strategies to manage levels of alertness. This program is fun for students and the adults working with them, and translates easily into real life. *$7.95*

863 Andy and His Yellow Frisbee
Woodbine House
6510 Bells Mill Rd
Bethesda, MD 20817-1636
301-897-3570
800-843-7323
Fax: 301-897-5838
http://www.woodbinehouse.com
info@woodbinehouse.com
Mary Thompson, Author
A heartwarming story about Andy, a boy with autism. Like many children with autism, Andy has a fascination with objects in motion. His talent for spinning his Frisbee and a new classmate's curiosity set this story in motion. Rosie, the watchful and protective sister, supplies backround on Andy and autism, as well as a sibling's perspective. *$14.95*
24 pages

864 Breakthroughs Manual: How to Reach Students with Autism
Therapro
225 Arlington St
Framingham, MA 01702-8773
508-872-9494
800-257-5376
Fax: 508-875-2062
http://www.therapro.com
info@therapro.com
Karen Sewell, Author
Karen Conrad, President
This manual features practical suggestions for everyday use with preschool through high school students. Covers communication, behavior, academics, self-help, life and social skills. Includes reproducible lesson plans and up to date listing of classroom materials and catalog supply companies. *$49.50*
243 pages

865 Busy Kids Movement
Therapro
225 Arlington St
Framingham, MA 01702-8773
508-872-9494
800-257-5376
Fax: 508-875-2062
http://www.therapro.com
info@therapro.com
Karen Conrad, President
Full of ideas for developing youngsters' gross motor skills. Games, dramatics, action songs, music and rythm activities. *$9.95*
64 pages

866 Calm Down and Play
Childswork
PO Box 1246
Wilkes-Barre, PA 18703-1246
800-962-1141
Fax: 800-262-1886
http://www.childswork.com
Sally Germain, Editor
Loretta Oleck Berger, Author
Filled with fun and effective activities to help children: calm down and control their impulses; focus, concentrate, and organize their thoughts; identify and verbalize feelings; channel and release excess energy appropriately; and build self-esteem and confidence. *$17.95*

867 Courageous Pacers Classroom Chart
Therapro
225 Arlington St
Framingham, MA 01702-8773
508-872-9494
800-257-5376
Fax: 508-875-2062
http://www.therapro.com
info@therapro.com
Karen Conrad, President
Tim Erson, Author
Highly recommended to accompany the Courageous Pacers Program. Assists in keeping record of 12 students' progress in walking and lifting. A great visual tool to view progress.

868 Courageous Pacers Program
Therapro
225 Arlington St
Framingham, MA 01702-8773
508-872-9494
800-257-5376
Fax: 508-875-2062
http://www.therapro.com
info@therapro.com
Karen Conrad, President
Tim Erson, Author
This fun and easy program was developed to help students become more active. Research shows that students who are more active, do better in school. The goal of the program is simple: get students to walk 100 miles and lift 10,000 pounds in a year.
92 pages

869 Face to Face: Resolving Conflict Without Giving in or Giving Up
820 S. Monaco Parkway
#255
Denver, CO 80224
602-633-4213
Fax: 202-667-8629
http://www.nafcm.org
mphillips@nafcm.org
Matt Phillips, Executive Director
Jan Bellard, Author
Jilda Gutierrez, Co-Author
Modular curriculum for training program for AmeriCorps members. Addresses conflict at the personal level, interpersonal level, and group collaboration. Includes workbook.

870 Forms for Helping the ADHD Child
Childswork
PO Box 1246
Wilkes-Barre, PA 18703-1246
800-962-1141
Fax: 800-262-1886
http://www.childswork.com
Sally Germain, Editor
Lawrence E. Shapiro, Author
Forms, charts, and checklists for treating children with Attention Deficit Hyperactivity Disorder cover a wide range of approaches. Includes effective aids in assessing, treating, and monitoring the progress of the ADHD child. *$ 31.95*
100 pages

871 Funsical Fitness With Silly-cise CD: Motor Development Activities
Therapro
225 Arlington St
Framingham, MA 01702-8773
508-872-9494
800-257-5376
Fax: 508-875-2062
http://www.therapro.com
info@therapro.com
Karen Conrad, President

This unique blending of developmentally appropriate gross motor, sensory integration, and aerobic activities is guaranteed to build children's strength, balance endurance, coordination, and self confidence. Leads children through four 15-minute classes of Wacky Walking, Grinnastics, Brain Gym, Warm Ups, Adventurobics, and Chill Out activities. *$15.00*

872 **Games we Should Play in School**
Therapro
225 Arlington St
Framingham, MA 01702-8773
508-872-9494
800-257-5376
Fax: 508-875-2062
http://www.therapro.com
info@therapro.com

Frank Aycox, Author
Karen Conrad, President
Includes over 75 interactive, fun, social games; describes how to effectively lead Social Play sessions in the classroom. Students become more cooperative, less antagonistic and more capable of increased attentiveness. Contains the secrets to enriching the entire school environment. *$16.50*
154 pages

873 **Jarvis Clutch: Social Spy**
Educators Publishing Service
PO Box 9031
Cambridge, MA 02139-9031
617-547-6706
800-225-5750
Fax: 617-547-3805
http://www.epsbooks.com
CustomerService.EPS@schoolspecialty.com

Melvin D Levine MD FAAP, Author
Rick Holden, President
Jeff Belanger, Regional Sales Manager
In Jarvis Clutch social spy, Dr. Mel Levine teams up with eight grader Jarvis Clutch for an insider's look at life on the middle school social scene. Jarvis's wry and insightful observations of student interactions at Eastern Middle School bring to light the myriad social challenges that adolescents face every day, including peer pressure, the need to seem cool, the perils of dating., Include the commentary in Jarivs' Spy Notes!

874 **Learning in Motion**
Therapro
225 Arlington St
Framingham, MA 01702-8773
508-872-9494
800-257-5376
Fax: 508-875-2062
http://www.therapro.com
info@therapro.com

Patricia Angermeir OTR BCP, Author
Joan Krzyzanowski OTR MS, Co-Author
Kristina Keller Moir OTR BCP, Co-Author
Written by 3 OTs, this book is for the busy therapist or teacher of preschoolers to second graders. Provides group activities using gross, fine andsensory motor skills in theme based curricula. Every lesson plan contains goals, objectives, materials and adaptations to facilitate inclusion and multilevel instructions. Includes 130 lesson plans with corresponding parent letters that explain the lesson and provide home follow-up activities. *$39.95*
379 pages

875 **New Language of Toys: Teaching Communication Skills to Children with Special Needs**
Therapro
225 Arlington St
Framingham, MA 01702-8773
508-872-9494
800-257-5376
Fax: 508-875-2062
http://www.therapro.com
info@therapro.com

Karen Conrad, President
Sue Schwarz PhD, Author
Joan Heller Miller EdM, Co-Author
Play time becomes a fun and educational experience with this revised hands-on approach for developing communication skills using everyday toys. Includes a fresh assortment of toys, books and new chapters on computer technology, language learning, videotapes and television. *$18.95*
289 pages

876 **Reaching Out, Joining In: Teaching Social Skills to Young Children with Autism**
Therapro
225 Arlington St
Framingham, MA 01702-8773
508-872-9494
800-257-5376
Fax: 508-875-2062
http://www.therapro.com
info@therapro.com

Mary Jane Weiss PhD BCBA, Author
Sandra Harris PhD, Co-Author
Karen Conrad, President
Describes how to help young children diagnosed within the autism spectrum with one of their most challenging areas of development, social behavior. Focuses on four broad topics: play skills; the language of social skills; undestanding another person's perspective; and using these skills in an inclusive classroom. The authors present concrete strategies to teach basic play skills, how to play with others, to recognize social cues and engage in social conversation. Practical and accessible. *$16.95*
215 pages

877 **Right from the Start: Behavioral Intervention for Young Children with Autism**
Therapro
225 Arlington St
Framingham, MA 01702-8773
508-872-9494
800-257-5376
Fax: 508-875-2062
http://www.therapro.com
info@therapro.com

Mary Jane Weiss PhD BCBA, Author
Sandra L Harris PhD, Co-Author
Karen Conrad, President
This informative and user-friendly guide helps parents and service providers explore programs that use early intensive behavioral intervention for young children with autism and related disorders. Within these programs, many children improve in intellectual, social and adaptive functioning, enabling them to move on to regular elementary and preschools. Benefits all children, but primarily useful for children age five and younger. *$16.95*
215 pages

878 **S'Cool Moves for Learning: A Program Designed to Enhance Learning Through Body-Mind**
Therapro
225 Arlington St
Framingham, MA 01702-8773
508-872-9494
800-257-5376
Fax: 508-875-2062
http://www.therapro.com
info@therapro.com

Debra M Heiberger MA, Author
Margot C Heiniger White MA OTR, Co-Author
Karen Conrad, President
The movement activities described in this book are organized in a way that is easy to integrate into the class routine throughout the day. The Minute Moves for the Classroom included in several chapters is a handy reference of movement activities which help make the transition from one activity to another fun and smooth. *$35.00*

879 Simple Steps: Developmental Activities for Infants, Toddlers & Two Year Olds
Therapro
225 Arlington St
Framingham, MA 01702-8773
508-872-9494
800-257-5376
Fax: 508-875-2062
http://www.therapro.com
info@therapro.com
Karen Miller, Author
Karen Conrad, President
Three hundred activities linked to the latest research in brain development. Outlines a typical developmental sequence in 10 domains: social/emotional, fine motor; gross motor; language; cognition; sensory; nature; music and movement; creativity and dramatic play. Chapters on curriculum development and learning environment also included. *$24.95*
293 pages

880 Solutions Kit for ADHD
Childswork
PO Box 1246
Wilkes-Barre, PA 18703-1246
800-962-1141
Fax: 800-262-1886
http://www.childswork.com
Sally Germain, Editor
Dana Regan, Author
Lawrence E Shapiro, Co-Author
This comprehensive kit is packed with hands-on materials for a multi-modal approach to working with ADHD kids aged 5 through 12. *$105.00*

881 Song Games for Sensory Integration
Therapro
225 Arlington St
Framingham, MA 01702-8773
508-872-9494
800-257-5376
Fax: 508-875-2062
http://www.therapro.com
info@therapro.com
Karen Conrad, President
Aubrey Carton, Author
Lois Hickman, Co-Author
For young children with sensory processing challenges, 15 play-along routines help remediate everything from bilateral skills to vestibular dysfunction. Narrative is helpful for parents. Includes an 81 page book filled with ideas for extending therapeutic value of these activites. 87 minute CD. *$21.00*
Audio Tape

882 Start to Finish: Developmentally Sequenced Fine Motor Activities for Preschool Children
Therapro
225 Arlington St
Framingham, MA 01702-8773
508-872-9494
800-257-5376
Fax: 508-875-2062
http://www.therapro.com
info@therapro.com
Nory Marsh, Author
Karen Conrad, President
Seventy stimulating activities target 4 areas of fine motor development normally acquired between 3 and 5: hand manipulation, pencil grasp, scissors skill and grasp, and visual motor skills. Each 30 minute activity has skills, projected goal, supplies needed, instructions and modifications provided and needs limited preparation time. *$59.50*

883 Stop, Relax and Think
Childswork
PO Box 1246
Wilkes Barre, PA 18703-1246
800-962-1141
Fax: 800-262-1886
http://www.childswork.com
Sally Germain, Editor
In this board game, active impulsive children learn motor control, relaxation skills, how to express their feelings, and how to problem-solve. Can be used both as a diagnostic and a treatment tool, and behaviors learned in the game can be generalized into the home or classroom. *$52.00*

884 Stop, Relax and Think Ball
Childswork
PO Box 1246
Wilkes-Barre, PA 18703-1246
800-962-1141
Fax: 800-262-1886
http://www.childswork.com
Sally Germain, Editor
This ball teaches children to control their impulsivity by helping them understand and control their actions. *$22.00*

885 Stop, Relax and Think Card Game
Childswork
PO Box 1246
Wilkes-Barre, PA 18703-1246
800-962-1141
Fax: 800-262-1886
http://www.childswork.com
Sally Germain, Editor
Becky Bridges, Author
Players are dealt Stop, Relax and Think cards and also Stressed Out, Confused, and Discouraged cards. As they acquire more cards, they must choose different self-control skills, and they learn the value of patience and cooperating with others to achieve a goal. *$21.95*

886 Stop, Relax and Think Scriptbook
Childswork
PO Box 1246
Wilkes-Barre, PA 18703-1246
800-962-1141
Fax: 800-262-1886
http://www.childswork.com
Sally Germain, Editor
Hennie Shore, Author
In this uniquely designed book, children can practice what to say and how to act in eight different scenarios common to children with behavioral problems. The counselor and the child sit across from each other and read the scripts. *$24.95*

887 Stop, Relax and Think Workbook
Childswork
PO Box 1246
Wilkes-Barre, PA 18703-1246
800-962-1141
Fax: 800-262-1886
http://www.childswork.com
Sally Germain, Editor
Lisa M. Schab, LCSW, Author
This new workbook contains more than 60 paper and pencil activities that teach children such important skills as: thinking about consequences, staying focused and completing a task, engaging in quiet activities without disturbing others, and more. *$19.95*

888 Successful Movement Challenges
Therapro
225 Arlington St
Framingham, MA 01702-8773
508-872-9494
800-257-5376
Fax: 508-875-2062
http://www.therapro.com
info@therapro.com
Jack Capon, Author
Karen Conrad, President
Extensive and exciting movement activities for children in preschool, elementary and special education. Includes movement exploration challenges using parachutes, balls, hoops, ropes, bean bags, rythm sticks, scarves and much more. This popular publication also includes body conditioning, mat activities and playground apparatus activities. Everyone enjoys the creative and carefully designed movement experiences. *$14.25*
127 pages

889 **Teaching Kids with Mental Health and Learning Disorders in the Regular Classroom**
Free Spirit Publishing
217 5th Ave N
Suite 200
Minneapolis, MN 55401-1299 800-735-7323
866-703-7322
Fax: 866-419-5199
http://www.freespirit.com
help4kids@freespirit.com
Judy Galbraith, Founder/President
Myles L. Cooley, Author
Generalized Anxiety Disorder (GAD), depression, Asperger's Syndrome, and ADHD. Many students have these and other mental health issues and learning problems. Written by a clinical psychologist, this guide describes mental health and learning disorders often observed in school children, explains how each might be exhibited in the classroom, and offers expert suggestions on what to do (and sometimes what not to do). *$34.95*
256 pages
ISBN 1-575420-89-9

890 **Understanding Argumentative Communication: How Many Ways Can You Ask for a Cookie?**
Therapro
225 Arlington St
Framingham, MA 01702-8773 508-872-9494
800-257-5376
Fax: 508-875-2062
http://www.therapro.com
info@therapro.com
Christine Derse MEd, Author
Janice Lopes MSEd, Co-Author
Karen Conrad, President
Ten uncomplicated lesson plans for classroom use. Teach a complete overview of all that Argumentative Communication encompasses or give students a brief awareness lesson about just one type of communication. Lessons can be used either consecutively or singly. Includes defining communication, gestures, sign language, object boards, picture boards, headsticks, eye pointing, scanning with picture boards, picture boards in sentence format and computers for argumentative communication. *$18.95*
142 pages

891 **Updown Chair**
R.E.A.L. Design
187 S Main St
Dolgeville, NY 13329-1455 315-429-3071
800-696-7041
Fax: 315-429-3071
http://www.realdesigninc.com
rdesign@twcny.rr.com
Kris Wohnsen, Co-Owner
Sam Camarello, Co-Owner
The updown chair is designed for children from 43-63 in height. It combines optimal positioning and sitting comfort with ease of adjustment. Changing the seat height can be done quickly and safely with our exclusive foot lever activation which uses a pneumatic cylinder assist. Children can be elevated to just the right position for floor or table top activities.

892 **Wikki Stix Hands On-Learning Activity Book**
Therapro
225 Arlington St
Framingham, MA 01702-8773 508-872-9494
800-257-5376
Fax: 508-875-2062
http://www.therapro.com
info@therapro.com
Karen Conrad, President
Loaded with great ideas for using Wikki Stix. For all ages and curriculums. *$3.50*

893 **Workbook for Verbal Expression**
PO Box 1579
Appleton, WI 54912-1579 419-589-1600
888-388-3224
Fax: 888-388-6344
http://www.schoolspecialty.com
orders@schoolspecialty.com
Joseph M. Yorio, President, CEO
Beth M Kennedy, Author
Kevin Baehler, Vice President, Acting CFO
A book of 100s of excercises from simple naming, automatic speech sequences, and repetition exercises to complex tasks in sentence formulation and abstract verbal reasoning. Item number 1435.

Social Studies

894 **American Government Today**
HMH Supplemental Publishers
222 Berkeley Street
Boston, MA 02116 617-351-5000
855-969-4642
Fax: 800-269-5232
http://www.hmhco.com
school.permissions@hmhco.com
Mark Sanders, Author
Linda K. Zecher, President, CEO & Director
Eric Shuman, Chief Financial Officer
Give limited readers unlimited access to social studies and citizenship topics! Whether applying for citizenship or studying for GED Test, learners need to know about our nation's capital and the democracy it hosts. In this series, even limited readers can get a clear picture of a complex system.
$52.00
ISBN 0-139822-03-9

895 **Calliope**
Cobblestone Publishing
30 Grove St
Suite C
Peterborough, NH 03458-1453 603-924-7209
800-821-0115
Fax: 603-924-7380
http://www.cobblestonepub.com
customerservice@caruspub.com
Rosalie Baker, Editor
Kid's world history magazine written for kids ages 9 to 14, goes beyond the facts to explore provocative issues. *$33.95*
9x/year

896 **Discoveries: Explore the Desert Ecosystem**
Sunburst Technology
1550 Executive Dr
Elgin, IL 60123-9311 800-321-7511
Fax: 888-608-0344
http://store.sunburst.com
service@sunburst.com
Michael Guillory, Channel Sales/Marketing Manager
This program invites students to explore the plants, animals, culture and georgraphy of the Sonoran Desert by day and by night.

897 **Discoveries: Explore the Everglades Ecosystem**
Sunburst Technology
1550 Executive Dr
Elgin, IL 60123-9311 800-321-7511
Fax: 888-608-0344
http://store.sunburst.com
service@sunburst.com
Michael Guillory, Channel Sales/Marketing Manager
This multi curricular research program takes students to the Everglades where they anchor their exploration photo realistic panaramas of the habitiat.

898 **Discoveries: Explore the Forest Ecosystem**
Sunburst Technology
1550 Executive Dr
Elgin, IL 60123-9311
800-321-7511
Fax: 888-608-0344
http://store.sunburst.com
service@sunburst.com
Michael Guillory, Channel Sales/Marketing Manager
This theme based CD-ROM enables students of all abilities to actively research a multitude of different forest ecosystems in the Appalachian National Park.

899 **Easybook Deluxe Writing Workshop: Colonial Times**
Sunburst Technology
1550 Executive Dr
Elgin, IL 60123-9311
800-321-7511
Fax: 888-608-0344
http://store.sunburst.com
service@sunburst.com
Michael Guillory, Channel Sales/Marketing Manager
Writing workshops combine theme-based activities with the award-winning EasyBook Deluxe.

900 **Easybook Deluxe Writing Workshop: Immigration**
Sunburst Technology
1550 Executive Dr
Elgin, IL 60123-9311
800-321-7511
Fax: 888-608-0344
http://store.sunburst.com
service@sunburst.com
Michael Guillory, Channel Sales/Marketing Manager
Writing workshops combine theme-based activities with the award-winning EasyBook Deluxe.

901 **Easybook Deluxe Writing Workshop: Rainforest & Astronomy**
Sunburst Technology
1550 Executive Dr
Elgin, IL 60123-9311
800-321-7511
Fax: 888-608-0344
http://store.sunburst.com
service@sunburst.com
Michael Guillory, Channel Sales/Marketing Manager
Writing workshops combine theme-based activities with the award-winning EasyBook Deluxe.

902 **Explorers & Exploration: Steadwell**
HMH Supplemental Publishers
222 Berkeley Street
Boston, MA 02116
617-351-5000
855-969-4642
Fax: 800-269-5232
http://www.hmhco.com
school.permissions@hmhco.com
Linda K. Zecher, President and CEO
Eric Shuman, Chief Financial Officer
John K. Dragoon, EVP and Chief Marketing Officer
Long ago adventures are still a thrill in these vividly illustrated titles. Maps, diagrams, and contemporary prints lend an authenic air. A time line and list of events in the appropriate century put history in perspective. *$44.40*
ISBN 0-739822-05-5

903 **First Biographies**
HMH Supplemental Publishers
222 Berkeley Street
Boston, MA 02116
617-351-5000
855-969-4642
Fax: 800-269-5232
http://www.hmhco.com
school.permissions@hmhco.com
Linda K. Zecher, President, CEO
Eric Shuman, CFO
John K. Dragoon, EVP and Chief Marketing Officer
True stories of true legends! Legendary figures triumph over tough challenges in these brief biographies. Beginning readers learn about favorite heroes and heroines in books they can read for themselves. *$98.80*
ISBN 0-817268-91-X

904 **Imagination Express Destination Time Trip USA**
Sunburst Technology
1550 Executive Dr
Elgin, IL 60123-9311
800-321-7511
Fax: 888-608-0344
http://store.sunburst.com
service@sunburst.com
Michael Guillory, Channel Sales/Marketing Manager
Student's travel through time to explore the history and development of a fictional New England town. An online scrapbook lets them learn about architecture, fashion, entertainment and events of the six major periods in U.S. history.

905 **Make-a-Map 3D**
Sunburst Technology
1550 Executive Dr
Elgin, IL 60123-9311
800-321-7511
Fax: 888-608-0344
http://store.sunburst.com
service@sunburst.com
Michael Guillory, Channel Sales/Marketing Manager
Students learn basic mapping, geography and navigation skills. Students design maps of their immediate surroundings by dragging and dropping roads and buildings and adding landmarks, land forms and traffic signs.

906 **Maps & Navigation**
Sunburst Technology
1550 Executive Dr
Elgin, IL 60123-9311
800-321-7511
Fax: 888-608-0344
http://store.sunburst.com
service@sunburst.com
Michael Guillory, Channel Sales/Marketing Manager
This exciting nautical simulation provides students with opportunities to use their math and science skills.

907 **Prehistoric Creaures Then & Now**
HMH Supplemental Publishers
222 Berkeley Street
Boston, MA 02116
617-351-5000
855-969-4642
Fax: 800-269-5232
http://www.hmhco.com
school.permissions@hmhco.com
K S Rodiguez, Author
Linda K. Zecher, President, CEO & Director
Eric Shuman, Chief Financial Officer
Now limited readers can dig into the details of dinosaurs! Each information-packed title includes a special spread with a project, a profile of a dinosaur expert, or a description of a recent dinosaur discovery.
ISBN 0-739821-47-4

908 **Story of the USA**
Educators Publishing Service
PO Box 9031
Cambridge, MA 02139-9031
617-547-6706
800-225-5750
Fax: 617-547-3805
http://www.epsbooks.com
CustomerService.EPS@schoolspecialty.com
Franklin Escher Jr, Author
Rick Holden, President
Jeff Belanger, Regional Sales Manager
A series of four workbooks for grades 4-8 which presents basic topics in American History: Book 1, Explorers and Settlers - Book 2, A Young Nation Solves Its Problems - Book 3, America Becomes A Giant - and Book 4, Modern America. A list of vocabulary words introduces each chapter and study questions test students' knowledge.

909 **Talking Walls Bundle**
Sunburst Technology
1550 Executive Dr
Elgin, IL 60123-9311
800-321-7511
Fax: 888-608-0344
http://store.sunburst.com
service@sunburst.com

Michael Guillory, Channel Sales/Marketing Manager
Broaden students' perspective of cultures around the world with this two program CD-ROM bundle. From the Great Wall of China to the Berlin Wall to the Vietnam Memorial, students explore 28 walls that represent examples of the greatest human achievements to the most intimate expressions of individuality.

910 **Test Practice Success: American History**
HMH Supplemental Publishers
222 Berkeley Street
Boston, MA 02116
617-351-5000
855-969-4642
Fax: 800-269-5232
http://www.hmhco.com
school.permissions@hmhco.com
Linda K. Zecher, President and CEO
Eric Shuman, Chief Financial Officer
John K. Dragoon, EVP and Chief Marketing Officer
When you are trying to meet history standards, standardized test preparation is hard to schedule. Now you can do both at the same time. Steck-Vaughn/Berrent Test Practice Success: American History refreshes basic skills, familiarizes students with test formats and directions, and teaches test-taking strategies, while drawing on the material students are studying in class. *$16.30*
ISBN 0-739831-31-3

911 **True Tales**
HMH Supplemental Publishers
222 Berkeley Street
Boston, MA 02116
617-351-5000
855-969-4642
Fax: 800-269-5232
http://www.hmhco.com
school.permissions@hmhco.com
Henry Billings, Author
Linda K. Zecher, President, CEO & Director
Eric Shuman, Chief Financial Officer
If you have been looking for reading comprehension materials for limiteed readers, your search is over. True Tales presents powerful real-lfe events with direct connections to geography and science at reading level 3. Gripping accounts of personal triumph and tragedy put geography and science in a very real context. Accompanying activities develop reading and language arts, science, and geography skills students need to boost test scores. *$205.00*
ISBN 0-739834-49-5

Study Skills

912 **Experiences with Writing Styles**
Harcourt Achieve
222 Berkeley Street
Boston, MA 02116
617-351-5000
855-969-4642
Fax: 800-269-5232
http://www.hmhco.com
school.permissions@hmhco.com
Linda K. Zecher, President and CEO
Eric Shuman, Chief Financial Officer
John K. Dragoon, EVP and Chief Marketing Officer
Give your students experience applying the writing process in nine relevant situations, from personal narratives to persuasive paragraphs to research reports. Units provide a clear definition of each genre and plenty of practice with prewriting, writing, revising, proofreading, and publishing. *$11.99*

913 **Keyboarding Skills**
Educators Publishing Service
PO Box 9031
Cambridge, MA 02139-9031
617-547-6706
800-225-5750
Fax: 617-547-3805
http://www.epsbooks.com
CustomerService.EPS@schoolspecialty.com
Diana Hanbury King, Author
Rick Holden, President
Jeff Belanger, Regional Sales Manager
This innovative touch typing method enables students of all ages to learn to type quickly and easily. After learning the alphabet, students can practice words, phrases, numbers, symbols and punctuation.

914 **Learning Strategies Curriculum**
Edge Enterprises
708 W 9th St
Suite 107
Lawrence, KS 66044-2846
785-749-1473
877-767-1487
Fax: 785-749-0207
http://www.edgeenterprisesinc.com
eeinfo@edgeenterprisesinc.com
Jean B. Schumaker Ph.D., President
Jacqueline Schafer, Editor
A learning strategy is an individual's approach to a learning task. It includes how a person thinks and acts when planning, executing and evaluating performance on the task and its outcomes. In short, learning strategy instruction focuses on how to learn and how to effectively use what has been learned. Manuals range from sentence writing to test taking. All require training. For information, contact the Kansas Center for Research on Learning, 3061 Dole Center, Lawrence 66045 (785-864-4780)

915 **Super Study Wheel: Homework Helper**
Therapro
225 Arlington St
Framingham, MA 01702-8773
508-872-9494
800-257-5376
Fax: 508-875-2062
http://www.therapro.com
info@therapro.com
Karen Conrad, President
The fun and simple way to find study tips. Developed by learning specialists and an occupational therapist, the Super Study Wheel is an idea-packed resource (with 101 tips) to improve study skills in 13 areas. As a visual, motor and kinesthetic tool, it is very helpful to students with unique learning styles. *$6.95*

Toys & Games, Catalogs

916 **Maxi Aids**
42 Executive Blvd
Farmingdale, NY 11735-4710
631-752-0521
800-522-6294
Fax: 631-752-0689
TTY: 631-752-0738
http://www.maxiaids.com
Elliot Zaretsky, President
Aids and appliances for independent living with products designed especially for the visually impaired, blind, hard of hearing, deaf, deaf-blind, arthritic and the physically challenged. New educational games and toys section.

917 **PCI Educational Publishing**
8700 Shoal Creek Boulevard
San Antonio, TX 78757-6897
512-451-3246
800-897-3202
Fax: 512-451-8542
http://www.pcieducation.com
jberger@pcieducation.com
Lee Wilson, President and CEO
Janie Haugen-McLane, Founder
Randy Pennington, Executive Vice President
Offers 14 programs in a gameboard format to improve life and social skills including Cooking Class, Community Skills, Looking Good, Eating Skills, Workplace Skills, Behavior Skills, Time Skills, Money Skills, Safety Skills, Household Skills, Social Skills, Health Skills, Survival Skills and Recreation Skills. Also offers a Life Skills catalog with over 140 additional products.

Toys & Games, Products

918 **Beads and Baubles**
Therapro
225 Arlington St
Framingham, MA 01702-8773
508-872-9494
800-257-5376
Fax: 508-875-2062
http://www.therapro.com
info@therapro.com
Karen Conrad, President
A basic stringing activity great for developing fine motor skills. Over 100 pieces in various shapes, colors, and sizes to string on a lace. Three laces included. *$7.99*

919 **Beads and Pattern Cards**
Therapro
225 Arlington St
Framingham, MA 01702-8773
508-872-9494
800-257-5376
Fax: 508-875-2062
http://www.therapro.com
info@therapro.com
Karen Conrad, President
Colorful wooden sphers, cubes, cylinders and laces provide pre-reading/early math practice and help develop shape/color sorting and recognition skills. *$27.95*

920 **Big Little Pegboard Set**
Therapro
225 Arlington St
Framingham, MA 01702-8773
508-872-9494
800-257-5376
Fax: 508-875-2062
http://www.therapro.com
info@therapro.com
Karen Conrad, President
Kids love to play with this set of 25 safe, brightly colored hardwood pegs and a durable foam rubber board. *$18.95*

921 **Busy Box Activity Centers**
Enabling Devices
50 Broadway
Hawthorne, NY 10532
914-747-3070
800-832-8697
Fax: 914-747-3480
http://www.enablingdevices.com
customer_support@enablingdevices.com
Steven E. Kanor PhD, President/Founder
With their bright colors and exciting variety of textures and shapes that are designed to invite exploration that results in rewards including buzzers, music box melodies, radio, vibrations, puffs of air, flashing lights, and even a model that talks. Encourages hand-eye coordination, fine motor skills, gross arm movement. A full line of activity centers are available to meet the needs of the learning disabled, hearing impaired, visually impaired and multisensory impaired. *$ 163.95*

922 **Colored Wooden Counting Cubes**
Therapro
225 Arlington St
Framingham, MA 01702-8723
508-872-9494
800-257-5376
Fax: 508-875-2062
http://www.therapro.com
info@therapro.com
Karen Conrad, President
100 cubes in 6 colors are perfect for counting, patterning, and building activities. Activity Guide included. *$19.95*

923 **Disc-O-Bocce**
Therapro
225 Arlington St
Framingham, MA 01702-8723
508-872-9494
800-257-5376
Fax: 508-875-2062
http://www.therapro.com
info@therapro.com
Karen Conrad, President
Requested by therapists working with adults, this item is also great for children. Hundreds of uses include tossing the discs onto the ground and stepping on them to follow their path, tossing and trying to hit the same color disc on the floor, or using the discs to toss in a game of tic-tac-toe on the floor. Includes 12 colorful bocce discs in a storage box with handle. *$29.95*

924 **Earobics® Clinic Version**
Abilitations Speech Bin
PO Box 1579
Appleton, W 54912-1579
419-589-1600
888-388-3224
Fax: 888-388-6344
http://www.schoolspecialty.com
orders@schoolspecialty.com
Joseph M. Yorio, President, CEO
Rick Holden, Executive Vice President
Kevin Baehler, Vice President, Acting CFO
Earobics features: Tasks and Level Counter with real time display, adaptive training technology for individualized programs and reporting to track and evaluate each individual's progress. Step 2 teaches critical language comprehension skills and trains the critical auditory skills children need for success in learning. Item number C484. *$298.99*

925 **Earobics® Home Version**
Abilitations Speech Bin
PO Box 1579
Appleton, W 54912-1579
419-589-1600
888-388-3224
Fax: 888-388-6344
http://www.schoolspecialty.com
orders@schoolspecialty.com
Joseph M. Yorio, President, CEO
Rick Holden, Executive Vice President
Kevin Baehler, Vice President, Acting CFO
Step 2 teaches critical language comprehension skills and trains the critical auditory skills children need for success in learning. It offers hundreds of levels of play, appealing graphics, and entertaining music to train the critical auditory skills young children need for success in learning. Item number C483. *$58.99*

926 **Earobics® Step 1 Home Version**
School Specialty
PO Box 1579
Appleton, WI 54912-1579
419-589-1600
888-388-3224
Fax: 888-388-6344
http://www.schoolspecialty.com
orders@schoolspecialty.com
Joseph M. Yorio, President, CEO
Rick Holden, Executive Vice President
Kevin Baehler, Vice President, Acting CFO
Step 1 offers hundreds of levels of play, appealing graphics, and entertaining music to train the critical auditory skills young children need for success in learning. Item number C481. *$58.99*

927 **Eye-Hand Coordination Boosters**
Therapro
225 Arlington St
Framingham, MA 01702-8723
508-872-9494
800-257-5376
Fax: 508-875-2062
http://www.therapro.com
info@therapro.com
Karen Conrad, President
L. Jay Lev, Author
A book of 92 masters that can be used over and over again with work sheets that are appropriate for all ages. These are perceptual motor activities that involve copying and tracing in the areas of visual tracking, discrimination and spatial relationships. *$21.50*

928 **Familiar Things**
Therapro
225 Arlington St
Framingham, MA 01702-8723
508-872-9494
800-257-5376
Fax: 508-875-2062
http://www.therapro.com
info@therapro.com
Karen Conrad, President
Identify and match shapes of common objects with these large square, rubber pieces. *$19.99*

929 **Flagship Carpets**
PO Box 1779
Calhoun, GA 30701
800-848-4055
http://www.flagshipcarpets.com
info@flagshipcarpets.com
Offers a variety of carpet games like hopscotch, the alphabet, geography maps, custom logo mats and more.

930 **GeoSafari Wonder World USA**
Educational Insights
152 W. Walnut St
Suite 201
Gardena, CA 90248
800-955-4436
Fax: 888-892-8731
http://www.educationalinsights.com
CS@educationalinsights.com
Navigate the United States in a thrilling, interactive tour across this giant, beautifully detailed 4' x 6' cloth map embroidered with state boundaries. As children learn about American geography, they will love attaching the 78 self-stick felt pieces that identify the states and their unique features. *$199.99*

931 **Geoboard Colored Plastic**
Therapro
225 Arlington St
Framingham, MA 01702-8723
508-872-9494
800-257-5376
Fax: 508-875-2062
http://www.therapro.com
info@therapro.com
Karen Conrad, President
Teach eye/hand coordination skills while strengthening pincher grasp with rubber bands. *$3.25*

932 **Geometrical Design Coloring Book**
Therapro
225 Arlington St
Framingham, MA 01702-8723
508-872-9494
800-257-5376
Fax: 508-875-2062
http://www.therapro.com
info@therapro.com
Karen Conrad, President
Spyros Horemis, Author
Color these 46 original designs of pure patterns and abstract shapes for a striking and beautiful result, regardless of skill level. Most designs are made of a combination of small and large areas. *$3.95*

933 **Get in Shape to Write**
Therapro
225 Arlington St
Framingham, MA 01702-8723
508-872-9494
800-257-5376
Fax: 508-875-2062
http://www.therapro.com
info@therapro.com
Karen Conrad, President
Phillip Bongiorno MA OTR, Author
Lorette Konezny, Editor
Practice the visual perceptual motor skills needed for writing with these colorful, fun, and engaging activities. The 23 reusuable activities will keep a student's interest while they learn to process auditory, visual, and motoor movement patterns. In addition, learn concepts of matching and sorting colors, shapes and familiar objects. *$12.95*

934 **Half 'n' Half Design and Color Book**
Therapro
225 Arlington St
Framingham, MA 01702-8723
508-872-9494
800-257-5376
Fax: 508-875-2062
http://www.therapro.com
info@therapro.com
Karen Conrad, President
Elaine Heller, Author
Geometric designs appropriate for all ages. The client draws over dotted lines to finish the other half of the printed design. *$15.00*

935 **Link N' Learn Activity Book**
Therapro
225 Arlington St
Framingham, MA 01702-8723
508-872-9494
800-257-5376
Fax: 508-875-2062
http://www.therapro.com
info@therapro.com
Karen Conrad, President
Carol A. Thornton, Author
A nice accompaniment to the color rings. There are great cognitive activities included. *$9.99*

936 **Link N' Learn Activity Cards**
Therapro
225 Arlington St
Framingham, MA 01702-8723
508-872-9494
800-257-5376
Fax: 508-875-2062
http://www.therapro.com
info@therapro.com
Karen Conrad, President
Learn patterning, sequencing and color discrimination and logic skills with this set of 20 cards that show life-sized links. An instructor's guide is included. *$7.99*

937 **Link N' Learn Color Rings**
Therapro
225 Arlington St
Framingham, MA 01702-8723
508-872-9494
800-257-5376
Fax: 508-875-2062
http://www.therapro.com
info@therapro.com
Karen Conrad, President
These easy to hook and separate colorful 1-1/2 inch plastic rings can be used in color sorting, counting, sequencing, and other perceptual/cognitive activities. *$5.99*

938 **Magicatch Set**
Therapro
225 Arlington St
Framingham, MA 01702-8723
508-872-9494
800-257-5376
Fax: 508-875-2062
http://www.therapro.com
info@therapro.com
Karen Conrad, President
This Velcro catch game offers a much higher degree of success and feeling of security than traditional ball tossing games. 7 1/2 inch neon catching paddles and 2 1/2 inch ball, in a mesh bag. No latex. *$7.50*

939 **Magnetic Fun**
Therapro
225 Arlington St
Framingham, MA 01702-8723
508-872-9494
800-257-5376
Fax: 508-875-2062
http://www.therapro.com
info@therapro.com
Karen Conrad, President
One swipe of the magic wand can pick up small objects without the need for a refined pincher grasp. *$13.95*

940 **Maze Book**
Therapro
225 Arlington St
Framingham, MA 01702-8723
508-872-9494
800-257-5376
Fax: 508-875-2062
http://www.therapro.com
info@therapro.com
Karen Conrad, President
Paul McCreary, Author
Significantly more challenging than the ABC Mazes; rich in perceptual activities. *$10.95*
32 pages

941 **Opposites Game**
Therapro
225 Arlington St
Framingham, MA 01702-8723
508-872-9494
800-257-5376
Fax: 508-875-2062
http://www.therapro.com
info@therapro.com
Karen Conrad, President
Children can explore the concept of opposites by matching and then joining these tiles. Self correcting feature allows for both independent and supervised play. Helps build observation and recognition skills. *$8.50*

942 **Parquetry Blocks & Pattern Cards**
Therapro
225 Arlington St
Framingham, MA 01702-8723
508-872-9494
800-257-5376
Fax: 508-875-2062
http://www.therapro.com
info@therapro.com
Karen Conrad, President
Encourages visual perceptual skills and challenges a person's sense of design and color with squares, triangles, and rhombuses in six colors. *$28.90*

943 **Pegboard Set**
Therapro
225 Arlington St
Framingham, MA 01702-8723
508-872-9494
800-257-5376
Fax: 508-875-2062
http://www.therapro.com
info@therapro.com
Karen Conrad, President
Encourage development of fine motor skills while teaching color, sorting, patterning and counting! Pegboard is 10.75 inches square and made of durable plastic featuring 100 holes in a 10 x 10 array. *$10.50*

944 **Plastic Cones**
Therapro
225 Arlington St
Framingham, MA 01702-8723
508-872-9494
800-257-5376
Fax: 508-875-2062
http://www.therapro.com
info@therapro.com
Karen Conrad, President
The 12-inch versions of the construction project cones are bright orange and made of lightweigth vinyl. Hole in top. *$8.25*

945 **Primer Pak**
Therapro
225 Arlington St
Framingham, MA 01702-8723
508-872-9494
800-257-5376
Fax: 508-875-2062
http://www.therapro.com
info@therapro.com
Karen Conrad, President
A challenging sampler of manipulatives. Four Fit-A-Space disk puzzles with basic shapes, an 8x8 Alphabet Puzzle, three Lacing Shapes for primary lacing, and 24 Locktagons to form structures. *$14.99*

946 **Rhyming Sounds Game**
Therapro
225 Arlington St
Framingham, MA 01702-8723
508-872-9494
800-257-5376
Fax: 508-875-2062
http://www.therapro.com
info@therapro.com
Karen Conrad, President
Introduces 32 different rhyming sounds as players match the ending sound of the picture tile to the corresponding object on the category boards. Includes sorting/storage tray, 56 picture tiles, and 4 category cards with self-checking feature. No reading required. *$9.99*

947 **Shape and Color Sorter**
Therapro
225 Arlington St
Framingham, MA 01702-8723
508-872-9494
800-257-5376
Fax: 508-875-2062
http://www.therapro.com
info@therapro.com
Karen Conrad, President
This simple and safe task of perception includes 25 crepe foam rubber pieces to sort by shape or color. Comes in five bright colors, each color representing a shape. Shapes fit nicely onto five large pegs. *$14.99*

948 **Shapes**
Therapro
225 Arlington St
Framingham, MA 01702-8723
508-872-9494
800-257-5376
Fax: 508-875-2062
http://www.therapro.com
info@therapro.com
Karen Conrad, President
Muncie Hendler, Author
This 8 1/2 x 11 inch high quality coloring book will help children learn to recognize shapes while improving their fine motor and perceptual skills. *$1.50*
30 pages

949 **Snail's Pace Race Game**
Therapro
225 Arlington St
Framingham, MA 01702-8723
508-872-9494
800-257-5376
Fax: 508-875-2062
http://www.therapro.com
info@therapro.com
Karen Conrad, President
This classic, easy color game is back and is fun for all to play. Roll the colored dice to see which wooden snail will move closer to the finish line. Promotes color recognition, understanding of taking turns, and sharing. *$ 19.95*

950 **Speak & Learn Communicator**
Enabling Devices
50 Broadway
Hawthorne, NY 10532
914-747-3070
800-832-8697
Fax: 914-747-3480
http://www.enablingdevices.com
customer_support@enablingdevices.com
Steven E. Kanor PhD, President/Founder
Memory game! Have fun individualizing this matching memory game. Pre-record your questions and answers and you're ready to play. This is an exciting way to reinforce identification and matching numbers, letters, shapes, and words. *$390.95*

951 **Spider Ball**
Therapro
225 Arlington St
Framingham, MA 01702-8723
508-872-9494
800-257-5376
Fax: 508-875-2062
http://www.therapro.com
info@therapro.com
Karen Conrad, President
Easy to catch, won't roll away! This foam rubber ball has rubber legs that make it incredibly easy to catch. Invented by a PE teacher to help children improve their ball playing skills. The Spiderball's legs act as brakes bringing it to a stop when rolled and minimizing the time needed to chase a missed ball. 2 1/4 inch diameter. *$4.50*

952 **Squidgie Flying Disc**
Therapro
225 Arlington St
Framingham, MA 01702-8723
508-872-9494
800-257-5376
Fax: 508-875-2062
http://www.therapro.com
info@therapro.com
Karen Conrad, President
This is a great flexible flying disc that is amazingly easy to throw and travels over long distances. It is soft and easy to catch. It will even float in the pool! *$5.50*

953 **String A Long Lacing Kit**
Therapro
225 Arlington St
Framingham, MA 01702-8723
508-872-9494
800-257-5376
Fax: 508-875-2062
http://www.therapro.com
info@therapro.com
Karen Conrad, President
A lacing activity that develops hand eye coordination and concentration as children create 2 colorful bead buddies. Each buddy has 4 laces attached to its painted heal now build the body with 23 beads! *$15.00*

954 **Things in My House: Picture Matching Game**
Therapro
225 Arlington St
Framingham, MA 01702-8723
508-872-9494
800-257-5376
Fax: 508-875-2062
http://www.therapro.com
info@therapro.com
Karen Conrad, President
Strengthen visual discrimination, sorting, and organizing skills. Young children enjoy finding correct matches in this fun first game. The colorful graphics depicting familiar household objects and activities encourage verbalization and imaginative play. *$9.99*

955 **Toddler Tote**
Therapro
225 Arlington St
Framingham, MA 01702-8723
508-872-9494
800-257-5376
Fax: 508-875-2062
http://www.therapro.com
info@therapro.com
Karen Conrad, President
Offers one Junior Fit-A-Space panel that has large geometric shapes; 4 Shape Squares providing basic shapes in a more challenging size; 2 Peg Play Vehicles and Pegs introducing early peg board skills; 3 Familiar Things and 2 piece puzzles and a handy take-along bag. *$14.99*

956 **Whistle Kit**
Therapro
225 Arlington St
Framingham, MA 01702-8723
508-872-9494
800-257-5376
Fax: 508-875-2062
http://www.therapro.com
info@therapro.com
Karen Conrad, President
The whistles in this collection are colorful and sturdy. Most feature moving parts as well as noise-makers to stimulate both ocular and oral motor skills. Includes nine whistles. Respiratory demand ranges from easy to difficult. *$18.95*

957 **Wikki Stix**
Therapro
225 Arlington St
Framingham, MA 01702-8723
508-872-9494
800-257-5376
Fax: 508-875-2062
http://www.therapro.com
info@therapro.com
Karen Conrad, President
Colorful, nontoxic waxed strings which are easily molded to create various forms, shapes and letters. Combine motor planning skill with fine motor skill by following simple shapes with Wikki Stix and then coloring in the shape. *$5.99*

958 **Windup Fishing Game**
Therapro
225 Arlington St
Framingham, MA 01702-8723
508-872-9494
800-257-5376
Fax: 508-875-2062
http://www.therapro.com
info@therapro.com
Karen Conrad, President
Encourages eye-hand coordination. Rubber hook safely catches velcro on chipboard fish. *$3.99*

959 **Wonder Ball**
Therapro
225 Arlington St
Framingham, MA 01702-8723
508-872-9494
800-257-5376
Fax: 508-875-2062
http://www.therapro.com
info@therapro.com
Karen Conrad, President
This 3 inch ball made of many small suction cups feels good in the palm of the hand and, when thrown against a smooth surface, will firmly stick. Pulling it from the surface requires strength, resulting in proprioceptive stimulation. *$5.99*

Writing

960 **ABC's, Numbers & Shapes**
Therapro
225 Arlington St
Framingham, MA 01702-8723
508-872-9494
800-257-5376
Fax: 508-875-2062
http://www.therapro.com
info@therapro.com
Karen Conrad, President
Do-A-Dot Activity Books are great for pre-writing skill books, printed on heavy paper stock, with each page perforated for easy removal. They promote eye-hand coordination and visual recognition. *$4.95*

961 **Author's Toolkit**
Sunburst Technology
1550 Executive Dr
Elgin, IL 60123-9311
800-321-7511
Fax: 888-608-0344
http://store.sunburst.com
service@sunburst.com

Students can use this comprehensive tool to organize ideas, make outlines, rough drafts, edit and print all their written work.

962 **Callirobics: Advanced Exercises**
Therapro
225 Arlington St
Framingham, MA 01702-8723
508-872-9494
800-257-5376
Fax: 508-875-2062
http://www.therapro.com
info@therapro.com

Karen Conrad, President
Liora Laufer, Author
Allows those who have finished earlier Callirobics programs to continue improving their handwriting in a fun and creative way. Callirobics Advanced lets one create shapes to popular music from around the world. *$29.95*
Book and CD

963 **Callirobics: Exercises for Adults**
Therapro
225 Arlington St
Framingham, MA 01702-8723
508-872-9494
800-257-5376
Fax: 508-875-2062
http://www.therapro.com
info@therapro.com

Karen Conrad, President
Liora Laufer, Author
Callirobics-for-Adults is a program designed to help adults regain handwriting skills to music. The music assists as an auditory cue in initiating writing movements, and will help develop a sense of rhythm in writing. The program consists of two sections: exercises of simple graphical shapes that help adults gain fluency in the writing movement, and exercises of various combinations of cursive letters. *$35.95*

964 **Callirobics: Handwriting Exercises to Music**
Therapro
225 Arlington St
Framingham, MA 01702-8723
508-872-9494
800-257-5376
Fax: 508-875-2062
http://www.therapro.com
info@therapro.com

Karen Conrad, President
Liora Laufer, Author
Ten structured sessions, each with 2 exercises and 2 pieces of music. Includes stickers and a certificate book. *$29.95*
Book and CD

965 **Callirobics: Prewriting Skills with Music**
Therapro
225 Arlington St
Framingham, MA 01702-8723
508-872-9494
800-257-5376
Fax: 508-875-2062
http://www.therapro.com
info@therapro.com

Karen Conrad, President
Liora Laufer, Author
These 11 handwriting exercises are a series of simple and enjoyable graphical patterns to be traced by the child while listening to popular melodies. *$29.95*
Book and CD

966 **Caps, Commas and Other Things**
Academic Therapy Publications
20 Leveroni Court
Novato, CA 94949-5746
415-883-3314
800-422-7249
Fax: 888-287-9975
http://www.academictherapy.com
sales@academictherapy.com

Jim Arena, President
Joanne Urban, Manager
Sheryl Pastorek, Author
A writing program for regular, remedial and ESL students in grades 3 through 12 and adults in basic education classes remedial ESL. Six levels on capitalization and punctuation, four levels on written expression. Specific lesson plans with reproducible worksheets. *$20.00*
264 pages
ISBN 0-878793-25-9

967 **Dysgraphia: Why Johnny Can't Write**
Therapro
225 Arlington St
Framingham, MA 01702-8723
508-872-9494
800-257-5376
Fax: 508-875-2062
http://www.therapro.com
info@therapro.com

Karen Conrad, President
Diane Walton Cavey, Author
Dysgraphia is a serious writing difficulty. This book provides guidelines for recognizing dysgraphic children and explains their special writing needs. Offers valuable tips, ideas and methods to promote success and self regard. *$ 13.95*

968 **Easybook Deluxe**
Sunburst Technology
1550 Executive Dr
Elgin, IL 60123-9311
800-321-7511
Fax: 888-608-0344
http://store.sunburst.com
service@sunburst.com
Designed to support the needs of a wide range of writers, this book publishing tool provides students with a creative environment to write, design and illustrate stories and reports, and to print their work in book formats.

969 **Easybook Deluxe Writing Workshop: Colonial Times**
Sunburst Technology
1550 Executive Dr
Elgin, IL 60123-9311
800-321-7511
Fax: 888-608-0344
http://store.sunburst.com
service@sunburst.com
Writing workshops combine theme-based activities with the award-winning EasyBook Deluxe.

970 **Easybook Deluxe Writing Workshop: Immigration**
Sunburst Technology
1550 Executive Dr
Elgin, IL 60123-9311
800-321-7511
Fax: 888-608-0344
http://store.sunburst.com
service@sunburst.com
Writing workshops combine theme-based activities with the award-winning EasyBook Deluxe.

971 **Easybook Deluxe Writing Workshop: Rainforest & Astronomy**
Sunburst Technology
1550 Executive Dr
Elgin, IL 60123-9311
800-321-7511
Fax: 888-608-0344
http://store.sunburst.com
service@sunburst.com
Writing workshops combine theme-based activities with the award-winning EasyBook Deluxe.

972 **Easybook Deluxe Writing Workshop: Whales & Oceans**
Sunburst Technology
1550 Executive Dr
Elgin, IL 60123-9311
800-321-7511
Fax: 888-608-0344
http://store.sunburst.com
service@sunburst.com
Writing workshops combine theme-based activities with the award-winning EasyBook Deluxe.

973 **Fonts 4 Teachers**
Therapro
225 Arlington St
Framingham, MA 01702-8723
508-872-9494
800-257-5376
Fax: 508-875-2062
http://www.therapro.com
info@therapro.com
Karen Conrad, President
A software collection of 31 True Type fonts for teachers, parents and students. Fonts include Tracing, lined and unlined Traditional Manuscript and Cursive (similar to Zaner Blouser and D'Nealian), math, clip art, decorative, time, American Sign Language symbols and more. The included manual is very informative, with great examples of lesson plans and educational goals. *$39.95*
Windows/Mac

974 **From Scribbling to Writing**
Therapro
225 Arlington St
Framingham, MA 01702-8723
508-872-9494
800-257-5376
Fax: 508-875-2062
http://www.therapro.com
info@therapro.com
Karen Conrad, President
Ideas, exercises and practice pages for all children preparing to write. Contains line drawing exercises, forms to complete, and forms for encouraging good flow of movement during writing. *$32.50*
99 pages

975 **Fun with Handwriting**
Therapro
225 Arlington St
Framingham, MA 01702-8723
508-872-9494
800-257-5376
Fax: 508-875-2062
http://www.therapro.com
info@therapro.com
Karen Conrad, President
One hundred and one ways to improve handwriting. Includes key to writing legibly, chalkboard activities, evaluation tips, and real world handwriting projects. *$16.00*
160 pages Spiral-bound

976 **Getting Ready to Write: Preschool-K**
Therapro
225 Arlington St
Framingham, MA 01702-8723
508-872-9494
800-257-5376
Fax: 508-875-2062
http://www.therapro.com
info@therapro.com
Karen Conrad, President
A wonderful little book for any handwriting program. Includes many basic skills needed for beginning writing such as matching like objects, finding differences, writing basic strokes, left to right sequence, etc. *$6.50*
97 pages

977 **Getting it Write**
Therapro
225 Arlington St
Framingham, MA 01702-8723
508-872-9494
800-257-5376
Fax: 508-875-2062
http://www.therapro.com
info@therapro.com
Karen Conrad, President
A 6-week course for individuals or groups of 4-10 children, 6-12 years. Weekly, 1/2 hour classes begin with a short orientation followed by 25 minutes of games and sensory motor activities, from prewriting to writing practice, from basic strokes to letter formation. Reproducible manuscript and cursive worksheets are included along with homework assignments. *$58.95*
215 pages

978 **Handwriting Without Tears**
806 W. Diamond Avenue
Suite 230
Gaithersburg, MD 20878
301-263-2700
Fax: 301-263-2707
http://www.hwtears.com
info@hwtears.com
Jan Z Olsen, OTR, Founder and Developer
An easy and fun method for children of all abilities to learn printing and cursive.

979 **Handwriting: Manuscript ABC Book**
Therapro
225 Arlington St
Framingham, MA 01702-8723
508-872-9494
800-257-5376
Fax: 508-875-2062
http://www.therapro.com
info@therapro.com
Karen Conrad, President
Illustrated rhymes, practice letters and words, coloring and tear out alphabet cards teach letter formation. *$11.95*
56 pages

980 **Home/School Activities Manuscript Practice**
Therapro
225 Arlington St
Framingham, MA 01702-8723
508-872-9494
800-257-5376
Fax: 508-875-2062
http://www.therapro.com
info@therapro.com
Karen Conrad, President
Directions for forming lower and upper case letters, and numbers, with space for practice. Activities use letters in words and sentences. *$11.95*
64 pages

981 **Let's Write Right: Teacher's Edition**
AVKO Educational Research Foundation
3084 Willard Rd
Birch Run, MI 48415-9404
810-686-9283
866-285-6612
Fax: 810-686-1101
http://www.avko.org
webmaster@avko.org
Don Mc Cabe, President/Research Director
Linda Heck, Vice-President
Michael Lane, Treasurer
This is a teacher's lesson plan book which uses an approach designed specifically for dyslexics to teach reading and spelling skills through the side door of penmanship exercises with an empasis on legibility. Student books are handy but are not required. *$19.95*

982 **Let's-Do-It-Write: Writing Readiness Workbook**
Therapro
225 Arlington St
Framingham, MA 01702-8723
508-872-9494
800-257-5376
Fax: 508-875-2062
http://www.therapro.com
info@therapro.com
Karen Conrad, President
A great variety of prewriting activities and exercises focusing on development of eye-hand coordination and motor, sensory and cognitive skills. Also, helps improve sitting posture, cutting skills, pencil grasp, spatial orientation and problem-solving. Written by an occupational therapist who is a special educator. *$19.95*
112 pages

983 **Making Handwriting Flow**
Oxton House Publishers
PO Box 209
Farmington, ME 04938
207-779-1923
800-539-7323
Fax: 207-779-0623
http://www.oxtonhouse.com
info@oxtonhouse.com
William Burlinghoff PhD, Owner
This packet inlcudes a 16-page booklet, 'Using Models and Drills for Fluency,' and 28 pages of tracing models of numerals, whole words, phrases, and sentences for both manuscript and cursive handwriting, along with a chart for tracking student progress. *$24.95*
ISBN 1-881929-15-9

984 **Media Weaver 3.5**
Sunburst Technology
1550 Executive Dr
Elgin, IL 60123-9311
800-321-7511
Fax: 888-608-0344
http://store.sunburst.com
service@sunburst.com
Publishing becomes a multimedia event with this dynamic word processor that contains hundreds of media elements and effective process writing resources.

985 **Middle School Writing: Expository Writing**
HMH Supplemental Publishers
222 Berkeley Street
Boston, MA 02116
617-351-5000
855-969-4642
Fax: 800-269-5232
http://www.hmhco.com
school.permissions@hmhco.com
Linda K. Zecher, President and CEO
Eric Shuman, Chief Financial Officer
John K. Dragoon, EVP and Chief Marketing Officer
An effective comprehensive review and reinforcement of the writing and research skills students will need. Effectively used in both school and home setting. Ideal for junior high or high school students in need of remediation. *$ 7.99*
ISBN 0-739829-28-9

986 **PAF Handwriting Programs for Print, Cursive (Right or Left-Handed)**
Educators Publishing Service
PO Box 9031
Cambridge, MA 02139-9031
617-547-6706
800-435-7728
Fax: 888-440-2665
http://www.epsbooks.com
CustomerService.EPS@schoolspecialty.com
Rick Holden, President
Eileen Perlman, Co-Author
These workbooks can be used in conjunction with the PAF curriculum or independently as a classroom penmanship program. They were specifically designed to accommodate all students including those with fine-motor, visual-motor and graphomotor weaknesses. The workbooks contain both large models for introducing motor patterns and smaller models to facilitate the transition to primary and loose-leaf papers. A detailed instruction booklet accompanies each workbook. *$25.00*

987 **StartWrite**
Therapro
225 Arlington St
Framingham, MA 01702-8723
508-872-9494
800-257-5376
Fax: 508-875-2062
http://www.therapro.com
info@therapro.com
Karen Conrad, President
With this easy-to-use software package, you can make papers and handwriting worksheets to meet individual student's needs. Type letters, words, or numbers and they appear in a dot format on the triple line guide. Change letter size, add shading, turn on or off guide lines and arrow strokes and place provided clipart. Fonts include Manuscript and Cursive, Modern Manuscript and Cursive and Italic Manuscript and Cursive. Useful manual included. *$42.50*
Windows/Mac

988 **Strategies for Success in Writing**
HMH Supplemental Publishers
222 Berkeley Street
Boston, MA 02116
617-351-5000
855-969-4642
Fax: 800-269-5232
http://www.hmhco.com
school.permissions@hmhco.com
Linda K. Zecher, President and CEO
Eric Shuman, Chief Financial Officer
John K. Dragoon, EVP and Chief Marketing Officer
Help your students gain success and master all the steps in writing through essay-writing strategies and exercises in proofreading, editing, and revising written work. This program also helps students approach tests strategically. *$16.60*
ISBN 0-739810-47-2

989 **Sunbuddy Writer**
Sunburst Technology
1550 Executive Dr
Elgin, IL 60123-9311
800-321-7511
Fax: 888-608-0344
http://store.sunburst.com
service@sunburst.com
An easy-to-use picture and word processor designed especially for young writers.

990 **Tool Chest: For Teachers, Parents and Students**
Therapro
225 Arlington St
Framingham, MA 01702-8723
508-872-9494
800-257-5376
Fax: 508-875-2062
http://www.therapro.com
info@therapro.com
Karen Conrad, President
Diana A. Henry, Author
Ideas for self-regulation and handwriting skills. 26+ activities, each on its own page, with rationale, supplies needed, instructions and related projects. Provides a fast way to prepare for OT activities. Supports the videotapes Tools for Teachers and Tools for Students. *$19.95*

991 **Type-It**
Educators Publishing Service
PO Box 9031
Cambridge, MA 02139-9031
617-547-6706
800-435-7728
Fax: 888-440-2666
http://www.epsbooks.com
CustomerService.EPS@schoolspecialty.com
Rick Holden, President
A linguistically oriented beginning 'touch-system' typing manual. A progress chart allows students to pace their progress in short, easily attainable units, often enabling them to proceed with little or no supervision.

992 **Write On! Plus: Beginning Writing Skills**
Sunburst Technology
1550 Executive Dr
Elgin, IL 60123-9311
800-321-7511
Fax: 888-608-0344
http://store.sunburst.com
service@sunburst.com
This classic process writing series teaches a wide range of core writing and literature skills through hundreds of motivating and challenging activities.

993 **Write On! Plus: Elementary Writing Skills**
Sunburst Technology
1550 Executive Dr
Elgin, IL 60123-9311
800-321-7511
Fax: 888-608-0344
http://store.sunburst.com
service@sunburst.com
This classic process writing series teaches a wide range of core writing and literature skills through hundreds of motivating and challenging activities.

994 **Write On! Plus: Essential Writing**
Sunburst Technology
1550 Executive Dr
Elgin, IL 60123-9311
800-321-7511
Fax: 888-608-0344
http://store.sunburst.com
service@sunburst.com
This classic process writing series teaches a wide range of core writing and literature skills through hundreds of motivating and challenging activities.

995 **Write On! Plus: Growing as a Writer**
Sunburst Technology
1550 Executive Dr
Elgin, IL 60123-9311
800-321-7511
Fax: 888-608-0344
http://store.sunburst.com
service@sunburst.com
This classic process writing series teaches a wide range of core writing and literature skills through hundreds of motivating and challenging activities.

996 **Write On! Plus: High School Writing Skills**
Sunburst Technology
1550 Executive Dr
Elgin, IL 60123-9311
800-321-7511
Fax: 888-608-0344
http://store.sunburst.com
service@sunburst.com
This classic process writing series teaches a wide range of core writing and literature skills through hundreds of motivating and challenging activities.

997 **Write On! Plus: Literature Studies**
Sunburst Technology
1550 Executive Dr
Elgin, IL 60123-9311
800-321-7511
Fax: 888-608-0344
http://store.sunburst.com
service@sunburst.com
This classic process writing series teaches a wide range of core writing and literature skills through hundreds of motivating and challenging activities.

998 **Write On! Plus: Middle School Writing Skills**
Sunburst Technology
1550 Executive Dr
Elgin, IL 60123-9311
800-321-7511
Fax: 888-608-0344
http://store.sunburst.com
service@sunburst.com
This classic process writing series teaches a wide range of core writing and literature skills through hundreds of motivating and challenging activities.

999 **Write On! Plus: Responding to Great Literature**
Sunburst Technology
1550 Executive Dr
Elgin, IL 60123-9311
800-321-7511
Fax: 888-608-0344
http://store.sunburst.com
service@sunburst.com
This classic process writing series teaches a wide range of core writing and literature skills through hundreds of motivating and challenging activities.

1000 **Write On! Plus: Spanish/ English Literacy Series**
Sunburst Technology
1550 Executive Dr
Elgin, IL 60123-9311
800-321-7511
Fax: 888-608-0344
http://store.sunburst.com
service@sunburst.com
This classic process writing series teaches a wide range of core writing and literature skills through hundreds of motivating and challenging activities.

1001 **Write On! Plus: Steps to Better Writing**
Sunburst Technology
1550 Executive Dr
Elgin, IL 60123-9311
800-321-7511
Fax: 888-608-0344
http://store.sunburst.com
service@sunburst.com
This classic process writing series teaches a wide range of core writing and literature skills through hundreds of motivating and challenging activities.

1002 **Write On! Plus: Writing with Picture Books**
Sunburst Technology
1550 Executive Dr
Elgin, IL 60123-9311
800-321-7511
Fax: 888-608-0344
http://store.sunburst.com
service@sunburst.com
This classic process writing series teaches a wide range of core writing and literature skills through hundreds of motivating and challenging activities.

1003 **Writer's Resources Library 2.0**
Sunburst Technology
1550 Executive Dr
Elgin, IL 60123-9311
800-321-7511
Fax: 888-608-0344
http://store.sunburst.com
service@sunburst.com
Students quickly access seven reference resources with this indispensable writing tool.

1004 **Writing Trek Grades 4-6**
Sunburst Technology
1550 Executive Dr
Elgin, IL 60123-9311
800-321-7511
Fax: 888-608-0344
http://store.sunburst.com
service@sunburst.com
Enhance your students' experience in your English language arts classroom with twelve authentic writing projects that build students' competence while encouraging creativity.

1005 **Writing Trek Grades 6-8**
Sunburst Technology
1550 Executive Dr
Elgin, IL 60123-9311
800-321-7511
Fax: 888-608-0344
http://store.sunburst.com
service@sunburst.com
Twelve authentic language arts projects, activities, and assignments develop your students' writing confidence and ability.

1006 **Writing Trek Grades 8-10**
Sunburst Technology
1550 Executive Dr
Elgin, IL 60123-9311
800-321-7511
Fax: 888-800-3028
http://store.sunburst.com
service@sunburst.com
Michael Guillory, Channel Sales/Marketing Manager
Help your students develop a concept of genre as they become familiar with the writing elements and characteristics of a variety of writing forms.

Learning Disabilities

1007 **ACA Conference**
American Counseling Association
6101 Stevenson Ave.
Suite 600
Alexandria, VA 22304 800-347-6647
Fax: 800-473-2329
http://www.counseling.org
membership@counseling.org
Simone Lambert, President
Heather Trepal, President-Elect
Thelma Duffey, Treasurer
Keynote speakers and workshops as well as exhibits are offered.
March

1008 **ACRES-American Council on Rural Special Education Conference**
West Virginia University
509 Allen Hall
P.O. Box 6122
Morgantown, WV 26506-6122 304-293-3450
http://www.acres-sped.org
acres-sped@mail.wvu.edu
Melinda Jones Ault, Chair
Tina Hudson, Chair Elect
Cathy Galyon Keramidas, Treasurer
Conference of special educators, teachers, and professors working with exceptional needs students. Keynote speakers, silent auction.
March

1009 **AHEAD Conference**
8015 W. Kenton Circle
Suite 230
Huntersville, NC 28078 704-947-7779
Fax: 704-948-7779
http://www.ahead.org
Stephan Smith, Executive Director
Carol Funckes, Chief Operations Officer
Oanh Huynh, Chief Financial Officer
A conference for new disability resource professionals that allows them to engage with others and develop a professional network.

1010 **AR-CEC Annual Conference**
Arkansas Council for Exceptional Children
1201 West Center
Beebe, AR 72012 479-967-6025
Fax: 479-967-6056
http://cec.k12.ar.us
arkansascec@gmail.com
Courtney Williams, President/Conference Liaison
Dee Dee Cain, Vice President
Ruth Eyres, President-Elect
The council is dedicated to meeting the needs of it's members through serving as an effective advocate, fostering involvement of the membership and advancing the professional and ethical growth of it's members. The conference is held annually at the Doubletree Hotel in Little Rock, AR.
Fall

1011 **ASHA Convention**
American Speech-Language-Hearing Association
2200 Research Blvd.
Rockville, MD 20850-3289 301-296-5700
800-498-2071
Fax: 301-296-8580
TTY: 301-296-5650
http://www.asha.org
Elise Davis-McFarland, President
Shari B. Robertson, President-Elect
Arlene A. Pietranton, Chief Executive Officer
ASHA is the nation's leading organization for speech-language pathologists, speech/language/hearing scientists, and audiologists. Topics addressed include hearing impairments, special education, and speech communication. There are approximately 16,000 attendees each year.
November

1012 **Active Parenting Publishers-Leader Training Workshops**
1220 Kennestone Circle
Suite 110
Marietta, GA 30066-6022 770-429-0565
800-825-0060
http://www.activeparenting.com
cservice@activeparenting.com
Michael H. Popkin, President/Founder
Provides parenting education curricula, including one for parents of ADD/ADHD children. Runs Leader Training Workshops for parents, educators, school counselors, and more.

1013 **Annual Postsecondary Disability Training Institute**
University of Connecticut
249 Glenbrook Rd.
Unit 2064
Storrs Mansfield, CT 06269-2064 860-486-3321
Fax: 860-486-5799
http://www.cped.uconn.edu
joseph.madaus@uconn.edu
Donna M. Korbel, Director
Assists concerned professionals to meet the unique needs of college students with disabilities.
June

1014 **Assistive Technology Certificate Program**
CSUN Center on Disabilities Training Program
18111 Nordhoff St.
Bayramian Hall 110
Northridge, CA 91330-8340 818-677-2578
Fax: 818-677-4929
http://www.csun.edu
conference@csun.edu
Sandy Plotin, Managing Director
Julia Santiago, Assistant Director
Barbara Towar, Operations Manager
Sponsor of national and international assistive technology training programs. The programs help to expand the knowledge of professionals and also introduces newcomers to the field. Participants learn about all forms of assistive technology and their potential areas of application.

1015 **Association Book Exhibit: Brain Research**
Association Book Exhibit
80 S. Early St.
Alexandria, VA 22304 703-619-5030
Fax: 703-684-4059
http://www.bookexhibit.com
info@bookexhibit.com
Mark Terotchi, President
Attendence is 800-1,000. Every serious publisher of Neuroscience material represented.

1016 **Behavioral Institute for Children and Adolescents**
203 Little Canada Rd. E
Suite 200
Little Canada, MN 55117 651-484-5510
Fax: 651-483-3879
http://www.behavioralinstitute.org
info@behavioralinstitute.org
Sheldon Braaten, Executive Director
Mitchell Yell, Director/President
Kathi Wilhite, Director/Treasurer
Promoting improved services for troubled children and youths. Provides a wide variety of supporting services to professionals and parents who work with children with emotional and behavioral challenges. Services include professional development, discounted publications and materials, conferences, workshops, consultation, program design and evaluation, a professional library, and scholarship program.

1017 **Butterflies for Change Workshops**
Darien, IL
630-323-5551
http://butterfliesforchange.org
deedyp@me.com
Nancy Brown, Inclusion Specialist/Founder
Bridget Brown, Founder/Speaker
Deedy Payne, Educational Consultant
Separate workshops that focus on person centered planning, self-determination, adapting educationcal curriculum to meet the needs of a diverse classroom, and other educational tools and strategies for persons with disabilities.

1018 **CACLD Spring & Fall Conferences**
Connecticut Assoc for Children and Adults with LD
25 Van Zant St.
Suite 15-5
East Norwalk, CT 06855-1719
203-838-5010
Fax: 203-866-6108
http://www.CACLD.org
cacld@optonline.net
Offers speakers, workshops, presentations, and more for professionals and parents of individuals with a learning disability or attention deficit disorder. CACLD has also donated hundreds of books and tapes to libraries, schools, and parent centers which help in training teachers and paraprofessionals.

1019 **CASE Conference**
Council of Administrators of Special Education
Osigian Office Centre
101 Katelyn Circle, Suite E
Warner Robbins, GA 31088
478-333-6892
Fax: 478-333-2453
http://www.casecec.org
lpurcell@casecec.org
Gary E. Myrah, President
Dr. Luann Purcell, Executive Director
Carrie Turner, Treasurer
International educational organization dedicated to the enhancement of worth, dignity, and the potential of each individual in society.
January

1020 **CEC Special Education Convention & Expo**
Council for Exceptional Children
2900 Crystal Dr.
Suite 100
Arlington, VA 22202-3557
888-232-7733
TTY: 866-915-5000
http://cecconvention.org
reneeg@cec.sped.org
Laurie VanderPloeg, President
Mary Lynn Boscardin, President Elect
Jim McCormick, Treasurer
The conference includes 20 stands, more than 400 sessions, Teacher2Teacher sessions, learning labs, and 20+ pre and post convention workshops.
January

1021 **CSUN Assistive Technology Conference**
California State University, Northridge
18111 Nordhoff St.
Bayramian Hall 110
Northridge, CA 91330-8340
818-677-2578
Fax: 818-677-4929
http://www.csun.edu
conference@csun.edu
Sandy Plotin, Managing Director
Julia Santiago, Assistant Director
Barbara Towar, Operations Manager
Comprehensive, international conference, where all technologies across all ages, disabilities, levels of education and training, employment and independent living are addressed. It is the largest conference of its kind with exhibit halls open free to public.

1022 **Closing the Gap Conference**
P.O. Box 68
Henderson, MN 56044
507-248-3294
Fax: 507-248-3810
http://www.closingthegap.com
info@closingthegap.com
Budd Hagen, Co-Founder
Dolores Hagen, Co-Founder
Megan Turek, Director
Annual international conference with over 100 exhibitors concerned with the use of assistive technology in special education and rehabilitation.
October

1023 **DFW Autism Conference**
FEAT-North Texas
7286 Glenview Dr.
Richland Hills, TX 76180
682-626-5000
Fax: 682-626-5001
http://www.dfwautismconference.com
Laurie Snyder, President
Gretchen Purnell, Secretary/Treasurer
A conference that allows experts to receive training that focuses on ways to improve the quality of life for those with special needs such as Autism, Asperger's, ADD/ADHD, and other learning disabilities.

1024 **EDU Therapeutics Training Program**
14401 Roland Canyon Rd.
Salinas, CA 93908
831-484-0994
Fax: 831-484-0998
http://www.edu-therapeutics.com
joan@EDU-Therapeutics.com
Terry McHenry, President
Dr. Joan Smith, Program Director
10 DVD training programs that aims to help children, youth, and adults with learning disabilities such as Dyslexia or ADD/ADHD.

1025 **Eden Autism Training Workshops**
Eden Autism
2 Merwick Rd.
Princeton, NJ 08540
609-987-0099
Fax: 609-987-0243
http://edenautism.org
info@edenservices.org
Michael K. Decker, President/CEO
Jennifer Bizub, Chief Operating Officer
David Napoleon, Chief Financial Officer
Provides year-round educational services, early intervention, parent training and workshops, respite care, outreach services, community based residential services, and employment opportunities for individuals with autism.

1026 **HELIX Conference**
PaTTAN
3190 William Pitt Way
Pittsburgh, PA 15238
412-826-2336
800-446-5607
http://www.pattan.net
James Palmiero, Director, Pittsburgh Office
Carol Good, Assistant Director
HELIX, or High Expectations for Students with Low Incidence Disabilities, is a conference for educational professionals to learn about strategies and supports for students with learning disabilities.

1027 **IDA Conference**
International Dyslexia Association
40 York Rd.
4th Fl.
Baltimore, MD 21204
410-296-0232
Fax: 410-321-5069
http://www.interdys.org
conference@dyslexiaida.org
Jennifer Topple, Chair
Elsa Cardenas-Hagan, Vice Chair
Rick Smith, Chief Executive Officer

The conference promotes effective teaching approaches and strives to pursue and provide the most comprehensive range of information and services that address dyslexia and related difficulties with learning to read and write.
Fall

1028 International Conference on Learning Disabilities
Council for Learning Disabilities
11184 Antioch Rd.
P.O. Box 405
Overland Park, KS 66210 913-491-1011
Fax: 913-491-1011
http://www.cldinternational.org
Sheri Berkeley, President
Brittany Hott, Vice President
Heather Haynes, Secretary
Focuses on all aspects pertaining to learning disabled individuals from a teaching and research perspective.
October

1029 LDA Annual International Conference
Learning Disabilities Association of America
4156 Library Rd.
Pittsburgh, PA 15234-1349 412-341-1515
Fax: 412-344-0224
http://www.LDAAmerica.org
info@ldaamerica.org
Beth McGaw, President
Jonathan Jones, First Vice President
Loreena Parks, Second Vice President
Topics addressed at the conference include advocacy, adult literacy, and classrooms for individuals with learning disabilities.
February

1030 Landmark School Outreach Program
Landmark School
429 Hale St.
P.O. Box 227
Prides Crossing, MA 01965 978-236-3216
Fax: 978-927-7268
http://www.landmarkoutreach.org
outreach@landmarkschool.org
Dan Ahearn, Director
Keryn Kewdor, Associate Director
Jenna Lanoue, Operations Manager
Provides consultation and professional development to schools, professional organizations, parent groups, and businesses on topics related to individuals with learning disabilities. Services are individually designed to meet the client's specific needs and can range from a two-hour workshop to a year-long collaboration.
1971

1031 Lindamood-Bell Learning Processes Professional Development
406 Higuera St.
San Luis Obispo, CA 93401 805-541-6383
Fax: 805-541-6383
http://www.lindamoodbell.com
Nanci Bell, Co-Founder/Director
Offers workshops nationwide for educators in the internationally acclaimed Lindamood-Bell teaching methods. Approximately 40 workshops hosted annually across the United State and Internationally. Inservices also available.

1032 NCFL Conference
National Center For Families Learning
325 W. Main St.
Suite 300
Louisville, KY 40202 502-584-1133
http://www.famlit.org
Sharon Darling, President/Founder
Comprehensive conference serving family literacy professionals and practitioners who are in the field of improving literacy skills and the lives of the parents and children. Attendees will learn about the latest research in the education industry, and hear from celebrity advocates and authors.
September

1033 National Head Start Association Parent Conference
1651 Prince St.
Alexandria, VA 22314 703-739-0875
866-677-8724
http://www.nhsa.org
Damon Carson, Chairman
Linda Meredith, Vice Chair
Yasmina S. Vinci, Executive Director
Newest information on enhancing parent involvement, child development, and sharpening parenting skills. More than 100 workshops.

1034 National Head Start Association Professional Development
1651 Prince St.
Alexandria, VA 22314 703-739-0875
866-677-8724
http://www.nhsa.org
Damon Carson, Chairman
Linda Meredith, Vice Chair
Yasmina S. Vinci, Executive Director
Health Services credentials are offered through a self study format. Family Services Credential Program is now offered at the Parent and Family Engagement Conference, and at the NHSA National Conference.

1035 North American Montessori Teachers' Association Conference
109106 Magnolia Dr.
Cleveland, OH 44106 216-721-3773
Fax: 216-721-3778
http://www.montessori-namta.org
David Kahn, Director
Montessori method of teaching is discussed as well as topics pertaining to all levels of special education. This and other conferences are held in different locations and months throughout the year.
Quarterly

1036 PDE Annual Conference
3190 William Pitt Way
Pittsburgh, PA 15238 412-826-2336
800-446-5607
TTY: 412-265-1002
http://www.pattan.net
James Palmiero, Director, Pittsburgh Office
Carol Good, Assistant Director
An annual conference designed by the Pennsylvania Training and Technical Assistance Network (PaTTAN), that allows educational professionals across the state to gather in order to network, listen to presentations, and learn about effective instructional design strategies for all students.

1037 Pacific Rim Conference on Disabilities
University of Hawaii Center on Disability Studies
1410 Lower Campus Rd.
#171F
Honolulu, HI 96822 808-956-5142
http://www.pacrim.hawaii.edu
prreg@hawaii.edu
Patricia Morissey, Director
Participants from the US and other Pacific Rim nations study such topics in disabilities as lifelong inclusion in education and community, new technology, family support, employment, and adult services.
March

1038 Pennsylvania Training and Technical Assistance Network Workshops
PaTTAN
6340 Flank Dr.
Harrisburg, PA 17112 717-541-4960
800-360-7282
TTY: 717-255-0869
http://www.pattan.net
Angela Kirby, Director
Victor Rodriguez-Diaz, Assistant Director
Chris Cherny, Assistant Director

Supports the Department of Education's efforts to lead and serve the educational community by offering professional development that builds the capacity of local educational agencies to meet students' needs. PaTTAN's primary focus is special education. However, services are also provided to support Early Intervention, student assessment, tutoring and other partnership efforts, all designed to help students succeed.

1039 **Reading 101: A Guide to Teaching Reading and Writing**
Reading Rockets
2775 S. Quincy St.
Arlington, VA 22206 http://www.readingrockets.org
readingrockets@weta.org
Noel Gunther, Executive Director
Christian Lindstrom, Director
Tina Chovanec, Director, Reading Rockets
A professional development course for K-3 teachers, developed by Reading Rockets in collaboration with the Center for Effective Reading Instruction and The International Dyslexia Association. Teachers can take the course at their own pace, while learning ways to support children struggling with reading and writing.

1040 **Son-Rise Program®**
Autism Treatment Center of America
2080 S. Undermountain Rd.
Sheffield, MA 01257 413-229-2100
877-766-7473
http://www.autismtreatment.com
Barry Neil Kaufman, Co-Founder
Raun K. Kaufman, Group Facilitator
Samahria Lyte Kaufman, Co-Founder
Since 1983, the Autism Treatment Center of America has provided innovative training programs and workshops for parents and professionals caring for children challenged by Autism, Autism Spectrum Disorders, Pervasive Developmental Disorder (PDD) and other developmental difficulties.
1983

1041 **TASH Annual Conference**
1875 Eye St. NW.
Suite 582
Washington, DC 20006 202-429-2080
Fax: 202-540-9019
http://www.tash.org
info@tash.org
Ruthie-Marie Beckwith, Executive Director
Bethany Alvare, Director, Marketing
Raquel Rosa, Special Projects Manager
Progressive international conference that focuses on strategies for achieving full inclusion for people with disabilities. This invigorating conference, which brings together the best hearts and minds in the disability movement, features over 450 breakout sessions, exhibits, roundtable discussions, poster sessions and much more.
Fall

1042 **Wilson Language Training**
47 Old Webster Rd.
Oxford, MA 01540 508-368-2399
800-899-8454
Fax: 508-368-2300
http://www.wilsonlanguage.com
info@wilsonlanguage.com
Barbara Wilson, Co-Founder/Co-President
Ed Wilson, Co-Founder/CFO
Our workshops instruct teachers, or other professionals in a related field, how to succeed with students who have not learned to read, write, and spell despite great effort. Established in order to provide training in the Wilson Reading System, the Wilson staff provides Two-Day Overview Workshops as well as certified Level I and II training.

1043 **Youth Change Workshops**
275 N. 3rd St.
Woodburn, OR 97071 503-982-4420
800-545-5736
Fax: 503-982-7910
http://www.youthchg.com
Ruth Herman Wells, Founder/Director
Provides general session, on-site, and online professional development workshops

Assistive Devices

1044 **AbleData National Institute on Disability & Rehab. Research**
U.S. Department of Education
103 West Broad St.
Suite 400
Falls Church, MD 22046
703-356-8035
800-227-0216
Fax: 703-356-8314
TTY: 703-992-8313
http://www.abledata.com
abledata@neweditions.net
Katherine Belknap, Project Director
Juanita Hardy, Information Specialist
David Johnson, Publications Director
AbleData is a free resource offering information on more than 40,000 assistive technology products for people with disabilities. Our listings include commercially available products and do-it-yourself solutions.

1045 **Ablenet**
2625 Patton Road
Roseville, MN 55113-1308
651-294-2200
800-322-0956
Fax: 651-294-2259
http://www.ablenetinc.com
customerservice@ablenetinc.com
Jennifer Thalhuber, President/CEO
Bill Sproull, Chairman
William Mills, Director
Dedicated to making a difference in the lives of people with disabilities.

1046 **Adaptive Device Locator System (ADLS)**
Academic Software
3504 Tates Creek Rd
Lexington, KY 40517-2601
859-552-1020
Fax: 253-799-4012
http://www.acsw.com
asistaff@acsw.com
Warren E Lacefield, President
Penelope D Ellis, COO/Dir Sales/Marketing
Sylvia B. Lacefield, Graphic Artist
System describes thousands of devices, cross references over 1000 vendors and illustrates devices graphically. The ADLS databases include a full spectrum of living aids, products ranging from specialized eating utensils to dressing aids, electronic switches, computer hardware and software, adapted physical education devices and much more. Now accessible on the internet through Adaptworld.com and Acsw.com *$195.00*

1047 **Alliance for Technology Access**
1119 Old Humboldt Road
Jackson, TN 38305
731-554-5282
800-914-3017
Fax: 731-554-5283
TTY: 731-554-5284
http://www.ataccess.org
atainfo@ataccess.org
James Allison, President
Mike Hewitt, Secretary/Treasurer
Bob Van der Linde, Vice President
The mission of the Alliance for Technology Access (ATA) is to increase the use of technology by children and adults with disabilities and functional limitations.

1048 **Braille Keyboard Sticker Overlay Label Kit**
Hooleon Corporation
PO Box 589
304 West Denby Ave
Melrose, NM 88124
575-253-4503
800-937-1337
Fax: 505-253-4299
http://www.hooleon.com
sales@hooleon.com
Joan Crozier, Founder
Bob Crozier, Founder
Transparent with raised braille allows both sighted and nonsighted users to use same keyboard.

1049 **Connect Outloud**
Freedom Scientific
11800 31st Ct N
St Petersburg, FL 33716-1805
727-803-8000
800-444-4443
Fax: 727-803-8001
http://www.freedomscientific.com
info@freedomscientific.com
John Blake, President, CEO
Designed to allow beginners through experienced blind or low vision computer users to access the Internet through speech and Braille output. Based on our JAWS for Windows technology, and offers additional access to Windows XP. *$ 249.00*

1050 **Controlpad 24**
Genovation
17741 Mitchell N
Irvine, CA 92614-6028
949-833-3355
800-822-4333
Fax: 949-833-0322
http://www.genovation.com
max@genovation.com
Fully programmable 24 key pad. Its principal purpose is to provide single keystroke macros.

1051 **Dyna Vox Technologies**
2100 Wharton St
Suite 400
Pittsburgh, PA 15203-1942
412-381-4883
866-396-2869
Fax: 412-381-5241
http://www.dynavoxtech.com
Ray.Merk@dynavoxtech.com
Sherry Bertner, Managing Director
DynaVox Technologies develops, manufactures, distributes and supports a variety of speech-output devices that allow individuals challenged by speech, lanugage and learning disabilities to make meaningful connections with their world. The company's products allow individuals of all ages and abilities to initiate and participate in conversations at home, work, in school and throughout the community. *$4500.00*

1052 **EZ Keys XP**
Words+
42505 10th St W
Lancaster, CA 93534-7059
661-723-7723
800-869-8521
Fax: 661-723-2114
http://www.words-plus.com
info@word-plus.com
Assistance program that provides keyboard control, dual word prediction, abbreviation-expansion and speech output while running standard software. *$695.00*

1053 **Enabling Devices**
50 Broadway
Hawthorne, NY 10532
914-747-3070
800-832-8697
Fax: 914-747-3480
http://www.enablingdevices.com
customer_support@enablingdevices.com
Steven E. Kanor PhD, President/Founder
A designer, manufacturer and distributor of unique and affordable assistive and adaptive technologies for the physically and mentally challenged, ED/TFSC's products are sought by parents, teachers, and professionals alike.

1054 **Genie Color TV**
TeleSensory
417 Cypress Street
Bakersfield, CA 93304
650-743-9515
800-804-8004
Fax: 661-327-2478
http://www.telesensory.com
info@telesensory.com
Brings clarity and comfort to reading and writing. Since many people with low vision find that specific color combinations enhance legibility, VersiColor offers 24 customized foreground and background color combinations to choose from in addition to a full color mode. Genie can also connect to a computer for use with Telesensory's Vista screen magnification system. *$2995.00*

1055 **Genovation**
17741 Mitchell N
Irvine, CA 92614-6028
949-833-3355
800-822-4333
Fax: 949-833-0322
http://www.genovation.com
max@genovation.com
Produces a wide variety of computer input devices for data-entry, and custom applications. Produces the Function Keypad 682 for people with limited dexterity. It is programmable, allowing the user to store macros (selected patterns of key strokes) into memory, and relegendable keys allow easy labeling of user-programmed functions. Additional options such as larger keys (1x2), allow reconfiguration to meet the user's needs. Call toll-free for pricing and availability.

1056 **Handbook of Adaptive Switches and Augmentative Communication Devices, 3rd Ed**
3504 Tates Creek Road
Lexington, KY 40517-2601
895-552-1020
Fax: 253-799-4012
http://www.acsw.com
asistaff@acsw.com
Warren E Lacefield, President
Penelope D Ellis, COO/Dir Sales/Marketing
Sylvia B. Lacefield, Graphic Artist
An essential sourcebook for assistive technology specialists, teacheers, therapists, and others who select adaptive swicthes and augmentative communication devices for persons with disabilities.

1057 **Home Row Indicators**
Hooleon Corporation
PO Box 589
304 West Denby Ave
Melrose, NM 88124
575-253-4503
800-937-1337
Fax: 505-253-4299
http://www.hooleon.com
sales@hooleon.com
Joan Crozier, Founder
Bob Crozier, Founder
Plastic adhesive labels with a raised bump in the center allowing the user to designate home row keys, or any other key, for quick recognition.

1058 **IntelliKeys**
IntelliTools
2625 Patton Road
Roseville, MN 55113-1308
651-294-2200
800-322-0956
Fax: 651-294-2259
http://www.ablenetinc.com
customerservice@ablenetinc.com
Jennifer Thalhuber, President/CEO
Bill Sproull, Chairman
William Mills, Director
Alternative, touch-sensitive keyboard. Plugs into any MAC, APPLE, or IBM compatible computer, no interface needed. *$395.00*

1059 **JAWS Screen Reading Software**
Freedom Scientific
11800 31st Ct N
St Petersburg, FL 33716-1805
727-803-8000
800-444-4443
Fax: 727-803-8001
http://www.freedomscientific.com
info@freedomscientific.com
John Blake, President, CEO
JAWS is a powerful accessibility solution for the blind & people with low vision that reads information from computer screens using synthesised speech. This advanced & versitile software was specifically designed to meet the needs of blind and visually impaired computer users. WIth JAWS, users can access their computer applications and the Internet via text-to-speech technology. Through the use of a refreshable braille display, JAWS can provide braille output in addition to or instead of speech

1060 **JAWS for Windows**
Freedom Scientific
11800 31st Ct N
St Petersburg, FL 33716-1805
727-803-8000
800-444-4443
Fax: 727-803-8001
http://www.freedomscientific.com
info@freedomscientific.com
John Blake, President, CEO
Works with your PC to provide access to today's software applications and the internet. With its internal software speech synthesizer and the computer's sound card, information from the screen is read aloud, providing technology to access a wide variety of information, education and job related applications.

1061 **Large Print Keyboard**
Hooleon Corporation
PO Box 589
304 West Denby Ave
Melrose, NM 88124
575-253-4503
800-937-1337
Fax: 505-253-4299
http://www.hooleon.com
sales@hooleon.com
Joan Crozier, Founder
Bob Crozier, Founder
Keyboard with 104 keys features large print on all the keys. *$49.95*

1062 **Large Print Lower Case Key Label Stickers**
Hooleon Corporation
PO Box 589
304 West Denby Ave
Melrose, NM 88124
575-253-4503
800-937-1337
Fax: 505-253-4299
http://www.hooleon.com
sales@hooleon.com
Joan Crozier, Founder
Bob Crozier, Founder
For children learning the keyboard. Made of durable rigid plastic and are die cut to fit exactly.

1063 **Lekotek of Georgia Shareware**
Lekotek of Georgia
1955 Cliff Valley Way NE
Suite 102
Atlanta, GA 30329-2437
404-633-3430
Fax: 404-633-1242
http://www.lekotekga.org
info@lekotekga.org
Helene Prokesch, Executive Director and Founder
Peggy McWilliams, Director of Technology Services
Ellen Lindemann, Assistant Director

Software created by our staff using Intellipics, Intellipics Studio or Hyperstudio. Players are included to run this shareware. Color overlays for intellemusic are included. Input methods are mouse, switch, touch window, head mouse and intellikeys if applicable. Subjects are colors and emotions, early childhood music in English and Spanish, shapes and sounds, pictures and letters.

1064 **Open Book**
Freedom Scientific
11800 31st Ct N
St Petersburg, FL 33716-1805 727-803-8000
800-444-4443
Fax: 727-803-8001
http://www.freedomscientific.com
info@freedomscientific.com
John Blake, President, CEO
Allows you to convert printed documents or graphic based text into an electronic text format using accurate optical character recognition and quality speech. The many powerful low vision tools allow you to customize how the document appears on your screen, while other features provide portability. *$995.00*

1065 **Phonic Ear Auditory Trainers**
Phonic Ear
2080 Lakeville Hwy
Petaluma, CA 94954-6713 707-769-1110
800-227-0735
Fax: 707-769-9624
http://www.phonicear.com
mail@phonicear.com
Paul Hickey, Director
A line of learning disabled communication equipment.

1066 **QuicKeys**
Startly Technologies
PO Box 65580
West Des Moines, IA 50265 515-221-1801
800-523-7638
Fax: 515-221-1806
http://www.startly.com
Assigns Macintosh & Windows functions to one keystroke.

1067 **Reading Pen**
Wizcom Technologies
Boston Post Rd W 33
Ste 320
Marlborough, MA 01752-1829 508-251-5388
888-777-0552
Fax: 508-251-5394
http://www.wizcomtech.com
usa.info@wizcomtech.com
Michael Kenan, President
Portable assistive reading device that reads words aloud and can be used anywhere. Scans a word from printed text, displays the word in large characters, reads the word aloud from built-in speaker or ear phones and defines the word with the press of a button. Displays syllables, keeps a history of scanned words, adjustable for left or right-handed use. Includes a tutorial video and audio cassette. Not recommended for persons with low vision or impaired fine motor control.

1068 **Switch Accessible Trackball**
Lekotek of Georgia
1955 Cliff Valley Way NE
Suite 102
Atlanta, GA 30329-2437 404-633-3430
Fax: 404-633-1242
http://www.lekotekga.org
info@lekotekga.org
Helene Prokesch, Executive Director and Founder
Peggy McWilliams, Director of Technology Services
Ellen Lindemann, Assistant Director
Universal to Mac or Windows, this device aids computer navigation where traditional devices are not used. Trackball guards available. *$125.00*

1069 **Unicorn Expanded Keyboard**
2625 Patton Road
Roseville, MN 55113-1308 651-294-2200
800-322-0956
Fax: 651-294-2259
http://www.ablenetinc.com
customerservice@ablenetinc.com
Jennifer Thalhuber, President/CEO
Bill Sproull, Chairman
William Mills, Director
Alternative keyboard with large, user-defined keys, requires interface. Smaller version is also available.

1070 **Unicorn Smart Keyboard**
2625 Patton Road
Roseville, MN 55113-1308 651-294-2200
800-322-0956
Fax: 651-294-2259
http://www.ablenetinc.com
customerservice@ablenetinc.com
Jennifer Thalhuber, President/CEO
Bill Sproull, Chairman
William Mills, Director
Works with any standard keyboard and offers seven overlays and a cable for one type of computer.

1071 **Universal Numeric Keypad**
Genovation
17741 Mitchell N
Irvine, CA 92614-6028 949-833-3355
800-822-4333
Fax: 949-833-0322
http://www.genovation.com
max@genovation.com
A 21 key numeric keypad that works with any laptop or portable computer.

1072 **Up and Running**
IntelliTools
2625 Patton Road
Roseville, MN 55113-1308 651-294-2200
800-322-0956
Fax: 651-294-2259
http://www.ablenetinc.com
customerservice@ablenetinc.com
Jennifer Thalhuber, President/CEO
Bill Sproull, Chairman
William Mills, Director
A custom overlay kit for the IntelliKeys Keyboard that provides instant access to a wide range of software including over 60 popular educational programs. *$69.95*

1073 **VISTA**
TeleSensory
417 Cypress Street
Bakersfield, CA 93304 650-743-9515
800-8048004
Fax: 661-327-2478
http://www.telesensory.com
info@telesensory.com
Image enlarging system that magnifies the print and graphics on the screen from three to 16 times. *$2495.00*

1074 **VisagraphIII Eye-Movement Recording System& Reading Plus**
Taylor Associated Communications
110 West Canal Street
Suite 301
Winooski, VT 05404 802-735-1942
800-732-3758
Fax: 802-419-4786
http://www.readingplus.com
info@readingplus.com
Mark Taylor, Chief Executive Officer
Kelly Scannell, Chief Operating Officer
Stan Taylor, Founder/Chairman
Measures reading performance efficiency, visual and functional proficiency, perceptual development, and information processing competence.

1075 **Window-Eyes**
GW Micro
725 Airport North Office Park
Fort Wayne, IN 46825-6707
260-489-3671
Fax: 260-489-2608
http://www.gwmicro.com
support@gwmicro.com
Erik Deckers, Director of Sales and Marketing
Screen reader that is adaptable to your specific needs and preferances. Works automatically so you can focus on your application program, not so much on operating the screen reader.

Books & Periodicals

1076 **AppleWorks Education**
AACE
P.O. Box 719
Waynesville, NC 28786
757-366-5606
Fax: 828-246-9557
http://www.aace.org
info@aace.org
Gary H. Marks, Executive Director
Tracy Jacobs, Office Manager
Covers educational uses of AppleWorks software. *$25.00*

1077 **Closing the Gap Magazine**
Closing the Gap Solutions
P.O. Box 68
Henderson, MN 56044
507-248-3294
Fax: 507-248-3810
http://www.closingthegap.com
info@closingthegap.com
Budd Hagen, Co-Founder
Dolores Hagen, Co-Founder
Megan Turek, Director
Bi-monthly magazine on the use of computer technology in special education and rehabilitation. CTG also sponsors an annual international conference.
40 pages

1078 **Computer Access-Computer Learning**
Special Needs Project
818-718-9900
Fax: 818-349-2027
http://www.specialneeds.com
Hod Gray, Editor
Ginny LaVine, Author
A resource manual in adaptive technology. *$22.50*
226 pages

1079 **MACcessories: Guide to Peripherals**
Western Illinois University: Macomb Projects
1 University Cir
Macomb, IL 61455-1367
309-298-1414
800-322-3905
Fax: 309-298-2305
http://www.wiu.edu
info@wiu.edu
Amanda B. Silberer, Audiology Clinic Coordinator
Joyce Johanson, Associate Director
Beverly Stuckwisch, Chief Clerk
Designed to help the Macintosh user understand peripheral devices. Includes descriptions of each device, advantages and disadvantages of each, procedures for installation, troubleshooting tips, suggested software and company resources. *$15.00*
41 pages

1080 **Switch to Turn Kids On**
Western Illinois University: Macomb Projects
Horrabin Hall 71b 1 University Cir
Macomb, IL 61455-1390
309-298-1414
800-322-3905
Fax: 309-298-2305
http://www.wiu.edu/users/micpc
info@wiu.edu
Amanda B. Silberer, Audiology Clinic Coordinator
Carrie Lowderman, Clerk
Beverly Stuckwisch, Chief Clerk
Guide to homemade switches gives information on conducting a switch workshop and constructing a battery interrupter as well as various kinds of switches (tread switches, ribbon switches, mercury switches, pillow switches). Contains illustrations and step-by-step instructions. *$12.00*
47 pages

Centers & Organizations

1081 **American Foundation for the Blind**
2 Penn Plaza
Suite 1102
New York, NY 10121
212-502-7600
800-232-5463
Fax: 888-545-8331
http://www.afb.org
afbinfo@afb.net
Carl R. Augusto, President/CEO
Kelly Bleach, Chief Administrative Officer
Rick Bozeman, Chief Financial Officer
Is a national nonprofit that expands possibilities for people with vision loss. AFB's priorities include broadening access to technology; elevating the quality of information and tools for the professionals who serve people with vision loss; and promoting independent and healthy living for people with vision loss by providing them and their families with relevant and timely resources.

1082 **Artificial Language Laboratory**
Michigan State University
405 Computer Ctr
East Lansing, MI 48824-1042
517-353-0870
Fax: 517-353-4766
http://www.msu.edu
John Eulenberg PhD, Director
Multidisciplinary teaching and research center involved in basic and applied research concerning the computer processing of formal linguistic structures.

1083 **Association for Educational Communications and Technology**
320 W. 8th St.
Ste 101
Bloomington, IN 47404-3745
812-335-7675
877-677-2328
Fax: 812-335-7678
http://www.aect.org
aect@aect.org
Stephen Harmon, President
Ellen Hoffman, Executive Secretary
Robert Maribe Branch, President-Elect
Provides leadership in educational communications and technology by linking professionals holding a common interest in the use of educational technology and its application to the learning process.

1084 **Birmingham Alliance for Technology Access Center**
Birmingham Independent Living Center
206 13th St S
Birmingham, AL 35233-1317
205-251-2223
Fax: 205-251-0605
TTY: 205-251-2223
http://www.ilrgb.org
bilc@bellsouth.net
Daniel G Kessler, Executive Director
Information dissemination, network, referral service, support services, and training. Disabilities served are cognitive, hearing, learning, physical, speech and vision.

1085 **Bluegrass Technology Center**
409 Southland Drive
Lexington, KY 40503
859-294-4343
800-209-7767
Fax: 866-576-9625
http://www.bluegrass-tech.org
office@bluegrass-tech.org

Bruce W. Turley, President
Robin Rice, Vice President
Odetta Carlisle, Secertary
Provides support to all persons with disabilities in their efforts to access technology and to increase awareness and understanding of how that technology can enhance their abilities to participate more fully in their community, assisting individuals directly or indirectly by working with their caregivers, therapists, vocational counselors, case managers, educators, employers, and community members.

1086 **CAST**
Center for Applied Special Technology
40 Harvard Mill Sq
Suite 3
Wakefield, MA 01880-3233
781-245-2212
Fax: 781-245-5212
TDD: 781-245-9320
http://www.cast.org
cast@cast.org

Stephen P. Crosby, Chairman
Sheldon H. Berman, Director
David Flink, Director
A nonprofit organization that works to expand learning opportunities for all individuals, especially those with disabilities, through the research and development of innovative, technology-based educational resources and strategies.

1087 **Center for Accessible Technology**
3075 Adeline
Suite 220
Berkeley, CA 97403
510-841-3224
Fax: 510-841-7956
http://www.cforat.org
info@cforat.org

Guy Thomas, President
Sara Armstrong Ph.D, Treasurer
Carol Cody, Executive Director
Resource center for parents, professionals, developers and individuals with disabilities, filled with computers, software, adapted toys and adaptive technology.

1088 **Center for Enabling Technology**
College of New Jersey
PO Box 7718
2000 Pennington Road
Ewing, NJ 08628-718
609-771-3016
Fax: 609-637-5172
TTY: 609-771-2309
http://www.tcnj.edu

R. Barbara Gitenstein, President
Lisa Angeloni, Vice President
Thomas Mahoney, General Counsel/VP
Ongoing projects that match assistive devices to the children who need them. Training and educational workshops.

1089 **Comprehensive Services for the Disabled**
PO Box 1605
Wall, NJ 07719-1605
732-681-5632
800-784-2919
Fax: 732-681-5632

Donald DeSanto, Executive Director
Helps special students realize their potential and bring college admission a step closer. Program designed to meet the needs and maximize the unique talents of each individual. The staff consists of highly qualified teachers who see beyond labels and reach the person inside. By pacing scholastics to each student's ability, the college increases understanding and makes learning a positive experience. Instruction is tailored to each individual.

1090 **Computer Access Center**
Empowertech
P.O. Box 12464
Albuquerque, NM 87195
505-242-9588
http://www.cac.org
info@cacradicalgrace.org

Richard Barlow, Director
Mark Cavanaugh, Director
Phil Robers, Director
Computer resource center serving primarily as a place where people with all types of disabilities can preview equipment. Workshops, seminars, after school clubs for children and individual consultations are provided.

1091 **Council for Exceptional Children Annual Convention & Expo**
Council for Exceptional Children
2900 Crystal Drive
Suite 1000
Arlington, VA 22202-3557
703-264-9454
800-224-6830
Fax: 703-620-2521
TDD: 866-915-5000
TTY: 866-915-5000
http://www.cec.sped.org
victore@cec.sped.org

Robin D. Brewer, President
James P. Heiden, President Elect
Christy A. Chambers, Immediate Past President
This database contains citations and abstracts of print and nonprint materials dealing with exceptional children, those who have disabilities and those who are gifted. Resources in all areas of special education and related services (including services provided by audiologists, speech therapists, occupational therapists, physical therapists, and educational psychologists) are covered in ECER.

1092 **Dialog Information Services**
2250 Perimeter Park Drive
Suite 300
Morrisville, NC 27560
919-804-6493
888-809-6193
Fax: 919-804-6410
http://www.proquest.com

Andy Snyder, Chairman
Kurt Sanford, CEO
Jonathan Collins, CFO
Offers access to over 390 data bases containing information on various aspects of disabling conditions and services to disabled individuals.

1093 **HEATH Resource Center**
2134 G St NW
Washington, DC 20052
http://www.heath.gwu.edu
AskHEATH@gwu.edu

Jessica Queener, Project Director
Reina Guartico, Research Assistant
Dr. Juliana Taymans, Professor
The HEATH Resource Center is an online clearinghouse on postsecondary education for individuals with disabilities. The HEATH Resource Center Clearinghouse has information for students with disabilities on educational disability support services, policies, procedures, adaptations, accessing college or university campuses, career-technical schools, and other postsecondary training entities.

1094 **High Tech Center Training Unit**
21050 McClellan Rd
Cupertino, CA 95014-4276
408-996-4636
800-411-8954
Fax: 408-996-6042
TTY: 408-252-4938
http://www.htctu.fhda.edu
info@htctu.net

Gaeir Dietrich, Director
Michael Fosnaugh, Administrative Assistant
Dale Kan, Network Specialist
Provides training for faculty and staff of the California community colleges in access technologies.

1095 **Iowa Program for Assistive Technology**
IA University Assistive Technology
100 Hawkins Dr
Iowa City, IA 52242-1011 800-779-2001
http://http://iowaat.org
IPAT@uiowa.edu
Jane Gay, Director
Gary Johnson, Coordinator, Community Program
Marlene Phipps, Office Clerk
Computer accesssed solutions for physically challenged students.

1096 **Learning Independence through Computers**
LINC
2301 Argonne Drive
Baltimore, MD 21218-4325 410-554-9134
Fax: 410-261-2907
http://www.linc.org
Theo Pinette, Executive Director
Jessica Robles, Volunteer Services Manager
Justin Creamer, Sr. Assistive Technology
Resource center that offers specially adapted computer technology to children and adults with a variety of disabilities. State-of-the-art systems allow consumers to achieve their potential for productivity and independence at home, school, work and in the community. Also offers a quarterly newsletter called Connections.

1097 **Lighthouse Central Florida**
215 E New Hampshire St
Orlando, FL 32804-6403 407-898-2483
Fax: 407-895-5255
http://www.lighthousecentralflorida.org
lighthouse@lcf-fl.org
Lee Nasehi, President/CEO
Donna Esbensen, VP/CFO
Provides life-changing services for children and adults who are blind and sight-impaired. Offers a comprehensive array of professional vision rehabilitation services in the Central Florida area.
1976

1098 **RESNA Technical Assistance Project**
1560 Wilson Blvd
Ste 850
Arlington, VA 22209 703-524-6686
Fax: 703-524-6639
http://www.resna.org
membership@resna.org
Michael Brogioli, Executive Director
Mary Ellen Buning, PhD, OTR/L, President
James Lenker, PhD, OTR/L, Treasurer
Provides technical assistance to states in the development and implementation of consumer responsive statewide programs of technology-related assistance under the Technology Related Assistance for Individuals with Disabilities Act of 1988.

1099 **Ruth Eason School**
648 Old Mill Rd
Millersville, MD 21108-1373 410-222-3815
Fax: 410-222-3817
http://www.aacps.org
schoolsite@aacps.org
Cathy Larner, Principal
Linda Abey, Principal
Tracy D Angelo, Secretary

1100 **Star Center**
1119 Old Humboldt Rd
Jackson, TN 38305-1752 731-668-3888
800-464-5619
Fax: 731-668-1666
TTY: 731-668-9664
http://www.starcenter.tn.org
information@starcenter.tn.org
Jane Gay, Executive Director
Johnson Gay, Coordinator
Marlene Phipps, Office Clerk
Technology center for people with disabilities. Some of the services are: music therapy, art therapy, augmentative communication evaluation and training, vocational evaluation, job placement, vision department, environmental controls.

1101 **Tech-Able**
1451 Klondike Road
Suite D
Conyers, GA 30094-5982 770-922-6768
Fax: 770-992-6769
http://www.techable.org
c.b.wright@techable.org
Cassandra Baker-Wright, Executive Director
Patricia Hanus, Program Assistant
Erika Ruffin-Mosley, Assistive Technology Trainer
Assistive technology demonstration and information center. Provides demonstrations of computer hardware and software specially designed to assist people with disabilities. Serves a wide range of disabilities and virtually all age groups. Also custom fabrication of key guards and switches.

1102 **Technology Access Center**
475 Metroplex Dr
Ste 301
Nashville, TN 37211-3142 615-248-6733
800-368-4651
Fax: 615-259-2536
TDD: 615-248-6733
http://www.tacnashville.org
techaccess@tacnashville.org
Bob Kibler, Director
Lynn Magner, Service Coordinator
Linda Judeich, Director of Services
Serves the community as a resource center and carries out specific projects related to assistive technology.

1103 **Technology Access Foundation**
605 SW 108th St
Seattle, WA 98146 206-725-9095
Fax: 206-725-9097
http://www.techaccess.org
taf@techaccess.org
Jill Scheuerman, President
Kelly Evans, Vice President
Harish Nanda, Treasurer
Provides information, consultation and technical assistance on assistive technology for people with disabilities, including computer hardware and software technology, and adaptive and assistive equipment.

1104 **Technology Assistance for Special Consumers**
1856 Keats Dr NW
Huntsville, AL 35810-4465 256-859-8300
Fax: 256-859-4332
http://www.ucptasc.org
tracyc@ucphuntsville.org
Cathy Scholl, President
Nicole Schroer, President Elect
Dr. Adam Hott, Secretary
Offers a computer resource center which has both computers and software for use at the center or for short-term.

1105 **Technology Utilization Program**
National Aeronautics and Space Administration
Suite 5K39
Washington, DC 20546 202-358-0000
Fax: 202-358-4338
http://www.nasa.gov
public-inquiries@hq.nasa.gov.
Charles F. Bolden, Jr., Administrator
David Radzanowski, Chief of Staff
Michael French, Deputy Administrator
Adapts aerospace technology to the development of equipment for the disabled, sick and elderly persons.

1106 **Technology for Language and Learning**
PO Box 327
East Rockaway, NY 11518
516-625-4550
Fax: 516-621-3321
ForTLL@aol.com
Joan Tanenhaus, Executive Director
An organization dedicated to advancing the use of computers and technology for children and adults with special language and learning needs. Public domain computer software for special education.

Games

1107 **A Day at Play**
Don Johnston
26799 W Commerce Dr
Volo, IL 60073-9675
847-740-0749
800-999-4660
Fax: 847-740-7326
http://www.donjohnston.com
info@donjohnston.com
Ruth Ziolkowski, President
A Day at Play and Out and About, programs in the UKanDu Little Books Series, are early literacy programs that consist of several create-your-own four-page animated stories that help build language experience for early readers. Students fill in the blanks to complete a sentence on each page and then watch the page come alive with animation and sound. After completing the story, students can print it out to make a book which can be read over and over again.

1108 **Academic Drill Builders: Wiz Works**
SRA Order Services
PO Box 182605
Columbus, OH 43218
800-334-7344
Fax: 614-860-1877
http://www.sraonline.com
SEG_CustomerService@mcgraw-hill.com
The McGraw-Hill Education Urban Advisory Resource works with large urban districts across the country to help them provide better quality instruction, curriculum, and assessment to their students. *$49.00*

1109 **Adaptive Physical Education Program**
2 Merwick Road
Princeton, NJ 08540-5711
609-987-0099
http://www.edenservices.org
Tom Mc Cool, Executive Director
Anne Holmes, Outreach/Support Director
This volume contains teaching programs in the area of sensory integration and adaptive physical education for students with autism. *$50.00*

1110 **Alpine Tram Ride**
Merit Software
121 W 27th St
Suite 603
New York, NY 10011-6262
212-675-8567
800-753-6488
Fax: 212-675-8607
http://www.meritsoftware.com
sales@meritsoftware.com
Ben Weintraub, CEO
Teaches cognitive redevelopment skills. *$12.95*

1111 **Blocks in Motion**
Don Johnston
26799 W Commerce Dr
Volo, IL 60073-9675
847-740-0749
800-999-4660
Fax: 847-740-7326
http://www.donjohnston.com
info@donjohnston.com
Ruth Ziolkowski, President
An art and motion program that makes drawing, creating and animating fun and educational for all users. Based on the Piagetian theory for motor-sensory development, this program promotes the concept that the process is as educational and as much fun as the end result. Good fine motor skills are not required for students to be successful and practice critical thinking. *$99.00*

1112 **CONCENTRATE! On Words and Concepts**
Laureate Learning Systems
110 E Spring St
Winooski, VT 05404-1898
802-655-4755
800-562-6801
Fax: 802-655-4757
http://www.laureatelearning.com
laureate-webmaster@laureatelearning.com
Mary Sweig Wilson Ph.D., President/CEO/Author
Bernard J. Fox, Vice President/Author
Marion Blank, Ph.D, Developmental Psychologist
A series of educational games that reinforces the lessons of the Words and Concepts Series while developing short term memory skills. *$105.00*

1113 **Camp Frog Hollow**
Don Johnston
26799 W Commerce Dr
Volo, IL 60073-9675
847-740-0749
800-999-4660
Fax: 847-740-7326
http://www.donjohnston.com
info@donjohnston.com
Ruth Ziolkowski, President
Camp Frog Hollow chronicles the further adventures of K.C. and Clyde as they head off to summer camp. This entertaining approach to reading, literacy and learning can be beneficial for individual reading lessons or large group activities. The journaling feature provides students the opportunity to record their thoughts and feelings while the tracking feature provides a record of progress for the teacher/parent.

1114 **Create with Garfield**
SRA Order Services
PO Box 182605
Columbus, OH 43218
800-843-8855
Fax: 972-228-1982
http://www.sraonline.com
SEG_CustomerService@mcgraw-hill.com
The McGraw-Hill Education Urban Advisory Resource works with large urban districts across the country to help them provide better quality instruction, curriculum, and assessment to their students.

1115 **Create with Garfield: Deluxe Edition**
SRA Order Services
PO Box 182605
Columbus, OH 43218
800-843-8855
Fax: 972-228-1982
http://www.sraonline.com
SEG_CustomerService@mcgraw-hill.com
The McGraw-Hill Education Urban Advisory Resource works with large urban districts across the country to help them provide better quality instruction, curriculum, and assessment to their students.

1116 **Dino-Games**
Academic Software
3504 Tates Creek Rd
Lexington, KY 40517-2601
859-552-1020
Fax: 253-799-4012
http://www.acsw.com
asistaff@acsw.com
Dr Warren E Lacefield, President
Penelope D Ellis, COO/Dir Sales/Marketing
Sylvia B. Lacefield, Graphic Artist
Single switch software programs designed for early switch practice. CD-ROM for Mac or PC. Visit web site for demonstrations. *$39.00*

1117 **Early Games for Young Children**
Software to Go-Gallaudet University
800 Florida Ave NE
Washington, DC 20002-3600 202-651-5220
Fax: 202-651-5109
http://www.gallaudet.edu
clerc.center@gallaudet.edu
Ken Kurlychek, Information Specialist
Ed Bosso, Vice President

1118 **Garfield Trivia Game**
SRA Order Services
PO Box 182605
Columbus, OH 43218 800-843-8855
Fax: 972-228-1982
http://www.sraonline.com
SEG_CustomerService@mcgraw-hill.com
The McGraw-Hill Education Urban Advisory Resource works with large urban districts across the country to help them provide better quality instruction, curriculum, and assessment to their students.

1119 **KC & Clyde in Fly Ball**
Don Johnston
26799 W Commerce Dr
Volo, IL 60073-9675 847-740-0749
800-999-4660
Fax: 847-740-7326
http://www.donjohnston.com
info@donjohnston.com
Ruth Ziolkowski, President
In the UKanDu Series of interactive software which is designed to promote learning, independence, and accommodate special needs. Word interaction and context are stressed as students progress through the story and make decisions on how the storyline will advance. Active interaction at the word level is encouraged by UKanDu the wordbird, the tour guide to language in this story. *$95.00*

1120 **Mind Over Matter**
World Class Learning
PO Box 639
Candler, NC 28715 800-638-6470
Fax: 800-638-6499
http://www.wclm.com
dealers@wclm.com
A game program that challenges students to solve 185 visual word puzzles or create their own puzzles, using symbols and graphics.

1121 **Monkey Business**
Merit Software
121 W 27th St
Suite 603
New York, NY 10001-6262 212-675-8567
800-753-6488
Fax: 212-675-8607
http://www.meritsoftware.com
sales@meritsoftware.com
Ben Weintraub, CEO
Choose one of the three levels of difficulty and play until a minimum score is reached. *$10.95*

1122 **Multi-Scan**
Academic Software
3504 Tates Creek Rd
Lexington, KY 40517-2601 859-552-1020
Fax: 253-799-4012
http://www.acsw.com
asistaff@acsw.com
Warren E Lacefield, President
Penelope D Ellis, COO/Dir Sales/Marketing
Sylvia B. Lacefield, Graphic Artist
Single switch activity center containing educational games such as numerical dot to dot, concentration, mazes, and matching, for PCs and Macintosh CD-ROM. Handbook for adaptive switches available. *$149.00*

1123 **On a Green Bus**
Don Johnston
26799 W Commerce Dr
Volo, IL 60073-9675 847-740-0749
800-999-4660
Fax: 847-740-7326
http://www.donjohnston.com
info@donjohnston.com
Ruth Ziolkowski, President
An early literacy program in the UKandDu Little Books Series consisting of several create-your-own four-page animated stories that help build language experience for early readers. Students fill in the blanks, completing sentences on each page. After completing the story, students can print it out to make a book which can be read over and over again.

1124 **Teddy Barrels of Fun**
SRA Order Services
PO Box 182605
Columbus, OH 43218 1-888-772-45
Fax: 972-228-1982
http://www.sraonline.com
SEG_CustomerService@mcgraw-hill.com
The McGraw-Hill Education Urban Advisory Resource works with large urban districts across the country to help them provide better quality instruction, curriculum, and assessment to their students. *$42.00*

Language Arts

1125 **Alphabet Circus**
SRA Order Services
PO Box 182605
Columbus, OH 43218 1-888-772-45
Fax: 972-228-1982
http://www.sraonline.com
SEG_CustomerService@mcgraw-hill.com
The McGraw-Hill Education Urban Advisory Resource works with large urban districts across the country to help them provide better quality instruction, curriculum, and assessment to their students. *$35.00*

1126 **American Sign Language Dictionary: Software**
Speech Bin
PO Box 1579
Appleton, WI 54912-1579 419-589-1600
888-388-3224
Fax: 888-388-6344
http://www.schoolspecialty.com
orders@schoolspecialty.com
Joseph M. Yorio, President, CEO
Rick Holden, Executive Vice President
Kevin Baehler, Vice President, Acting CFO
The CD includes captivating video clips that show 2,500+ words, phrases, and idioms in sign language. The videos may be played at normal speed, slow motion, and stop action. Animations explain origins of selected signs; drills and games are provided to reinforce learning. Item number M545 for Windows $24.95 Item number M540 for MAC. *$29.95*

1127 **American Sign Language Video Dictionary & Inflection Guide**
Harris Communications
15155 Technology Dr
Eden Prairie, MN 55344-2273 952-906-1180
800-825-6758
Fax: 952-906-1099
TTY: 800-825-9187
http://www.harriscomm.com
info@harriscomm.com
Dr. Robert Harris, President
Darla Hudson, Customer Service
Lori Foss, Marketing Director

Combines text, video, and animation to create a leading interactive reference tool that makes learning ASL easy and fun. Contains 2700 signs, searching capabilities in 5 languages, new learning games, and expanded sections in fingerspelling. Part #CD 144. *$49.95*
448 pages Video

1128 AtoZap!
Sunburst Technology
3150 W Higgins Rd
Suite 140
Hoffman Estates, IL 60619 800-321-7511
http://www.sunburst.com
Service@sunburst.com
When users select an A, little airplanes that fly madly about appear. Users select T and students have their own telephone to talk to any one of nine animated friends. This program for prereaders has an activity for every letter.

1129 Auditory Skills
Psychological Software Services
3304 W 75th St
Indianapolis, IN 46268 317-257-9672
Fax: 317-257-9674
http://www.neuroscience.cnter.com
nsc@neuroscience.cnter.com
Odie L Bracy, Clinical Neuropsychologist
Nancy Bracy, Office Manager
Andrea Oakes, Clinical Assistant
Four computer programs designed to aid in the remediation of auditory discrimination problems. *$50.00*

1130 Basic Skills Products
EDCON Publishing Group
P.O. Box 383759
Waikoloa, HI 96738 415-580-0953
888-553-3266
Fax: 877-597-6376
http://www.edconpublishing.com
Deals with basic math and language arts. Free catalog available.

1131 Challenging Our Minds
Psychological Software Services
3304 W 75th St
Indianapolis, IN 46268 317-257-9672
Fax: 317-257-9674
http://www.challenging-our-minds.com
info@challenging-our-minds.com
Odie L Bracy, President
Nancy Bracy, Office Manager
Challenging our Minds (COM) is a cognitive enhancement system designed by a neuropsychologist to develop and enhance cognitive functions across the domains of attention, executive skills, memory, visuospatial skills, problem solving skills, communication and psychosocial skills. COM is a subscription website providign online cognitive enhancement applications for all children.

1132 Character Education:Life Skills Online Education
Phillip Roy Inc.
PO Box 130
Indian Rocks Beach, FL 33785 727-593-2700
800-255-9085
Fax: 727-595-2685
http://www.philliproy.com
info@philliproy.com
Ruth Bragman, President
Includes 77 CDs, 77 books and unlimited interactive online access, per purchasing site. All print materials are also available to be Brailled and all CDs come with complete audio components along with interactive graphics. Pre/post tests included along with teacher's guide and lesson plans. All materials can be duplicated at purchasing site. No yearly fees. *$3950.00*

1133 Cognitive Rehabilitation
Technology for Language and Learning
PO Box 327
East Rockaway, NY 11518 516-625-4550
Fax: 516-621-3321
A series of public domain programs that strengthen cognitive skills, memory, language and visual motor skills. *$20.00*

1134 Construct-A-Word I & II
SRA Order Services
PO Box 182605
Columbus, OH 43218 800-334-7344
Fax: 800-953-8691
http://www.mheducation.com
SEG_CustomerService@mheducation.com
David Levin, President/CEO
David Stafford, SVP/General Counsel
Maryellen Valaitis, SVP, Human Resources
The McGraw-Hill Education Urban Advisory Resource works with large urban districts across the country to help them provide better quality instruction, curriculum, and assessment to their students. *$99.00*

1135 Crypto Cube
Software to Go-Gallaudet University
800 Florida Ave NE
Washington, DC 20002-3695 202-651-5031
Fax: 202-651-5109
TTY: 202-651-5855
http://clerccenter.gallaudet.edu
clerc.center@gallaudet.edu
Ed Bosso, Vice President
Ken Kurlychek, Electronic Information

1136 Curious George Pre-K ABCs
Sunburst Technology
3150 W Higgins Rd
Suite 140
Hoffman Estates, IL 60619 800-321-7511
http://www.sunburst.com
service@sunburst.com
Children go on a lively adventure with Curious George visiting six multi level activities that provide an animated introduction to letters and their sounds. Students discover letter names and shapes, initial letter sounds, letter pronunciations, the order of the alphabet and new vocabulary words during the fun exursions with Curious George. Mac/Win CD-ROM

1137 Eden Institute Curriculum: Classroom
2 Merwick Road
Princeton, NJ 08540 609-987-0099
Fax: 609-987-0243
http://edenautism.org
Peter H. Bell, President/CEO
John Inzilla, Chief Financial Officer
Jennifer Bizub, Chief Operating Officer
This volume is geered toward students with autism who have mastered some basic academic skills and are able to learn in a small group setting. Teaching programs include academics, domestic and social skills. *$100.00*

1138 Elephant Ears: English with Speech
Ballard & Tighe
471 Atlas Street
PO Box 219
Brea, CA 92822-0219 714-990-4332
800-321-4332
Fax: 714-255-9828
http://www.ballard-tighe.com
info@ballard-tighe.com
Dorothy Roberts, Chairperson
Dr. Sari Luoma, Vice President, Assessment
Fred Tan, VP, Information Technology
Features instruction and assessment of prepositions in a 3-part diskette. *$49.00*

1139 **Emerging Literacy**
Technology for Language and Learning
PO Box 327
East Rockaway, NY 11518 516-625-4550
Fax: 516-621-3321

A five-volume set of stories. *$25.00*

1140 **Essential Learning Systems**
Creative Education Institute
4567 Lake Shore Driveÿ
P.O. Box 7306ÿ
Waco, TX 76710 254-751-1188
800-234-7319
Fax: 888-475-2402
http://www.ceilearning.com
info@ceilearning.com

Enables special education, learning disabled and dyslexic students to develop the skills they need to learn. Using computer exercises to appropriately stimulate the brain's language areas, the lagging learning skills can be developed and patterns of correct language taught.

1141 **First Phonics**
Sunburst Technology
3150 W Higgins Rd
Suite 140
Hoffman Estates, IL 60619 800-321-7511
http://www.sunburst.com
service@sunburst.com

Targets the phonics skills that all children need to develop, sounding out the first letter of a word. This program offers four different engaging activities that you can customize to match each child's specific need.

1142 **Gremlin Hunt**
Merit Software
121 West 27th Street
Suite 1200
New York, NY 10001 212-675-8567
800-753-6488
Fax: 800-918-9336
http://www.meritsoftware.com
sales@meritsoftware.com

Ben Weintraub, CEO
Gremlins test visual discrimination and memory skills at three levels. *$9.95*

1143 **High Frequency Vocabulary**
Technology for Language and Learning
PO Box 327
East Rockaway, NY 11518 516-625-4550
Fax: 516-621-3321

Each volume of the series has 10 stories that teach specific vocabulary. *$35.00*

1144 **Hint and Hunt I & II**
SRA Order Services
PO Box 182605
Columbus, OH 43218 800-334-7344
Fax: 800-953-8691
http://www.mheducation.com
SEG_CustomerService@mheducation.com

David Levin, President/CEO
David Stafford, SVP/General Counsel
Maryellen Valaitis, SVP, Human Resources
The McGraw-Hill Education Urban Advisory Resource works with large urban districts across the country to help them provide better quality instruction, curriculum, and assessment to their students. *$99.00*

1145 **HyperStudio Stacks**
Technology for Language and Learning
PO Box 327
East Rockaway, NY 11518 516-625-4550
Fax: 516-621-3321

Offers various volumes in language arts, social studies and reading. *$10.00*

1146 **IDEA Cat I, II and III**
Ballard & Tighe
471 Atlas Street
PO Box 219
Brea, CA 92822-0219 714-990-4332
800-321-4332
Fax: 714-255-9828
http://www.ballard-tighe.com
info@ballard-tighe.com

Dorothy Roberts, Chairperson
Dr. Sari Luoma, Vice President, Assessment
Fred Tan, VP, Information Technology
Computer-assisted teaching of English language lessons reinforces skills of Level I, II, and III of the IDEA Oral Program. *$142.00*

1147 **Improving Reading/Spelling Skills via Keyboarding**
AVKO Educational Research Foundation
3084 Willard Road
Birch Run, MI 48415-9404 810-686-9283
866-285-6612
Fax: 810-686-1101
http://www.avko.org
webmaster@avko.org

Don McCabe, President, Research Director
Linda Heck, Vice President, Clio, Michigan
Michael Lane, Treasurer, Clio, Michigan
Students learn spelling patterns and acquire important word recognition skills as they slowly and methodically learn proper fingering and keystrokes on a typewriter or computer keyboard. *$12.95*
ISBN 1-564004-01-5

1148 **Katie's Farm**
Lawrence Productions
6146 West Main St.
Suite A
Kalamazoo, MI 49009 269-903-2395
http://www.lpi.com
sales@lpi.com

Karen Morehouse, Operations Manager
Designed to encourage exploration and language development. *$29.95*

1149 **Kid Pix**
Riverdeep
222 Berkeley Street
Boston, MA 02116 617-351-5000
888-242-6747
Fax: 877-892-9820
http://www.hmhco.com
IIEcustomerservice@hmhpub.com

Linda K. Zecher, President, CEO, Director
James G. Nicholson, President, Riverside Publishing
William Bayers, EVP, General Counsel
Houghton Mifflin Harcourt offers a wide array of technology-driven pre-k-12 solutions that inspire excellence and innovation in education, and raise student achievement. *$59.95*

1150 **Kids Media Magic 2.0**
Sunburst Technology
3150 W Higgins Rd
Suite 140
Hoffman Estates, IL 60619 800-321-7511
http://www.sunburst.com
service@sunburst.com

The first multimedia word processor designed for young children. Help your child become a fluent reader and writer. The Rebus Bar automatically scrolls over 45 vocabulary words as students type.

1151 **Language Carnival I**
SRA Order Services
PO Box 182605
Columbus, OH 43218 800-334-7344
Fax: 800-953-8691
http://www.mheducation.com
SEG_CustomerService@mheducation.com

David Levin, President/CEO
David Stafford, SVP and General Counsel
Maryellen Valaitis, SVP Human Resources
The McGraw-Hill Education Urban Advisory Resource works with large urban districts across the country to help them provide better quality instruction, curriculum, and assessment to their students.

1152 **Language Carnival II**
SRA Order Services
PO Box 182605
Columbus, OH 43218 800-334-7344
Fax: 800-953-8691
http://www.mheducation.com
SEG_CustomerService@mheducation.com
David Levin, President/CEO
David Stafford, SVP and General Counsel
Maryellen Valaitis, SVP Human Resources
The McGraw-Hill Education Urban Advisory Resource works with large urban districts across the country to help them provide better quality instruction, curriculum, and assessment to their students.

1153 **Language Master**
Franklin Learning Resources
2 Manhattan Drive
Burlington, NJ 08016 609-386-2500
800-266-5626
Fax: 609-239-5950
http://www.franklin.com
service@franklin.com
A language master without speech defining over 83,000 words, spelling correction capability, pick/edit feature, vocabulary enrichment activities and advanced word list. *$79.95*

1154 **Learn to Match**
Technology for Language and Learning
PO Box 327
East Rockaway, NY 11518 516-625-4550
Fax: 516-621-3321
Joan Tanenhaus, Founder
Ten volume set of picture-matching disks. *$50.00*

1155 **Letter Sounds**
Sunburst Technology
3150 W Higgins Rd
Suite 140
Hoffman Estates, IL 60619 800-321-7511
http://www.sunburst.com
service@sunburst.com
Students develop phonemic awareness skills as they make the connection between consonant letters and their sounds.

1156 **Letters and First Words**
C&C Software
5713 Kentford Cir
Wichita, KS 67220-3131 316-683-6056
800-752-2086
Carol Clark, President
Helps children learn to identify letters and recognize their associated sounds. *$30.00*

1157 **Lexia Phonics Based Reading**
Lexia Learning Systems
200 Baker Avenue Ext
Concord, MA 01742 978-405-6200
800-435-3942
Fax: 978-287-0062
http://www.lexialearning.com
info@lexialearning.com
Nicholas C Gaehde, President
Collin Earnst, Vice President of Marketing
Peter Koso, Vice President of Operations
Five activity areas with 64 branching units and practice with 535 one-syllable words and 90 two-syllable words, sentences and stories. *$250.00*

1158 **Look! Listen! & Learn Language!**
Abilitations Speech Bin
PO Box 1579
Appleton, WI 54912-1579 419-589-1425
888-388-3224
Fax: 888-388-6344
http://www.schoolspecialty.com
orders@schoolspecialty.com
Joseph M. Yorio, President, CEO
Patrick T. Collins, EVP, Distribution
Rick Holden, EVP
Interactive activities for children with autism, PDD, Down syndrome, language delay, or apraxia include: hello; Match Same to Same; Quack; Let's talk About It; visual scanning/attention and match ups! Item number L177. *$98.99*

1159 **M-ss-ng L-nks Single Educational Software**
Sunburst Technology
3150 W Higgins Rd
Suite 140
Hoffman Estates, IL 60619 800-321-7511
http://www.sunburst.com
service@sunburst.com
This award-winning program is an engrossing language puzzle. A passage appears with letters or words missing. Students complete it based on their knowledge of word structure, spelling, grammar, meaning in context, and literary style.

1160 **Max's Attic: Long & Short Vowels**
Sunburst Technology
3150 W Higgins Rd
Suite 140
Hoffman Estates, IL 60619 800-321-7511
http://www.sunburst.com
service@sunburst.com
Filled to the rafters with phonics fun, this animated program builds your students' vowel recognition skills.

1161 **Memory I**
Psychological Software Services
3304 W 75th St
Indianapolis, IN 46268 317-257-9672
Fax: 317-257-9674
http://www.neuroscience.cnter.com
nsc@neuroscience.cnter.com
Odie L Bracy, PhD, HSPP, Clinical Neuropsychologist
Nancy Bracy, Office Manager
Andrea Oakes, Clinical Assistant
Consists of four computer programs designed to provide verbal and nonverbal memory exercises. *$110.00*

1162 **Memory II**
Psychological Software Services
3304 W 75th St
Indianapolis, IN 46268 317-257-9672
Fax: 317-257-9674
http://www.neuroscience.cnter.com
nsc@neuroscience.cnter.com
Odie L Bracy, PhD, HSPP, Clinical Neuropsychologist
Nancy Bracy, Office Manager
Andrea Oakes, Clinical Assistant
These programs allow for work with encoding, categorizing and organizing skills. *$150.00*

1163 **Microcomputer Language Assessment and Development System**
Laureate Learning Systems
110 East Spring Street
Winooski, VT 05404-1898 802-655-4755
800-562-6801
Fax: 802-655-4757
http://www.laureatelearning.com
laureate-webmaster@laureatelearning.com
Dr. Mary Sweig Wilson Ph.D., President/CEO, Founder
Bernard J. Fox, Co-Founder, Vice President
Marion Blank, Ph.D, Developmental Psychologist

A series of seven diskettes designed to teach over 45 fundamental syntactic rules. Students are presented two or three pictures, depending on the grammatical construction being trained with optional speech and/or text and asked to select the picture which represents the correct construction. *$775.00*

1164 Mike Mulligan & His Steam Shovel
Sunburst Technology
3150 W Higgins Rd
Suite 140
Hoffman Estates, IL 60619
800-321-7511
http://www.sunburst.com
service@sunburst.com

This CD-ROM version of the Caldecott classic lets students experience interactive book reading and participate in four skills-based extension activities that promote memory, matching, sequencing, listening, pattern recognition and map reading skills.

1165 My Own Bookshelf
Soft Touch
12301 Central Ave NE Ste 205
P.O. Box 490215
Blaine, MN 55449
763-502-0440
888-755-1402
Fax: 763-862-2920
http://www.marblesoft.com
support@marblesoft.com

Joyce Meyer, President
Mark Larson, CEO, Product Development

Research indicates that when students select their own books to read, their literacy levels improve. My Own Bookshelf gives students the ability to select their own books and to read them as often as they wish. *$30.00*

1166 Optimum Resource
1 Mathews Drive
Suite 107
Hilton Head Island, SC 29926
843-689-8000
888-784-2592
Fax: 843-689-8008
http://www.stickybear.com
info@stickybear.com

Richard Hefter, President

An educational software publishing company for grades K-12. Our software titles are available in Consumer, School, Labpack or Site License versions. Please call for further details. Prices range from $59.95 for Consumer to $699.95 for Site Licenses.

1167 Phonology: Software
Abilitations Speech Bin
PO Box 1579
Appleton, WI 54912-1579
419-589-1425
888-388-3224
Fax: 888-388-6344
http://www.schoolspecialty.com
orders@schoolspecialty.com

Joseph M. Yorio, President, CEO
Patrick T. Collins, EVP, Distribution
Rick Holden, EVP

This unique software gives you six entertaining games to treat children's phonological disorders. The program uses target patterns in a pattern cycling approach to phonological processess. Item number L183. *$98.99*

1168 Python Path Phonics Word Families
Sunburst Technology
3150 W Higgins Rd
Suite 140
Hoffman Estates, IL 60619
800-321-7511
http://www.sunburst.com
service@sunburst.com

Your child improves their word-building skills by playing three fun strategy games that involve linking one-or two-letter consonant beginnings to basic word endings.

1169 Read, Write and Type! Learning System
Talking Fingers
830 Rincon Way
San Rafael, CA 94903
415-472-3103
800-674-9126
http://www.readwritetype.com
contact@talkingfingers.com

Jeannine Herron, Developer
Leslie Grimm, Developer

This 40-lesson adventure is a powerful tool for 6-8 year-olds just learning to read, for children of other cultures learning to read and write in English, and for students of any age who are struggling to become successful readers and writers.

1170 Same or Different
Merit Software
121 West 27th Street
Suite 1200
New York, NY 10001
212-675-8567
800-753-6488
Fax: 800-918-9336
http://www.meritsoftware.com
sales@meritsoftware.com

Ben Weintraub, CEO

Requires students to make important visual discriminations which involve shape, color and whole/part relationships. *$9.95*

1171 Sequencing Fun!
Sunburst Technology
3150 W Higgins Rd
Suite 140
Hoffman Estates, IL 60619
800-321-7511
http://www.sunburst.com
service@sunburst.com

Text, pictures, animation and video clips provide a fun filled program that encourages critical thinking skills.

1172 Show Time
Software to Go-Gallaudet University
800 Florida Ave NE
Washington, DC 20002-3695
202-651-5031
Fax: 202-651-5109
http://clerccenter.gallaudet.edu
clerc.center@gallaudet.edu

Ed Bosso, Vice President
Ken Kurlychek, EI Specialist

1173 Soft Tools
Psychological Software Services
3304 W 75th St
Indianapolis, IN 46268-1664
317-257-9672
Fax: 317-257-9674
http://www.neuroscience.cnter.com
nsc@neuroscience.cnter.com

Odie L Bracy, PhD, HSPP, Clinical Neuropsychologist
Nancy Bracy, Office Manager
Andrea Oakes, Clinical Assistant

Menu-driven disk versions of the computer programs published in the Cognitive Rehabilitation Journal. *$50.00*

1174 Sound Match
Enable/Schneier Communication Unit
1603 Court Street
Syracuse, NY 13208
315-455-7591
Fax: 315-455-5989
TTY: 315-455-1794
http://www.enablecny.org
info@enablecny.orgÿÿ

Michael Wolfson, Chief Financial Officer
Prudence York, Executive Director
Mary DiBiase, Program Director

Presents a variety of sounds/noises requiring gross levels of auditory discrimination and matching. *$25.00*

1175 **Speaking Language Master Special Edition**
Franklin Learning Resources
2 Manhattan Drive
Burlington, NJ 08016
609-386-2500
800-266-5626
Fax: 609-239-5950
http://www.franklin.com
service@franklin.com

A language master with speech defining over 110,000 words, spelling correction capability, pick/edit feature, vocabulary enrichment activities and advanced word list. *$79.95*

1176 **Spell-a-Word**
RJ Cooper & Associates
22600 Lambert St.
Ste 708A
Lake Forest, CA 92630
800-752-6673
Fax: 949-582-3169
http://www.rjcooper.com
info@rjcooper.com

R J Cooper, Owner

A large print, talking, spelling program. It uses an errorless learning method. It has both a drill and test mode, which a supervisor can set. Letters, words or phrases are entered by a supervisor and recorded by supervisor, peer, or sibling. Available for Mac, Windows. *$59.00*

1177 **Spellagraph**
Software to Go-Gallaudet University
800 Florida Ave NE
Washington, DC 20002-3695
202-651-5031
Fax: 202-651-5109
http://clerccenter.gallaudet.edu
clerc.center@gallaudet.edu

Ed Bosso, Vice President
Ken Kurlychek, EI Specialist

1178 **Spelling Ace**
Franklin Learning Resources
2 Manhattan Drive
Burlington, NJ 08016
609-386-2500
800-266-5626
Fax: 609-239-5950
http://www.franklin.com
service@franklin.com

The basic spelling corrector with 80,000 words. Sound-Alikes feature identifies commonly confused words. *$25.00*

1179 **Spelling Mastery**
SRA/McGraw-Hill
PO Box 182605
Columbus, OH 43218
800-334-7344
Fax: 800-953-8691
http://www.mheducation.com
SEG_CustomerService@mheducation.com

David Levin, President/CEO
David Stafford, SVP and General Counsel
Maryellen Valaitis, SVP, Human Resources

The McGraw-Hill Education Urban Advisory Resource works with large urban districts across the country to help them provide better quality instruction, curriculum, and assessment to their students.

1180 **Stanley Sticker Stories**
Riverdeep
222 Berkeley Street
Boston, MA 02116
617-351-5000
855-969-4642
Fax: 877-892-9820
http://www.hmhco.com
IIEcustomerservice@hmhpub.com

Linda K. Zecher, President, CEO, Director
James G. Nicholson, President, Riverside Publishing
John K. Dragoon, EVP, Chief Marketing Officer

Houghton Mifflin Harcourt offers a wide array of technology-driven pre-k-12 solutions that inspire excellence and innovation in education, and raise student achievement. *$59.95*

1181 **Sunken Treasure Adventure: Beginning Blends**
Sunburst Technology
3150 W Higgins Rd
Suite 140
Hoffman Estates, IL 60619
800-321-7511
http://www.sunburst.com
service@sunburst.com

Focus on beginning blends sounds and concepts with three high-spirited games that invite students to use two letter consonant blends as they build words.

1182 **Syllasearch I, II, III, IV**
SRA Order Services
PO Box 182605
Columbus, OH 43218
800-334-7344
Fax: 800-953-8691
http://www.mheducation.com
SEG_CustomerService@mheducation.com

David Levin, President/CEO
David Stafford, SVP and General Counsel
Maryellen Valaitis, SVP, Human Resources

The McGraw-Hill Education Urban Advisory Resource works with large urban districts across the country to help them provide better quality instruction, curriculum, and assessment to their students. *$99.00*

1183 **Talking Nouns II: Sterling Edition**
Laureate Learning Systems
110 East Spring Street
Winooski, VT 05404-1898
802-655-4755
800-562-6801
Fax: 802-655-4757
http://www.laureatelearning.com
laureate-webmaster@laureatelearning.com

Dr. Mary Sweig Wilson Ph.D., President/CEO, Founder
Bernard J. Fox, Co-Founder, Vice President
Marion Blank, Ph.D, Developmental Psychologist

Designed to build expressive language and augmentative communication skills. *$130.00*

1184 **Talking Nouns: Sterling Edition**
Laureate Learning Systems
110 East Spring Street
Winooski, VT 05404-1898
802-655-4755
800-562-6801
Fax: 802-655-4757
http://www.laureatelearning.com
laureate-webmaster@laureatelearning.com

Dr. Mary Sweig Wilson Ph.D., President/CEO, Founder
Bernard J. Fox, Co-Founder, Vice President
Marion Blank, Ph.D, Developmental Psychologist

An interactive communication product that helps build expressive language and augmentative communication skills. *$130.00*

1185 **Talking Verbs Sterling Edition**
Laureate Learning Systems
110 East Spring Street
Winooski, VT 05404-1898
802-655-4755
800-562-6801
Fax: 802-655-4757
http://www.laureatelearning.com
laureate-webmaster@laureatelearning.com

Dr. Mary Sweig Wilson Ph.D., President/CEO, Founder
Bernard J. Fox, Co-Founder, Vice President
Marion Blank, Ph.D, Developmental Psychologist

Builds expressive language and augmentative communication skills. *$130.00*

1186 **Twenty Categories**
Laureate Learning Systems
110 East Spring Street
Winooski, VT 05404-1898
802-655-4755
800-562-6801
Fax: 802-655-4757
http://www.laureatelearning.com
laureate-webmaster@laureatelearning.com
Dr. Mary Sweig Wilson Ph.D., President/CEO, Founder
Bernard J. Fox, Co-Founder, Vice President
Marion Blank, Ph.D, Developmental Psychologist
Designed to use with children and adults, these two diskettes provide instruction in both abstracting the correct category for a noun and placing a noun in the appropriate category. *$100.00*

1187 **Type to Learn 3**
Sunburst Technology
3150 W Higgins Rd
Suite 140
Hoffman Estates, IL 60619
800-321-7511
http://www.sunburst.com
service@sunburst.com
With the 25 lessons in this animated update of Type to Learn, students embark on time travel missions to learn keyboarding skills.

1188 **Type to Learn Jr**
Sunburst Technology
3150 W Higgins Rd
Suite 140
Hoffman Estates, IL 60619
800-321-7511
http://www.sunburst.com
service@sunburst.com
One of the first steps to literacy is learning how to use the keyboard. Age appropriate instruction and three practice activities help students use the computer with greater ease.

1189 **Type to Learn Jr New Keys for Kids**
Sunburst Technology
3150 W Higgins Rd
Suite 140
Hoffman Estates, IL 60619
800-321-7511
http://www.sunburst.com
service@sunburst.com
With new keys to learn, your early keyboarders focus on using the letter and number keys, the shift key, home row and are introduced to selected internet symbols.

1190 **Vowel Patterns**
Sunburst Technology
3150 W Higgins Rd
Suite 140
Hoffman Estates, IL 60619
800-321-7511
http://www.sunburst.com
service@sunburst.com
Some vowels are neither long nor short. In this investigation, students explore and learn to use abstract vowels.

1191 **Word Invasion: Academic Skill Builders in Language Arts**
SRA Order Services
PO Box 182605
Columbus, OH 43218
800-334-7344
Fax: 800-953-8691
http://www.mheducation.com
SEG_CustomerService@mheducation.com
David Levin, President/CEO
David Stafford, SVP and General Counsel
Maryellen Valaitis, SVP, Human Resources
The McGraw-Hill Education Urban Advisory Resource works with large urban districts across the country to help them provide better quality instruction, curriculum, and assessment to their students. *$49.00*

1192 **Word Master: Academic Skill Builders in Language Arts**
SRA Order Services
PO Box 182605
Columbus, OH 43218
800-334-7344
Fax: 800-953-8691
http://www.mheducation.com
SEG_CustomerService@mheducation.com
David Levin, President/CEO
David Stafford, SVP and General Counsel
Maryellen Valaitis, SVP, Human Resources
The McGraw-Hill Education Urban Advisory Resource works with large urban districts across the country to help them provide better quality instruction, curriculum, and assessment to their students. *$49.00*

1193 **Word Wise I and II: Better Comprehension Through Vocabulary**
SRA Order Services
PO Box 182605
Columbus, OH 43218
800-334-7344
Fax: 800-953-8691
http://www.mheducation.com
SEG_CustomerService@mheducation.com
David Levin, President/CEO
David Stafford, SVP and General Counsel
Maryellen Valaitis, SVP, Human Resources
The McGraw-Hill Education Urban Advisory Resource works with large urban districts across the country to help them provide better quality instruction, curriculum, and assessment to their students.

Life Skills

1194 **Bozons' Quest**
110 East Spring Street
Winooski, VT 05404-1898
802-655-4755
800-562-6801
Fax: 802-655-4757
http://www.laureatelearning.com
laureate-webmaster@laureatelearning.com
Dr. Mary Sweig Wilson Ph.D., President/CEO, Founder
Bernard J. Fox, Co-Founder, Vice President
Marion Blank, Ph.D, Developmental Psychologist
A computer game designed to teach cognitive skills and strategies and left/right discrimination skills.

1195 **Calendar Fun with Lollipop Dragon**
SVE & Churchill Media
700 Indian Springs Drive
Lancaster, PA 17601
888-892-3484
Fax: 877-324-6830
http://store.discoveryeducation.com
education_info@discovery.com
Young students learn the calendar basics. *$84.00*

1196 **Comparison Kitchen**
SRA Order Services
PO Box 182605
Columbus, OH 43218
800-334-7344
Fax: 800-953-8691
http://www.mheducation.com
SEG_CustomerService@mheducation.com
David Levin, President/CEO
David Stafford, SVP and General Counsel
Maryellen Valaitis, SVP, Human Resources
The McGraw-Hill Education Urban Advisory Resource works with large urban districts across the country to help them provide better quality instruction, curriculum, and assessment to their students. *$35.00*

1197 **Early Learning: Preparing Children for School, Phillip Roy, Inc.**
PO Box 130
Indian Rocks Beach, FL 33785
727-593-2700
800-255-9085
Fax: 727-595-2685
http://www.philliproy.com
info@philliproy.com
Ruth Bragman, President
This program includes unlimited online access to 42 interactive lessons per individual. This pre-kindergarten curriculum has over 250 activities which include: Math, Problem-Solving, Reading, Language Development, Physical Skills, Self-Esteem, Your Community, and Healthy Habits. Includes audio and interactive graphics. Allows parents to work with their children at home or any place. Can be duplicated at the purcashing school. No yearly fees.

1198 **Electric Crayon**
Merit Software
121 West 27th Street
Suite 1200
New York, NY 10001
212-675-8567
800-753-6488
Fax: 800-918-9336
http://www.meritsoftware.com
sales@meritsoftware.com
Ben Weintraub, CEO
A tool to help preschool and primary aged children learn about and enjoy the computer. *$14.95*

1199 **First Categories Sterling Edition**
Laureate Learning Systems
110 East Spring Street
Winooski, VT 05404-1898
802-655-4755
800-562-6801
Fax: 802-655-4757
http://www.laureatelearning.com
laureate-webmaster@laureatelearning.com
Dr. Mary Sweig Wilson Ph.D., President/CEO, Founder
Bernard J. Fox, Co-Founder, Vice President
Marion Blank, Ph.D, Developmental Psychologist
A computer program that trains 6 early categories using 60 nouns. Eleven innovative, activities, hundreds of drawings, and photographs and exciting 3-D animation make this program fun and effective. *$230.00*

1200 **First R**
Milliken Publishing
501 East Third Street
Box 802
Dayton, OH 45401-0802
937-228-6118
800-444-1144
Fax: 937-223-2042
http://www.lorenzeducationalpress.com
lep@lorenz.com
Thomas Moore, President
Evan Gould, Author
Barbara Meeks, Author
A phonetically-based word recognition program with emphasis on comprehension. *$325.00*

1201 **First Verbs Sterling Edition**
Laureate Learning Systems
110 East Spring Street
Winooski, VT 05404-1898
802-655-4755
800-562-6801
Fax: 802-655-4757
http://www.laureatelearning.com
laureate-webmaster@laureatelearning.com
Dr. Mary Sweig Wilson Ph.D., President/CEO, Founder
Bernard J. Fox, Co-Founder, Vice President
Marion Blank, Ph.D, Developmental Psychologist
A computer program that trains and tests 40 early developing verbs using animated pictures and a natural sounding female voice. *$225.00*

1202 **First Words II Sterling Edition**
Laureate Learning Systems
110 East Spring Street
Winooski, VT 05404-1898
802-655-4755
800-562-6801
Fax: 802-655-4757
http://www.laureatelearning.com
laureate-webmaster@laureatelearning.com
Dr. Mary Sweig Wilson Ph.D., President/CEO, Founder
Bernard J. Fox, Co-Founder, Vice President
Marion Blank, Ph.D, Developmental Psychologist
Continues the training of First Words with training and testing of an additional 50 early developing nouns presented within the same 10 categories as used in First Words. *$235.00*

1203 **First Words Sterling Edition**
Laureate Learning Systems
110 East Spring Street
Winooski, VT 05404-1898
802-655-4755
800-562-6801
Fax: 802-655-4757
http://www.laureatelearning.com
laureate-webmaster@laureatelearning.com
Dr. Mary Sweig Wilson Ph.D., President/CEO, Founder
Bernard J. Fox, Co-Founder, Vice President
Marion Blank, Ph.D, Developmental Psychologist
A talking program that trains and tests 50 early developing nouns presented within 10 categories. *$235.00*

1204 **Fish Scales**
SRA Order Services
PO Box 182605
Columbus, OH 43218
800-334-7344
Fax: 800-953-8691
http://www.mheducation.com
SEG_CustomerService@mheducation.com
David Levin, President/CEO
David Stafford, SVP and General Counsel
Maryellen Valaitis, SVP, Human Resources
The McGraw-Hill Education Urban Advisory Resource works with large urban districts across the country to help them provide better quality instruction, curriculum, and assessment to their students. *$35.00*

1205 **Following Directions: Left and Right**
Laureate Learning Systems
110 East Spring Street
Winooski, VT 05404-1898
802-655-4755
800-562-6801
Fax: 802-655-4757
http://www.laureatelearning.com
laureate-webmaster@laureatelearning.com
Dr. Mary Sweig Wilson Ph.D., President/CEO, Founder
Bernard J. Fox, Co-Founder, Vice President
Marion Blank, Ph.D, Developmental Psychologist
This computer program uses ten activities to improve your ability to follow directions and develop left/right discrimination skills. *$125.00*

1206 **Following Directions: One and Two-Level Commands**
Laureate Learning Systems
110 East Spring Street
Winooski, VT 05404-1898
802-655-4755
800-562-6801
Fax: 802-655-4757
http://www.laureatelearning.com
laureate-webmaster@laureatelearning.com
Dr. Mary Sweig Wilson Ph.D., President/CEO, Founder
Bernard J. Fox, Co-Founder, Vice President
Marion Blank, Ph.D, Developmental Psychologist
Designed for a broad range of students experiencing difficulty in processing, remembering and following oral commands, a program of exercises on short and long-term memory highlighting specific spatial, directional and ordinary terms. *$175.00*

1207 **Functional Skills System and MECA**
Conover Company
4 Brookwood Court
Appleton, WI 54914
800-933-1933
Fax: 800-933-1943
http://www.conovercompany.com
sales@conovercompany.com
Functional Skills System software assists in the transition from school to the community and workplace. Functional literary, functional life skills, functional social skills, functional work skills. MECA - The system for creating post-secondary transition outcomes and the instructional services to support them. *$2535.00*

1208 **Information Station**
SVE & Churchill Media
700 Indian Springs Drive
Lancaster, PA 17601
888-892-3484
Fax: 877-324-6830
http://store.discoveryeducation.com
education_info@discovery.com
Students who boot up this software will find themselves floating miles above the earth orbiting the planet in an information station satellite. *$144.00*

1209 **Lion's Workshop**
Merit Software
121 West 27th Street
Suite 1200
New York, NY 10001
212-675-8567
800-753-6488
Fax: 800-918-9336
http://www.meritsoftware.com
sales@meritsoftware.com
Ben Weintraub, CEO
Presents various objects with parts missing or with like objects to be matched. *$9.95*

1210 **Marsh Media**
Marshware
PO Box 8082
Shawnee Mission, KS 66208-0082
800-821-3303
Fax: 866-333-7421
http://www.marshmedia.com
info@marshmedia.com
Joan K Marsh, President
Marsh Media publishes closed captioned health and guidance videos for the classroom and school library. Catalog available.

1211 **Math Spending and Saving**
World Class Learning
PO Box 639
Candler, NC 28715
800-638-6470
Fax: 800-638-6499
http://www.wclm.com
jdash@wclm.com
Designed for secondary students and adults, this program focuses on personal financial management, comparison shopping and calculation of essential banking transactions.

1212 **Money Skills**
MarbleSoft
12301 Central Ave NE Ste 205
P.O. Box 490215
Blaine, MN 55449
763-502-0440
888-755-1402
Fax: 763-862-2920
http://www.marblesoft.com
support@marblesoft.com
Joyce Meyer, President
Mark Larson, CEO, Product Development
Vicki Larson, Sales
Money Skills 2.0 includes five activities that teach counting money and making change: Coins and Bills; Counting Money; Making Change; how much change? and the Marblesoft Store. Teaches American, Canadian and European money using clear, realistic pictures of the money. Single and dual-switch scanning options on all difficulty levels. Runs on Macintosh and Windows computers. *$60.00*

1213 **My House: Language Activities of Daily Living**
Laureate Learning Systems
110 East Spring Street
Winooski, VT 05404-1898
802-655-4755
800-562-6801
Fax: 802-655-4757
http://www.laureatelearning.com
laureate-webmaster@laureatelearning.com
Dr. Mary Sweig Wilson Ph.D., President/CEO, Founder
Bernard J. Fox, Co-Founder, Vice President
Marion Blank, Ph.D, Developmental Psychologist
Train over 300 functional vocabulary items, increase understanding of objects and their functions while building independence in the home, community, and school. *$150.00*

1214 **Optimum Resource**
1 Mathews Drive
Suite 107
Hilton Head Island, SC 29926
843-689-8000
888-784-2592
Fax: 843-689-8008
http://www.stickybear.com
info@stickybear.com
Richard Hefter, President
An educational software publishing company for grades K-12. Our software titles are available in Consumer, School, Labpack or Site License versions. Please call for further details. Prices range from $59.95 for Consumer to $699.95 for Site Licenses.

1215 **PAVE: Perceptual Accuracy/Visual Efficiency**
Software to Go-Gallaudet University
800 Florida Ave NE
Washington, DC 20002-3695
202-651-5031
Fax: 202-651-5109
http://clerccenter.gallaudet.edu
clerc.center@gallaudet.edu
Ed Bosso, Vice President
Ken Kurlychek, EI Specialist

1216 **Print Shop Deluxe**
Riverdeep
222 Berkeley Street
Boston, MA 02116
617-351-5000
855-969-4642
Fax: 877-892-9820
http://www.hmhco.com
IIEcustomerservice@hmhpub.com
Linda K. Zecher, President, CEO, Director
James G. Nicholson, President, Riverside Publishing
John K. Dragoon, EVP, Chief Marketing Officer
Houghton Mifflin Harcourt offers a wide array of technology-driven pre-k-12 solutions that inspire excellence and innovation in education, and raise student achievement.

1217 **Quiz Castle**
Software to Go-Gallaudet University
800 Florida Ave NE
Washington, DC 20002-3695
202-651-5031
Fax: 202-651-5109
http://clerccenter.gallaudet.edu
clerc.center@gallaudet.edu
Ed Bosso, Vice President
Ken Kurlychek, EI Specialist

1218 **Secondary Print Pack**
Failure Free
140 Cabarrus Ave W
Concord, NC 28025-5150
704-786-7838
800-542-2170
Fax: 704-785-8940
http://www.failurefree.com
info@failurefree.com
Joseph Lockavitch, President
Thousands of independent activities teaching over 750 words. *$1929.00*

1219 **Stickybear Software**
Optimum Resource
1 Mathews Drive
Suite 107
Hilton Head Island, SC 29926
843-689-8000
888-784-2592
Fax: 843-689-8008
http://www.stickybear.com
info@stickybear.com
Richard Hefter, President
An educational software publishing company for grades K-12. Our software titles are available in Consumer, School, Labpack or Site License versions. Please call for further details. Prices range from $59.95 for Consumer to $699.95 for Site Licenses.

1220 **Teenage Switch Progressions**
RJ Cooper & Associates
22600 Lambert St.
Ste 708A
Lake Forest, CA 92630
800-752-6673
Fax: 949-582-3169
http://www.rjcooper.com
info@rjcooper.com
R J Cooper, Owner
Five activities for teenage persons working on switch training, attention training, life skills simulation and following directions. *$59.00*

1221 **TeleSensory**
417 Cypress Street
Bakersfield, CA 93304
650-743-9515
800-804-8004
Fax: 661-327-2478
http://www.telesensory.com
info@telesensory.com
Helps visually impaired people become more independent with the most comprehensive products available anywhere for reading, writing, taking notes and using computers.

Math

1222 **Access to Math**
Don Johnston
26799 West Commerce Drive
Volo, IL 60073
847-740-0749
800-999-4660
Fax: 847-740-7326
http://www.donjohnston.com
info@donjohnston.com
Don Johnston, Founder
Ruth Ziolkowski, President
The Macintosh talking math worksheet program that's two products in one. For teachers, it makes customized worksheets in a snap. For students who struggle, it provides individualized on-screen lessons.

1223 **Algebra Stars**
Sunburst Technology
3150 W Higgins Rd
Suite 140
Hoffman Estates, IL 60619
800-321-7511
http://www.sunburst.com
service@sunburst.com
Students build their understanding of algebra by constructing, categorizing, and solving equations and classifying polynomial expressions using algebra tiles.

1224 **Alien Addition: Academic Skill Builders in Math**
SRA Order Services
PO Box 182605
Columbus, OH 43218
800-334-7344
Fax: 800-953-8691
http://www.mheducation.com
SEG_CustomerService@mheducation.com
David Levin, President/CEO
David Stafford, SVP and General Counsel
Maryellen Valaitis, SVP, Human Resources
The McGraw-Hill Education Urban Advisory Resource works with large urban districts across the country to help them provide better quality instruction, curriculum, and assessment to their students. *$49.00*

1225 **Awesome Animated Monster Maker Math**
Sunburst Technology
3150 W Higgins Rd
Suite 140
Hoffman Estates, IL 60619
800-321-7511
http://www.sunburst.com
service@sunburst.com
With an emphasis on building core math skills, this humorous program incorporates the monstrous and the ridiculous into a structured learning environment. Students choose from six skill levels tailored to the 3rd to 8th grade.

1226 **Awesome Animated Monster Maker Math and Monster Workshop**
Sunburst Technology
3150 W Higgins Rd
Suite 140
Hoffman Estates, IL 60619
800-321-7511
http://www.sunburst.com
service@sunburst.com
Students develop money and strategic thinking skills with this irresistable game that has them tinker about making monsters.

1227 **Awesome Animated Monster Maker Number Drop**
Sunburst Technology
3150 W Higgins Rd
Suite 140
Hoffman Estates, IL 60619
800-321-7511
http://www.sunburst.com
service@sunburst.com
Your students will think on their mathematical feet estimating and solving thousands of number problems in an arcade-style game designed to improve their performance in numeration, money, fractions, and decimals.

1228 **Basic Math Competency Skill Building**
Educational Activities Software
PO Box 220790
Saint Louis, MO 63122
866-243-8464
Fax: 239-225-9299
http://www.ea-software.com
jwest@siboneylg.com
Jan West, Sales Director
Michael Conlon, Author
An interactive, tutorial and practice program to teach competency with arithmetic operations, decimals, fractions, graphs, measurement and geometric concepts. (stand alone version) MA02 *$369.00*

1229 **Basic Skills Products**
EDCON Publishing Group
30 Montauk Blvd
Oakdale, NY 11769
631-567-7227
888-553-3266
Fax: 631-567-8745
http://www.edconpublishing.com
Deals with basic math and language arts. Free catalog available.

1230 **Building Perspective**
Sunburst Technology
3150 W Higgins Rd
Suite 140
Hoffman Estates, IL 60619 800-321-7511
http://www.sunburst.com
service@sunburst.com
Develop spatial perception and reasoning skills with this award-winning program that will sharpen your students' problem-solving abilities.

1231 **Building Perspective Deluxe**
Sunburst Technology
3150 W Higgins Rd
Suite 140
Hoffman Estates, IL 60619 800-321-7511
http://www.sunburst.com
service@sunburst.com
New visual thinking challenges await your students as they engage in three spacial reasoning activities that develop their 3D thinking, deductive reasoning and problem solving skills

1232 **Combining Shapes**
Sunburst Technology
3150 W Higgins Rd
Suite 140
Hoffman Estates, IL 60619 800-321-7511
http://www.sunburst.com
service@sunburst.com
Students discover the properties of simple geometric figures through concrete experience combining shapes. Measurements, estimating and operation skills are part of this fun program.

1233 **Conceptual Skills**
Psychological Software Services
3304 W 75th St
Indianapolis, IN 46268-1664 317-257-9672
Fax: 317-257-9674
http://www.neuroscience.cnter.com
nsc@neuroscience.cnter.com
Odie L Bracy, PhD, HSPP, Clinical Neuropsychologist
Nancy Bracy, Office Manager
Andrea Oakes, Clinical Assistant
Twelve programs designed to enhance skills involved in relationships, comparisons and number concepts. *$50.00*

1234 **Concert Tour Entrepreneur**
Sunburst Technology
3150 W Higgins Rd
Suite 140
Hoffman Estates, IL 60619 800-321-7511
http://www.sunburst.com
service@sunburst.com
Your students improve math, planning and problem solving skills as they manage a band in this music management business simulation.

1235 **Counters**
Software to Go-Gallaudet University
800 Florida Ave NE
Washington, DC 20002-3695 202-651-5031
Fax: 202-651-5109
http://clerccenter.gallaudet.edu
clerc.center@gallaudet.edu
Ed Bosso, Vice President
Ken Kurlychek, EI Specialist

1236 **Counting Critters**
Software to Go-Gallaudet University
800 Florida Ave NE
Washington, DC 20002-3695 202-651-5031
Fax: 202-651-5109
http://clerccenter.gallaudet.edu
clerc.center@gallaudet.edu
Ed Bosso, Vice President
Ken Kurlychek, EI Specialist

1237 **DLM Math Fluency Program: Addition Facts**
SRA Order Services
PO Box 182605
Columbus, OH 43218 800-334-7344
Fax: 800-953-8691
http://www.mheducation.com
SEG_CustomerService@mheducation.com
David Levin, President/CEO
David Stafford, SVP and General Counsel
Maryellen Valaitis, SVP, Human Resources
The McGraw-Hill Education Urban Advisory Resource works with large urban districts across the country to help them provide better quality instruction, curriculum, and assessment to their students. *$32.00*

1238 **DLM Math Fluency Program: Division Facts**
SRA Order Services
PO Box 182605
Columbus, OH 43218 800-334-7344
Fax: 800-953-8691
http://www.mheducation.com
SEG_CustomerService@mheducation.com
David Levin, President/CEO
David Stafford, SVP and General Counsel
Maryellen Valaitis, SVP, Human Resources
The McGraw-Hill Education Urban Advisory Resource works with large urban districts across the country to help them provide better quality instruction, curriculum, and assessment to their students.

1239 **DLM Math Fluency Program: Multiplication Facts**
SRA Order Services
PO Box 182605
Columbus, OH 43218 800-334-7344
Fax: 800-953-8691
http://www.mheducation.com
SEG_CustomerService@mheducation.com
David Levin, President/CEO
David Stafford, SVP and General Counsel
Maryellen Valaitis, SVP, Human Resources
The McGraw-Hill Education Urban Advisory Resource works with large urban districts across the country to help them provide better quality instruction, curriculum, and assessment to their students. *$32.00*

1240 **DLM Math Fluency Program: Subtraction Facts**
SRA Order Services
PO Box 182605
Columbus, OH 43218 800-334-7344
Fax: 800-953-8691
http://www.mheducation.com
SEG_CustomerService@mheducation.com
David Levin, President/CEO
David Stafford, SVP and General Counsel
Maryellen Valaitis, SVP, Human Resources
The McGraw-Hill Education Urban Advisory Resource works with large urban districts across the country to help them provide better quality instruction, curriculum, and assessment to their students. *$32.00*

1241 **Data Explorer**
Sunburst Technology
3150 W Higgins Rd
Suite 140
Hoffman Estates, IL 60619 800-321-7511
http://www.sunburst.com
service@sunburst.com
This easy-to-use CD-ROM provides the flexibility needed for eleven different graph types including tools for long-term data analysis projects.

1242 **Dragon Mix: Academic Skill Builders in Math**
SRA Order Services
PO Box 182605
Columbus, OH 43218 800-334-7344
Fax: 800-953-8691
http://www.mheducation.com
SEG_CustomerService@mheducation.com

David Levin, President/CEO
David Stafford, SVP and General Counsel
Maryellen Valaitis, SVP, Human Resources
The McGraw-Hill Education Urban Advisory Resource works with large urban districts across the country to help them provide better quality instruction, curriculum, and assessment to their students. *$49.00*

1243 **Elementary Math Bundle**
Sunburst Technology
3150 W Higgins Rd
Suite 140
Hoffman Estates, IL 60619 800-321-7511
http://www.sunburst.com
service@sunburst.com
Number sense and operations are the focus of the Elementary Math Bundle. Students engage in activities that reinforce basic addition and subtraction skills. This product comes with Splish Splash Math, Ten Tricky Tiles and Numbers Undercover.

1244 **Equation Tile Teasers**
Sunburst Technology
3150 W Higgins Rd
Suite 140
Hoffman Estates, IL 60619 800-321-7511
http://www.sunburst.com
service@sunburst.com
Students develop logic thinking and pre-algebra skills solving sets of numbers equations in three challenging problem-solving activities.

1245 **Equations**
Software to Go-Gallaudet University
800 Florida Ave NE
Washington, DC 20002-3695 202-651-5031
Fax: 202-651-5109
http://clerccenter.gallaudet.edu
clerc.center@gallaudet.edu
Ed Bosso, Vice President
Ken Kurlychek, EI Specialist

1246 **Factory Deluxe**
Sunburst Technology
3150 W Higgins Rd
Suite 140
Hoffman Estates, IL 60619 800-321-7511
http://www.sunburst.com
service@sunburst.com
Five activities explore shapes, rotation, angles, geometric attributes, area formulas, and computation. Includes journal, record keeping, and on-screen help. This program helps sharpen geometry, visual thinking and problem solving skills.

1247 **Fast-Track Fractions**
SRA Order Services
PO Box 182605
Columbus, OH 43218 800-334-7344
Fax: 800-953-8691
http://www.mheducation.com
SEG_CustomerService@mheducation.com
David Levin, President/CEO
David Stafford, SVP and General Counsel
Maryellen Valaitis, SVP, Human Resources
The McGraw-Hill Education Urban Advisory Resource works with large urban districts across the country to help them provide better quality instruction, curriculum, and assessment to their students. *$46.00*

1248 **Fraction Attraction**
Sunburst Technology
3150 W Higgins Rd
Suite 140
Hoffman Estates, IL 60619 800-321-7511
http://www.sunburst.com
service@sunburst.com
Build the fraction skills of ordering, equivalence, relative sizes and multiple representations with four, multi-level, carnival style games.

1249 **Fraction Fuel-Up**
SRA Order Services
PO Box 182605
Columbus, OH 43218 800-334-7344
Fax: 800-953-8691
http://www.mheducation.com
SEG_CustomerService@mheducation.com
David Levin, President/CEO
David Stafford, SVP/General Counsel
Maryellen Valaitis, SVP Human Resources
The McGraw-Hill Education Urban Advisory Resource works with large urban districts across the country to help them provide better quality instruction, curriculum, and assessment to their students. *$46.00*

1250 **Get Up and Go!**
Sunburst Technology
3150 W Higgins Rd
Suite 140
Hoffman Estates, IL 60619 800-321-7511
http://www.sunburst.com
service@sunburst.com
Students interpret and construct timelines through three descriptive activities in the animated program. Students are introduced to timelines as they participate in an interactive story.

1251 **Learning About Numbers**
C&C Software
5713 Kentford Cir
Wichita, KS 67220-3131 316-683-6056
800-752-2086
Carol Clark, President
Three segments use computer graphics to provide students with an experience in working with numbers. *$25.00*

1252 **Math Machine**
Software to Go-Gallaudet University
800 Florida Ave NE
Washington, DC 20002-3695 202-651-5031
Fax: 202-651-5109
http://clerccenter.gallaudet.edu
clerc.center@gallaudet.edu
Ed Bosso, Vice President
Ken Kurlychek, EI Specialist

1253 **Math Masters: Addition and Subtraction**
SRA Order Services
PO Box 182605
Columbus, OH 43218 800-334-7344
Fax: 800-953-8691
http://www.mheducation.com
SEG_CustomerService@mheducation.com
David Levin, President/CEO
David Stafford, SVP/General Counsel
Maryellen Valaitis, SVP Human Resources
The McGraw-Hill Education Urban Advisory Resource works with large urban districts across the country to help them provide better quality instruction, curriculum, and assessment to their students.

1254 **Math Masters: Multiplication and Division**
SRA Order Services
PO Box 182605
Columbus, OH 43218 800-334-7344
Fax: 800-953-8691
http://www.mheducation.com
SEG_CustomerService@mheducation.com
David Levin, President/CEO
David Stafford, SVP/General Counsel
Maryellen Valaitis, SVP Human Resources
The McGraw-Hill Education Urban Advisory Resource works with large urban districts across the country to help them provide better quality instruction, curriculum, and assessment to their students.

1255 **Math Shop**
Software to Go-Gallaudet University
800 Florida Ave NE
Washington, DC 20002-3695 202-651-5031
Fax: 202-651-5109
http://clerccenter.gallaudet.edu
clerc.center@gallaudet.edu
Ed Bosso, Vice President
Ken Kurlychek, EI Specialist

1256 **Math Skill Games**
Software to Go-Gallaudet University
800 Florida Ave NE
Washington, DC 20002-3695 202-651-5031
Fax: 202-651-5109
http://clerccenter.gallaudet.edu
clerc.center@gallaudet.edu
Ed Bosso, Vice President
Ken Kurlychek, EI Specialist

1257 **Math for Everyday Living**
Educational Activities Software
PO Box 87
Baldwin, NY 11510 800-797-3223
Fax: 516-623-9282
http://www.edact.com
learn@edact.com
Rose Falco, Educational Activities
Designed for secondary students, a tutorial and practice program with simulated activities for applying math skills in making change, working with sales slips, unit pricing, computing gas mileage and sales tax. *$89.00*

1258 **Mighty Math Astro Algebra**
Riverdeep
222 Berkeley Street
Boston, MA 02116 617-351-5000
855-969-4642
Fax: 877-892-9820
http://www.hmhco.com
IIEcustomerservice@hmhpub.com
Linda K. Zecher, President, CEO, Director
James G. Nicholson, President, Riverside Publishing
John K. Dragoon, EVP, Chief Marketing Officer
Houghton Mifflin Harcourt offers a wide array of technology-driven pre-k-12 solutions that inspire excellence and innovation in education, and raise student achievement. *$59.95*

1259 **Mighty Math Calculating Crew**
Riverdeep
222 Berkeley Street
Boston, MA 02116 617-351-5000
855-969-4642
Fax: 877-892-9820
http://www.hmhco.com
IIEcustomerservice@hmhpub.com
Linda K. Zecher, President, CEO, Director
James G. Nicholson, President, Riverside Publishing
John K. Dragoon, EVP, Chief Marketing Officer
Houghton Mifflin Harcourt offers a wide array of technology-driven pre-k-12 solutions that inspire excellence and innovation in education, and raise student achievement. *$59.95*

1260 **Mighty Math Carnival Countdown**
Riverdeep
222 Berkeley Street
Boston, MA 02116 617-351-5000
855-969-4642
Fax: 877-892-9820
http://www.hmhco.com
IIEcustomerservice@hmhpub.com
Linda K. Zecher, President, CEO, Director
James G. Nicholson, President, Riverside Publishing
John K. Dragoon, EVP, Chief Marketing Officer
Houghton Mifflin Harcourt offers a wide array of technology-driven pre-k-12 solutions that inspire excellence and innovation in education, and raise student achievement. *$59.95*

1261 **Mighty Math Cosmic Geometry**
Riverdeep
222 Berkeley Street
Boston, MA 02116 617-351-5000
855-969-4642
Fax: 877-892-9820
http://www.hmhco.com
IIEcustomerservice@hmhpub.com
Linda K. Zecher, President, CEO, Director
James G. Nicholson, President, Riverside Publishing
John K. Dragoon, EVP, Chief Marketing Officer
Houghton Mifflin Harcourt offers a wide array of technology-driven pre-k-12 solutions that inspire excellence and innovation in education, and raise student achievement. *$59.95*

1262 **Mighty Math Number Heroes**
Riverdeep
222 Berkeley Street
Boston, MA 02116 617-351-5000
855-969-4642
Fax: 877-892-9820
http://www.hmhco.com
IIEcustomerservice@hmhpub.com
Linda K. Zecher, President, CEO, Director
James G. Nicholson, President, Riverside Publishing
John K. Dragoon, EVP, Chief Marketing Officer
Houghton Mifflin Harcourt offers a wide array of technology-driven pre-k-12 solutions that inspire excellence and innovation in education, and raise student achievement. *$59.95*

1263 **Mighty Math Zoo Zillions**
Riverdeep
222 Berkeley Street
Boston, MA 02116 617-351-5000
855-969-4642
Fax: 877-892-9820
http://www.hmhco.com
IIEcustomerservice@hmhpub.com
Linda K. Zecher, President, CEO, Director
James G. Nicholson, President, Riverside Publishing
John K. Dragoon, EVP, Chief Marketing Officer
Houghton Mifflin Harcourt offers a wide array of technology-driven pre-k-12 solutions that inspire excellence and innovation in education, and raise student achievement. *$59.95*

1264 **Millie's Math House**
Riverdeep
222 Berkeley Street
Boston, MA 02116 617-351-5000
855-969-4642
Fax: 877-892-9820
http://www.hmhco.com
IIEcustomerservice@hmhpub.com
Linda K. Zecher, President, CEO, Director
James G. Nicholson, President, Riverside Publishing
John K. Dragoon, EVP, Chief Marketing Officer
Houghton Mifflin Harcourt offers a wide array of technology-driven pre-k-12 solutions that inspire excellence and innovation in education, and raise student achievement. *$59.95*

1265 **Number Farm**
Software to Go-Gallaudet University
800 Florida Ave NE
Washington, DC 20002-3695 202-651-5031
Fax: 202-651-5109
http://clerccenter.gallaudet.edu
clerc.center@gallaudet.edu
Ed Bosso, Vice President
Ken Kurlychek, EI Specialist

1266 **Number Please**
Merit Software
121 West 27th Street
Suite 1200
New York, NY 10001
212-675-8567
800-753-6488
Fax: 800-918-9336
http://www.meritsoftware.com
sales@meritsoftware.com
Ben Weintraub, CEO
Students are challenged to remember combinations of 4, 7 and 10 digit numbers. *$9.95*

1267 **Number Sense and Problem Solving**
Sunburst Technology
3150 W Higgins Rd
Suite 140
Hoffman Estates, IL 60619
800-321-7511
http://www.sunburst.com
service@sunburst.com
Build number and operation skills with these three programs: How the West Was One + Three x Four, Divide and Conquer and Puzzle Tank.

1268 **Number Stumper**
Software to Go-Gallaudet University
800 Florida Ave NE
Washington, DC 20002-3695
202-651-5031
Fax: 202-651-5109
http://clerccenter.gallaudet.edu
clerc.center@gallaudet.edu
Ed Bosso, Vice President
Ken Kurlychek, EI Specialist

1269 **Race Car 'rithmetic**
Software to Go-Gallaudet University
800 Florida Ave NE
Washington, DC 20002-3695
202-651-5031
Fax: 202-651-5109
http://clerccenter.gallaudet.edu
clerc.center@gallaudet.edu
Ed Bosso, Vice President
Ken Kurlychek, EI Specialist

1270 **Read and Solve Math Problems #1**
Educational Activities
PO Box 87
Baldwin, NY 11510
800-797-3223
Fax: 516-623-9282
http://www.edact.com
learn@edact.com
Rose Falco, Educational Activities
A tutorial and practice program for students which focuses on recognition of key words in solving arithmetic word problems, writing equations and solving word problems. *$109.00*

1271 **Read and Solve Math Problems #2**
Educational Activities
PO Box 87
Baldwin, NY 11510
800-797-3223
Fax: 516-623-9282
http://www.edact.com
learn@edact.com
Rose Falco, Educational Activities
A tutorial and practice program for students which focuses on recognition of key words in solving two-step arithmetic problems, writing equations and solving two-step word problems. *$109.00*

1272 **Read and Solve Math Problems #3**
Educational Activities
PO Box 87
Baldwin, NY 11510
800-797-3223
Fax: 516-623-9282
http://www.edact.com
learn@edact.com
Rose Falco, Educational Activities
Designed for students, this tutorial and practice program provides initial instruction and experience in critical thinking and problem-solving using fractions and mixed numbers. *$109.00*

1273 **Shape Up!**
Sunburst Technology
3150 W Higgins Rd
Suite 140
Hoffman Estates, IL 60619
800-321-7511
http://www.sunburst.com
service@sunburst.com
Students actively create and manipulate shapes to discover important ideas about mathematics in an electronic playground of two and three dimensional shapes.

1274 **Spatial Relationships**
Sunburst Technology
3150 W Higgins Rd
Suite 140
Hoffman Estates, IL 60619
800-321-7511
http://www.sunburst.com
service@sunburst.com
Your students will strenghten their spatial perception, spatial reasoning and problem-solving skills with three great programs now on one CD-ROM.

1275 **Splish Splash Math**
Sunburst Technology
3150 W Higgins Rd
Suite 140
Hoffman Estates, IL 60619
800-321-7511
http://www.sunburst.com
service@sunburst.com
Students learn and practice basic operation skills as they engage in this high interest program that keeps them motivated. Great visual rewards and three levels of difficulty keep students challanged.

1276 **Tenth Planet: Combining & Breaking Apart Numbers**
Sunburst Technology
3150 W Higgins Rd
Suite 140
Hoffman Estates, IL 60619
800-321-7511
http://www.sunburst.com
service@sunburst.com
Students explore part-whole relationships and develop number sense by combining and breaking apart numbers in a variety of problem-solving situations.

1277 **Tenth Planet: Comparing with Ratios**
Sunburst Technology
3150 W Higgins Rd
Suite 140
Hoffman Estates, IL 60619
800-321-7511
http://www.sunburst.com
service@sunburst.com
Students learn that ratio is a way to compare amounts by using multiplication and division. Through five engaging activities, students recognize and describe ratios, develop proportional thinking skills, estimate ratios, determine equivalent ratios, and use ratios to analyze data.

1278 **Tenth Planet: Equivalent Fractions**
Sunburst Technology
3150 W Higgins Rd
Suite 140
Hoffman Estates, IL 60619
800-321-7511
http://www.sunburst.com
service@sunburst.com
This exciting investigation develops students' conceptual understanding that every fraction can be named in many different but equivalent ways.

1279 **Tenth Planet: Fraction Operations**
Sunburst Technology
3150 W Higgins Rd
Suite 140
Hoffman Estates, IL 60619
800-321-7511
http://www.sunburst.com
service@sunburst.com
Students build on their concepts of fraction meaning and equivalence as they learn how to perform operations with fractions.

1280 **World Class Learning Materials**
World Class Learning
PO Box 639
Candler, NC 28715
800-638-6470
Fax: 800-638-6499
http://www.wclm.com
jdash@wclm.com
Designed for secondary students and adults, this program focuses on personal financial management, comparison shopping and calculation of essential banking transactions.

1281 **Zap! Around Town**
Sunburst Technology
3150 W Higgins Rd
Suite 140
Hoffman Estates, IL 60619
800-321-7511
http://www.sunburst.com
service@sunburst.com
Students develop mapping and direction skills in this easy-to-use, animated program featuring Shelby, your friendly Sunbuddy guide.

Preschool

1282 **Creature Series**
Laureate Learning Systems
110 East Spring Street
Winooski, VT 05404-1898
802-655-4755
800-562-6801
Fax: 802-655-4757
http://www.laureatelearning.com
laureate-webmaster@laureatelearning.com
Dr. Mary Sweig Wilson Ph.D., President/CEO, Founder
Bernard J. Fox, Co-Founder, Vice President
Marion Blank, Ph.D, Developmental Psychologist
Six different computer programs designed to improve visual and auditory attention and teach cause and effect, turn taking, and switch use. *$95.00*

1283 **Curious George Visits the Library**
Software to Go-Gallaudet University
800 Florida Ave NE
Washington, DC 20002-3695
202-651-5031
Fax: 202-651-5109
http://clerccenter.gallaudet.edu
clerc.center@gallaudet.edu
Ed Bosso, Vice President
Ken Kurlychek, EI Specialist

1284 **Early Discoveries: Size and Logic**
Software to Go-Gallaudet University
800 Florida Ave NE
Washington, DC 20002-3695
202-651-5031
Fax: 202-651-5109
http://clerccenter.gallaudet.edu
clerc.center@gallaudet.edu
Ed Bosso, Vice President
Ken Kurlychek, EI Specialist

1285 **Early Emerging Rules Series**
Laureate Learning Systems
110 East Spring Street
Winooski, VT 05404-1898
802-655-4755
800-562-6801
Fax: 802-655-4757
http://www.laureatelearning.com
laureate-webmaster@laureatelearning.com
Dr. Mary Sweig Wilson Ph.D., President/CEO, Founder
Bernard J. Fox, Co-Founder, Vice President
Marion Blank, Ph.D, Developmental Psychologist
Three programs that introduce early developing grammatical constructions and facilitate the transition from single words to word combinations. *$175.00*

1286 **Early Learning I**
MarbleSoft
12301 Central Ave NE Ste 205
P.O. Box 490215
Blaine, MN 55449
763-502-0440
888-755-1402
Fax: 763-862-2920
http://www.marblesoft.com
support@marblesoft.com
Joyce Meyer, President
Mark Larson, CEO, Product Development
Vicki Larson, Sales
Early Learning 2.0 includes four activities that teach prereading skills. Single and dual-switch scanning are built in and special prompts allow blind students to use all levels of difficulty. Includes Matching Colors, Learning Shapes, Counting Numbers and Letter Match. Runs on Macintosh and Windows computers. *$70.00*

1287 **Early and Advanced Switch Games**
RJ Cooper & Associates
22600 Lambert St.
Ste 708A
Lake Forest, CA 92630
800-752-6673
Fax: 949-582-3169
http://www.rjcooper.com
info@rjcooper.com
R J Cooper, Owner
Thirteen single switch games that start at cause/effect, work through timing and selection and graduate with matching and manipulation tasks. *$59.00*

1288 **Edustar's Early Childhood Special Education Programs**
Edustar America
Ste 186
6220 S Orange Blossom Trl
Orlando, FL 32809-4627
561-638-8733
800-952-3041
Fax: 561-330-0849
http://www.orlandomedicalinstitute.com
info@omi.edu
David Zeldin, Marketing Manager
Stewart Holtz, Curriculum Director
Integrated software program that incorporates manipulatives and special tables for learning early childhood subjects. Features include an illuminated six key keyboard. A special U-shaped touch table for the physically challenged and changeable mats and keys for different subject areas.

1289 **Joystick Games**
Technology for Language and Learning
PO Box 327
East Rockaway, NY 11518
516-625-4550
Fax: 516-621-3321
Joan Tanenhaus, Founder
Five volumes of public domain joystick programs. *$28.50*

1290 **Kindercomp Gold**
Software to Go-Gallaudet University
800 Florida Ave NE
Washington, DC 20002-3695
202-651-5031
Fax: 202-651-5109
http://clerccenter.gallaudet.edu
clerc.center@gallaudet.edu
Ed Bosso, Vice President
Ken Kurlychek, EI Specialist

1291 **Old MacDonald's Farm Deluxe**
KidTECH
12301 Central Ave NE Ste 205
P.O. Box 490215
Blaine, MN 55449
763-502-0440
888-755-1402
Fax: 763-862-2920
http://www.marblesoft.com
support@marblesoft.com
Joyce Meyer, President
Mark Larson, CEO, Product Development
Vicki Larson, Sales
Utilizes the all-time favorite children's song to teach vocabulary and animal sounds to young children. *$30.00*

1292 **Shape and Color Rodeo**
SRA Order Services
PO Box 182605
Columbus, OH 43218
800-334-7344
Fax: 800-953-8691
http://www.mheducation.com
SEG_CustomerService@mheducation.com
David Levin, President/CEO
David Stafford, SVP/General Counsel
Maryellen Valaitis, SVP Human Resources
The McGraw-Hill Education Urban Advisory Resource works with large urban districts across the country to help them provide better quality instruction, curriculum, and assessment to their students. *$35.00*

1293 **Trudy's Time and Place House**
Riverdeep
222 Berkeley Street
Boston, MA 02116
617-351-5000
855-969-4642
Fax: 877-892-9820
http://www.hmhco.com
IIEcustomerservice@hmhpub.com
Linda K. Zecher, President, CEO, Director
James G. Nicholson, President, Riverside Publishing
John K. Dragoon, EVP, Chief Marketing Officer
Houghton Mifflin Harcourt offers a wide array of technology-driven pre-k-12 solutions that inspire excellence and innovation in education, and raise student achievement. *$59.95*

1294 **Word Pieces**
Software to Go-Gallaudet University
800 Florida Ave NE
Washington, DC 20002-3695
202-651-5031
Fax: 202-651-5109
http://clerccenter.gallaudet.edu
clerc.center@gallaudet.edu
Ed Bosso, Vice President
Ken Kurlychek, EI Specialist

Problem Solving

1295 **Captain's Log**
BrainTrain
727 Twinridge Lane
North Chesterfield, VA 23235
804-320-0105
800-822-0538
Fax: 804-320-2491
http://www.braintrain.com
info@braintrain.com
Joseph A Sandford, Ph.D., Founder
Virginia Sandford, VP, Sales & Marketing
A comprehensive, multilevel computerized mental gym to help people with brain injuries, learning disabilities, developmental disabilities, ADD, ADHD and psychiatric disorders improve their cognitive skills. *$2695.00*
ISBN 3-490019-95-0

1296 **Changes Around Us CD-ROM**
222 Berkeley Street
Boston, MA 02116
617-351-5000
855-969-4642
Fax: 877-892-9820
http://www.hmhco.com
IIEcustomerservice@hmhpub.com
Linda K. Zecher, President, CEO, Director
James G. Nicholson, President, Riverside Publishing
John K. Dragoon, EVP, Chief Marketing Officer
Nature is the natural choice for observing change. By observing and researching dramatic visual sequences such as the stages of development of a butterfly, children develop a broad understanding of the concept of change. As they search this multimedia database for images and information about plant and animal life cycles and seasonal change, students strengthen their abilities in research, analysis, problem-solving, critical thinking and communication.

1297 **Factory Deluxe: Grades 4 to 8**
Sunburst Technology
3150 W Higgins Rd
Suite 140
Hoffman Estates, IL 60619
800-321-7511
http://www.sunburst.com
service@sunburst.com
Five activities explore shapes, rotation, angles, geometric attributes, area formulas, and computation. Includes journal, record keeping, and on-screen help. This program helps sharpen geometry, visual thinking and problem solving skills.

1298 **Freddy's Puzzling Adventures**
SRA Order Services
PO Box 182605
Columbus, OH 43218
800-334-7344
Fax: 800-953-8691
http://www.mheducation.com
SEG_CustomerService@mheducation.com
David Levin, President/CEO
David Stafford, SVP/General Counsel
Maryellen Valaitis, SVP Human Resources
The McGraw-Hill Education Urban Advisory Resource works with large urban districts across the country to help them provide better quality instruction, curriculum, and assessment to their students. *$34.00*

1299 **Guessing and Thinking**
Software to Go-Gallaudet University
800 Florida Ave NE
Washington, DC 20002-3695
202-651-5031
Fax: 202-651-5109
http://clerccenter.gallaudet.edu
clerc.center@gallaudet.edu
Ed Bosso, Vice President
Ken Kurlychek, EI Specialist

1300 **High School Math Bundle**
Sunburst Technology
3150 W Higgins Rd
Suite 140
Hoffman Estates, IL 60619
800-321-7511
http://www.sunburst.com
service@sunburst.com
Each program in this bundle focuses on a specific area to ensure that your students master the math skills they need. This bundle allows students to master basics of Algebra, explore equations and graphs, practice learning with algebra graphs, use trigonometric functions, apply math concepts to practical situations and improve problem solving and data analysis skills.

1301 **Ice Cream Truck**
Sunburst Technology
3150 W Higgins Rd
Suite 140
Hoffman Estates, IL 60619
800-321-7511
http://www.sunburst.com
service@sunburst.com

Elementary students learn important problem solving, strategic planning and math operation skills, as they become owners of a busy ice cream truck.

1302 **Memory Match**
Software to Go-Gallaudet University
800 Florida Ave NE
Washington, DC 20002-3695 202-651-5031
Fax: 202-651-5109
http://clerccenter.gallaudet.edu
clerc.center@gallaudet.edu
Ed Bosso, Vice President
Ken Kurlychek, EI Specialist

1303 **Memory: A First Step in Problem Solving**
Software to Go-Gallaudet University
800 Florida Ave NE
Washington, DC 20002-3695 202-651-5031
Fax: 202-651-5109
http://clerccenter.gallaudet.edu
clerc.center@gallaudet.edu
Ed Bosso, Vice President
Ken Kurlychek, EI Specialist

1304 **Merit Software**
Merit Software
121 West 27th Street
Suite 1200
New York, NY 10001 212-675-8567
800-753-6488
Fax: 800-918-9336
http://www.meritsoftware.com
sales@meritsoftware.com
Ben Weintraub, CEO
Deductive logic and problem solving are the primary skills developed in the variation of the game MASTERMIND. *$9.95*

1305 **Middle School Math Bundle**
Sunburst Technology
3150 W Higgins Rd
Suite 140
Hoffman Estates, IL 60619 800-321-7511
http://www.sunburst.com
service@sunburst.com
This bundle helps improve student's logical thinking, number sense and operation skills. This product comes with Math Arena, Building Perspective Deluxe, Equation Tile Teasers and Easy Sheet.

1306 **Nordic Software**
P.O. Box 5403
Lincoln, NE 68505 402-489-1557
800-306-6502
Fax: 402-489-1560
http://www.nordicsoftware.com
webmaster@nordicsoftware.com
Develops and publishes entertaining, educational software. Children ages three and up can build math skills, expand their vocabulary and increase proficiency in spelling, among other subjects. *$59.95*

1307 **Number Sense & Problem Solving CD-ROM**
Sunburst Technology
3150 W Higgins Rd
Suite 140
Hoffman Estates, IL 60619 800-321-7511
http://www.sunburst.com
service@sunburst.com
Build number and operation skills with these three programs: How the West Was One + Three x Four, Divide and Conquer and Puzzle Tank.

1308 **Problem Solving**
Psychological Software Services
3304 W 75th St
Indianapolis, IN 46268-1664 317-257-9672
Fax: 317-257-9674
http://www.neuroscience.cnter.com
nsc@neuroscience.cnter.com
Odie L Bracy, PhD, HSPP, Clinical Neuropsychologist
Nancy Bracy, Office Manager
Andrea Oakes, Clinical Assistant
Nine computer programs designed to challenge high functioning patients/students with tasks requiring logic. *$150.00*

1309 **Single Switch Games**
MarbleSoft
12301 Central Ave NE Ste 205
P.O. Box 490215
Blaine, MN 55449 763-502-0440
888-755-1402
Fax: 763-862-2920
http://www.marblesoft.com
support@marblesoft.com
Joyce Meyer, President
Mark Larson, CEO, Product Development
Vicki Larson, Sales
There's a lot of educational software for single switch users, but how about something that's just for fun? We've taken some games similar to the ones you enjoyed as a kid and made them work just right for single switch users. Includes Single Switch Maze, A Frog's Life, Switching Lanes, Switch Invaders, Slingshot Gallery and Scurry. Runs on Macintosh and Windows computers. *$30.00*

1310 **Sliding Block**
Merit Software
121 West 27th Street
Suite 1200
New York, NY 10001 212-675-8567
800-753-6488
Fax: 800-918-9336
http://www.meritsoftware.com
sales@meritsoftware.com
Ben Weintraub, CEO
Learners rearrange one of the four pictures which can be scrambled at five separate levels to test visual discrimination and problem solving skills. *$9.95*

1311 **SmartDriver**
BrainTrain
727 Twinridge Lane
North Chesterfield, VA 23235 804-320-0105
800-822-0538
Fax: 804-320-2491
http://www.braintrain.com
info@braintrain.com
Joseph A Sandford, Ph.D., Founder
Virginia Sandford, VP, Sales & Marketing
Visual attention building software where you 'win' by driving defensively and following the rules of the road. Children love this driving game that teaches visual attention, visual tracking, patience, following the rules, planning, and hand-eye coordination.

1312 **SoundSmart**
BrainTrain
727 Twinridge Lane
North Chesterfield, VA 23235 804-320-0105
800-822-0538
Fax: 804-320-2491
http://www.braintrain.com
info@braintrain.com
Joseph A Sandford, Ph.D., Founder
Virginia Sandford, VP, Sales & Marketing
Auditory Attention Building software to help improve phonenic awareness, listening skills, working memory, mental processing speech and self-control. *$549.00*

1313 **Strategy Challenges Collection: 1**
Riverdeep
222 Berkeley Street
Boston, MA 02116
617-351-5000
855-969-4642
Fax: 877-892-9820
http://www.hmhco.com
IIEcustomerservice@hmhpub.com
Linda K. Zecher, President, CEO, Director
James G. Nicholson, President, Riverside Publishing
John K. Dragoon, EVP, Chief Marketing Officer
Houghton Mifflin Harcourt offers a wide array of technology-driven pre-k-12 solutions that inspire excellence and innovation in education, and raise student achievement.
$39.95

1314 **Strategy Challenges Collection: 2**
Riverdeep
222 Berkeley Street
Boston, MA 02116
617-351-5000
855-969-4642
Fax: 877-892-9820
http://www.hmhco.com
IIEcustomerservice@hmhpub.com
Linda K. Zecher, President, CEO, Director
James G. Nicholson, President, Riverside Publishing
John K. Dragoon, EVP, Chief Marketing Officer
Houghton Mifflin Harcourt offers a wide array of technology-driven pre-k-12 solutions that inspire excellence and innovation in education, and raise student achievement.
$39.95

1315 **Thinkin' Things Collection: 3**
Riverdeep
222 Berkeley Street
Boston, MA 02116
617-351-5000
855-969-4642
Fax: 877-892-9820
http://www.hmhco.com
IIEcustomerservice@hmhpub.com
Linda K. Zecher, President, CEO, Director
James G. Nicholson, President, Riverside Publishing
John K. Dragoon, EVP, Chief Marketing Officer
Houghton Mifflin Harcourt offers a wide array of technology-driven pre-k-12 solutions that inspire excellence and innovation in education, and raise student achievement.

1316 **Thinkin' Things: All Around Frippletown**
Riverdeep
222 Berkeley Street
Boston, MA 02116
617-351-5000
855-969-4642
Fax: 877-892-9820
http://www.hmhco.com
IIEcustomerservice@hmhpub.com
Linda K. Zecher, President, CEO, Director
James G. Nicholson, President, Riverside Publishing
John K. Dragoon, EVP, Chief Marketing Officer
Houghton Mifflin Harcourt offers a wide array of technology-driven pre-k-12 solutions that inspire excellence and innovation in education, and raise student achievement.

1317 **Thinkin' Things: Collection 1**
Riverdeep
222 Berkeley Street
Boston, MA 02116
617-351-5000
855-969-4642
Fax: 877-892-9820
http://www.hmhco.com
IIEcustomerservice@hmhpub.com
Linda K. Zecher, President, CEO, Director
James G. Nicholson, President, Riverside Publishing
John K. Dragoon, EVP, Chief Marketing Officer
Houghton Mifflin Harcourt offers a wide array of technology-driven pre-k-12 solutions that inspire excellence and innovation in education, and raise student achievement.

1318 **Thinkin' Things: Collection 2**
Riverdeep
222 Berkeley Street
Boston, MA 02116
617-351-5000
855-969-4642
Fax: 877-892-9820
http://www.hmhco.com
IIEcustomerservice@hmhpub.com
Linda K. Zecher, President, CEO, Director
James G. Nicholson, President, Riverside Publishing
John K. Dragoon, EVP, Chief Marketing Officer
Houghton Mifflin Harcourt offers a wide array of technology-driven pre-k-12 solutions that inspire excellence and innovation in education, and raise student achievement.

1319 **Thinkin' Things: Sky Island Mysteries**
Riverdeep
222 Berkeley Street
Boston, MA 02116
617-351-5000
855-969-4642
Fax: 877-892-9820
http://www.hmhco.com
IIEcustomerservice@hmhpub.com
Linda K. Zecher, President, CEO, Director
James G. Nicholson, President, Riverside Publishing
John K. Dragoon, EVP, Chief Marketing Officer
Houghton Mifflin Harcourt offers a wide array of technology-driven pre-k-12 solutions that inspire excellence and innovation in education, and raise student achievement.

Professional Resources

1320 **Accurate Assessments**
18047 Oak Street
Omaha, NE 68130
402-341-8880
800-324-7966
Fax: 402-341-8911
http://www.myaccucare.com
info@orionhealthcare.com
Accurate Assessments offers a full range of superior innovative technological services and expertise to the behavioral health industry. Our premier product, AccuCare Behavioral Healthcare System, was developed by teams of experts in their respective fields, insuring our products are truly useful to clinicians and are easy to use. This innovative software program is a comprehensive and adaptable approach to the behavioral health practice environment.

1321 **Beyond Drill and Practice: Expanding the Computer Mainstream**
Council for Exceptional Children
Suite 500
655 Tyee Road
Victoria, BC
250-412-3258
http://www.abebooks.com
sellbooks@abebooks.com
Susan Jo Russell, Author
Rebecca Corwin, Author
Janice R. Mokros, Author
Provides informative guidelines and examples for teachers who want to expand the use of the computer as a learning tool. *$10.00*
120 pages

1322 **CE Software**
PO Box 65580
West Des Moines, IA 50265
515-221-1801
800-523-7638
Fax: 515-221-1806
http://startly.com
International software developer. Many products for adaptive technology.

1323 **Compass Learning**
203 Colorado Street
Austin, TX 78701
512-478-9600
800-678-1412
Fax: 512-492-6193
http://www.compasslearning.com
support@compasslearning.com
Tammy Deal, Vice President, Human Resources
Arthur Vanderveen, VP, Development
Eileen Shihadeh, VP, Marketing
Educational software for teachers of K-12.

1324 **Computer Retrieval of Information on Scientific Project (CRISP)**
National Institute of Health
9000 Rockville Pike
Building 12A
Bethesda, MD 20892
301-496-5703
866-319-4357
TTY: 301-496-8294
http://cit.nih.gov
commons@od.nih.gov
Andrea T. Norris, Director
Alfred H. Whitley, Deputy Director of Admin
A major scientific information system containing data on the research programs supported by the US Public Health Service.

1325 **Conover Company**
4 Brookwood Court
Appleton, WI 54914
920-882-1272
800-933-1933
Fax: 800-933-1943
http://www.conovercompany.com
sales@conovercompany.com
Becky Schmitz, President
Mike Schmitz, Vice President of Operations
Provides off-the-shelf as well as custom sales and marketing, training, presentation, and application programs that connect learning to the workplace. Delivery platforms include workshops, print, custom software, CD-ROM, multimedia, internet, and intranet.

1326 **Developmental Profile**
Western Psychological Services
625 Alaska Avenue
Torrance, CA 90503-5124
424-201-8800
800-648-8857
Fax: 424-201-6950
http://www.wpspublish.com
customerservice@wpspublish.com
Jeffrey Manson, President, CEO
Dave Herzberg, Ph.D., VP, Research & Development
Amanda Wynn, Marketing Director
This computer program substantially reduces the time educators spend on preparing Individualized Educational Plans (IEPs). The system allows the user to use any IEP format. Simply type the format into the computer, and the program will customize the system to your district's specifications. *$115.00*

1327 **FileMaker Inc.**
5201 Patrick Henry Drive
Santa Clara, CA 95054
408-987-7000
800-325-2747
Fax: 408-987-3002
http://www.filemaker.com
filemaker_pr@filemaker.com
Dominique Goupil, President
Bill Epling, SVP/CAO
Frank Lu, Vice President of Engineering
Company that produces a variety of Macintosh Documentation.

1328 **International Society for Technology in Education (ISTE)**
University of Oregon
180 West 8th Ave
Suite 300
Eugene, OR 97401-2916
541-302-3777
800-336-5191
Fax: 541-302-3778
http://www.iste.org
iste@iste.org
Brian Lewis,ÿM.A.,ÿC.A.E., CEO
Tracee Aliotti, Chief Marketing Officer
Anne Tully, Chief Operating Officer
A nonprofit professional organization dedicated to promoting appropriate uses of information technology to support and improve learning, teaching, and administration in K-12 education and teacher education.

1329 **KidDesk**
Riverdeep
222 3rd Ave SE
4th Floor
Cedar Rapids, IA 52401
319-395-9626
800-825-4420
Fax: 319-395-0217
http://web.riverdeep.net/portal/page?_pageid=81
info@riverdeep.net
Barry O'Callaghan, Executive Chairman & CEO
Tony Mulderry, EVP, Corporate Development
Jim Ruddy, Chief Revenue Officer
A hard disk security program, KidDesk makes it easy for kids to launch their programs, but impossible for them to access adult programs. Includes interactive desktop accessories including desktop-to-desktop electronic mail, and voice mail. *$24.95*

1330 **KidDesk: Family Edition**
Riverdeep
222 3rd Ave SE
4th Floor
Cedar Rapids, IA 52401
319-395-9626
800-825-4420
Fax: 319-395-0217
http://web.riverdeep.net/portal/page?_pageid=81
info@riverdeep.net
Barry O'Callaghan, Executive Chairman & CEO
Tony Mulderry, EVP, Corporate Development
Jim Ruddy, Chief Revenue Officer
Now kids can launch their programs, but can't access yours! With KidDesk Family Edition, you can give your children the keys to the computer without putting your programs and files at risk! The auto-start option provides constant hard drive security — any time your computer is turned on, KidDesk will appear. *$24.95*

1331 **Laureate Learning Systems**
110 East Spring Street
Winooski, VT 05404-1898
802-655-4755
800-562-6801
Fax: 802-655-4757
http://www.laureatelearning.com
laureate-webmaster@laureatelearning.com
Dr. Mary Sweig Wilson Ph.D., President/CEO, Founder
Bernard J. Fox, Co-Founder, Vice President
Marion Blank, Ph.D, Developmental Psychologist
Provides resources for people with learning disabilities.

1332 **Learning Company**
Riverdeep
100 Pine Street
Suite 1900
San Francisco, CA 94111
415-659-2000
800-825-4420
Fax: 415-659-2020
http://web.riverdeep.net/portal/page?_pageid=81
info@riverdeep.net
Barry O'Callaghan, Executive Chairman & CEO
Tony Mulderry, EVP, Corporate Development
Jim Ruddy, Chief Revenue Officer

1333 **Microsoft Corporation**
1 Microsoft Way
Redmond, WA 98052-6399
425-882-8080
800-642-7676
Fax: 425-936-7329
http://www.microsoft.com
Steve Ballmer, CEO
Lisa Brummel, Chief People Officer
Tony Bates, President
Our mission is to enable people and businesses throughout the world to realize their full potential.

1334 **Print Module**
Failure Free
140 Cabarrus Ave West
Concord, NC 28025
704-786-7838
888-233-READ
Fax: 704-785-8940
http://www.failurefree.com
info@failurefree.com
Dr. Joseph Lockavitch, Author and President
Joe Lockavitch, VP Sales and Marketing
Includes teacher's manual, instructional readers, flashcards, independent activities and illustrated independent reading booklets. *$499.00*

1335 **PsycINFO Database**
American Psychological Association
750 First St. NE
Washington, DC 20002-4242
202-336-5500
800-374-2721
Fax: 202-336-5997
TDD: 202-336-6123
TTY: 202-336-6123
http://www.apa.org
mis@apa.org
Norman B. Anderson, PhD, EVP, Chief Executive Officer
Archie Turner, VP, Chief Financial Officer
Tony Habash, DSc, Chief Information Officer
An online abstract database that provides access to citations to the international serial literature in psychology and related disciplines from 1887 to present. Available via PsycINFO Direct at www.psycinfo.com.

1336 **Public Domain Software**
Kentucky Special Ed TechTraining Center
229 Taylor Education Building
UK College of Education
Lexington, KY 40506-0017
859-257-6076
Fax: 859-257-1325
TDD: 859-257-4714
http://2b.education.uky.edu
amanda.nelson@uky.edu
Mary John O'Hair, Dean and Professor
Parker Fawson, Associate Dean
Steve R. Parker, Associate Professor
Entire collections of Macintosh, MS-DOS or Apple II software.

1337 **Riverdeep**
100 Pine Street
Suite 1900
San Francisco, CA 94111
415-659-2000
800-825-4420
Fax: 415-659-2020
http://web.riverdeep.net/portal/page?_pageid=81
info@riverdeep.net
Barry O'Callaghan, Executive Chairman & CEO
Tony Mulderry, EVP, Corporate Development
Jim Ruddy, Chief Revenue Officer
Developer of educational software, including software for mathematics instruction.

1338 **Scholastic**
2931 E McCarty St
Jefferson City, MO 65101-4468
573-636-5271
800-724-6527
Fax: 573-636-0549
http://www.scholastic.com
custserv@scholastic.com
Faye Edwards, Executive VP/CAO/CEO
Larry Holland, Human Resources Director
Dick Robinson, President & CEO
For more than 90 years, Scholastic has been delivering outstanding books, magazines and educational programs directly to schools and families through channels that have become childhood traditions - Scholastic Book Fairs, monthly Book Clubs, and Scholastic News classroom magazines.

1339 **Speech Bin Abilitations**
PO Box 1579
Appleton, WI 54912-1579
419-589-1425
888-388-3224
Fax: 888-388-6344
http://www.schoolspecialty.com
orders@schoolspecialty.com
Joseph M. Yorio, President, CEO
Patrick T. Collins, EVP, Distribution
Rick Holden, Executive Vice President
The Speech Bin offers materials to help persons of all ages who have special needs. We specialize in products for children and adults who have communication disorders.

1340 **Sunburst**
3150 W Higgins Rd
Suite 140
Hoffman Estates, IL 60619
800-321-7511
http://www.sunburst.com
service@sunburst.com
Dan Figurski, President
Michael Guillroy, Channel Sales/Marketing Manager

Reading

1341 **Adaptive Technology Tools**
Freedom Scientific
11800 31st Court North
St Petersburg, FL 33716-1805
727-803-8000
800-444-4443
Fax: 727-803-8001
http://www.freedomscientific.com
info@FreedomScientific.com
John Blake, President, CEO
Peggy Dalton, Director, Professional Services
Bryan Carver, Inside Sales Director
A wide variety of adaptive technology tools for the visually or reading impaired person.

1342 **An Open Book**
Freedom Scientific
11800 31st Court North
St Petersburg, FL 33716-1805
727-803-8000
800-444-4443
Fax: 727-803-8001
http://www.freedomscientific.com
info@FreedomScientific.com
John Blake, President, CEO
Peggy Dalton, Director, Professional Services
Bryan Carver, Inside Sales Director
The stand-alone reading machine, An Open Book, is an easy-to-use appliance for noncomputer users that comes equipped with a Hewlett Packard ScanJet IIP scanner, DECtalk PC speech synthesizer and a 17 key keypad. An Open Book uses Calera WordScan optical character recognition (OCR) to convert pages into text, then reads it aloud with a speech synthesizer.

1343 **An Open Book Unbound**
Freedom Scientific
11800 31st Court North
St Petersburg, FL 33716-1805
727-803-8000
800-444-4443
Fax: 727-803-8001
http://www.freedomscientific.com
info@FreedomScientific.com
John Blake, President, CEO
Peggy Dalton, Director, Professional Services
Bryan Carver, Inside Sales Director
PC-based OCR and reading software. Together with a scanner and a speech synthesizer, this software provides everything needed to make an IBM-compatible PC into a talking reading machine. The system includes automatic page orientation, automatic contrast control, decolumnization of multicolumn documents and recognition of a wide variety of type fonts and sizes. *$995.00*

1344 **Bailey's Book House**
Riverdeep
222 3rd Ave SE
4th Floor
Cedar Rapids, IA 52401
319-395-9626
800-825-4420
Fax: 319-395-0217
http://web.riverdeep.net/portal/page?_pageid=81
info@riverdeep.net
Barry O'Callaghan, Executive Chairman & CEO
Tony Mulderry, EVP, Corporate Development
Jim Ruddy, Chief Revenue Officer
The award-winning Bailey's Book House now features 2 new activities! Bailey and his friends encourage young children to build important literacy skills while developing a love for reading. In seven activities, kids explore the sounds and meanings of letters, words, sentences, rhymes and stories. No reading skills are required: all directions and written words are spoken. *$59.95*

1345 **Comprehension Connection**
Milliken Publishing
501 East Third Street
Box 802
Dayton, OH 45401-0802
937-228-6118
800-444-1144
Fax: 937-223-2042
http://www.lorenzeducationalpress.com
lep@lorenz.com
Thomas Moore, President
Comprehension Connection improves reading comprehension by stressing basic skills that combine the reading process with relevant activities and interesting, thought-provoking stories. This award-winning software package spans six reading levels that increase in difficulty. Passages range from 150-300 words. *$150.00*

1346 **Cosmic Reading Journey**
Sunburst Technology
3150 W Higgins Rd
Suite 140
Hoffman Estates, IL 60619
800-321-7511
http://www.sunburst.com
service@sunburst.com
Michael Guillroy, Channel Sales/Marketing Manager
Dan Figurski, President
This reading comprehension program provides meaningful summary and writing activities for the 100 books that early readers and their teachers love most.

1347 **Don Johnston Reading**
Don Johnston
26799 West Commerce Drive
Volo, IL 60073
847-740-0749
800-999-4660
Fax: 847-740-7326
http://www.donjohnston.com
info@donjohnston.com
Don Johnston, Founder
Ruth Ziolkowski, President
Mindy Brown, Marketing Director
Don Johnston Inc. is a provider of quality products and services that enable people with special needs to discover their potential and experience success. Products are developed for the areas of computer access and for those who struggle with reading and writing.

1348 **Failure Free Reading**
140 Cabarrus Ave West
Concord, NC 28025
704-786-7838
888-233-READ
Fax: 704-785-8940
http://www.failurefree.com
info@failurefree.com
Dr. Joseph Lockavitch, Author and President
Joe Lockavitch, VP Sales and Marketing
Curriculum areas covered: reading for those with learning disabilities and moderate mentally disabled/emotionally disabled.

1349 **Judy Lynn Software**
PO Box 373
East Brunswick, NJ 08816
732-390-8845
Fax: 732-390-8845
http://www.judylynn.com
techsupt@judylynn.com
Elliot Pludwinski, Founder/President
Offers switch computer programs for windows. The programs are geared towards students with a cognitive age level from 9 months and up. Programs are reasonably priced from $39-$79. Recipient of a Parents' Choice Honor.

1350 **Kurzweil 3000**
Kurzweil Educational Systems
24 Prime Parkway
Suite 303
Natick, MA 01760
508-647-1340
800-894-5374
Fax: 781-276-0650
http://www.kurzweiledu.com
customerservice@cambiumtech.com
Mike Sokol, President/CEO
Kurzweil Educational's flagship product for struggling readers and writers. It is widely recognized as the most comprehensive and integrated solution for addressing language and literacy difficulties. The software uses a multisensory approach — presenting printed or electronic text on the computer screen with added visual and audible accessibility. The product incorporates a host of dynamic features including powerful decoding, study skills tools and test taking tools.

1351 **Lexia Cross-Trainer**
Lexia Learning Systems
200 Baker Avenue Ext
Concord, MA 01742
978-405-6200
800-435-3942
Fax: 978-287-0062
http://www.lexialearning.com
info@lexialearning.com
Nick Gaehde, President
Paul More, Vice President, Finance
Collin Earnst, Vice President of Marketing
Interactive software with an engaging video-gme interface that is designed to strengthen cognitive skills. Activities that advance visual-spatial and logical reasoning skills are designed to improve the memory, critical thinking, and problem solving abilities necessary for academic success in all subjects. *$250.00*

1352 **Lexia Early Reading**
Lexia Learning Systems
200 Baker Avenue Ext
Concord, MA 01742
978-405-6200
800-435-3942
Fax: 978-287-0062
http://www.lexialearning.com
info@lexialearning.com
Nick Gaehde, President
Paul More, Vice President, Finance
Collin Earnst, Vice President of Marketing

Engaging, interactive software fochildren aged four to six that introduces and develops proficiency with phonological principles and the alphabet - both proven indicators of later reading success.

1353 **Lexia Primary Reading**
Lexia Learning Systems
200 Baker Avenue Ext
Concord, MA 01742
978-405-6200
800-435-3942
Fax: 978-287-0062
http://www.lexialearning.com
info@lexialearning.com
Nick Gaehde, President
Paul More, Vice President, Finance
Collin Earnst, Vice President of Marketing
Interactive software designed to ensure mastery of basic phonological skills and introduce more advanced phonics priciples. five levels of engaging activities deliver practice in phonemic awareness, sight-word recognition, word attack strategies, sound-symbol correspondence, listening and reading comprehension. *$50.00*

1354 **Lexia Strategies for Older Students**
Lexia Learning Systems
200 Baker Avenue Ext
Concord, MA 01742
978-405-6200
800-435-3942
Fax: 978-287-0062
http://www.lexialearning.com
info@lexialearning.com
Nick Gaehde, President
Paul More, Vice President, Finance
Collin Earnst, Vice President of Marketing
Reading skills software program specifically designed for ages 9-adult. Five levels of activities provide extensive practice in everything from basic phonological awareness to advanced word attack strategy and vocabulary development based on Greek and Laitn word roots. *$250.00*

1355 **Mike Mulligan & His Steam Shovel**
Sunburst Technology
3150 W Higgins Rd
Suite 140
Hoffman Estates, IL 60619
800-321-7511
http://www.sunburst.com
service@sunburst.com
Dan Figurski, President
Michael Guillory, Channel Sales/Marketing Manager
This CD-ROM version of the Caldecott classic lets students experience interactive book reading and participate in four skills-based extension activities that promote memory, matching, sequencing, listening, pattern recognition and map reading skills.

1356 **Optimum Resource**
1 Mathews Drive
Suite 107
Hilton Head Island, SC 29926
843-689-8000
888-784-2592
Fax: 843-689-8008
http://www.stickybear.com
info@stickybear.com
Richard Hefter, President
An educational software publishing company for grades K-12. Our software titles are available in Consumer, School, Labpack or Site License versions. Please call for further details. Prices range from $59.95 for Consumer to $699.95 for Site Licenses.

1357 **Polar Express**
Sunburst Technology
3150 W Higgins Rd
Suite 140
Hoffman Estates, IL 60619
800-321-7511
http://www.sunburst.com
service@sunburst.com
Dan Figurski, President
Michael Guillory, Channel Sales/Marketing Manager
Share the magic and enchantment of the holiday season with this CD-ROM version of Chris Van Allsburg's Caldecott-winning picture book.

1358 **Prolexia**
4726 13th Ave NW
Rochester, MN 55901-2631
507-780-1859
888-776-5394
Fax: 507-252-0131
http://www.prolexia.com
info@prolexia.com
John Rylander, President
UltraPhonics Tutor software teaches reading, spelling, handwriting, & pronunication to beginners and those with dyslexia via multisensory structured phonics.

1359 **Read On! Plus**
Sunburst Technology
3150 W Higgins Rd
Suite 140
Hoffman Estates, IL 60619
800-321-7511
http://www.sunburst.com
service@sunburst.com
Dan Figurski, President
Michael Guillory, Channel Sales/Marketing Manager
Promote skills and strategies that improve reading comprehension, and build appreciation for literature and the written word.

1360 **Read, Write and Type! Learning Systems**
Talking Fingers
830 Rincon Way
San Rafael, CA 94903
415-472-3103
800-674-9126
Fax: 415-472-7812
TDD: 415-472-3106
http://www.readwritetype.com
contact@talkingfingers.com
Dr. Jeannine Herron, Co-Founder
Dr. Leslie Grimm, Co-Founder
A 40-level software adventure providing highly motivating instruction and practice in phonics, reading, writing, spelling and typing. This multisensory program includes 9 levels of assessment and reports. Classroom packs available.

1361 **Reading Power Modules Books**
Steck-Vaughn Company
9400 Southpark Center Loop
Orlando, FL 32819
407-345-2000
800-225-5425
Fax: 800-699-9459
http://www.hmhco.com
IIEcustomerservice@hmhpub.com
Linda K. Zecher, President, CEO, Director
James G. Nicholson, President, Riverside Publishing
John K. Dragoon, EVP, Chief Marketing Officer
Supplementary reading based on 4 decades of reading research. Companion books give students and teachers a choice of formats. High interest stories reinforce reading comprehension skills while building vocabulary, spelling skills, reading fluency, and speed.

1362 **Reading Skills Bundle**
Sunburst Technology
3150 W Higgins Rd
Suite 140
Hoffman Estates, IL 60619
800-321-7511
http://www.sunburst.com
service@sunburst.com
Dan Figurski, President
Michael Guillory, Channel Sales/Marketing Manager
Teach beginning reading with teacher-developed programs that sequentially present phonics, phonemic awareness, word recognition, and reading comprehension concepts.

1363 **Reading Who? Reading You!**
Sunburst Technology
3150 W Higgins Rd
Suite 140
Hoffman Estates, IL 60619
800-321-7511
http://www.sunburst.com
service@sunburst.com
Dan Figurski, President
Michael Guillory, Channel Sales/Marketing Manager
Teach beginning reading skills effectively with phonics instruction built into engaging games and puzzles that have children asking for more.

1364 **Sentence Master: Level 1, 2, 3, 4**
Laureate Learning Systems
110 East Spring Street
Winooski, VT 05404-1898
802-655-4755
800-562-6801
Fax: 802-655-4757
http://www.laureatelearning.com
laureate-webmaster@laureatelearning.com
Dr. Mary Sweig Wilson Ph.D., President/CEO, Founder
Bernard J. Fox, Co-Founder, Vice President
Marion Blank, Ph.D, Developmental Psychologist
A revolutionary way to teach beginning reading. Avoiding the confusing rules of phonics and the complexity of whole language, The Sentence Master focuses on the most frequently-used words of our language; i.e. the, is, but, and, etc., by truly teaching these little words, The Sentence Master gives students control over the majority of text they will ever encounter. *$495.00*

1365 **Simon Sounds It Out**
Don Johnston
26799 West Commerce Drive
Volo, IL 60073
847-740-0749
800-999-4660
Fax: 847-740-7326
http://www.donjohnston.com
info@donjohnston.com
Don Johnston, Founder
Ruth Ziolkowski, President
Mindy Brown, Marketing Director
Struggling students who can recite the alphabet and recognize letters on a page may still have trouble making connections between letters and sounds. This creates a barrier to recognizing and learning words which prevents your students from reading and writing successfully. Simon Sounds It Out provides the vital practice and repetition they need to overcome the letter-to-sound barrier. *$59.00*

1366 **Stickybear Software**
Optimum Resource
1 Mathews Drive
Suite 107
Hilton Head Island, SC 29926
843-689-8000
888-784-2592
Fax: 843-689-8008
http://www.stickybear.com
info@stickybear.com
Richard Hefter, President
An educational software publishing company for grades K-12. Our software titles are available in Consumer, School, Labpack or Site License versions. Please call for further details. Prices range from $59.95 for Consumer to $699.95 for Site Licenses.

1367 **Tenth Planet Roots, Prefixes & Suffixes**
Sunburst Technology
3150 W Higgins Rd
Suite 140
Hoffman Estates, IL 60619
800-321-7511
http://www.sunburst.com
service@sunburst.com
Dan Figurski, President
Michael Guillory, Channel Sales/Marketing Manager
Students learn to decode difficult and more complex words as they engage in six activities where they construct and dissect words with roots, prefixes and suffixes.

1368 **Time for Teachers Online**
Stern Center for Language and Learning
183 Talcott Road
Suite 101
Williston, VT 05495
802-878-2332
800-544-4863
Fax: 802-878-0230
http://www.sterncenter.org
learning@sterncenter.org
Blanche Podhajski, Ph.D., President
Janna Osman, M.Ed., VP, Programs
Michael Shapiro, M.B.A., Chief Financial Officer
A 45 hour course completed entirely on the internet, designed to help teachers implement research-based best practices in reading instruction. *$525.00*

Science

1369 **Changes Around Us CD-ROM**
9400 Southpark Center Loop
Orlando, FL 32819
407-345-2000
800-225-5425
Fax: 800-699-9459
http://www.hmhco.com
IIEcustomerservice@hmhpub.com
Linda K. Zecher, President, CEO, Director
James G. Nicholson, President, Riverside Publishing
John K. Dragoon, EVP, Chief Marketing Officer
Nature is the natural choice for observing change. By observing and researching dramatic visual sequences such as the stages of development of a butterfly, children develop a broad understanding of the concept of change. As they search this multimedia database for images and information about plant and animal life cycles and seasonal change, students strengthen their abilities in research, analysis, problem-solving, critical thinking and communication.

1370 **Exploring Heat**
TERC
2067 Massachusetts Ave
Cambridge, MA 02140
617-873-9600
Fax: 617-873-9601
http://www.terc.edu
contactus@terc.edu
Arthur Nelson, Founder
George E. Hein, Chairman
Chris Dede, Board Member
A combination of lessons, software, temperature probes and activity sheets, specifically designed for the learning disabled child. *$160.00*

1371 **Field Trip Into the Sea**
Sunburst Technology
3150 W Higgins Rd
Suite 140
Hoffman Estates, IL 60619
800-321-7511
http://www.sunburst.com
service@sunburst.com
Dan Figurski, President
Michael Guillory, Channel Sales/Marketing Manager
Visit a kelp forest and the rocky shore with this information packed guide that lets your students learn about the plants, animals and habitats of coastal environments.

1372 **Field Trip to the Rain Forest**
Sunburst Technology
3150 W Higgins Rd
Suite 140
Hoffman Estates, IL 60619
800-321-7511
http://www.sunburst.com
service@sunburst.com
Dan Figurski, President
Michael Guillory, Channel Sales/Marketing Manager
Visit a Central American rainforest to learn more about its plants and animals with this dynamic research program that includes a useful information management tool.

1373 Learn About Life Science: Animals
Sunburst Technology
3150 W Higgins Rd
Suite 140
Hoffman Estates, IL 60619 800-321-7511
http://www.sunburst.com
service@sunburst.com
Dan Figurski, President
Michael Guillory, Channel Sales/Marketing Manager
Learn about animal classification, adaptation to climate, domestication and special relationships between humans and animals.

1374 Learn About Life Science: Plants
Sunburst Technology
3150 W Higgins Rd
Suite 140
Hoffman Estates, IL 60619 800-321-7511
http://www.sunburst.com
service@sunburst.com
Dan Figurski, President
Michael Guillory, Channel Sales/Marketing Manager
Students explore the world of plants. From small seeds to tall trees students learn what plants are and what they need to grow.

1375 Milliken Science Series: Circulation and Digestion
Milliken Publishing
501 East Third Street
Box 802
Dayton, OH 45401-0802 937-228-6118
800-444-1144
Fax: 937-223-2042
http://www.lorenzeducationalpress.com
lep@lorenz.com
Thomas Moore, President
Delores Boufard, Author
A program designed to introduce students to two subsystems of the human body. Provides practice using the correct terms for the various organs that make up each system, illustrating how the parts of each subsystem work together, and ensuring that students can explain the functions of the subsystems and their parts.

1376 Sammy's Science House
Riverdeep
222 3rd Ave SE
4th Floor
Cedar Rapids, IA 52401 319-395-9626
800-825-4420
Fax: 319-395-0217
http://web.riverdeep.net/portal/page?_pageid=81
info@riverdeep.net
Barry O'Callaghan, Executive Chairman & CEO
Tony Mulderry, EVP, Corporate Development
Jim Ruddy, Chief Revenue Officer
Developed by early learning experts, the award-winning Sammy's Science House builds important early science skills, encourages wonder and joy as children discover the world of science around them. Five engaging activities help children practice sorting, sequencing, observing, predicting and constructing. They'll learn about plants, animals, minerals, fun seasons and weather, too! *$59.95*

1377 Talking Walls
Riverdeep
222 3rd Ave SE
4th Floor
Cedar Rapids, IA 52401 319-395-9626
800-825-4420
Fax: 319-395-0217
http://web.riverdeep.net/portal/page?_pageid=81
info@riverdeep.net
Barry O'Callaghan, Executive Chairman & CEO
Tony Mulderry, EVP, Corporate Development
Jim Ruddy, Chief Revenue Officer
The Talking Walls Software Series is a wonderful springboard for a student's journey of exploration and discovery. This comprehensive collection of researched resources and materials enables students to focus on learning while conducting a guided search for information.

1378 Talking Walls: The Stories Continue
Riverdeep
222 3rd Ave SE
4th Floor
Cedar Rapids, IA 52401 319-395-9626
800-825-4420
Fax: 319-395-0217
http://web.riverdeep.net/portal/page?_pageid=81
info@riverdeep.net
Barry O'Callaghan, Executive Chairman & CEO
Tony Mulderry, EVP, Corporate Development
Jim Ruddy, Chief Revenue Officer
Using the Talking Walls Software Series, students discover the stories behind some of the world's most fascinating walls. The award-winning books, interactive software, carefully chosen Web sites, and suggested classroom activities build upon each other, providing a rich learning experience that includes text, video, and hands-on projects.

Social Studies

1379 Discoveries: Explore the Desert Ecosystem
Sunburst Technology
3150 W Higgins Rd
Suite 140
Hoffman Estates, IL 60619 800-321-7511
Fax: 888-800-3028
http://www.sunburst.com
service@sunburst.com
Dan Figurski, President
Michael Guillory, Channel Sales/Marketing Manager
This program invites students to explore the plants, animals, culture and georgraphy of the Sonoran Desert by day and by night.

1380 Discoveries: Explore the Everglades Ecosystem
Sunburst Technology
3150 W Higgins Rd
Suite 140
Hoffman Estates, IL 60619 800-321-7511
Fax: 888-800-3028
http://www.sunburst.com
service@sunburst.com
Dan Figurski, President
Michael Guillory, Channel Sales/Marketing Manager
This multi curricular research program takes students to the Everglades where they anchor their exploration photo realistic panaramas of the habitiat.

1381 Discoveries: Explore the Forest Ecosystem
Sunburst Technology
3150 W Higgins Rd
Suite 140
Hoffman Estates, IL 60619 800-321-7511
Fax: 888-800-3028
http://www.sunburst.com
service@sunburst.com
Dan Figurski, President
Michael Guillory, Channel Sales/Marketing Manager
This theme based CD-ROM enables students of all abilities to actively research a multitude of different forest ecosystems in the Appalachian National Park.

1382 Imagination Express Destination: Castle
Riverdeep
222 3rd Ave SE
4th Floor
Cedar Rapids, IA 52401 319-395-9626
800-825-4420
Fax: 319-395-0217
http://web.riverdeep.net/portal/page?_pageid=81
info@riverdeep.net

Barry O'Callaghan, Executive Chairman & CEO
Tony Mulderry, EVP, Corporate Development
Jim Ruddy, Chief Revenue Officer
Kids enter a medieval kingdom where knights, jesters, wild boars and falconers become actors in their own interactive stories. As kids cast characters, develop plots, narrate and write and record dialogue, they become enthusiastic writers, editors, producers and publishers! *$59.95*

1383 **Imagination Express Destination: Neighborhood**
Riverdeep
222 3rd Ave SE
4th Floor
Cedar Rapids, IA 52401
319-395-9626
800-825-4420
Fax: 319-395-0217
http://web.riverdeep.net/portal/page?_pageid=81
info@riverdeep.net
Barry O'Callaghan, Executive Chairman & CEO
Tony Mulderry, EVP, Corporate Development
Jim Ruddy, Chief Revenue Officer
In Destination: Neighborhood, familiar settings and characters encourage kids to write about actual or imagined adventures. Kids enjoy developing creativity, writing and communication skills as they explore the neighborhood and all the people who live there. As kids select scenes, choose and animate stickers, write, narrate, add music and record dialogue, their stories, journals, letters and poems come alive! *$59.95*

1384 **Imagination Express Destination: Ocean**
Riverdeep
222 3rd Ave SE
4th Floor
Cedar Rapids, IA 52401
319-395-9626
800-825-4420
Fax: 319-395-0217
http://web.riverdeep.net/portal/page?_pageid=81
info@riverdeep.net
Barry O'Callaghan, Executive Chairman & CEO
Tony Mulderry, EVP, Corporate Development
Jim Ruddy, Chief Revenue Officer
The fascinating shores and depths of Destination: Ocean inspire kids to create interactive stories and movies. Using exciting new technology, kids make stickers move across each scene: sharks swim through the sea kelp while dolphins leap above waves! With Destination: Ocean, your child's writing and creativity will soar! *$59.95*

1385 **Imagination Express Destination: Pyramids**
Riverdeep
222 3rd Ave SE
4th Floor
Cedar Rapids, IA 52401
319-395-9626
800-825-4420
Fax: 319-395-0217
http://web.riverdeep.net/portal/page?_pageid=81
info@riverdeep.net
Barry O'Callaghan, Executive Chairman & CEO
Tony Mulderry, EVP, Corporate Development
Jim Ruddy, Chief Revenue Officer
Kids can create interactive electronic books and movies featuring pharaohs, mummies and life on the Nile. Builds writing, creativity and communication skills as they learn about and explore this captivating destination. Kids select scenes, choose and animate characters, plan plots, write stories, narrate pages and add music, dialogue and sound effects to make their own adventures. *$59.95*

1386 **Imagination Express Destination: Rain Forest**
Riverdeep
222 3rd Ave SE
4th Floor
Cedar Rapids, IA 52401
319-365-6108
800-825-4420
Fax: 319-395-0217
http://web.riverdeep.net/portal/page?_pageid=81
info@riverdeep.net
Barry O'Callaghan, Executive Chairman & CEO
Tony Mulderry, EVP, Corporate Development
Jim Ruddy, Chief Revenue Officer
Rain Forest invities kids to step into a Panamanian rain forest, where they craft exciting, interactive adventures filled with exotic plants, insects, waterfalls and Kuna Indians. Kids build essential communication skills as they select scenes and characters, plan plots, write, narrate, animate and record dialogue to create remarkable adventures! *$59.95*

1387 **Imagination Express Destination: Time Trip USA**
Riverdeep
222 3rd Ave SE
4th Floor
Cedar Rapids, IA 52401
319-395-9626
800-825-4420
Fax: 319-395-0217
http://web.riverdeep.net/portal/page?_pageid=81
info@riverdeep.net
Barry O'Callaghan, Executive Chairman & CEO
Tony Mulderry, EVP, Corporate Development
Jim Ruddy, Chief Revenue Officer
Children will love traveling through time to create interactive electronic books and movies set in a fictional New England town. As students select scenes, cast charcters, develop plots, narrate, write and record dialogue, they'll bring the town's history to life through their own exciting adventures. *$59.95*

Speech

1388 **Eden Institute Curriculum: Speech and Language**
2 Merwick Road
Princeton, NJ 08540-5711
609-987-0099
Fax: 609-987-0243
http://www.edenservices.org
info@edenservices.org
Dr. Tom Mc Cool, President/CEO
Melinda McAleer, Chief Development Officer
Anne Holmes, M.S., C.C.C.,, Chief Clinical Officer
Peceptive, expressive and pragmatic language skills programs for students with autism. *$170.00*

1389 **Spectral Speech Analysis: Software**
Speech Bin
PO Box 1579
Appleton, WI 54912-1579
419-589-1425
888-388-3224
Fax: 888-388-6344
http://www.schoolspecialty.com
orders@schoolspecialty.com
Joseph M. Yorio, President, CEO
Patrick T. Collins, EVP, Distribution
Rick Holden, Executive Vice President
This exciting new software uses visual feedback as an effective speech treatment tool. Speech-language pathologists can record speech and corresponding visual displays for clients who then try to match either auditory or visual targets. These built-in visual patterns can be displayed as either sophisticated spectrograms or real-time waveforms. Item number P227. *$159.95*

Word Processors

1390 **Dr. Peet's TalkWriter**
Interest Driven Learning
Apt 303
446 Bouchelle Dr
New Smyrna Beach, FL 32169-5429
816-478-4824
800-245-5733
Fax: 816-478-4824
http://www.drpeet.com
lpeet@drpeet.com
Bill William Peet, PhD, CEO
Libby Peet EdD, Adaptive Access Specialist

A talking, singing word processor designed to meet the needs of young learners from three to eight. Runs on Windows.

1391 **Kids Media Magic 2.0**
Sunburst Technology
3150 W Higgins Rd
Suite 140
Hoffman Estates, IL 60619
800-321-7511
Fax: 888-800-3028
http://www.sunburst.com
service@sunburst.com
Dan Figurski, President
Michael Guillory, Channel Sales/Marketing Manager
The first multimedia word processor designed for young children. Help your child become a fluent reader and writer. The Rebus Bar automatically scrolls over 45 vocabulary words as students type.

1392 **Media Weaver 3.5**
Sunburst Technology
3150 W Higgins Rd
Suite 140
Hoffman Estates, IL 60619
800-321-7511
Fax: 888-800-3028
http://www.sunburst.com
service@sunburst.com
Dan Figurski, President
Michael Guillory, Channel Sales/Marketing Manager
Publishing becomes a multimedia event with this dynamic word processor that contains hundreds of media elements and effective process writing resources.

1393 **Sunbuddy Writer**
Sunburst Technology
3150 W Higgins Rd
Suite 140
Hoffman Estates, IL 60619
800-321-7511
Fax: 888-800-3028
http://www.sunburst.com
service@sunburst.com
Dan Figurski, President
Michael Guillory, Channel Sales/Marketing Manager
An easy-to-use picture and word processor designed especially for young writers.

1394 **Write: Outloud to Go**
Don Johnston
26799 West Commerce Drive
Volo, IL 60073
847-740-0749
800-999-4660
Fax: 847-740-7326
http://www.donjohnston.com
info@donjohnston.com
Don Johnston, Founder
Ruth Ziolkowski, President
Mindy Brown, Marketing Director
A flexible and user-friendly talking word processor that offers multisensory learning and positive reinforcement for writers of all ages and ability levels. Powerful features include a talking spell checker, on-screen speech and file management and color capabilities that allow for customization to meet individual needs or preferences. Requires Macintosh computer. Voted Best Special Needs Product by the Software Publishers Association. *$99.00*

Writing

1395 **Abbreviation/Expansion**
Zygo Industries
48834 Kato Road
Suite 101-A
Fremont, CA 94538
510-249-9660
800-234-6006
Fax: 510-770-4930
http://www.zygo-usa.com
zygo@zygo-usa.com
Lawrence H. Weiss, President
Adam D. Weiss, VP, Sales & Marketing
Allows the individual to define and store word/phrase abbreviations to achieve efficiency and accelerated entry rate of text. *$95.00*

1396 **Author's Toolkit**
Sunburst Technology
3150 W Higgins Rd
Suite 140
Hoffman Estates, IL 60619
800-321-7511
Fax: 888-800-3028
http://www.sunburst.com
service@sunburst.com
Dan Figurski, President
Michael Guillory, Channel Sales/Marketing Manager
Students can use this comprehensive tool to organize ideas, make outlines, rough drafts, edit and print all their written work.

1397 **Dr. Peet's Picture Writer**
Interest Driven Learning
Apt 303
446 Bouchelle Dr
New Smyrna Beach, FL 32169-5429
386-427-4473
800-245-5733
Fax: 816-478-4824
http://www.drpeet.com
lpeet@drpeet.com
Bill William Peet, PhD, CEO
Libby Peet EdD, Adaptive Access Specialist
A talking picture-writer. It guides novice writers, regardless of age, motivation or ability, in creating simple talking picture sentences about things that are interesting and important to them. *$500.00*

1398 **Easybook Deluxe**
Sunburst Technology
3150 W Higgins Rd
Suite 140
Hoffman Estates, IL 60619
800-321-7511
Fax: 888-800-3028
http://www.sunburst.com
service@sunburst.com
Dan Figurski, President
Michael Guillory, Channel Sales/Marketing Manager
Designed to support the needs of a wide range of writers, this book publishing tool provides students with a creative environment to write, design and illustrate stories and reports, and to print their work in book formats.

1399 **Fonts4Teachers**
Therapro
225 Arlington Street
Framingham, MA 01702-8723
508-872-9494
800-257-5376
Fax: 508-875-2062
http://www.theraproducts.com
info@therapro.com
Karen Conrad, President
A software collection of 31 True Type fonts for teachers, parents and students. Fonts include Tracing, lined and unlined Traditional Manuscript and Cursive (similar to Zaner Blouser and D'Nealian), math, clip art, decorative, time, American Sign Language symbols and more. The included manual is very informative, with great examples of lesson plans and educational goals. *$39.95*
Windows/Mac

1400 **Great Beginnings**
Teacher Support Software
5600 West 83rd Street
Suite 300, 8200 Tower
Bloomington, MN 55437
888-351-4199
800-447-5286
Fax: 800-896-1760
http://www.edmentum.com
info@edmentum.com

Vin Riera, President, CEO
Dan Juckniess, Senior Vice President
Stacey Herteux, Vice President, Human Resources
From a broad selection of topics and descriptive words, students may create their own stories and illustrate them with colorful graphics. *$69.95*

1401 **Language Experience Recorder Plus**
Teacher Support Software
5600 West 83rd Street
Suite 300, 8200 Tower
Bloomington, MN 55437
888-351-4199
800-447-5286
Fax: 800-896-1760
http://www.edmentum.com
info@edmentum.com

Vin Riera, President, CEO
Dan Juckniess, Senior Vice President
Stacey Herteux, Vice President, Human Resources
This program provides students with the opportunity to read, write and hear their own experience stories. Analyzes student writing. Cumulative word list, word and sentence counts and readability estimate. *$99.95*

1402 **Mega Dots 2.3**
Duxbury Systems
270 Littleton Rd
Unit 6
Westford, MA 01886-3523
978-692-3000
Fax: 978-692-7912
http://www.duxburysystems.com
info@duxsys.com

Joe Sullivan, President
Peter Sullivan, VP of Software Development
Neal Kuniansky, Marketing Director
MegaDots is a mature DOS braille translator with powerful features for the volume transcriber and producer. Its straightforward, style based system and automated features let you create great braille with only a few keystrokes, yet it is sophisticated enough to please the fussiest braille producers. You can control each step MegaDots follows to format, translate and produce braille documents. *$540.00*

1403 **Once Upon a Time Volume I: Passport to Discovery**
Compu-Teach
16541 Redmond Way
Suite C
Redmond, WA 98052
425-885-0517
800-448-3224
Fax: 425-883-9169
http://www.compu-teach.com
info@compu-teach.com

David Urban, President
Features familiar objects associated with three unique themes. These graphic images offer limitless possibilities for new stories and illustrations. As children author books from one to hundreds of pages, they can either display them on screen or print them out. Themes: Farm Life; Down Main Street; and On Safari. *$59.95*

1404 **Once Upon a Time Volume II: Worlds of Enchantment**
Compu-Teach
16541 Redmond Way
Suite C
Redmond, WA 98052
425-885-0517
800-448-3224
Fax: 425-883-9169
http://www.compu-teach.com
info@compu-teach.com

David Urban, President
Makes writing, reading and vocabulary skills easy to learn. While building their illustrations, children experiment with perspective and other spatial relationships. This volume features familiar objects associated with three unique themes: Underwater; Dinosaur Age; and Forest Friends. *$59.95*

1405 **Once Upon a Time Volume III: Journey Through Time**
Compu-Teach
16541 Redmond Way
Suite C
Redmond, WA 98052
425-885-0517
800-448-3224
Fax: 425-883-9169
http://www.compu-teach.com
info@compu-teach.com

David Urban, President
Makes writing, reading and vocabulary skills easy to learn. With imagination as a youngster's only guide, the important concepts of story creation and illustration are naturally discovered. Themes: Medieval Times, Wild West and Outer Space. *$59.95*

1406 **Once Upon a Time Volume IV: Exploring Nature**
Compu-Teach
16541 Redmond Way
Suite C
Redmond, WA 98052
425-885-0517
800-448-3224
Fax: 425-883-9169
http://www.compu-teach.com
info@compu-teach.com

David Urban, President
The latest in award-winning creative writing series. Kids just hear, click and draw as the state of the art graphics and digitized voice make writing, reading and vocabulary skills easy to learn. Themes: Rain Forest; African Grasslands; Ocean; Desert; and Forest. *$59.95*

1407 **Read, Write and Type Learning System**
Talking Fingers, California Neuropsych Services
830 Rincon Way
San Rafael, CA 94903
415-472-3103
800-674-9126
Fax: 415-472-7812
TDD: 415-472-3106
http://www.readwritetype.com
contact@talkingfingers.com

Dr. Jeannine Herron, Co-Founder
Dr. Leslie Grimm, Co-Founder
A 40-level software adventure providing highly motivating instruction and practice in phonics, reading, writing, spelling and typing. This multisensory program includes 9 levels of assessment and reports. Classroom packs available.

1408 **StartWrite Handwriting Software**
Therapro
225 Arlington Street
Framingham, MA 01702-8723
508-872-9494
800-257-5376
Fax: 508-875-2062
http://www.theraproducts.com
info@therapro.com

Karen Conrad, President
With this easy-to-use software package, you can make papers and handwriting worksheets to meet individual student's needs. Type letters, words, or numbers and they appear in a dot format on the triple line guide. Change letter size, add shading, turn on or off guide lines and arrow strokes and place provided clipart. Fonts include Manuscript and Cursive, Modern Manuscript and Cursive and Italic Manuscript and Cursive. Useful manual included. *$39.95*
Windows/Mac

1409 **Writing Trek Grades 4-6**
Sunburst Technology
3150 W Higgins Rd
Suite 140
Hoffman Estates, IL 60619
800-321-7511
Fax: 888-800-3028
http://www.sunburst.com
service@sunburst.com

Dan Figurski, President
Michael Guillory, Channel Sales/Marketing Manager
Enhance your students' experience in your English language arts classroom with twelve authentic writing projects that build students' competence while encouraging creativity.

1410 **Writing Trek Grades 6-8**
Sunburst Technology
3150 W Higgins Rd
Suite 140
Hoffman Estates, IL 60619
800-321-7511
Fax: 888-800-3028
http://www.sunburst.com
service@sunburst.com

Dan Figurski, President
Michael Guillory, Channel Sales/Marketing Manager
Twelve authentic language arts projects, activities, and assignments develop your students' writing confidence and ability.

1411 **Writing Trek Grades 8-10**
Sunburst Technology
3150 W Higgins Rd
Suite 140
Hoffman Estates, IL 60619
800-321-7511
Fax: 888-800-3028
http://www.sunburst.com
service@sunburst.com

Dan Figurski, President
Michael Guillory, Channel Sales/Marketing Manager
Help your students develop a concept of genre as they become familiar with the writing elements and characteristics of a variety of writing forms.

General

1412 **AFS Intercultural Programs**
71 West 23rd St.
6th Fl.
New York, NY 10010-4120
212-807-8686
Fax: 212-807-1001
http://afs.org
info@afs.org
Dr. Vishaka N. Desai, Chair
J. Brian Atwood, Vice Chair
AFS offers a variety of exchange programs, including High School Study Abroad, Langage Learning, Volunteer Abroad, Adult Study Abroad, Internships Abroad, Teacher Exchanges, Summer/Short-term Study Abroad, and more.

1413 **Academic Programs International (API)**
301 Camp Craft Rd.
Suite 100
Austin, TX 78746
512-600-8900
800-844-4124
Fax: 512-600-8999
http://apiabroad.com
api@apiabroad.com
Jennifer Attal Allen, President/Executive Director
Brittany Norman, Executive Vice President
Provides academic and cross-cultural experiences for students that promotes cultural sensitivity and understanding of the global nature of the world.

1414 **American Institute for Foreign Study**
1 High Ridge Park
Stamford, CT 06905
203-399-5000
866-906-2437
Fax: 203-399-5590
http://www.aifs.com
info@aifs.com
Sir Cyril Taylor, Founder
William L. Gertz, President/CEO & Chairman
Organizes cultural exchange programs throughout the world for more than 50,000 students each year, and arranges insurance coverage for participantsin their program as well as those of other organizations. Also provides summer travel programs overseas and in the U.S. ranging from 1 week to a full academic year.

1415 **American-Scandinavian Foundation**
58 Park Ave.
New York, NY 10016
212-779-3587
http://www.scandinaviahouse.org
info@amscan.org
Edward P. Gallagher, President/CEO
Lynn Carter, EVP/Corporate Secretary
Lynda Selde, Director, Development
Promotes international understanding through educational and cultural exchange between the United States and Denmark, Finalnd, Iceland, Norway and Sweden.

1416 **Andeo International Homestays**
620 S.W. 5th Ave.
Suite 625
Portland, OR 97204
503-274-1776
http://www.andeo.org
info@andeo.org
Melinda Samis, Executive Director
Sara Bruckner, Deputy Director
Kellie Irish, College Programs Manager
Formerly International Summerstays, an international network of families, students, teachers, independent travelers, and homestay specialists who are dedicated to exploring cross-cultural friendship and understanding.
1981

1417 **Arcadia University: College of Global Studies**
450 South Easton Rd.
Glenside, PA 19038-3295
215-572-2901
866-927-2234
Fax: 215-572-2174
http://www.arcadia.edu/abroad
educationabroad@arcadia.edu
Lorna Stern, VP
Colleen Burke, Chief Operating Officer
The College offers study abroad programs for undergraduate and graduate students, internship and research opportunities, student and faculty exchanges, and service learning programs, all ranging in length from semester, year, and short-term study/research abroad programs.

1418 **CEA**
2999 N. 44th St.
Suite 200
Phoenix, AZ 85018-7248
480-448-6013
800-266-4441
Fax: 480-557-7926
http://www.ceastudyabroad.com
info@ceaStudyAbroad.com
Brian J. Boubek, CEO/Chairman
Deborah Keely, Senior VP, Finance/Operations
Caroline Walsh, Senior VP, Program Development
Offers exchange programs across 12 countries that allows students to earn credits that count toward graduation.

1419 **Council on International Educational Exchange**
300 Fore St.
Portland, ME 04101
207-553-4000
http://www.ciee.org
contact@ciee.org
James P. Pellow, President/CEO
Brenda Majeski, Chief Marketing Officer
Tim Propp, Chief Operating Officer
CIEE creates and administers programs that allow high school and university students and educators to study and teach abroad. Programs and literature address participants with disabilities.

1420 **Cross-Cultural Solutions**
P.O. Box 102075
Pasadena, CA 91189
914-632-0022
http://www.crossculturalsolutions.org
Lauren Maitland, Director, Programs
Steven C. Rosenthal, Founder/Advisor
Cassandra Tomkin, Chief Operating Officer
Offers exchange programs for volunteers, university students, high school students, and groups.

1421 **Cultural Vistas**
233 Broadway
Suite 2120
New York, NY 10279
212-497-3500
http://culturalvistas.org
info@culturalvistas.org
Jennifer Clinton, President/CEO
Linda Boughton, COO/Chief Engagement Officer
Dan Ewert, VP, Program Research
Non-profit organization dedicated to encouraging and facilitating the exchange of qualified individuals between the US and other countries so they may gain practical work experience and improve international understanding.

1422 **Earthstewards Network**
1425 Cowgill Ave.
Bellingham, WA 98225
800-561-2909
http://www.earthstewards.org
outreach@earthstewards.org
Danaan Parry, Co-Founder
Bruce Haley, Director
Charlie Olson, Director
A network of people who participate in projects that promote conflict resolution, citizen diplomacy, and global communication.
1979

1423 **Education First High School Exchange Year**
1 Education St.
Cambridge, MA 02141 800-447-4273
http://www.efexchangeyear.org
exchangeyear@ef.com
Offers an opportunity to study and live for a year in a foreign country for students between the ages of 15 and 18.

1424 **Higher Education Consortium for Urban Affairs**
2233 University Ave. W.
Suite 210
Saint Paul, MN 55114 651-287-3300
Fax: 651-659-9421
http://www.hecua.org
hecua@hecua.org
Andrew Williams, Executive Director
Jim Sauder, Director, Finance/Operations
Laney Ohmans, Director, Development
Consortium of 15 Midwest colleges and universities offering undergraduate, academic programs, both international and domestic that incorporate field study and internships in the examination of urban and global issues.

1425 **IES Abroad**
33 W. Monroe St.
Suite 2300
Chicago, IL 60603 312-944-1750
800-995-2300
http://www.iesabroad.org
info@iesabroad.org
Signore Ezio Vergani, Chair
James E. Crawford III, Vice Chair
Dr. Mary M. Dwyer, President/CEO
Offers experiential learning opportunities to students through study abroad and internship programs.

1426 **IPSL**
4110 S.E. Hawthorne Blvd.
Suite 200
Portland, OR 97214 503-395-4775
Fax: 503-954-1881
http://www.ipsl.org
info@ipsl.org
Thomas Winston Morgan, President
Arianne Newton, Director of Programs
Dr. Erin Barnhart, IPSL Academic Officer
A not-for-profit educational organization incorporated in NYS serving students, collegs, universities, service agencies, and related organizations around the world by fostering programs that link volunteer service to the community and academic study.

1427 **Institute of International Education**
809 United Nations Plaza
New York, NY 10017 212-883-8200
Fax: 212-984-5452
http://www.iie.org
Allen E. Goodman, President/CEO
Maxmillian Angerholzer III, Executive Vice President
Jason Czyz, Chief Financial Officer
Helps enable people to travel abroad in order to build connections and learn about other cultures.

1428 **Lions Club International**
300 West 22nd St.
Oak Brook, IL 60523-8842 630-571-5466
http://www.lionsclub.org
districtadministration@lionsclub.org
Gudrun Biort-Yngvadottir, International President
Jung-Yul Choi, First Vice President
Haynes ÿ Townsend, Second Vice President
Over 46,000 individual clubs in over 190 countries and geographical areas, providing community service and promoting improved international relations. Clubs work with local communities to provide needed and useful programs for sight, diabetes and hearing, and aid in study abroad.

1429 **Lisle**
P.O. Box 1932
Leander, TX 78646 512-259-4404
http://www.lisleinternational.org
office@lisleinternational.org
Bill Kinney, President
Mark Kinney, Executive Director
Barbara Bratton, Operations Manager
Educational organization which works toward world peace and a better quality of human life through increased understanding between persons of similar and different cultures.

1430 **Mobility International (MIUSA)**
132 E. Broadway
Suite 343
Eugene, OR 97401 541-343-1284
Fax: 541-343-6812
TTY: 541-343-1284
http://www.miusa.org
Susan Sygall, CEO/Co-Founder
Susan Dunn, Program Manager
Cindy Lewis, Director of Programs
MIUSA offers short-term international exchange programs in the US and abroad for people with and without disabilities, including non-apparent disabilities.

1431 **National Society for Experimental Education**
19 Mantua Rd.
Mount Royal, NJ 08061 856-423-3427
Fax: 856-423-3420
http://www.nsee.org
nsee@talley.com
Stephanie Thomason, President
Marianna Savoca, Vice President
Haley Brust, Executive Director
A non-profit membership association of educators, businesses, and community leaders. Also serves as a national resource center for the development and improvement of experimental education programs nationwide.
1971

1432 **No Barriers USA**
224 Canyon Ave.
Suite 207
Fort Collins, CO 80521 970-484-3633
http://www.nobarriersusa.org
info@nobarriersusa.org
David Shurna, Executive Director
Cindy Bean, Chief Development Officer
Summer Clowers, Project Coordinator
No Barriers USA offers exchange programs for youth and veterans with a disability.

1433 **Peace Corps**
1111 20th St., NW.
Washington, DC 20526 855-855-1961
http://www.peacecorps.gov
Josephine K. Olson, Director
Kathy Stroker, Deputy Chief Executive Officer
Michelle K. Brooks, Chief of Staff
A volunteer opportunity for individuals wishing to enact change and immerse themselves in a community abroad. The Peace Corps is committed to providing accomocations in its programs, activities, and volunteer service for indsiviuals with disabilities.

1434 **People to People International**
2405 Grand Blvd.
Suite 500
Kansas City, MO 64108 816-531-4701
800-676-7874
Fax: 816-561-7502
http://www.ptpi.org
ptpi@ptpi.org
Merrill Eisenhower Atwater, Chief Executive Officer
John Maloney, Vice President, Opertions
Nicole Randall, Director, Public Relations

Nonpolitical, non-profit organization working outside the government to advance the cause of international understanding through international contact.

1435 **Rotary International**
1560 Sherman Ave.
Evanston, IL 60201-3698
847-866-3000
866-976-8279
http://my.rotary.org
Barry Rassin, President
Ron Burton, Trustee Chair
John Hewko, General Secretary
A program for volunteers that offers the opportunity to travel abroad and help promote peace, fight disease, support education, provide clearn water, grow local economies, and more.

1436 **SUNY Buffalo Office of International Education**
1300 Elmwood Ave.
South Wing 430
Buffalo, NY 14222
716-878-4620
Fax: 716-878-3054
http://studyabroad.buffalostate.edu/
intleduc@buffalostate.edu
Melissa Holland, Director
International exchange office for students who wish to study abroad for a semester.

1437 **Semester at Sea**
Colorado State University
2243 Centre Ave.
Suite 300
Fort Collins, CO 80526
970-491-3500
800-854-0195
Fax: 970-237-3207
http://www.semesteratsea.org
info@semesteratsea.org
Gary Ransdell, President/CEO
Larry D. Grant, Vice President, Finance/CFO
Robert Kling, Senior Academic Advisor
A non-profit organization that offers an exchange program for students on board a ship. Administered in conjunction with Colorado State University, Semester at Sea will take students to multiple countries in order to educate them with a global understanding.

1438 **Servas United States**
1125 16th St.
Suite 201
Arcata, CA 95521-5585
707-825-1714
Fax: 707-825-1762
http://usservas.org
info@usservas.org
Chris-Ann Lauria, Chair
Dennis Mogerman, Vice Chair
Steve Kanters, Treasurer
US Servas offers exchanges programs for people of all ages and abilities. They provide volunteer opportuites, host local gatherings, and sponsors conferences.

1439 **Sister Cities International**
915 15th St., N.W.
4th Fl.
Washington, DC 20005
202-347-8630
Fax: 202-393-6524
http://www.sister-cities.org
info@sistercities.org
Roger-Mark De Souza, President/CEO
Adam Kaplan, Vice President
Leletha Marshall, Director, Development
A non-profit citizen diplomacy network; creating and strengthening partnerships between the US and international communities in an effort to increase global cooperation at the municipal level, to promote cultural understanding, and to stimulate economic development. Encourages local community development and volunteer action by motivating and empowering private citizens, municipal officials, and business leaders to conduct long-term programs of mutual benefit, including exchange situations.

1440 **Study Abroad**
Davidson College
P.O. Box 7155
Davidson, NC 28035
704-894-2250
Fax: 704-894-2120
http://www.davidson.edu
abroad@davidson.edu
Naomi Otterness, Director
Abbie Naglosky, Assistant Director
An educational exchange program for students of Davidson College. Echange periods range from one scool year, one semester, or a summer program.

1441 **The Fullbright Program**
Institute of International Education
809 United Nations Plaza
New York, NY 10017
212-883-8200
Fax: 212-984-5452
http://www.iie.org
Allan E. Goodman, President/CEO
Maxmillian Angerholzer III, Executive Vice President
Jason Czyz, Chief Financial Officer
An international exchange program run by the Institute of International Education and sponsored by the US government, for US students to go abroad and for non-US citizens to come to the united states.

1442 **United Planet**
256 Marginal St.
East Boston, MA 02128
617-874-8041
Fax: 617-874-8941
http://www.unitedplanet.org
longterm@unitedplanet.org
Dave Santulli, Founder/President
Jonathan Hass, Human Resources Manager
Gretchen Dobson, Board Chair
United Planted is a non-profit organization that aims to create a global community through exchange programs. They are affiliated with the International Cultural Youth Exchange.

1443 **World Experience**
2440 S. Hacienda Blvd.
Suite 116
Hacienda Heights, CA 91745
626-330-5719
http://www.worldexperience.org
info@worldexperience.org
Kerry Gonzales, President
Marge Archambault, President
Offers a quality and affordable program for over three decades and continues to provide students and host families a youth exchange program based on individual attention, with the help of an international network of overseas directors and USA coordinators

1444 **Youth for Understanding USA**
641 S St., N.W.
Suite 200
Washington, DC 20001
240-774-5200
800-833-6243
Fax: 202-588-7571
http://online.yfuusa.org
Daryl Weinert, Chairman
Laurence Wohlers, Vice Chairman
Scott J. Messing, President/CEO

Non-profit international exchange program, prepares young people for their responsibilities and opportunities in todays changing, interdependent world through homestay exchange programs. Offers year, semester, and summer study abroad and scholarship opportunities in 40 countries worldwide.

Federal

1445 **ABLE DATA**
USDE National Institution on Disability/Rehab
103 W Broad St
Ste 400
Falls Church, VA 22046
800-227-0216
Fax: 703-356-8314
TTY: 703-992-8313
http://abledata.gov
abledata@neweditions.net
Robert Jaeger, NIDILRR Director
Kristi Hill, Deputy Director
Sponsored by the National Institute on Disability, Independent Living and Rehabilitation Research (NIDILRR) of the US Department of Education; provides information on more than 46,000 assistive technology products, including detailed descriptions of each product, price and company information.

1446 **ADA Information Line**
US Department of Justice
950 Pennsylvania Avenue, NW
Washington, DC 20530
800-514-0301
TTY: 800-514-0383
http://www.ada.gov/infoline
Rebecca B. Bond, Chief
Christina Gallindo-Walsh, Deputy Chief
Kevin Kijewski, Deputy Chief
Answers questions about Title II (public services) and Title III (public accommodations) of the Americans with Disabilities Act (ADA). Provides materials and technical assistance on the provisions of the ADA.

1447 **ADA Technical Assistance Programs**
US Department of Justice
950 Pennsylvania Avenue NW
Washington, DC 20530
800-514-0301
TTY: 800-514-0383
http://www.ada.gov
Rebecca B. Bond, Chief
Christina Gallindo-Walsh, Deputy Chief
Kevin Kijewski, Deputy Chief
Federally funded regional resource centers that provide information and referral, technical assistance, public awareness, and training on all aspects of the Americans with Disabilities Act (ADA).

1448 **Americans with Disabilities Act (ADA) Resource Guide**
National Center for State Courts
300 Newport Ave
Williamsburg, VA 23185
800-616-6164
Fax: 757-220-0449
http://www.ncsc.org
Mary McQueen, President
Deborah Smith, NCSC Contact
Blake P. Kavangh, NCSC Contact
Disseminates information on ADA compliance to state and local court systems. Will develop a diagnostic checklist and strategies for compliance specifically relevant to the state and local courts.

1449 **Civil Rights Division: US Department of Justice**
Office of the Assistant Attorney General
950 Pennsylvania Avenue NW
Washington, DC 20530-0001
202-514-2000
TDD: 800-877-8339
TTY: 800-877-8339
http://www.justice.gov
Jeff Sessions, Attorney General
The program institution within the federal government responsible for enforcing federal statutes prohibiting discrimination on the basis of race, sex, disability, religion, and national origin.

1450 **Clearinghouse on Disability Information**
Office of Special Education/Rehabilitative Service
550 12th St SW
Room 5133
Washington, DC 20202-2550
202-245-7307
Fax: 202-245-7636
TDD: 202-205-5637
http://www.ed.gov
Betsy DeVos, Secretary of Education
Carolyn Corlett, Contact
Provides information to people with disabilities, or anyone requesting information, by doing research and providing documents in response to inquiries. Information provided includes areas of federal funding for disability-related programs. Staff is trained to refer requests to other sources of disability-related information, if necessary.

1451 **Division of Adult Education and Literacy (DAEL)**
US Department of Education
400 Maryland Avenue, SW
Washington, DC 20202
800-872-5327
Fax: 202-401-0689
TTY: 800-437-0833
http://www.ed.gov
Betsy DeVos, Secretary of Education
Provides information which deals with state administered adult education programs funded under the Adult Education and Family Literacy Act, and provide resources that support adult education activities.

1452 **Employment and Training Administration: US Department of Labor**
200 Constitution Ave NW
Washington, DC 20210
866-487-2365
TTY: 866-487-2365
http://www.doleta.gov
R. Alexander Acosta, Secretary of Labor
Patrick Pizzella, Deputy Secretary of Labor
Nicholas C. Geale, Chief of Staff
Administers federal government job training and worker dislocation programs, federal grants to states for public employment service programs, and unemployment insurance benefits. These services are primarily provided through state and local workforce development systems.

1453 **Equal Employment Opportunity Commission**
Washington, DC
800-669-4000
TTY: 202-669-6820
http://www.eeoc.gov
info@eeoc.gov
Milton A. Mayo Jr., Inspector General
Victoria A. Lipnic, Acting Chair
Enforces Section 501 which prohibits discrimination on the basis of disability in Federal employment, and requires that all Federal agencies establish and implement affirmative action programs for hiring, placing and advancing individuals with disabilities. Also oversees Federal sector equal employment opportunity complaint processing system.

1454 **Eunice Kennedy Shriver National Institute of Child Health and Human Development (NICHD)**
National Institutes of Health
PO Box 3006
Rockville, MD 20847
800-370-2943
Fax: 866-760-5947
TTY: 888-320-6942
http://www.nichd.nih.gov
NICHDInformationResourceCenter@mail.nih.gov
Diana W. Bianchi, MD, Director
The mission of the Eunice Kennedy Shriver National Institute of Child Health and Human Development (NICHD) is to ensure that every person is born healthy and wanted, that women suffer no harmful effects from the reproductive process, that all children have the chance to fulfill their potential to live healthy and productive lives free from disease or disability, and to ensure the health, productivity, independence and well-being of all people through optimal rehabilitation.

1455 **National Council on Disability**
1331 F St NW
Ste 850
Washington, DC 20004
202-272-2004
Fax: 202-272-2022
TTY: 202-272-2074
http://www.ncd.gov
ncd@ncd.gov
Lisa Grubb, Executive Director
Joan M. Durocher, General Counsel
An independent federal agency comprised of 15 members appointed by the President and confirmed by the Senate.
1978

1456 **National Institute of Mental Health**
Science Policy, Planning & Communications
6001 Executive Blvd
Room 6200, MSC 9663
Bethesda, MD 20892-9663
866-615-6464
Fax: 301-443-4279
TTY: 301-443-8431
http://www.nimh.nih.gov
nimhinfo@nih.gov
Joshua A. Gordon, Director
Mission is to diminish the burden of mental illness through research. This public health mandate demands that we harness powerful scientific tools to achieve better understanding, treatment and eventually prevention of mental illness.

1457 **National Institute on Disability, Independent Living, and Rehabilitation Research**
US Department of Health & Human Services
330 C St SW
Room 1304
Washington, DC 20201
202-795-7398
Fax: 202-205-0392
http://about-acl.gov
raina.mcdowell@acl.hhs.gov
Robert Jaeger, Director
Kristi Hill, Deputy Director
Ruth Brannon, Director, Research Sciences
Provides leadership and support for a comprehensive program of research related to the rehabilitation of individuals with disabilities. All of the programmatic efforts are aimed to improving the lives of individuals with disabilities from birth through adulthood.

1458 **National Library Services for the Blind and Physically Handicapped**
1291 Taylor St NW
Washington, DC 20542
202-707-5100
800-424-8567
Fax: 202-707-0744
TDD: 202-707-0744
http://www.loc.gov/nls
nls@loc.gov
Karen Keninger, Director
Kristen Fernekes, Head of Publications & Media
Michael Katzmann, Chief of Materials Development
Administers a national library service that provdies braille and recorded books and magazines on free loan to anyone who cannot read standard print because of visual or physical disabilities.
1931

1459 **National Technical Information Service: US Department of Commerce**
5301 Shawnee Rd
Alexandria, VA 22312
703-605-6050
800-363-2068
Fax: 703-605-6880
TDD: 703-487-4639
http://www.ntis.gov
info@ntis.gov
Avi Bender, Director
Greg Capella, Deputy Director
Serves the nation as the largest central resource for government-funded scientific, technical, engineering, and business related information available today.

1460 **Office for Civil Rights: US Department of Health and Human Services**
200 Independence Ave SW
Room 509F, HHH Bldg
Washington, DC 20201
800-368-1019
TDD: 800-537-7697
http://www.hhs.gov/ocr
Roger Severino, Director
Promotes and ensures that people have equal access to an opportunity to participate in and receive services from all HHS programs without facing unlawful discrimination, and that the privacy of their health information is protectec while ensuring access to care.

1461 **Office for Civil Rights: US Department of Education**
400 Maryland Ave SW
Washington, DC 20202-1100
800-421-3481
Fax: 202-453-6012
TTY: 800-877-8339
http://www.ed.gov/ocr
ocr@ed.gov
Kenneth L. Marcus, Assistant Secretary
Earl Morgan, Executive Officer
To ensure equal access to education and to promote educational excellence throughout the nation through vigourous enforcement of civil rights.

1462 **Office of Disability Employment Policy: US Department of Labor**
200 Constitution Ave NW
Washington, DC 20210
866-487-2365
TTY: 866-487-2365
http://www.dol.gov/odep
webmaster@dol.gov
R. Alexander Acosta, Secretary of Labour
Patrick Pizella, Deputy Secretary of Labor
Nicholas C. Geale, Chief of Staff
Provides national leadership by developing and influencing disability-related employment policy as well as practice affecting the employment of people with disabilities.

1463 **Office of Federal Contract Compliance Programs: US Department of Labor**
200 Constitution Ave NW
Washington, DC 20210
866-487-2365
TTY: 866-487-2365
http://www.dol.gov/ofccp
webmaster@dol.gov
Ondray T. Harris, Director
Marika Litras, Acting Deputy Director
Kelley Smith, Chief of Staff
Responsible for ensuring that employers doing business with the Federal government comply with the laws and regulations requiring nondiscrimination and affirmative action in employment.

1464 **Office of Personnel Management**
1900 E St NW
Washington, DC 20415-1000
202-606-1800
TTY: 800-877-8339
http://www.opm.gov
Jeff T.H. Pon, Director
Michael J. Rigas, Deputy Director
Michael D. Dovilla, Chief of Staff
The central personnel agency of the federal government. Provides information on the selective placement program for persons with disabilities.

1465 **Rehabilitation Services Administration State Vocational Program**
US Department of Education
400 Maryland Avenue SW
Washington, DC 20202
800-872-5327
http://www.ed.gov
Betsy DeVos, Secretary of Education

State and local vocational rehabilitation agencies provide comprehensive services of rehabilitation, training and job-related assistance to people with disabilities and assist employers in recruiting, training, placing, accommodating and meeting other employment-related needs of people with disabilities.

1466 **Social Security Administration**
Office of Public Inquiries
5 Park Center Court
Owings Mills, MD 21117
800-772-1213
TTY: 800-325-0778
http://www.ssa.gov
Nancy A. Berryhill, Acting Commissioner
Beatrice M. Disman, Chief of Staff
Provides financial assistance to those with disabilities who meet eligibility requirements.

1467 **US Census Bureau**
4600 Silver Hill Rd
Washington, DC 20233
301-763-4636
800-923-8282
TTY: 800-877-8339
http://www.census.gov
pio@census.gov
Enrique Lamas, Deputy Director and COO
Ron Jarmin, Director
The principal statistical agency of the federal government. It publishes data on persons with disabilities, as well as other demographic data derived from censuses and surveys.

1468 **US Department of Health & Human Services**
200 Independence Ave SW
Room 509F, HHH Bldg
Washington, DC 20201
877-696-6775
http://www.hhs.gov
Alex M. Azar II, Secretary
Eric D. Hargan, Deputy Secretary
Peter Urbanowicz, Chief of Staff
Councils in each state provide training and technical assistance to local and state agencies, employers and the public, improving services to people with developmental disabilities.

Alabama

1469 **Alabama Council for Developmental Disabilities**
100 N Union St
PO Box 301410
Montgomery, AL 36130
334-242-3976
http://www.acdd.org
myra.jones@mh.alabama.gov
Elmyra Jones-Banks, Executive Director
Sophia Wright-Dixon, Fiscal Manager
Holli C. Zukowski, Contracts Manager
Serves as an advocate for Alabama's citizens with developmental disabilities and their families; to empower them with the knowledge and opportunity to make informed choices and exercise control over their own lives; and to create a climate for positive social change to enable them to be respected, independent and productive integrated members of society.

1470 **Alabama Department of Industrial Relations**
649 Monroe St
Montgomery, AL 36131
334-242-8055
http://labor.alabama.gov
Vivian Handy, Labor Administrator
Fitzgerald Washington, Secretary & Executive
To effectively use tax dollars to provide state and federal mandated workforce protection programs promoting a positive economic environment for Alabama employers and workers and to produce and disseminate information on the Alabama economy.

1471 **Alabama Disabilities Advocacy Program**
624 Paul W Bryant Dr
5th Fl, Martha Parham Hall W
Tuscaloosa, AL 35487
205-348-4928
800-826-1675
Fax: 205-348-3909
http://www.adap.ua.edu
adap@adap.ua.edu
James A. Tucker, Director
Nancy E. Anderson, Associate Director
Angie Allen, Senior Case Advocate
To provide quality, legally-based advocacy services to Alabamians with disabilities in order to protect, promote and expand their rights.

1472 **Alabama Prison Arts & Education Project**
Alabama Department of Corrections
301 S Ripley St
PO Box 301501
Montgomery, AL 36130-1501
334-353-3883
http://www.doc.state.al.us
Constituent.Services@doc.alabama.gov
Kyes Stevens, Founder & Director
Jefferson S. Dunn, Commissioner
A program sponsored by Auburn University to provide educational opportunities to inmates across the state. The program offers classes in the arts, humanities, hard sciences, and human sciences. Classes are introductory college level.

1473 **Alabama State Department of Education**
50 N Ripley St
PO Box 302101
Montgomery, AL 36104
334-242-9700
Eric G. Mackey, State Superintendent
Dr. Daniel Boyd, Deputy State Superintendent
Michael Sibley, Director of Communications

1474 **Division of Developmental Disabilities**
Alabama Department of Mental Health
100 North Union St
PO Box 301410
Montgomery, AL 36130-1410
334-242-3454
800-367-0955
Fax: 334-242-0725
http://www.mh.alabama.gov
Jeff Williams, Interim Associate Commissioner
Offers services and support programs for persons with developmental disabilities and their families.

1475 **GED Testing Program**
Alabama Community College System
135 S Unition St
Montgomery, AL 36130-2130
334-293-4500
Fax: 334-293-4504
http://www.accs.cc
Kay Ivey, Governor/President of the Board
Jimmy H. Baker, Chancellor
Erika Rhodes, Administrative Assistant
The Alabama Community College System is the official administrator of the GED testing program throughout the state.

Alaska

1476 **Alaska State Commission for Human Rights**
800 A St
Ste 204
Anchorage, AK 99501-3669
907-274-4692
800-478-4692
Fax: 907-278-8588
TTY: 800-478-4692
http://humanrights.alaska.govs
Brandon H. Nakasato, Chair
Christa J. Bruce-Kotrc, Vice Chair
The state agency which enforces the Alaska Human Rights Law. Consists of seven persons appointed by the governor and confirmed by the legislature.

1477 **Assistive Technology of Alaska (ATLA)**
3330 Arctic Blvd
Ste 101
Anchorage, AK 99503
907-563-2599
800-723-2852
Fax: 907-563-0699
http://www.atlaak.org
atla@atlaak.org
Kathy Privratsky, Executive Director
To enhance the quality of life for Alaskans through education, demonstration, consultation, acquisition and implementation of assistive technologies. ATLA is Alaska's only assistive technology project for the Tech Act.

1478 **Center for Community**
700 Katlian
Ste B
Sitka, AK 99835
907-747-6960
800-478-6970
Fax: 907-747-4868
http://cfc.org
info@cfc.org
Bryan O'Callaghan, Executive Director
Patrick Hughes, President
Barbara Stocker, Vice President
Center for Community is a multiservice agency that provides early intervention, respite, futures planning, functional skills training, and vocational assistance and personal care for people with disabilities.

1479 **Correctional Education Division: Alaska**
Department of Corrections/Division of Institutions
550 West 7th Avenue
Suite 1700
Anchorage, AK 99501
907-269-7397
Fax: 907-269-7390
http://www.correct.state.ak.us/
anna.herzberger@alaska.gov
Dean Williams, Commissioner
Clare Sullivan, Dep. Commissioner, Institutions
Karen Cann, Dep. Comm., Transitional Svcs
The Alaska Department of Corrections offers educational programs such as GED classes and testing, English as a Second Language, high school Refresher courses, and computer instruction courses.

1480 **Disability Law Center of Alaska**
3330 Arctic Blvd
Ste 103
Anchorage, AK 99503
907-565-1002
800-478-1234
Fax: 907-565-1000
http://www.dlcak.org
akpa@dlcak.org
Tracy Barbee, President
Kim Rion, VP, Corporate Compliance
Sarah Randolph-Andrew, Secretary
An independent non-profit organization that provides legal advocacyservices for people with disabilities anywhere in Alaska. To promote and protect the legal and human rights of individuals with physical and/or mental disabilities.

1481 **Employment and Training Services**
Alaska Department of Labor & Workforce Development
PO Box 115509
Juneau, AK 99811-5509
907-465-2712
Fax: 907-465-4537
http://labor.state.ak.us
esd.director@alaska.gov
Patsy Westcott, Director
Promotes employment, economic stability, and growth by operating a no-fee labor exchange that meets the needs of employers, job seekers, and veterans.

1482 **State Department of Education & Early Development**
State of Alaska
801 W 10th St, Ste 200
PO Box 110500
Juneau, AK 99811-0500
907-465-2800
Fax: 907-465-4156
TTY: 907-465-2800
http://www.eed.state.ak.us
eed.webmaster@alaska.gov
James K. Fields, State Board Chair
Barbara A. Thompson, First Vice Chair
Melissa McCormick, Executive Secretary
State education agency.

1483 **State GED Administration: GED Testing Program**
Alaska Department of Education
801 W 10th St, Ste 200
PO Box 110500
Juneau, AK 99811-0500
907-465-2800
Fax: 907-465-4156
TTY: 907-465-2800
http://www.eed.state.ak.us
eed.webmaster@alaska.gov
James K. Fields, State Board Chair
Barbara A. Thompson, First Vice Chair
Melissa McCormick, Executive Secretary
GED courses and testing administered by the State education agency.

Arizona

1484 **Arizona Center for Disability Law**
5025 E Washington St
Ste 202
Phoenix, AZ 85034
602-274-6287
800-927-2260
Fax: 602-274-6779
TTY: 602-274-6287
http://www.azdisabilitylaw.org
center@azdisabilitylaw.org
Sami Hamed, President
Sherri Collins, Secretary
Floyd Galloway, Treasurer
Advocates for the legal rights of persons with disabilities to be free from abuse, neglect and discrimination; and to have access to education, healthcare, housing and jobs, and other services in order to maximize independence and achieve equality.

1485 **Arizona Center for Law in the Public Interest**
514 W Roosevelt St
Phoenix, AZ 85003
602-258-8850
Fax: 602-258-8757
http://www.aclpi.org
Stacy Gabriel, President
Daniel J. Adelman, Executive Director
Adriane Hofmeyr, Secretary
A nonprofit law firm dedicated to ensuring government accountability and protecting the legal rights of Arizonans.

1486 **Arizona Department of Economic Security**
Rehabilitation Services Administration
11526 W Bell Rd
Surprise, AZ 85378
602-771-1850
800-563-1221
http://des.az.gov
Doug Ducey, Governor
Michael Trailor, Director
Tasya Peterson, Communications Director
Promotes the safety, well-being, and self sufficiency of children, asults and families.

1487 **Arizona Department of Education**
1535 W Jefferson St
Phoenix, AZ 85007
602-542-5393
800-352-4558
http://www.azed.gov
adeinbox@azed.gov
Alissa Trollinger, Deputy Associate Superintendent
To serve Arizona's local communities to ensure every child has access to education.

1488 **Arizona Developmental Disabilities Planning Council (ADDPC)**
3839 N 3rd St
Ste 306
Phoenix, AZ 85012
602-542-8970
877-665-3176
Fax: 602-542-8978
TTY: 602-542-8979
http://addpc.az.gov
addpc@azdes.gov
Erica McFadden, Executive Director
Marcella Cran, Grants Manager
Lani St. Cyr, Fiscal Manager
To work in partnership with individuals with developmental disabilities and their families through systems change, advocacy and capacity building activities that promote indpendence, choice and the ability to pursue their own dreams.

1489 **Correctional Education**
Arizona Department of Corrections
1601 W Jefferson St
Phoenix, AZ 85007
602-364-3234
http://corrections.az.gov
Charles L. Ryan, Director
Educational programs include GED preparation, functional literacy, and work/employment skills.

1490 **Division of Adult Education**
Arizona Department of Education
1535 W Jefferson St
Phoenix, AZ 85007
602-258-2410
Fax: 602-542-0031
http://www.azed.gov/adultedservices
adulted@azed.gov
Alissa Trollinger, Deputy Associate Superintendent
To ensure that learners 16 years of age and older have access to quality educational opportunities.

1491 **Fair Employment Practice Agency**
Office of the Arizona Attorney General
2005 N Central Ave
Phoenix, AZ 85004
602-542-5263
800-352-8431
Fax: 602-542-8885
TTY: 602-542-5002
http://www.azag.gov
AGInfo@azag.gov
Mark Brnovich, Attorney General
Michael Bailey, Chief Deputy/Chief of Staff

1492 **GED Testing Services**
Arizona Department of Education
1535 W Jefferson St
Phoenix, AZ 85007
602-542-5393
800-352-4558
http://www.azed.gov
adeinbox@azed.gov
Alissa Trollinger, Deputy Associate Superintendent

Arkansas

1493 **Arkansas Department of Corrections**
PO Box 8707
Pine Bluff, AR 71611-8707
870-267-6999
http://adc.arkansas.gov
adc.webmaster@arkansas.gov
Wendy Kelley, Director
Benny Magness, Chair
Bobby Glover, Vice Chair
To provide public safety by carrying out the mandates of the courts; provide a safe humane environment for staff and inmates; provide programs to strengthen the work ethic; and provide opportunities for spiritual, mental, and physical growth.

1494 **Arkansas Department of Education**
Four Capitol Mall
Room 403-A
Little Rock, AR 72201
501-682-4475
http://www.arkansased.gov
Johnny Key, Commissioner
Ivy Pfeffer, Deputy Commissioner
Lori Freno, General Counsel
Strives to ensure that all children in the state have access to a quality education by providing educators, administrators and staff with leadership, resources and training.

1495 **Arkansas Department of Special Education**
1401 West Capitol Ave
Victory Bldg., Suite 450
Little Rock, AR 72201
501-682-4221
Fax: 501-682-5159
TTY: 501-682-4222
http://www.arkansased.gov
Johnny Key, Commissioner
Ivy Pfeffer, Deputy Commissioner
Lori Freno, General Counsel
The Special Education Unit works with local school districts to ensure all children with disabilities have access to and recieve Free Appropriate Public Education.

1496 **Arkansas Department of Workforce Services**
#2 Capitol Mall
PO Box 2981
Little Rock, AR 72203
501-682-2121
855-225-4440
Fax: 501-682-8845
TDD: 501-296-1669
http://www.dws.arkansas.gov
ADWS.info@arkansas.gov
Daryl Bassett, Director
Ron Snead, Deputy Director
Kristopher Jones, Assistant Director
Offers a variety of services for employers and job seekers in the state of Arkansas.

1497 **Arkansas Governor's Developmental Disabilities Council**
1515 W 7th St
Ste 320-330
Little Rock, AR 72201
501-682-2897
http://gcdd.ark.org
ddcstaff@dfa.arkansas.gov
Eric Munson, Executive Director
Diana Wilson, Program Manager
Melissa Trostle-Hall, Operations Coordinator
Supports people with developmental disabilities in the achievement of independence, productivity, integration and inclusion in the community.

1498 **Assistive Technology Project**
Increasing Capabilities Access Network (ICAN)
900 W 7th St
Little Rock, AR 72201
501-666-8868
800-828-2799
Fax: 501-666-5319
TTY: 800-828-2799
http://ar-ican.org
A consumer responsive statewide program promoting assistive technology devices and resources for persons of all ages and all disabilities.

1499 **Client Assistance Program (CAP) Disability Rights Center of Arkansas**
400 W Capitol
Ste 1200
Little Rock, AR 72201
501-296-1775
800-482-1174
Fax: 501-296-1779
TTY: 800-482-1174
http://disabilityrightsar.org
info@disabilityrightsar.org
Julie Petty, President
Mark George, Vice President
Scott Hall, Treasurer
The purpose of CAP is to protect the rights of persons receiving or seeking services funded under the federal Rehabilitation Act. According to thise law, CAP services are available for all clients or applicants of the following services: Vocational Rehabilitation Services, Independent Living Services, Supported Employment, Independent Living Centers, and Projects with Industry.

1500 **Increasing Capabilities Access Network**
900 W 7th St
Little Rock, AR 72201
501-666-8868
800-828-2799
Fax: 501-666-5319
TTY: 800-828-2799
http://ar-ican.org
A federally funded program of Arkansas Rehabilitation Services, is designed to make technology available and accessible for all who need it. ICAN is a funding information resource and provides information on new and existing technology free to any person regardless of age or disability.

1501 **Office of the Governor**
500 Woodlane St
Ste 250
Little Rock, AR 72201
501-682-2345
http://www.governor.arkansas.gov
Asa Hutchinson, Governor
Bruce Campbell, Director
Alison Williams, Chief of Staff

1502 **Protection & Advocacy for Individuals with Developmental Disabilities (PADD)**
Disability Rights Center
400 W Capitol
Ste 1200
Little Rock, AR 72201
501-296-1775
800-482-1174
Fax: 501-296-1779
TTY: 800-482-1174
http://disabilityrightsar.org
info@disabilityrightsar.org
Julie Petty, President
Mark George, Vice President
Scott Hall, Treasurer
Carry out activities under several Federal programs to provide a range of services to adocate for and protect the rights of persons with disabilities throughout the state.

1503 **State GED Administration**
Arkansas Department of Career Education
3 Capitol Mall
Little Rock, AR 72201
501-682-1500
http://arcareereducation.org
ACECommunications@arkansas.gov
Asa Hutchinson, Governor
Charisse Childers, PhD, Director
Maria Lorna Claudio, Chief Financial Officer
Serves all Arkansans who are 16 years or older, not enrolled in or graduated from high school, and who meet other state requirements regarding residency and testing eligibility.

California

1504 **California Department of Fair Employment and Housing**
2218 Kausen Dr
Ste 100
Elk Grove, CA 95758
800-884-1684
TDD: 800-700-2320
http://www.dfeh.ca.gov
contact.center@dfeh.ca.gov
Kevin Kish, Director
Joan Keegan, Chief Deputy Director
DeLesa Swanigan, Deputy Director, Administration
To protect the people of California from unlawful discrimination in employment, housing and public accomodations, and from the perpetration of acts of hate violence.

1505 **California Department of Rehabilitation**
721 Capitol Mall
Sacramento, CA 95814
916-324-1313
800-952-5544
TTY: 844-729-2800
http://www.rehab.cahwnet.gov
externalaffairs@dor.ca.gov
Joe Xavier, Director
Works in partnership with consumers and other stakeholders to provide services and advocacy resulting in employment, independent living and equality for individuals with disabilities.

1506 **California Department of Special Education**
1430 N St
Sacramento, CA 95814-5901
916-319-0800
http://www.cde.ca.gov
scheduler@cde.ca.gov
Tom Torlakson, Executive Officer
Information and reesources to serve the unique needs of persons with disabilities so that each person will meet or exceed high standards of achivement in academic and nonacademic skills.

1507 **California Employment Development Department**
PO Box 826880, MIC 83
Sacramento, CA 94280-0001
http://www.edd.ca.gov
Edmund G. Brown, Jr., Governor
David M. Lanier, Secretary
Patrick W. Henning, Director
Promotes California's economic growth by providing services to keep employers, employees, and job seekers competitive.

1508 **California State Board of Education**
1430 N St
Sacramento, CA 95814-5901
916-319-0827
Fax: 916-319-0175
TTY: 916-445-4556
http://www.cde.ca.gov/be
sbe@cde.ca.gov
Dr. Michael Kirst, President
Dr. Ilene Straus, Vice President
Karen Stapf Walters, Executive Director
The State Board of Education (SBE) is the governing and policy making body of the California Department of Education. The SBE sets K-12 education policy in the areas of standards, instructional materials, accessment, and accountability.

1509 **California State Council on Developmental Disabilities**
1507 21st St
Ste 210
Sacramento, CA 95811
916-322-8481
866-802-0514
Fax: 916-443-4957
TTY: 916-324-8420
http://www.scdd.ca.gov
council@dcdd.ca.gov
Aaron Carruthers, Executive Director

Advocates, promotes and implements policies and practices that achieve self-determination, independence, productivity and inclusion in all aspects of community life for Californians with developmental disabilities and their families.

1510 **Clearinghouse for Specialized Media and Technology**
California Department of Education
1430 N St
Sacramento, CA 95814-5901 916-319-0881
http://www.cde.ca.gov
csmt@cde.ca.gov
Tom Torlakson, Executive Officer
Provides accessible formats of adopted curriculum to qualified students with disabilities in California.

1511 **DBTAC: Pacific ADA Center**
555 12th St
Ste 1030
Oakland, CA 94607-4046 510-285-5600
800-949-4232
Fax: 510-285-5614
TTY: 800-949-4232
http://www.adapacific.org
Erica C. Jones, MPH, Director
To build a partnership between the disability and business communities and to promote full and unrestricted participation in society for persons with disabilities through education and technical assistance.

1512 **Disability Rights California (California's Protection and Advocacy System)**
1831 K St
Sacramento, CA 95811-4114 916-504-5800
Fax: 916-504-5802
http://www.disabilityrightsca.org
legalmail@disabilityrightsca.org
Catherine Blakemore, Executive Director
Karen Keene, Finance Director
Steve Haas, Human Resources Director
A private, nonprofit organization that protects the legal, civil and service rights of Californians with disabilities.
1978

1513 **Employment Development Department: Employment Services Woodland**
PO Box 826880, MIC 83
Sacramento, CA 94280-0001 http://www.edd.ca.gov
Patrick W. Henning, Jr., Director
Edmund G. Brown, Jr., Governor
David M. Lanier, LWDA Secretary
The Employment Development Department promote's California's economic growth by providing services to keep employers, employees, and job seekers competitive.

1514 **Office of Civil Rights: California**
US Department of Education
400 Maryland Ave, SW
Washington, DC 20202-1100 800-421-3481
Fax: 202-453-6012
TDD: 800-877-8339
http://www.ed.gov
ocr@ed.gov
Betsy DeVos, Secretary of Education
The mission of the OCR of California is to ensure all children have access to public education.

1515 **Office of Correctional Education (OCE)**
Sacramento, CA 916-324-7308
http://www.cdcr.ca.gov
Edmund G. Brown, Jr., Governor
Scott Kernan, CDCR Secretary
Offers academic and education programs for all California state prisons.

1516 **Region IX: US Department of Health and Human Services**
200 Independence Ave, SW
Washington, DC 20201 877-696-6775
http://www.hhs.gov
Alex M. Azar II, Scretary

1517 **Sacramento County Office of Education**
PO Box 269003
Sacramento, CA 95826-9003 916-228-2500
http://www.scoe.net
David W. Gordon, Superintendent
The mission of the SCOE is to help students prepare for college, entering the workforce and engaging in the community.

Colorado

1518 **Assistive Technology Partners**
601 East 18th Avenue
Pearl Plaza, Suite 130
Denver, CO 80203 303-315-1280
Fax: 303-315-1270
http://www.ucdenver.edu
generalinfo@AT-Partners.org
Bill Caileÿ, Chair
Cathy Bodine, Ph.D., CCC-SLP, Executive Director
Mike Dino, Advisory Council Member
Designed to support capacity building and advocacy activities, and to assist states in maintaining permanent, comprehensive statewide programs of technology related assistance for all people with disabilities living in Colorado.

1519 **Colorado Civil Rights Division**
Colorado Department of Regulatory Agencies
1560 Broadway
Ste 825
Denver, CO 80202 303-894-2997
Fax: 303-894-7570
http://www.dora.state.co.us
dora_ccrd@state.co.us
Aubrey Elenis, Esq., Director
The mission of the CCRD is to enforce Colorado's anti-discrimination laws within the fields of employment, housing and public accommodations.

1520 **Colorado Department of Labor and Employment**
633 17th St
Ste 201
Denver, CO 80202-3660 303-318-8000
800-388-5515
http://www.colorado.gov/pacific/cdle
Sam Walker, Executive Director
Provides current information on the state's economy and job market. Assists employees and job seekers through unemployment benefits, worker's compensation, and other services.

1521 **Colorado Disabilities Services**
Colorado Department of Human Services
1575 Sherman St
8th Fl
Denver, CO 80203-1714 303-866-5700
Fax: 303-866-5563
http://www.colorado.gov/pacific/cdhs
cdhs_communications@state.co.us
Reggie Bicha, Executive Director
Katie McLoughlin, Chief Legal Director
Laura Morsch-Babu, Director of Communication
Provides leadership for the direction, funding, and operation of services to persons with disabilities within Colorado.

1522 **Disability Law Colorado**
455 Sherman St
Ste 130
Denver, CO 80203
303-722-0300
800-288-1376
Fax: 303-722-0720
http://disabilitylawco.org
dlcmail@disabilitylawco.org
Mary Anne Harvey, Executive Director
Alison L. Butler, Esq., Director of Legal Services
Mike Robbins, Director of Development/Mktg
Formerly known as the Legal Center, Disability Law Colorado protects and promotes the rights of people with disabilities and older people in Colorado through direct legal representation, advocacy, education and legislative analysis.
1977

1523 **Offender Education Division**
Colorado Department of Corrections
Ste 400
1250 Academy Park Loop
Colorado Springs, CO 80910
719-226-4569
http://www.colorado.gov/pacific/cdoc
cdoc@state.co.us
Rick Raemisch, Executive Director
Renae Jordan, Dir., Clinic & Correctional Svcs
Travis Trani, Director of Prisons
To meet the diverse educational needs of inmates through the provision of quality academic, vocational, life skills, and transitional services whereby inmates can successfully integrate into society, gain and maintain employment and become responsible, productive individuals.

1524 **Region VIII: US Department of Education**
Office of Civil Rights
Cesar E Chavez Memorial Bldng
1244 Speer Blvd, Ste 310
Denver, CO 80204-3582
303-844-5695
Fax: 303-844-4303
TDD: 800-877-8339
http://www.ed.gov
ocr.denver@ed.gov
Kenneth L. Marcus, Assistant Secretary
Earl Morgan, Executive Officer
Kristine Minami, Senior Counsel
This office covers the states of Arizona, Colorado, New Mexico, Utah, and Wyoming.

1525 **Region VIII: US Department of Health and Human Services**
1961 Stout St
Room 08-148
Denver, CO 80294
800-368-1019
Fax: 202-619-3818
TDD: 800-537-7697
http://www.hhs.gov
ocrmail@hhs.gov
Alex M. Azar II, Secretary
Eric D. Hargan, Deputy Secretary
Peter Urbanowicz, Chief of Staff

1526 **Region VIII: US Department of Labor-Office of Federal Contract Compliance**
US Department of Labor
525 S Griffin St
Room 840
Dallas, TX 75202-5092
972-850-2550
Fax: 972-850-2552
TTY: 877-889-5627
http://www.dol.gov/ofccp
OFCCP-SW-CC4@dol.gov
Melissa L. Speer, Regional Director
Aida Collins, Deputy Regional Director
Allen Boyd, Regional Outreach Coordinator
These regional offices of agencies enforce laws prohibiting employment discrimination on the basis of disability.

1527 **State Department of Education**
201 E Colfax Ave
Denver, CO 80203
303-866-6600
Fax: 303-830-0793
http://www.cde.state.co.us
Katy Anthes, PhD, Commissioner
Alyssa Pearson, Deputy Commissioner
Jennifer Okes, Chief Operating Officer
The administrative arm of the Colorado Board of Education. CDE serves colorado's 178 local school districts, providing them with leadership, consultation and administrative services on a statewide and regional basis.

Connecticut

1528 **Bureau of Education & Services for the Blind**
184 Windsor Ave
Windsor, CT 06095
860-602-4000
800-842-4510
Fax: 860-602-4020
TDD: 860-602-4221
http://www.ct.go/besb
brian.sigman@ct.gov
Alan Sylvestre, Chair
Brian S. Sigman, Executive Director
Provide quality educational and rehabilitative service to all people who are legally blind or deaf-blind and children who are visually impaired.

1529 **Bureau of Special Education & Pupil Services**
Department of Education
PO Box 2219
Hartford, CT 06145-2219
860-713-6910
Fax: 860-713-7051
http://portal.ct.gov/sde
Bryan Klimkiewicz, Chief, Bureau of Special Edu.
Melissa K. Wlodarczyk Hickey, Reading & Literacy Director
Offers information on educational programs and services. The Complaint Resolution Process Office answers and processes parent complaints regarding procedural violations by local educational agencies and facilities. The Due Process Office is responsible for the management of special education and due process proceedings which are available to parents and school districts.

1530 **CHILD FIND of Connecticut**
Connecticut Parent Advocacy Center
338 Main Street
Niantic, CT 06357
860-739-3089
800-445-2722
http://www.cpacinc.org/hot-topics/child-find
Child Find is part of the Individuals with Disabilities Education Improvement Act that requires each state to establish a system for identifying and evaluting children with disabilities who have to special education needs.

1531 **Connecticut Bureau of Rehabilitation Services**
Department of Social Services
55 Farmington Ave
12th Floor
Hartford, CT 06105-3730
860-424-4844
800-537-2549
Fax: 860-424-4850
TDD: 860-920-7163
http://www.ct.gov/brs
dors.brs.contactus@ct.gov
David Doukas, Director
Creates opportunities that enable individuals with significant disabilities to work competitively and live independently. Strive to provide appropriate, individualized services, develop effective partnerships, and share sufficient information so that consumers and their families may make informed choices about the rehabilitation process and employment options.

1532 **Connecticut Department of Social Services**
55 Farmington Ave
Hartford, CT 06105-3730
855-626-6632
TDD: 800-842-4524
TTY: 800-842-4524
http://portal.ct.gov/DSS
Roderick L. Bremby, Commissioner
Provides a broad range of services to the elderly, disabled, families and individuals who need assistance in maintaining or achieving their full potential for self-director, self-reliance and independent living.

1533 **Connecticut Office of Protection and Advocacy for Persons with Disabilities**
60-B Weston St
Hartford, CT
860-297-4345
800-842-7303
http://www.ct.gov/brs
David Doukas, Director
The Client Assistance Program (CAP) supports families and individuals who are affected by developmental disabilities through advice, advocacy and legal representation.

1534 **Connecticut State Department of Education**
450 Columbus Boulevard
Hartford, CT 06103
860-713-6543
http://portal.ct.gov/SDE
Dianna R. Wentzell, Commissioner of Education
The adminstrative arm of the Connecticut State Board of Education. Through leadership, curriculum, research, planning, evaluation, assessment, data analyses and other assistance, the Department helps to ensure equal opportunity and excellence in education for all Connecticut students.

1535 **Connecticut Tech Act Project**
Department of Rehabilitation Services (DORS)
55 Farmington Ave
12th Fl
Hartford, CT 06105
860-424-4881
800-537-2549
Fax: 860-424-4850
TTY: 860-424-4839
http://www.cttechact.com
Erin Soli, Advisory Council Chair
The mission of the Connecticut Tech Art Project is to increase independence and improve the lives of individuals with disabilities through access to Assistive Technology for work, school and community living.
1992

1536 **Correctional Education Division: Connecticut**
Department of Correction
24 Wolcott Hill Rd
Wethersfield, CT 06109
860-692-7537
Fax: 860-692-7538
http://portal.ct.gov/DOC
Maria Pirro, Acting Superintendent
Mike Nunes, Dir., Special Education
Caryn McCarthy, Dir., Career Tech Education
Provides opportunities that will support an offender's successful community reintegration. Education programming is available to inmates through the Unified School District (USD)#l, a legally vested school district within the Department of Correction (DOC).

1537 **Disability Rights Connecticut**
846 Wethersfield Ave
Hartford, CT 06114
860-297-4300
800-842-7303
Fax: 860-296-0055
http://www.disrightsct.org
info@disrightsct.org
Gretchen Knauff, Executive Director
Cathy Cushman, Legal Director
Edwin Evarts, President
Advocacy group dedicated to improving the lives of persons with disabilities and their families by eliminating barriers and allowing them to exercise their civil, legal, and human rights.

1538 **State GED Administration**
Bureau of Adult Education and Training
450 Columbus Blvd
Ste 508
Hartford, CT 06103-1841
860-807-2110
877-392-6433
http://portal.ct.gov/Services/Education
ged@ct.gov
Dianna R. Wentzell, Commissioner of Education
The primary aid of the GED testing program in Connecticut is to provide a second opportunity for individuals to obtain their high school diplomas.

Delaware

1539 **Client Assistance Program (CAP)**
United Cerebral Palsy of Delaware, Inc.
700A River Rd
Wilmington, DE 19809-2746
302-764-2400
Fax: 302-764-8713
http://ucpde.org/programs
ucpde@ucpde.org
Linda J. Royal, President
D. Bruce McClenathan, Vice President
Provides free services to consumers and applicants for projects, programs and facilities funded under the Rehabilitation Act.

1540 **Community Legal Aid Society**
100 W 10th St
Ste 801
Wilmington, DE 19801
302-575-0660
800-292-7980
Fax: 302-575-0840
TDD: 302-575-0696
TTY: 302-575-0696
http://www.declasi.org
Thomas B. Strayer, CAO & CFO
Daniel G. Atkins, Esq., Executive Director
Jason D. Stoehr, Director of Development
Community Legal Aid Society is a private, non-profit law firm dedicated to equal justice for all. Prodive civil legal services to assist clients in becoming self sufficient and meeting basic needs with dignity. Clients include members of the community who have low incomes, who have disabilities, or who are age 60 and over.

1541 **Correctional Education Division**
Department of Corrections
245 McKee Rd
Dover, DE 19904
302-739-5601
http://doc.delaware.gov
Perry Phelps, Commissioner

1542 **Delaware Assistive Technology Initiative (DATI)**
University of Delaware
461 Wyoming Rd
Newark, DE 19716
302-831-0354
TDD: 302-831-4689
http://www.cds.udel.edu/at/dati
cds-info@udel.edu
Beth Mineo, Director
Loretta McLaren, Staff Assistant
DATI connects Delawareans who have disabilities with the tools they need in order to learn, work, play, and participate in community life safely and independently. DATI also operates Assistive Technology Resource Centers that offer training as well as no-cost equipment demonstrations and loans. DATI also provides funding information, develops partnerships with state agencies and organizations, and publishes resource materials and event calendars.

1543 Delaware Department of Education
401 Federal St, Ste 2
The Townsend Building
Dover, DE 19901-3639 302-735-4000
http://www.doe.k12.de.us
Dorrell Green, Dir., Innovation & Improvement
Emily Cunningham, Chief of Staff
Susan Bunting, Secretary
Committed to promoting the highest quality education for every Delaware student by providing visionary leadership and superior service.

1544 Delaware Department of Labor
4425 N Market St
Wilmington, DE 19802 http://www.delawareworks.com
dlabor@state.de.us
Cerron Cade, Secretary
Connects people to jobs, resources, monetary benefits, workplace protections and labor market information to promote financial independence, workplace justice and a strong economy.

1545 Developmental Disabilities Services
Delaware Department of Health & Social Security
1056 S Governor's Ave
Ste 101
Dover, DE 19904 302-744-9600
866-552-5758
http://dhss.delaware.gov/dhss/ddds
Marie Nonnenmacher, Director
Nicole Lawless, Executive Secretary
Marissa Catalon, Deputy Director
Delaware's DDS program offers services to persons with developmental disabilities and their families, including assistance in navigating federal and state service systems, family support, employment information, transition services, and residential services.

1546 State GED Administration: Delaware
Department of Education
401 Federal St, Ste 2
The Townsend Building
Dover, DE 19901-3639 302-735-4000
http://www.doe.k12.de.us
Dorrell Green, Dir., Innovation & Improvement
Emily Cunningham, Chief of Staff
Susan Bunting, Secretary
The primary aid of the GED testing program in Delaware is to provide a second opportunity for individuals to obtain their high school diplomas.

District of Columbia

1547 Client Assistance Program (CAP): District of Columbia
University Legal Services
220 I St NE
Ste 130
Washington, DC 20002 202-547-0198
Fax: 202-547-2083
http://www.uls-dc.org
Jane M. Brown, Esq., Executive Director
Sandy Bernstein, Esq., Legal Director
Alicia C. Johns, AT Program Director
A federally funded program authorized under the amended Rehabilitation Act of 1973. University Legal Services administers the CAP program in the District of Columbia under contract with the District of Columbia Rehabilitation Services Administration. The goal of CAP is to identify, explain, and resolve the problems residents of the District of Columbia may be having with the rehabilitation program as quickly as possible.

1548 DC Department of Employment Services
4058 Minnesota Ave, NE
Washington, DC 20019 202-724-7000
Fax: 202-673-6993
TDD: 202-673-6994
TTY: 202-673-6994
http://does.dc.gov
does@dc.gov
Dr Unique N. Morris-Hughes, Director
The mission of the Department of Employment Services is to plan, develop and administer employment-related services to all segments of the Washington, DC metropolitan population.

1549 DC Developmental Disabilities Council
One Judiciary Square
441 4th St NW 729 N
Washington, DC 20001 202-724-8612
Fax: 202-727-9484
TTY: 202-724-8612
http://ddc.dc.gov
Alison Whyte, Executive Director
Lisa Matthew, Chair
Ricardo Thornton, Vice Chair
The District of Columbia's Developmental Disabilities Council advocates on behalf of people with developmental disabilities and their families in order to provide support, empowerment, and allow them to achieve independence, inclusion and equality.

1550 DC Office of Disability Rights
441 4th St NW 729 N
Washington, DC 20001 202-724-9484
Fax: 202-727-9484
TTY: 202-727-3363
http://odr.dc.gov
odr@dc.gov
Matthew McCollough, Director
The District of Columbia's Office of Disability Rights is dedicated to ensuring that programs, services, benefits, and facilities are fully accessible and usable by people with disabilities. ODR aims to include all residents of DC and provide support to those in need.

1551 DC State Board of Education
441 4th St NW 530 S
Washington, DC 20001 202-741-0888
Fax: 202-741-0879
TTY: 202-741-0888
http://sboe.dc.gov
sboe@dc.gov
John-Paul C. Hayworth, Executive Director
The mission of District of Columbia's State Board of Education is to provide leadership in policy, student support, and advocacy. The board oversees the public education system and ensures the value of every student.

1552 District of Columbia Department of Corrections
2000 14th St NW
7th Fl
Washington, DC 20009 http://doc.dc.gov
doc@dc.gov
Quincy L. Booth, Director
Maria Amato, General Counsel
Sallie Thomas, Executive Assistant
Provides public safety by ensuring the safe, secure, and human confinement of pertrial detainees and sentenced misdemeanant prisoners.

1553 District of Columbia Department on Disability Services
250 E St SW
Washington, DC 20024 202-730-1700
Fax: 202-730-1843
http://dds.dc.gov
dds@dc.gov
Andrew Reese, Director

Provides information and coordination of services for persons with disabilities and their families within the District of Columbia. Services include employement assistance, vocational rehabilitation, residential aid, and family support.

1554 **District of Columbia Fair Employment Practice Agencies**
DC Office of Human Rights
441 4th St NW
Ste 570
Washington, DC 20001
202-727-4559
Fax: 202-727-9589
TTY: 202-727-9589
http://ohr.dc.gov
ohr@dc.gov
Monica Palacio, Director
The DC Office of Human Rights is an agency of the District of Columbia government that seeks to eradicate discrimination, increase equal opportunity, and protect human rights in the city. The Office is also the advocate for the practice of good human relations and mutual understanding among the various racial ethnic and religious groups in the District of Columbia.

1555 **Office of Civil Rights: District of Columbia**
US Department of Education
400 Maryland Ave SW
Washington, DC 20202-1100
800-421-3481
Fax: 202-453-6012
TDD: 800-877-8339
http://www.ed.gov.
ocr@ed.gov
This office covers the states of District of Columbia, North Carolina, South Carolina and Virginia.

1556 **Office of Human Rights: District of Columbia**
Government of the District of Columbia
441 4th St NW
Ste 570 N
Washington, DC 20001
202-727-4559
Fax: 202-727-9589
http://ohr.dc.gov
ohr@dc.gov
Monica Palacio, Director
The DC Office of Human Rights is an agency of the District of Columbia government that seeks to eradicate discrimination, increase equal opportunity, and protect human rights in the city.

1557 **Protection and Advocacy Program: Districtof Columbia**
University Legal Services
220 I St NE
Ste 130
Washington, DC 20002
202-547-4747
Fax: 202-547-2083
TTY: 202-547-2657
http://www.uls-dc.org
info@uls-dc.org
Jane M. Brown, Esq., Executive Director
Sandy Bernstein, Esq., Legal Director
Alicia C. Johns, AT Program Director
A program authorized by federal law to help the District of Columbia residents with developemntal disabilities exercise their full rights as citizens.

Florida

1558 **Agency for Persons with Disabilities**
4030 Esplanade Way
Ste 380
Tallahassee, FL 32399-0950
850-488-4257
866-273-2273
Fax: 850-922-6456
http://apd.myflorida.com
apd.info@apdcares.org
Barbara Palmer, Director
The Agency partners with local communities and private service providers to assist people with developmental disabilities and their familes across the state of Florida.
1904

1559 **Client Assistance Program (CAP): Advocacy Center for Persons with Disabilities**
Disability Rights Florida
2473 Care Dr
Ste 200
Tallahassee, FL 32308
850-488-9071
800-342-0823
Fax: 850-488-8640
TDD: 800-346-4127
http://www.disabilityrightsflorida.org
Stephanie Preshong Brown, Chair
Alan Quiles, Vice Chair
Cherie Hall, Executive Director (Interim)
Assists anyone with a disability that is interested in applying for and receiving services from rehabilitation programs, projects or facilities funded under the Rehabilitation Act.

1560 **Disability Rights Florida**
2473 Care Dr
Ste 200
Tallahassee, FL 32308
850-488-9071
800-342-0823
Fax: 850-488-8640
TDD: 800-346-4127
http://www.disabilityrightsflorida.org
Cherie Hall, Interim Executive Director
Ann Siegel, Dir., Advocacy & Education
Amanda Heystek, Dir., Systems Reform
Advocacy group dedicated to improving the lives of persons with disabilities and their families by eliminating barriers and allowing them to exercise their civil, legal, and human rights.

1561 **Division of Vocational Rehabilitation**
Florida Department of Education
4070 Esplanade Way
Tallahassee, FL 32399-7016
850-245-3399
800-451-4327
http://www.rehabworks.org
Allison Flanagan, Director
Offers employment assistance for people with physical or mental disabilities in order to encourage and enhance independence. Specialized programs include Transition Youth, Deaf Hard of Hearing and Deaf-Blind services, Supported Employment, Independent Living, Migrant and Seaonal Farmworkers, and Florida Alliance for Assistive Services and Technology.

1562 **Florida Department of Education**
325 W Gaines St
Tallahassee, FL 32399
850-245-0505
Fax: 850-245-9667
http://www.fldoe.org
commissioner@fldoe.org
Pam Stewart, Commissioner
Kathy Hebda, Chief of Staff
Hershel Lyons, Chancellor of Public Schools

1563 **Florida Department of Labor and Employment Security**
800-860-9467
http://flworkcomp.com
Provides worker's compensation insurance.

1564 **Florida Developmental Disabilities Council, Inc.**
124 Marriott Dr
Ste 203
Tallahassee, FL 32301
850-488-4180
800-580-7801
Fax: 850-922-6702
TDD: 888-488-8633
http://www.fddc.org
fddc@fddc.org

Valerie Breen, Executive Director
Sheila Griz-Swift, Deputy Director of Programs
Cindy Tan, Special Projects Manager
A nonprofit organization sponsored by the Department of Health and Human Services Administration on Developmental Disabilities of Florida. DDC offers family support for people with disabilities and oversees administration of services and programs.
1971

1565 **Florida Fair Employment Practice Agency**
Florida Commission on Human Relations
4075 Esplanade Way
Unit 100
Tallahassee, FL 32399
850-488-7082
http://fchr.myflorida.com
fchrinfo@fchr.myflorida.com
Michelle Wilson, Executive Director
To prevent unlawful discrimination by ensuring people in Florida are treated fairly and are given access to opportunities in employment, housing, and certain public accommodations; and to promote mutual respect among groups through education and partnerships.

Georgia

1566 **Client Assistance Program (CAP): Georgia Division of Persons with Disabilities**
123 N McDonough St
Decatur, GA 30030
800-822-9727
Fax: 404-373-4110
TTY: 404-373-2040
http://www.georgiacap.com
acarraway@georgiacap.com
Charles L. Martin, Director
Ashley Carraway, Assistant Director
Jennifer Page, Counselor
Advocacy counseling and other services for persons with disabilities.

1567 **Georgia Advocacy Office**
Decatur, GA
404-885-1234
800-537-2329
Fax: 404-378-0031
TDD: 800-537-2329
http://www.thegao.org
info@thegao.org
Ruby Moore, Executive Director
Julie Kegley, Sr Staff Attorney/Progam Dir.
Olwyn DeMarco, Chief Operating Officer
Our mission is to work with and for oppressed and vulnerable individuals in Georgia who are labeled as disabled of mentally ill of secure their protection and advocacy.

1568 **Georgia Department of Behavioral Health and Developmental Disabilities**
Two Peachtree St NW
24th Fl
Atlanta, GA 30303
404-657-2252
http://dbhdd.georgia.gov
Judy Fitzgerald, Commissioner
Jeff Minor, Deputy Commissioner/COO
Ron Wakefield, Dir., Developmental Disabilities
Provides services and support to persons with developmental disabilities. The department's mission is to help persons with disabilities achieve independence.

1569 **Georgia Department of Technical & Adult Education**
Technical College System of Georgia
1800 Century Pl NE
Ste 400
Atlanta, GA 30345
404-679-1600
http://tcsg.edu
Ben Copeland, Chair
Shirley Smith, Vice Chair
The Georgia Department of Technical and Adult Education oversees the state's system of technical colleges, the adult literacy program, and a host of economic and workforce development programs.

1570 **Governor's Council on Developmental Disabilities**
2 Peachtree St NW
Ste 26-246
Atlanta, GA 30303
404-657-2126
888-275-4233
Fax: 404-657-2132
TDD: 404-657-2133
http://www.gcdd.org
eric.jacobson@gcdd.ga.gov
Hilary Hibben, Media Relations Director
Eric Jacobson, Executive Director
Dawn Alford, Public Policy Director
To collaborate with Georgia citizens, public and private advocacy organizations, and policy makers to positively influence ppublic policies that enhance the quality of life for people with developmental disabilities and their families.

1571 **Office of Civil Rights: Georgia**
US Department of Education
400 Maryland Ave SW
Washington, DC 20202-1100
800-421-3481
Fax: 202-453-6012
TDD: 800-877-8339
http://www.ed.gov
ocr@ed.gov
Earl Morgan, Executive Director
Brittany Bull, Attorney Advisor
Kristine Minami, Senior Consel
This office covers the states of Florida, Georgia and Tennessee.

1572 **State Department of Education**
Department of Technical and Adult Education
205 Jesse Hill Jr. Dr SE
Atlanta, GA 30334
404-656-2800
800-311-3627
Fax: 404-651-8737
http://www.gadoe.org
askdoe@gadoe.org
Richard Woods, Superintendent

1573 **State GED Administration: Georgia**
GA Department of Technical and Adult Education
205 Jesse Hill Jr. Dr SE
Atlanta, GA 30334
404-656-2800
800-311-3627
Fax: 404-651-8737
http://www.gadoe.org
Richard Woods, Superintendent
The primary aid of the GED testign program in Georgia is to provide a second opportunity for individuals to obtain their high school diplomas.

1574 **Tools for Life, the Georgia Assistive Technology Act Program**
Georgia Institute of Technology/AMAC
512 Means St
Ste 250
Atlanta, GA 30318
404-894-0541
http://www.gatfl.org
info@gatfl.org
Carolyn P. Phillips, Program Director
Ben Jacobs, Accommodations Specialist
Liz Persaud, Program & Outreach Manager
The Tools for Life lists local and national training opportunities coming to Georgia.

Hawaii

1575 **Correctional Education**
Department of Public Safety
919 Ala Moana Blvd
4th Fl
Honolulu, HI 96814 808-587-1258
Fax: 808-587-2568
http://dps.hawaii.gov
Nolan Espinda, Director of Public Safety
Jodie Maesaka, Deputy Director of Corrections

1576 **Developmental Disabilities Division**
Hawaii Department of Health
1250 Punchbowl St
Rm 463
Honolulu, HI 96813 808-586-5840
Fax: 808-586-5844
http://health.hawaii.gov/ddd
Bruce S. Anderson, PhD, Director of Health
Keith Y. Yamamoto, Deputy Director
Janice Okubo, Public Information Officer
Offers services for people with developmental disabilities and oversees programs accross the state of Hawaii.

1577 **Division of Vocational Rehabilitation**
Hawaii Department of Human Services
1390 Miller St
Rm 209
Honolulu, HI 96813 808-586-4993
Fax: 808-586-4890
http://humanservices.hawaii.gov/vocationalrehab
dhs@dhs.hawaii.gov
Pankaj Bhanot, Director
Cathy Betts, Deputy Director
Provides employement services to people with physical or cognitive disabilities. Services include training, support and career placement.

1578 **Hawaii Disability Rights Center**
1132 Bishop St
Ste 2102
Honolulu, HI 96813 808-949-2922
800-882-1057
Fax: 808-949-2928
TTY: 808-949-2922
http://www.hawaiidisabilityrights.org
info@hawaiidisabilityrights.org
Andrew Grant, President
Mary Ellen Markley, Vice President
Louis Erteschik, Executive Director

1579 **Hawaii State Council on Developmental Disabilities**
1010 Richards St
Ste 122
Honolulu, HI 96813 808-586-8100
http://health.hawaii.gov
Bruce S. Anderson, PhD, Director of Health
Lynn N. Fallin, Director, Health Svcs Admin.
Janice Okubo, Public Information Officer
To support people with developmental disabilities to control their own destiny and determine the quality of life they desire.

1580 **Hawaii State Department of Education**
1390 Miller St
Honolulu, HI 96813 808-586-3230
http://www.hawaiipublicschools.org
doe_info@hawaiideo.org
Christina Kishimoto, Superintendent
Phyllis Unebasami, Deputy Superintendent
Heidi Armstrong, Student Support Services

1581 **State GED Administration: Hawaii**
Community Education Office
475 22nd Ave
Room 202
Honolulu, HI 96816 808-203-5511
http://www.hawaiipublicschools.org
inquiry@hawaiidoe.k12.hi.us

Idaho

1582 **Disability Rights Idaho**
Comprehensive Advocacy (Co-Ad)
4477 Emerald St
Ste B-100
Boise, ID 83706-2066 208-336-5353
800-632-5125
Fax: 208-336-5396
http://www.disabilityrightsidaho.org
info@disabilityrightsidaho.org
James R. Baugh, Executive Director
Amy Cunningham, Legal Director
Dina Flores-Brewer, Advocacy Director
Comprehensive Advocacy, Inc is the designated Protection and Advocacy System for Idaho. Co-Ad provides advocacy for people with disabilities who have been abused/neglected; denied services or benefits; have experienced rights violations or discrimination because of their disability; or have voting accessibility problems. Co-Ad provides information & referral; negotitation & mediation; short term & technical assistance; legal advice/representation.

1583 **Idaho Assistive Technology Project**
1187 Alturas Dr
Moscow, ID 83843 800-432-8324
Fax: 208-885-6102
http://www.idahoat.org
idahoat@uidaho.edu
Janice Carson, Project Director
Dan Dyer, Technical Assistance Coordinator
Sue House, Statewide Program Specialist
The Idaho Assistive Technology Project (IATP) is a federally funded program managed by the Center on Disabilities and Human Development at the University of Idaho. The goal of IATP is to increase the availability of assistive technology devices and services for Idahoans with disabilities. The IATP offers free trainings and technical assistance, a low-interest loan program, assistive technology assessments for children and agriculture workers, and free informational materials.

1584 **Idaho Career & Technical Education**
650 W State St
Len B. Jordan Bldg, Room 324
Boise, ID 83720-0095 208-334-3216
Fax: 208-334-2365
http://cte.idaho.gov
Tammy Ackerland, Manager
Andrew Armstrong, Administrator Support
Cruz Gallegos, State Coordinator
The primary aid of the GED testing program in Idaho is to provide a second opportunity for individuals to obtain their high school equivalency certificate.

1585 **Idaho Department of Education**
650 W State St
Boise, ID 83720 208-332-6800
Fax: 208-334-2228
http://www.sde.idaho.gov
info@sde.idaho.gov
Sherri Ybarra, Superintendent
Determined to create a customer-driven education system that meets the needs of every student in Idaho and prepares them to live, work and succeed in the 21st century.

1586 **Idaho Division of Vocational Rehabilitation**
650 W State St
Room 150
Boise, ID 83720
208-334-3390
Fax: 208-334-5305
http://www.vr.idaho.gov
Jane Donnellan, Administrator
A state-federal program whose goal is to assist people with disabilities to prepare for, secure, retain or regain employment.

1587 **Idaho Fair Employment Practice Agency**
Idaho Human Rights Commission
317 W Main St
2nd Fl
Boise, ID 83735-0660
208-334-2873
888-249-7025
Fax: 208-334-2664
http://humanrights.idaho.gov
inquiry@ihrc.idaho.gov
Benjamin Earwicker, Administrator
Doug Werth, Deputy Attorney General
Rick Rhodes, Senior Civil Rights Investigator

1588 **Idaho Human Rights Commission**
317 W Main St
2nd Fl
Boise, ID 83735-0660
208-334-2873
888-249-7025
Fax: 208-334-2664
TDD: 208-334-4751
TTY: 208-334-4751
http://humanrights.idaho.gov
inquiry@ihrc.idaho.gov
Benjamin Earwicker, Ph.D., Director/Administrator
Brian Scigliano, President of the Commission
Rick Rhodes, Senior Civil Rights Investigator
To administer state and federal andti-discrimination laws in Idaho in a manner that is fair, accurate, and timely; and to work towards ensuring that all people within the state are treated with dignity and respect in their places of employment, housing, education and public accommodations.

1589 **State Department of Education: Special Education**
650 W State St
Boise, ID 83720
208-332-6800
Fax: 208-334-2228
http://www.sde.idaho.gov
info@sde.idaho.gov
Sherri Ybarra, Superintendent
To enable all students to achieve high academic standards and quality of life. The Special Education Team works collaboratively with districts, agencies, and parents to ensure students receive quality, meaningful, and needed services.

Illinois

1590 **Chicago Board of Education**
Office of the Board of Education
42 W Madison St
Chicago, IL 60602
773-553-1600
http://www.cpsboe.org
Frank M. Clark, President
Jaime Guzman, Vice President
Offers instruction and information services, curriculum information and government relations advocacy.

1591 **Client Assistance Program (CAP): Illinois Department of Human Services**
100 South Grand Ave E
Springfield, IL 62762
800-843-6154
TTY: 866-324-5553
http://www.dhs.state.il.us
James T. Dimas, Secretary
Provides free services to consumers and applicants for projects, programs and facilities funded under the Rehabilitation Act.

1592 **Correctional Education**
Illinois Department of Corrections
1301 Concordia Court
PO Box 19277
Springfield, IL 62794-9277
217-558-2200
http://www.illinois.gov/idoc
Bruce Rauner, Governor
John R. Baldwin, Acting Director
Jared Brunk, Chief Financial Officer

1593 **DBTAC: Great Lakes ADA Center**
University of Illinois at Chicago
1640 W Roosevelt Rd
Room 405
Chicago, IL 60608
312-413-1407
800-949-4232
Fax: 312-413-1856
TTY: 312-413-1407
http://www.adagreatlakes.org
adata@adagreatlakes.org
Increases awareness and knowledge with the ultimate goal of achieving voluntary compliance with the Americans with Disabilities Act. This is accomplished within targeted audiences through provision of customized training, expert assistance, and dissemination of information developed by various sources, including the federal agencies responsible for enforcement of the ADA.

1594 **Illinois Assistive Technology**
1020 S Spring St
Springfield, IL 62704
217-522-7985
800-852-5110
Fax: 217-522-8067
TTY: 212-522-9966
http://www.iltech.org
iatp@iltech.org
Horacio Esparza, President
Rita Howells, Vice President
Rian Dowd, Treasurer
The primary focus is on education, employment, community living, information technology and telecommunications. The mission is to enable people iwth disabilities so they can fully participate in all aspects of life.

1595 **Illinois Council on Developmental Disabilities**
207 State House
Springfield, IL 62706
217-782-0244
TTY: 888-261-3336
http://www.illinois.gov
vanessa.morris@illinois.gov
Kimberly Mercer-Schleider, Director
Mariel R. Hamer, Ass. Dir., Program & Policy
Vanessa Morris, Administrative Assistant
Dedicated to improving the lives of people with developmental disabilities through advocacy, systemic change and capacity building. Focuses its efforts across a person's life span so that people with developmental disabilities can enjoy life as any other Illinoisan. The Council completes its work through a variety of methods including grant awards, technical assistance and collaboration.

1596 **Illinois Department of Commerce and Economic Opportunity**
500 E Monroe St
Springfield, IL 62701
217-782-7500
TTY: 800-785-6055
http://www.illinois.gov/dceo
Sean McCarthy, Director
Amberly Zwiener, Assistant Director
Jared Walkowitz, Chief Operating Officer
Provides opportunities for businesses, entrepreneurs, and residents of Illinois in order to improve quality of life.

1597 **Illinois Department of Employment Security**
33 S State St
Chicago, IL 60603
800-244-5631
TTY: 866-488-4016
http://www.ides.illinois.gov
Jeff Mays, Director

IDES helps job seekers find jobs and employers find workers. IDES also publishes information on careers across the state and the Illinois economy.

1598 Illinois Department of Human Rights
100 W Randolph St
10th Fl, Intake Unit
Chicago, IL 60601 312-814-6200
Fax: 312-814-1436
TTY: 866-740-3953
http://www.illinois.gov/dhr
Janice Glenn, Director
Civil rights enforcement agency covering employment, housing, financial credit, public accomodation, sexual harassment in education in the State of Illinois.

1599 Illinois Department of Rehabilitation Services
100 South Grand Ave E
Springfield, IL 62762 800-843-6154
TTY: 866-324-5553
http://www.dhs.state.il.us
James T. Dimas, Secretary
Fred Flather, Chief of Staff
Khari Hunt, Chief Operating Officer
DHS' Office of Rehabilitation Services is the state's lead agency serving individuals with disabilities.

1600 Illinois State Board of Education
100 N 1st St
Springfield, IL 62777 217-782-4321
866-262-6663
http://www.isbe.net
Tony Smith, PhD, State Superintendent, Education
James T. Meeks, Chair
Eligio Cerda Pimentel, Vice Chair
Sets educational policies and guidelines for public and private schools, preschool through grade 12, as well as vocational education. Analyzes the aims, needs and requirements of edcuation and recommends legislation to the General Assembly and Governor for the benefit of the more than 2 million school children in Illinois.

1601 Office of Civil Rights: Illinois
US Department of Education
400 Maryland Ave SW
Washington, DC 20202 800-872-5327
http://www.ed.gov
Betsy DeVos, Secretary of Education
This office covers the states of Illinois, Indiana, Iowa, Minnesota, North Dakota, and Wisconsin.

1602 Protection & Advocacy Agency
Equip for Equality
20 N Michigan Ave
Ste 300
Chicago, IL 60602 312-341-0022
800-537-2632
TTY: 800-610-2779
http://www.equipforequality.org
Zena Naiditch, President & CEO
John K. Holto, PhD, Chair
Sue Suter, Vice Chair
The mission of Equip for Equality is to advance the human and civil rights of children and adults with physical and mental disabilities. The only state-wide cross-disability, comprehensive advocacy organization providing self-advocacy assistance, legal services, and disability rights education while also engaging in publi policy and legislative advocacy and conducting abuse investigation and other oversight activities.

1603 Region V: Civil Rights Office
US Department of Health & Human Services
200 Independence Ave SW
Washington, DC 20201 877-696-6775
http://www.hhs.gov
Alex M. Azar II, Secretary of Health & Human Svcs

1604 Region V: US Small Business Administration
500 W Madison St
Ste 1150
Chicago, IL 60661 312-353-0357
Fax: 312-353-3426
http://www.sba.gov
Robert Scott, Regional Administrator
Andrea Roebker, Regional Communications Director
These regional offices of agencies enforce laws prohibiting employment discrimination on the basis of disability. Serving Illinois, Indiana, Michigan, Minnesota, Ohio, and Wisconsin.

Indiana

1605 Bureau of Developmental Disabilities Services
Family and Social Services Administration
402 W Washington St
PO Box 7083
Indianapolis, IN 46207-7083 800-545-7763
Fax: 317-232-1240
http://www.in.gov/fssa/ddrs
BQIS.Help@fssa.IN.gov
Provides services for people with developmental disabilities in order to achieve independence and higher quality of life.

1606 Education Division: Indiana Department of Correction
302 W Washington
Ste E334
Indianapolis, IN 46204 317-233-3111
http://www.in.gov/idoc
John Nally, Director
Offers educational programs such as GED classes and testing, English as a Second Language, high school Refresher courses, and computer instruction courses.

1607 Indiana Department of Correction
Rm E334
302 W Washington St
Indianapolis, IN 46204 317-232-5711
http://www.in.gov/idoc
mauxier@idoc.in.gov
Randy Koester, Chief of Staff
Margaux Auxier, Administrative Assistant
Christina Emberson-Reagle, Chief Financial Officer
To maintain public safety and provide offenders with self improvement programs, job skills and family values in an efficient and cost effective manner for a successful return to the community as law-abiding citizens.

1608 Indiana Department of Workforce Development Disability Program Navigator
10 N Senate Ave
Indianapolis, IN 46204 800-891-6499
http://www.in.gov/dwd
Frederick D. Payne, Commissioner
Josh Richardson, Chief of Staff
Bill Nonte, Chief Financial Officer
Provides guideance to employers on the hiring of individuals with disabilities as well as additional tax credits and assistance for their employers. Also provide assistance to schools on transition to work needs of students with disabilities. Guides individuals with disabilities through the career services available in our WorkOne Centers as they obtain employment.

1609 Indiana Disability Rights
4701 N Keystone Ave
Ste 222
Indianapolis, IN 46205 317-722-5555
800-622-4845
TTY: 800-838-1131
http://www.indianadisabilityrights.org
info@indianadisabilityrights.org
Dawn Adams, Executive Director
Kathy Chu, Chief Financial Officer
Melissa Keyes, Legal Director

A nonprofit organization dedicated to improving the quality of life for people with learning disabilities and developmental disabilities.

1610 **Indiana Division of Youth Services: Juvenile Education Program**
302 W Washington St
Rm E334
Indianapolis, IN 46204 317-232-5711
http://www.in.gov/idoc/dys
Robert Carter, Commissioner
Christine Blessinger, Executive Director
Natalie Walker, Assistant Director
Offers educational programs such as GED classes and testing, English as a Second Language, high school Refresher courses, and computer instruction courses.

1611 **Indiana Protection & Advocacy Services**
Indiana Disability Rights
Ste 222
4701 N Keystone Ave
Indianapolis, IN 46205 317-722-5555
800-622-4845
Fax: 317-722-5564
TTY: 800-838-1131
http://www.in.gov/idr
info@IndianaDisabilityRights.org
Dawn Adams, Executive Director
Melissa Keyes, Legal Director
Created to protect and advocate the rights of people with disabilities and is Indiana's federally designated Protection and Advocacy system and client assistance program. An independent state agency, which recieves no state funding and is independent from all service providers, as required by federal and state law.

1612 **State Department of Education**
115 W Washington St
South Tower, Ste 600
Indianapolis, IN 46204 317-232-6610
Fax: 317-232-8004
http://www.doe.in.gov
webmaster@doe.in.gov
Dr. Jennifer McCormick, Superintendent
Mike Brown, Director of Legislative Affairs
Dr. Kenneth Folks, Chief Acadmeic Officer
Mission is to fulfill its statutory responsibilty by establishing policies that promote excellence in learning for all students.

1613 **State GED Administration**
Office of Adult Education
115 W Washington St
South Tower, Ste 600
Indianapolis, IN 46204 317-232-6610
Fax: 317-232-8004
http://www.doe.in.gov
webmaster@doe.in.gov
Dr. Jennifer McCormick, Superintendent
Mike Brown, Director of Legislative Affairs
Dr. Kenneth Folks, Chief Academic Officer

1614 **UITS Assistive Technology & Accessibility Centers**
Indianapolis, IN 812-856-4112
http://atac.iu.edu
atac@iu.edu
Brian Richwine, Manager
ATAC works with Indiana University to offer assistive technology and IT consultations, training, and support.

Iowa

1615 **Client Assistance Program (CAP): Iowa Division of Persons with Disabilities**
321 E 12th St
Lucas State Office Bldng
Des Moines, IA 50319 800-652-4298
Fax: 515-242-6119
http://humanrights.iowa.gov
dhr.disabilites@iowa.gov
San Wong, Director
Exists to promote the employment of Iowans with disabilities and reduce barriers to employment by providing information, referral, assessment and guidance, training and negotiation services to employers and citizens with disabilities.

1616 **Governor's Council on Developmental Disabilities**
700 2nd Ave
Ste 101
Des Moines, IA 50309 515-288-0463
http://iddcouncil.idaction.org
Brooke Lovelace Hundling, Executive Director
Rik Shannon, Public Policy Manager
Steve Crew, Chair
Identifies, develops and promotes public policy and support practices through capacity building, advocacy, and systems change activities. The purpose is to ensure that people with developmental disabilities and their families are included in planning, decision making, and development of policy related to services and supports that affect their quality of life and full participation in communities of their choice.

1617 **Iowa Department of Corrections: Education Division**
515-725-5701
http://doc.iowa.gov
doc.information@iowa.gov
Jerry Bartruff, Director
Cord Overton, Communications Director
Offers educational programs such as GED classes and testing, English as a Second Language, high school Refresher courses, and computer instruction courses.

1618 **Iowa Department of Education**
400 E 14th St
Des Moines, IA 50319-0146 515-281-5294
Fax: 515-242-5988
http://www.educateiowa.gov
ryan.wise@iowa.gov
Ryan Wise, Director
Nicole Proesch, Legal Director
Staci Hupp, Chief Bureau Communications
Champion excellence in education through superior leadership and services. Committed to high levels of learning, achievement and performance for all students, so they will become successful members of their community and the workforce.

1619 **Iowa Welfare Programs**
Iowa Department of Human Services
2309 Euclid Ave
Des Moines, IA 50314 515-725-2600
Fax: 515-564-4148
http://www.dhs.iowa.gov
Jerry R. Foxhoeven, Director
Mikki Stier, Deputy Director
Kim Reynolds, Governor
To provide assistance to families in need in the Des Moines area.

1620 **Iowa Workforce Development**
200 Army Post Rd
Des Moines, IA 50315 515-281-9619
Fax: 515-281-9640
http://www.iowaworkforcedevelopment.gov
region11.web@iwd.iowa.gov

Beth Townsend, Director
Myron Linn, Deputy Director
Ryan West, Admin., Operations Division
A state agency dedicated to providing employment services to job seekers across Iowa.

1621 **Iowa Workforce Innovation & Opportunity Act (WIOA)**
Iowa Workforce Development
200 Army Post Rd
Des Moines, IA 50315 515-281-9619
Fax: 515-281-9640
http://www.iowaworkforcedevelopment.gov
Beth Townsend, Executive Director
Myron Linn, Deputy Director
Ryan West, Admin., Operations Division
WIOA replaced the Workforce Investment Act in 2015. The program provides job placement and training services. Especially for those workers who have been laid off, or have other barriers to steady employment.

1622 **Learning Disabilities Association of Iowa**
5665 Greendale Rd
Ste D
Johnston, IA 50131 515-280-8558
888-690-5324
Fax: 515-243-1902
http://www.lda-ia.org
kathylda@askresource.org
Dedicated to identifying causes and promoting prevention of learning disabilities and to enhancing the quality of life for all individuals with learning disabilities and their families.

1623 **Protection & Advocacy Services**
Disability Rights Iowa
200 E Court Ave
Ste 300
Des Moines, IA 50309 515-278-2502
800-779-2502
TTY: 515-278-0571
http://disabilityrightsiowa.org
info@driowa.org
Jane Hudson, JD, Executive Director
Cyndy Miller, Legal Director
A federally funded program that will protect and advocate for the human and legal rights that ensure individuals with disabilities and/or mental illness a free, appropriate public education, employment opportunities and residence or treatment in the least restricitve environment or method and for freedom from stigma.

Kansas

1624 **Disability Rights Center of Kansas**
214 SW 6th Ave
Ste 100
Topeka, KS 66603 785-273-9661
877-776-1541
Fax: 785-273-9414
TDD: 877-335-3725
http://www.drckansas.org
Rocky Nichols, M.P.A., Executive Director
Nick Cobos, Office Assistant
Bev Masters, Administrative Assistant
Formerly Kansas Advocacy & Protection Services, a public interest legal advocacy agency empowered by federal law to advocate for the civil and legal rights of Kansans with disabilities.

1625 **Kansas Adult Education Association**
Barton County Community College
Barton Community Collegeÿ
245 NE 30 Rd
Great Bend, KS 67530 620-792-2701
800-748-7594
http://www.bartonccc.edu
Tana Cooper, Director of Admissions
Wendy Rodriguez, Admissions Secretary
The Kansas Adult Education Association has been the professional association for adult educators at community colleges, school districts, and non-profit organizations.

1626 **Kansas Department of Labor**
401 SW Topeka Blvd
Topeka, KS 66603 785-575-1460
http://www.dol.ks.gov
Lana Gordon, Secretary
Formerly the Kansas Department of Human Resources, advances the economic well being of all Kansans through responsive workforce services.

1627 **Kansas Human Rights Commission**
900 SW Jackson
Ste 568-S
Topeka, KS 66612-1258 785-296-3206
Fax: 785-296-0589
http://www.khrc.net
khrc@ks.gov
Ruth Glover, Executive Director
To prevent and eliminate discrimination and assure equal opportunities in all employment relations, to eliminate profiling in conjunction with traffic stops, to eliminate and prevent discrimination, segregation or separation, and assure equal opportunities in all places of public accommodations an in housing.

1628 **Kansas Rehabilitation Services Program**
Department for Children & Families
555 S Kansas Ave
Topeka, KS 66603 785-296-3271
http://www.dcf.ks.gov
Gina Meier-Hummel, Secretary
To protect children and promote adult self-sufficiency.

1629 **Kansas State Department of Education**
900 SW Jackson St
Landon State Office Bldng
Topeka, KS 66612-1212 785-296-3201
http://www.ksde.org
contact@ksde.org
Randy Watson, Commissioner
Promotes the mission of the Kansas State Board of Education through leadership and support for student learning in Kansas.

1630 **Kansas State GED Administration**
Kansas Board of Regents
1000 SW Jackson St
Ste 520
Topeka, KS 66612-1368 785-430-4240
Fax: 785-430-4233
http://www.kansasregents.org
Blake Flanders, President & CEO
Sue Grosdidier, State GED Administrator
The Kansas Board of Regents is the state's GED administrator.

1631 **Office of Disability Services**
Wichita State University
1845 Fairmount
Grace Wilkie, Room 203
Wichita, KS 67260-0132 316-978-3309
Fax: 316-978-3114
TDD: 316-854-3032
http://www.wichita.edu
John Bardo, President
Werner Golling, VP, Finance & Administration
Teri Hall, VP, Student Affairs
To enable students, staff, faculty and guests of Wichita State University to achieve their educational goals, both personal and academic, to the fullest of their abilities by providing and coordinating accessibility services which afford individuals with learning, mental or physical disabilities the equal opportunity to attain these goals.

Kentucky

1632 **Assistive Technology Office**
8412 Westport Rd
Louisville, KY 40242 800-327-5287
http://www.katsnet.org
info@katsnet.org
To make assistive technology information, devices and services easily obtainable for people of any age and/or disability.

1633 **Kentucky Adult Education**
Council on Postsecondary Education
1024 Capital Center Dr
Ste 250
Frankfort, KY 40601 502-573-5114
Fax: 502-573-5436
TTY: 502-573-5114
http://www.kyae.ky.gov
toni.quire@ky.gov
Toni Quire, Executive Secretary
To provide a responsive and innovative adult education system that enables students to acheive and prosper.

1634 **Kentucky Client Assistance Program**
Education & Workforce Development Cabinet
300 Sower Blvd
4th Fl
Frankfort, KY 40601 502-564-8035
800-633-6283
Fax: 502-564-1566
http://kycap.ky.gov
Provides advocacy for persons with disabilities who are clients or applicants of the Office of Vocational Rehabilitation or the Office for the Blind and are having problems receiving services.

1635 **Kentucky Department of Corrections**
Health Services Building
275 E Main St
PO Box 2400
Frankfort, KY 40602-2400 502-564-4726
Fax: 502-564-5037
http://www.corrections.ky.gov
Jim Erwin, Commissioner
Hilarye Dailey, Deputy Commissioner
Randy White, Deputy Commissioner
To protect the citizens of the Commonwealth and to provide a safe, secure and human environment for staff and offenders in carrying out the mandates of the legislative and judicial processes; and to provide opportunities for offenders to acquire skills which facilitate non-criminal behavior.

1636 **Kentucky Department of Education**
300 Sower Blvd
5th Fl
Frankfort, KY 40601 502-564-3141
http://www.education.ky.gov
webmaster@education.ky.gov
Dr. Wayne D. Lewis, Jr., Interim Commissioner

1637 **Kentucky Protection and Advocacy**
5 Mill Creek Park
Frankfort, KY 40601 502-564-2967
800-372-2988
Fax: 502-695-6764
http://www.kypa.net
kypandainquiry@gmail.com
Marsha Hockensmith, Executive Director
An independent state agency that was designated by the Governor as the protection and advocacy agency for Kentucky. To protect and promote the rights of Kentuckians with disabilities through legally based individuals and systemic advocacy, and education.

1638 **Learning Disabilities Association of Kentucky**
2210 Goldsmith Ln
Ste 118
Louisville, KY 40218 502-473-1256
http://www.ldaofky.org
LDAofKY@yahoo.com
Tim Woods, Executive Director
A non-profit organization of individuals with learning differences and attention difficulties, their parents, educators, and other service providers.

Louisiana

1639 **Client Assistance Program (CAP): Louisiana HDQS Division of Persons with Disabilities**
Advocacy Center
8325 Oak St
New Orleans, LA 70118 800-960-7705
Fax: 504-522-5507
http://www.advocacyla.org
advocacycenter@advocacyla.org
Bob Whitney, Interim Executive Director
Jason Kehoe, Chief Financial Officer
Sarah Voigt, Legal Director
Advocacy services to applicants and clients of Louisiana Rehabilitation Services (LRS) and American Indian Rehabilitation Services (AIRS). No fee. Committed to the belief in the dignity of every life and the freedom of everyone to experience the highest degree of self-determination. Exists to protect and advocate for human and legal rights of the elderly and disabled. Umbrella organization for Advocacy Centers in Baton Rouge, Lafayette, Shreveport, Monroe, Pineville, Jackson, and Mandeville.

1640 **Correctional Education**
Louisiana Department of Public Safety & Correction
PO Box 94304
Baton Rouge, LA 70804-9304 225-342-6740
Fax: 225-342-3095
http://doc.la.gov/education
James M. Le Blanc, Secretary
Promotes quality correctional education.

1641 **Louisiana Assistive Technology Access Network**
3042 Old Forge Dr
Ste D
Baton Rouge, LA 70808 225-925-9500
800-270-6185
http://www.latan.org
info@latan.org
Yakima Black, President & CEO
Assists individuals with disabilities to achieve a higher quality of life and greater independence through increased access to assistive technology as part of their daily lives.

1642 **Louisiana Department of Children & Family Services**
627 N 4th St
Baton Rouge, LA 70802 888-524-3578
http://www.dcfs.la.gov
LAHelpU.dcfs@la.gov
John Bel Edwards, Governor
The Louisiana Department of Children and Family Services is responsible for the state's foster care system, child protection investigations, family services, Family Independence Temporary Assistance Prgram (FITAP), disability determination, and more.

1643 **State Department of Education**
Department of Education
1201 N 3rd St
Baton Rouge, LA 70802-5243 877-453-2721
http://www.louisianabelieves.com
John White, Superintendent

1644 **State GED Administration**
Louisiana Department of Education
2888 Brightside Dr
Baton Rouge, LA 70804
225-763-5515
877-453-2721
http://www.louisianabelieves.com
John White, Superintendent
Promotes quality adult education.

Maine

1645 **Adult Education Program**
Maine Department of Education
23 State House Station
Augusta, ME 04333-0023
207-624-6000
Fax: 207-624-6700
http://www.maine.gov/doe/adulted
Robert Hasson, Commissioner
Gail Senese, Director, Even Start Coordinator
Amy Poland, Director, Adult Edu. Specialist
Offers courses in literacy and basic education, GED testing, college transition assistance, career preperation, and distance learning.

1646 **Bureau of Rehabilitation Services**
Department of Labor
150 State House Station
Augusta, ME 04333-0150
207-623-6799
800-760-1573
Fax: 207-287-5292
TTY: 207-623-6799
http://www.maine.gov/rehab
John Butera, Commissioner
Works to bring about full access to employment, independence and community integration for people with disabilities.

1647 **Client Assistance Program (CAP)**
C.A.R.E.S., Inc.
134 Main St
Ste 2C
Winthrop, ME 04364
207-377-7055
800-773-7055
Fax: 207-377-7057
http://www.caresinc.org
kathy.despres@caresin.org
Stephen Beam, Executive Director
Kathy Despres, Program Director
Jenny Ardito, Advocate
A federally funded program that provides information, assistance and advocacy to people with disabilities who are applying for or receiving services under the Rehabilitation Act.
1988

1648 **Developmental Disabilities Council**
225 Western Ave
Ste 4
Augusta, ME 04330
207-287-4213
800-244-3990
Fax: 207-287-8001
http://www.maineddc.org
nancy.e.cronin@maine.gov
Nancy Cronin, Executive Director
Rachel Dyer, Associate Director
Angela Burgess, Program Associate
A partnership of people with developmental disabilities, family memebers, and state and local agencies and organizations. The purpose is to assure that individuals with disabilities and their families participate in the design of, and have access to needed community services, individualized supports, and other forms of assistance thqat promote-self determination, independence, productivity, integration, and inclusion in all facets of family and community life.

1649 **Maine Human Rights Commission**
51 State House Station
Augusta, ME 04333
207-624-6290
Fax: 207-624-8729
http://www.maine.gov/mhrc
amy.sneirson@mhrc.maine.gov
Amy Sneirson, Executtive Director
Barbara Archer Hirsch, Commission Counsel
Alice Neal, Chief Investigator
Holds the responsibility of enforcing Maine's anti-discrimination laws. The Commission investigates complaints of unlawful discrimination in employmen, housing, education, access to public accommodatoins, extension of credit, and offensive names.

1650 **Protection & Advocacy Agency**
Disability Rights Center
24 Stone St
Ste 204
Augusta, ME 04330
207-626-2774
800-452-1948
Fax: 207-621-1419
TTY: 800-452-1948
http://www.drcme.org
advocate@drcme.org
Kim Moody, Executive Director
Rick Langley, Deputy Director
Peter M. Rice, Esq., Legal Director
The Disability Rights Center is Maine's protection and advocacy agency for people with disabilities. To enhance and promote the equality, self-determination, independence, productivity, integratio, and inclusion of people with disabilities through education, strategoc advocacy and legal intervention.

1651 **Security and Employment Service Center**
Dept of Administrative and Financial Services
108 State House Station
Augusta, ME 04333-0108
207-623-6700
Fax: 207-287-8394
http://www.maine.gov/sesc
Katharine Wiltuck, Director
Marilyn Leimbach, Deputy Director
Susan Bell, Director of Human Resources
Provides financial and human resource services to the Departments of Defense, Veterans, and Emergency Management; Labor; Professional and Financial REgulation; and, Public Safety.

Maryland

1652 **Client Assistance Program (CAP) Maryland Division of Rehabilitation Services**
2301 Argonne Drive
Baltimore, MD 21218
410-554-9442
888-554-0334
TDD: 443-798-2840
http://dors.maryland.gov
dors@maryland.gov
Thomas Laverty, Director
Megan Glaze-Keller, Staff Specialist
Helps individuals who have concerns or difficulties when applying or receiving rehabiliation services funded under the Rehabilitation Act.

1653 **Disability Law Center**
1500ÿUnion Ave
Ste 2000
Baltimore, MD 21211
410-727-6352
800-233-7201
Fax: 410-727-6389
TTY: 410-235-5387
http://disabilityrightsmd.org
feedback@DisabilityRightsMD.org
Robin Murphy, Executive Director
Meghan Marsh, Director of Operations
Charmaine Glass, Director of Finance

A provate, non-profit organization staffed by attorneys and paralegals. MDLC is the Protection and Advocacy organization for Maryland. MDLC's mission is to endure that people with disabilities are accorded the full rights and entitlements afforded to them by state and federal law.

1654 **Disability Rights Maryland**
1500 Union Ave
Ste 2000
Baltimore, MD 21211
410-727-6352
800-233-7201
Fax: 410-727-6389
TTY: 410-235-5387
http://www.disabilityrightsmd.org
feedback@DisabilityRightsMD.org
Robin Murphy, Executive Director
Charmaine Glass, Director of Finance
Meghan Marsh, Director of Operations
A nonprofit organization dedicated to improving the quality of life for people with learning disabilities and developmental disabilities.

1655 **Maryland Developmental Disabilities Council**
217 E Redwood St
Ste 1300
Baltimore, MD 21202
410-767-3670
800-305-6441
Fax: 410-333-3686
http://www.md-council.org
info@md-council.org
Brian Cox, Executive Director
Rachel London, Esq., Deputy Director
Faye Bell-Boulware, Administrative Coordinator
A public policy organization comprised of people with disabilities and family memebers who are joined by state officials, service providers an dother designated partners. Also an independent, self-governing organization that represents the interests of people with developmental disabilities and their families.

1656 **Maryland Technology Assistance Program**
Department of Disabilities
Rm T-17
2301 Argonne Dr
Baltimore, MD 21218
410-554-9230
800-832-4827
Fax: 410-554-9237
TTY: 866-881-7488
http://mdod.maryland.gov/mdtap
mdtap@mdtap.org
James McCarthy, Executive Director
Provides tools to help people who are disabled or elderly enjoy the same rights and opportunities as other citizens.

1657 **State Department of Education**
200 W Baltimore St
Baltimore, MD 21201-2595
410-767-0100
888-246-0016
TDD: 410-333-6442
http://www.marylandpublicschools.org
info.msde@maryland.gov
Mirya Simpson, Executive Director
Dr. Karen B. Salmon, State Superintendent
To provide leadership, support, and accountability for effective systems of public education, library services, and rehabilitation services.

Massachusetts

1658 **Autism Support Center: Northshore Arc**
6 Southside Rd
Danvers, MA 01923
978-777-9135
http://ne-arc.org/services/autism-services
asc@ne-arc.org
Jo Ann Simons, Chief Executive Officer
Joanne Plourde, Chief Operating Officer
Cyndi Gavlick, Chief Financial Officer
Created to support parents and professionals who expressed a need for assistance finding information and support about autism, pervasive developmental disorder (PDD) and Asperger's Disorder. Empowers families who have a member with autism or related disorder by providing current, accurate, and unbiased information about autism, services, referrals, resources and research trends.
1991

1659 **Department of Corrections**
50 Maple St
Milford, MA 01757
508-422-3300
http://www.mass.gov
Charlie Baker, Governor
Promote public safety by incarcerating offenders while providing opportunities for participation in effective programs.

1660 **Massachusetts Commission Against Discrimination**
1 Ashburton Place
Boston, MA 02108
617-994-6000
Fax: 617-994-6024
TTY: 617-994-6196
http://www.mass.gov
assistanttochairman@state.ma.us
Thomas Gallitano, Chair
Tani Sapirstein, Vice Chair
The state's chief civil rights agency that works to eliminate discrimination on a variety of bases and areas, and strives to advance the civil rights of the people of the Commonwealth through law enforcement, outreach and training.

1661 **Massachusetts General Education Development (GED)**
MA Department of Elementary & Secondary Education
75 Pleasant St
Malden, MA 02148-4906
781-338-3000
TTY: 800-439-2370
http://www.doe.mass.edu
eoewebservices@doe.mass.edu
Tom Mechem, State GED Chief Examiner
Jeff C. Riley, Commissioner
Twelve test centers operate state-wide to serve the needs of the adult population in need of a high school credential.

1662 **Massachusetts Office on Disability**
One Ashburton Pl
Room 1305
Boston, MA 02108
617-727-7440
800-322-2020
Fax: 617-727-0965
TTY: 617-727-7440
http://www.mass.gov
David D'Arcangelo, Director
To bring about full and equal participation of people with disabilities in all aspects of life. It works to assure the advancement of legal rights and for the promotion of maximum opportunities, supportive services, accommodations and accessibility in a manner which fosters dignity and self determination.

1663 **Massachusetts Rehabilitation Commission**
600 Washington St
Boston, MA 02211
617-204-3600
800-245-6543
Fax: 617-727-1354
TDD: 800-245-6543
http://www.mass.gov/mrc
commissioner@mrc.state.ma.us
Toni A. Wolf, Commissioner
Promotes dignity for individuals with disabilities through employment and independent living in the community.

1664 **Office of Civil Rights: Massachusetts**
US Department of Education
400 Maryland Ave SW
Washington, DC 20202
800-421-3481
Fax: 202-453-6012
TDD: 800-877-8339
http://www.ed.gov
ocr@ed.gov

Earl Morgan, Executive Officer
Kristine Minami, Senior Counsel
Kenneth L. Marcus, Assistant Secretary
This office covers the states of Connecticut, Maine, Massachusetts, New Hampshire, Rhode Island and Vermont.

1665 **Office of Federal Contract Compliance**
US Department of Labor
201 Varick St
Room 750
New York, NY 10014-4800 646-264-3170
Fax: 646-264-3009
TTY: 877-889-5627
http://www.dol.gov/ofccp
OFCCP-NE-CC4@dol.gov
Ondray T. Harris, Director
Craig E. Leen, Deputy Director
Kelley Smith, Chief of Staff
Enforces laws prohibiting employment discrimination on the basis of disability. This office represents New Jersey, New York, Puerto Rico, Virgin Islands, Connecticut, Maine, Massachusetts, New Hampshire, Rhode Island, and Vermont.

1666 **Protection & Advocacy Agency**
Disability Law Center
11 Beacon St
Ste 925
Boston, MA 02108 617-723-8455
800-872-9992
Fax: 617-723-9125
TTY: 617-892-4404
http://www.dlc-ma.org
mail@dlc-ma.org
Joseph Ambash, Esq., President
Scott Semel, Esq., Vice President & Treasurer
Shey Jaboin, Secretary
A private, non-profit organization responsible for providing protection and advocacy for the rights of Massachusetts residents with disabilities. Provides legal advocacy on disability issues that promote the fundamental rights of all people with disabilities to participate fully and equally in the social and economic life of Massachusetts.

1667 **Region I: Office for Civil Rights**
US Department Health & Human Services
200 Independence Ave SW
Washington, DC 20201 877-696-6775
http://www.hhs.gov
Alex M. Azar II, Secretary
Eric D. Hargan, Deputy Secretary
Peter Urbanowicz, Chief of Staff

1668 **Region I: US Small Business Administration**
Massachusetts District Office
10 Causeway St
Ste 265A
Boston, MA 02222 617-565-8416
Fax: 617-565-8420
http://www.sba.gov/offices/regional/i
Wendell G. Davis, Regional Administrator
Elizabeth Moisuk, Regional Communications Director
These regional offices of agencies enforce laws prohibiting employment discrimination on the basis of disability. Region I represents Connecticut, Maine, Massachusetts, New Hampshire, Rhode Island, and Vermont.

1669 **State Department of Adult Education**
Adult and Community Learning Services
75 Pleasant St
Malden, MA 02148-4906 781-338-3000
TTY: 800-439-2370
http://www.doe.mass.edu/acls/#
acls@doe.mass.edu
Tom Mechem, State GED Chief Examiner
Jeff C. Riley, Commissioner
Adult and Community Learning Services, a unit at the MA Department of Education, oversees and improves no-cost basic educational services (ABE) for adults in Masssachusetts. ACLS's mission is to provide each and every adult with opportunities to develop literacy skills needed to qualify for further education, job training, and better employment, and to reach his/her full potential as a family member, productive worker, and citizen.

Michigan

1670 **Client Assistance Program (CAP): Michigan Department of Persons with Disabilities**
4095 Legacy Pkwyÿ
Ste 500
Lansing, MI 48911-4264 517-487-1755
800-288-5923
Fax: 517-487-0827
TTY: 517-374-4687
http://www.mpas.org
John McCulloch, President, Royal Oak
Veda A. Sharp. MSW, First VP, Detroit
Elmer L. Cerano, Executive Director
Assists people who are seeking or receiving services from Michigan Rehabilitation Services, Consumer Choice Programs, Michigan Commission for the Blind, Centers for Independent Living, and Supported Employment and Transition Programs.

1671 **Michigan Correctional Educational Division**
Department of Corrections
206 E Michigan Ave, Grandview Plz
PO Box 30003
Lansing, MI 48909 517-335-1426
http://www.michigan.gov/corrections
mdoc-cfa-admin@michigan.gov
Ken McKee, Correctional Facilities Director
Rick Snyder, Governor
The Michigan Department of Corrections offers an education program for inmates in order to help them develop their academic, work and social competence. Program includes Employment Readiness, ABE, GED, and ELS classes, Career and Technical education, Career and Technical Counseling, as well as college courses.

1672 **Michigan Developmental Disabilities Council**
Department of Health & Human Services
320 S Walnut St
Lansing, MI 48913 517-335-3158
Fax: 517-335-2751
TDD: 517-335-3171
http://www.michigan.gov/mdhhs
mdhhs-dd-council@michigan.gov
Vendella M. Collins, Executive Director
The Michigan Developmental Disabilities Council is an advocacy organization for people with developmental disabilities. Promotes equal opportunities.

1673 **Michigan Disability Resources**
234 W Baraga Ave
Marquette, MI 49855 906-228-2850
http://www.michigan.gov/disabilityresources
Rick Snyder, Governor
An online resources center for all information pertaining to programs and services for people with physical and developmental disabilities.

1674 **Michigan Protection and Advocacy Service**
4095 Legacy Pkwyÿ
Ste 500
Lansing, MI 48911-4264 517-487-1755
800-288-5923
Fax: 517-487-0827
TTY: 517-374-4687
http://www.mpas.org
John McCulloch, President, Royal Oak
Veda A. Sharp, MSW, First VP, Detroit
Elmer L. Cerano, Executive Director

Advocates for people with disabilities and gives information and advice about their rights as a person with disabilities.

1675 **Michigan Rehabilitation Services**
Department of Health & Human Services
333 S Grand Ave
PO Box 30195
Lansing, MI 48909 517-373-3740
http://www.michigan.gov/mdhhs
Rick Snyder, Governor
Provides employment and educational services and training for teenagers and adults with disabilities. MRS works in collaboration with local school systems, Michigan Career and Technical Institute, community colleges, and other postsecondary institutions.

1676 **State Department of Adult Education**
Michigan Department of Education
608 W Allegan St
PO Box 30008
Lansing, MI 48909 833-633-5788
Fax: 517-355-4565
http://www.michigan.gov/mde
adulted@michigan.gov
Shella Allese, Interim Superintendent
Randy Riley, Director, Library of Michigan
Promotes quality adult education.

1677 **State GED Administration**
Michigan Department of Education
608 W Allegan St
PO Box 30008
Lansing, MI 48909 833-633-5788
Fax: 517-355-4565
http://www.michigan.gov
adulted@michigan.gov
Shella Allese, Interim Superintendent
Randy Riley, Director, Library of Michigan
Promotes adult education.

Minnesota

1678 **Education Division: Minnesota Department of Corrections**
1450 Energy Park Dr
Ste 200
St. Paul, MN 55108-5219 651-361-7200
Fax: 651-642-0223
http://mn.gov/doc
Marcie Koetke, Education Director
Tom Roy, Commissioner
Sarah J. Fitzgerald, Communications Director
Offers educational programs such as GED classes and testing, English as a Second Language, high school Refresher courses, and computer instruction courses.

1679 **Health Services Minneapolis**
University of St Thomas
Brady Residence Hall
Lower Level
St. Paul, MN 651-962-6750
http://www.stthomas.edu/healthservices
healthservices@stthomas.edu
Madonna McDermott, MS, MPA, Exec. Dir., Health & Wellness
Marilee Votel-Kvall, MD, Medical Director
Dena Abrahamson, Systems Specialist
Provides special services and resources to meet the unique needs of graduate students, education students (both graduate and undergraduate), and alumni/ae.

1680 **Minnesota Department of Early Childhood Family Education (ECFE)**
Department of Education
1500 Highwayÿ36 W
Roseville, MN 55113-4266 651-582-8200
http://www.education.state.mn.us
Dr. Brenda Cassellius, Commissioner
Jessie Montano, Deputy Commissioner
A public school program for Minnesota families with children between infancy to kindergarten entrance. ECFE's goal is to assist parents in providing early education.

1681 **Minnesota Department of Education**
1500 Highway 36 W
Roseville, MN 55113 651-582-8200
http://education.mn.gov
mde.commissioner@state.mn.us
Brenda Cassellius, Commissioner
Charlene Briner, Deputy Commissioner
Josh Collins, Communications Director

1682 **Minnesota Department of Human Rights**
625 Robert St N
Freeman Building
St. Paul, MN 55155 651-539-1100
800-657-3704
Fax: 651-296-9042
TTY: 800-627-3529
http://mn.gov/mdhr
info.MDHR@state.mn.us
Kevin M. Lindsey, Commissioner
Rowzat Shipchandler, Deputy Commissioner
Christine Dufour, Communications
The Minnesota Department of Human Rights (MDHR) is a neutral state agency that investigates charges of illegal discrimination, ensures that businesses seeking state contracts are in compliance with equal opportunity requirements, and trives to eliminate discrimination by educating Minnesotans about their rights and responsibilities under the state Human Rights Act.

1683 **Minnesota Governor's Council on Developmental Disabilities**
658 Cedar St
370 Centennial Office Building
St. Paul, MN 55155 651-296-4018
877-348-0505
Fax: 651-297-7200
TTY: 800-627-3529
http://mn.gov/mnddc
admin.dd@state.mn.us
Colleen Wieck, PhD, Executive Officer
Michelle Albeck, Council Member
Ashley Bailey, Council Member
To provide information, education, and training to build knowledge, develop skills, and change attitudes that will lead to increased independence, productivity, self determination, integration and inclusion for all people with developmental disabilities and their families.

1684 **Minnesota's Assistive Technology Act Program**
Minnesota STAR Program
658 Cedar St
358 Centennial Office Building
St. Paul, MN 55155 651-201-2640
888-234-1267
Fax: 651-282-6671
TTY: 800-627-3529
http://mn.gov/admin/star
star.program@state.mn.us
Kim Moccia, Program Director
Joan Gillum, Contracts Coordinator
STAR's mission is to help all Minnesotans with disabilities gain access to and acquire the assistive technology they need to live, learn, work and play. The Minnesota STAR Program is federally funded by the Rehabilitation Services Administration in assordance with the Assistive Technology Act of 1998.

1685 **Protection & Advocacy Agency**
Minnesota Disability Law Center
430 1st Avenue N
Minneapolis, MN 55401 612-334-5970
http://mylegalaid.org

Drew Schaffer, Executive Director
Lisa Cohen, Deputy Director for Operations
Andrea Kaufman, Director of Development
To advance the dignity, self-determination and equality of individuals with disabilities.

1686 **State Department of Adult Basic Education**
Department of Education
1500 Highwayÿ36 W
Roseville, MN 55113
651-582-8200
Fax: 651-582-8202
http://education.mn.gov
mde.commissioner@state.mn.us
Dr. Brenda Cassellius, Commissioner
Charlene Brinder, Deputy Commissioner
Josh Collins, Communications Director
Offered through Minnesota's public school system, provides opportunities to obtain academic, interpersonal and problem-solving skills necessary to live self-sufficient lives.

Mississippi

1687 **Adult Career & Technical Education**
Mississippi Department of Education
359 North West St
PO Box 771ÿ
Jackson, MS 39205
601-359-3974
Fax: 601-359-6619
http://www.mde.k12.ms.us/cte/pa/adult_learners
Carey M. Wright, EdD, Superintendent
Promotes adult education through training courses.

1688 **Disability Rights Mississippi**
5 Old River Pl
Ste 101
Jackson, MS 39202
601-968-0600
800-772-4057
Fax: 601-968-0665
http://www.drms.ms
ptribble@drms.ms
Polly Tribble, Executive Director
Beverly Sheriff, Chief Financial Officer
Micah Dutro, Legal Director
A nonprofit organization dedicated to improving the quality of life for people with learning disabilities and developmental disabilities.

1689 **Mississippi Department of Corrections**
633 N State St
Jackson, MS 39202
601-359-5600
http://www.mdoc.ms.gov
officeofcommunications@mdoc.state.ms.us
Pelicia E. Hall, Commissioner
Grace Fisher, Communications Director
To provide and promote public safety through efficient and effective offender custody, care, control and treatment consistent with sound correctional prinicipals and constitutional standards.

1690 **Mississippi Department of Employment Security**
1235 Echelon Prkwy
PO Box 1699
Jackson, MS 39215-1699
601-321-6000
http://www.mdes.ms.gov
comments@mdes.ms.gov
Mark Henry, Executive Director
A state agency to help citizens find jobs through the Job Centers. Temporary unemployment benefits are also available.

1691 **Mississippi Project START**
PO Box 1698
Jackson, MS 39215-1698
601-853-5249
800-852-8328
Fax: 601-853-5218
http://www.msprojectstart.org
nsimmons@mdrs.ms.gov
Patsy Galtelli, Project Director
Nekeba Simmons, Administrative Assistant
Quincy Walker, Program Coordinator
To ensure the provision of appropriate Technology-Related services for Mississippians with disabilities by increasing the awareness of and access to Assistive Technology and by helping the existing service systems to become more consumer repsonsive so that all Mississippians with disabilities will receive appropriate Technology-related services and devices.

1692 **Mississippi Vocational Rehabilitation**
Department of Rehabilitation Services
1281 Highway 51
Madison, MS 39110
800-443-1000
http://www.mdrs.ms.gov/vocationalrehab
ccirrequests@mdrs.ms.gov
Lavonda Hart, Director
A federal state program that works with people who have physical or mental disabilities to prepare for, gain or retain employment.

1693 **State Department of Education**
359 North West St
PO Box 771ÿ
Jackson, MS 39205
601-359-3513
http://www.mde.k12.ms.us
Carey M. Wright, EdD, Superintendent
Dr. Jason S. Dean, Chair
Buddy Bailey, Vice Chair
Promotes quality education.

Missouri

1694 **Assistive Technology**
1501 NW Jefferson St
Blue Springs, MO 64015
816-655-6700
http://at.mo.gov
info@mo-at.org
David Baker, Director
Michael L. Parson, Governor
Eileen Belton, Program Coordinator
To increase access to assistive technology for Missourians with all types of disabilities, of all ages.

1695 **EEOC St. Louis District Office**
Robert A Young Federal Building
1222 Spruce St
Rm 8.100
Saint Louis, MO 63103
800-669-4000
Fax: 314-539-7894
TDD: 844-234-5122
TTY: 800-669-6820
http://www.eeoc.gov
James R. Neely, Jr., Director
Andrea Baran, Regional Attorney
These regional offices of agencies enforce laws prohibiting employment discrimination on the basis of disability.

1696 **Governor's Council on Disability (GCD)**
301 W High St, Rm 840
PO Box 1668
Jefferson City, MO 65102
573-751-2600
800-877-8249
Fax: 573-526-4109
http://disability.mo.gov/gcd
gcd@oa.mo.gov
Michael L. Parson, Governor
Claudia Browner, Executive Director
Yvonne Wright, Chair
GCD promotes the inclusion of Missourians with disabilities in all aspects of community life by education residents, employers, schools and universities of their rights and responsibilities under the Americans with Disabilities Act. Educational seminars and training are available.

1697 **Great Plains Disability and Business Technical Assistance Center (DBTAC)**
100 Corporate Lake Dr
Columbia, MO 65203
573-882-3600
800-949-4232
Fax: 573-884-4925
TTY: 573-882-3600
http://www.gpadacenter.org
adacenter@missouri.edu
Jim de Jong, Executive Director
Chuck Graham, Associate Director
Espoir Mabengo, Information Specialist
To provide information, materials and technical assistance to individuals and entities that are covered by the Americans with Disabilities Act. In addition to the ADA, Great Plains ADA Center provides the ADA and disability-related legislation such as the Family Medical Leave Act, Workforce Investment Act and the Telecommunications Act.

1698 **Missouri Department of Elementary & Secondary Education**
205 Jefferson St
Jefferson City, MO 65101
573-751-4212
http://dese.mo.gov
Michael L. Parson, Governor
Dr. Roger Dorson, Interim Commissioner

1699 **Missouri Developmental Disabilitis Council**
1706 E Elm St
PO Box 687
Jefferson City, MO 65102
573-751-8611
800-500-7878
Fax: 573-526-2755
http://www.moddcouncil.org
cholterman@moddcouncil.org
Vicky Davidson, Executive Director
Dolores Sparks, Program Coordinator/Advocate
Katheryne Staeger-Wilson, Program Coordinator/Outreach
Works in partnership with state and federal agencies to help develop, improve and expand services and programs that support people with developmental disabilities.

1700 **Missouri Protection & Advocacy Services**
925 S Country Club Dr
Jefferson City, MO 65109
573-659-0678
800-392-8667
Fax: 573-659-0677
TDD: 800-735-2966
http://www.moadvocacy.org
app.unit@mo-pa.org
Sharon Williams, Chair, Lee's Summit
Jason Mize, Vice Chair, Columbia
Katharine Kinder, Secretary/Treasurer, Columbia
A federally mandated system in the state of Missouri which provides protection of the rights of persons with disabilities through leagally-based avocacy

1701 **Office of Civil Rights: Missouri**
US Department of Education
400 Maryland Ave SW
Washington, DC 20202
800-421-3481
Fax: 202-453-6012
TDD: 800-877-8339
http://www.ed.gov
ocr@ed.gov
Kenneth L. Marcus, Assistant Secretary
Earl Morgan, Executive Director
Kristine Minami, Senior Counsel
This office covers the states of Kansas, Missouri, Nebraska, Oklahoma and South Dakota.

1702 **Region VII: US Department of Health and Human Services**
Office For Civil Rights
601 East 12th St
Room S1801
Kansas City, MO 64106
816-426-2821
http://www.hhs.gov
Jeff Kahrs, JD, Regional Director
Timothy Noonan, Regional Manager

Montana

1703 **Assistive Technology Project**
University of Montana Rural Institute
MonTECH Program
29 McGill Hall
Missoula, MT 59812
406-243-5751
877-243-5511
Fax: 406-243-4730
http://montech.ruralinsitute.umt.edu
montech@ruralinstitute.umt.edu
Anna Margaret Goldman, Prgram Director
Dave Gentry, Assistive Technology Resources
Shawn Hanson, Outreach Coordinator
This statewide program at the University of Montana promotes assistive devices and services for persons of all ages with disabilities.

1704 **Correctional Education**
Montana Department of Corrections
5 S Last Chance Gulch
PO Box 201301
Helena, MT 59620-1301
406-444-3930
Fax: 406-444-4920
http://cor.mt.gov
Reginald D. Michael, Director
Cynthia L. Wolken, Deputy Director
Judy Beck, Communications Director
Provides education programs for inmates.

1705 **Disability Rights Montana**
1022 Chestnut St
Helena, MT 59601
406-449-2344
800-245-4743
Fax: 406-449-2418
http://disabilityrightsmt.org
advocate@disabilityrightsmt.org
Bernadette Franks-Ongoy, Executive Director
Christine Simonich, Advocate Specialist
Faun Pullin, Office Coordinator
A nonprofit organization dedicated to improving the quality of life for people with learning disabilities and developmental disabilities.

1706 **Montana Council on Developmental Disabilities (MCDD)**
2714 Billings Ave
Helena, MT 59601
406-443-4332
866-443-4332
Fax: 406-443-4192
http://www.mtcdd.org
deborah@mtcdd.org
Deborah Swingley, CEO/Executive Director
Dee Burrell, Contract Manager
The goal of the Council is to increase the indpendence, productivity, inclusion and integration into the community of people with developmental disabilities through systemic change, capacity building and advocacy activities.

1707 **Montana Department of Labor & Industry**
PO Box 1728
Helena, MT 59624-1728
406-444-2840
Fax: 406-444-1419
TTY: 406-444-0532
http://dli.mt.gov
dliquestions@mt.gov

Galen Hollenbaugh, Commissioner
Jake Troyer, Communications Director
Rende Mackay, Human Resources Director
Promotes the well-being of Montana's workers, employers, and all citizens, and upholds their rights and responsibilities. Committed to being responsive to communities and businesses at the local level.

1708 **Montana Developmental Services Division**
Department of Public Health & Human Services
111 Sanders
Rm 305
Helena, MT 59604
406-444-2995
Fax: 406-444-0230
http://dphhs.mt.gov/dsd
Novelene Martin, Bureau Chief
Sheila Hogan, Director
Offers additional services for people with developmental disabilities and their families seperate from programs provided through schools, Medicaid, private insurance and social security.

1709 **Montana Disability Employment & Transition**
Department of Public Health & Human Services
111 Sanders St
Helena, MT 59604
406-444-2995
Fax: 406-444-0230
http://dphhs.mt.gov/detd
Sheila Hogan, Director
Dedicated to helping people with disabilities gain and sustain employment in order to enhance independence and allow for further opportunity.

1710 **Montana Office of Public Instruction**
PO Box 202501
Helena, MT 59620-2501
406-444-3095
888-231-9393
http://opi.mt.gov
Elsie Arntzen, Superintendent
Phoebe Williams, Executive Office Administrator
Dylan Klapmeier, Communications Director
Supports local schools, students and parents across the state of Montana in order to achieve quality education.

1711 **Office of Adult Basic and Literacy Education**
Montana Office of Public Instruction
PO Box 202501
Helena, MT 59620-2501
406-444-4443
http://opi.mt.gov
katie.madsen@mt.gov
Katie Madsen, Manager
Adult education programs include basic literacy, workplace literacy, family literacy, preparation for GED, English as a Second Language and other services that provide adults and out of school youth opportunities at enhancing skills, improving parenting, and youth assistance related to employment and self-sufficiency.

1712 **University of Montana's Rural Institute - MonTECH Program**
29 McGill Hall
Missoula, MT 59812
406-243-5751
877-243-5511
Fax: 406-243-4730
http://montech.ruralinstitute.umt.edu
montech@ruralinstitute.umt.edu
Anna Margaret Goldman, Program Director
Bobby Dutreix, Technical Support
Shawna Hanson, Outreach Coordinator
A program of the University of Montana Rural Institute: Center for Excellence in Disability, Education, Research and Service. Specialize in Assistive Technology and oversee a variety of AT related grants and contracts. The overall goal is to develop a comprehensive, statewide system of assistive technology related assistance.

Nebraska

1713 **Answers4Families: Center on Children, Families and the Law**
206 S 13th St
Ste 1000
Lincoln, NE 68588-0227
402-472-0844
800-746-8420
http://www.answers4families.org
A project of the Center on Children, Families and Law at University of Nebraska. Mission is to provide info, opportunities, education and support to Nebraskans through Internet resources. The Center serves individuals with special needs and mental health disorders, foster families, caregivers, assisted living, and school nurses.
1994

1714 **Assistive Technology Partnership**
3901 N 27th St
Ste 5
Lincoln, NE 68521
402-471-0734
877-713-4002
Fax: 402-471-6052
http://atp.nebraska.gov
Chris Gaspari, Chair
Dedicated to helping Nebraskans with disabilities, their families and professionals obtain assistive technology devices and services.
1989

1715 **Client Assistance Program (CAP): Nebraska Hotline for Disability Services**
301 Centennial Mall S
Box 94987
Lincoln, NE 68509
402-471-0801
800-742-7594
http://www.cap.nebraska.gov
shari.bahensky@nebraska.gov
Shari Bahensky, Executive Director
The Client Assistance Program helps individuals who have concerns or difficulties when applying for or receiving rehabilitation services funded under the Rehabilitation Act.

1716 **Nebraska Advocacy Services**
Center for Disability Rights, Law & Advocacy
134 S 13th St
Ste 600
Lincoln, NE 68508
402-474-3183
800-422-6691
Fax: 402-474-3274
http://www.disabilityrightsnebraska.org
info@disabilityrightsnebraska.org
Eric Evans, Chief Executive Officer
Judy Sinner, Fiscal & HR Director
Tania Diaz, Legal Services Director
Created to assist individuals with disabilities and their families in protecting and advocating for their rights. From its beginning, NAS has promoted the principles of equality, self-determination, and dignity of persons with disabilities.

1717 **Nebraska Department of Labor**
Lincoln, NE
402-471-9000
http://www.dol.nebraska.gov

1718 **Nebraska Equal Opportunity Commission**
301 Centennial Mall S
5th Fl, PO Box 94934
Lincoln, NE 68509-4934
402-471-2024
800-642-6112
Fax: 402-471-4059
http://www.neoc.ne.gov
Marna Munn, Executive Director
Eric Drumheller, Chair
Rita Griess, Vice Chair
A state agency that investigates complaints of discrimination in employment, housing and public accomodations.

1719 **Nebraska Vocational Rehabilitation**
Nebraska Department of Education
P.O. Box 94987
Lincoln, NE 68509
402-471-3644
877-637-3422
Fax: 402-471-0788
http://www.vr.nebraska.gov
marketingteam.vr@nebraska.gov
Lindy Foley, Director
Nebraska VR helps people with disabilities prepare for, obtain, and maintain employment while helping businesses recruit, train, and retain employees with disabilities.

1720 **State Department of Education**
301 Centennial Mall S
PO Box 94987
Lincoln, NE 68509-4987
402-471-2295
Fax: 402-471-8127
http://www.education.ne.gov
Dr. Matthew Blomstedt, Commissioner
Brian Halstead, Chief of Staff
Dean Folkers, Chief Information Officer
Organized into teams that interact to operate the agency and carry out the duties assigned by state and federal statutes and the policy directions of the State Board of Education.

1721 **State GED Administration: Nebraska**
Nebraska Department of Education
301 Centennial Mall S
PO Box 94987
Lincoln, NE 68509-4987
402-471-2295
Fax: 402-471-0117
http://www.education.ne.gov
Dr. Matthew Blomstedt, Commissioner
Brian Halstead, Chief of Staff
Dean Folkers, Chief Information Officer
To provide educational opportunities for adults to improve their literacy skills to a level requisite for effective citizenship and productive employment. This includes preparation for and successful completion of the high school equivalency program.

Nevada

1722 **Assistive Technology for Independent Living (AT/IL) Program**
Nevada Aging & Disability Services Division
3416 Goni Rd
Ste D-132
Carson City, NV 89706
775-687-4210
http://adsd.nv.gov
adsd@adsd.nv.gov
Dena Schmidt, Administrator
Lisa Sherych, Deputy Administrator
Jennifer Frischmann, Manager, Quality Assurance
Promotes independent living through technology. Includes home and vehicle modifications, durable medical equipment, visual aids, mobility devices and personal communication technology.

1723 **Client Assistance Program (CAP): Nevada Division of Persons with Disability**
Dpt of Employment, Training and Rehabilitation
2820 W Charleston Blvd
Ste 11
Las Vegas, NV 89102
702-257-8150
888-349-3843
Fax: 702-257-8170
TTY: 888-349-3843
http://www.detr.state.nv.us
lasvegas@ndalc.org
Shelley Hendren, Rehabilitation Administrator
To assist and advocate for clients and applicants in their relationships with projects, programs, and community rehabilitation programs that provide services under the Act. The program is also responsible for informing individuals with disabilities in Nevada, of the services and benefits available to them.

1724 **Correctional Education and Vocational Training**
Nevada Department of Corrections
5500 Snyder Ave, Bldng 17
PO Box 7011
Carson City, NV 89702
775-887-3285
http://doc.nv.gov
Kim Petersen, Education Division Coordinator
James Dzurenda, Corrections Department Director
To continue and expand an educational training program which contains literacy, ESL, numeracy, community outreach, and vocational training that will provide long-term benefits to both inmates and the Nevada community in general.

1725 **Department of Employment, Training and Rehabilitation**
2800 E St. Louis Ave
Las Vegas, NV 89104
http://www.detr.state.nv.us
detradmn@nvdetr.org
Comprised of four divisions with numerous bureaus programs, and services housed in offices throughout Nevada to provide citizens the state's premier source of employment, training, and rehabilitative programs.

1726 **Nevada Bureau of Disability Adjudication**
Department of Employment, Training & Rehab
500 E Third St
Carson City, NV 89713
775-885-3700
800-882-4430
TTY: 800-882-4430
http://detr.state.nv.us
detradmn@nvdetr.org
Shelley Hendren, Rehabilitation Administrator
Evaluates applications from individuals with permanent disabilities to determine if they are eligible for federal Supplemental Security Income or Social Security Disability Insurance (SSDI).

1727 **Nevada Disability Advocacy and Law Center**
2820 W Charleston Blvd
Ste 11
Las Vegas, NV 89102
702-257-8150
888-349-3843
Fax: 702-257-8170
TTY: 702-257-8150
http://www.ndalc.org
lasvegas@ndalc.org
Jack Mayes, Executive Director
William Heaivilin, Supervising Rights Attorney
A private, nonprofit organization and serves as Nevada's federally mandated protection and advocacy system for the human, legal, and service rights of individuals with disabilities.

1728 **Nevada Equal Rights Commission**
Department of Employment, Training & Rehab
1820 E Sahara Ave
Ste 314
Las Vegas, NV 89104
702-486-7161
800-326-6868
Fax: 702-486-7054
TTY: 800-326-6868
http://www.nvdetr.org
detradmn@nvdetr.org
To foster the rights of all persons to seek, obtain and maintain employment, and to access services in places of public accomodation without discrimination, distinction, exclusion or restriction because of race, religion creed, color, age, sex (gender and/or orientation), disability, national origin, or ancestry.

1729 **Nevada Governor's Council on Developmental Disabilities**
896 W Nye Lane
Ste 202
Carson City, NV 89703
775-684-8619
Fax: 775-684-8626
http://www.nevadaddcouncil.org
elmarquez@dhhs.nv.gov

Kari Horn, Executive Director
Catherine Nielsen, Projects Manager
Ellen Marquez, Executive Assistant
To provide resources at the community level which promote equal opportunity and life choices for people with disabilities through which they may positively contribute to Nevada society.

1730 **Nevada State Rehabilitation Council**
Nevada Rehabilitation Division
2800 E St. Louis Ave
Las Vegas, NV 89104 702-486-5230
TTY: 702-486-1018
http://www.detr.state.nv.us
detradmn@nvdetr.org
Shelley Hendren, Rehabilitation Administrator
To help insure vocational rehabilitation programs are consumer oriented, driven and result in employment outcomes for Nevadans with disabilities. Funding for innovation and expansions grants.

1731 **State Department of Adult Education**
Nevada Department of Education
755 N Roop St
Ste 201
Carson City, NV 89701 775-687-5980
Fax: 775-687-5978
http://www.doe.nv.gov
Steve Canavero, PhD, Supt, Public Instruction
Brett Barley, Dep. Supt., Student Achievment
Roger Rahming, Dep. Supt., Business/Support Svc
To provide leadership and resources to enable all learners to gain knowledge and skills needed to achieve career and employment goals, meet civic duties and accomplish educational objective.

1732 **State Department of Education**
700 E Fifth St
Carson City, NV 89701 775-687-9200
Fax: 775-687-9101
http://www.doe.nv.gov
Steve Canavero, PhD, Supt., Public Intruction
Brett Barley, Dep. Supt., Student Achievement
Roger Rahming, Dep. Supt., Business/Support Svs
The Nevada State Board of Education acts as an advocate and visionary for all children and sets the policy that allows every child equal access to educational services, provides the vision for a premier educational system and works in partnership with other stakeholders to ensure high levels of success for all in terms of job readiness, graduation, ability to be lifelong learners, problem solvers, citizens able to adapt to a changing world and contributing members of a society.

New Hampshire

1733 **Granite State Independent Living**
21 Chenell Dr
Concord, NH 03301 603-228-9680
800-826-3700
Fax: 603-225-3304
http://www.gsil.org
info@gsil.org
Clyde E. Terry, JD, Chief Executive Officer
Debora Krider, EdD, Chief Operating Officer
Linda Tsantoulis, PHR, VP, Human Resources
A statewide non-profit, service and advocacy organization that provides tools for living life on your terms. To promote life with independence for people with disabilities through the four core services of advocacy, information, education and support.

1734 **Institute on Disability**
University of New Hampshire
10 West Edge Dr
Ste 101
Durham, NH 03824 603-862-4320
Fax: 603-862-0555
TTY: 800-735-2964
http://iod.unh.edu
contact.iod@unh.edu
Linda Bimbo, Acting Director
Jennifer Donahue, Finance Manager
Tobey Partch-Davies, PhD, Project Director
Established to provide a coherent university-based focus for the improvement of knowledge, policies, and practices related to the lives of persons with disabilities and their families. Also advances policies and systems changes, promising practices, education, and research that strengthen communities and ensure full access, equal opportunities, and participation for all persons.

1735 **New Hampshire Commission for Human Rights**
2 Industrial Park Dr
Concord, NH 03301 603-271-2767
http://www.nh.gov/hrc
humanrights@nh.gov
Matt Mayberry, Chair
Enforcement of RSA 354-A, the Law Against Discrimination and the ADA Title I, Employment, and Housing. Private School/Pre-and After School program enrollees, not public school. All employees covered regardless of public/private distinction if 6 or more employees (NH) 15 or more (Federal).

1736 **New Hampshire Developmental Disabilities Council**
1 1/2 Beacon St
Concord, NH 03301-4447 603-271-3236
Fax: 603-271-1156
http://www.nhddc.org
NHCDD.Director@ddc.nh.gov
Isadora Rodriguez-Legendre, Executive Director
Karen Blake, Chair
Chris Rueggeberg, Policy Director
A federally funded agency that supports public policies and initiatives that remove barriers and promote opportunities in all areas of life.

1737 **New Hampshire Disabilities Right Center**
64 N Main St
Ste 2, 3 Fl
Concord, NH 03301-4913 603-228-0432
800-834-1721
Fax: 603-225-2077
TTY: 800-834-1721
http://www.drcnh.org
advocacy@drcnh.org
Lisa DiMartino, President
John Tobin, Vice President
Cynthia Trottier, Treasurer
Dedicated to eliminating barriers existing in New Hampshire to the full an dequal enjoyment of civil and other legal rights by people with disabilities.

1738 **New Hampshire Employment Security**
45 S Fruit St
Concord, NH 03301-2410 603-228-4100
Fax: 603-229-4353
http://www.nhes.nh.gov
Carol.A.Aubut@nhes.nh.gov
George N. Copadis, Commissioner
Chris Sununu, Governor
Refers individuals with disabilities to organizations and agencies that assist people with disabilities without charge.

1739 **New Hampshire Governor's Commission on Disability**
121 S Fruit St
Ste 101
Concord, NH 03301
603-271-2773
800-852-3405
Fax: 603-271-2837
http://www.nh.gov/disability
disability@gcd.nh.gov

Chris Sununu, Governor
Paul Van Blarigan, Chair
H. Dee Clanton, Commission Member
Serves people with cross-disabilities, provides assistance and advocacy with the Americans with Disability Act and other disability law compliance. The Commission advives the Governor, the Legislature, and all state agencies in regards to disability-related compliance.

1740 **Parent Information Center**
54 Old Suncook Rd
Concord, NH 03301
603-224-7005
800-947-7005
Fax: 603-224-4365
http://www.picnh.org

Michelle Lewis, Executive Director
Tracy Messing, Office Manager
James Butterfield, Accountant
A recognized leader in building strong family/school partnerships. PIC provides information, support, and educational programs for parents, family members, educators, and the community. PIC is a pioneer in promoting effective parent involvment in the special education process.

1741 **ServiceLink**
Concord, NH 03301
http://www.nh.gov
disability@nh.gov

Chris Sununu, Governor
Provides community supportive information and referral assistance to Edlers, their families and Adults with Disabilities in accessing services for caregivee support, financial and legal concerns, home care services, housing information and assistance, recreational and social events, information about applying for Medicaid and Medicaid programs such as Choices For Independence program.

1742 **State Department of Education: Division of Career Technology & Adult Learning-Vocational Rehab**
101 Pleasant St
Concord, NH 03301-3494
603-271-3494
Fax: 603-271-1953
TTY: 603-271-3494
http://www.education.nh.gov
info@doe.nh.gov

Frank Edelblut, Commissioner
Christine Brennan, Deputy Commissioner
Provides services to both individuals with disabilities and employers. People with disabilities can work and take advantage of the opportunities available to the citizens of New Hampshire. A joint State/Federal program that seeks to empower people to make informed choices, build viable careers, and live more independently in the community.

New Jersey

1743 **Assistive Technology Center (ATAC)**
Disability Rights New Jersey
210 S Broad St
3rd Fl
Trenton, NJ 08608
609-292-9742
800-922-7233
Fax: 609-777-0187
TTY: 609-633-7106
http://www.drnj.org
advocate@drnj.org

Joseph Young, Executive Director
Ellen Catanese, Director of Administration
Assists individuals in overcoming barriers in the system and making assistive technology more accessible to individuals with disabilities throughout the state.

1744 **Disability Rights New Jersey**
210 S Broad St
3rd Floor
Trenton, NJ 08608
609-292-9742
800-922-7233
Fax: 609-777-0187
TTY: 609-633-7106
http://www.drnj.org
advocate@drnj.org

Joseph Young, Executive Director
Ellen Catanese, Director of Administration
To protect, advocate for and advance the rights of persons with disabilites in pursuit of a society in which persons with disabilities exercise self-determination and choice, and are treated with dignity.

1745 **New Jersey Attorney General's Office Department of Law and Public Safety**
PO Box 080
Trenton, NJ 08625-0080
609-292-4925
Fax: 609-292-3508
http://www.nj.gov/oag

Gurbir S. Grewal, Attorney General
The Division on Civil Rights enforces the New Jersey Law Against Discrimination which prohibits discrimination in employment, housing and public accommodations because of race, creed, color, national origin, ancestry, sex, affectional and sexual orientation, marital status, nationality or handicap.

1746 **New Jersey Department of Special Education**
New Jersey Department of Education
PO Box 500
Trenton, NJ 08625-0500
609-376-9060
Fax: 609-984-8422
http://www.nj.gov/education/specialed

Phil Murphy, Governor
Sheila Oliver, Lt. Governor
The office is resonsible for administering all federal funds received for educating people with disabilities ages 3 through 21. Also monitors the delivery of special education programs operated under state authority, provides mediation services to parents and school districts, processes hearings and conducts complaint investigations. Also funds four learning resource centers (LRCs) that provide information, circulate materials, offer technical assistance/consultation and production services.

1747 **New Jersey Programs for Infants and Toddlers with Disabilities: Early Intervention System**
New Jersey Department of Health
PO Box 360
Trenton, NJ 08625-0360 http://www.nj.gov/health/fhs/eis

Phil Murphy, Governor
Sheila Oliver, Lt. Governor
The New Jersey Early Intervention System provides a comprehensive system of services for children, birth to age three, with developmental delays or disabilities and their families.

1748 **State Department of Adult Education**
Department of Education
PO Box 500
Trenton, NJ 08625-0500
609-777-1050
Fax: 609-292-3768
http://www.state.nj.us/education
adulted@doe.nj.gov

Dr. Lamont Repollet, Acting Commissioner

1749 **State GED Administration: Office of Specialized Populations**
New Jersey Department of Education
PO Box 500
Trenton, NJ 08625 609-777-1050
Fax: 609-292-3768
http://www.state.nj.us/education
adulted@doe.nj.gov
Dr. Lamont Repollet, Acting Commissioner

New Mexico

1750 **Client Assistance Program (CAP): New Mexico Disability Rights**
3916 Juan Tabo Blvd NE
Albuquerque, NM 87111 505-256-3100
800-432-4682
Fax: 505-256-3184
TTY: 505-256-3100
http://www.drnm.org
info@drnm.org
Jeanne A. Hamrick, President
John Foley, Vice President
Jonathan Toledo, Secretary Treasurer
Helps persons with disabilities who have concerns about agencies in New Mexico that provide rehabilitation or independent living services. The kind of help may be information or advocacy. For questions about Division of Vocational Rehabilitation, Commission for the Blind, Independent Living Centers and Preojects With Industsry CAP can help.

1751 **Disability Rights New Mexico**
3916 Juan Tabo Blvd NE
Albuquerque, NM 87111 505-256-3100
800-432-4682
Fax: 505-256-3184
http://www.drnm.org
info@drnm.org
Jeanne A. Hamrick, President
John Foley, Vice President
Jonathan Toledo, Secretary/Treasurer
A nonprofit organization dedicated to improving the quality of life for people with learning disabilities and developmental disabilities.

1752 **New Mexico Department of Workforce Solutions**
401 Broadway NE
Albuquerque, NM 87102 877-664-6984
Fax: 505-841-8491
TTY: 505-841-8617
http://www.dws.state.nm.us
Serves the workforce of New Mexico, offering resources for job seekers, unemployment insurance, work compensation, trational services for veterans, and resources for businesses. The agency also makes information on the labor market accessable.

1753 **New Mexico Human Rights Commission**
490 Old Santa Fe Trail
Room 400
Santa Fe, NM 87501
http://www.governor.state.nm.us/human_rights
Susana Martinez, Governor
To eliminate discrimination across the state of New Mexico.

1754 **New Mexico Public Education Department**
300 Don Gaspar Ave
Santa Fe, NM 87501 505-827-1436
http://webnew.ped.state.nm.us
Christopher Ruszkowski, Secretary
Icela Pelayo, Dep. Secretary,Teaching/Learning
To provide leadership, technical assistance and quality assurance to improve student performance and close the achievement gap.

1755 **New Mexico State GED Testing Program**
New Mexico Public Education Department
300 Don Gaspar Ave
Santa Fe, NM 87501 505-827-5800
http://webnew.ped.state.nm.us
Christopher Ruszkowski, Secretary
Icela Pelayo, Dep. Secretary,Teaching/Learning
The primary aid of the GED testing program in New Mexico is to proive a second opportunity for individuals to obtain their high school diplomas.

1756 **New Mexico Technology Assistance Program**
Family Caregiver Alliance
625 Silver Ave SW
Ste 100B
Albuquerque, NM 87102 505-841-4464
877-696-1470
Fax: 505-841-4467
http://www.caregiver.org
A statewide program to assist people with disabilities through technology and communication devices. The goal of the program to help people with disabilities live independently and engage with their community.

1757 **State Department of Adult Education**
Department of Education
300 Don Gaspar Ave
Santa Fe, NM 87501 505-827-5800
http://webnew.ped.state.nm.us
Christopher Ruszkowski, Secretary
Icela Pelayo, Dep. Secretary,Teaching/Learning

New York

1758 **DBTAC: Northeast ADA Center**
Cornell University
201 Dolgen Hall
Ithaca, NY 14853 607-255-6686
800-949-4232
Fax: 607-255-2763
TTY: 800-949-4232
http://www.northeastada.org
northeastada@cornell.edu
Wendy Strobel-Gower, Director
Joe Zesski, Assistant Director
Vicki Chang, Research Support Specialist
Provides information, referrals, resources, and raining on equal opportunity for people with disabilities and on the Americans with Disabilities Act. Serve businesses, employers, government entities, individuals with disabilities, and the media in NY, NJ, PR, and the US Virgin Islands.

1759 **Department of Corrections and Communnity Supervision**
1220 Washington Ave
Bldg 2
Albany, NY 12226-2050 *Fax:* 518-457-4966
http://www.doccs.ny.gov
Andrew M. Cuomo, Governor
Anthony J. Annucci, Commissioner
To provide for public protection by administering a network of correctional facilities that: retain inmates in safe custody until released by law; offer inmates an opportunity to improve their rmployment potential and their ability to function in a non-criminal fashion; offer staff a variety of opportunities for career enrichment and advancement; and, offer stable and humane community environments in which all participants, staff anf inmates can perform their required tasks.

1760 **Disability Rights New York**
725 Broadway
Ste 450
Albany, NY 12207
518-432-7861
800-993-8982
Fax: 518-427-6561
TTY: 518-512-3448
http://www.drny.org
mail@DRNY.org
Andrew M. Cuomo, Governor
Timothy A. Clune, Esq., Exeutive Director
Jennifer J. Monthie, Esq., Legal Director
The protection and advocacy program for people with disabilities in the state of New York.

1761 **NYS Developmental Disabilities Planning Council**
99 Washington Ave
Ste 1230
Albany, NY 12210
800-395-3372
http://ddpc.ny.gov
information@ddpc.ny.gov
Andrew M. Cuomo, Governor
James Traylor, Chair
Timothy A. Clune, Esq., Executive Director
In partnership with individuals with developmental disabilities, their families and communities provides leadership by promoting policies, plans and practices.

1762 **New York Department of Labor: Division of Employment and Workforce Solutions**
W.A. Harriman Campus
Bldng 12
Albany, NY 12240
518-457-9000
888-469-7365
TDD: 800-662-1220
TTY: 800-662-1220
http://www.labor.ny.gov
nysdol@labor.state.ny.us
Andrew M. Cuomo, Governor
Provides leadership concerning policies, programs, and administration of the workforce investment system. Services for adults, dislocated workers, youth, and minorities.

1763 **Office of Civil Rights: New York**
US Department of Education
32 Old Slip
26th Fl
New York, NY 10005-2500
646-428-3900
Fax: 646-428-3843
TDD: 800-877-8339
http://www.ed.gov
ocr.newyork@ed.gov
Kenneth L. Marcus, Assistant Secretary
Earl Morgan, Executive Officer
Kristine Minami, Senior Counsel
This office covers the states of New Jersey and New York.

1764 **Office of Instructional Support**
New York State Department of Education
89 Washington Ave
Rm 875 EBA
Albany, NY 12234
518-474-5915
Fax: 518-486-2233
http://www.nysed.gov
MaryEllen Eliaÿ, Commissioner
Supports quality instruction, career and technical education, adult and famiy literacy, middle-level education, professional development for teachers, and promote workforce development.

1765 **Programs for Children with Special Health Care Needs**
Bureau of Child & Adolescent Health Dept of Health
112 State St
Room 300
Albany, NY 12207
518-447-4820
Fax: 518-447-4855
http://www.health.ny.gov
Andrew M. Cuomo, Governor
Howard Zucker, MD, Commissioner
To achieve a statewide system of care for children with special healthcare needs and their families that link them to appropriate health and related services, identifies gaps and barriers and assists in their resolution, and assures access to quality healthcare.

1766 **Programs for Infants and Toddlers with Disabilities**
Bureau of Early Intervention
Corning Tower Building, Rm 287
Empire State Plz
Albany, NY 12237-0660
518-473-7016
http://www.health.ny.gov
bei@health.ny.gov
Andrew M. Cuomo, Governor
Howard Zucker, MD, Commissioner
The Early Intervention Program offers a variety of therapeutic and support services to eligible infants and toddlers with disabilities and their families.

1767 **Region II: US Department of Health and Human Services**
26 Federal Plz
Ste 3312
New York, NY 10278
800-368-1019
Fax: 202-619-3818
http://www.hhs.gov
ocrmail@hhs.gov
Alex M. Azar II, Secretary
Eric D. Hargan, Deputy Secretary
Peter Urbanowicz, Chief of Staff
The United States government's principal agency for protecting the health of all Americans and providing essential human services, especially for those who are least able to help themselves.

1768 **State GED Administration**
State Department of Education
89 Washington Ave
Albany, NY 12234
518-474-3852
http://www.nysed.gov
ged@mail.nysed.gov
MaryEllen Eliaÿ, Commissioner
Instruction and testing for those over the age of 16 to earn the General Educational Development diploma.

1769 **Vocational & Educational Services for Individuals with Disabilities (VESID)**
231 W Main St
Malone, NY 12953
800-882-2803
http://www.vesid.nysed.gov
To promote educational equality and excellence for students with disabilities while ensuring that they receive civil rights and protection; assure appropriate continuity between the child and adult services systems; and provide the highest quality vocational rehabilitation and independent living services to all eligible persons as quickly as those services are required to enable them to work and live independent, self-directed lives.

North Carolina

1770 **Assistive Technology Program**
North Carolina Vocational Rehabilitation Services
2801 Mail Service Center
Raleigh, NC 27699-2801
919-855-3500
Fax: 919-715-1776
http://www.ncdhhs.gov
Rae Bachus, Assistive Technologist
Lynne Deese, Media and Training Coordinator
Sonya Clark, Information Specialist
A state and federally funded program that provides assistive technology services statewide to people of all ages and abilities.

1771 **Client Assistance Program (CAP): North Carolina Division of Vocational Rehabilitation Services**
2801 Mail Service Center
Raleigh, NC 27699-2801
919-855-3500
800-689-9090
TDD: 919-324-1500
TTY: 919-855-3579
http://www.ncdhhs.gov/divisions/dvrs
John Marens, Director
Tami Andrews, Administrative Assistant
Karen Martin, Client Advocate
The Client Assistance Program helps people understand and use rehabilitation services.

1772 **Disability Rights North Carolina**
3724 National Dr
Ste 100
Raleigh, NC 27612
919-856-2195
877-235-4210
Fax: 919-856-2244
TTY: 888-268-5535
http://www.disabilityrightsnc.org
info@disabilityrightsnc.org
Vicki Smith, Executive Director
Brad Spivey, Chief Financial Officer
Janice Willmott, Chief Administrative Officer
A nonprofit organization dedicated to improving the quality of life for people with learning disabilities and developmental disabilities.

1773 **NCWorks Commission**
North Carolina Department of Commerce
301 N Wilmington St
Raleigh, NC 27601-1058
919-814-4600
http://www.nccommerce.com
info@nccommerce.com
Roy Cooper, Governor
Anthony M. Copeland, Secretary of Commerce
George Sherrill, Chief of Staff
Created under the federal Workforce Innovation and Opportunity Act, NCWorks Commission includes representatives from local businesses, workforce agencies, educations, and community leaders who aspire to enable the state's workforce and help businesses grow.

1774 **North Carolina Council on Developmental Disabilities**
3125 Poplarwood Court
Ste 200
Raleigh, NC 27604
919-850-2901
800-357-6916
Fax: 919-850-2915
TDD: 800-357-6916
TTY: 800-357-9616
http://nccdd.org
info@nccdd.org
Alexandra McArthur, Council Chairperson
Aldea LaParr, Secretary
To ensure that people with developmental disabilities and their families participate in the design of and have access to culturally competent services and supports, as well as other assistance and opportunities, which promote inclusive communities.

1775 **North Carolina Division of Employment Security**
Department of Commerce
700 Wade Ave
Raleigh, NC 27605
888-737-0259
Fax: 919-250-4315
http://des.nc.gov/des
assistantsecretary@nccommerce.com
Roy Cooper, Governor
Anthony M. Copeland, Secretary of Commerce
Lockhart Taylor, Assistant Secretary

1776 **North Carolina Division of Vocational Rehabilitation**
2801 Mail Service Ctr
Raleigh, NC 27699-2801
919-324-1500
800-689-9090
TDD: 919-324-1500
http://www.ncdhhs.gov/divisions/dvrs
Baldwin Keith Renner, Chair
To promote employment and independence for people with disabilities through customer partnership and community leadership.

1777 **North Carolina Office of Administrative Hearings: Civil Rights Division**
1711 New Hope Church Rd
Raleigh, NC 27609
919-431-3000
http://www.oah.state.nc.us
Responsible for charges alleging discrimination in the basis of race, color, sex, religion, age, national origin or disability in employment, or charges alleging retaliation for opposition to such discrimination brought by previous and current state employees or applicants for employment for positions covered by the State Personnel Act, including county government employees.

1778 **State Department of Adult Education**
North Carolina Community College
200 West Jones St
Raleigh, NC 27603
919-807-7100
http://www.nccommunitycolleges.edu
webmaster@nccommunitycolleges.edu

North Dakota

1779 **Client Assistance Program (CAP): North Dakota**
Wells Fargo Bank Building
400 East Broadway, Ste 409
Bismarck, ND 58501-4071
701-328-2950
800-472-2670
Fax: 701-328-3934
http://www.ndpanda.org/cap
panda@nd.gov
David Boeck, Director of Legal Services
Corinne Hofmann, Director of Policy and Operation
Teresa Larsen, Executive Director
Assists clients and client applicants of North Dakota Vocational Rehabilitation services, Tribal Vocational Rehabilitation, or Independent Living services.

1780 **North Dakota Department of Human Services**
600 E Boulevard Ave
Dept 325
Bismarck, ND 58505-0250
701-328-2310
800-472-2622
Fax: 701-328-2359
TTY: 800-366-6888
http://www.nd.gov/dhs
dhseo@nd.gov
Christopher Jones, Executive Director
To provide quality, efficient, and effective human services, which improve the lives of people.

1781 **North Dakota Department of Labor: Fair Employment Practice Agency**
600 E Boulevard Ave
Dept. 406
Bismarck, ND 58505-0340
701-328-2660
800-582-8032
Fax: 701-328-2031
TTY: 800-366-6888
http://www.nd.gov/labor
Michelle Kommer, Commissioner of Labor
Provides information and enforces laws related to labor standards and discrimination in employment, housing, public services, public accommodations and lending. The department also issues sub minimum wage certificates, verifies independent contractor status and licenses employment agencies.

1782 **North Dakota Department of Public Instruction**
600 E Boulevard Ave
Dept. 201
Bismarck, ND 58505-0440
701-328-2660
Fax: 701-328-2461
http://www.nd.gov/dpi
dpi@nd.gov
Kirsten Baesler], State Superintendent
Patty Carmichael, Executive Assistant
To ensure a uniform, statewide system for effective learning.

1783 **North Dakota Division of Vocational Rehab**
1237 W Divide Ave
Ste 1B
Bismark, ND 58501-1208
701-328-8950
800-755-2745
Fax: 701-328-8969
http://www.nd.gov/dhs/dvr
dhsvr@nd.gov
Robyn Throlson, Acting State Director
Patty Wanner, Operations Administrator
Barbara Burghart, Transition Services Program
Dedicated to helping people with disabilities improve upon their vocational skills and assist businesses across North Dakota develop solutions to disability-related issues.

1784 **North Dakota Early Intervention Program**
Department of Human Services
151 S 4th St
Ste 204
Grand Forks, ND 58201-4735
701-795-3000
Fax: 701-795-3050
TTY: 701-795-3060
http://www.nd.gov/dhs/services
dhsds@nd.gov
Amanda Carlson, Program Administrator
The Early Intervention Program works to identify children at risk in the early stages of a developmental disability.

1785 **North Dakota State Council On Developmental Disabilities**
1500 E Capitol Ave
Bismarck, ND 58501
701-328-4847
http://www.nd.gov/scdd
Julie Horntvedt, Executive Director
Kaelee Knoell, Program Assistant
Represents the voice of all persons with developmental disabilities in North Dakota.

1786 **Protection & Advocacy Project**
Disability Rights North Dakota
400 E Broadway
Ste 409
Bismarck, ND 58501-4071
701-328-2950
800-472-2670
Fax: 701-328-3934
http://www.ndpanda.org
panda@nd.gov
Teresa Larsen, Executive Director
Denise Harvey, Director of Program Services
Corinne Hofmann, Dir., Policy and Operations
A nonprofit organization dedicated to improving the quality of life for people with learning disabilities, physical or developmental disabilities.

1787 **Special Education North Dakota**
Department of Public Instruction
600 East Boulevard Ave
Dept 201
Bismark, ND 58505-0440
701-328-2277
http://www.nd.gov/dpi
cindy_wilcox@bismarkschools.org
Cindy Wilcox, Director
Special Education is dedicated to improving results for infants, toddlers and children with disabilities through financial support in local schools.

Ohio

1788 **Assistive Technology of Ohio**
Area 299
1314 Kinnear Rd
Columbus, OH 43212
614-292-2390
800-784-3425
http://atohio.engineering.osu.edu
atohio@osu.edu
William Darling, Executive Director
Eric Rathburn, Legislative Liaison
Marilyn Spetka, Program Manager
To help Ohioans with disabilities acquire assistive technology. Offer several programs and services to achieve that goal. Also keep up with current legislative activity that affects persons with disabilities.

1789 **Client Assistance Program (CAP)**
Disability Rights Ohio
200 Civic Center Dr
Ste 300
Columbus, OH 43215
614-466-7264
800-282-9181
Fax: 614-644-1888
TTY: 614-728-2553
http://www.disabilityrightsohio.org
Michael Kirkman, Executive Director
Kerstin Sjoberg, Asst. Exec. Dir./Dir., Advocacy
Paul Koehler, Chief Financial Officer
Advocates for and protects the rights of individuals with disabilities who are applying for or receiving rehabilitation services from the Ohio Bureau of Vocational Rehabilitation (BVR) or the Ohio Bureau of Services for the Visually Impaired (BSVI).

1790 **Correctional Education**
Department of Rehabilitation & Correction
770 W Broad St
Columbus, OH 43222
614-387-0588
http://www.drc.ohio.gov
Gary C. Mohr, Director
Protects and supports Ohioans by ensuring that adult felony offenders are effectively supervised in environments that are safe, humane, and appropriately secure.

1791 **Office of Civil Rights: Ohio**
US Department of Education
1350 Euclid Ave
Ste 325
Cleveland, OH 44114-1812
216-522-4970
Fax: 216-522-2573
TDD: 800-877-8339
http://www.ed.gov
ocr.cleveland@ed.gov
Kenneth L. Marcus, Assistant Secretary
Earl Morgan, Executive Officer
Kristine Minami, Senior Counsel
This office covers the states of Michigan and Ohio.

1792 **Ohio Adult Basic and Literacy Education**
25 S Front St
Columbus, OH 43215
877-644-6338
http://education.ohio.gov
contact.center@education.ohio.gov
John R. Kasich, Governor
Paolo DeMaria, Superintendent
Provides quality leadership for the establishment, improvement an dexpansion of lifelong learning opportunities for adults in their family, community and work roles.

1793 **Ohio Civil Rights Commission**
30 E Broad St
Columbus, OH 43215
614-466-7900
http://crc.ohio.gov
G. Michael Payton, Executive Directorÿÿ

To enforce state laws against discrimination. OCRC receives and investigates charges of discrimination in employment, public accommodations, housing, credit and higher education on the bases of race, colo, religion, sex, national origin, disability, age, ancestry or familial status.

1794 **Ohio Developmental Disabilities Council**
899 E Broad St
Ste 203
Columbus, OH 43205
614-466-5205
800-766-7426
http://ddc.ohio.gov
kimberly.crishbaum@dodd.ohio.gov
Jo Haney Spargo, Chair
Ken Latham, Executive Director
John Kashich, Governor
To create change that improves independence, productivity and inclusion for people with developmental disabilities and their families in community life.

1795 **Ohio Office of Workforce Development**
Ohio Department of Job & Family Services
Fl 32
30 E Broad St
Columbus, OH 43215
614-466-6282
http://jfs.ohio.gov
workforce@jfs.ohio.gov
Cynthia C. Dungey, Director
The role of OWD is to work in partnership with the U.S. Department of Labor, Governor's Office and a variety of stakeholders in order to provide administration and operational management for several federal programs and to offer specific services in support of the programs. OWD's primary responsibility is to promote job creation and to advance Ohio's workforce.

1796 **Protection & Advocacy Agency**
Disability Rights Ohio
200 Civic Center Dr
Ste 300
Columbus, OH 43215
614-466-7264
800-282-9181
Fax: 614-644-1888
TTY: 614-728-2553
http://www.disabilityrightsohio.org
Michael Kirkman, Executive Director
Kerstin Sjoberg, Asst. Exec. Dir./Dir., Advocacy
Paul Koehler, Chief Financial Officer
To protect and advocate, in partnership with people with disabilities, for their human, civil and legal rights.

1797 **State Department of Education**
25 S Front St
Columbus, OH 43215
877-644-6338
http://education.ohio.gov
contact.center@education.ohio.gov
John R. Kasich, Governor
Debe Terhar, President
Dr. Lonny J. Rivera, Interim Superintendent

1798 **State GED Administration**
State Department of Education
25 S Front St
Rm 309
Columbus, OH 43215
877-644-6338
http://education.ohio.gov
contact.center@education.ohio.gov
John R. Kasich, Governor
Debe Terhar, President
Dr. Lonny J. Rivera, Interim Superintendent

Oklahoma

1799 **Client Assistance Program (CAP): Oklahoma Division**
Office of Disability Concerns
1111 N Lee Ave
Ste 500
Oklahoma City, OK 73103
405-521-3756
800-522-8224
http://www.ok.gov/odc
doug.macmillan@odc.ok.gov
Doug MacMillan, Director
William Ginn, Disability Program Specialist
Valencia Stiggers, Disability Program Specialist
The purpose of this program is to advise and inform clients and client applicants of all services and benefits available to them through programs authorized under the Rehabilitation Act of 1973. Assist and advocates for clients and client applicants in their relationships with projects, programs, and community rehabilitation programs providing services under the Act.

1800 **Correctional Education**
Department of Corrections
PO Box 11400
Oklahoma City, OK 73136-0400
405-425-2500
Fax: 405-425-2500
http://doc.ok.gov
webmaster@doc.ok.gov
Dr. Jeana Ely, Superintendent of Schools
Joe M. Allbaugh, Director
Scott Crow, Chief of Operations

1801 **Oklahoma State Department of Education**
2500 N Lincoln Blvd
Oklahoma City, OK 73105
405-521-3301
Fax: 405-521-6205
http://www.ok.gov/sde
sdeservicedesk@sde.ok.gov
Bill Connolly, Executive Director
Joy Hofmeister, State Superintendent
Treasure Morgan, Executive Assistant
Improve student success through: service to schools, parents and students; leadership for education reform; and regulation/deregulation of state and federal laws to provide accountability while removing any barriers to student success.

1802 **Oklahoma's Assistive Technology Act Program**
Oklahoma ABLE Tech
405-744-9748
800-257-1705
http://www.okabletech.org
abletech@okstate.edu
Linda Jaco, Director of Sponsored Programs
Milissa Gofourth, Program Manager
Brenda Dawes, Program Manager
A clearinghouse for resources relating to assistive technology for people with disabilities and their families.

1803 **Protection & Advocacy Agency**
Disability Law Center
2915 Classen Blvd
Ste 300
Oklahoma City, OK 73106
405-525-7755
800-880-7755
Fax: 405-525-7759
http://okdlc.org
Melissa K. Sublett, Executive Director
Brian Wilkerson, Director of Litigation/Legal Svs
Heather Moorhead, Fiscal Manager
Helps people with disabilities achieve equality, inclusion in society and personal independence without regard to disabling conditions.

1804 **State Department of Adult Education**
Department of Education
2500 N Lincoln Blvd
Oklahoma City, OK 73105
405-377-2000
800-522-5810
http://sde.ok.gov
sdeservicedesk@sde.ok.gov
Bill Connolly, Executive Director
Joy Hofmeister, State Superintendent
Treasure Morgan, Executive Assistant

1805 **State GED Administration**
Department of Education
2500 N Lincoln Blvd
Oklahoma City, OK 73105
405-377-2000
800-522-5810
http://sde.ok.gov
sdeservicedesk@sde.ok.gov
Bill Connolly, Executive Director
Joy Hofmeister, State Superintendent
Treasure Morgan, Executive Assistant

Oregon

1806 **Assistive Technology Program**
Access Technologies
2225 Lancaster Drive NE
Salem, OR 97305
503-361-1201
http://www.accesstechnologiesinc.org
info@accesstechnologiesinc.org
Laurie Brooks, President
Davey Hulse, Chair
A statewide program promoting services and assistive devices for people with disabilities.

1807 **Department of Community Colleges and Workforce Development**
255 Capitol St NE
3rd Fl
Salem, OR 97310
503-947-2414
http://www.oregon.gov
info.hecc@state.or.us
Patrick Crane, Director
Donna Lewelling, Deputy Director
Contribute leadership and resources to increase skills, knowledge and carrier opportunities.

1808 **Disability Rights Oregon**
511 SW 10th Ave
Ste 200
Portland, OR 97205
503-243-2081
800-452-1694
Fax: 503-243-1738
http://www.droregon.org
Michael Bailey, Chair
Jan Campbell, Vice Chair
Bob Joondeph, Executive Director
An independent non-profit organization which provides legal advocacy services for people with disabilities anywhere in Oregon. OAC offers free legal assistance and other advocacy services to individuals who are considered to have physical or mental disabilities. OAC works only on legal problems which relate directly to the disability.

1809 **Office of Vocational Rehabilitation Services**
Department of Human Services
500 Summer St NE E-15
Salem, OR 97301
503-945-5880
877-277-0513
http://www.oregon.gov
vr.info@state.or.us
Fariborz Pakseresht, DHS Director
Jeannine Beatrice, Cheif of Staff
Eric Moore, Chief Financial Officer
Helps Oregonians with disabilities to prepare for, finad and retain jobs.

1810 **Oregon Bureau of Labor and Industry: Fair Employment Practice Agency**
800 NE Oregon St
Ste 1045
Portland, OR 97232
971-673-0761
Fax: 971-673-0762
TTY: 971-673-0761
http://www.oregon.gov/BOLI/
mailb@boli.state.or.us
Brad Avakian, Commissioner
Protects labor rights, works to advance employment opportunities, and protects housing and public accomodations.

1811 **Oregon Council on Developmental Disabilities**
2485 SE Ladd Ave
Ste 231
Portland, OR 97214
503-235-0369
http://www.ocdd.org
info@ocdd.org
Jamie Daignault, Executive Director
Carrie Salehiamin, Operations Manager
Ryley Newport, Communications Director
To create change that improves the lives of Oregonians with developmental disabilities.

1812 **Oregon Department of Education: Work-Based Learning**
255 Capitol St NE
Salem, OR 97310-0203
503-947-5600
Fax: 503-378-5156
http://www.oregon.gov/ode
Marc.Siegel@state.or.us
Colt Gill, Director of Education
Marcus Siegel, Communications Director
An applied learning program to assist students to prepare for college and the workforce.

1813 **Oregon Department of Human Services: Children and Youth Division**
500 Summer St NE
E15
Salem, OR 97301
503-945-5600
Fax: 503-581-6198
http://www.oregon.gov/dhs
Fariborz Pakseresht, DHS Director
Jeannine Beatrice, Chief of Staff
Eric Moore, Chief Financial Officer
Administration for Oregon's foster care system, Child Protective Services program, adoptation, child care assistance, the Independent Living Program, and more.

1814 **Oregon Employment Department**
875 Union St NE
Salem, OR 97311
503-947-1394
800-237-3710
Fax: 503-947-1472
http://www.oregon.gov/EMPLOY/
Kay Erickson, Director
Supports economic stability for Oregonians and communities during times of unemployment through the payment of unemployment benefits. Serves businesses by recruiting and referring the best qualified applicants to jobs, and provides resources to diverse job seekers in support of their employment needs.

Pennsylvania

1815 **Bureau of Adult Basic & Literacy Education**
333 Market St
Harrisburg, PA 17126
717-783-6788
http://www.education.pa.gov/Postsecondary-Adult
Tom Wolf, Governor
Pedro Rivera, Secretary
Provides instructional services for Pennsylvanians to develop basic skills necessary to sustain employment and/or further their education.

1816 **Client Assistance Program (CAP): Pennsylvania Division**
1515 Market St
Ste 1300
Philadelphia, PA 19102 215-557-7112
888-745-2357
Fax: 215-557-7602
TDD: 215-557-7112
http://www.equalemployment.org
info@equalemployment.org
Stephen S. Pennington, Esq., Executive Director
Lanette D. Suarez, Case Manager/Advocate
Margaret Passio-McKenna, Senior Advocate
CAP is an advocacy program for people with disabilities administered by the Center for Disability Law and Policy. CAP helps people who are seeking services from the Office of Vocational Rehabilitation, Blindness and Visual Services, Centers for Independent Living and other programs funded under federal law. CAP services are provided at no charge.

1817 **Disability Rights Network of Pennsylvania**
301 Chestnut St
Ste 300
Harrisburg, PA 17101 717-236-8110
800-692-7443
Fax: 717-236-0192
TDD: 877-375-7139
TTY: 800-692-7443
http://www.disabilityrightspa.org
Jeniece Davis, Chair
Charles Giambrone, Vice Chair
Peri Jude Radecic, Chief Executive Officer
A statewide, non-profit corporation designated as the federally-mandated organization to advance and protect the civil rights of adults and children with disabilities. DRN works with people with disabilities and their families, their organizations, and their advocates to ensure their rights to live in their communities with the services they need, to receive a full and inclusive education, to live free of discrimination, abuse and neglect.

1818 **Office of Civil Rights: Pennsylvania**
US Department of Education
100 Penn Sq E
Ste 515
Philadelphia, PA 19107-3323 215-656-8541
Fax: 215-656-8605
TDD: 800-877-8339
http://www.ed.gov
ocr.philadelphia@ed.gov
Kenneth L. Marcus, Assistant Secretary
Earl Morgan, Executive Officer
Kristine Minami, Senior Counsel
This office covers the states of Delaware, Kentucky, Maryland, Pennsylvania and West Virginia.

1819 **Pennsylvania Department of Corrections**
1920 Technology Parkway
Mechanicsburg, PA 17050 717-728-2573
http://www.cor.pa.gov
ra-contactdoc@pa.gov
John E. Wetzel, Secretary
Daniel McIntyre, Director
Provides basic education and vocational programs to inmates to provide them with opportunities to acquire the skills and values necessary to become productive law-abiding citizens; while respecting the rights of crime victims.

1820 **Pennsylvania Developmental Disabilities Council**
605 South Dr
Room 561 Forum Building
Harrisburg, PA 17120 717-787-6057
877-685-4452
TTY: 717-705-0819
http://www.paddc.org
Graham Mulholland, Executive Director
Sandra Amador Dusek, Deputy Director
Engages in advocacy, systems change and capacity building for people with disabilities and their families in order to: support people with disabilities in taking control of their own lives; ensure access to goods, services, and supports; build inclusive communities; pursue a cross-disability agenda; and to change negative societal attitudes towards people with disabilities.

1821 **Pennsylvania Human Rights Commission**
333 Market St
8th Fl
Harrisburg, PA 17101-2210 717-787-4410
TTY: 717-787-7279
http://www.phrc.pa.gov
Chad Dion Lassiter, Executive Director
M. Joel Bolstein, Interim Chair
Tom Wolf, Governor
To administer and enforce the PHRAct and the PFEOA of the Commonwealth of the Pennsylvania for the identification and elimination of discrimination and the providing of equal opportunity for all persons.

1822 **Pennsylvania's Initiative on Assistive Technology**
1755 N 13th St
Student Center, Rm 411 S
Philadelphia, PA 19122 215-204-1356
800-204-7428
TTY: 215-204-1805
http://www.temple.edu/instituteondisabilities
ATinfo@temple.edu
Celia Feinstein, Executive Director
Susan Fullam, Director of Communication
Jule Ann Lieberman, Program Coordinator
Strives to enhance the lives of Pennsylvanians with disabilities, older Pennsylvanians, and their families, through access to and acquisition of assitive technology devices and services, which allow for choice, control and independence at home, work, school, play and in their neighborhoods.

1823 **Region III: US Department of Health and Human Services Civil Rights Office**
US Department of Health & Human Services
801 Market St
Ste 9300
Philadelphia, PA 19107-3134 800-368-1019
Fax: 202-619-7697
TDD: 800-537-7697
http://www.hhs.gov
ocrmail@hhs.gov
Barbara Holland, Regional Manager
Alex M. Azar, II, Secretary
Eric D. Hargan, Deputy Secretary

1824 **State Department of Education**
333 Market St
Harrisburg, PA 17126 717-783-6788
http://www.education.pa.gov
ra-edhse@pa.gov
Tom Wolf, Governor
Pedro A. Rivera, Secretary
To lead and serve the educational community to enable each individual to grow into an inspired, productive, fulfilled lifelong learner.

1825 **State GED Administration**
Pennsylvania Department of Education
333 Market St
Harrisburg, PA 17126 717-783-6788
717-787-5532
http://www.education.pa.gov
ra-edhse@pa.gov
Tom Wolf, Governor
Pedro A. Rivera, Secretary

Rhode Island

1826 **Correctional Education**
Rhode Island Department of Corrections
40 Howard Avenue
Cranston, RI 02920
401-462-1000
http://www.doc.ri.gov
doc.director@doc.ri.gov
Patricia A. Coyne-Fague, Acting Director
Susan Perez, Programming Services Officer
Kathleen Kelly, Chief Legal Counsel

1827 **Protection & Advocacy Agency**
Rhode Island Disability Law Center
275 Westminster St
Ste 401
Providence, RI 02903-3434
401-831-3150
800-733-5332
Fax: 401-274-5568
TTY: 401-831-5335
http://www.ridlc.org
info@ridlc.org
Raymond L. Bandusky, Executive Director
Darby Castigliego, Dir., Finance & Administration
To assist people with differing abilities in their efforts to achieve full inclusion in society and to exercise their civil and human rights through the provision of legal advocacy.

1828 **Rhode Island Assistive Technology Access Partnership (ATAP)**
Department of Health & Human Services
401-462-7917
http://www.atap.ri.gov
melanie.sbardella@ors.ri.gov
Melanie Sbardella, Program Director
Works in partnership with organizations across the state of Rhode Island to improve access and usage of assistive technology for persons with disabilities. Initiatives include: demonstrations, training, public awareness, and loans.

1829 **Rhode Island Commission for Human Rights**
180 Westminster St
3rd Fl
Providence, RI 02903
401-222-2661
Fax: 401-222-2616
TTY: 402-222-2661
http://www.richr.ri.gov
John B. Susa, PhD, Chair
Michael Evora, Esq., Executive Director
Betsy Ross, Chief Clerk
A state agency that enforces civil rights law.

1830 **Rhode Island Department of Elementary and Secondary Education**
Rhode Island Department of Education
255 Westminster St
Providence, RI 02903
401-222-4600
http://www.ride.ri.gov
EQAC@ride.ri.gov
Barbara S. Cottam, Chair
Mary Ann Snider, Deputy Commissioner
Brian Darrow, Chief of Staff

1831 **Rhode Island Department of Labor & Training**
1511 Pontiac Ave
Cranston, RI 02920
401-462-8000
Fax: 401-462-8872
TTY: 401-462-8000
http://www.dlt.state.ri.us
Scott R. Jensen, Director
Providing workforce protection and development services with courtesy, responsiveness and effectiveness.

1832 **Rhode Island Developmental Disabilities Council**
400 Bald Hill Rd
Ste 515
Warwick, RI 02886
401-737-1238
Fax: 401-737-3395
TDD: 401-732-1238
http://www.riddc.org
riddc@riddc.org
Kevin Nerney, Associate Director
Sue Babin, Special Projects Coordinator
Promotes the ideas that will enhance the lives of people with developmental disabilities.

1833 **State Department of Adult Education**
255 Westminster St
Providence, RI 02903
401-222-4600
http://www.ride.ri.gov
Barbara S. Cottam, Chair
Administer grant funded programs in Adult Basic Education, GED, and English for Speakers of Other Languages. Promote stronger families, upward mobility, and active citizenship through effective adult basic education services. The classes support adults who wish to advance their education towards a high school credential, training, and/or post secondary degrees.

1834 **TechACCESS of Rhode Island**
Technology Services for People with Disabilities
161 Comstock Pkwy
Cranston, RI 02921
401-463-0202
Fax: 401-463-3433
TTY: 401-463-0202
http://www.techaccess-ri.org
techaccess@techaccess-ri.org
Kelly Charlebois, Executive Director
Randy Conroy, Assistive Technology Consultant
Offers services to both children and adults through technology; includes evaluations and training sessions.

South Carolina

1835 **Assistive Technology Program**
South Carolina Developmental Disabilities Council
1205 Pendleton St
Ste 461
Columbia, SC 29201
803-734-0465
TTY: 803-734-1147
http://www.scddc.state.sc.us
Valarie.Bishop@admin.sc.gov
Valarie Bishop, Executive Director
Cheryl English, Program Information Coordinator
Esther Williams, Administrative Specialist
A statewide project established to provide an opportunity for individuals with disabilities to lead the fullest, most productive lives possible.

1836 **Protection & Advocacy for People with Disabilities**
3710 Landmark Dr
Ste 208
Columbia, SC 29204
803-782-0639
866-275-7273
TTY: 866-232-4525
http://www.pandasc.org
info@pandasc.org
Dana Lang, Chair
Barbara Cullum, Vice Chair
Gloria Prevost, Executive Director
To protect the legal, civil, and human rights of people with disabilities in South Carolina by enabling individuals to advocate for themselves, speaking in their behalf when they have been discriminated against or denied a services to which they are entitled, and promoting policies and services which respect their choices.

1837 **South Carolina Developmental Disabilities Council**
1205 Pendleton St
Ste 461
Columbia, SC 29201
803-734-0465
TTY: 803-734-1147
http://www.scddc.state.sc.us
Valarie.Bishop@admin.sc.gov
Valarie Bishop, Executive Director
Cheryl English, Program Information Coordinator
Esther Williams, Administrative Specialist
To provide leadership in advocating, funding and implementing initiatives which recognize the inherent dignity of each individual, and promote independence, productivity, respect and inclusion for all persons with disabilities and their families.

1838 **South Carolina Employment and Workforce**
1550 Gadsden St
PO Box 995
Columbia, SC 29202
803-737-2400
TTY: 803-737-2400
http://dew.sc.gov
Cheryl M. Stanton, Executive Director
Government division responsible for unemployment insurance benefits, unemployment taxes, and assisting people find employment opportunities.

1839 **South Carolina Human Affairs Commission**
1026 Sumter St
Columbia, SC 29201
803-737-7800
800-521-0725
TDD: 803-253-4125
http://www.schac.gov
information@schac.state.sc.us
John A. Oakland, Chair
Cheryl F.C. Ludlam, Vice Chair
To eliminate and prevent unlawful discrimination in employment, housing, and public accommodations on the basis of race, color, national origin and religion.

1840 **State Department of Adult Education**
South Carolina Department of Education
1429 Senate St
Columbia, SC 29201
803-734-8347
http://ed.sc.gov
ged@ed.sc.gov
Molly Spearman, State Superintendent
Betsy Carpentier, Chief of Staff & COO
Mike King, Director, Adult Education
Provides the opportunity for adults with low literacy skills (less than eighth grade level), to work with materials to be taught in an environment conducive to their level, and to improve their reading, math, and writing skills.

1841 **State GED Administration**
South Carolina Department of Education
1429 Senate St
Columbia, SC 29201
803-734-8347
http://ed.sc.gov
ged@ed.sc.gov
Molly Spearman, State Superintendent
Betsy Carpentier, Chief of Staff & COO
Mike King, Director, Adult Education

South Dakota

1842 **Client Assistance Program (CAP): South Dakota Division**
South Dakota Disability Rights
221 S Central Ave
Ste 38
Pierre, SD 57501
605-224-8294
800-658-4782
Fax: 605-224-5125
TTY: 800-658-4782
http://drsdlaw.org
Provides free services to eligible consumers and applicants for projects, programs and facilities funded under the rehabilitation act.

1843 **Department of Correction: Education Coordinator**
3200 E Hwy 34
Pierre, SD 57501
605-773-3478
Fax: 605-773-3794
http://doc.sd.gov
Provides basic education and vocational programs to inmates to provide them with opportunities to acquire the skills and values necessary to become productive law-abiding citizens; while respecting the rights of crime victims.

1844 **South Dakota Council on Developmental Disabilities**
Department of Human Services
500 E Capitol Ave
Pierre, SD 57501-5007
605-773-6369
http://dhs.sd.gov
infoddc@state.sd.us
Arlene Poncelet, Executive Director
The SD Council is authorized under federal law to address the unmet needs of people with developmental disabilities through advocacy, capacity building and systems change activities. The mission is to assist people with developmental disabilities and their families in achieving the quality of life they desire.

1845 **South Dakota Disability Rights**
221 S Central Ave
Ste 38
Pierre, SD 57501
605-224-8294
800-658-4782
Fax: 605-224-5125
TTY: 800-658-4782
http://drdslaw.org
To protect and advocate the rights of South Dakotans with disabilities through legal, administrative, and other remedies.

1846 **South Dakota Division of Human Rights**
South Dakota Department of Labor & Regulation
123 W Missouri Ave
Pierre, SD 57501
605-773-3681
Fax: 605-773-4211
http://dlr.sd.gov/human_rights
To promote equal opportunity through the administration and enforcement of the Human Relations Act of 1972. The act is designed to protect the public from discrimination because of race, color, creed, religion, sex, disability, ancestry or national origin.

1847 **South Dakota Division of Special Education**
Department of Education
800 Governors Dr
Pierre, SD 57501
605-773-3134
Fax: 605-773-6139
http://doe.sd.gov/sped
Holly.Robling@state.sd.us
Mary Stadick Smith, Interim Secretary of Education
Marta Neuman, Senior Secretary
The Office of Special Education advocates for the availability of the full range of personnel, programming, and placement options, including early intervention and transition services, required to assure that all individuals with disabilities are able to achieve maximum independence upon exiting from school.

1848 **South Dakota Governor's Office of Economic Development**
Pierre, SD 57501
605-773-4633
http://www.sdreadytowork.com
Scott.Stern@sdreadytowork.com
Dennis Daugaard, Governor
Scott Stern, Commissioner
Aaron Scheibe, Deputy Commissioner
Job training programs provide an important framework for developing public-private sector partnerships. Programs funded by the Community Development Block Grants.

1849 **South Dakota Rehabilitation Services: Assistive Technology**
Department of Human Services
3800 E Highway 34
Pierre, SD 57501-5070
605-773-5484
605-773-5483
http://dhs.sd.gov/rehabservices/AT.aspx
Ensures that persons with disabilities have access to assistive technology.

1850 **State GED Administration**
Department of Labor
123 W Missouri Ave
Pierre, SD 57501
605-773-5017
Fax: 605-773-6184
http://www.sdjobs.org
barb.unruh@state.sd.us
Marcia Hultman, Labor Secretary
Barb Unruh, GED Administrator

Tennessee

1851 **Department of Human Services: Division of Rehabilitation Services**
400 Deaderick St
Nashville, TN 37243-1403
615-313-4891
800-270-1349
TTY: 615-313-5695
http://www.tn.gov/humanservices
Danielle W. Barnes, Commissioner
Trevor Lauri, Executive Assistant
To improve the well-being of economically disadvantaged, disabled or vulnerable Tennesseans through a network of financial, employment, rehabilitative and protective services.

1852 **Disability Rights Tennessee**
2 International Plz
Ste 825
Nashville, TN 37217
615-298-1080
800-342-1660
Fax: 615-298-2046
http://www.disabilityrightstn.org
GetHelp@disabilityrightstn.org
Lisa Primm, Executive Director
Susan Mee, Legal Director
Shelia Mullis, Director of Finance & HR
A nonprofit organization dedicated to improving the quality of life for people with learning disabilities and developmental disabilities.

1853 **State Department of Education**
710 James Robertson Pkwy
Nashville, TN 37243
615-741-5158
http://www.tn.gov/education
Candice McQueen, Commissioner of Education
Sara Gast, Director of Communications
Kathleen Airhart, Deputy Commissioner & COO
The department is reponsible for ensuring equal, safe, and quality learning opportunities for all students, pre-kindergartern through 12th grade.

1854 **State GED Administration**
State Department of Education
710 James Robertson Pkwy
Nashville, TN 37243
615-741-5158
http://www.tn.gov/education
Candice McQueen, Commissioner of Education
Sara Gast, Director of Communications
Kathleen Airhart, Deputy Commissioner & COO

1855 **Tennessee Correctional Education**
Department of Correction
320 6th Ave N
Nashville, TN 37243-0465
615-741-1000
http://www.tn.gov/correction
TDOC.webmaster@tn.gov
Tony C. Parker, Commissioner
Offers educational programs to inmates such as Adult Basic Education and Career and Technical Education. College programs are also available through partnership with THEI and Lipscomb University.

1856 **Tennessee Council on Developmental Disabilities**
500 James Robertson Pkwy
Davy Crockett Tower, 1st Fl
Nashville, TN 37243
615-532-6615
http://www.tn.gov/cdd
tnddc@tn.gov
Wanda Willis, Executive Director
Lynette Porter, Deputy Director
Mildred Sparkman, Administrative Secretary
A State office that promotes public policies to increase and support the inclusion of individuals with developmental disabilities in their communities.

1857 **Tennessee Technology Access Project**
400 Deadrick St
12th Fl
Nashville, TN 37243-1403
615-313-5183
800-732-5059
TTY: 615-313-5695
http://www.tn.gov/humanservices/ds/ttap.html
tn.ttap@tn.gov
Danielle Barnes, Commissioner
Gena Lewis, Deputy Commissioner
Tony Mathews, Deputy Commissioner Operations
A statewide program designed to increase access to, and acquisition of, assisitve technology devices and services.

Texas

1858 **Disability Rights Texas**
2222 W Braker Lane
Austin, TX 78758
512-454-4816
866-362-2851
Fax: 512-323-0902
http://www.disabilityrightstx.org
Mary Faithfull, Executive Director
Nonprofit legal organization that provides services and advances the rights of people with disabilities.

1859 **Learning Disabilities Association of America Texas**
PO Box 831392
Richardson, TX 75083
512-458-8234
800-604-7500
Promotes the educational and general welfare of individuals with learning disabilities.

1860 **Office of Civil Rights: Texas**
US Department of Education
1999 Bryan St
Ste 1620
Dallas, TX 75201-6810
214-661-9600
Fax: 214-661-9587
TDD: 800-877-8339
http://www.ed.gov
ocr.dallas@ed.gov
Kenneth L. Marcus, Assistant Secretary
Earl Morgan, Executive Officer
Kristine Minami, Senior Counsel
The Dallas office covers the states of Alabama, Arkansas, Louisiana, Mississippi and Texas.

1861 **Southwest ADA Center: Region VI**
ÿ
Houston, TX 77030
586-573-5951
http://www.swdbtac.org
elinor@swdbtac.org
One of ten DBTACs funded by the National Institute on Disability and Rehabilitation Research. The DBTAC serves a wide range of audiences who are interested in or impacted by these laws, including employers, businesses, government agencies, schools and people with disabilities.

1862 **State GED Administration**
Texas Education Agency
1701 N Congress Ave
Austin, TX 78701
512-463-9734
http://www.tea.texas.gov
Mike Morath, Commissioner
A.J. Crabill, Deputy Commissioner
To build capacity for consistent testing services throughout the state in order that all eligible candidates may have an oportunity to earn high school equivalency credentials based on the General Educational Development (GED) Tests.

1863 **Texas Assistive Technology Network (TATN)**
7145 W Tidwell
Region 4 ESC
Houston, TX 77092
713-744-6831
http://www.texasat.net
tatn@esc4.net
Angela Standridge, Director
Formed out of representatives from each Texas Education Services Centers and the Texas Education Agency, TATN provides leadership and fosters collaboration with education institutions. The mission of TATN is to improve access and usage of assistive technology for students with disabilities.

1864 **Texas Council for Developmental Disabilities**
6201 E Oltorf St
Ste 600
Austin, TX 78741-7509
512-437-5432
800-262-0334
Fax: 512-437-5434
http://www.tcdd.texas.gov
tcdd@tcdd.texas.gov
Mary Durheim, Chair
John W. Thomas, Vice Chair
Beth Stalvey, Executive Director
To create change so that all people with disabilities are fully included in their communities and exercise control over their own lives.

1865 **Texas Department of Criminal Justice**
PO Box 99
Huntsville, TX 77342-0099
936-295-6371
http://www.tdcj.state.tx.us
To provide public safety, promote positive change in offender behavior, reintegrate offenders into society, and assist victims of crime.

1866 **Texas Education Agency**
1701 N Congress Ave
Austin, TX 78701
512-463-9734
http://tea.texas.gov
Mike Morath, Commissioner
A.J. Crabill, Deputy Commissioner
To provide leadership, guidance, and resources to help schools meet the educational needs of all students.

1867 **Texas Workforce Commission: Civil Rights Division**
101 E 15th St
Rm 370
Austin, TX 78778-0001
800-628-5115
http://twc.texas.gov
ombudsman@twc.state.tx.us
Ruth Ruggero, Chair
Enforces the Texas Commission on Human Rights Act and the Texas Fair Housing Act. The Human Rights Act prohibits discrimination in regards to employment, housing, and public accommodations based on race, color, religion, sex, national origin, mental or physical disability, familial status and retaliation.

Utah

1868 **Assistive Technology Program**
6855 Old Main Hill
Logan, UT 84322-6855
800-524-5152
http://www.uatpat.org
Sachin Pavithran, Program Director
Marilyn Hammond, UATF Executive Director
Lois Summers, Staff Assistant
Serve individuals with disabilities of all ages in Utah and the intermountain region. Provide AT devices and services, and train university students, parents, children with disabilities and professional services providers about AT. Also coordinate the services with community organizations and others who provide independence-related support to individuals with disabilities.

1869 **Center for Persons with Disabilities**
Utah State University
6800 Old Main Hl
Logan, UT 84322-6800
435-797-1981
http://www.cpdusu.org
Utah's University Center for excellence in developmental disabilities education, research, and services.

1870 **Department of Workforce Services**
PO Box 45249
Salt Lake City, UT 84145-0249
801-526-9675
http://jobs.utah.gov
dwscontactus@utah.gov
Jon Pierpont, Executive Director
Casey Cameron, Deputy Director
Greg Paras, Deputy Director
Provides employment and support services for our customers to improve their economic opportunities.

1871 **Disability Law Center**
205 N 400 W
Salt Lake City, UT 84103
800-662-9080
Fax: 801-363-1437
http://www.disabilitylawcenter.org
Juliette P. White, President
Anthony Bake, Vice President
Jan Brock, Treasurer
A private non-profit organization designated as the Protection and Advocacy agency for the state of Utah to protect the rights of people with disabilities in Utah. To enforce and strengthen laws that protect the opportunities, choices and legal rights of people with disabilities in Utah.

1872 **Utah Antidiscrimination and Labor Division**
Utah Labor Commission
160 East 300 South, 3rd Fl
PO Box 146640
Salt Lake City, UT 84114-6640
801-530-6801
800-222-1238
http://laborcommission.utah.gov
discrimination@utah.gov
Investigates and resolves employment and housing discrimination complaints and enforces Utah's minimum wage, wage payment requirements, laws which protect youth in employment and the requirement that private employeemnt agencies be licensed. The Division also conducts public awareness and educational presentations.

1873 **Utah Center for Assistive Technology**
Workforce Services Rehabilitation
PO Box 45249
Salt Lake City, UT 84145-0249
801-526-9675
http://jobs.utah.gov
dwscontactus@utah.gov
Jon Pierpont, Executive Director
Casey Cameron, Deputy Director
Greg Paras, Deputy Director
To enhance human potential through facilitating the application of assistive technologies for persons with disabilities.

1874 **Utah Developmental Disabilities Council**
155 S 300 W
Ste 100
Salt Lake City, UT 84101
801-245-7350
Fax: 801-533-3968
http://www.utahddcouncil.org
Ddilley@utah.gov

Libby Oseguera, Executive Director
Lindsey Hunter, Administrative Secretary
Rickie Crandall, Program Support Specialist

The mission of the Utah DD council is to be the states leading source of critical innovative and progressive knowledge, advocacy, leadership and collaboration to enhance the life of individuals with developmental disabilities.

1875 **Utah State Office of Education**
PO Box 144200
Salt Lake City, UT 84114-4200
801-538-7500
http://www.schools.utah.gov
mark.peterson@schools.utah.gov

Brian Olmstead, State GED Administrator
Brenda Jacobsen, GED Testing Assistant

Promotes adult education and GED Testing in Utah.

Vermont

1876 **Disability Rights Vermont**
141 Main St
Ste 7
Montpelier, VT 05602
802-229-1355
800-834-7890
Fax: 802-229-1359
http://www.disabilityrightsvt.org
info@disabilityrightsvt.org

Sarah Wendell-Launderville, President
David LaCroix, Vice President
Charlie Crocker, Treasurer

Dedicated to addressing problems, questions and complaints brought to it by Vermonters with disabilities. Mission is to promote the equality, dignity, and self-determination of people with disabilities. Provides information, referral and advocacy services, in cluding legal representation when appropriate, to individuals with disabilities throughout Vermont. Also advocates to promote positive systematic responses to issues affecting people with disabilities.

1877 **Vermont Assistive Technology Program**
Department of Health & Human Services
NOB 1 North
280 State Dr
Waterbury, VT 05671-1090
800-750-6355
Fax: 802-241-0341
http://atp.vermont.gov

Graham Dewyea, Program Director

The program assists persons of all ages with disabilities access assistive technology and provide them with solutions to overcome barriers at home, work, and in the local community.

1878 **Vermont Client Assistance Program**
Vermont Law Help
800-889-2047
http://vtlawhelp.org

Advocacy group dedicated to improving the lives of persons with disabilities and their families by eliminating barriers and allowing them to exercise their civil, legal, and human rights.

1879 **Vermont Department of Children & Families**
280 State Dr
HC 1 N
Waterbury, VT 05671-1080
http://dcf.vermont.gov

To promote the social, emotional, physical and economic well being and the safety of Vermont's children and families.

1880 **Vermont Department of Education**
219 N Main St
Ste 402
Barre, VT 05641
802-479-1030
http://www.education.vermont.gov
aoe.edinfo@vermont.gov

Daniel M. French, Secretary

Provide leadership and support to help all Vermont students achieve excellence.

1881 **Vermont Department of Labor**
5 Green Mountain Dr
PO Box 488
Montpelier, VT 05601-0488
802-828-4000
Fax: 802-828-4022
TDD: 800-650-4152
http://labor.vermont.gov
labor.webinput@vermont.gov

Lindsay H. Kurrle, Commissioner

To improve and enhance services to the public by combining under one department: employment security, employment-related services, labor market information, safety and training for Vermont workers, and employers, workers compensation, and wage and hour.

1882 **Vermont Developmental Disabilities Council**
322 Industrial Ln
Berlin, VT 05633-0206
802-828-1310
888-317-2006
Fax: 802-828-1321
http://www.ddc.vermont.gov
vtddc@vermont.gov

Kirsten Murphy, Executive Director
Susan Aranoff, Senior Planner & Policy Analyst
Chelsea Hayward, Administrative Assistant

Statewide board that works to increase public awareness about critical issues affecting Vermonters with developmental disabilities and their families.

1883 **Vermont Governor's Office**
109 State St
Pavilion
Montpelier, VT 05609
802-828-3333
Fax: 802-828-3339
TTY: 800-649-6825
http://www.governor.vermont.gov

Phil Scott, Governor

1884 **Vermont Special Education**
Vermont Department of Education
219 N Main St
Ste 402
Barre, VT 05641
802-479-1030
http://education.vermont.gov
aoe.edinfo@vermont.gov

Daniel M. French, Secretary

Provides technical assistance to schools and other organization to help ensure that schools understand and comply with federal and state laws and regulations related to providing special education services.

Virginia

1885 **Assistive Technology System**
Department for Aging & Rehabilitative Services
2001 Mayvill St
Ste 202
Richmond, VA 23230
804-662-9990
800-552-5019
TTY: 800-464-9950
http://www.vats.org

Elizabeth Flaherty, Chair
Kelly Lum, Vice Chair
Peggy Fields, PhD, Council Secretary

To ensure that Virginians of all ages and abilities can acquire the appropriate, affordable assistive and information technologies and services they need to participate in society as active citizens.

1886 **Department of Correctional Education**
PO Box 26963
Richmond, VA 23261-6963 804-674-3000
http://vadoc.virginia.gov
Harold W. Clarke, Director
Scott Richeson, Dep. Dir., Programs/Education
A. David Robinson, Chief of Corrections Operations
Provides quality educational programs that enable incarcerated youth and adults to become responsible, productive, tax-paying members of their community.

1887 **Diasbility Law Center of Virginia**
1512 Willow Lawn
Ste 100
Richmond, VA 23230 804-225-2042
800-552-3962
Fax: 804-662-7057
http://dlcv.org
info@dlcv.org
Colleen Miller, Executive Director
Tina King, Operations Coordinator
Dana Traynham, Senior Staff Attorney
To protect and advance legal, human, and civil rights of persons with disabilities; combat and prevent abuse, neglect, and discrimination; and to promote independence, choice, and self determination by persons with disabilities.

1888 **Office of Adult Education and Literacy**
Virginia Department of Education
PO Box 2120
Richmond, VA 23218 804-225-2023
http://www.doe.virginia.gov
Dr. James F. Lane, Superintendent
Laura Jennings, Senior Administrative Assistant
Becky Marable, Director of Human Resources
Operates as the designated agency to coordinate all secondary adult education and literacy services in the commonwealth.

1889 **State Department of Education**
PO Box 2120
Richmond, VA 23218 804-225-2023
http://www.doe.virginia.gov
Dr. James F. Lane, Superintendent
Laura Jennings, Senior Administrative Assistant
Becky Marable, Director of Human Resources
Promotes quality education.

1890 **State GED Administration**
Office of Adult Education and Literacy
PO Box 2120
Richmond, VA 23218 804-225-2023
http://www.doe.virginia.gov
Dr. James F. Lane, Superintendent
Laura Jennings, Senior Administrative Assistant
Becky Marable, Director of Human Resources
Promotes quality education for adults.

1891 **Virginia Board for People with Disabilities**
1100 Bank St
7th Fl
Richmond, VA 23219 804-786-0016
http://www.vaboard.org
info@vbpd.virginia.gov
Mary McAdam, Chair
Rachel Laughlin, Vice Chair
Heidi Lawyer, Executive Director
To enrich the lives of Virginians with disabilities by providing a voice for their concerns.

Washington

1892 **Correctional Education**
Washington Department of Corrections
PO Box 41100
Olympia, WA 98504-1100 360-725-8213
http://www.doc.wa.gov
DOCCorrespondenceUnit@doc.wa.gov
Stephen Sinclair, Secretary
Julie Martin, Deputy Secretary
The Department of Corrections, in collaboration with its criminal justice partners, will contribute to staff and community safety and hold offenders accountable through administration of criminal sanctions and effective re-entry programs.

1893 **Disability Rights Washington**
315 5th Ave S
Ste 850
Seattle, WA 98104 206-324-1521
800-562-2702
Fax: 206-957-0729
TTY: 206-324-1521
http://www.disabilityrightswa.org
info@dr-wa.org
Mark Stroh, Executive Director
A private non-profit organization that protects the rights of people with disabilities statewide. To advance the dignity, equality, and self-determination of people with disabilities. Also work to pursue justice on matters related to human and legal rights.

1894 **Region X: Office of Federal Contract Compliance**
US Department of Labor
90 7th St
Ste 18-300
San Francisco, CA 94103-1516 415-625-7800
Fax: 415-625-7799
TTY: 877-889-5627
http://www.dol.gov/ofccp
OFCCP-Public@dol.gov
Janette Wipper, Regional Director
Jane Suhr, Deputy Regional Director
Administers Federal Law requiring recipients of Federal Contract dollars to uphold affirmative action and equal employment pooprtunity for all workers, including but not limited to minorities, women, veterans and disabled employees.

1895 **Region X: US Department of Education Office for Civil Rights**
US Department of Education
915 2nd Ave
Room 3310
Seattle, WA 98174-1099 206-607-1600
Fax: 206-607-1601
TDD: 800-877-8339
http://www.ed.gov
ocr.seattle@ed.gov
Kenneth L. Marcus, Assistant Secretary
Earl Morgan, Executive Officer
Kristine Minami, Senior Counsel
This office covers the states of Alaska, Hawaii, Idaho, Montana, Nevada, Oregon, and Washington.

1896 **Region X: US Department of Health and Human Services, Office of Civil Rights**
US Department of Health & Human Services
90 7th St
Ste 4-100
San Francisco, CA 94103 800-368-1019
Fax: 202-619-7697
TTY: 800-537-7697
http://www.hhs.gov
ocrmail@hhs.gov
Alex M. Azar II, Secretary
Eric D. Hargan, Deputy Secretary
Peter Urbanowicz, Chief of Staff

1897 **WA State Board for Community and Technical Colleges**
PO Box 42495
1300 Quince Street SE, 4th Fl
Olympia, WA 98504-2495
360-704-4400
Fax: 360-704-4415
http://www.sbctc.edu
support@sbctc.edu

Larry Brown, Chair
Anne Fennessy, Vice Chair
Jan Yoshiwara, Executive Director
Promotes adult education.

1898 **Washington Human Rights Commission**
711 S Capitol Way
Ste 402
Olympia, WA 98504
800-233-3247
http://www.hum.wa.gov

Sharon Ortiz, Executive Director
Charlene Strong, Commission Chair
Guadalupe Gamboa, Commissioner
The Washington State Human Rights Commission enforces the Washington Law Against Discrimination, the broadest civil rights statute in the United States. It provides technical assistance and training. It also does studies and writes white papers on issues of social justice.

1899 **Washington State Board for Community and Technical Colleges**
Office of Adult Basic Education
1300 Quince St SE
4th Fl
Olympia, WA 98504-2495
360-704-4400
Fax: 360-704-4415
http://www.sbctc.ctc.edu
support@sbctc.edu

Larry Brown, Chair
Anne Fennesy, Vice Chair
Jan Yashiwara, Executive Director
Promotes the quality of adult education.

1900 **Washington State Client Assistance Program**
2531 Rainier Ave S
Seattle, WA 98144
206-721-5999
800-544-2121
TTY: 888-721-6072
http://www.washingtoncap.org
info@washingtoncap.org

Jerry Johnsen, Director
Provides information and advocacy for persons seeking services from the Department of Services for the Blind and the Division of Vocational Rehabilitation. Approximately 25 percent of cases involve assistive technology issues.

1901 **Washington State Developmental Disabilities Council**
PO Box 48314
Olympia, WA 98504-8314
360-586-3560
800-634-4473
Fax: 360-586-2424
http://www.ddc.wa.gov
Ed.Holen@ddc.wa.gov

Ed Holen, Executive Director
Aziz Aladin, Budget Director
Donna Patrick, Public Policy Director
Holds that individuals with developmental disabilities, including those with the most severe disabilities, have the right to achieve independence, productivity, integration and inclusion into the community.

1902 **Washington State Governor's Committee on Disability Issues & Employment**
PO Box 9046
Olympia, WA 98507
360-902-9500
800-318-6022
http://esd.wa.gov

Suzan LeVine, Commissioner
Janelle Guthrie, Director of Communications
Tim Probst, Director, Workforce Initiatives
Information about disability rights programs and services.

West Virginia

1903 **Client Assistance Program (CAP): West Virginia Division**
Disability Rights West Virginia
1207 Quarrier St
Ste 400
Charleston, WV 25301
304-346-0847
800-950-5250
Fax: 304-346-0867
http://www.drofwv.org

Susan Given, Executive Director
Barbara Griner, Administrative Director
Josh Stricker, System Administrator
Mandated in 1984, to provide advocacy to individuals seeking services under the federal Rehabilitation Act (such as services from the West Virginia Division of Rehabilitation Services, Centers for Independent Living, supported employment programs and sheltered workshops).

1904 **Disability Rights West Virginia**
1207 Quarrier St
Ste 400
Charleston, WV 25301
304-346-0847
800-950-5250
Fax: 304-346-0867
http://www.drofwv.org

Susan Given, Executive Director
Taniua Hardy, Program Director
Barbara Criner, Administrative Director
A nonprofit organization dedicated to improving the quality of life for people with learning disabilities and developmental disabilities.

1905 **Office of Diversion and Transition Programs**
State Department of Education
Building 6, Room 728
1900 Kanawha Blvd East
Charleston, WV 25305-0330
304-558-8833
Fax: 304-558-3946
http://wvde.state.wv.us/odtp

Steven L. Paine, EdD, Superintendent
David G. Perry, President
Provides educational services to over 6,000 institutionalized juveniles and adults. It protects the constitutional rights of institutionalized persons by providing programs and services that help change their lives.

1906 **State Department of Education**
1900 Kanawha Blvd E
Building 6
Charleston, WV 25305
304-558-2681
http://wvde.state.wv.us

Steven L. Paine, EdD, State Superintendent
David G. Perry, President
Promotes quality education.

1907 **State GED Administration**
1900 Kanawha Blvd E
Building 6
Charleston, WV 25305
304-558-2681
http://wvde.state.wv.us/tasc

Steven L. Paine, EdD, Superintendent
David G. Perry, President
Ellen Killion, Administrator
To provide accommodations to qualifying GED candidates.

1908 **West Virginia Adult Basic Education**
West Virginia Department of Education
1900 Kanawha Blvd E
Building 6
Charleston, WV 25305
304-558-2681
800-642-2670
http://wvde.us/adult-education

Mendy Marshall, Executive Director
Cyndy Sundstrom, Manager
Sandra Adkins, Coordinator

To enable adult learners to be literate, productive, and successful in the workplace, home and community by delivering responsive adult education programs and services.

1909 **West Virginia Assistive Technology System**
WVU Center for Execellence In Disabilities
959 Hartman Run Rd
Morgantown, WV 26505 800-841-8436
http://wvats.cedwvu.org
wvats@hsc.wvu.edu
Jessi Wright, Program Manager
Jamie Church, Program Coordinator
Jack Stewart, Assistant Director
Provides access to Assistive Technology through information and referral, technical assistance training, device demonstration, loan & exchange.

Wisconsin

1910 **Correctional Education Association of Wisconsin**
http://www.ceawisconsin.org
jerrybednarowski@new.rr.com
David Hines, President
Margaret Done, Secretary
Timothy Malchow, Treasurer
A nonprofit, professional education association dedicated to providing quality education to correctional sites in Wisconsin.
1984

1911 **Department of Public Instruction**
125 S Webster St
Madison, WI 53703 608-266-3390
800-441-4563
http://dpi.wi.gov
webadmin@dpi.wi.gov
Tony Evers, State Superintendent
Dawn B. Crim, Assistant State Superintendent
Debra Gaffney-Dilley, Executive Staff Assistant
Promotes quality education.

1912 **Disability Rights Wisconsin**
131 W Wilson St
Ste 700
Madison, WI 53703 608-267-0214
800-928-8778
http://www.disabilityrightswi.org
Dan Idzikowski, Executive Director
DRW challenges systems and society to achieve positive changes in the lives of people with disabilities and their families.

1913 **State GED Administration**
Department of Public Instruction
125 S Webster St
Madison, WI 53703 608-266-3390
800-441-4563
http://dpi.wi.gov
Tony Evers, State Superintendent
Dawn B. Crim, Assistant State Superintendent
Debra Gaffney-Dilley, Executive Staff Assistant
Promotes quality adult education.

1914 **WisTech**
Wisconsin Department of Health Services
1 W. Wilson St, Rm 650
PO Box 7850
Madison, WI 53703 608-266-9622
http://www.dhs.wisconsin.gov
Linda Seemeyer, Secretary
Tom Engels, Deputy Secretary
Wisconsin's Assistive Technology Program provides information on selecting, funding, installing and using assistive technology.

1915 **Wisconsin Board for People with Developmental Disabilities**
101 E Wilson St
Room 219
Madison, WI 53703 608-266-7826
http://www.wi-bpdd.org
Pam Malin, Chair
Beth Swedeen, Executive Director
Jeremy Gundlach, Communications Specialist
Established to advocate on behalf of individuals with developmental disabilities, foster welcoming and inclusive communities, and improve the disability service system. To help people with developmental disabilities become independent, productive, and included in all facets of community life.

1916 **Wisconsin Department of Workforce Development**
PO Box 7946
Madison, WI 53707-7946 608-266-3131
Fax: 608-266-1784
http://dwd.wisconsin.gov
sec@dwd.wisconsin.gov
Ray Allen, Secretary
Christopher Hagerup, Deputy Secretary
Chytania Brown, Administrator
A state agency charged with building and strengthening Wisconsin's workforce in the 21st century and beyond. The Departmen's primary responsibilities include providing job services, training and employment assistance to people looking for work, at the same time as itworks with employers on finding the necessary workers to fill current job openings.

1917 **Wisconsin Equal Rights Division**
Department of Workforce Development
201 E Washington Ave.
Room A100
Madison, WI 53703 608-266-6860
Fax: 608-267-4592
TTY: 608-264-8752
http://dwd.wisconsin.gov/er
erinfo@dwd.wisconsin.gov
Robert A. Rodriguez, Division Administrator
Jim Chiolino, Deputy Division Administrator
To protect the rights of all people in Wisconsin under the civil rights and labor standards laws and to achieve compliance through education, outreach, and enforcement by empowered and committed employees.

1918 **Wisconsin Governor's Committee for People with Disabilities**
1 W Wilson St
Madison, WI 53703 608-266-1865
TTY: 800-947-3529
http://dhs.wisconsin.gov
DHSwebmaster@dhs.wisconsin.gov
Linda Seemeyer, Secretary
Tom Engels, Deputy Secretary
Jennifer Malcore, Assistant Deputy Secretary
Established to improve employment opportunities for people with disabilities.

Wyoming

1919 **Adult Basic Education**
Wyoming Community College Commission
2300 Capitol Ave, 5th Fl
Ste B
Cheyenne, WY 82002 307-777-7763
http://communitycolleges.wy.edu
Matt Mead, Governor
Jillian Balow, Superintendent
Saundra Meyer, Commission Chair
Focuses on strengthening basic reading, writing, and math skills for adults.

1920 **Client Assistance Program (CAP): Wyoming**
Protection & Advocacy System Wyoming
7344 Stockmann St
Cheyenne, WY 82009
307-632-3496
Fax: 307-638-0815
http://www.wypanda.com
wypanda@wypanda.com
Jeanne Thobro, Chief Executive Officer
Provides free services to consumers and applicants for projects, programs and facilities funded under the rehabilitation act.
1977

1921 **Correctional Education: Wyoming Women's Center**
1000 W Griffith
PO Box 300
Lusk, WY 82225
307-334-3693
Fax: 307-334-2254
http://corrections.wyo.gov
chris.thayer@wyo.gov
Matt Mead, Governor
Robert Lampert, Director
The Wyoming Women's Center is a full service, secure correctional facility for female offenders and the sole adult female facility in the State of Wyoming. In October 2000, WWC opened a self-contained 16 bed intensive addiction treatment unit, a is highly structured long term 7-9 month program based upon the therapeutic community treatment model. It is tailored to provide gender specific services and is funded with a combination of state and federal resources.

1922 **Protection & Advocacy System**
7344 Stockmann St
Cheyenne, WY 82009
307-632-3496
Fax: 307-638-0815
http://www.wypanda.com
wypanda@wypanda.com
Jeanne Thobro, Chief Executive Officer
It is the goal of Wyoming's Protection & Advocacy System, Inc. to ensure that all of its web resources are accessible to all who use the website.

1923 **State Department of Education**
122 W 25th St
Ste 5200
Cheyenne, WY 82002
307-777-7675
Fax: 307-777-6234
http://edu.wyoming.gov
Jillian Balow, Superintendent
Dicky Shanor, Chief of Staff
Dianne Bailey, Chief Financial Officer
Dedicated to accessible education.

1924 **State GED Administration**
State Department of Education
122 W 25th St
Ste 5200
Cheyenne, WY 82002
307-777-7675
Fax: 307-777-6234
http://edu.wyoming.gov
Jillian Balow, Superintendent
Dicky Shanor, Chief of Staff
Dianne Bailey, Chief Financial Officer
Promotes quality adult education.

1925 **Wyoming Department of Workforce Services**
350 S Washington St
Afton, WY 83110
307-886-9260
Fax: 307-886-2969
http://www.wyomingworkforce.org
John Cox, Director
John Ysebaert, Deputy Director
Employment training for persons working in Wyoming.

1926 **Wyoming Technology Access Program**
Wyoming Institute for Disabilities
1000 E University Ave
Dept. 4298
Laramie, WY 82071
307-766-2761
888-989-9463
Fax: 307-766-2763
TTY: 800-908-7011
http://www.uwyo.edu/wind/watr/wytap.html
wytap@wilr.org
Sandy Root-Elledge, Executive Director
Canyon Hardesty, Deputy Director
Felicia Arce, AT Program Specialist
Wyoming Assistive Technology Resources (WATR) and Wyoming Independent Living (WIL) partnered with First Interstate Bank of Laramie to offer a program that assists people with disabilities to finance assistive technology devices and services.

National Programs

1927 **Academic Institute**
2495 140th Ave NE
Suite D-210
Bellevue, WA 98005
425-401-6844
Fax: 425-556-6972
http://www.academicinstitute.com
sherrill@academicinstitute.com
Sherrill O'Shaughnessy, Founder/Executive Director
To prepare students for success in college and their lives beyond by helping them cultivate: a sense of capability, determination, resilience, self-advocacy and a love of learning.

1928 **American Association for Adult and Continuing Education**
10111 Martin Luther King Jr Hwy
Ste 200C
Bowie, MD 20720
301-459-6261
Fax: 301-459-6241
http://www.aaace.org
office@aaace.org
Steven Schmidt, President
Jonathan Taylor, Secretary
Jim Berger, Treasurer
Provides leadership for the field of adult and continuing education by expanding opportunities for adult growth and development; unifying adult educators; fostering the development and dissemination of theory, research, informaiton and best practices; promoting identity and standards for the profession; and advocating relevant public policy and social change initiatives.

1929 **American Literacy Council**
1441 Mariposa Avenue
Boulder, CO 80302
303-440-7385
http://www.americanliteracy.com
presidentalc3@americanliteracy.com
Alan Mole, President
Roberta Mahoney, Vice President
Joe Little, Director
Conveys information on new solutions, innovative technologies and tools for engaging more boldly in the battle for literacy.

1930 **Association of Educational Therapists**
7044 S. 13th St.
Oak Creek, WI 53154
414-908-4949
http://www.aetonline.org
customercare@AETOnline.org
Judith Brennan, President
Polly Brophy, Treasurer
Kaye Ragland, Secretary
A national professional organization dedicated to establishing ethical professional standards, defining the roles and responsibilities of the educational therapist, providing opportunities for professional growth, and to studying techniques and technologies, philosophies, and research related to the practice of educational therapy.
1979

1931 **Association on Higher Education and Disability (AHEAD)**
8015 West Kenton Circle
Suite 230
Huntersville, NC 28078
704-947-7779
Fax: 704-948-7779
http://www.ahead.org
Jamie Axelrod, President
Gaeir Dietrich, Treasurer
Stephan Smith, Executive Director
A professional membership organization for individuals involved in the development of policy and in the provision of quality services to meet the needs of persons with disabilities involved in all areas of higher education.
3,000 members 1977

1932 **Career College Association (CCA)**
1101 Connecticut Ave NW
Ste 900
Washington, DC 20036
202-336-6700
866-711-8574
Fax: 202-336-6828
http://www.career.org
cca@career.org
Robert Herzog, Chair
Jeffery Cooper, Vice Chair
Steve Gunderson, President and CEO
A voluntary membership organization of accredited, private, postsecondary schools, institutes, colleges and universities that provide career-specific educational programs.
1,400 members

1933 **Center for the Improvement of Early Reading Achievement (CIERA)**
University of Michigan School of Education
610 E University Ave
Rm 2002 SEB
Ann Arbor, MI 48109-1259
734-647-6940
Fax: 734-615-4858
http://www.ciera.org
ciera@umich.edu
Karen Wixon, Former Director
Joanne Carlisle, Former Co-Director
Deanna Birdyshaw, Former Associate Director
To improve the reading achievement of America's youth by generating and disseminating theoretical, empirical, and practical solutions to the learning and teaching of beginning reading.

1934 **Council for Educational Diagnostic Services**
Council for Exceptional Children
2900 Crystal Drive
Suite 1000
Arlington, VA 22202-3557
888-232-7733
888-232-7733
Fax: 703-264-9494
TTY: 866-915-5000
http://www.cec.sped.org
Robin D. Brewer, President
Alexander T. Graham, Secretary
Benjamin White, Student Member
Ensures the highest quality of diagnostic and prescriptive procedures involved in the education of individuals with disabilities and/or who are gifted.

1935 **Distance Education and Training Council (DETC)**
1601 18th St NW
Ste 2
Washington, DC 20009
202-234-5100
Fax: 202-332-1386
http://www.detc.org
detc@detc.org
Leah K. Matthews, Executive Director
Charles Baldwin, CFO
Sally R. Welch, Associate Director
A voluntary, non-governmental, educational organization that operates a nationally recognized accrediting association. Fosters and preserves high quality, educationally sound and widely accepted distance education and independent learning solutions.
1926

1936 **Division for Children's Communication Development**
Council for Exceptional Children
2900 Crystal Drive
Suite 1000
Arlington, VA 22202-3557
888-232-7733
888-232-7733
Fax: 703-265-9494
TTY: 866-915-5000
http://www.cec.sped.org
service@cec.sped.org
Robin D. Brewer, President
Alexander T. Graham, Secretary
Benjamin White, Student Member

Dedicated to improving the education of children with communication delays and disorders and hearing loss. Members include professionals serving individuals with hearing, speech and language disorders in the areas of receptive and expressive, verbal and nonverbal spoken, written and sign communication. Members receive a quarterly journal and newsletter three times a year.

1937 **Division for Culturally and Linguistically Diverse Learners**
Council for Exceptional Children
2900 Crystal Drive
Suite 1000
Arlington, VA 22202-3557
888-232-7733
888-232-7733
Fax: 703-264-9494
TTY: 866-915-5000
http://www.cec.sped.org

Robin D. Brewer, President
Alexander T. Graham, Secretary
Benjamin White, Student Member
Advances educational opportunities for culturally and linguistically diverse learners with disabilities and/or who are gifted, their families and the professionals who serve them.

1938 **Division for Research**
Council for Exceptional Children
2900 Crystal Drive
Suite 1000
Arlington, VA 22202-3557
888-232-7733
888-232-7733
Fax: 703-264-9494
TTY: 866-915-5000
http://www.cec.sped.org

Robin D. Brewer, President
Alexander T. Graham, Secretary
Benjamin White, Student Member
Devoted to the advancement of research related to the education of individuals with disabilities and/or who are gifted.

1939 **Educational Advisory Group**
2222 Eastlake Ave E
Seattle, WA 98102-3419
206-323-1838
Fax: 206-267-1325
http://www.eduadvisory.com

Yvonne Jones, Director
Specializes in matching children with the learning environments that are best for them and works with families to help them identify concerns and establish priorities about their child's education.

1940 **Institute for Educational Leadership**
4301 Connecticut Ave., NW
Suite 100
Washington, DC 20008
202-822-8405
Fax: 202-872-4050
http://www.iel.org
iel@iel.org

Johan Uvin, President
Karen Mapp, Chair
Sara A. Sneed, Vice Chair
The Institute aims to improve education and the lives of children and their families through positive and visionary change.

1941 **Institute for Human Centered Design (ICHD)**
200 Portland St.
Suite 1
Boston, MA 02114
617-695-1225
800-949-4232
Fax: 617-482-8099
TTY: 617-695-1225
http://humancentereddesign.org
info@HumanCenteredDesign.org

Ralph Jackson, President
Gabriela Bonome-Sims, Director, Administration
Valerie Fletcher, Executive Director
Founded as Adaptive Environments, committed to advancing the role of design in expanding opportunity and enhancing experience for people of all ages and abilities through excellence in design.

1942 **Institute for the Study of Adult Literacy**
Pennsylvania State Univ. College of Education
226 Chambers Building
University Park, PA 16802
814-865-0488
Fax: 814-863-6108
http://www.ed.psu.edu/isal
isal@psu.edu

David H. Monk, Co-Director
Emily Martell, Finance Office
Suzanne Wayne, Public Relations
Experienced staff assista providers with: program design and delivery; customized instructional materials and assessment development; professional development (including distance learning); and program evaluations.

1943 **International Dyslexia Association**
40 York Rd.
4th Fl.
Baltimore, MD 21204
410-296-0232
Fax: 410-321-5069
http://www.dyslexiaida.org
info@ydslexiaida.org

Rick Smith, Chief Executive Officer
Newton Guerin, Chief Operating Officer
David Holste, Chief Financial Officer
The International Dyslexia Association is an international organization that concerns itself with the complex issues of dyslexia. The IDA membership consists of a variety of professionals in partnership with people with dyslexia and their families and all others interested in The Association's mission.

1944 **Learning Resource Network**
P.O. Box 9
River Falls, WI 54022
800-678-5376
Fax: 888-234-8633
http://www.lern.org
info@lern.org

William A. Draves, President
Julie Coates, SVP, Information Services
Greg Marsello, SVP, Organizational Development
An organization dedicated to offering informational resources and consultative expertise on continuing education and lifelong learning. Disseminates publications, newsletters, webinars, and conferences that provide strategies and methodologies for professionals in educational institutions.
1974

1945 **National Adult Education Professional Development Consortium**
444 N. Capitol St., NW
Suite 422
Washington, DC 20001
202-624-5250
Fax: 202-624-1947
http://www.naepdc.org
ptyler@naepdc.org

Patricia H. Tyler, Executive Director
Reecie Stagnolia, Chair
Gene Sofer, Director, Government Relations
An organization dedicated to enhancing adult education through professional development and dissemination of information and assistive resources.

1946 **National Adult Literacy & Learning Disabilities Center (NALLD)**
FHI360
359 Blackwell Street
Suite 200
Durham, NC 27701
919-544-7040
Fax: 919-544-7262
http://www.fhi360.org
media@fhi360.org

Parick c. Fine, Chief Executive Officer
Robert S. Murphy, CFO
Deborah Kennedy, COO
The center is a national resource for information on learning disabilities in adults and on the relationship between learning disabilities and low-level literacy skills.

1947 **National Association for Adults with Special Learning Needs (NAASLN)**
P.O. Box 716
Bryn Mawr, PA 19010 http://www.naasln.org
Richard Cooper, President
Joan Hudson-Miller, Co-President
Frances A. Holthaus, Vice President
An association for those who serve adults with special learning needs. Members include educators, trainers, employers, and human service providers. Aims to ensure that adults with special learning needs have opportunities necessary to become successful lifelong learners.

1948 **National Association of Private Special Education Centers**
601 Pennsylvania Ave., NW
Suite 900 - South Building
Washington, DC 20004 202-434-8225
http://www.napsec.org
napsec@napsec.org
Tom Dempsey, President
Dr. Tom McCool, Vice President
Tom Celli, Treasurer
A non-profit association whose mission is to ensure access for individuals to private special education as a vital component of the continuum of appropriate placement and services in American education. The association consists solely of private special education programs that serve both both privately and publicly placed individuals of all ages with disabilities.
1971

1949 **National Center for Family Literacy**
325 W Main St
Ste 300
Louisville, KY 40202 502-584-1133
Fax: 502-584-0172
http://www.famlit.org
notify@familieslearning.org
George Siemens, Board Member
Sharon Darling, Board Member
Jason Falls, Board Member
Mission is to not only provide every family with the opportunity to learn, but the ability to learn anf grow together. Ensures the cycle of learning and progress passes from generation to generation.

1950 **National Center for Learning Disabilities (NCLD)**
32 Laight St.
2nd Fl.
New York, NY 10013 888-575-7373
http://www.ncld.org
Frederic M. Poses, Chair
Mimi Corcoran, President/CEO
Rashonda Ambrose, Director, Strategic Partnerships
Works to ensure that the nation's 15 million children, adolescents, and adults with learning disabilities have every opportunity for succees in school, work, and life. NCLD also provides essential information to parents, professionals, and individuals with learning disabilities; promotes research and programs to foster effective learning; and advocates for policies to protect and strengthen educational rights and opportunities.

1951 **National Center for the Study of Adult Learning & Literacy**
Harvard Graduate School of Education
Appian Way
Cambridge, MA 02138 617-495-3414
Fax: 617-495-4811
http://www.gse.harvard.edu
webeditor@gse.harvard.edu
James E. Ryan, Dean
The National Center for the Study of Adult Learning & Literacy both informs and learns from practice. Its rigorous, high quality research increases knowledge and gives those teaching, managing, and setting policy in adult literacy education a sound basis for making decisions.

1952 **National Center on Adult Literacy (NCAL)**
University of Pennsylvania
3700 Walnut Street
Philadelphia, PA 19104-6216 215-898-9803
Fax: 215-573-2115
http://www.literacy.org/
boyle@literacy.upenn.edu
Daniel A. Wagner, Founder and Director
Mohamed Maamouri, Associate Director
Ruth Boyle, Administrative Assistant
NCAL's mission incorporates three primary goals: to improve understanding of youth and adult learning; to foster innovation and increase effectiveness in youth and adult basic education and literacy work; and to expand access to information and build capacity for literacy and basic skills service.
1990

1953 **National Education Association (NEA)**
1201 16th St., NW
Washington, DC 20036-3290 202-833-4000
Fax: 202-822-7974
http://www.nea.org
Lily Eskelsen Garc¡a, President
Becky Pringle, Vice-President
John C. Stocks, Executive Director
Advocates for education professionals and seeks to unite members and the nation to fulfill the promise of public education to prepare every student to succeed in a diverse and interdependent world.

1954 **National Lekotek Center**
2001 N Clybourn
Chicago, IL 60614 773-528-5766
Fax: 773-537-2992
TTY: 773-973-2180
http://www.lekotek.org
lekotek@lekotek.org
Elaine D. Cottey, Chair
Kevin Limbeck, President & CEO
Carol Neiger, Secretary
The central source on toys and play for children with special needs.

1955 **Office of Special Education Programs**
US Department of Education
400 Maryland Avenue, SW
Washington, DC 20202 202-208-5815
800-872-5327
http://www2.ed.gov
Melody Musgrove, Director
Dedicated to improving results for infants, toddlers, children and youth with disabilities ages birth through 21 by providing leadership and financial support to assist states and local districts.

1956 **ProLiteracy**
104 Marcellus Street
Syracuse, NY 13204 315-422-9121
888-528-2224
Fax: 315-422-6369
http://www.proliteracy.org
info@proliteracy.org

John Ward, Chair
Nikki Zollar, Vice Chair
Kevin Morgan, President/CEO
Champions the power of literacy to improve the lives of adults and their families, communities, and societies. Works with its members and partners, and the adult learners they serve, along with local, national, and international organizations. Helps build the capacity and quality of programs that are teaching adults to read, write, compute, use technology and learn English as a new language.

1957 **Thinking and Learning Connection**
Parents Helping Parents
1400 Parkmoor Avenue
Suite 100
San Jose, CA 95126
408-727-5775
855-727-5775
Fax: 408-286-1116
http://www.php.com
Hitesh Shah, Chair
Mary Ellen Peterson, Executive Director/CEO, PHP
Paul Schutz, CFO
A group of independent associates committed to teaching learning different students. The primary focus is working with dyslexia and dyscalculia. The individualized education programs utilize extensive multisensory approaches to teach reading, spelling, handwriting, composition, comprehension and mathematics.

Alabama

1958 **Alabama Commission on Higher Education**
PO Box 302000
Montgomery, AL 36130-2000
334-242-1998
Fax: 334-242-0268
http://www.ache.state.al.us
Gregory G Fitch PhD, Executive Director
Jacinta Whitehurst, Administrative Assistant
Margaret Gunter, Director
Ths state agency responsible for the overall statewide planning and coordination of higher education in Alabama. Seeks to provide reasonable access to quality collegiate and university education for the citizens of Alabama.

1959 **South Baldwin Literacy Council**
21441 U.S. Hwy 98 East
Foley, AL 36535
251-943-7323
Fax: 251-970-3578
http://www.southbaldwinliteracycouncil.org/
literacy@gulftel.com
Keith Cardwell, President
Jan Taylor, Vice President
Rosalie Wolfe, Treasurer
Provides instruction by trained volunteer tutors in a one-on-one or small group setting to residents of South Baldwin County. Instruction is centered around the learners' individual goals and capabilities and is designed to improve basic reading, writing and life skills.

1960 **The Literacy Council**
2301 1st Ave N
Ste 102
Birmingham, AL 35203
205-326-1925
888-448-7323
http://www.literacy-council.org
info@literacy-council.org
Leigh Hancock, Chairman
Jordan DeMoss, Vice Chair
Beth Wilder, President & Executive Director
A non-profit organization which serves a five-county area, is dedicated to reducing literacy. Efforts include providing resources and referrals by maintaining a toll-free literacy helpline which serves as a primary point of contact for individuals seeking literacy assistance.

Alaska

1961 **Alaska Adult Basic Education**
SERRC
210 Ferry Eay
Juneau, AK 99801
907-586-6806
Fax: 907-463-3811
http://www.serrc.org
info@serrc.org
Eugene Avey, Board Member
Robert Boyle, Board Member
Steve Bradshaw, Board Member
The mission of the Adult Basic Education program is to provide instruction in the basic skills of reading, writing, and mathematics to adult learners in order to prepare them for transitioning into the labor market or higher academic or vocational training.

1962 **Anchorage Literacy Project**
Ste 104
1345 Rudakof Cir
Anchorage, AK 99508
907-337-1981
Fax: 907-338-3105
http://www.alaskaliteracyprogram.org
akliteracy@alaskaliteracyprogram.org
Linda Gerwin, President
Anne Newell, Vice President
Polly Smith, Executive Director
Dedicated to improving the lives of adults and their families by helping to build their literacy skills. Offer direct literacy skills for adults-native born citizens and recent immigrants alike-through on-site classes and one-on-one tutoring.

1963 **Literacy Council of Alaska**
517 Gaffney Rd
Fairbanks, AK 99701
907-456-6212
Fax: 907-456-4302
http://www.literacycouncilofalaska.org
lca@literacycouncilofalaska.org
Lisa Baker, Chairman
Mike Kolsa, Executive Director
Becky Magowan, Business Manager
Promotes literacy for people of all ages in Fairbanks and the Interior. The goals are to help community members achieve individual educational goals and to raise public awareness about literacy.

Arizona

1964 **Chandler Public Library Adult Basic Education**
PO Box 4008
Mail Stop 601
Chandler, AZ 85244-4008
480-782-2800
http://www.chandlerlibrary.org
marybeth.gardner@chandleraz.gov
Dolly Franco, President
Chris Loschiavo, Secretary
Marybeth Gardner, Library Development
Provides adult basic education classes for learners who need to improve their basic skills in reading, writing, and math. Gives GED preparation classes to help students prepare to take the GED exam.

1965 **Literacy Volunteers of Maricopa County**
1616 East Indian School Road
Suite 200
Phoenix, AZ 85016
602-274-3430
Fax: 602-274-6831
http://www.literacyvolunteers-maricopa.org
lvmc@lvmc.net
John Faulds, President
Jesus Love, Vice President
Brenda Church, Secretary

A non-profit organization dedicated to teaching adults 16 years and older how to read, write, speak English and prepare for the GED. Also offer computer literacy which includes the basics of using a computer, accessing the Internet and using basic Microsoft programs.

1966 **Literacy Volunteers of Tucson A Program of Literacy Connects**
200 E. Yavapai Road
Tucson, AZ 85705 520-882-8006
http://www.literacyconnects.org
info@literacyconnects.org
Sylvia Lee, Chairman
Cliff Bowman, Vice Chair
Betty Stauffer, Executive Director
Recruits, trains and matches tutors with adults (age 16 and up) in need of basic literacy (reading and writing) skills and/or English Language Acquisition for Adults (ELAA). Provides a friendly non-threatening environment that appeals to adult learners in all walks of life.

1967 **Yuma Reading Council**
2951 S. 21st Dr.
Yuma, AZ 85364-3846 928-782-1871
Fax: 928-782-9420
http://www.yumalibrary.org
greg.ferguson@yumacountyaz.go
Gregory Ferguson, Chairman
Brian D. Ewing, President
Provides one to one tutoring for basic literacy and english as a second language, and converstaion classes for beginning, intermediate and advanced levels for English as a second language students.

Arkansas

1968 **Arkansas Adult Learning Resource Center**
3905 Cooperative Way
Ste D
Little Rock, AR 72209 877-963-4433
Fax: 501-907-2492
http://www.aalrc.org/
info@aalrc.org
Marsha Talyor, Director
The Arkansas Adult Learning Resource Center was established in 1990 to provide a source for identification, evaluation, and dissemination of materials and information to adult education/literacy programs within the state.

1969 **Arkansas Literacy Council**
801 South Louisiana Street
Little Rock, AR 72201 501-907-2490
800-264-7323
Fax: 501-907-2492
http://www.arkansasliteracy.org
info@arkansasliteracy.org
Barbara Hanley, Chairman
Joe Burkett, Vice Chair
Nancy Leonhardt, Executive Director
Provides structure to a network of local literacy councils. These councils recruit and train volunteers to tutor adults who either need help with basic reading, writing, and math skills, or who want to learn English as a Second Language

1970 **Drew County Literacy Council**
801 South Louisiana Street
Little Rock, AR 72201 501-907-2490
800-264-7323
Fax: 501-907-2492
http://www.arkansasliteracy.org
info@arkansasliteracy.org
Barbara Hanley, Chairman
Joe Burkett, Vice Chair
Nancy Leonhardt, Executive Director
Formed by citizens that were concerned about the adult illiteracy rate reported in the 1980 census. Strives to recruit, train and match volunteer tutors with illiterate adults in the county using The Laubach Way to Reading and Laubach Way to English.

1971 **Faulkner County Literacy Council**
615 E Robins St
PO Box 2106
Conway, AR 72033 501-329-7323
http://www.faulknercoliteracy.org
fclc@conwaycorp.net
Emily Maggion, Executive Director
Provides free instruction through trained volunteers to adults in Faulkner County who lack basic reading, writing, mathematics, English as a second language and life skills.

1972 **Literacy Action of Central Arkansas**
P.O. Box 900
Little Rock, AR 72203 501-372-7323
Fax: 501-371-9888
http://www.literacylittlerock.org
ca@literacylittlerock.org
Dan Boland, President
Lee Hartz, Vice President
Bill Foster, Treasurer
A non-profit organization that teaches reading skills to adults and English skills to non-native adults.
1986

1973 **Literacy Council of Arkansas County**
801 South Louisiana Street
Little Rock, AR 72201 501-907-2490
800-264-7323
Fax: 501-907-2492
http://www.arkansasliteracy.org
info@arkansasliteracy.org
Barbara Hanley, Chairman
Joe Burkett, Vice Chair
Nancy Leonhardt, Executive Director

1974 **Literacy Council of Benton County**
205 NW A St
Bentonville, AR 72712 479-273-3486
Fax: 479-273-7545
http://goliteracy.org
readlcbc@sbcgloabl.net
Andy Gottman, President
Martha Walsh, Vice President
Vicki Ronald, Executive Director
A non-profit agency that increases Adult English literacy by developing volunteer tutors to teach students because Literacy Changes Lives. Empowers people to improve their wuality of lives within the community we all share by increasing adult English Literacy.

1975 **Literacy Council of Crittenden County**
2000 W Broadway St
West Memphis, AR 72301 870-733-6760
Fax: 870-733-6737
http://www.arkansasliteracy.org
jkfluker@midsouthcc.edu
Kim Fluker, Director

1976 **Literacy Council of Garland County**
119 Hobson Ave
Hot Springs, AR 71901 501-624-7323
Fax: 501-624-2994
http://www.arkansasliteracy.org
literacylady@sbcglobal.net
Pat McClaran, Director

1977 **Literacy Council of Grant County**
201 S Rose St
PO Box 432
Sheridan, AR 72150
870-942-5711
Fax: 870-942-7228
http://www.arkansasliteracy.org
literacy@windstream.net
Jo Ann Click, Director

1978 **Literacy Council of Hot Spring County**
122 E Page
PO Box 1485
Malvern, AR 72104
501-304-6679
Fax: 501-332-4043
http://www.readhelp.com
readhelp@sbcglobal.net
Jane Goodwin, Director
Offers a variety of educational services at no charge that range from literacy for adults to peer-tutoring for children; English as a second language to Learning Differences screening.

1979 **Literacy Council of Jefferson County**
402 E 5th
PO Box 7066
Pine Bluff, AR 71611
920-675-0500
Fax: 870-850-0984
http://www.jclc.us/
Karyn at kcable@jclc.us
Lynn Forseth, Executive Director

1980 **Literacy Council of Lonoke County**
306 N Center
PO Box 234
Lonoke, AR 72086
501-676-7478
Fax: 501-676-7478
http://www.arkansasliteracy.org
lonokeliteracy@sbcglobal.net
Claire Rogers, Director

1981 **Literacy Council of Monroe County**
234 W Cedar St
Brinkley, AR 72021
870-734-3333
Fax: 870-734-3333
http://www.arkansasliteracy.org
lcmc1992@gmail.com
Martha Pineda, Director

1982 **Literacy Council of North Central Arkansas**
PO Box 187
Leslie, AR 72645
870-447-3241
800-264-7323
Fax: 870-447-3241
http://www.arkansasliteracy.org
pogocatwoman26@gmail.com
Susan Vorwald, Director

1983 **Literacy Council of Western Arkansas**
PO Box 423
Fort Smith, AR 72902
479-783-2665
Fax: 479-783-5332
http://www.arkansasliteracy.org
helptoread@sbcglobal.net
Bruce Singleton, Director

1984 **Literacy League of Craighead County**
324 W Huntington Ave
PO Box 9251
Jonesboro, AR 72403
870-910-6511
Fax: 870-910-0552
http://www.arkansasliteracy.org
acbutts2006@yahoo.com
Amy Butts, Director

1985 **Ozark Literacy Council**
2596 Keystone Crossing
Fayetteville, AR 72703
479-521-8250
Fax: 479-582-0846
http://www.ozarkliteracy.org
info@ozarkliteracy.org
Don Moore, Chairman
Margot Jackson, Executive Director
Mina Phebus, Progarm Director
Provides quality basic literacy and language instruction enabling people to learn and communicate effectively.

1986 **Pope County Literacy Council**
1000 S Arkansas Ave
PO Box 1276
Russellville, AR 72811
479-967-7323
Fax: 479-968-6248
http://www.arkansasliteracy.org
popecoliteracy@centurytel.net
Jennifer Merkey, Director

1987 **St. John's ESL Program**
583 W Grand Ave
Hot Springs, AR 71901
501-624-3171
Fax: 501-624-3171
http://www.sjshs.org
aisaacs@sjshs.org
Angela Issacs, Principal
Jamie Cardenas, President
Lori Hinson, Secretary

1988 **Twin Lakes Literacy Council**
1318 Bradley Dr
Ste 14
Mountain Home, AR 72653
870-425-7323
Fax: 870-424-3646
http://www.twinlakesliteracycouncil.org
twinlakeslc@yahoo.com
Nancy Tester, Executive Director
To promote and enhance literacy efforts and to encourage volunteers to participate in all phases of this endeavor.

1989 **Van Buren County Literacy Council**
Clinton, AR 72031
501-745-6440
Fax: 501-745-6440
http://www.arkansasliteracy.org
dogwood@artelco.com
Brenda Wood, Director

California

1990 **Butte County Library Adult Reading Program**
25 County Center Dr.
Suite 200
Oroville, CA 95965
530-538-7631
888-538-7198
Fax: 530-538-7120
http://www.buttecounty.net
literacy@buttecounty.net
Paul Hahn, CAO/Clerk of the Board
Kathleen Sweeney, Assistant Clerk of the Board
Tutoring at no charge in reading, writing and math. Participants will learn the basics and more with one-on-one tutoring. A volunteer tutor will meet with participants at any branch library in Butte County.

1991 **California Association of Private Special Education Schools (CAPSES)**
921 11th St
Ste 501
Sacramento, CA 95814
916-447-7061
Fax: 916-447-1320
http://www.capses.com
director@capses.com

Teresa Malekzadeh, President
Rebecca Foo, Secretary
Susan Lane, Executive Director
A statewide professional association of nonpublic schools, agencies, organizations and individuals who specialize in the delivery of special education programs to students with learning disabilities.
1973

1992 **California Department of Education**
Office of the Secretary for Education
1430 N Street
Sacramento, CA 95814 916-323-0611
Fax: 916-323-3753
http://www.cde.ca.gov/
Tom Torlakson, State Superintendent
The Office of the Secretary for Education is responsible for advising and making policy recommendations to the Governor on education issues.

1993 **California Literacy**
PO Box 70916
Pasadena, CA 91117-7916 626-395-9989
Fax: 626-356-9327
http://www.caliteracy.org
office@caliteracy.org
Archana Carey, Director
California Literacy was founded in 1956 and is the nation's oldest and largest statewide adult volunteer literacy organization. Its purpose is to establish literacy programs and to support them through tutor training, consulting, and ongoing education.

1994 **Lake County Literacy Coalition**
1425 N High St
Lakeport, CA 95453 707-263-8817
Fax: 707-263-6796
http://www.co.lake.ca.us
Jim Comstock, 1st District
Jeff Smith, 2nd District
Denise Rushing, 3rd District
A non-profit volunteer organization that sponsors and supports the Adult Literacy Program of Lake County Library. Also offer special training sessions on specific topics, such as ESL, learning disabilities and teaching grammar.

1995 **Literacy Program: County of Los Angeles Public Library**
Rm 208
7400 E. Imperial Hwy
Downey, CA 90242-3375 562-940-8400
http://www.colapublib.org
mdtodd@library.lacounty.gov
William T Fujioka, CEO
J. Tyler McCauley, Auditor/Controller
The Literacy Centers of the County of Los Angeles Public Library offer a variety of literacy services for adults and families at no charge. Literacy services include one-to-one basic literacy tutoring, English as a Second Language group instruction, Family Literacy and self-help instruction on audio cassettes, videocassettes and computer-based training. The literacy program is an affiliate of Literacy Volunteers of America, Inc.

1996 **Literacy Volunteers of America: Willits Public Library**
501 Low Gap Road
Ukiah, CA 95482 707-459-5908
http://www.mendolibrary.org
lvawillits@pacific.net
Carre Brown, 1st District
John McCowen, 2nd District
John Pinches, 3rd District
The Literacy program offers one-on-one reading, writing and tutoring for adults in the area.

1997 **Marin Literacy Program**
San Rafael Public Library
1100 E St
San Rafael, CA 94901 415-485-3318
Fax: 415-485-3112
http://www.marinliteracy.org
readandwrite@marinliteracy.org
Paul Cummins, President
Robin Carpenter, Executive Director
David Sason, Secretary
Provides Marin County adults with free student-centered instruction in reading, writing, and speaking to help them reach their full potential at work, at home, and in the community.

1998 **Merced Adult School**
3430 A Street
Atwater, CA 95301 209-385-6400
Fax: 209-385-6442
http://www.muhsd.k12.ca.us
dglass@muhsd.k12.ca.us
Sam Spangler, President
Dave Honey, Vice President
William G. Snyder, Clerk
To empower adult students to discover their own unique, productive places in our dynamic world and encourage them to be lifelong learners.

1999 **Metropolitan Adult Education Program**
760 Hillsdale Ave
San Jose, CA 95136 408-723-6400
http://www.metroed.net
Daniel Bobay, President
Matthew Dean, Vice President
Lan Nguyen, Clerk
A unit of the Metropolitan Education and offers adult education classes for free or at a very low-cost. Classes are convenient, accessible, and have flexible schedules to meet the family and work needs of adults. Courses range from basic skills in math, reading and writing, ESL Citizenship, 50+ Program to Career Technical (Vocational) certificate programs.

2000 **Mid City Adult Learning Center**
Belmont Community Adult School
1510 Cambria St
Los Angeles, CA 90017 213-483-5256
Fax: 213-413-1356
http://www.literacynet.org/slrc/la/home.html
midcity@otan.dni.us
Judy Griffin, Resource Manager
Fernando Dejo, Technical Assistant
Elanie Svensson, ESL Resource Teacher
Provides adult education on ESL, basic reading, language and literacy programs.

2001 **Newport Beach Public Library Literacy Services**
1000 Avocado Ave
Newport Beach, CA 92660 949-717-3800
Fax: 949-640-5681
http://www.newportbeachlibrary.org/literacy
Robyn Grant, Chair
John Prichard, Vice Chair
Eleanor M. Palk, Secretary
Provides free literacy instruction to adults who live or work in the Newport Beach area.

2002 **Sacramento Public Library Literacy Service**
828 I St
Sacramento, CA 95814 916-264-2920
800-561-4636
http://www.saclibrary.org
director@saclibrary.org
Mary Ellen Shay, President
April Butcher, Executive Director
Yolanda Torrecillas, Development Manager

The Literacy Service is committed to helping adults attain the skills they need to achieve their goals and develop their knowledge and potential. Free one-on-one tutoring is provided to English speaking adults who want to improve their basic reading and writing skills.

2003 **Sweetwater State Literacy Regional Resource Center**
Adult Resource Center
458 Moss St
Chula Vista, CA 91911-1726 619-691-5791
Fax: 619-425-8728
http://www.literacynet.org/slrc/sweetwater/home
hurley@otan.dni.us
Alice Hurley, Director
The Sweetwater State Literacy Resource Center is located at the Adult and Continuing Education Division of the Sweetwater Union High School District. The Division is the fourth largest adult education program in the State of California, serving over 32,000 adult learners yearly.

2004 **Vision Literacy of California**
Pro Literacy Worldwide
540 Valley Way
Bldg 4
Milpitas, CA 95035 408-676-7323
Fax: 408-956-9384
http://www.visionliteracy.org
info@visionliteracy.org
Steven C. Toy, President
Candace Levers, Secretary
Kathleen Campbell, Treasurer
Vision Literacy is dedicated to enriching the community in which we live by helping adults improve their literacy skills.

Colorado

2005 **Adult Literacy Program**
PO Box 4856
Basalt, CO 81621 970-963-9200
Fax: 970-963-9200
http://www.englishinaction.org
info@englishinaction.org
Julie Fox-Rubin, Founder
Lara Beaulieu, Executive Director
Viviana Gonzalez, Program Coordinator/Case Manager
Building community through language and leadership development.

2006 **Archuleta County Education Center**
P.O.Box 1079
Pagosa Springs, CO 81147-1079 970-264-2835
http://www.archuletacountyeducationcenter.com
Lynell Wiggers, Adult Education Program Director
A non-profit organization, that through fundraising, grants and strategic partnerships with other organizations and agencies, provides a wide variety of learning experiences and services for children, youth and adults as well as providing a fundamental infrastructure asset that supports the economic development priorities of the communities it serves.

2007 **Colorado Adult Education and Family Literacy**
Colorado Department of Education
201 E Colfax Ave
Denver, CO 80203 303-866-6600
Fax: 303-866-6599
http://www.cde.state.co.us
Margaret Kirkpatrick, State Director
To assist adults to become literate in English and obtain the knowledge and skills necessary for employment and self-sufficiency.

2008 **Durango Adult Education Center**
701 Camino del Rio
Suite 301
Durango, CO 81301 970-385-4354
Fax: 970-385-7968
http://www.durangoaec.org
info@durangoedcenter.org
Lon Erwin, President
Teresa Malone, Executive Director
Christine Imming, Director, Finance
A private, non-profit organization that has been dedicated to providing educational resources for adults, seniors and youth in the duragno area.

2009 **Learning Source**
455 South Pierce Streetÿ
Lakewood, CO 80226 303-922-4683
Fax: 303-742-9929
http://www.coloradoliteracy.org
info@thelearningsource.orgÿ
Joshua Evans, Executive Director
Harry Chan, Family Literacy Program Manager
Daun Miller Barr, Assistant to Executive Director
Provides opportunities for motivated adult learners and families to attain their educational goals through adult and family literacy, GED preparation and English Language instruction.

2010 **Pine River Community Learning Center**
535 Candelaria Dr
Ignacio, CO 81137 970-563-0681
http://www.prclc.org
lowen@prclc.org
Susan Visser, Executive Director
Cathy Calderwood, Director
Tish Nelson, Education Coordinatorÿ
A nonprofit educational organization dedicated to the principle that life is learning, to the unparalleled welath of cultures in the rural Southwest and the unique gifts of its people.

Connecticut

2011 **Connecticut Literacy Resource Center**
111 Charter Oak Avenue
Hartford, CT 06106 860-247-2732
Fax: 860-246-3304
http://www.crec.org
tjohnsonsmith@crec.org
Sandy Cruz Serrano, COO, Interim CFO
Dr. Bruce E. Douglas, Ph.D., Executive Director
Mason Thrall, Director of Operations
The Literacy Center offers services that foster literacy development from early childhood to adult. Technical assistance and training are available in the following areas: School Readiness; k-12; and Family Literacy.

2012 **LEARN: Regional Educational Service Center**
44 Hatchetts Hill Road
Old Lyme, CT 06371 860-434-4800
Fax: 860-434-4837
http://www.learn.k12.ct.us
ehowley@learn.k12.ct.us
Eileen S. Howley, Executive Director
Doreen Marvin, Director of Development
Jean Paul LeBlanc, Director of Business/Finance
LEARN initiates, supports and provides a wide range of programs and services that enhance the quality and expand the opportunities for learning in the educational community.

2013 **Literacy Center of Milford**
Fannie Beach Community Center
16 Dixon Street
Milford, CT 06460 203-878-4800
Fax: 203-878-1080
http://www.literacycenterofmilford.com
director@literacycenterofmilford.com

Martin O'Neill, President
Sheila Hageman, VP
Pam Reiss, Treasurer
Serves people from other countries who want to learn the English language and it helps people in need of mastering basic reading, writing and math skills. Provides a quality program where people can find the help and support they require to meet their basic literacy needs.

2014 Literacy Volunteers of Central Connecticut
20 High Street
New Britain, CT 06051
860-229-7323
Fax: 860-223-6729
http://www.literacycentral.org
lvcctraining@gmail.com
Cassandra Crowal, President
Sumakshi Vali, VP
Lynne Prairie, Associate Director
Provides small group and one-on-one literacy tutoring to over 350 adults with flexible hours, individual attention, student centered learning, and high quality, caring volunteer tutors. Provide free, high quality training to adults who would like to become Literacy Volunteers.

2015 Literacy Volunteers of Eastern Connecticut
106 Truman Street
OIC Building - 3rd Floor
New London, CT 06320
860-443-4800
Fax: 860-443-4880
http://www.englishhelp.org
office@englishhelp.org
Jerold A. Sinnamon, President
Edward G. Perkins, VP
Terrence Hickey, Treasurer
A not-for-profit, volunteer-based organization whose mission is to help people communicate in English and thrive in American culture, as consumers and as workers.

2016 Literacy Volunteers of Greater Hartford
30 Arbor Street
First Floor South Building
Hartford, CT 06106
860-233-3853
Fax: 860-838-6442
http://www.lvgh.org
cj.hauss@lvgh.org
Carol DeVido Hauss, Executive Director
Mark Briggs, Program Development Director
Shannon Houston, Assistant Director
Improves the ability of Greater Hartford adults to read, write and speak English. Trains volunteers to provide English literacy instruction to over 600 Hartford area adults per year.

2017 Literacy Volunteers of Greater New Haven
4 Science Park
New Haven, CT 06511
203-776-5899
Fax: 203-745-4629
http://www.lvagnh.org
info@lvagnh.org
Bernadette Holodak, VP
Nicholas Iwanec, CPA, Treasurer
Doss Venema, Executive Director
A non-profit educational organization that trains and supports volunteer tutors who provide free literacy tutoring for adults who need to improve their reading, writing, and oral communication skills.

2018 Literacy Volunteers of Northern Connecticut
Asnuntuck CC B-131
1010 Enfield Street
Enfield, CT 06082-3873
860-253-3038
http://connecticut.networkofcare.org
Brain J Mc Cartney, Executive Director

2019 Literacy Volunteers-Valley Shore
61 Goodspeed Drive
Westbrook, CT 06498
860-399-0280
Fax: 860-767-1038
http://www.vsliteracy.org
info@vsliteracy.org
Gina Calabro, President
Sharon Colvin, VP
John Ferrara, Executive Director

2020 Literacy Volunteers: Stamford/Greenwich
60 Palmer's Hill Road
Stamford, CT 06902
203-324-3167
Fax: 203-358-2327
http://www.lvsg.org
barnold@familycenters.org
Bob Arnold, President, CEO
Carole Elias, EVP
Bob Short, VP
A community-based organization that utilizes the services of trained volunteers to provide free, high-quality reading, writing and English language programs to adults, both American and foreign born, for the purpose of enabling them to acquire the literacy skills necessary to achieve personal and occupational goals.

2021 Mercy Learning Center
637 Park Avenue
Bridgeport, CT 06604
203-334-6699
Fax: 203-332-6852
http://www.mercylearningcenter.org
info@mercylearningcenter.org
Jane E Ferreira, President/CEO
Nicole Cassidy, Development Directorÿ
Cathy Alfandre, Vocational Counselorÿ
Provides basic literacy and life skills training to low-income women using a holistic approach within a compassionate, supportive environment.

Delaware

2022 Delaware Department of Education: Adult Community Education
Department of Public Instruction
401 Federal Street
John G. Townsend Building
Dover, DE 19901
302-735-4000
Fax: 302-739-4654
http://www.doe.k12.de.us
Jack Markell, Governor
Mike Barlow, Chief of Staff
James Collins, Deputy Chief of Staff
Provides students with opportunities to develop skills needed to qualify for further education, job training, and better employment.

2023 Literacy Council of Prince George's County
17527 Nassau Commons
Suite 213
LewesHyattsville, DE 19958
302-645-7177
Fax: 301-699-9707
http://www.technogoober.com
info@technogoober.com
Frank Payton, Uber Goober
Nathan Bradshaw, Code Goober
Chad Lane, Network Gobber
The primary non-profit organization for the advocacy and implementation of literacy programs in the county. Provides services for adult learners in acquiring, improving and applying basic literacy skills includinf reading, writing, math and oral communication.

2024 Literacy Volunteers Serving Adults: Northern Delaware
PO Box 2083
Wilmington, DE 19899-2083
302-658-5624
Fax: 302-654-9132
http://www.litvolunteers.org
c.shermeyer@verizon.net
Bob Hurka, Chair
Cynthia E. Shermeyer, Executive Director
Alyssa Almond, Program Coordinator

Helps adults improve literacy skills and thereby realize their potential to be confident, self sufficient and productive employees and community members. Deliver services and programs in reading, writing, English language, math, workplace and computer skills.

2025 Literacy Volunteers of America: Wilmington Library
10 E 10th Street
Wilmington, DE 19801
302-571-7400
Fax: 302-654-9132
http://www.wilmlib.org
wilmref@lib.de.us
H. Rodney Scott, President
Samuel A. Nolen, VP
John R. Matlusky, Chief of Staff
An organization of volunteers that provide a variety of services locally to enable people to achieve personal goals through literacy programs.

2026 NEW START Adult Learning Program
115 High Street
Odessa, DE 19730
302-378-8838
Fax: 302-378-7803
http://corbitlibrary.org
corbitlibrary@gmail.com
Susan Menei, Coordinator
A non-profit educational organization whose mission is to enable adults to acquire the listening, speaking, reading, writing, mathematics and technology skills they need to solve problems they encounter in daily life.

2027 State of Delaware Adult and Community Education Network
516 W. Loockerman St.
Dover, DE 19904
302-739-7080
800-464-4357
Fax: 302-739-5565
http://www.acenetwork.org
Joanne Heaphy, Director
The ACE Network is a service agency that supports adult education and literacy providers through training and resource development.

District of Columbia

2028 Academy of Hope
601 Edgewood St NE
Suite 25
Washington, DC 20017
202-269-6623
Fax: 202-269-6632
http://www.aohdc.org
Brian McNamee, COO
Lecester Johnson, Executive Director
Adriana Kao, Senior Director, Development
Changes lives and improves community by providing high-quality adult education in a supportive and empowering environment.

2029 Carlos Rosario International Public Charter School
1100 Harvard St NW
Washington, DC 20009
202-797-4700
Fax: 202-232-6442
http://www.carlosrosario.org
info@carlosrosario.org
Sonia Gutierrez, President, Emeritus
Allison R. Kokkoros, CEO, Executive Director
Dr. Ryan Monroe, Principal, Harvard Campus
Offers an array of classes integrated within award-winning adult education programs which are considered models at the national and international level.

2030 District of Columbia Public Schools
1200 First Street NE
Washington, DC 20002
202-442-5885
Fax: 202-442-5026
http://dcps.dc.gov
Kaya Henderson, Chancellor
The public school system is committed to constant improvements in the achievement of all students today in preparation for their world tomorrow.

2031 Literacy Volunteers of the National Capital Area
635 Edgewood Street NE
Washington, DC 20017
202-387-1772
Fax: 202-588-0714
http://www.lvanca.org
info@lvanca.org
Patricia Evans, President
LaMar Hortman, Treasurer
Rita Daniels, Executive Director
Empowers adults and families by providing literacy instruction and skills-based education, thereby enriching all aspects of their personal and professional lives.

2032 U.S. Department Of Education
400 Maryland Avenue, SW
Washington, DC 20202
202-842-0973
800-872-5327
Fax: 202-205-8748
http://www.ed.gov
ovae@ed.gov
Emma Vadehra, Chief of Staff
Eric Waldo, Senior Advisor
John Easton, Director
To help all people achieve the knowledge and skills to be lifelong learners, to be successful in their chosen careers, and to be effective citizens.

2033 Washington Literacy Council
1918 18th St NW
Ste B2
Washington, DC 20009-1794
202-387-9029
Fax: 202-387-0271
http://www.washingtonliteracycouncil.org
info@washlit.org
Terry Algire, Executive Director
The Washinton Literacy Council trains volunteers to use reading redmediation approaches when tutoring and leading small groups.

Florida

2034 Adult Literacy League
345 W Michigan St
Ste 100
Orlando, FL 32806
407-422-1540
Fax: 407-422-1529
http://www.adultliteracyleague.org
info@adultliteracyleague.org
Joyce Whidden, Executive Director
Gina Solomon, Chief Development Officer
Stacy McKenna, Program Manager
Develops readers to build a strong and literate community. Serves as the premier literacy resource providing education, training and information in Central Florida.

2035 Advocacy Center for Persons with Disabilities
National Disability Rights Network
2728 Centerview Drive
Ste 102
Tallahassee, FL 32301
850-488-9071
800-342-0823
Fax: 850-488-8640
TDD: 800-346-4127
http://www.advocacycenter.org
Hubert Grissom, President
To advance the quality of life, dignity, equality, and freedom of choice of persons with disabilities through collaboration, education, advocacy, as well as legal and legislative strategies.

2036 **Florida Coalition**
250 N. Orange Avenue
Suite 1110
Orlando, FL 32801
407-246-7110
800-237-5113
Fax: 407-246-7104
http://www.floridaliteracy.org
info@floridaliteracy.org
Gregory Smith, Executive Director
Annie Schmidt, Resource Specialist
Jessica Ward, Education &Training Coordinator
A nonprofit organization funded through private and corporate donations, state of Florida grants, and a diverse membership. Supports Florida's adult literacy volunteers and their programs. Provides information and services to literacy volunteers and providers in communications and networking, technical assistance and training, public affairs, advocacy, and student leadership.

2037 **Florida Literacy Resource Center**
283 Trojan Trail
Tallahassee, FL 32311
850-922-5343
Fax: 850-922-5352
http://www.ace-leon.org
aceinfo@leonschools.net
Regina Browning, Principal
As part of the State Library, the State Resource Center provides electronic and print resources.

2038 **Florida Vocational Rehabilitation Agency: Division of Vocational Rehabilitation**
4070 Esplanade Wayÿ
Tallahassee, FL 32399-7016
850-245-3399
800-451-4327
TDD: 800-451-4327
http://www.rehabworks.org
Aleisa McKinlay, Division Director
Patrick Cannon, Council Member
Don Chester, Council Member
A federal state program that works with people who have physical or mental disabilities to prepare for, gain or retain employment.

2039 **Learn to Read**
303 N. Laura St.
P.O. Box 2178
Jacksonville, FL 32202
904-399-8894
Fax: 904-399-2508
http://www.learntoreadinc.org
learntoread.jax@gmail.com
Judy Bradshaw, Executive Director
Sherri Jackson, Literacy Program Manager
Alicia Harris, Literacy Program Coordinator
Dedicated to improving adult literacy in Duval County. Serves adults 16 years of age and older in Northeats Florida who want to improve reading skills or learn to read.

2040 **Learning Disabilities Association of Florida**
7100 W. Camino Real
Suite 215
Boca Raton, FL 33433
561-247-0221
Fax: 561-327-2633
http://www.lda-florida.org
cathyeldafl@gmail.com
Mark Halpert, Co-President
Cathy Einhorn, Co-President
Dale King, Board Member
The Learning Disabilities Association of Florida is a nonprofit volunteer organization of parents, professionals and LD adults.

2041 **Literacy Florida**
2981 South Lookout Blvd
Port St Lucie, FL 34984
http://www.[illegible]o.freeservers.com/whats_new.htm
havenpsl@adelphia.net
Jim Wilder, President
Sandy Newell, VP
Glenda Norvell, Secretary

Georgia

2042 **Gainesville Hall County Alliance for Literacy**
4-1/2 Stallworth Street
Gainesville, GA 30501
770-531-4337
Fax: 770-531-6406
http://allianceforliteracy.org
all4lit@bellsouth.net
Dorothy W. Shinafelt, Executive Director
Serves as the Umbrella agency for all literacy concerns in the community. Provides free educational programs for adults 16 years and older who have not graduated from high school or whose native language is not English.

2043 **Georgia Department of Education**
Department of Technical & Adult Education
Ste 400
1800 Century Pl NE
Atlanta, GA 30345-4304
404-679-1625
Fax: 404-679-1630
http://www.dtae.org
mdelaney@dtae.org
Ron Jackson, Director
To oversee the state's system of technical colleges, the adult literacy program, and a host of economic workforce development programs.

2044 **Georgia Department of Technical & Adult Education**
Ste 400
1800 Century Pl NE
Atlanta, GA 30345-4304
404-679-1625
Fax: 404-679-1630
http://www.dtae.org
mdelaney@dtae.org
Ron Jackson, Director
The Georgia Department of Technical and Adult Education oversees the state's system of technical colleges, the adult literacy program, and a host of economic and workforce development programs

2045 **Georgia Literacy Resource Center: Office of Adult Literacy**
Ste 400
1800 Century Pl NE
Atlanta, GA 30345-4304
404-679-1625
Fax: 404-679-1630
http://www.dtae.org
mdelaney@dtae.org
Ron Jackson, Director
The mission of the adult literacy programs is to enable every adult learner in Georgia to acquire the necessary basic skills in reading, writing, computation, speaking, and listening to compete successfully in today's workplace, strengthen family foundations, and exercise full citizenship.

2046 **Literacy Volunteers of America: Forsyth County**
PO Box 1097
Cumming, GA 30028-1097
770-887-0074
http://www.litreacyforsyth.org
focolit@sellsouth.net
Eddith DeVeau, Executive Director
Dianne Anth, Director
Dedicated to teaching adults to read in the Forsyth County region.

2047 **Literacy Volunteers of Atlanta**
246 Sycamore Street
Suite 110
Decatur, GA 30030
404-377-7323
Fax: 404-377-8662
http://www.lvama.org
kprovence@literacyaction.org
Michele Henry, Executive Director
Kelley Provence, Site Director
Angela Green, Basic Literacy Coordinator
To increase adult and family literacy primarily through volunteer tutoring. The goal is to provide all of the literacy skills crucial for more productive, prosperous and confident lives, thus improving the quality of life of all Georgians.

2048 **Newton County Reads**
8134 Geiger St
Box 5
Covington, GA 30014
678-342-7943
Fax: 678-342-7964
http://www.newtonreads.org
newtoncountyreads@earthlink.net
Renee' Jones, Director
Helps adults improve their literacy skills and/or earn a GED certificate through an active volunteer tutoring program; maintain an ever-expanding list of literacy resources available in Newton County; helps adults find and get started in the literacy programs that most effectively meet their needs.

2049 **North Georgia Technical College Adult Education**
1500 Hwy 197 N
PO Box 65
Clarkesville, GA 30523
706-754-7700
Fax: 706-754-7777
http://www.northgatech.edu/adulted
info@northgatech.edu
Steve Dougherty, President
Designed for adults who have different needs, backgrounds, and skill levels. Provide a full range of services for adults who need to acquire or improve basic reading, math, and/or written communication skills in order to prepare them to enter or succeed in the workplace or postsecondary educational programs.

2050 **Okefenokee Regional Library System**
401 Lee Avenue
Waycross, GA 31501
912-287-4978
Fax: 912-284-2533
http://www.okrls.org
ikeaton@okrls.org
Pat Prevatt, Chair
Charles Eames, Vice Chair
John Miller, Manager
Public library

2051 **Toccoa/Stephens County Literacy Council**
P.O.Box 63
Toccoa, GA 30577-1400
706-886-6082
Fax: 706-282-7633
mwalters3@yahoo.com
Michelle Austin, Director

2052 **Volunteers for Literacy of Habersham County**
555 Monroe St.
Unit 20
Clarkesville, GA 30523
706-839-0200
Fax: 706-754-1014
http://www.habershamga.com

Hawaii

2053 **CALC/Hilo Public Library**
300 Waianuenue Ave
Hilo, HI 96720-2447
808-933-8893
Fax: 808-933-8895
http://literacynet.org
calchilo@gte.net
Kit Holz, Project Manager
Mission is to provide access to learning resources and tutoring services to help adults acquire and/or improve their skills in reading, writing, math, English as a Second Language and computer use.

2054 **Hawaii Literacy**
245 N. Kukui St.
Suite 202
Honolulu, HI 96817
808-537-6706
Fax: 808-528-1690
http://www.hawaiiliteracy.org
info@hawaiiliteracy.org
R. Scott Simon, President
Brandon Kurisu, VP
Suzanne Skjold, Executive Director
Helps people gain knowledge and skills by providing literacy and lifelong learning services.

2055 **Hui Malama Learning Center**
375 Mahalani Street
Wailuku, HI 96793
808-244-5911
Fax: 808-242-0762
http://www.mauihui.org
huimalama@mauihui.org
Pualani Enos, J.D., Executive Director
Deanna Kramer, Finance & HR Manager
Robyn Delima, Operations Manager
Provides middle school, high-school, and GED-preparation programs, as well as tutoring and educational enrichment programs to public and private school students grades K-12.

Idaho

2056 **ABE:College of Southern Idaho**
Adult Basic Education
315 Falls Ave
P.O. Box 1238
Twin Falls, ID 83303
208-732-6221
800-680-0274
Fax: 208-736-4705
http://www.csi.edu
info@csi.edu
Dr. Jeff Fox, President
Dr. Todd Schwarz, EVP, Chief Academic Officer
Mike Mason, VP, Administration
Designed to improve the educational level of adults, out-of-school youth and non-English speaking persons in our eight-county service area.

2057 **Idaho Adult Education Office**
650 West State Street
P.O. Box 83720
Boise, ID 83720-0027
208-332-6800
800-432-4601
Fax: 208-334-2228
http://www.sde.idaho.gov
MRMcGrath@sde.idaho.gov
Tom Luna, State Superintendant
Luci Willits, Chief of Staff
Melissa McGrath, Public Information officer

2058 **Idaho Coalition for Adult Literacy**
325 W State St
Boise, ID 83702
208-334-2150
800-458-3271
Fax: 208-334-4016
http://www.lili.org
lili@libraries.idaho.gov
Ann Joslin, Coordinator
An nonprofit organization which raise public awareness about the importance of a literate society.

2059 **Idaho State Library**
325 W State St
Boise, ID 83702
208-334-2150
800-458-3271
Fax: 208-334-4016
http://www.lili.org
lili@isl.state.id.us
Ann Joslin, Director
Offers a history of pioneering new frontiers in library services.

2060 **Learning Lab**
308 E 36th St
Garden City, ID 83714
208-344-1335
Fax: 208-344-1171
http://www.learninglabinc.org
info@learninglabinc.org
Ann Heilman, Executive Director
Monique Smith, Education Director
Martha Strong, Adult Education Coordinator
A computer-assisted learning center for adults and families with birth to six-year-old children. Students receive basic skills instruction including mathematics, reading, writing, spelling, GED preparation and workplace skills in a comfortable, confidential environment.

Illinois

2061 **Adult Literacy at People's Resource Center**
201 S Naperville Rd
Wheaton, IL 60187
630-682-5402
Fax: 630-682-5412
http://www.peoplesrc.org
Mark Demich, President
Henry Davis, Jr., VP
Kim Perez, Executive Director
Exists to respond to basic human needs, promote dignity and justice, and create a future of hope and opportunity for the residents of DuPage County, IL through discovering and sharing personal and community resources.

2062 **Aquinas Literacy Center**
3540 S Hermitage Ave
Chicago, IL 60609
773-927-0512
Fax: 773-927-8980
http://www.aquinasliteracycenter.org
aquinaslit@aol.com
Alison Altmeyer, Executive Director
Meg Green, Program Director
Lori Rogers, Volunteer Coordinator
A nonprofit, community-based literacy center serving the residents of McKinley Park and other south and southwest side Chicago neighborhoods. Offers individualized English language instruction, group conversation classes, and group computer classes at not cost to students.

2063 **C.E.F.S. Literacy Program**
1805 S Banker
PO Box 928
Effingham, IL 62401-0928
217-342-2193
Fax: 217-342-4701
http://www.cefseoc.org
learningcenter@cefseoc.org
Helps adults and families meet their literacy goals in reading, writing, math and English language skills and to promote education and lifelong learning as the key to personal, economic, and social success.

2064 **Carl Sandburg College Literacy Coalition**
2400 Tom L. Wilson Blvd.ÿ
Galesburg, IL 61401
309-344-2518
855-468-6272
Fax: 309-344-1395
http://www.sandburg.edu
kavalos@sandburg.edu
Improves the reading and basic math skills of adults and their families by offering one-on-one and small group tutoring services.

2065 **Common Place Family Learning Center**
514 S Shelley St
Peoria, IL 61605
309-674-3315
Fax: 309-674-0627
http://www.commonplacepeoria.org
commonplace@sbcglobal.net
Cheryl Dawson, Chair
Connie Voss, Executive Director
Wayne Cannon, Director of Adult Programs
A non-profit, social service agency located on the south side of Peoria, IL. Strive to eliminate poverty and injustice through education. The youth and adult programs are based on education and literacy.

2066 **Dominican Literacy Center**
260 Vermont Avenue
Aurora, IL 60505
630-898-4636
Fax: 630-898-4636
http://www.dominicanliteracycenter.org
domlitctr@sbcglobal.net
David Cox, Advisory Board
Laura Martinez, Advisory Board
Mary Kennedy, Advisory Board
Helps women learn to read, write and speak English within an atmosphere of mutual respect and dignity.

2067 **Equip for Equality**
20 N Michigan Ave
Ste 300
Chicago, IL 60602
312-341-0022
800-537-2632
TTY: 800-610-2779
http://www.equipforequality.org
Zena Naiditch, President & CEO
John K.ÿ Holton, PhD, Chair
Sue Suter, Vice Chair
Advances the human and civil rights of children and adults with physical and mental disabilities in Illinois. The only statewide, cross-disability, comprehensive advocacy organization prodiving self-advocacy assistance, legal services, and disability rights education while also engaging in public policy and legislative advocacy and conducting abuse investigations and other oversight activities.

2068 **Equip for Equality: Carbondale**
300 East Main Street
Suite 18
Carbondale, IL 62901
618-457-7930
800-758-0559
Fax: 618-457-7985
TTY: 800-610-2779
http://www.equipforequality.org
contactus@equipforequality.org
Duane C. Quaini, Chairperson
Jeannine M.ÿ Cordero, Vice Chairperson
Zena Naiditch, President/CEO
Independent, private, not-for-profit organization that provides free legal services and self advocacy assistance to people with disabilities in the areas of discrimination, assistive technology, special education, guardianship defense, abuse and neglect, and community integration.

2069 **Equip for Equality: Moline**
1515 Fifth Avenue
Suite 420
Moline, IL 61265
309-786-6868
800-758-6869
Fax: 309-797-8710
TTY: 800-610-2779
http://www.equipforequality.org
contactus@equipforequality.org
Duane C. Quaini, Chairperson
Jeannine M.ÿ Cordero, Vice Chairperson
Zena Naiditch, President/CEO
Independent, private, not-for-profit organization that provides free legal services and self advocacy assistance to people with disabilities in the areas of discrimination, assistive technology, special education, guardianship defense, abuse and neglect, and community integration.

2070 **Equip for Equality: Springfield**
1 West Old State Capitol Plaza
Suite 816
Springfield, IL 62701
217-544-0464
800-758-0464
Fax: 217-523-0720
TTY: 800-610-2779
http://www.equipforequality.org
contactus@equipforequality.org
Duane C. Quaini, Chairperson
Jeannine M.ÿ Cordero, Vice Chairperson
Zena Naiditch, President/CEO
Independent, private, not-for-profit organization that provides free legal services and self advocacy assistance to people with disabilities in the areas of discrimination, assistive technology, special education, guardianship defense, abuse and neglect, and community integration.

2071 **Illinois Library Association**
33 West Grand Avenue
Suite 401
Chicago, IL 60654-6799
312-644-1896
Fax: 312-644-1899
http://www.ila.org
ila@ila.org
Jeannieÿ Dilger, President
Betsy Adamowskiÿÿ, Vice President/President-Elect
Leora Siegel, Treasurer
The Illinois Library Association is the voice for Illinois Libraries and the millions who depend on them. It provides leadership for the development, promotion, and improvement of library services in Illinois and for the library community.

2072 **Illinois Literacy Resource Development Center**
209 W Clark St
Ste 15
Champaign, IL 61820-4640
217-355-6068
Fax: 217-355-6347
http://www.champaign.illinoiscircle.com/c-15597
Suzanne Knell, Executive Director
The Illinois Literacy Resource Development Center is dedicated to improving literacy policy and practice at the local, state, and national levels. It is a nonprofit organization supporting literacy and adult education efforts throughout Illinois and the nation. One key to its success has been its ability to build partnerships among the organizations, individuals and agencies working in the literacy arena from the local to the national level.

2073 **Illinois Office of Rehabilitation Services**
Illinois Department of Human Services
100 South Grand Avenue East
Springfield, IL 62762
217-557-1601
800-843-6154
TTY: 217-557-2134
http://www.dhs.state.il.us
Carol Kraus, CFO, Operations
Grace Hong Duffin, Chief of Staff
Tom Green, Director, Communications
DHS' Office of Rehabilitation Services is the state's lead agency serving individuals with disabilities.

2074 **Literacy Chicago**
17 North State Street
Suite 1010
Chicago, IL 60602
312-870-1100
Fax: 312-870-4488
http://www.literacychicago.org
info@literacychicago.org
Richard Dominguez, Executive Director
June C. Porter, Director of Adult Literacy
John Mosman, Administrative Assistant
A nonprofit organization that empowers individuals to achieve greater self sufficiency through language and literacy instruction.

2075 **Literacy Connection**
270 North Grove Ave.
Elgin, IL 60120
847-742-6565
Fax: 847-742-6599
http://www.elginliteracy.org
info@elginliteracy.org
Chris Awe, President
Deborah Giardina, VP
Karen Oswald, Executive Director
A non-profit, community-based organization helping individuals acquire fundamental literacy skills and learn to read, write, speak and understand English.

2076 **Literacy Council**
982 N Main St
Rockford, IL 61103
815-963-7323
Fax: 815-963-7347
http://www.theliteracycouncil.org
read@theliteracycouncil.org
Cindy Waddick, Executive Director
Heather Tucker, Finance Director
Debra Lindley, Program Director
Provides literacy instruction to individuals and families to strengthen communities.

2077 **Literacy Volunteers of America: Illinois**
30 East Adams Streetÿ
Suite 1130ÿ
Chicago, IL 60603
312-857-1582
Fax: 312-857-1586
http://www.literacyvolunteersillinois.org
info@lvillinois.org
Dorothy M Miaso, Executive Director
Chamala Travis, Program Coordinator
Trudye Connolly, Program Associate
A statewide organization committed to developing and supporting volunteer literacy programs that help families, adults and out-of-school teens increase their literacy skills.

2078 **Literacy Volunteers of DuPage**
24W500 Maple Ave
Ste 217
Naperville, IL 60540-6057
630-416-6699
Fax: 630-416-9465
http://www.literacyvolunteersdupage.org
info@literacydupage.org
Rick Lochner, President
Bernie Steiger, Executive Director
Carol Garcia, Program Director
A nonprofit, community-based organization that provides accessible and customized tutoring in reading, writing, speaking, and understanding English to help adults achieve independence.

2079 **Literacy Volunteers of Fox Valley**
One South Sixth Avenue
Saint Charles, IL 60174
630-584-2811
Fax: 630-584-3448
http://www.lvfv.org
info@lvfv.org

Peg Coker, Executive Director
Maureen Powelson, Program Coordinator
Angelo Cobo, Office Assistant
Helps individuals in the region acquire and validate the literacy skills that they need to function more effectively in contemporary U.S. society.

2080 **Literacy Volunteers of Lake County**
128 N County St
Waukegan, IL 60085 847-623-2041
Fax: 847-623-2092
http://www.adultlearningconnection.org
Mission is to extend educational opportunities to Lake COunty adult students and their families.

2081 **Literacy Volunteers of Western Cook County**
1010 West Lake Street, Suite 603B
PO Box 4502
Oak Park, IL 60301 708-848-8499
Fax: 708-848-9564
http://www.lvwcc.org
info@lvwcc.org
Esther Chase, President, Acting Exe. Director
Mario K. Medina, Treasurer
Jasmine Brown, Partnerships Specialist
Helps adults reach their literacy goals through customized one-on-one tutoring by trained volunteers.

2082 **Project CARE**
Morton College
3801 S Central Ave
Cicero, IL 60804 708-656-8000
Fax: 708-656-3186
http://www.morton.edu
projectcare@morton.edu
Dr. Dana A. Grove, President
Marlena A. Thompson, Director, Student Development
Kenneth Stock, SPHR, Director, HR
A volunteer adult literacy program that uses trained tutors to teach adult students seeking assistance with reading and writing, and/or adults who are learning English as a second language.

2083 **Project READ**
5800 Godfrey Road
Benjamin Godfrey Campus
Godfrey, IL 62035 618-468-7000
800-YES-LCCC
Fax: 618-468-7820
http://www.lc.cc.il.us
lartis@lc.edu
Robert Watson, Chairman
Brenda W. McCain, Vice Chairman
Walter S. Ahlemeyer, Secretary
Goal is to increase literacy throughout the area with one-on-one tutoring. Project READ Community Service Coordinators are available to provide information to community groups, arrange free training for volunteers and distribute materials and support to tutor-learner pairs.

Indiana

2084 **Adult Literacy Program of Gibson County**
232 W Broadway
P.O. Box 1134
Princeton, IN 47670 812-386-9100
http://www.gibsonadultliteracy.org
literacy@gibsoncounty.net
Sharen Buyher, President
Cynthia Schrodt, Secretary
Ruth Jones, Board Member
Provides an opportunity for any adult in Gibson County to attain basic English Language literacy skills.

2085 **Indy Reads: Indianapolis/Marion County Public Library**
PO Box 211
Indianapolis, IN 46206-0211 317-275-4100
http://www.indypl.org
jnytes@indypl.org
Joanne M. Sanders, President
Rev. T.D. Robinson, Vice President
Jackie Nytes, Chief Executive Officer
Indy Reads, a nationally recognized not-for-profit affiliate of the Indianapolis-Marion County Public Library, exists to improve the reading and writing skills of adults in Marion County who read at or below the sixth grade level.

2086 **Literacy Alliance**
709 Clay St
Ste 100
Fort Wayne, IN 46802-2019 260-426-7323
Fax: 260-424-0371
http://www.tria.org
trlafw@yahoo.com
Judith Stabelli, Executive Director
Adult education

2087 **Morrisson/Reeves Library Literacy Resource Center**
80 North 6th Street
Richmond, IN 47374 765-966-8291
Fax: 765-962-1318
http://www.mrlinfo.org
library@mrlinfo.org
Paris Pegg, Library Director
Sue King, Adult Services Manager
Sarah Morey, Technical Services Manager
The Literacy Resource Center provides free training for volunteers to tutor adults in Wayne County who want to learn to read, write and do basic math.

2088 **Steuben County Literacy Coalition**
1208 S Wayne St
Angola, IN 46703 260-665-1414
Fax: 260-665-3357
http://www.steubenliteracy.org
Dolores Tichenor, President
Lon Keyes, President-Elect
Breann Fink, Executive Director
Mission shall be to foster lifelong leraning and improved literacy through high quality and accessible educational opportunities for children and adults in Steuben County.

Iowa

2089 **Adult Basic Education and Adult Literacy Program**
Kirkwood Community College
6301 Kirkwood Blvd SW
Cedar Rapids, IA 52404 319-398-5411
800-332-2055
http://www.kirkwood.edu
ask@kirkwood.edu
Dr. Mick Starcevich, President
Bill Lamb, VP, Academic Affairs
John Henik, Associate VP, Academic Affairs
Provides instruction to enable adults to increase self-sufficiency, improve employability, prepare for continued learning and better meet their responsibilities. Recruits volunteers, trains them in literacy teaching techniques and matches them with adults wanting instruction in reading skills development.

2090 **Iowa Department of Education: Iowa Literacy Council Programs**
400 E 14th Street
Grimes State Office Buliding
Des Moines, IA 50319-0146 515-281-5294
Fax: 515-242-5988
http://www.educateiowa.gov
jason.glass@iowa.gov

Brad Buck, Director
Nicole Proesch, Legal Director
Ryan Wise, Deputy Director, Policy
Helps adults and families develop their potential through improved literacy, education, and training.

2091 **Iowa Literacy Resource Center**
415 Commercial St
Waterloo, IA 50701-1317
319-233-1200
800-772-2023
Fax: 319-233-1964
http://www.readiowa.org
riesberg@neilsa.org
Eunice Riefberg, Director
The Center provides a link to resource materials in Iowa and at a regional and national level for adult literacy practitioners and students. These resources are available in many formats: including print, audio, video and online.

2092 **Iowa Vocational Rehabilitation Agency**
Department of Education
510 East 12th Street
Jessie Parker Building
Des Moines, IA 50319-0240
515-281-4211
Fax: 515-281-7645
TTY: 515-281-4211
http://www.ivrs.iowa.gov
David.Mitchell@iowa.gov
David Mitchell, Administrator

2093 **Iowa Workforce Investment Act**
200 East Grand Avenue
Des Moines, IA 50309
515-725-3000
Fax: 515-725-3010
http://www.iowaeconomicdevelopment.com
info@iowa.gov
Debi Durham, Director
Tina Hoffman, Media
Job placement and training services. Especially for those workers who have been laid off, or have other barriers to steady employment.

2094 **Learning Disabilities Association of Iowa**
5665 Greendale Rd
Ste D
Johnston, IA 50131
515-280-8558
888-690-5324
Fax: 515-243-1902
http://www.lda-ia.org
kathylda@askresource.org
Vicki Goshon, President
Kim Miller, 1st VP
Patty Beyer, 2nd VP
Dedicated to identifying causes and promoting prevention of learning disabilities and to enhancing the quality of life for all individuals with learning disabilities and their families.

2095 **Library Literacy Programs: State Library of Iowa**
1112 E Grand Ave
Miller Building
Des Moines, IA 50319
515-281-4105
800-248-4483
Fax: 515-281-6191
http://www.statelibraryofiowa.org
helpdesk@silo.lib.ia.us
Mary Wegner, Director/State Librarian

2096 **Southeastern Community College:Literacy Program**
200 North Main
Mt Pleasant, IA 52641
319-385-8012
http://www.scciowa.edu
jcouch@scciowa.edu
Dr. Michael Ash, President
Dr. Carole Richardson, VP, Academic Affairs
Jeff Ebbing, Director, Marketing & Comm.
Provides information to students who need to get their GED, and helps them to read and write.

2097 **Western Iowa Tech Community College**
4647 Stone Avenue
P.O. Box 5199
Sioux City, IA 51102-5199
712-274-6400
800-352-4649
http://www.witcc.edu
info@witcc.edu
Dr. Robert Rasmus, Board President
Russell Wray, Board VP
Neal Adler, District I
Recruits volunteer mentors and adult learners throughout the year, and arranges for them to meet and work together.

Kansas

2098 **Arkansas City Literacy Council**
Arkansas City Public Library
120 E 5th Ave
Arkansas City, KS 67005
620-442-1280
http://www.arkcity.org
literacy@acpl.org
Lianne Flax, Adult Services Director
A non-profit, volunteer organization that provides literacy and English language tutoring to adults and older youth so they may gain the listening, speaking, and reading skills needed to be successful in life.

2099 **Butler Community College Adult Education**
901 S. Haverhill Rd
El Dorado, KS 67042
316-321-2222
Fax: 316-322-8450
http://www.butlercc.edu
kallen2@butlercc.edu
Kimberley Krull, President
Kirsten Allen, Director, Admissions
Todd Carter, Athletic Director
Mission is to produce students who make measurable gains in educational skill, workplace readiness, and technology skills.

2100 **Emporia Literacy Program**
3301 West 18th Avenue
Flint Hills Technical College
Emporia, KS 66801
620-343-4600
800-711-6947
Fax: 620-343-4610
http://www.fhtc.edu
askus@fhtc.edu
Mary Beth Voorhees, Chair
Mark Remmert, Vice Chair
Dr. Dean Hollenbeck, President

2101 **Hutchinson Public Library: Literacy Resources**
901 N Main St
Hutchinson, KS 67501
620-663-5441
Fax: 620-663-1583
http://www.hutchpl.org
info@hutchpl.org
Sandra Gustafson, Coordinator
Dianne Brown, Head of Circulation
Ruth Heidebrecht, Head of Collection Development
Provides staff to help adults improve their reading, writing and language skills.

2102 **Kansas Adult Education Association**
Barton County Community College
Barton Community College
245 NE 30 Rd
Great Bend, KS 67530
620-792-2701
800-748-7594
http://www.bartonccc.edu
quinnp@bartonccc.edu
Dr. Penny Quinn, VP, Student Services
Mike Johnson, Trustee
Marsha Miller, Assistant to the Vice President

The Kansas Adult Education Association has been the professional association for adult educators at community colleges, school districts, and non-profit organizations.

2103 Kansas Correctional Education
714 SW Jackson
Suite 300
Topeka, KS 66603
785-296-3317
888-317-8204
http://www.doc.ks.gov
kdocpub@doc.ks.gov
Keith Bradshaw, Director, Fiscal Services
Jan Clausing, Director of Human Resources
Ray Roberts, Secretary of Corrections
The provision of correctional education programming to inmates.

2104 Kansas Department of Corrections
714 SW Jackson
Suite 300
Topeka, KS 66603
785-296-3317
888-317-8204
Fax: 785-296-0014
http://www.doc.ks.gov
kdocpub@doc.ks.gov
Keith Bradshaw, Director, Fiscal Services
Jan Clausing, Director of Human Resources
Ray Roberts, Secretary of Corrections
State corrections agency/department.

2105 Kansas Department of Social & Rehabilitation Services
915 SW Harrison St
Topeka, KS 66612-1505
785-296-3959
888-369-4777
Fax: 785-296-2173
TTY: 785-296-1491
http://www.dcf.ks.gov
Phyllis Gilmore, Secretary
Wm. Jeff Kahrs, Chief of Staff
Angela de Rocha, Communications Director
To assist people with disabilities achieve suitable employment and independence.

2106 Kansas Literacy Resource Center
1000 SW Jackson St
Ste 520
Topeka, KS 66612-1368
785-296-3421
Fax: 785-296-0983
http://www.kansasregents.org
dglass@ksbor.org
Andy Tompkins, President & CEO
Connie Bollig, Executive Assistant
Julene Miller, General Counsel
Enhances systems, both public and private, which provide basic skills education across Kansas. The Center serves as the catalyst for collaborative efforts that address the needs of undereducated adults in Kansas.

2107 Kansas State Department of Adult Education
900 SW Jackson Street
Topeka, KS 66612-1212
785-296-3201
Fax: 785-296-7933
http://www.ksde.org
contact@ksde.org
Lori Adams, Education Program Consultant
Kayeri Akweks, Education Program Consultant
Evelyn Alden, Web editor
To assist adults to become literate and obtain the knowledge and skills necessary for employment and self-sufficiency.

2108 Kansas State Literacy Resource Center: Kansas State Department of Education
1000 SW Jackson St
Ste 520
Topeka, KS 66612-1368
785-296-3421
Fax: 785-296-0983
http://www.kansasregents.org
dglass@ksbor.org
Andy Tompkins, President & CEO
Connie Bollig, Executive Assistant
Julene Miller, General Counsel
The State Literacy Resource Center can assist adult education practitioners across the nation in locating and accessing the most current materials in their issue area.

2109 Preparing for the Future: Adult Learning Services
230 W 7th St
Junction City, KS 66441-3097
785-238-4311
Fax: 785-238-7873
http://www.jclib.org
jclibrary@jclib.org
Susan Moyer, Director
Cheryl Jorgensen, Assistant Director
Sarah Jones, Head of Circulation

Kentucky

2110 Ashland Adult Education
Ashland Community & Technical College
1400 College Drive
Ashland, KY 41101-3617
606-326-2000
800-928-4256
http://ashland.kctcs.edu
joan.flanery@kctcs.edu
Kay Adkins, President and CEO
Richard Adams, Custodial Worker II
Linda Adkins, Office Support Asst
Provides education services that prepare adults with the essential skills they need to function as workers, citizens and family members of the 21st century. The program enables them to develop essential skills for living and wage earning and to better their self-concepts.

2111 Kentucky Laubach Literacy Action
1024 Capital Center Dr
Suite 250
Frankfort, KY 40601-7514
502-573-5114
800-928-7323
Fax: 502-573-5436
TTY: 800-928-7323
http://kyae.ky.gov
dvislisel@mail.state.ky.us
Elizabeth Arauz, Business Specialist
D.J. Begley, Senior Associate
Gayle Box, Senior Associate
Dedicated to helping adults of all ages improve their lives and their communities by learning reading, writing, match and problem-solving skills.

2112 Kentucky Literacy Volunteers of America
1024 Capital Center Dr
Suite 250
Frankfort, KY 40601-7514
502-573-5114
800-928-7323
Fax: 502-573-5436
TTY: 800-928-7323
http://kyae.ky.gov
dvislsel@mail.state.ky.us
Elizabeth Arauz, Business Specialist
D.J. Begley, Senior Associate
Gayle Box, Senior Associate
Promotes literacy for people of all ages.

2113 Operation Read
470 Copper Drive
Lexington, KY 40507-0235
859-254-9964
866-774-4872
Fax: 859-254-5834
http://bluegrass.kctcs.edu
opread@gx.net
Nicholas Mueller, Executive Director
Helping adults learn to read to help imrove their lives, the lives of their children and the lives in their community.

2114 **Simpson County Literacy Council**
231 S College St
Franklin, KY 42134-1809
270-586-7234
Fax: 270-598-0906
http://www.readtobefree.org
read@readtobefree.org
Debra Thompson, Director
A private, non-profit organization that provides a variety of services to enable people to achieve personal goals through literacy, basic reading & math, GED prep, computer classes, math & reading for college and more.

2115 **Winchester Adult Education Center**
52 N Maple St
Winchester, KY 40391
859-744-1975
Fax: 859-744-1424
http://www.winchesteradulteducation.org
mwells_cae@roadrunner.com
Victor Brown, Staff
Bill Baber, Staff
Beekie Denton, Staff
For those 16 years of age and older and out of school, provides facilities, materials, and services in order to improve lifelong learning skills leading to economic independence and quality of life.

Louisiana

2116 **Adult Literacy Advocates of Baton Rouge**
460 North 11th Street
Baton Rouge, LA 70802-4607
225-383-1090
Fax: 225-387-5999
http://www.adultliteracyadvocates.org
info@adultliteracyadvocates.org
Pam Creighton, Executive Director

2117 **Literacy Council of Southwest Louisiana**
Central School Arts & Humanities Center
809 Kirby St
Ste 126
Lake Charles, LA 70601
337-494-7000
Fax: 337-494-7915
http://www.literacyswla.org
info@literacyswla.org
Vicky Hand, President
Tommeka Semien, Executive Director
Alvin Joseph, President-Elect
A community-based, non-profit organization that provides instructional programs to improve educational skill levels in Southwest Louisiana and works to increase public awareness of literacy-related issues.

2118 **Literacy Volunteers Centenary College**
2911 Centenary Boulevard
PO Box 41188
Shreveport, LA 71134-1188
318-869-2411
Fax: 318-869-2474
http://www.literacyconnections.com
lvecent@bellsouth.net
Sue Lee, Executive Director

2119 **VITA (Volunteer Instructors Teaching Adults)**
905 Jefferson St
Ste 404
Lafayette, LA 70501-7913
337-234-4600
Fax: 337-234-4672
http://www.vitalaf.org
vitala@bellsouth.net
Bill Bowers, President
Jeff Ackermann, Vice -Chairman
Gene Cole, Secretary
Specially trained volunteers learn to teach reading and writing using easy to follow manuals and to also provide goal-oriented, one on one or in small group. VITA provides the professional training, materials, and support that enable the volunteers to assist adults in acquiring basic reading and writing skills.

Maine

2120 **Biddeford Adult Education**
64 West Street
PO Box 624
Biddeford, ME 04005
207-282-3883
Fax: 207-286-9581
http://biddeford.maineadulted.org
adulted@biddefordschooldepartment.org
Paulette Bonneau, Director
Sue De Cesare, Community Adult Education Leader
Anne Beaulieu, Administrative Assistant

2121 **Center for Adult Learning and Literacy: University of Maine**
Pro Literacy Worldwide
5749 Merrill Hall
Orono, ME 04469-5749
207-581-1865
877-486-2364
Fax: 207-581-1517
http://www.umaine.edu
president@umaine.edu
Paul W. Ferguson, President
The Center for Adult Learning and Literacy offers quality, research-based professional development and resources, based on funded initiatives to improve the quality of services within the Maine Adult Education System.

2122 **Literacy Volunteers of Androscoggin**
15 Sacred Heart Place
Auburn, ME 04210
207-333-4785
http://www.literacyvolunteersandro.org
literacy@literacyvolunteersandro.org
Tahlia Chamberlain, Executive Director
Providing free one-on-one tutoring and other educational services to help adults in Androscoggin County acquire the basic reading, writing and math skills they need to enhance their lives and achieve their personal goals.

2123 **Literacy Volunteers of Aroostook County**
Caribou Learning Center
75 Bennett Drive
Caribou, ME 04736
207-325-3490
Fax: 207-325-8916
http://rsu39.maineadulted.org
lvaroostook@gmail.com
Lyn Michaud, Director
Provides free, confidential services to any Aroostokk COunty adult with the desire to increase their literacy skill.

2124 **Literacy Volunteers of Bangor**
200 Hogan Rd
Bangor, ME 04401-5604
207-947-8451
Fax: 207-942-1391
http://lvbangor.org
admin@lvbangor.org
Audrey Braccio, President
Brendan Trainor, Vice President
Tina Dowling, Treasurer
A group of people who are dedicated to improving literacy in the community one person at a time. Many of the volunteers choose to become a tutor and teach another adult to read or speak English.

2125 **Literacy Volunteers of Greater Augusta**
12 Spruce St
Ste 2
Augusta, ME 04330
207-626-3440
Fax: 207-626-3440
http://www.lva-augusta.org
info@lva-augusta.org
Mark Flight, Chairperson
Lori Gray, Vice-Chairperson
Virginia Marriner, Affiliate Director
Promote and foster increased literacy for adults who have low literacy skills or those for whom English is not their native language through volunteer tutoring.

2126 **Literacy Volunteers of Greater Portland**
PO Box 8585
Portland, ME 04104
207-775-0105
Fax: 207-780-1701
http://www.lvaportland.org
lvportland@learningworks.me
Kristen Stevens, Executive Director
Offers, free, confidential, student-centered, individual and small group tutoring to adults seeking to develop the literacy skills they need to reach important life goals like reading their first books, obtaining citizenship, helping their children with homework, taking care of personal bills and finding employment.

2127 **Literacy Volunteers of Greater Saco/Biddeford**
841 North Road
Dover Foxcroft, ME 04426
207-283-2954
http://www.maineadulted.org
info@maineadulted.org
Brenda Gagne, Director
Bernadette Farrar, Asst. Director
Lisa Robertson, ABE Coordinator
Trains volunteers to provide educational programs and services that improve reading, writing and related literacy skills, and to empower adults by enhancing their life skills in the area of family, work, health and community.

2128 **Literacy Volunteers of Greater Sanford**
883 Main St
Ste 4
Sanford, ME 04073
207-324-2486
Fax: 207-324-2486
http://www.sanfordliteracy.org
lvgsanford@gmail.com
Kimberley Moran, Executive Director
Supports the literacy needs of local adults with free, confidential, one-on-one tutoring and small group instruction in reading, math, computers, studying for the GED, licenses, and other life skills by trained adult volunteers.

2129 **Literacy Volunteers of Maine**
142 High St
Ste 526
Portland, ME 04101
207-773-3191
Fax: 207-221-1123
http://www.lvmaine.org
info@lvmaine.org
Chip Brewer, Co-President
Benjamin Smith, Co-President
Dedicated to providing increased access to literacy services for Maine adults who wish to acquire or improve their literacy skills.

2130 **Literacy Volunteers of Mid-Coast Maine**
28 Lincoln St
Rockland, ME 04841
207-594-5154
Fax: 207-594-5154
http://lvmidcoast.maineadulted.org
bgifford@msad5.org
Beth A Gifford, Program Director
Dedicated to improving the literacy skills of adults in our community. Deliver instruction using a dedicated corps of well trained volunteer tutors.

2131 **Literacy Volunteers of Waldo County**
5 Stephenson Ln
Belfast, ME 04915
207-338-2200
Fax: 207-338-1652
http://www.broadreachmaine.org
info@brmaine.org
Kate Quinn Finlay, Executive Director
Karla Edney, Financial Director
Deborah Schilder, Director of Development
Helps children and families to develop the skills they need to lead healthy and productive lives. Share the knowledge and experience with child-and-family serving organizations across the state and nation.

2132 **Maine Literacy Resource Center**
University of Maine
5749 Merrill Hall
Orono, ME 04469-5749
207-581-1865
877-486-2364
Fax: 207-581-1517
http://www.umaine.edu
president@umaine.edu
Susan J. Hunter, President
Jeffery Hecker, EVP
Jake Ward, VP
As part of the State Library, the State Resource Center provides electronic and print resources.

2133 **Tri-County Literacy**
2 Sheridan Rd
Bath, ME 04530
207-443-6384
877-885-7441
http://www.tricountyliteracy.org
tricountyliteracy@tricountyliteracy.org
Darlene Marciniak, Executive Director
A non-profit organization dedicated to improving people's lives through three literacy programs; Adult Literacy, Read With Me (Family Literacy), and Reading For Better Business.

Maryland

2134 **Anne Arundel County Literacy Council**
80 West St.
Suite A
Annapolis, MD 21401
410-269-4419
http://www.icanread.org
director@aaclc.org
Lisa Vernon, Executive Director
JoAnn Cook, Student coordinator
Jane Seiss, Tutor Coordinator
Free, convenient, and individualized reading, writing, math, and speaking English instruction for low-income adults in Anne Arundel County. Books, tutoring, and assessments are free and students can meet for lessons with their tutors in any public location in Anne Arundel County and at convenient days and times for their schedules.

2135 **Calvert County Literacy Council**
37600 New Market Road
P.O. Box 459
Charlotte, MD 20622-2508
301-934-9442
Fax: 301-884-0438
http://smrla.org
calvertliteracy@somd.lib.md.us
Maria Isle Birnkammer, Director
Provides volunteers to help with one-on-one tutoring or small group tutoring.

2136 **Center for Adult and Family Literacy: Community College of Baltimore County**
7200 Sollers Point Rd
Building E, Ste 104
Baltimore, MD 21222-4649
443-840-3692
http://www.ccbcmd.edu
abonner@ccbcmd.edu
Sandra Kurtinitis, President
Classes to provide training and instruction for adults with literacy problems.

2137 **Charles County Literacy Council**
United Way Bldg
10250 La Plata Rd
La Plata, MD 20646
301-934-6488
Fax: 301-392-9286
http://www.charlescountyliteracy.org
charlescountyliteracy@comcast.net
Valerie Kettner, President
Lisa Hackley, Vice President
Kathy Joy, Treasurer

A not-for-profit organization, provides free community-based one-on-one adult literacy tutoring to ensure that all adults have the access to quality education needed to fully realize their potential as individuals, parents and citizens

2138 **Howard University School of Continuing Education**
2400 Sixth Street, NW
Suite 440
Washington, DC 20059-5603
202-806-6100
Fax: 301-585-8911
http://www.howard.edu
csnell@howard.edu

Stacey J. Mobley, Chairman
Wayne A.I. Frederick, President
Larkin Arnold, Founder
Howard University Continuing Education was established in April 1986 to meet the education and training needs of professionals, administrators, entrepreneurs, technical personnel, paraprofessionals and other adults on an individual or group basis.

2139 **Literacy Council of Frederick County**
110 E Patrick St
Frederick, MD 21701
301-600-2066
http://www.fredericklireracy.org
info@fredericklireracy.org

Caroline Gaver, President
Beth Lowe, 1st Vice President
Sandy Doggett, 2nd Vice President
A non-profit, non-secretarian, educational organization dedicated to helping non-literate and semi-literate adult residents in the county improve their language skills through one-on-one tutoring.

2140 **Literacy Council of Montgomery County**
21 Maryland Ave
Ste 320
Rockville, MD 20850
301-610-0030
Fax: 301-610-0034
http://www.literacycouncilmcmd.org
info@literacycouncilmcmd.org
Marty Stephens, Executive Director
Danielle Verbiestÿ, Deputy Director
Patrickÿ Salami, Development Director
A non-profit organization founded to help adults living or working in the county who want to achieve functional levels of reading, writing, and speaking English so that they may improve the quality of their life and their ability to participate in the community.

2141 **Maryland Adult Literacy Resource Center**
UMBC, Department of Education
1000 Hilltop Circle
Baltimore, MD 21250-2029
410-455-6725
888-464-3346
Fax: 410-455-1139
http://www.umbc.edu
ira@umbc.edu
Freeman A. Hrabowski, President
As part of the State Library, the State Resource Center provides resources and information for adult literacy providers and students in Maryland.

Massachusetts

2142 **A Legacy for Literacy**
330 Homer St
Newton Center, MA 02459
617-796-1360
TTY: 617-552-7154
http://www.newtonfreelibrary.net
legacyforliteracy@yahoo.com
Barbara Lietzke, President
Robert Klivans, Treasurer
Audrey Cooper, Trustee
Provides free tutoring services for adults of limited English proficiency.

2143 **Adult Center at PAL**
Curry College
1071 Blue Hill Ave
Milton, MA 02186
617-333-0500
Fax: 617-333-2114
http://www.curry.edu
lhubbard@curry.edu
Kennet K. Quigley, President
Offers adults with learning disabilities or attention deficits a safe, supportive place to work on developing their strengths. Serves adult students enrolled in courses at Curry College or at other institutions of higher education.

2144 **ESL Center**
43 Amity St
Amherst, MA 01002
413-259-3090
Fax: 413-256-4096
http://www.joneslibrary.org
esl@joneslibrary.org
Austin Sarat, President
Chris Hoffmann, Vice President
Tamson Ely, Secretary
Provides volunteer tutors, tutoring space, study materials, computer-assisted instruction, citizenship classes, English classes and referrals to adult immigrants in the Amherst area.

2145 **Eastern Massachusetts Literacy Council**
English at Large
800 West Cummings Park
Suite 5550
Woburn, MA 01801-3608
781-395-2374
TTY: 781-395-2374
http://www.englishatlarge.org
info@englishatlarge.org
Catherine Corliss, President
Laura Henry, Vice President
Evan Fitzpatrick, Treasurer
The Eastern Massachusetts Literacy Council is a private non-profit affiliate of ProLiteracy Worldwide, the largest nonprofit volunteer adult literacy organization in the world. The EMLC trains volunteers to assist adults who are learning English as another language and adults who wish to strengthen their basic reading skills.

2146 **JOBS Program: Massachusetts Employment Services Program**
19 Staniford St
Charles F. Hurley Building
Boston, MA 02114-1704
617-626-5300
Fax: 617-348-5191
http://www.mass.gov
DCSCustomerfeedback@detma.org
Deval Patrick, Governer
Glen Shor, Secretary
Matthew H. Malone, Secretary of Education
The Employment Services Program is a joint federal and state funded program whose primary goal is to provide a way to self-sufficiency for TAFDC families ESP is an employment-oriented program that is based on a work-first approach.

2147 **Literacy Network of South Berkshire**
100 Main St
Lee, MA 01238-1614
413-243-0471
Fax: 413-243-6754
http://www.litnetsb.org
info@litnetsb.org
Lucy Prashker, President
Bill Dunlaevy, Treasurer
Laura Qualliotine, Executive Director
Serving the 15 towns of Southern Berkshire County in Massachusetts. Providing free one-on-one tutoring to adults in reading, GED preparation, ESL, and citizenship preparation.

2148 Literacy Volunteers of Greater Worcester
3 Salem Sq
Rm 332
Worcester, MA 01608
508-754-8056
Fax: 508-754-8056
http://www.lvgw.org
info@lvgw.orgÿ

Hank Stolz, President
Harold Jones, Vice President
Lionel Carbonneau, Trasurer
Provides confidential, free, individualized, year-round tutoring in either basic reading or English for speakers of other languages.

2149 Literacy Volunteers of Massachusetts
8 Faneuil Hall Marketplace
3rd floor
Boston, MA 02108
617-367-1313
Fax: 617-367-8894
TTY: 888-466-1313
http://www.lvm.org
kgriffiths@lvm.org

Kristin Griffiths, Director
Literacy Volunteers of Massachusetts helps adults learn to read and write or speak English by matching them with trained volunteer tutors.

2150 Literacy Volunteers of Methuen
305 Broadway
Methuen, MA 01844-6806
978-686-4080
Fax: 978-686-8669
http://www.nevinslibrary.org
litvolmeth@gmail.com

James H. Smith, Chairman
Ralph Prolman, Vice chairman
Kritika McLeod, Director
Brings free, private, flexible, individualized instruction to adults in the community who are struggling everyday with basic reading and language problems.

2151 Literacy Volunteers of the Montachusett Area
610 Main St
Fitchburg, MA 01420
978-343-8184
Fax: 978-343-4680
http://www.literacyvolunteersmontachusett.org
literacy26@aol.com

Shirley Shirley, President
Gloria Maybury, Program Coordinator
Laura Beauregard, Secretary
Promotes and fosters increased literacy in the Montachusett Area through trained volunteer tutoring and to empower adults for whom English is a second language. Encourage and aid individuals, groups or organizations desiring to increase literacy through voluntary programs.

2152 Massachusetts Correctional Education: Inmate Training & Education
PO Box 71
Hodder House, Two Merchant Road
Framingham, MA 01704
508-935-0901
Fax: 508-935-0907
http://www.mass.gov
cvicari@doc.state.ma.us

Carolyn J. Vicari, Director
To establish departmental policy regarding inmates' involvement in academic and vocational training programs.

2153 Massachusetts Family Literacy Consortium
MA Dept of Elementary & Secondary Education
75 Pleasant St
Malden, MA 02148
781-338-3102
Fax: 781-338-3770
http://www.doe.mass.edu
boe@doe.mass.edu

Maura o. Banta, Chairman
Donald Willyard, Chairman
Vanessa Calderon Rosado, Cheif Executive officer
A statewide initiative with the mission of forging effective partnerships among state agencies, community organizations, and other interested parties to expand and strengthen family literacy and support.

2154 Massachusetts GED Administration: Massachusetts Department of Education
75 Pleasant St
Malden, MA 02148
781-338-3102
Fax: 781-338-3770
http://www.doe.mass.edu
boe@doe.mass.edu

Maura o. Banta, Chairman
Donald Willyard, Chairman
Vanessa Calderon Rosado, Cheif Executive officer
Thirty-three test centers operate state-wide to serve the needs of the adult population in need of a high school credential.

2155 Massachusetts Job Training Partnership Act: Department of Employment & Training
19 Staniford St
Boston, MA 02114-2502
617-626-5400
Fax: 617-570-8581
http://www.detma.org
mstonge@detma.org

Edward Malmberg, Executive Director
Supplies information on the local labor market and assists companies in locating employees.

2156 Pollard Memorial Library Adult Literacy Program
401 Merrimack St
Lowell, MA 01850-5999
978-970-4120
Fax: 978-970-4117
TDD: 978-970-4129
http://www.pollardml.org

Victoria Woodley, Director
Susan Fougstedt, Assistant Director
Mollyÿ Hancock, Coordinator of Youth Services
Offers free, confidential, private and flexibly scheduled tutoring to adults with little or no reading or writing skills, and those who wish to become more fluent English speakers, readers or writers.

Michigan

2157 Capital Area Literacy Coalition
1028 E Saginaw
Lansing, MI 48906-5518
517-485-4949
Fax: 517-485-1924
http://www.thereadingpeople.org
mail@thereadingpeople.org

Lois Bader, Executive Director
Di Clark, Assistant Director
Sarah Crockett, Administrative Assistant
The Capital Area Literacy Coalition helps children and adults learn to read, write and speak English with an ultimate goal of helping individuals achieve self-sufficiency.

2158 Kent County Literacy Council
111 Library St NE
Grand Rapids, MI 49503-3268
616-459-5151
Fax: 616-245-8069
http://www.kentliteracy.org
info@kentliteracy.org

Susan Ledy, Executive Director
A non-profit organization founded in 1986 that provides literacy services to over 1,000 adults in reading and english communication. In addition to the adult tutoring programs, we also serve area counties through the Customized Workplace English Program providing fee-based customized Workplace English Language, accent modification, and multicultrual training to area companies; and the Family Literacy Program which offers literacy and ESL instruction, workshops, and events.

2159 **Michigan Assistive Technology: Michigan Rehabilitation Services**
119 Pere Marquette Dr
Suite 1C
Lansing, MI 48912-1231 517-485-4477
Fax: 517-485-4488
http://www.publicpolicy.com
ppa@publicpolicy.com
Jeffrey D. Padden, President
Nancy Hewat, Executive Director
Chris Andrews, Senior Communications Consultant
Solves information and policy-development problems for clients.

2160 **Michigan Libraries and Adult Literacy**
PO Box 30007
702 W. Kalamazoo St.
Lansing, MI 48909-7507 517-373-1300
877-479-0021
Fax: 517-373-5700
TDD: 517-373-1592
http://www.michigan.gov
librarian@michigan.gov
Nancy Robertson, Director
Rick Snyder, Governor
Allison Scott, Exe Director to the Governor

2161 **Michigan Workforce Investment Act**
119 Pere Marquette Dr
Suite 1C
Lansing, MI 48912-1231 517-485-4477
Fax: 517-485-4488
http://www.publicpolicy.com
ppa@publicpolicy.com
Jeff Padden, President
Colleen E. Graber, Director
Dr. Paul Elam, Dirctor of Safety and Justice

Minnesota

2162 **Adult Basic Education**
Minnesota Department of Education
1500 Highway 36 W
Roseville, MN 55113 651-582-8200
Fax: 651-634-5154
http://www.education.state.mn.us
Alice Seagren, Commissioner
Barry Shaffer, Director
Mark Dayton, Office of Governor
Available statewide at no cost to adult learners and is administered through the Minnesota Department of Education. To be eligible for ABE services, a person must be 16 years old or older, not enrolled in K-12 public or private school and lack basic academic skills in one or more of the following areas: reading, writing, speaking and mathematics.

2163 **Alexandria Literacy Project**
1204 Hwy 27 W
Room 907
Alexandria, MN 56308 320-762-3312
Fax: 320-762-3313
http://www.thealp.org
rfinke@alexandria.k12.mn.us
Rollie Finke, Coordinator
Purpose is to recruit and tutor adults who want to improve their basic reading, writing, spelling and/or math skills; to tutor adults originally from other countries who want to improve their English listening, speaking, reading and writing skills; to train volunteer tutors and literacy leaders; to promote and encourage this teaching and training.

2164 **English Learning Center**
Our Saviour's Outreach Ministries
2315 Chicago Ave S
Minneapolis, MN 55404 612-871-5900
Fax: 612-871-0017
http://www.osom-mn.org
Michaelÿ Kuchta, Chairman
Colleen Whalen, Vice-Chairman
Justin Kappel, Secretary
Educationally empowering immigrant and refugee adults and their families towards self-determination.

2165 **Learning Disabilities Association of Minnesota**
6100 Golden Valley Rd
Golden Valley, MN 55422 952-582-6000
Fax: 952-582-6031
http://www.ldaminnesota.org
info@ldaminnesota.org
Jeff Fox, President
Sherry Holtz, Vice President
Jerry Golden, Treasurer
A nonprofit agency providing programs and services for learners of all ages, specializing in learning disabilities or other learning difficulties such as ADHD.

2166 **Minnesota Department of Employment and Economic Development**
Minnesota Workforce Center
332 Minnesota St
Suite E-200
Saint Paul, MN 55101-1351 651-259-7114
800-657-3858
TTY: 651-296-3900
http://mn.gov/deed
deed.lmi@state.mn.us
Mark R. Phillips, Commisioner
Bonnie Elsey, Director
The Department of Employment and Economic Development is Minnesota's principal economic development agency, with programs promoting business expansion and retention, workforce development, international trade, community development and tourism.

2167 **Minnesota LINCS: Literacy Council**
700 Raymond Avenue
Suite 180
Saint Paul, MN 55114 651-645-2277
800-225-7323
Fax: 651-645-2272
http://www.mnliteracy.org
email@mnliteracy.org
Jewelie Grape, President
Rudy Brynolfson, Treasurer
Carla Engstrom, Executive Committee Chair
Makes information available to literacy and other educators throughout Minnesota. The system is a result of cooperation between numerous agencies and organizations in Minnesota that realize the benefit of using the internet to provide information to the public. The system allows literacy and other educators to locate information at one central site or follow links to connect to wherever the information resides.

2168 **Minnesota Life Work Center**
University of St Thomas
1000 LaSalle Ave
Ste 110
Minneapolis, MN 55403 651-962-4763
http://www.stthomas.edu/lifeworkcenter
lifework@stthomas.edu
Provides special services and resources to meet the needs of all students, especially those on the Minneapolis campus.

2169 **Minnesota Literacy Training Network**
University of St Thomas
2115 Summit Avenue
Minneapolis, MN 55105-2025 651-962-5000
800-328-6819
Fax: 651-962-4014
http://www.stthomas.edu
webmaster@stthomas.edu
Julie H. Sullivan, Ph.D., President
Deborah Simmons, Director
Literacy Training Network offers noncredit learning opportunities for adult basic education and literacy training staff in Minnesota.

2170 **Minnesota Vocational Rehabilitation Services**
332 Minnesota St
Ste E-200
Saint Paul, MN 55101-1805
651-259-7366
800-328-9095
Fax: 651-297-5159
TTY: 651-296-3900
http://mn.gov/deed
deed.lmi@state.mn.us
Kimberley Pack, Director
Provides basic vocational rehabilitation services to consumers including vocational counseling, planning, guidance and placement, as well as certain special services based on individual circumstances.

Mississippi

2171 **Corinth-Alcorn Literacy Council**
1023 N Fillmore St
Corinth, MS 38834-4100
662-286-9759
Fax: 662-286-8010
http://www.alcornliteracy.com
literacy38834@yahoo.com
Cheryl Meints, President
Tommy Hardwick, Treasurer
Becky Williams, Secretary

Missouri

2172 **Joplin NALA Read**
ProLiteracy America
123 S. Main Street
Joplin, MO 64801-0447
417-782-2646
Fax: 417-782-2648
http://www.joplinnala.org
joplinnala@123mail.org
Marj Boudreaux, Director
Joan Doner, Program Coordinator
Gail Brown, Administrative Assistant
An adult literacy council, serving adults 17 years and older in the areas of Math, ESL, and reading. Trains volunteers to tutor and furnish all books for the tutors and students. A not-for-profit organization, that receives funding from United Way and the state Adult Education & Literacy department.

2173 **LIFT: St. Louis**
815 Olive St
Ste 22
Saint Louis, MO 63101
314-678-4443
800-729-4443
Fax: 314-678-2938
http://www.lift-missouri.org
todea@webster.edu
Dawnÿ Kitchell, President
Doug Crews, Vice President
Del Doss Hemsley, Trasurer
Serves as Missouri's Literacy Resource Center, provides training, technical assistance, and materials for educators and family literacy programs.

2174 **Literacy Kansas City**
211 W Armour Blvd
Third Fl
Kansas City, MO 64111
816-333-9332
Fax: 816-444-6628
http://www.literacykc.org
info@literacykc.org
Lynne O'Connell, Vice President
Judy Pfannenstiel, Secretary
Julee Fox, Trasurer
To advance literacy through direct services, advocacy and collaboration.

2175 **Literacy Roundtable**
YMCA Literacy Council
2635 Gravois Ave
Saint Louis, MO 63118
314-776-7102
Fax: 314-776-6872
http://www.literacyroundtable.org
cmithcell@ymcastlouis.org
Caroline Mitchell, Coordinator
A consortium of literacy providers throughout the St. Louis-Metro East area whose mission is to support literacy efforts in the Missouri and Illinois bi-state region.

2176 **Parkway Area Adult Education and Literacy**
13157 N Olive Spur
Saint Louis, MO 63141
314-415-4940
Fax: 314-415-4938
http://www.edline.net
pkwyael@yahoo.com
Sally Sandy, Director
Adult basic skills, literacy, GED prep, work readiness, transition to post-secondary, ESL, citizenship, TOFEL prep for those 17 years of age and no longer enrolled in school.

2177 **St Louis Public Schools Adult Education and Literacy**
801 N. 11th Street
Saint Louis, MO 63101
314-231-3720
Fax: 314-367-3057
http://www.slps.org
Supt@slps.org
Dr. Kevin Adams, Superintendent
Dr. Nicole Williams, Chief Academics Officer
Provides opportunities for adults to participate in the GED; ESOL; Workforce Development; Life Skills; Literacy Enhancement and Family Literacy programs.

Montana

2178 **LVA Richland County**
121 3rd Ave NW
Sidney, MT 59270
406-480-1971
http://www.richlandlva.org
info@richlandlva.org
Sue Zimmerman, Program Coordinator
A non-profit, community-based organization working to help adults improve their basic literacy skills, and learn other skills needed for today's modern life.

2179 **Montana Literacy Resource Center**
1515 E 6th Avenue
PO Box 201800
Helena, MT 59620-1800
406-444-3115
800-338-5087
Fax: 406-444-0266
TDD: 406-444-4799
TTY: 406-444-4799
http://www.msl.mt.gov
msl@mt.gov
Jennie Stapp, State Librarian
Kris Schmitz, Central Service Manager
Stacy Bruhn, GIS Web Developer
A state-wide literacy support network.

Nebraska

2180 **Answers4Families: Center on Children, Families, Law**
206 S 13th St
Ste 1000
Lincoln, NE 68508-0227
402-472-0844
800-746-8420
Fax: 402-472-8412
http://www.answers4families.org

A project of the Center on Children, Families and Law at University of Nebraska. Mission is to provide info, opportunities, education and support to Nebraskans through Internet resources. The Center serves individuals with special needs and mental health disorders, foster families, caregivers, assisted living, and school nurses.

2181 **Client Assistance Program (CAP): Nebraska Division of Persons with Disabilities**

301 Centennial Mall S
Box 94987
Lincoln, NE 68509
402-471-3656
800-742-7594
Fax: 402-471-0117
http://www.cap.state.ne.us
victoria.rasmussen@nebraska.gov

Frank Lloyd, Executive Director

The Client Assistance Program helps individuals who have concerns or difficulties when applying for or receiving rehabilitation services funded under the Rehabilitation Act.

2182 **Lincoln Literacy Council**

745 S 9th St
Lincoln, NE 68508
402-476-7323
Fax: 402-476-2122
http://www.lincolnliteracy.org
info@lincolnliteracy.org

David Bargen, President
Cynthia Martinez, First Vice President
Kelly Neil, Second Vice President

To assist people of all cultures and strengthen the community by teaching English language and literacy skills.

2183 **Literacy Center for the Midlands**

1823 Harney St
Ste 204
Omaha, NE 68102
402-342-7323
Fax: 402-345-9045
http://www.midlandsliteracy.org
btodd@midlandsliteracy.org

Beverly Todd, Executive Director

To empower adults and families by helping them acquire the literacy skills and practices to be active and contributing members of their communities.

2184 **Platte Valley Literacy Association**

P.O. Box 159
Columbus, NE 68602
402-562-5904
Fax: 402- 564-944
http://www.megavision.net
literacy@megavision.com

Jolene Hake, Executive Director

Organization that collaborates with Central Community College Adult Basic Education to respond to the educational needs of our community.

Nevada

2185 **Nevada Department of Adult Education**

755 N Roop St
Carson City, NV 89701
775-687-7289
Fax: 775-687-8636
http://nde.doe.nv.gov

Brad Deeds, ABE/ESL/GED Programs

provides adult basic education and literacy services in order to assist adults to become literate and obtain the knowledge and skills necessary for employment and self-sufficiency; to assist adults who are parents to obtain the educational skills necessary to become full partners in the education of their children; and to assist adults in the completion of a secondary school education.

2186 **Nevada Economic Opportunity Board: Community Action Partnership**

330 W. Washington Ave
Suite 7
Las Vegas, NV 89106
702-647-3307
Fax: 702-647-0803
http://www.eobccnv.org
Info@eobccnv.org

Lawrence Weekly, President
Aaron Ford, Secretary
Fred Haron, Treasurer

Located in one of the fastest growing and most diverse communities in the United States, the Economic Opportunity Board of Clark County is a highly innovative Community Action Agency. Our mission is to eliminate poverty by providing programs, resources, services, and advocacy for self-sufficiency and economic empowerment.

2187 **Nevada Literacy Coalition: State Literacy Resource Center**

100 N Stewart St
Carson City, NV 89701-4285
775-885-1010
800-445-9673
Fax: 775-684-3344
http://www.nevadaculture.org
sfgraf@clan.lib.nv.us

Claudia Vechio, Director
Larry Friedman, Deputy Director
Greg Fine, Marketing and Advertising

The Nevada State Literacy Resource Center has books, newsletters and a wide variety of multi-media resources such as videos, audiotapes and games for literacy instruction and programs for literacy students, trainers and tutors.

2188 **Northern Nevada Literacy Council**

1400 Wedekind Rd
Reno, NV 89512-2465
775-356-1007
Fax: 775-356-1009
http://www.nnlc.org
director@nnlc.org

Susan Robinson, Executive Director
Mike Benson, Data Manager
Katie Plaz, Bookkepper and Office Manager

Provides English as a second language, adult basic skills, and GED preparatory instructions for adults, 18 years of age and over, who lack a high school diploma or GED or essential basic skills to function successfully in the workplace.

New Hampshire

2189 **New Hampshire Literacy Volunteers of America**

405 Pine St
Manchester, NH 03104-6106
603-624-6550
Fax: 603-624-6559
http://www.manchesternh.gov

Mark Brewer, Director
Robert Gagne, Chairman
Wesley Anderson, Director

This program is the only nationally accredited adult literacy program in New Hampshire. Provides free confidential one-to-one tutoring for adults who want to learn to write and read for lifelong learning.

New Jersey

2190 **Jersey City Library Literacy Program**

472 Jersey Ave
Jersey City, NJ 07302-3456
201-547-4526
Fax: 201-435-5746
http://www.jclibrary.org
literacy@jclibrary.org

Sondra E. Buesing Riley, President
John A. Mehos, Treasurer
Esther Wintner, Secretary

Provides free one-on-one basic reading instruction for Jersey City residents aged sixteen and older. Work with students ranging from non-readers through the fifth grade level. Offers small conversation group classes for immigrants striving to learn to speak, read and write English.

2191 **Literacy Volunteers in Mercer County**
224 Main St.
Ste 104
Metuchen, NJ 08840
732-906-5456
800- 848-004
Fax: 609-587-6137
http://literacynj.org
lvmercer@verizon.net
Perrine Robinson Geller, President
Elizabeth Gloeggler, CEO
Jessica Tomkins, COO
Trains, coordinates and supports the efforts of a dedicated group of volunteer literacy tutors. Volunteers provide free, confidential literacy tutoring services to adult residents in Mercer COunty at a variety of locations including the public libraries, workplace sites, churches and retirement homes.

2192 **Literacy Volunteers of America Essex/Passaic County**
Passaic Public Library
195 Gregory Ave
Passaic, NJ 07005
973-470-0039
Fax: 973-470-0098
http://www.lvanewark.org
lvanewark@verizon.net
Sally Rice, President
Kathy Mollica, Vice President
Jordan Fried, Treasury
Provides free literacy services to adults who have been identified as needing instruction in reading and/or English conversation; and to families who are experiencing literacy and/or learning difficulties.

2193 **Literacy Volunteers of Camden County**
203 Laurel Rd
3rdÿfloor
Voorhees, NJ 08043-2349
856-772-1636
Fax: 856-772-2761
http://lva.camden.lib.nj.us
literacy@camdencountylibrary.org
Denise Weinberg, Director
An adult literacy organization that tutors Camden County, NJ adults (18 years or over) residents who are at the lowest levels of literacy and who need help speaking or understanding English (ESL) or who need help with elementary reading or math skills.

2194 **Literacy Volunteers of Cape-Atlantic**
743 N Main St
Pleasantville, NJ 08232-1541
609-383-3377
Fax: 609-383-0234
http://www.lvacapeatlantic.com
literacyvolunteers@comcast.net
Pamela Grites, Executive Director
Katherine Micale, Program Director
Patrica Epps, Administrative Assistant
Helps individuals in Atlantic and Cape May Counties improve their English language skills so they can participate more fully in family, workplace and community life.

2195 **Literacy Volunteers of Englewood Library**
31 Engle St
Englewood, NJ 07631-2903
201-568-2215
Fax: 201-568-6895
http://www.englewoodlibrary.org
ctaylor@bccls.org
Katharine Glynn, President
Frank Huttle, Mayor
Catherine Wolverton, Library Director
Offers three tutor-training workshops each year with an extensive collection of books, workbooks, and cassettes for tutors and students to borrow with a current library card.

2196 **Literacy Volunteers of Gloucester County**
PO Box 1106
Turnersville, NJ 08012
856-218-4743
http://www.literacyvgc.org
info@literacyvgc.org
Trudy Lawrence, Executive Director
Providing free, one-on-one adult tutoring to those with the lowest level of literacy - below a 5th grade level.

2197 **Literacy Volunteers of Middlesex**
Suite F
380 Washington Road
Sayreville, NJ 08872
732-432-8000
Fax: 732-432-8189
http://www.lpnj.org
info@lpnj.org
Mary Ellen Firestone, President
Christine Sienkielewski, Director
Trained volunteers that provide free tutoring services to adults with limited literacy skills, enabling them to achieve their personal goals and to enhance their contributions to the community.

2198 **Literacy Volunteers of Monmouth County**
213 Broadway
Long Branch, NJ 07740
732-571-0209
Fax: 732-571-2474
http://www.lvmonmouthnj.org
lvmonmouth@brookdalecc.edu
Chris Vecere, President
Manuel J. Alarez, Vice President
Thomas J. White, Secretary
Mission is to promote increased literacy for adults in Monmouth County through the effetive use of volunteers and in collaboration with individuals, groups and organizations desiring to foster increased literacy.

2199 **Literacy Volunteers of Morris County**
10 Pine St
Morristown, NJ 07960
973-984-1998
Fax: 973-971-0291
http://www.lvamorris.org
lvamorris@yahoo.com
Debbie Leon, Director
Promotes increased literacy and fluency in English for adult learners in this area through the effective use of volunteers, the provisions of support services for volunteers and learners, and through collaboration with individuals, groups and any organization desirous of fostering increased literacy.

2200 **Literacy Volunteers of Plainfield Public Library**
800 Park Ave
Plainfield, NJ 07060-2517
908-757-1111
Fax: 908-754-0063
http://www.plainfieldlibrary.info
literacy@plfdpl.info
Joseph Hugh Da Rold, Director
Mary Ellen Rogan, Assistant Director
Scott Kuchinsky, Coordinator
Mission is to develop the literacy skills of adults with minimum reading skills.

2201 **Literacy Volunteers of Somerset County**
120 Finderne Ave
Box 7
Bridgewater, NJ 08807
908-725-5430
Fax: 908-707-2077
http://www.literacysomerset.org
info@literacysomerset.org
Martha Davis, President
Phil Areminio, Vice President
Steve Cummins, Trasurer
Promotes literacy through a network of community volunteers.

2202 **Literacy Volunteers of Union County**
224 Main St.
Metuchen, NJ 08840
732-906-5456
Fax: 800-848-0048
http://literacynj.org
literacyinfo@lvaunion.org
Perrine Robinson Geller, President
Elizabeth Gloeggler, CEO
Jessica Tomkins, COO
A non-profit organization that improves the lives of adults in the county by teaching them to read, write and speak English so they can participate more fully in family, workplace and community life.

2203 **People Care Center**
120 Finderne Avenue
Bridgewater, NJ 08807
908-725-2299
Fax: 908-725-2607
http://www.peoplecarecenter.org
info@peoplecarecenter.org
Joseph Antico, President
Jay Perantoni, VP
Marie Hughes, Executive Director

New Mexico

2204 **Adult Basic Education Division of Dona Ana Community College**
2800 N. Sonoma Ranch Blvd
Las Cruces, NM 88011
575-527-7500
800-903-7503
Fax: 575-528-7300
http://dabcc-www.nmsu.edu
sdegiuli@nmsu.edu
Renay Scott, President
Andrew Burke, VP, Business & Finance
Monica Torres, Interim VP, Academic Affairs

2205 **Carlsbad Literacy Program**
Ann Wood Literacy Center
511 N 12th Street
P.O. Box 3112
Carlsbad, NM 88221
575-885-1752
Fax: 575-885-7980
http://www.carlsbadliteracyprogram.com
literacy1@valornet.com
Delora Elizondo, Coordinator
Provides opportunities for adult community members to learn to read and to improve their reading and writing abilities.

2206 **Curry County Literacy Council**
Clovis Community College
417 Schepps Blvd
Rm 171
Clovis, NM 88101
575-769-2811
800-769-1409
Fax: 575-769-4190
http://www.clovis.edu
curry.literacy@clovis.edu
Dr. Becky Rowley, President
Dr. Robin Jones, VP
Tom Drake, VP, Administration
Goal is to provide one with a sense of security to gain employment, have life skills, and assist in language development.

2207 **Deming Literacy Program**
PO Box 1932
2301 South Tin St.
Deming, NM 88031-1932
575-546-7571
Fax: 505-546-1356
http://www.centerfornonprofitexcellence.org
dlpdeming@gmail.com
Marisol D. Perez, Director
The Literacy Home Mentoring and After School Project will encourage parents to read to their children at home, as well as provide mentors to help children with their reading skills after school.

2208 **Literacy Volunteers of America: Dona Ana County**
MSC 3DA
P.O. Box 30001
Las Cruces, NM 88003-8001
575-527-7544
800-903-7540
Fax: 575-528-7065
http://www.readwritenow.org
sdegiuli@nmsu.edu
Linda Coshenet, Chair
Anita C. Hernandez, Ph.D., Vice Chair
Jackie Kiefer, Treasurer, Secretary
The Literacy Volunteers of America is designed to help people who cannot read or write the English language. This program gives adults a new opportunity to learn reading through the sixth-grade level.

2209 **Literacy Volunteers of America: Las Vegas, San Miguel**
Box 9000
Las Vegas, NM 87701
505-425-7511
877-850-9064
http://www.nmhu.edu
president_office@nmhu.edu
James Fries, President
Gilbert D. Rivera, Vice President
Darlene Chavez, Development Finance Officer
Las Vegas/San Miquel Literacy Volunteers are a part of the national non-profit organization Literacy Volunteers of America, which is dedicated to promoting literacy throughout the country.

2210 **Literacy Volunteers of America: Socorro County**
PO Box 1431
Socorro, NM 87801-1431
505-835-4659
Fax: 505-835-1182
http://www.volunteermatch.org
lva_socorro@hotmail.com
Joyce Aguilar, Executive Director
Promotes literacy for people of Socorro County.

2211 **Literacy Volunteers of Santa Fe**
6401 Richards Avenue
Room 514A
Santa Fe, NM 87508
505-428-1353
Fax: 505-428-1338
http://www.lvsf.org
lvsf@sfcc.edu
Letty Naranjo, Executive Director
Israel Garcia, Program Assistant
Dedicated to providing free tutoring and encouragement for adults and their families who want to read, write and speak English.

2212 **New Mexico Coalition for Literacy**
3209 Mercantile Ct
Suite B
Santa Fe, NM 87507
505-982-3997
800-233-7587
Fax: 505-982-4095
http://www.nmcl.org
info@nmcl.org
Heather Heunermund, Executive Director
Encourages and supports community-based literacy programs and is the New Mexico affiliate and coordinator for the national program of ProLiteracy America, overseeing certification and coordination of its volunteer, tutor trainers.

2213 **Read West**
2900 Grande Blvd
PO Box 44508
Rio Rancho, NM 87124
505-892-1131
Fax: 505-896-3780
http://www.readwest.org
readwest@readwest.org

Linda Stokes, President
Kitty McMahon, VP
Gwenevere Johnson, Treasurer
Targets adults with low literacy or whose first language is not English. Provides free, customized, one-to-one, tutoring to help adults improve. their reading, writing and English language.
1989

2214 Roswell Literacy Council
609 West 10th Street
Roswell, NM 88201 575-625-1369
Fax: 575-622-8280
http://www.roswell-literacy.org
literacy@dfn.com
Andrae England, Director
Dedicated to adult learning in Chaves County.

2215 Valencia County Literacy Council
280 La Entrada
Los Lunas, NM 87031 505-925-8926
Fax: 505-925-8924
http://www.valencialiteracy.org
joglesby@valencialiteracy.org
Dolores Padilla, President
Roberta Scott, VP
Paul Baca, Executive Director
To enable adults to achieve personal goals and very young children to achieve pre-literacy skills through literacy services provided to families free of charge.

New York

2216 Literacy Volunteers of America: Middletown
70 Fulton Street
Middletown, NY 10940 845-341-5460
Fax: 845-343-7191
http://www.literacyorangeny.org
info@LiteracyOrangeNY.com
Christine Rolando, Executive Director
An organization of volunteers that provides a variety of services to enable people to achieve personal goals through literacy. Their belief is that the ability to read is critical to personal freedom and maintenance of a democratic society. These beliefs have led to the following commitments: the personal growth of their students; the effective use of their volunteers; the improvement of society and strengthening and improving the organization.

2217 Literacy Volunteers of Oswego County
45 E. Schuyler Street
Bldg. 31, Fort Ontario
Oswego, NY 13126 315-342-8839
Fax: 315-342-3489
http://www.lvoswego.org
lvoswego@oco.org
Jane Murphy, Executive Director
Beth Kazel, Director of Education Services
Meg Henderson, Program Coordinator
A non-profit community-based educational organization that provides quality tutoring in basic literacy skills and conversational English.

2218 Literacy Volunteers of Otsego & Delaware Counties
Oneonta Adult Education
31 Center Street
Oneonta, NY 13820-3510 607-433-3645
800-782-3858
http://oneontaadulteducation.org
lvodc@oneonta.edu
To change lives of courageous, motivated adults who do not possess functional skills needed to perform ordinary, everyday tasks in an ever-changing global society.

2219 New York Literacy Assistance Center
39 Broadway
Suite 1250
New York, NY 10006 212-803-3300
Fax: 212-785-3685
http://www.lacnyc.org
elyser@lacnyc.org
Elizabeth Horton, Chair
John Gordon, Associate VP, Programs
J. David Nelson, Chief Operating Officer
A nonprofit organization dedicated to supporting and promoting the expansion of quality literacy services in New York.

2220 New York Literacy Resource Center
State University of New York
1400 Washington Ave
Albany, NY 12222 518-442-3300
800-331-0931
Fax: 518-442-5383
http://www.albany.edu
Robert J. Jones, President
Miriam Trementozzi, Associate VP
Daniel Butterworth, Program Director
State Literacy Resource Center is a statewide literacy information network throughout the state.

2221 New York Literacy Volunteers of America
149 Central Ave.
Lancaster, NY 14086 716-651-0465
Fax: 716-651-0542
http://literacynewyork.org
info@literacynewyork.org
Janice Cuddahee, Executive Director
Kathy Houghton, Director of Program Services
Chip Carlin, Associate Executive Director
Provides technical program, and training assistance and workshops to a network of 36 local, community-based affiliates who annually provide over 400,000 hours of reading and basic skills instruction to adult learners.

2222 Resources for Children with Special Needs
116 E. 16th Street
5th Floor
New York, NY 10003 212-677-4650
Fax: 212-254-4070
http://www.resourcesnyc.org
info@resourcesnyc.org
Rachel Howard, Executive Director
Stephen Stern, Director, Finance
Todd Dorman, Director, Communications
Independent nonprofit organization that works for families and children with all special needs, across all boroughs, to understand, navigate, and access the services needed to ensure that all children have the opportunity to develop their full potential.

North Carolina

2223 Blue Ridge Literacy Council
PO Box 1728
Hendersonville, NC 28793 828-696-3811
Fax: 828-696-3887
http://www.litcouncil.org
skirkland@litcouncil.org
Judy Hansen, President
Rickey Parker, Vice President
Steve Kirkland, Executive Director
Provides adults in Henderson County the English communication and literacy skills they need to reach their full potential as individuals, parents, workers and citizens.

2224 **Durham Literacy Center**
1905 Chapel Hill Road
P.O. Box 52209
Durham, NC 27707
919-489-8383
Fax: 919-489-7637
http://www.durhamliteracy.org
info@durhamliteracy.org
Reginald Hodges, Executive Director
Shondra Brewer, Administrative Assistant
Gardy Perard, Coordinator
Works to assist Durham County teenagers and adults achieve personal goals and experience positive life change through increased literacy. Helps teenagers and adults gain the reading and writing skills, English language skills, and educational credentials (GED) needed to earn a living wage.

2225 **Gaston Literacy Council**
116 South Marietta Street
Gastonia, NC 28052
704-868-4815
Fax: 704-867-7796
http://www.gastonliteracy.org
literacy@gastonliteracy.org
Gayle Kersh, Chair
Tim Efird, Vice Chair
Kaye Gribble, Executive Director
A progressive organization dedicated to helping individuals improve their reading, writing, mathematics, listening, speaking, and technology skills.

2226 **Literacy Council Of Buncombe County**
31 College Place
Suite B-221
Asheville, NC 28801
828-254-3442
Fax: 828-254-1742
http://www.litcouncil.com
info@litcouncil.com
Ashley Lasher, Executive Director
Brantlee Eisenman, Development Director
Erin Sebelius, ESOL Director
Promotes increased adult literacy in Buncombe County through effective use of trained tutors; to provide support services for tutors and learners; and to collaborate with individuals, groups, or other community organizations desiring to foster increased adult literacy.

2227 **Literacy Volunteers of America: Pitt County**
3107 S Evans Street
Suite E
Greenville, NC 27858
252-353-6578
Fax: 252-353-6868
http://www.pittliteracy.org
info@pittliteracy.org
Lynn Pischke, Executive Director
To promote literacy in Pitt County through trained volunteer tutors who provide one on one and small group tutoring to adults with limited reading, writing or English speaking/literacy skills.

2228 **North Carolina Literacy Resource Center**
North Carolina Community College
200 West Jones Street
Raleigh, NC 27603
919-807-7100
Fax: 919-807-7165
http://www.nccommunitycolleges.edu
allenb@ncccs.cc.nc.us
Dr. R. Scott Ralls, President
Lisa Tolley, Program Manager
North Carolina Community College Literacy Resource Center collects and disseminates information about literacy resources and organizations.

2229 **Reading Connections of North Carolina**
122 N. Elm Street
Suite 920
Greensboro, NC 27401
336-230-2223
Fax: 336-230-2203
http://www.readingconnections.org
info@readingconnections.org
Jennifer Gore, Executive Director
Roberta Hawthorne, Program Manager
Alexana Garcia, ABE Coordinator
To provide and advocate for free, individualized adult literacy services to promote life changes for Guilford County residents and surrounding communities.

North Dakota

2230 **North Dakota Adult Education and Literacy Resource Center**
600 E. Boulevard Avenue
Dept. 201, Floors 9, 10, and 11
Bismarck, ND 58505-0440
701-328-2260
Fax: 701-328-2461
http://www.dpi.state.nd.us
dpi@nd.gov
Kirsten Baesler, State Superintendent
Valerie Fischer, State Director
Jolli Marcellais, Administrative Assistant
Promotes and supports free programs that help adults over the age of 16 obtain the basic academic and educational skills they need to be productive workers, family members, and citizens.

2231 **North Dakota Department of Career and Technical Education**
State Capitol 15th Floor
600 E Boulevard Ave
Bismarck, ND 58505
701-328-3180
Fax: 701-328-1255
http://www.nd.gov
cte@nd.us
Wayne Kutzer, Director
The mission of the Board for Vocational and Technical Education is to work with others to provide all North Dakota citizens with the technical skills, knowledge, and attitudes necessary for successful performance in a globally competitive workplace.

2232 **North Dakota Department of Human Services: Welfare & Public Assistance**
600 East Boulevard Avenue
Dept. 325
Bismarck, ND 58505-0250
701-328-2310
800-472-2622
Fax: 701-328-2359
TTY: 800-366-6888
http://www.nd.gov/dhs
dhseo@nd.gov
Carol K Olson, Executive Director
To provide services and support for poor, disabled, ill, elderly or juvenile clients in North Dakota.

2233 **North Dakota Department of Public Instruction**
600 E. Boulevard Avenue
Dept. 201, Floors 9, 10, and 11
Bismarck, ND 58505-0440
701-328-2260
Fax: 701-328-2461
http://www.dpi.state.nd.us
dpi@nd.gov
Kirsten Baesler, State Superintendent
Valerie Fischer, State Director
Jolli Marcellais, Administrative Assistant
This unit provides funding and technical assistance to local programs and monitors progress of each funded project. This unit is also responsible for the administration of the GED Testing Program.

2234 **North Dakota Reading Association**
2420 2nd Ave SW
Minot, ND 58701-3332
701-857-4642
Fax: 701-857-8761
http://ndreadon.utma.com
Paula.Rogers@sendit.nodak.edu
Joyce Hinman, State Coordinator

To provide a variety of professional development opportunities; to increase the building of partnerships with other organizations; to actively promote literacy locally and globally; to assist in the strengthening of local councils and their services to members; and to promote writing with young authors.

2235 **North Dakota Workforce Development Council**
1600 E Century Ave, Suite 2
P.O. Box 2057
Bismarck, ND 58503 701-328-5300
Fax: 701-328-5320
TTY: 800-366-6888
http://www.commerce.nd.gov
commerce@nd.gov
Al Anderson, Commissioner, Dept. of Commerce
Paul Lucy, Director, Finance
Wayde Sick, Director, Workforce Development
The role of the North Dakota Workforce Development Council is to advise the Governor and the Public concerning the nature and extent of workforce development in the context of North Dakota's economic development needs, and how to meet these needs effectively while maximizing the efficient use of available resources and avoiding unnecessary duplication of effort.

Ohio

2236 **Central/Southeast ABLE Resource Center**
Ohio University
338 McCracken Hall
Athens, OH 45701 740-593-4419
800-753-1519
Fax: 740-593-2834
http://www.ouliteracycenter.org
literacy@ohio.edu
Sharon Reynolds, Director
Committed to the development of literacy in southeastern Ohio and to research in all areas of literacy.

2237 **Clark County Literacy Coalition**
137 East High Street
Springfield, OH 45502-1215 937-323-8617
Fax: 937-328-6911
http://www.clarkcountyliteracy.org
david.smiddy@clarkcountyliteracy.org
Lisa Holmes, President
Dedicated to increasing the level of functional literacy and self-sufficiency among the people in Clark County.

2238 **Columbus Literacy Council**
195 N Grant Ave
Columbus, OH 43215-2607 614-221-5013
Fax: 614-221-5892
http://www.columbusliteracy.com
jwatson@columbusliteracy.org
Joy D Watson, Executive Director
A volunteer-based organization dedicated to increasing the level of functional literacy of adults in Central Ohio through teaching the English language skills of listening, speaking, reading and writing.

2239 **Literacy Council of Clermont/Brown Counties**
745 Center St
Ste 300
Milford, OH 45150 513-831-7323
Fax: 513-831-7324
http://www.clermontbrownliteracy.org
susan.vilardo@clermontbrownliteracy.org
Joann Kiser, President
Rebecca Proud, Vice President
Susan M. Vilardo, Executive Director
Offers one-on-one volunteer tutor education in reading, writing, spelling and comprehension to adults 18 years of age and older with low-level reading skills or who cannot read. One-on-one tutor education in English speaking reading and writing for adults 18 and older who seek ESL/ESOL.

2240 **Miami Valley Literacy Council**
333 West First St
Ste 130
Dayton, OH 45402 937-223-4922
Fax: 937-223-0271
http://www.discoverliteracy.org
rgilmore@discoverliteracy.org
Russ Gilmore, Executive Director
Offers classes, one-to-one tutoring, and independent study options to adults in the Miami Valley who have low-level literacy of English language skills. Also works with school-aged children and teens below grade level in reading and math in the after-school program The Learning Club.

2241 **Ohio Literacy Network**
6161 Busch Blvd
Ste 84
Columbus, OH 43229 614-505-0716
800-228-7323
Fax: 614-505-0718
http://www.ohioliteracynetwork.org
atoops@ohioliteracynetworking.org
Allen Toops, Executive Director
Mission is to build Ohio's workforce by strengthening adult and family literacy education accomplished by connecting learners, educators and volunteers to a wide variety of educational resources.

2242 **Ohio Literacy Resource Center**
Kent State University
Research 1-1100 Summit Street, Kent
PO Box 5190
Kent, OH 44242-0001 330-672-2007
800-765-2897
Fax: 330-672-4841
http://literacy.kent.edu
olrc@literacy.kent.edu
Marty Ropog, Director
Tim Ponder, LINCS coordinator
Susie Lockhart, Office Manager
The OLRC Mission is to stimulate joint planning and coordination of literacy services at the local, regional and state levels, and to enhance the capacity of state and local organizations and services delivery systems.

2243 **Project LEARN of Summit County**
60 South High Street
Akron, OH 44326 330-434-9461
866-934-7323
Fax: 330-643-9195
http://www.projectlearnsummit.org
info@projectlearnsummit.org
Rick Mc Intosh, Executive Director
Stephanie Norris, Admissions Assistant
Rose Austin, Data Manager
Project LEARN is a nonprofit, community-based organization providing Summit County's nonreading adult population with free, confidential, small group classes and tutoring. Helps adults reach their goals of self-sufficiency, independence and job retention.

2244 **Project LITE**
6th And Reid Ave
Lorain, OH 44052 440-244-1192
800-322-READ
Fax: 440-244-1733
http://www.lorain.lib.oh.us
contact-lite@lorain.lib.oh.us
Linda Pierce, Director

2245 **Project: LEARN**
105 W. Liberty Street
Medina, OH 44256 330-723-1314
http://www.projectlearnmedina.org
projectlearn.medina@gmail.com
Linda Smalley, Executive Director
Provides one-on-one tutoring to adults in reading, math and English as a second language.

2246 **Seeds of Literacy Project: St Colman Family Learning Center**
3104 W. 25th Street
3rd Floor
Cleveland, OH 44109
216-661-7950
Fax: 216-661-7952
http://www.seedsofliteracy.org
bonnieentler@seedsofliteracy.org
Bonnie Entler, Executive Director
Rachel Cotton, Site Coordinator
Daniel McLaughlin, Program Officer
Helping adults in need of assistance in reading, writing and mathematical skills and to improve their ability to function, compete, and advance in society in an atmosphere of Christian care and compassion.

Oklahoma

2247 **Center for Study of Literacy**
Northeastern State University
2400 W. Shawnee
PO Box 549
Muskogee, OK 74401
918-683-0040
Fax: 918-781-5425
http://www.nsuok.edu
mcelroyt@nsuok.edu
Dr. Steve Turner, President
Dr. Laura Boren, VP, Student Affairs
David Koehn, VP, Finance & Business
Provides the illiterate or undereducated adult with training; provides instructional support for the Northeastern State University's faculty and pre-service teachers participate in computer literacy training to gain an understanding of computer assisted instruction; to serve as a reesource unit for other social agencies, teachers, administrators and public school students; to serve as the clearinghouse for literacy for the state of Oklahoma; to initiate research on literacy.

2248 **Community Literacy Center**
5131 N. Classen Circle
Suite 204
Oklahoma City, OK 73118-4420
405-524-7323
Fax: 405-608-0533
http://www.communityliteracy.com
okcread@caol.com
Becky O'Dell, Executive Director
Laura Taylor, Coordinator
Tara Beall, Communications Coordinator
A private, non-profit organization dedicated to teaching adults to read.

2249 **Creek County Literacy Program**
27 W Dewey Ave
Sapulpa, OK 74066-3909
918-224-9647
Fax: 918-224-3546
http://www.creeklit.okpls.org
creeklit@yahoo.com
Barbara Belk, Executive Director
Provides free reading instruction to functionally illiterate adults who live or work in Creek County, to prepare families to manage their health care needs and to be effectively involved in the education of their children, to tutor children/youth who may have different learning styles, and to provide reading improvement programs county-wide

2250 **Great Plains Literacy Council**
Southern Prairie Library System
421 North Hudson
Altus, OK 73521
580-477-2890
888-302-9053
Fax: 580-477-3626
http://www.spls.lib.ok.us
literacy1@spls.lib.ok.us
Ida Fay Winters, Director
Helps to increase the awareness of the illiteracy problem and offers a viable solution. Recruits dedicated, tutors who help to motivate those who are considered illiterate and give them the opportunity to become contributing members of the community.

2251 **Guthrie Literacy Program**
201 N Division Street
Guthrie, OK 73044
405-282-0050
Fax: 405-282-2804
http://www.guthrie.okpls.org
co@cityofguthrie.com
Linda Gens, Library Services Director
Utilizes curriculum that focuses on the individual student's interests and needs, then tutors help the student set the goals and work with them to achieve those goals.

2252 **Junior League of Oklahoma City**
1001 NW Grand Boulevard
Oklahoma City, OK 73118
405-843-5668
Fax: 405-843-0994
http://www.jloc.org
info@jloc.org
Kristi Leonard, President
Nazette Zuhdi, President Elect
Jenifer Randle, Administrative VP
Organization of women committed to promoting volunteerism, developing the potential of women and to improving the community through the effective action and leadership of trained volunteers. The purpose is exclusively educational and charitable.

2253 **Literacy & Evangelism International**
1800 S Jackson Ave
Tulsa, OK 74107
918-585-3826
Fax: 918-585-3224
http://www.literacyevangelism.org
general@literacyevangelism.org
A missionary fellowship desiring to see the Church in every nation effectively reaching the illiterate, bringing them the Living Word Jesus Christ, through enabling them to read the written Word of God.

2254 **Literacy Volunteers of America: Tulsa City County Library**
400 Civic Center
Tulsa, OK 74103
918-549-7323
Fax: 918-596-7907
http://www.tulsalibrary.org
jgreb@tccl.lib.ok.us
Linda Saferite, Executive Director
Sally Frasier, Commission Member
Rebecca Marks, Commission Member
We offer one-on-one tutoring to adults and young adults who wish to improve their reading and writing skills.

2255 **Muskogee Area Literacy Council**
801 West Okmulgee
Muskogee, OK 74401-6840
918-682-6657
888-291-8152
Fax: 918-682-9466
http://www.eok.lib.ok.us
muskpublib@eodls.org
Penny Chastain, Coordinator
Jan Bryant, Head of Muskogee Public Library
Debbie Goodwin, Head of Circulation

2256 **Northwest Oklahoma Literacy Council**
1500 Main St
Woodward, OK 73801-3044
580-254-8582
Fax: 580-254-8546
nwoklitcouncil@woodward.lib.ok.us
Cathy Johnson, Director
Mission is to break the intergenerational cycle of illiteracy by broadening the learner and service base to include family members. Services include literacy and parenting instruction, as a compliment to ESL, adult basic education, and learning disabilities programs.

2257 Oklahoma Literacy Council
300 Park Ave
Oklahoma City, OK 73102-3600 405-232-3780
Fax: 405-606-3722
http://www.literacyokc.org
director@literacyokc.org
Millonn Lamb, Executive Director
Promotes literacy in adults who are in need of improving literacy skills to function successfully in society.

2258 Oklahoma Literacy Resource Center
200 N.E. 18th St.
Oklahoma City, OK 73105 405-521-2502
800-522-8116
Fax: 405-525-7804
http://www.odl.state.ok.us
lgelders@oltn.state.ok.us
Leslie Gelders, Literacy Administrator
Susan C. McVey, Director
Vicki Sullivan, Deputy Director
Provides leadership, resources, training, and information to Oklahoma;s library and community-based literacy network.

2259 Opportunities Industrialization Center of Oklahoma County
400 N Walnut Ave
Oklahoma City, OK 73104-2207 405-235-2651
Fax: 405-235-2653
http://oicofoklahomacounty.org
oicoc@sbcglobal.net
Jerry Day, Chairman
Monique Jackson, Vice Chairman
Patricia Kelly, Executive Director
Empowers individuals through Academic and Career education to become more productive citizens in the community.

Oregon

2260 Oregon Department of Human Resource Adult & Family Services Division
500 Summer St NE
Salem, OR 97301 503-945-5944
Fax: 503-378-2897
TTY: 503-945-6214
http://www.oregon.gov
dhr.info@state.or.us
John Kitzhaber, Governor
Carolyn Ross, Director
Ellen F. Rosenblum, Attorney General
This group combines programs from the former Adult & Family Services Division and the State Office for Services to Children and Families.

2261 Oregon Employment Department
875 Union St NE
Salem, OR 97311 877-517-5627
800-237-3710
Fax: 503-947-1472
http://www.workinginoregon.org
Laurie Warner, Director
Supports economic stability for Oregonians and communities during times of unemployment through the payment of unemployment benefits. Serves businesses by recruiting and referring the best qualified applicants to jobs, and provides resources to diverse job seekers in support of their employment needs.

2262 Oregon GED Administrator: Office of Community College Services
255 Capitol St NE
Salem, OR 97310-1300 503-378-8648
Fax: 503-378-3365
http://www.oregon.gov
sharlene.walker@state.or.us
John Kitzhaber, Governor
Carolyn Ross, Director
Ellen F. Rosenblum, Attorney General
Mission is to contribute leadership and resources to increase the skills, knowledge and career opportunities of Oregonians.

2263 Oregon State Library
250 Winter St NE
Salem, OR 97301-3950 503-378-4243
Fax: 503-585-8059
http://www.oregon.gov
leann.bromeland@state.or.us
John Kitzhaber, Governor
Carolyn Ross, Director
Ellen F. Rosenblum, Attorney General
Mission is to provide quality information services to Oregon state government, to provide reading materials to blind and print-disabled Oregonians, and to provide leadership, grants, and other assistance to improve local library service for all Oregonians.

Pennsylvania

2264 Delaware County Literacy Council
2217 Providence Avenue
Chester, PA 19013 610-876-4811
Fax: 610-876-5414
http://www.delcoliteracy.org
khyzer@delcoliteracy.org
Kate Hyzer, Executive Director
Susan Keller, Comm & Technology Specialist
Deb Charley, Adult Education Coordinator
Dedicated to providing free, individual and small group literacy instruction to non-and low-reading adults residing in Delaware County, through a county-wide network of trained volunteer tutors and instructors.

2265 Learning Disabilities Association of Pennsylvania
4751 Lindle Rd
Ste 114
Harrisburg, PA 17111 717-939-3731
888-775-3272
http://www.ldapa.org
ldapaininfo@aol.com
Deborah Rodes, President
An advocacy organization dedicated to helping children and adults with learning disabilities and other related neurological disorders.

2266 Literacy Council of Lancaster/Lebanon
24ÿSouth Queen Street
Lancaster, PA 17603 717-295-5523
Fax: 717-295-5342
http://www.adultlit.org
info@adultlit.org
Cheryl Hiester, Executive Director
Jenny Bair, Program Director
Bobbi Hurst, Student Coordinator, Lancaster
A private, non-profit education agency that provides high quality basic education to adults in Lancaster and Lebanon Counties. Promotes literacy and help adults reach their reading, writing, math and English communication goalsthrough personalized instruction.

2267 Pennsylvania Literacy Resource Center
12th Floor
333 Market St
Harrisburg, PA 17126 717-783-6788
800-992-2283
Fax: 717-783-5420
TTY: 717-783-8445
http://www.portal.state.pa.us
alubrecht@pa.gov
Alice Lubrecht, Director
As part of the State Library, the State Resource Center provides electronic and print resources.

2268 **York County Literacy Council**
800 E King St
York, PA 17403
717-845-8719
Fax: 717-699-5620
http://www.yorkliteracy.org
exec.dir@yorkliteracy.org
Bobbi Anne DeLeo, Executive Director
Rita Hewitt, Community Relations Manager
Lezlie Phillips, Adult Reading Coordinator
Dedicated to advancing adult literacy in York County. Client services are provided confidentially and free of charge to York County residents

Rhode Island

2269 **Literacy Volunteers of America: Rhode Island**
Ste 106
260 W Exchange St
Providence, RI 02903
401-861-0815
Fax: 401-861-0863
http://www.literacyvolunteers.org
lvaricindy@aol.com
Yvette Kenner, Executive Director
The mission of LVA-RI is to advance adult literacy in Rhode Island by: providing training and support services to local LVA-RI affiliates, volunteer tutors and adult literacy services; providing the state with information about adult literacy and with appropriate referral services; collaborating with other organizations to promote adult literacy in Rhode Island.

2270 **Literacy Volunteers of Kent County**
1672 Flat River Road
Route 117
Coventry, RI 02816
401-822-9100
Fax: 401-822-9133
http://www.coventrylibrary.org
AskReference@coventrylibrary.org
John Ball, Chair
Patricia Pare, VP
Colleen Duffy-Golec, Secretary
Receive intensive tutor training through a series of workshops that will prepare you to teach one-on-one or in small groups.

2271 **Literacy Volunteers of Providence County**
P.O.Box 72611
Providence, RI 02907-0611
401-351-0511
http://www.lvari.org
chris@lvari.org
Christine Hedenberg, Executive Director
Provides critical support services to local literacy volunteer affiliates, volunteer tutors and adult literacy students; collaborating with organizations to promote adult literacy in Rhode Island; partnering with companies and employers to improve workforce literacy skills; and acting as a state-wide resource for awareness and information about adult literacy, and for adult learner referrals to educational programs.

2272 **Literacy Volunteers of South County**
1935 Kingstown Rd
Wakefield, RI 02879
401-225-1068
http://www.211ri.org
info@uwri.org
David Henley, President
Volunteer-based literacy agent that provides services in Narragansett, North Kingstown and South Kingstown. Provides free, one-on-one tutoring to sdults who request Basic English Skills or English as a Second Language.

2273 **Literacy Volunteers of Washington County**
93 Tower Street
Units 25 & 26
Westerly, RI 02891
401-596-9411
http://www.literacywashingtoncounty.org
litwashcty@verizon.net
Ramon Garcia, President
Terence J. Malaghan, CPA, Treasurer
Ruth Tureckova, Executive Director
Assists adults interested in improving their literacy skills through free programs based on a participant's individual goals.

2274 **Literary Resources Rhode Island**
Brown University
PO Box 1974
Providence, RI 02912
401-863-1000
Fax: 401-863-3094
http://www.brown.edu
president@brown.edu
Christina H. Paxson, President
Elizabeth Huidekoper, EVP, Finance & Administration
David Savitz, VP, Research
Literacy Resources Rhode Island was established in 1997. Its goals include: expand existing professional capacity within the state's adult education community; increase educator and learner capacity to use and interact with online technology; and assist in improving delivery of services to adult learners, thereby strengthening adult education provision across the state.

2275 **Rhode Island Human Resource Investment Council**
1511 Pontiac Avenue
Building 72-2
Cranston, RI 02920
401-462-8860
Fax: 401-462-8865
http://www.rihric.com
rbrooks@dlt.ri.gov
Constance Howes, Chair
Rick Brooks, Executive Director
Amelia Anne Roberts, Office Manager

2276 **Rhode Island Vocational and Rehabilitation Agency**
40 Fountain Street
Providence, RI 02903
401-421-7005
Fax: 401-421-9259
TDD: 401-421-7016
http://www.ors.ri.gov
rcarroll@ors.state.ri.us
John Microulis, Administrator
Ronald Racine, Acting Associate Director
Roberta Greene Whittemore, Assistant Administrator of VR
Assists people with disabilities to become employed and to live independently in the community. In order to achieve this goal, we work in partnership with the State Rehabilitation Council, our customers, staff and community.

2277 **Rhode Island Workforce Literacy Collaborative**
260 W Exchange St
Ste 201
Providence, RI 02903-1047
401-861-0815
Fax: 401-861-0863
http://www.riwlc.org
Yvette Kenner, Executive Director
A group of non-profit agencies and other companies funded by the Human Resource Investment Council to provide workforce or worksite literacy services to adults in Rhode Island. These services are designed to upgrade the skills of those who are employed or seeking employment, in order to help Rhode Island achieve a high-performance workforce.

South Carolina

2278 **Greater Columbia Literacy Council Turning Pages Adult Literacy**
4840 Forest Dr
Ste 6-B, PMB 267
Columbia, SC 29206-2412
803-240-2441
Fax: 803-782-1210
http://www.literacycolumbia.org
literacycolumbia@earthlink.net
Deborah W Yoho, Executive Director

Mission is to enable adults, through customized learning programs, to improve English language and reading skills.

2279 **Greenville Literacy Association**
225 S Pleasantburg Dr
Ste C-10
Greenville, SC 29607-2533 864-467-3456
Fax: 864-467-3558
http://www.greenvilleliteracy.org
thomas@greenvilleliteracy.org
Jane Thomas, Executive Director
Leah Clark, ABE Training
Cheryl Bentley, Book Sale
To empower adults to participate more effectively in the community by providing quality instruction in reading, writing, math and speaking English

2280 **Greenwood Literacy Council**
1855 Calhoun Road
P.O. Box 248
Greenwood, SC 29648-0248 864-941-5400
Fax: 864-941-5427
http://www.gwd50.org
kjennings12@gwd50.org
Kathy Jennings, Director
Ken Cobb, Board Member
Claude Wright, Board Member
Provides ongoing, comprehensive adult literacy programs in Greenwood, for illiterate adults and their families.

2281 **Literacy Volunteers of the Lowcountry**
Pro Literacy America
1-B Kittie's Landing Way
P.O. Box 3725
Bluffton, SC 29910 843-815-6616
Fax: 843-686-6949
http://www.lowcountryliteracy.org
nwilliams@lowcountryliteracy.org
Jean Heyduck, Executive Director
Marie Lewis, Program Manager
Phil Lindstrom, Finance Director
To increase adult literacy in the greater Beaufort County area by providing leadership, creating awareness, and offering quality instructional services.

2282 **Oconee Adult Education**
414 South Pine Streetÿ
Walhalla, SC 29691ÿ 864-886-4429
Fax: 864-886-4430
http://www.oconee.k12.sc.us
mthorsland@oconee.k12.sc.us
Dr. Michael Thorsland, Superintendent
Maxine Pettit, Administrative Assistant
Deb Wickliffe, Communications Specialist
To assist adults in becoming literate, to assist adults in the completion of a secondary school education, and to assist adults in improving their knowledge and skills relating to employment and parenting.

2283 **South Carolina Adult Literacy Educators**
297 Pascallas Street
Blackville, SC 29817 803-284-5605
Fax: 803-284-4417
http://www.barnwell19.k12.sc.us
leah.bias@barnwell19.k12.sc.us
Teresa L. Pope, Superintendent
Rebecca Grubbs, Director, Finance
Leah Bias, Director, Special Education

2284 **South Carolina Department of Education**
1429 Senate Street
Columbia, SC 29201 803-734-8500
Fax: 803-734-4426
http://www.ed.sc.gov
sc.supfed@ed.sc.gov
Mick Zais, State Superintendent
Scott English, Chief Operating Officer
Mr. Don Cantrell, Chief Information Officer
Provides people of all ages and backgrounds who are blind, visually impaired or reading disabled with free books, magazines, and special publications in Braille, Large Print and Audio formats.

2285 **South Carolina Literacy Resource Center**
1722 Main Street
Suite 104
Columbia, SC 29201 803-929-2563
800-277-7323
Fax: 803-929-2571
http://www2.ed.gov/pubs/TeachersGuide/slrc.html
SCLRC@aol.com
Peggy May, Director
The mission of the South Carolina Resource Center is to provide leadership in literacy to South Carolina's adults and their families, in conjunction with state and local public and private nonprofit efforts. The Center serves as a site for training for adult literacy providers, as a reciprocal link with the National Institute for Literacy for the purpose of sharing information to service providers, and as a clearinghouse for state-of-the-art literacy materials and technology.

2286 **Trident Literacy Association**
5416-B Rivers Avenue
North Charleston, SC 29406 843-747-2223
Fax: 843-744-2970
http://www.tridentlit.org
echepenik@tridentlit.org
Eileen Chepenik, Executive Director
Stella Necker, Program Director
Judianne Schmenk, Development Director
To increase literacy in Charleston, Berkeley, and Dorchester counties by offering instruction, using a self-paced, individualized curriculum in reading, writing, mathematics, English as a second language, GED preparation, and basic computer use.

South Dakota

2287 **Adult Education and Literacy Program**
South Dakota Department of Labor
Kneip Bldg
700 Governors Dr
Pierre, SD 57501 605-773-3101
Fax: 605-773-6185
http://www.state.sd.us
marcia.hess@state.sd.us
Marcia Hess, State Administrator
Adult Education & Literacy instruction is designed to teach persons 16 years of age or older to read and write English and to substantially raise their educational level. The purpose of the program is to expand the educational opportunities for adults and to establish programs that will enable all adults to acquire basic skills necessary to function in society and allow them to continue their education to at least the level of completion of secondary school.

2288 **South Dakota Literacy Council**
816 Samara Ave
Volga, SD 57071 605-627-5138
Fax: 605-627-5138
http://www.readsd.org
jberglund@blackhills.com
John Berglund, President
Alma McClanahan, VP
Betty VanderZee, Treasurer
Goal is to help people receive educational help in a confidential setting.

2289 **South Dakota Literacy Resource Center**
700 Governors Drive
Pierre, SD 57501 605-773-3101
800-423-6665
Fax: 605-773-6184
http://wdcrobcolp01.ed.gov/programs/EROD
marcia.hess@state.sd.us

Marcia Hess, State Administrator
The mission of the SD Literary Resource Center is to establish a state wide on-line computer catalog of all existing literacy materials within South Dakota and a South Dakota Literacy Resource Center home page with links to other literacy sites within South Dakota, regionally and nationally.

Tennessee

2290 **Adult Education Foundation of Blount County**
1500 Jett Rd
Maryville, TN 37804-3359
865-982-8998
Fax: 865-983-8848
http://www.blountk12.org/adult_ed/index.htm
blountliteracy@gmail.com
Carol Ergenbright, Coordinator
Serving as an advocate for adult literacy by partnering with Adult Education programs and staff; promoting community involvement and providing assistance with funding.

2291 **Center for Literary Studies**
University of Tennessee
600 Henley St
Suite 312
Knoxville, TN 37996
865-974-4109
Fax: 865-974-3857
http://www.cls.utk.edu
Geri Mulligan, Director
Aaron Kohring, Interim Director
Gail Cope, Program Coordinator
To support and advance literacy education across the lifespan. Works with providers of literacy edcuation to strengthen their capacity to help individuals build knowledge and improve skills needed to be life-long learners and active members of families, communities, and workplaces.

2292 **Claiborne County Adult Reading Experience**
Claiborne County Schools
1403 Tazewell Road
P.O. Box 179
Tazewell, TN 37879
423-626-3543
Fax: 423-626-5945
http://www.claibornecountyschools.com
swilliams3@k12tn.net
Michelle Huddleston, Chairman
Tim Duncan, Vice Chairman
Connie Holdway, Director of Schools

2293 **Collierville Literacy Council**
167 Washington Street
Collierville, TN 38017
901-854-0288
http://www.colliervilleliteracy.org
colliervilleliteracy@earthlink.net
John Barrios, President
Annette Key, Immediate Past President
Wanda Chism, Secretary
A non-profit organization dedicated to providing opportunities for adults to attain educational goals that enhance individual growth and benefit families, the work place and the community.

2294 **Learning Center for Adults and Families**
833 N Ocoee St
Cleveland, TN 37311-2254
423-478-1117
Fax: 423-478-1153
http://www.learningcenter.ws
clewis@learningcenter.ws
Candace Lewis, Executive Director

2295 **Literacy Council of Kingsport**
326 Commerce Street
Kingsport, TN 37660
423-392-4643
http://www.literacycouncilofkingsport.org
admin@literacycouncilofkingsport.org
Nada J. Weekley, Executive Director
Pat Mattingly, Program/Volunteer Coordinator
A non-profit organization dedicated to serving citizens in Kingsport and Sullivan County. Offers free, one-on-one tutoring for adults and qualified children who want to learn to read or to improve their reading skills.

2296 **Literacy Council of Sumner County**
260 W Main Street
City Square Shopping Center
Hendersonville, TN 37075
615-822-8112
Fax: 615-822-3665
http://www.literacysumner.org
info@literacysumner.org
Margie Anderson, Director
To provide resources, counseling, and tutoring to children, youth, and adults to enhance their skills in all academic areas.

2297 **Literacy Mid-South**
2158 Union Ave., Suite 515
P.O. Box 111229
Memphis, TN 38104
901-327-6000
Fax: 901-458-4969
http://www.literacymidsouth.org
kdean@literacymidsouth.org
Kevin Dean, Executive Director
Jeff Rhodin, Director, Collaborative Action
Heather Nordtvedt, Director of Development

2298 **Nashville Adult Literacy Council**
Cohn Adult Learning Center
4805 Park Ave
Suite 305
Nashville, TN 37209
615-298-8060
Fax: 615-298-8444
http://www.nashvilleliteracy.org
info@nashvilleliteracy.org
Meg Nugent, Director
Jill Mora, Marketing Director
Patty Swartzbaugh, Program Manager
Teaches reading to U.S.-born adults and English skills to adult immigrants.

2299 **Read To Succeed**
200 East Main Street
PO Box 12161
Murfreesboro, TN 37130
615-738-7323
http://www.readtosucceed.org
info@readtosucceed.org
Steve Daniel, President
Brian Coleman, VP
Lisa Mitchell, Executive Director
The community literacy collaborative in Rutherford County, will promote reading, with an emphasis on family literacy. This non-profit initiative supports literacy programs and fosters awareness of the importance of reading.

2300 **Tennessee Department of Education**
710 James Robertson Parkway
Andrew Johnson Tower, 6th Floor
Nashville, TN 37243-0382
615-741-2731
800-531-1515
http://www.state.tn.us
education.comments@tn.gov
Timothy K Webb, Commissioner
Mission is to take Tennessee to the top in education. Guides administration of the state's K-12 public schools.

2301 **Tennessee School-to-Work Office**
14th Floor, Citizens Plaza State Of
400 Deaderick Street
Nashville, TN 37243
615-313-4981
http://www.state.tn.us
maryjane.ware@tn.gov
Bill Haslam, Governor

Texas

2302 **Commerce Library Literacy Program**
1210 Park Street
Commerce, TX 75429
903-886-6858
Fax: 903-886-7239
http://www.commercepubliclibrary.org
commerce@koyote.com
Pricilla Donovan, Director

2303 **Greater Orange Area Literacy Services**
PO Box 221
520 W Decatur Ave
Orange, TX 77631
409-886-4311
Fax: 409-886-0149
goalsliteracy@sbcglobal.net
Sharon LeBlanc, Executive Director
Adult literacy program

2304 **Irving Public Library Literacy Program**
825 W Irving Blvd
PO Box 152288
Irving, TX 75060
972-721-2411
Fax: 972-721-3733
http://cityofirving.org
Customer-Service@cityofirving.org
Tracy Bearden, Manager
Charles Anderson, City Attorney
Promotes literacy among people of all ages.

2305 **Literacy Austin**
2222 Rosewood Ave
Austin, TX 78702
512-478-7323
Fax: 512-479-7323
TDD: 512-478-7323
http://www.literacyaustin.org
info@literacyaustin.org
Gail Harmon, Program Director
Melinda Mitchiner, Program Services Coordinator
Mission is to provide instruction for basic literacy and English as a Second Language (ESL) to adults, age 17 and older, who read below the fifth-grade leve. Vision is to improve the quality of an adult's life through improved literacy skills.

2306 **Literacy Center of Marshall: Harrison County**
700 W. Houston Street
P.O. Box 148
Marshall, TX 75670
903-935-0962
http://www.marshallliteracy.org
kdeluca23@gmail.com
Karla DeLuca, Executive Director

2307 **Literacy Volunteers of America: Bastrop**
1201 Church St
Bastrop, TX 78602-2909
512-321-6686
http://www.main.org/lva-bastrop/
suemunster@aol.com
Sue Steinbring, Director
Provides literacy training and pre-GED for students, English as a Second Language, tutoring and tutor training.

2308 **Literacy Volunteers of America: Bay City Matagorda County**
PO Box 1596
Bay City, TX 77404-1596
979-244-9544
Fax: 979-244-9566
http://www.literacymc.org
lva_mc@yahoo.com
Linda Brown, Director
Sandy Thomas, Program Coordinator
Promotes literacy for people of all ages.

2309 **Literacy Volunteers of America: Laredo**
P 10 Fort McIntosh
LCC Main Campus
Laredo, TX 78040
956-724-5207
Fax: 956-725-4253
http://www.lvalaredo.org
lvlaredo@grandecom.net
Doroteo Sandoval, Executive Director
Promotes literacy for people of all ages.

2310 **Literacy Volunteers of America: Montgomery County**
412 W. Phillips, Suite 125
P.O. Box 2704
Conroe, TX 77305-2704
936-494-0635
888-878-9400
http://lvamc.org
literacymc@yahoo.com
Linda Ricketts, Director
Laura Davis, Program Manager
Ranak Amin, Office Volunteer
As part of the national literacy organization, combats illiteracy in Montgomery County through volunteer tutoring.

2311 **Literacy Volunteers of America: Port Arthur Literacy Support**
4615 9th Avenue
Port Arthur, TX 77642-5818
409-985-8838
Fax: 409-985-5969
http://www.pap.lib.tx.us
jmartine@paplibrary.org
Jose Martinez, Director
Debra Lawrence, Administrative Assistant
LaTrice Gallow, Senior Library Clerk
A library based umbrella group which works with three primary programs: ono-on-one tutoring for those who cannot read or read at a very low level; GED Computer Lab assistance for adults who are striving to get their General Equivalency Diploma - in cooperation with Port Arthur Independent School District; and English-as-a-Second Language (ESL) in cooperation with the Port Arthur Independent School District.

2312 **Literacy Volunteers of America: Wimberley Area**
14100 Ranch Road 12
P.O. Box 12
Wimberley, TX 78676
512-847-2201
Fax: 701-254-4313
http://www.wimberley.org
trailsend@anvilcom.com
Linda Mueller, Director
Nonprofit, volunteer organization which exists to improve the reading, writing, speaking, cultural and life skills of adults reading at or below the sixth grade level and/or those for whom English is not their native language. Provides GED instruction. All services are free.

2313 **Texas Families and Literacy**
1006 C, Junction Hwy.
Kerrville, TX 78028
830-896-8787
Fax: 830-896-3639
http://www.familiesandliteracy.org
famandlit1@hctc.net
Mike Hunter, Executive Director
Annette Kurtz, Operations Coordinator
Anita Rios, Administrative Assistant

2314 **Texas Family Literacy Center**
601 University Drive
College of Education, EDU Room 2112ÿ
San Marcos, TX 78666
512-245-9600
Fax: 512-245-8151
http://www.tei.education.txstate.edu/famlit
yr01@txstate.edu
Ysabel Ramirez, Grant Directror
Gloria Rodriguez, Grant Secretary
Dr. Emily Miller Payne, Director

Mission is to strengthen family literacy programs and enhance the knowledge skills, instructional practices and resources available to family literacy educators statewide.

2315 **Victoria Adult Literacy**
802 E. Crestwood Drive
Victoria, TX 77901
361-582-4273
Fax: 361-582-4348
http://www.victorialiteracycouncil.org
valcsm@yahoo.com
Stacey Milberger, Executive Director
Eden Casal, VALC Program Coordinator
Dani Clowers, Program Assistant

2316 **Weslaco Public Library**
525 S Kansas Ave
Weslaco, TX 78596
956-968-4533
Fax: 956-968-8922
http://www.weslaco.lib.tx.us
webmaster@weslaco.lib.tx.us
Michael Fisher, Executive Director

Utah

2317 **Bridgerland Literacy**
1301 N 600 W
Logan, UT 84321
435-750-3262
http://www.bridgerlandliteracy.org
bridgerland.literacy@gmail.com
Alex Stoddard, Director
Linda Fretwell, Student Coordinator
Melissa Allen, Outreach Coordinator

2318 **Project Read**
550 N University Avenue
Suite 215
Provo, UT 84601
801-852-6654
Fax: 801-852-7663
http://www.project-read.com
projectreadutah@gmail.com
Shauna K Brown, Director
Chelsea Hansen, Program Coordinator
Seeks to prevent and alleviate adult illiteracy in Utah County. Provides one-on-one tutoring services to help improve reading and writing skills sufficiently to meet personal goals, function well in society, and become more productive citizens.

2319 **Utah Literacy Action Center**
3595 South Main Street
Salt Lake City, UT 84115-4434
801-265-9081
Fax: 801-265-9643
http://www.literacyactioncenter.org
lac@literacyactioncenter.org
Margaret Griffin, Treasurer
Deborah Young, Ed.D., Executive Director
Charles Curtin, Secretary
Transforms English-speaking adults, who enter the program with limited reading, writing, or math skills, into skilled, passionate, habitual, critical readers, writers, and mathematicians.

Vermont

2320 **ABE Career and Lifelong Learning: Vermont Department of Education**
120 State St
Montpelier, VT 05620-2501
802-828-3135
800-881-1561
Fax: 802-828-3146
http://women.vermont.gov/resource-directory/edu
srobinson@doe.state.vt.us
Cary Brown, Executive Director
Lilly Talbert, Coordinator
Claire Greene, Executive Staff Assistant
Promotes quality education.

2321 **Central Vermont Adult Basic Education**
46 Washington Street
Suite 100
Barre, VT 05641
802-476-4588
Fax: 802-476-5860
http://www.cvabe.org
info@cvabe.org
Sydney Lea, President, Treasurer
Jon Bourgo, VP
Carol Shults-Perkins, Executive Director
Provides free adult education and literacy instruction for adults, out of school youth, and immigrants and refugees in the belief that a person who is literate has the essential key for self understanding and for full and active membership in the world.

2322 **Tutorial Center**
208 Pleasant Street
Bennington, VT 05201
802-447-0111
Fax: 802-447-7607
http://tutoringvermont.org
Jack Glade, Executive Director
Provides tutoring to improve success for 200 children; prevents 20 teenagers at risk of dropping out from doing so; helps 80 high school dropouts to earn a high school diploma or GED; builds literacy skills of 400 adults; helps 20 adults transition into college or post-secondary career paths; and transforms 50 computer-illiterate adults into competent computer users.

2323 **Vermont Assistive Technology Project: Dept of Aging and Disabilities**
103 South Main Street
Weeks Building
Waterbury, VT 05671-1601
802-241-2620
800-750-6355
Fax: 802-241-2174
TTY: 802-241-1464
http://dail.vermont.gov
julie.tucker@ahs.state.vt.us
Julie L Tucker, Program Director
Provides information and referrals, training for service providers and others, equipment and software demonstrations, tryouts, and technical assistance.

2324 **Vermont Division of Vocational Rehabilitation**
VocRehab Of Vermont
103 South Main Street
Weeks 1A
Waterbury, VT 05671-2303
866-879-6757
TTY: 802-241-1455
http://www.vocrehab.vermont.gov
jana.sherman@ahs.state.vt.us
Diane Dalmasse, Director of VocRehab Division
VocRehab's mission is to assist Vermonters with disabilities, find and maintain meaningful employment in their communities. VocRehab Vermont works in close partnership with the Vermont Association of Business, Industry and Rehabilitation. Contact local VocRehab office for information about services.

2325 **Vermont Literacy Resource Center: Dept of Education**
120 State St
Montpelier, VT 05602-2703
802-828-5148
Fax: 802-828-0573
http://www.state.vt.us
wross@doe.state.vt.us
Wendy Ross, Director
The Vermont Literacy Resource Center links Vermont to national, regional, and state literacy organizations, provides staff development and serves as a clearinghouse for the literacy community. The Vermont Literacy Resource Center is located at the Vermont Department of Education.

Virginia

2326 Adult Learning Center
4160 Virginia Beach Blvd
Virginia Beach, VA 23452 757-648-6050
Fax: 757-306-0999
http://www.adultlearning.vbschools.com
ppalombo@vbschools.com
Paul Palombo, Director
Heather Lamb, Coordinator
Joseph Panchik, Coordinator
To respond to the needs of the adult population by offering a comprehensive educational program to the community.

2327 Charlotte County Literacy Program
395 Thomas Jefferson Hwy, Suite B
P.O. Box 286
Charlotte Court House, VA 23923 434-542-5782
http://www.charlotte-learning.org
charlit@pure.net
Tonya Pulliam, Director
Offers basic and family literacy programs, ESL and computer, parenting and work skills.

2328 Citizens for Adult Literacy & Learning
PO Box 123
Monroe, VA 24574 434-929-2630
http://www.callamherst.org
marcia.swain@callamherst.org
Marcia Swain, Program Coordinator
Aim is to help adults improve their quality of life by mastering basic reading, writing and math skills.

2329 Eastern Shore Literacy Council
29300 Lankford Highway
White Building
Melfa, VA 23410 757-789-1761
Fax: 757-442-6517
http://www.shoreliteracy.org
esliteracy@gmail.com
Laura Chuquin-Naylor, Executive Director
Janet Booth, Director
Renee Beall, Program Coordinator
Providing literacy tutoring without charge to adult residents of the Eastern Shore so they may acquire the skills needed to improve their particiaption in society and enrich their lives.

2330 Highlands Educational Literacy Program
13168 Meadowview Square
Meadowview, VA 276-944-5144
Fax: 276-676-0677
http://www.helpliteracyofwc.org
helplit2@gmail.com
Christy Hicks, Chairperson
Beth Hilton, Executive Director
Tina Mitchell, Volunteer Coordinator
To provide basic literacy instruction for adults in Washington County, changing lives one word at a time.

2331 Literacy Council of Northern Virginia
2855 Annandale Road
Falls Church, VA 22042 703-237-0866
Fax: 703-237-2863
http://www.lcnv.org
info@lcnv.org
Patricia Donnelly, Executive Director
Carole Vinograd Bausell, Director of Tutoring Programs
Nathan Caruso, Program Assistant
To teach adults the basic skills of reading, writing, speaking and understanding English in order to empower them to participate more fully and confidently in their communities.

2332 Literacy Volunteers of America: Nelson County
PO Box 422
Lovingston, VA 22949 434-996-0485
http://www.nelsoncountyliteracy.org
nanamump@aol.com
Charles Strauss, Director

2333 Literacy Volunteers of America: New River Valley
195 West Main Street
Christiansburg, VA 24073 540-382-7262
Fax: 540-382-7262
http://www.lvnrv.org
lvnrv@verizon.net
Dr. Toni Cox, President
C. Barry Anderson, President Elect
Janet Kester, Program Coordinator
The empowerment of every adult in the New River Valley through the provision of opportunities to achieve independence through literacy.

2334 Literacy Volunteers of America: Prince William
4326 Dale Blvd
Suite 6
Woodbridge, VA 22193 703-670-5702
Fax: 703-583-0703
http://www.lvapw.org
lvapw@aol.com
Ken Ikeda, President
Vicki Gross, Executive Director
Deborah Abbott, Program Director
Mission is to teach adults to read. Takes volunteers from the community, train them to be tutors and then match them with adults with low literacy skills. Provides the professional training, materials, and support that enable the volunteers to be effective tutors.

2335 Literacy Volunteers of America: Shenandoah County
PO Box 303
Woodstock, VA 22664 540-459-2446
http://www.lv-sc.org
inquiries@lv-sc.org
Paula Gould, Director

2336 Literacy Volunteers of Charlottesville/Albemarle
233 4th Street NW
PO Box 1156
Charlottesville, VA 22903 434-977-3838
http://literacyforall.org
info@literacyforall.org
Jean Kollar, President
Mary Jane King, VP
Ellen Moore Osborne, Executive Director
Provides one-on-one, confidential tutoring in basic literacy and English as a second language to adults living ot working in Charlottesville and Albemarle County.

2337 Literacy Volunteers of Roanoke Valley
706 S Jefferson St
Roanoke, VA 24016-5104 540-265-9339
877-582-7323
Fax: 540-265-4814
http://www.lvarv.org
info@lvarv.org
Annette Loschert, Executive Director
To teach English literacy skills to adults and to raise literacy awareness throughout the Roanoke Valley.

2338 Literacy Volunteers: Campbell County Public Library
PO Box 310
Rustburg, VA 24588-0310 434-332-9561
Fax: 434-332-9697
http://www.campbellcountylibraries.org
lpwheeler@co.campbell.va.us
Nan Carmack, Program Manager
Provides free, confidential instruction for adults who live or work in Campbell COunty, VA. Adult Basic Education and English for Speakers of other languages.

2339 **Loudoun Literacy Council**
17 Royal Street SW
Leesburg, VA 20175
703-777-2205
Fax: 703-777-7260
http://www.loudounliteracy.org
info@loudounliteracy.org
Sean Jordan, President
David Bruce, VP
Leslie Mazeska, Executive Director
A community-based, nonprofit, educational organization dedicated to improving literacy throughout Loudoun County. Recruit and train volunteers to teach adults, both native-speakers and speakers of other languages, to read, speak, write and understand English. Also provides early literacy enrichment for at-risk preschool children and children who reside in local homeless shelters, while supporting their parents as their child's first teacher.

2340 **READ Center Reading & Education for Adult Development**
2000 Bremo Road
Suite 102
Richmond, VA 23226
804-288-9930
Fax: 804-288-9915
http://www.readcenter.org
frontdesk@readcenter.org
Helps low-level reading adults develop basic reading and communication skills through one-to-one tutoring so they can fulfill their goals and their roles as citizens, workers and family members.

2341 **Skyline Literacy Coalition**
975 S. High Street
Harrisonburg, VA 22801
540-433-0505
Fax: 540-433-0955
http://skylineliteracy.org
skylineliteracy@gmail.com
Laura Zarrugh, President
Charlette McQuilkin, VP
Elizabeth Girvan, Executive Director
A nonprofit organization dedicated to promoting learning and literacy throughout the Shenandoah Valley.

2342 **Virginia Adult Learning Resource Center**
3600 W Broad St, Suite 112
PO Box 842037
Richmond, VA 23230-4930
804-828-6521
800-237-0178
Fax: 804-828-7539
http://www.valrc.org
vdesk@vcu.edu
Barbara Gibson, Manager
Katie Bratisax, Technology & Support Specialist
Hillary Major, Communications Specialist
To equip the field of adult education and literacy with essential skills and resources by delivering innovative and effective training, publications, curriculum design, and prgram development.

2343 **Virginia Council of Administrators of Special Education**
1110 N Glebe Rd
Ste 300
Arlington, VA 22201-5704
703-264-9454
800-224-6830
Fax: 703-264-9494
http://www.vcase.org
marylwall@aol.com
Jim Gallagher, President
Dr. Jessica McClung, Secretary
Leorie K Mallory, Treasurer
A professional organization that promotes professional leadership through the provision of collegial support and current information on recommended instructional practices as well as local, state and national trends in Special Education for professionals who serve students with disabilities in order to improve the quality and delivery of special education services in Virginia's public schools.

2344 **Virginia Literacy Foundation**
413 Stuart Circle
Executive Suite 303
Richmond, VA 23220
804-237-8909
Fax: 804-237-8901
http://www.virginialiteracy.org
vlilv@earthlink.net
Jeannie P Baliles, Founder/Chairperson
Mark E Emblidge, Ph.D., Founding Director
Jane Bassett Spilman, Vice Chairperson
Provides funding and technical support to private, volunteer literacy organizations throughout Virginia via challenge grants, training and direct consulting.

Washington

2345 **Division of Vocational Rehabilitation**
PO Box 45340
Olympia, WA 98504-5340
360-725-3636
800-367-5621
Fax: 360-407-8007
http://www.dshs.wa.gov
Serves people with disabilities who want to work but face a substantial barrier to finding or keeping a job. Provides individualized employment services and counseling to people with disabilites and also provides technical assistance and training to employers about the employment of people with disabilities.

2346 **Literacy Council of Kitsap**
616 5th Street
Bremerton, WA 98337-1416
360-373-1539
Fax: 360-373-6859
http://www.kitsapliteracy.org
info@kitsapliteracy.org
Carol Rainey, Chair
Terry Schroeder, Treasurer
Winnie Flores-Logan, Board Member
Dedicated to Adult Basic Education (ABE) and GED testing preparation, along with English as a Second Language. Promote and provide literacy services to the residents of Kitsap County.

2347 **Literacy Council of Seattle**
8500 14th Ave NW
Crown Hill UMC
Seattle, WA 98117
206-233-9720
http://www.literacyseattle.org
info@literacyseattle.org
Kristen Holway, President
Jennifer Collins-Friedrichs, Executive Director
Valerie Margulis, Treasurer
Volunteers teach adults the English skills they need to be successful in their jobs, families, and the community.

2348 **Literacy Source: Community Learning Center**
720 N 35th St
Suite # 103
Seattle, WA 98103
206-782-2050
Fax: 206-781-2583
http://www.literacy-source.org
info@literacy-source.org
Jack Kuester, President
Theresa Verwey, Vice President
Ann Dalton, Secretary
Builds a literate community and promote self-sufficiency by providing learner-centered instruction to adults in English literacy and basic life skills.

2349 **Sound Learning of Mason & Thurston County**
133 W Railroad Ave
P.O. Box 2529
Shelton, WA 98584
360-426-9733
Fax: 360-426-9789
http://www.masoncountyliteracy.org

Pamela Farr, Chair
Toby Kevin, Vice Chair
Ross Wiggins, Secretary
Provides free instruction to adults to improve reading, writing and math skills, study for a GED, or learn English as a second language.

2350 **St. James ESL Program**
St. James Cathedral
804 Ninth Avenue
Seattle, WA 98104-1265 206-622-3559
Fax: 206-622-5303
http://www.stjames-cathedral.org
esl@stjames-catherdral.org
Chris Koehler, Director
Helping adult refugees and immigrants learn English and become U.S. citizens.

2351 **Whatcom Literacy Council**
3028 Lindbergh Ave
Building A
Bellingham, WA 98225 360-752-8678
Fax: 360-752-6770
http://www.whatcomliteracy.org
info@whatcomliteracy.org
Valerie Lagen, President
Mike Henniger, Vice President
Joyce Eschliman, Treasurer
Helping adults in Whatcom County improve their literacy skills or learn to use English as a second language. Through customized, individual tutoring, students learn critical skills needed to become self-sufficient.

West Virginia

2352 **Division of Technical & Adult Education Services: West Virginia**
1900 Kanawha Boulevard East
Charleston, WV 25305 304-558-2000
Fax: 304-342-7025
http://careertech.k12.wv.us
gparsons@access.k12.wv.us
Kathy D'Antoni EdD, Asst State Superintendent
Gigi Parsons, Division Secretary
Better prepare students for the world of work and higher education through education programs and training offered at the career and technical education sites throughout the state.

2353 **W Virginia Regional Education Services**
501 22nd St
Dunbar, WV 25064-1711 304-766-7655
800-642-2670
Fax: 304-766-2824
Chuck Nichols, Executive Director
Offers services for literacy and adult basic education including literacy hotline, networks newsletter, resources for English as a second language, beginning literacy, learning disabilities and other special learning needs.

2354 **West Virginia Department of Education**
1900 Kanawha Blvd E
Bldg 6, Rm 351
Charleston, WV 25305-0330 304-558-3660
800-642-2670
Fax: 304-558-0198
http://wvde.state.wv.us

Wisconsin

2355 **ADVOCAP Literacy Services**
W911 State Highway 44
Markesan, WI 53946 920-398-3907
800-631-6617
Fax: 920-398-2103
http://www.advocap.org
mikeb@advocap.org
Michael Bonertz, Executive Director
Tony Beregszazi, Deputy Director
Tanya Marcoe, Finance Director

2356 **Fox Valley Literacy Council**
130 E. Franklin St.
Appleton, WI 54911 920-991-9840
Fax: 920-991-1012
http://www.fvlc.net
foxvalleylit@tds.net
James Frascona, President
Craig Gagnon, Vice Chair
Cindy Darling, Secretary
Provides English literacy education to adults with the help of trained volunteers. The Fox Valley Literacy Council shares the power of learning to transform lives and enrich the community.

2357 **Jefferson County Literacy Council**
112 S Main St
Jefferson, WI 53549 920-675-0500
Fax: 920-675-0510
http://www.jclc.us
jottow@jclc.us
Lynn Forseth, Executive Director
Karyn Cable, Operations Manager
Jessica Hellenbrand, Educational Coordinator
Committed to building communities that are strong in literacy, language and cultural understandings through information and resource sharing, referral, assessment and instructional services.

2358 **Literacy Council of Greater Waukesha**
217 Wisconsin Ave
Ste 16
Waukesha, WI 53186 262-547-7323
http://www.waukeshaliteracy.org
drunning@waukeshaliteracy.org
Debra Running, Executive Director
Cathy Kozlowicz, Program Coordinator
Provides, confidential, one-on-one tutoring and mentoring services to individuals who need help with reading, writing, spelling, math and English as a second language.

2359 **Literacy Network**
701 Dane St.
Madison, WI 53713 608-244-3911
http://www.litnetwork.org/
info@litnetwork.org
Donna Hurd, President
Jeff Burkhart, Executive Director
Teachers reading, writing, communication, and computer skills to Dane County adults so they can achieve financial security, well-being, and deeper engagement with their families and the community.

2360 **Literacy Services of Wisconsin**
2724 W Wells St
Milwaukee, WI 53208-3597 414-344-5878
Fax: 414-344-1061
http://www.literacyservices.org
india@literacyservices.org
David Hanson, President
Ginger Duivon, Executive Director
Mary Tobin, Treasurer

Provides literacy education motivated adults through the efforts of dedicated volunteers, the support of th ecommunity and the use of specialized curriculum to meet the individual and community needs.

2361 **Literacy Volunteers of America: Chippewa Valley**
770 Scheidler Rd
Chippewa Falls, WI 54729
715-738-3857
Fax: 715-967-2445
http://www.lvcv.org
Paul Kulig, President
Laurie Klinkhammer, Vice President
Greta Heike, Treasurer
A community-based literacy program that trains and supports volunteers to educate adults and their families, helping them acquire the skills necessary to achieve economic self-sufficiency and function effectively in their roles as citizens, workers, and family members.

2362 **Literacy Volunteers of America: Eau Claire**
800 Wisconsin St #70
Bldg D02, Ste 301
Eau Claire, WI 54703
715-834-0222
Fax: 715-834-2546
http://www.lvcv.org
Paul Kulig, President
Laurie Klinkhammer, Vice President
Greta Heike, Treasurer
A community-based literacy program that trains and supports volunteers to educate adults and their families, helping them acquire the skills necessary to achieve economic self-sufficiency and function effectively in their roles as citizens, workers, and family members.

2363 **Literacy Volunteers of America: Marquette County**
PO Box 671
Montello, WI 53949-0671
608-297-8900
Fax: 608-297-2673
http://www.mcreads.org
literacyvmc@yahoo.com
Vicki Huffman, President
Luann Zieman, Vice President
Mary Faltz, Secretary
Promotes literacy for people of all ages.

2364 **Marathon County Literacy Council**
300 1st St
Wausau, WI 54403
715-261-7292
Fax: 715-261-7232
http://wvls.lib.wi.us
info@mcliteracy.us
Tom Bobrofsky, President
Douglas Lay, Vice President
Michael Otten, Treasurer
A nonprofit organization dedicated to improving literacy throughout Marathon County. Offers tutoring services for all Marathon County adults in need of assistance.

2365 **Milwaukee Achiever Literacy Services**
5566 N 69th St
Milwaukee, WI 53218
414-463-7389
Fax: 414-463-9484
http://milwaukeeachiever.org
ssterling@milwaukeeachiever.org
Tracy Loken Webber, President
Dan Berton, Chair
Brenda Thompson, Secretary
Provides education, life skills training and workforce development instruction for adult learners in an atmosphere of mutual acceptance and respect.

2366 **Racine Literacy Council**
734 Lake Ave
Racine, WI 53403
262-632-9495
Fax: 262-632-9502
http://www.racineliteracy.com
kgregor@racineliteracy.com
Don Cress, President
Sandy Brosseau, Secretary
Mary Biesack, Treasurer
A volunteer-based organization whose mission is to provide adult literacy programs in Racine County and to bring awareness to the community about the importance and impact of literacy.

2367 **Walworth County Literacy Council**
1000 E Centralia St
Elkhorn, WI 53121
262-957-0142; *Fax:* 262-741-5275
http://www.walworthcoliteracy.com
wclc@walworthcoliteracy.com
Abby Baker, Coordinator
Provides student-centered instruction in basic literacy skills and English as a second language. Promotes awareness of literacy issues and seeks support from the community to develop literacy programs.

2368 **Winnebago County Literacy Council**
106 Washington Ave
Oshkosh, WI 54901-4985
920-236-5185
Fax: 920-236-5227
http://www.winlit.org
traska@winlit.org
Natalie Johnson, President
Donna Altepeter, Vice President
Becky Srubas, Secretary
To increase literacy skills of adults and families so they can make informed decisions in order to function effectively in society.

2369 **Wisconsin Literacy Resource Center**
211 S Paterson St
Ste 310
Madison, WI 53703
608-257-1655; *Fax:* 608-661-0208
http://www.wisconsinliteracy.orgs
info@wisconsinliteracy.org
Dave Endres, President
Greg Simmons, Vice President
Lorie Zantow, Treasurer
A statewide agency that was formed as a coalition of adult, family and workplace literacy providers for the purpose of supporting one another through resource development, information and referrals, training and advocacy.

Wyoming

2370 **Pomona Public Library Literacy Services**
2300 Capitol Ave
Hathaway Building, 2nd Floor
Cheyenne, WY 82002-2060
307-777-7690
Fax: 307-777-6234
TTY: 307-777-7744
http://www.k12.wy.us
Cindy Hill, State Superintendant
Deb Lindsey, Assesment
Tiffany Dobler, Special Programs
The Pomona Literacy Service provides free adult literacy services to the City of Pomona. Volunteers provide tutorial programs to adults (16 years and older) who do not have basic literacy skills or whose literacy skills are so limited that they are not able to function independently in daily life or acquire employment or higher education.

2371 **Teton Literacy Program**
1715 High School Rd, Ste 260
PO Box 465
Jackson, WY 83001
307-733-9242; *Fax:* 307-733-9086
http://www.tetonliteracy.org
info@tetonliteracy.org
Bill Maloney, President
Jim Thorburn, Vice President
Petria Fossel, Secretary
Serves Teton County with educational resources to better reading, writing, and language skills of the diverse community.

Adults

2372 **A Mind At A Time**
Simon & Schuster
1230 Avenue of the Americas
New York, NY 10020-1513 212-698-7000
http://www.simonandschuster.biz
shop.feedback@simonsays.com
Mel Levine, Author
Written by Melvin Levine, and published in 2003. It shows parents and others how to identify the individual learning patterns, explaining how to strenghten a child's abilities and either bypasss or overcome the child's weakness, producing positive results instead of reapeated frustration and failure. *$15.00*
352 pages
ISBN 0-743202-23-6

2373 **A Miracle to Believe In**
Option Indigo Press
2080 S Undermountain Rd
Sheffield, MA 01257-9643 413-229-8727
800-714-2779
Fax: 413-229-8727
http://www.optionindigo.com
indigo@bcn.net
Barry Neil Kaufman, Author
A group of people from all walks of life come together and are transformed as they reach out, under the direction of Kaufman, to help a little boy the medical world had given up as hopeless. This heartwarming journey of loving a child back to life will not only inspire, but presents a compelling new way to deal with life's traumas and difficulties. *$7.99*
388 pages Yearly

2374 **All Kinds of Minds: Young Student's Book About Learning Disabilities & Disorders**
Educators Publishing Service
PO Box 9031
Cambridge, MA 02139-9031 617-547-6706
800-225-5750
Fax: 888-440-2665
http://eps.schoolspecialty.com/
CustomerService.EPS@schoolspecialty.com
Melvin Levine, Author
Alana Trisler, Author
Carol Einstein, Author
Written by Melvin Levine, and published in 1992. Helps children with learning disabilities to come to terms with it. Shows them how to get around or just work out any problems with their disabilities.
283 pages paperback
ISBN 0-838820-90-5

2375 **Closer Look: Perspectives & Reflections on College Students with LD**
Curry College Bookstore
1071 Blue Hill Ave
Milton, MA 02186-2302 617-333-0500
Fax: 617-333-6860
http://www.curry.edu
dgoss@curry.edu
Diane Goss, Editor/Author
Jane Adelizzi, Co-Author
This book is a collection of personal accounts by teachers and learners. It's a sensitive portrayal of the real world of teaching and learning, particularly as it impacts on those with learning differences. Topics include connections between theory and practice, emotions and learning disabilities, classroom trauma, learning disabilities and social deficits, metacognitive development, ESL and learning disabilities, models for inclusion and practical strategies. *$ 24.95*
241 pages paperback
ISBN 0-964975-20-3

2376 **Diverse Learners in the Mainstream Classroom: Strategies for Supporting ALL Students Across Areas**
Heinemann
PO Box 6926
Portsmouth, NH 03802-6926 603-431-7894
800-225-5800
Fax: 877-231-6980
http://www.heinemann.com
custserv@heinemann.com
Yvonne S Freeman, Author
Davide E Freeman, Co-Author
Reynaldo Ramirez, Co-Author
A comprehensive book offering strategies and practices teachers can use from PreK-through high school. Provides everything from the big picture to the everyday details teachers want. *$27.00*
272 pages
ISBN 0-325013-13-8

2377 **Dyslexia in Adults: Taking Charge of Your Life**
Taylor Publishing
7211 Circle S Road
Austin, TX 78745 512-444-0571
800-225-3687
Fax: 512-440-2160
http://www.balfour.com
Rings@balfour.com
Kathleen Nosek, Author
Adult dyslexics are experts at hiding reading, writing, and spelling difficulties long after high school. Dyslexia in Adults is a perfect guidebook for adult dyslexias to use in coping with day-to-day problems that are complicated by their learning disability. *$12.95*
206 pages Paperback
ISBN 0-878339-48-5

2378 **Faking It: A Look into the Mind of a Creative Learner**
Heinemann
PO Box 6926
Portsmouth, NH 03802-6926 603-431-7894
800-225-5800
Fax: 877-231-6980
http://www.heinemann.com
custserv@heinemann.com
Christopher Lee, Author
Rosemary Jackson, Co-Author
Engage in professional dialog with Heinemann's celebrated authors and colleagues! *$17.95*
200 pages paperback
ISBN 0-867092-96-3

2379 **From Disability to Possibility: The Powerof Inclusive Classrooms**
Heinemann
PO Box 6926
Portsmouth, NH 03802-6926 603-431-7894
800-225-5800
Fax: 877-231-6980
http://www.heinemann.com
custserv@heinemann.com
Patrick Schwarz, Author
Offers a meaningful, practical and doable alternative to traditional special education practice both during the school years and after. *$15.00*
112 pages
ISBN 0-325009-93-3

2380 **How to Get Services by Being Assertive**
Family Resource Center on Disabilities
Room 300
20 E Jackson Blvd
Chicago, IL 60604-2265 312-939-3513
800-952-4199
Fax: 312-854-8980
TDD: 312-939-3519
http://www.frcd.org
info@frcd.org

Charlotte Jardins, Author
Myra Christian, Contact
Gloria Mikucki, Contact
A 100 page manual that demonstrates positive assertiveness techniques. Price includes postage and handling. *$12.00*
100 pages

2381 **Inclusion-Classroom Problem Solver; Structures and Supports to Serve ALL Learners**
Heinemann
PO Box 6926
Portsmouth, NH 03802-6926 603-431-7894
800-225-5800
Fax: 877-231-6980
http://www.heinemann.com
custserv@heinemann.com
Constance McGrath, Author
Provides proven ways to create a classroom that replaces frustrating temporary accommodations with and inclusive, joyous environment designed to work for every student. *$17.50*
144 pages
ISBN 0-325012-70-4

2382 **Kids Behind the Label: An Inside at ADHD for Classroom Teachers**
Heinemann
PO Box 6926
Portsmouth, NH 03802-6926 603-431-7894
800-225-5800
Fax: 877-231-6980
http://www.heinemann.com
custserv@heinemann.com
Trudy Knowles, Author
Students with Attention-Deficit/Hyperactivity Disorder (ADHD) tell you what they experience coming to class each day. Their descriptions will forever change how you approach ADHD students, allowing you to contrast their frustrating in-school behavior with the frustration they feel trying to complete their work and make sense of their world. *$18.50*
160 pages
ISBN 0-325009-67-4

2383 **Myth of Laziness**
Simon & Schuster
1230 Avenue of the Americas
New York, NY 10020-1513 212-698-7000
http://www.simonandschuster.biz
shop.feedback@simonsays.com
Mel Levine, Author
Written by Melvin Levine and published in 2003. It shows parents how to nurture their children's strength's and improve their classroom productivity. Also, it shows how correcting these problems early will help children live a fulfilling and productive adult life.
288 pages
ISBN 0-743213-68-8

2384 **New Horizons Information for the Air Traveler with a Disability**
Office of Aviation Enforcement and Proceedings
1200 New Jersey Ave SE
Washington, DC 20590 http://www.dot.gov/airconsumer
This guide is designed to offer travelers with disabilities a brief but authoritative source of information about Air Carrier Access rules; the accommodations, facilities, and services that are now required to be available.

2385 **No Easy Answer**
Bantam Partners
1745 Broadway
New York, NY 10019-4305 212-782-9000
http://www.randomhouse.com
bdpublicity@randomhouse.com
Rob Meritt, Author
Brooker Brown, Co-Author
Parents and teachers of learning disabled children have turned to No Easy Answer for information, advice, and comfort. This completely updated edition contains new chapters on Attention Deficit Disorder and Attention Deficit Hyperactivity Disorder, and on the public laws that guarantee an equal education for learning disabled children. *$23.00*
416 pages paperback
ISBN 0-553354-50-7

2386 **Out of Darkness**
Connecticut Assoc for Children and Adults with LD
Ste 15-5
25 Van Zant St
Norwalk, CT 06855-1729 203-838-5010
Fax: 203-866-6108
http://www.cacld.org
cacld@optonline.net
Russell Freedman, Author
Article by an adult who discovers at age 30 that he has ADD. *$1.00*
4 pages

2387 **Painting the Joy of the Soul**
Learning Disabilities Association of America
4156 Library Rd
Pittsburgh, PA 15234-1349 412-341-1515
Fax: 412-344-0224
http://www.ldanatl.org
info@LDAAmerica.org
Peter Rippe, Author
P Buckley Moss, Co-Author
The first comprehensively researched and written book on the art and life of America's beloved artist, P. Buckley Moss, whose passion for painting is equal only to her passion for people, especially those with learning disabilities. Inspirational book about a woman who succeeded not in spite of her disability, but because of it. Contains 168 full color pages, over 100 art images. *$50.00*
168 pages
ISBN 0-964687-09-7

2388 **Rethinking the Education of Deaf Students: Theory and Practice from a Teacher's Perspective**
Heinemann
PO Box 6926
Portsmouth, NH 03802-6926 603-431-7894
800-225-5800
Fax: 877-231-6980
http://www.heinemann.com
custserv@heinemann.com
Sue Livingston, Author
Offers alternatives and demonstrates how American Sign Language (ASL) and English can coexist in the same classroom, embedded in the context of what is being taught. *$23.00*
180 pages
ISBN 0-435072-36-0

2389 **Son-Rise: The Miracle Continues**
Option Indigo Press
2080 S Undermountain Rd
Sheffield, MA 01257-9643 413-229-2100
800-714-2779
Fax: 413-229-8727
http://www.optionindigo.com
indigo@bcn.net
Barry Neil Kaufman, Author
Raun Kaufman, Co-Author
This book documents Raun Kaufman's astonishing development from a lifeless, autistic, retarded child into a highly verbal, lovable youngster with no traces of his former condition. It includes details of Raun's extraordinary progress from the age of four into young adulthood. It also shares moving accounts of five families that successfully used the Son-Rise Program to reach their own special children. An awe-inspiring reminder that love moves mountains. *$14.95*
372 pages
ISBN 0-915811-61-8

2390 **The Eight Ball Club: Ocean of Fire**
ESOL Publishing LLC
10305 Colony View Dr
Fairfax, VA 22032-3222 703-250-7097
http://www.theeightballclub.com
esolpublishing@cox.net; mcpuginrodas@aol.com
MC Pugin-Roads, Author
Publisher of novels designed for Special Ed and ESL students and activity books that go with the novel. These novels can be enjoyed by mainstream students as well. The Eight Ball Club: Ocean of Fire has vocac words in bold print, photographic illustrations, academic science terms, and a glossary. It's a teen-interest, easy reading adventure. *$18.95*
144 pages

2391 **What About Me? Strategies for Teaching Misunderstood Learners**
Heinemann
PO Box 6926
Portsmouth, NH 03802-6926 603-431-7894
800-225-5800
Fax: 877-231-6980
http://www.heinemann.com
custserv@heinemann.com
Christopher Lee, Author
Rosemary Jackson, Co-Author
A practical yet personal book on how to help special learners grow into self-sufficient responsible adults who can recognize their strengths and manage their weeknesses. *$19.50*
166 pages
ISBN 0-325003-48-1

2392 **You're Welcome: 30 Innovative Ideas for the Inclusive Classroom**
Heinemann
PO Box 6926
Portsmouth, NH 03802-6926 603-431-7894
800-225-5800
Fax: 877-231-6980
http://www.heinemann.com
custserv@heinemann.com
Patrick Schwarz, Author
Paula Kluth, Co-Author
Three handbooks; 30 key ideas-all the information you need to start making inclusion work effectively. *$18.00*
ISBN 0-325012-04-9

Children

2393 **An Alphabet of Animal Signs**
Harris Communications
15155 Technology Dr
Eden Prairie, MN 55344-2273 952-906-1180
800-825-6758
Fax: 952-906-1099
TDD: 952-906-1198
TTY: 800-825-9187
http://www.harriscomm.com
info@harriscomm.com
S Harold Collins, Author
Darla Hudson, Customer Service
A fun sign language starter book that presents an animal sign for each letter of the alphabet. Part #B816. *$4.95*
16 pages Paperback
ISBN 0-931993-65-2

2394 **Basic Vocabulary: American Sign Language Basic Vocabulary: American Sign Language for Parents**
Harris Communications
15155 Technology Dr
Eden Prairie, MN 55344-2273 952-906-1180
800-825-6758
Fax: 952-906-1099
TDD: 952-906-1198
TTY: 800-825-9187
http://www.harriscomm.com
info@harriscomm.com
Terrance K O'Rourke, Author
Darla Hudson, Customer Service
A child's first dictionary of signs. Arranged alphabetically, this book incorporates developmental lists helpful to both deaf and hearing children with over 1,000 clear illustrations. Part #B294. *$8.95*
228 pages Paperback
ISBN 0-932666-00-0

2395 **Beginning Signing Primer**
Harris Communications
15155 Technology Dr
Eden Prairie, MN 55344-2273 952-906-1180
800-825-6758
Fax: 952-906-1099
TDD: 952-906-1198
TTY: 800-825-9187
http://www.harriscomm.com
info@harriscomm.com
Darla Hudson, Customer Service
A set of 100 cards designed especially for beginning signers. The cards present seven topics with words and signs. The topics: Color; Creatures; Family; Months; Days; Time and Weather. Part #B398. *$7.95*

2396 **Christmas Bear**
Teddy Bear Press
Suite 67
3703 S. Edmunds Street
Seattle, WA 98118 206-402-6947
866-870-7323
Fax: 866-870-7323
http://www.teddybearpress.net
fparker@teddybearpress.net
Fran Parker, President/Author
An 11x17 big book with color illustrations and a large print format uses the same simple sentence structure fount in I Can Read and Reading Is Fun programs. This story adds seasonal words to the developing sight vocabulary found in our reading programs. *$19.95*
12 pages
ISBN 1-928876-11-0

2397 **Don't Give Up Kid**
Verbal Images Press
46 Duncott Rd.
Fairport, NY 14450-8602 585-746-7239
Fax: 585-264-1448
http://verbalimagespress.com
jeanne@verbalimagespress.com
Victoria Harmison, Marketing Director
Jeanne Gehret MA, Author
Like a river overflowing its banks, Ben wreaks havoc until he learns to recognize his Attention Deficit Disorder (ADD). By the end of this tale, Ben's family wonders how they could have gotten along without his specia way of seeing the world. *$9.95*
40 pages Paperback
ISBN 1-884281-10-9

2398 **Fischer Decoding Mastery Test**
Oxton House Publishers
124 Main Street
Suite 203
Farmington, ME 04938 207-779-1923
800-539-7323
Fax: 207-779-0623
http://www.oxtonhouse.com
info@oxtonhouse.com
William Berlinghoff PhD, Managing Editor
Cheryl Martin, Marketing
Debra Richards, Office Manager
This powerful, flexible diagnostic tool tells you precisely which decoding skills have been mastered (don't need to be taught), which skills are in transition (need some attention), and which skills need to be taught from scratch. Based on more than 40 years of clinical experience, it is a highly reliable way to pinpoint each beginning reader's exact needs and to measure progress against previous performance.

2399 **Fundamentals of Autism**
Slosson Educational Publications
PO Box 280
538 Buffalo Road
East Aurora, NY 14052
888-756-7766
Fax: 800-655-3840
http://www.slosson.com
slosson@slosson.com

Steven Slosson, President
Georgina Moynihan, TTFM
A handbook for those who work with children diagnosed as autistic.

2400 **Funny Bunny and Sunny Bunny**
Teddy Bear Press
Suite 67
3703 S. Edmunds Street
Seattle, WA 98118
206-402-6947
866-870-7323
Fax: 866-870-7323
http://www.teddybearpress.net
fparker@teddybearpress.net

Fran Parker, President/Author
An 11x17 big book with color illustrations and a large print format uses the same simple sentence structure fount in I Can Read and Reading Is Fun programs. This story adds seasonal words to the developing sight vocabulary found in our reading programs. *$19.95*
17 pages
ISBN 1-928876-14-5

2401 **Halloween Bear**
Teddy Bear Press
Suite 67
3703 S. Edmunds Street
Seattle, WA 98118
206-402-6947
866-870-7323
Fax: 866-870-7323
http://www.teddybearpress.net
fparker@teddybearpress.net

Fran Parker, President/Author
An 11x17 big book with color illustrations and a large print format uses the same simple sentence structure fount in I Can Read and Reading Is Fun programs. This story adds seasonal words to the developing sight vocabulary found in our reading programs. *$19.95*
13 pages
ISBN 1-928876-15-3

2402 **Handmade Alphabet**
Harris Communications
15155 Technology Dr
Eden Prairie, MN 55344-2273
952-906-1180
800-825-6758
Fax: 952-906-1099
TDD: 952-906-1198
TTY: 800-825-9187
http://www.harriscomm.com
info@harriscomm.com

Laura Rankin, Author
Darla Hudson, Customer Service
An alphabet book which celebrates the beauty of the manual alphabet. Each illustration consists of the manual representation of the letter linked with an item beginning with that letter. Part #B310SC. *$6.99*
32 pages Paperback
ISBN 0-803709-74-9

2403 **I Can Read Charts**
Teddy Bear Press
Suite 67
3703 S. Edmunds Street
Seattle, WA 98118
206-402-6947
866-870-7323
Fax: 866-870-7323
http://www.teddybearpress.net
fparker@teddybearpress.net

Frank Babaloni, President/Author
Designed to accompany the I Can Read program is an 11x17 big book containing 54 charts which can be used to assist in introducing new words to students. These charts also provide review for previously taught words with either individual student or a small group. *$59.95*
54 pages

2404 **I Can Sign My ABC's**
Harris Communications
15155 Technology Dr
Eden Prairie, MN 55344-2273
952-906-1180
800-825-6758
Fax: 952-906-1099
TDD: 952-906-1198
TTY: 800-825-9187
http://www.harriscomm.com
info@harriscomm.com

Darla Hudson, Customer Service
The Sign with Me alphabet book is a book for all children. It is designed to teach the 26 letters of the alphabet and the corresponding manual alphabet in sign language. The book provides early exposure to letter recognition plus a unique opportunity to introduce sign language to young children. Part #B132. *$11.95*
52 pages Hardcover
ISBN 0-939849-00-3

2405 **Jumpin' Johnny Get Back to Work: A Child's Guide to ADHD/Hyperactivity**
Connecticut Assoc for Children and Adults with LD
Ste 15-5
25 Van Zant St
Norwalk, CT 06855-1729
203-838-5010
Fax: 203-866-6108
http://www.CACLD.org
cacld@juno.com

Michael Gordon PhD, Author
Written primarily for elementary age youngsters with ADHD, this book helps them to understand their disability. Also valuable as an educational tool for parents, siblings, friends and classmates. The author's text reflects his sensitivity toward children with ADHD. *$12.50*
24 pages

2406 **Leo the Late Bloomer**
Connecticut Assoc for Children and Adults with LD
Ste 15-5
25 Van Zant St
Norwalk, CT 06855-1729
203-838-5010
Fax: 203-866-6108
http://www.CACLD.org
cacld@juno.com

Beryl Kaufman, Executive Director
Robert Kraus, Author
A wonderful book for the young child who is having problems learning. Children follow along with Leo as he finally blooms. *$6.50*

2407 **My First Book of Sign**
Harris Communications
15155 Technology Dr
Eden Prairie, MN 55344-2273
952-906-1180
800-825-6758
Fax: 952-906-1099
TDD: 952-906-1198
TTY: 800-825-9187
http://www.harriscomm.com
info@harriscomm.com

Pamela J Baker, Author
Darla Hudson, Customer Service

This book is an excellent source to teach children and even adults sign language. The illustrations are accurate in their representation of sign. It is colorful and visually attractive which makes it easy to read. The black and white manual alphabet, the fingerspelling, and aspects of sign provide exellent directions and pointers to signing correctly. The sign descriptions are a great supplement to the illustrations. Part #B147. *$22.95*
76 pages Hardcover
ISBN 0-930323-20-3

2408 **My Signing Book of Numbers**
Harris Communications
15155 Technology Dr
Eden Prairie, MN 55344-2273 952-906-1180
800-825-6758
Fax: 952-906-1099
TDD: 952-906-1198
TTY: 800-825-9187
http://www.harriscomm.com
info@harriscomm.com
Patricia Bellan Gillen, Author
Darla Hudson, Customer Service
Learn signs for numbers 0 through 20, and 30 through 100 by tens. *$22.95*
56 pages Hardcover
ISBN 0-930323-37-8

2409 **Rosey: The Imperfect Angel**
Special Needs Project
Ste H
324 State St
Santa Barbara, CA 93101-2364 818-718-9900
800-333-6867
Fax: 818-349-2027
http://www.specialneeds.com
books@specialneeds.com
Sandra Lee Peckinpah, Author
Rosie, an angel with a cleft palate, works hard in her heavenly garden after the Boss Angel declares her disfigured mouth as lovely as a rose petal. Her reward is to be born on earth, as a baby with a cleft. *$15.95*
28 pages
ISBN 0-962780-60-8

2410 **Scare Bear**
Teddy Bear Press
3703 S. Edmunds Street
Suite 67
Seattle, WA 98118 206-402-6947
866-870-7323
Fax: 866-870-7323
http://www.teddybearpress.net
fparker@teddybearpress.net
Fran Parker, President/Author
An 11x17 big book with color illustrations and a large print format uses the same simple sentence structure fount in I Can Read and Reading Is Fun programs. This story adds seasonal words to the developing sight vocabulary found in our reading programs. *$19.95*
13 pages
ISBN 1-928876-16-1

2411 **Signing is Fun: A Child's Introduction to the Basics of Sign Language**
Harris Communications
15155 Technology Dr
Eden Prairie, MN 55344-2273 952-906-1180
800-825-6758
Fax: 952-906-1099
TDD: 952-906-1198
TTY: 800-825-9187
http://www.harriscomm.com
info@harriscomm.com
Mickey Flodin, Author
Darla Hudson, Customer Service
The author of Signing for Kids offers children their first glimpse at a whole new world. Starting with the alphabet and working up to everyday phrases, this volume uses clear instructions on how to begin using American Sign Language and features an informative introduction to signing and its importance. One hundred and fifty illustrations. Part #B496
$9.00
95 pages Paperback
ISBN 0-613720-18-0

2412 **Sixth Grade Can Really Kill You**
Penquin Putnam Publishing Group
375 Hudson St
New York, NY 10014-3658 212-366-2000
800-847-5515
Fax: 212-366-2666
http://www.penguingroup.com
ecommerce@us.penguingroup.com
Barthe DeClements, Author
Helen's learning difficulties cause her to act up and are threatening to keep her from passing sixth grade.
160 pages Paperback
ISBN 0-142413-80-1

2413 **Snowbear**
Teddy Bear Press
Suite 67
3703 S. Edmunds Street
Seattle, WA 98118 206-402-6947
866-870-7323
Fax: 866-870-7323
http://www.teddybearpress.net
fparker@teddybearpress.net
Fran Parker, President/Author
An 11x17 big book with color illustrations and a large print format uses the same simple sentence structure fount in I Can Read and Reading Is Fun programs. This story adds seasonal words to the developing sight vocabulary found in our reading programs. *$19.95*
13 pages
ISBN 1-928876-12-9

2414 **Someone Special, Just Like You**
Special Needs Project
Ste H
324 State St
Santa Barbara, CA 93101-2364 818-718-9900
800-333-6867
Fax: 818-349-2027
http://www.specialneeds.com
books@specialneeds.com
Tricia Brown, Author
A handsome photo-essay including a range of youngsters with disabilities at four preschools in the San Francisco Bay area. *$7.95*
64 pages

2415 **Study Skills: A Landmark School Student Guide**
429 Hale St
Prides Crossing
Prides Crossing, MA 01965 978-236-3216
Fax: 978-927-7268
http://www.landmarkoutreach.org
outreach@landmarkschool.org
Robert Broudo, Principal

2416 **Unicorns Are Real!**
Learning Disabilities Association of America
4156 Library Rd
Pittsburgh, PA 15234-1349 412-341-1515
Fax: 412-344-0224
http://www.ldanatl.org
ldanatl@usaor.net
Barbara Meister Vitale, Author

This mega best-seller provides 65 practical, easy-to follow-lessons to develop the much ignored right brain tendencies of children. These simple yet dramatically effective ideas and activities have helped thousands with learning difficulties. Includes an easy-to-administer screening checklist to determine hemisphere dominance, engaging instructional activities that draw on the intuitive, nonverbal abilities of the right brain, a list of skills associated with each brain hemisphere and more. *$14.95*
174 pages
ISBN 0-446323-40-3

2417 **Valentine Bear**
Teddy Bear Press
Suite 67
3703 S. Edmunds Street
Seattle, WA 98118 206-402-6947
866-870-7323
Fax: 866-870-7323
http://www.teddybearpress.net
fparker@teddybearpress.net
Fran Parker, President/Author
An 11x17 big book with color illustrations and a large print format uses the same simple sentence structure fount in I Can Read and Reading Is Fun programs. This story adds seasonal words to the developing sight vocabulary found in our reading programs. *$19.95*
13 pages
ISBN 1-928876-13-7

2418 **Visual Perception and Attention Workbook**
Therapro
225 Arlington St
Framingham, MA 01702-8723 508-872-9494
800-257-5376
Fax: 508-875-2062
http://www.therapro.com
info@therapro.com
Karen Conrad, Owner
Kathleen Anderson MS CCC-SP, Author
Pamela Crow Miller, Co-Author
Simple mazes, visual discrimination and visual form constancy task, telling time and much more.

Law

2419 **Dispute Resolution Journal**
American Arbitration Association
Fl 10
1633 Broadway
New York, NY 10019-6708 212-716-5800
800-778-7879
Fax: 212-716-5905
http://www.adr.org
zuckermans@adr.org
William K Slate Ii, CEO
Susan Zuckerman, Author
Provides information on mediation, arbitration and other dispute resolution alternatives. *$150.00*
96 pages Quarterly

2420 **Education of the Handicapped: Laws**
William Hein & Company
1285 Main St
Buffalo, NY 14209-1987 716-882-2600
800-828-7571
Fax: 716-883-8100
http://www.wshein.com
mail@wshein.com
Kevin Marmion, President
Bernard D Reams Jr, Author
Focuses on elementary and secondary Education Act of 1965 and its amendment, Education For All Handicapped Children Act of 1975 and its amendments and acts providing services for the disabled.
ISBN 0-899411-57-6

2421 **Ethical and Legal Issues in School Counseling**
American School Counselor Association
Ste 625
1101 King St
Alexandria, VA 22314-2957 703-683-2722
800-306-4722
Fax: 703-683-1619
http://www.schoolcounselor.org
asca@schoolcounselor.org
Wayne C Huey, Author
Theodore Phant Remley, Editor
Perhaps the increase in litigation involving educators and mental health practitioners is a factor. Certainly the laws are changing or at least are being interpreted differently, requiring counselors to stay up-to-date. The process of decision-making and some of the more complex issues in ethical and legal areas are summarized in this digest. *$40.50*
341 pages
ISBN 1-556200-55-2

2422 **Individuals with Disabilities: Implementing the Newest Laws**
Corwin Press
2455 Teller Rd
Thousand Oaks, CA 91320-2218 805-499-9734
800-233-9936
Fax: 805-499-5323
http://www.corwin.com
order@corwin.com
Joan L Curcio, Author
Patricia F First, Co-Author
Aimed at school administrators, this highly readable book covers the three major pieces of legislation: Americans with Disabilities Act of 1990; Individuals with Disabilities Education Act; and the Rehabilitation Act of 1973. Suitable for lay public use, anyone needing an overview of the laws affecting education and disabilities. *$12.95*
64 pages
ISBN 0-803960-55-7

2423 **Learning Disabilities and the Law in Higher Education and Employment**
JKL Communications
Ste 707
2700 Virginia Ave NW
Washington, DC 20037-1909 202-321-4100
Fax: 850-233-3350
lathamlaw@gmail.com
Peter S Latham JD, Director
Patricia Horan Latham JD, Director
Deals with issues in education and employment. Covers: Section 504, the IDEA, and ADA. Reviews court cases. *$15.00*
ISBN 1-883560-13-6

2424 **Least Restrictive Environment**
State Education Resource Center
100 Roscommon Dr
Middletown, CT 06457-1520 860-632-1485
Fax: 860-632-8870
http://www.ctserc.org
info@ctserc.org
A self-assessment resource to determine if the policies, practices and procedures in place at schools are in line with the requirements of the Individuals with Disabilities Education Improvement Act.

2425 **Legal Notes for Education**
Oakstone Business Publishing
136 Madison Avenue
8th Floor
New York, NY 10016 212-209-0500
Fax: 212-209-0501
http://www.haightscross.com
info@haightscross.com
Steven B. Epstein, Chairman
Summaries of court decisions dealing with education law. *$122.00*

2426 **Legal Rights of Persons with Disabilities: An Analysis of Federal Law**
LRP Publications
360 Hiatt Drive
Palm Beach Gardens
Florida, FL 33418
800-341-7874
Fax: 561-622-2423
http://www.lrp.com
custserv@lrp.com
Bonnie P Tucker, Author
This book will provide professionals working with the disabled a comprehensive analysis of the rights accorded individuals with disabilities under federal law. *$185.00*
2226 pages
ISBN 0-934753-46-6

2427 **National Association of State Directors of Developmental Disabilities (NASDDDS)**
301 N Fairfax St
Ste 101
Alexandria, VA 22314
703-683-4202
Fax: 703-684-1395
http://www.nasddds.org
ksnyder@nasddds.org
Mary Lee Fay, Executive Director
Community Services Reporter (CSR) is the only monthly newsletter in the U.S. reporting exclusively on state and local efforts in supporting and serving individuals with developmental disabilities and their families. Topics covered in CSR include state service initiatives such as new service designs, financial management strategies, supports for self-advocacy; key state legislation; facility closures; litigation summaries; research developments, and budget overviews. *$145.00*
12 issues subs.

2428 **Numbers that add up to Educational Rights for Children with Disabilities**
Children's Defense Fund
25 E Street N.W.
Washington, DC 20001-1522
202-628-8787
800-233-1200
http://www.childrensdefense.org
cdfinfo@childrensdefense.org
Ellen Mancuso, Author
Information on the laws 94-142 and 504. *$4.75*
68 pages
ISBN 0-938008-73-0

2429 **Parent's Guide to the Social Security Administration**
The Eden Family of Services
2 Merwick Rd
Princeton, NJ 08540-5711
609-987-0099
Fax: 609-987-0243
http://www.edenautism.org
info@edenau.orgtism
Tom Mc Cool, President
A parents' guide to the Social Security Administration and Social Security Work Incentive Programs. *$16.00*

2430 **Purposeful Integration: Inherently Equal**
Federation for Children with Special Needs
Suite 1102
529 Main Street
Boston, MA 02109
617-236-7210
800-331-0688
Fax: 617-241-0330
http://www.fcsn.org
fcsninfo@fcsn.org
James F. Whalen, President
Michael Weiner, Treasurer
This publication covers integration, mainstreaming, and least restrictive environments. *$8.00*
55 pages

2431 **Section 504: Help for the Learning Disabled College Student**
Connecticut Assoc for Children and Adults with LD
Ste 15-5
25 Van Zant St
Norwalk, CT 06855-1729
203-838-5010
Fax: 203-866-6108
http://www.cacld.org
cacld@juno.com
Beryl Kaufman, Executive Director
Joan Sedita, Author
Provides a review of Section 504 of the Vocational Rehabilitation Act as it relates specifically to the learning disabled. *$3.25*

2432 **So You're Going to a Hearing: Preparing for Public Law 94-142**
Learning Disabilities Association of America
4156 Library Rd
Pittsburgh, PA 15234-1349
412-341-1515
Fax: 412-344-0224
http://www.ldanatl.org
ldanatl@usaor.net
A public informational source offering legal advice to children and youth with learning disabilities. *$5.50*

2433 **Special Education Law Update**
Data Research
Ste 3100
4635 Nicols Rd
Eagan, MN 55122-3337
651-452-8267
800-365-4900
Fax: 651-452-8694
http://www.dataresearchinc.com
Monthly newsletter service. Cases, legislation, administrative regulations and law review articles dealing with special education law. Annual index and binder included. *$159.00*

2434 **Special Education in Juvenile Corrections**
Council for Exceptional Children
Suite 1000
2900 Crystal Drive
Arlington, VA 22202-3557
703-620-3660
866-509-0218
Fax: 703-264-9494
TTY: 866-915-5000
http://www.cec.sped.org
service@cec.sped.org
Margaret J. McLaughin, President
James P. Heiden, Treasurer
This topic is of increasing concern. This book describes the demographics of incarcerated youth and suggests some promising practices that are being used. *$8.90*
25 pages
ISBN 0-865862-03-6

2435 **Special Law for Special People**
Gray,Rust, St. Amand, Moffett & Brieske LLP
950 E Paces Ferry Rd NE
1700 Atlanta Plaza
Atlanta, GA 30326-1180
404-870-7373
Fax: 404-870-7374
http://www.grsmb.com
James T. Brieske, Attorney
Matthew A. Ericksen, Attorney
A ten-tape video series that is designed to assist in educating regular education personnel as to the legal requirements of IDEA and Section 504. *$5.95*

2436 **Statutes, Regulations and Case Law**
Center for Education and Employment Law
PO Box 3008
Malvern, PA 19355
800-365-4900
Fax: 610-647-8089
http://www.ceelonline.com
curt_brown@pbp.com
Curt Brown Esq, Group Publisher
Steve McEllistrem Esq, Senior Editor

Provides summaries of recent court cases impacting disability issues as well as reports on legislation and administrative regulations that are of importance to you. *$259.00*
Monthly

2437 **Stories Behind Special Education Case Law**
Special Needs Project
Ste H
324 State St
Santa Barbara, CA 93101-2364
818-718-9900
800-333-6867
Fax: 818-349-2027
http://www.specialneeds.com
books@specialneeds.com

Reed Martin, Author
The personal stories behind ten leading court cases that shaped the basic principles of special education law. *$12.95*
119 pages Paperback
ISBN 0-878223-32-0

2438 **Students with Disabilities and Special Education**
Center for Education and Employment Law
PO Box 3008
Malvern, PA 19355
800-365-4900
Fax: 610-647-8089
http://www.ceelonline.com
curt_brown@pbp.com

Curt Brown Esq, Group Publisher
Steve McEllistrem Esq, Senior Editor
A desk reference that helps you determine if your program conforms to IDEA statutes and regulations in a comprehensive and concise format. We bring you analyses of recent court cases across the country that will help you safeguard your legal rights, and educate your colleagues in the law so they too are better qualified to identify and deal with developing legal issues. *$294.00*
500+ pages
ISBN 0-939675-44-7

2439 **Technology, Curriculum, and Professional Development**
Corwin Press
2455 Teller Rd
Thousand Oaks, CA 91320-2218
805-499-9734
800-233-9936
Fax: 805-499-5323
http://www.corwin.com
order@corwin.com

John Woodward, Author/Editor
Larry Cuban, Co-Author/Editor
Adapting schools to meet the needs of students with disabilities. The history of special education technologies, the requirements of IDEA'97, and the successes and obstacles for special education technology implementation. *$76.95*
264 pages
ISBN 0-761977-42-2

2440 **Testing Students with Disabilities**
Corwin Press
2455 Teller Rd
Thousand Oaks, CA 91320-2218
805-499-9734
800-233-9936
Fax: 805-499-5323
http://www.corwin.com
order@corwin.com

Martha Thurlow, Author
James Ysseldyke, Co-Author
Judy Elliot, Co-Author
Practical strategies for complying with district and state requirements. Helps translate the issues surrounding state and district testing of students with disabilities, including IDEA, into what educators need to know and do. *$ 80.95*
344 pages
ISBN 0-761938-08-7

2441 **US Department of Justice: Disabilities Rights Section**
950 Pennsylvania Ave NW
Washington, DC 20530
202-307-0663
800-514-0301
Fax: 202-307-1197
TTY: 800-514-0383
http://www.ada.gov
askdoj@usdoj.gov

Rebecca B. Bond, Chief
Zita Jhonson Betts, Deputy Chief
Roberta Kirkendall, Special Councel
Information concerning the rights people with learning disabilities have under the Americans with Disabilities Act.

2442 **US Department of Justice: Disability Rights Section**
950 Pennsylvania Ave NW
Washington, DC 20530
202-307-0663
800-514-0301
Fax: 202-307-1197
TTY: 800-514-0383
http://www.ada.gov
askdoj@usdoj.gov

Rebecca B. Bond, Chief
Zita Jhonson Betts, Deputy Chief
Roberta Kirkendall, Special Councel
The primary goal of the Disability Rights Section is to achieve equal opportunity for people with disabilities in the United States by implementing the Americans with Disabilities Act (ADA).

Parents & Professionals

2443 **125 Brain Games for Babies**
Therapro
225 Arlington St
Framingham, MA 01702-8723
508-872-9494
800-257-5376
Fax: 508-875-2062
http://www.therapro.com
info@therapro.com

Jackie Silberg, uthor
Packed with everyday opportunities to enhance brain development of children from birth to 12 months. Each game includes notes on recent brain research in practical terms.
$14.95
143 pages
ISBN 0-876591-99-3

2444 **A Miracle to Believe In**
Option Indigo Press
2080 S Undermountain Rd
Sheffield, MA 01257-9643
413-229-8727
800-562-7171
Fax: 413-229-8727
http://www.optionindigo.com
indigo@bcn.net

Barry Kausman, Author
A group of people from all walks of life come together and are transformed as they reach out, under the direction of Kaufman, to help a little boy the medical world had given up as hopeless. This heartwarming journey of loving a child back to life will not only inspire, but presents a compelling new way to deal with life's traumas and difficulties. *$7.99*
388 pages
ISBN 0-449201-08-2

2445 **A Practical Parent's Handbook on Teaching Children with Learning Disabilities**
Charles C Thomas
2600 S 1st St
Springfield, IL 62704-4730
217-789-8980
800-258-8980
Fax: 217-789-9130
http://www.ccthomas.com
books@ccthomas.com

Shelby Holley, Author

Publisher of Education and Special Education books.
308 pages
ISBN 0-398061-50-5

2446 **ADHD in Adolescents: Diagnosis and Treatment**
Guilford Publications
72 Spring St
New York, NY 10012-4019 212-431-9800
800-365-7006
Fax: 212-966-6708
http://www.guilford.com
info@guilford.com
Arthur L Robin, Author
Here Dr. Robin teaches us not only about the facts of the disorder, but also about its nature and the proper means of clinically evaluating it. Includes numerous reproducible forms for clinicians and clients, among them rating scales and detailed checklists for psychological testing, interviewing, treatment planning, and school and family interventions. *$35.00*
461 pages Paperback
ISBN 1-572303-91-3

2447 **About Dyslexia: Unraveling the Myth**
Connecticut Assoc for Children and Adults with LD
Ste 15-5
25 Van Zant St
Norwalk, CT 06855-1729 203-838-5010
Fax: 203-866-6108
http://www.cacld.org
cacld@optonline.net
Beryl Kaufman, Executive Director
Priscilla Vail, Author
This book focuses on the communication patterns of strength and weaknesses in dyslexic people from early childhood through adulthood. *$7.95*
49 pages
ISBN 1-864010-55-8

2448 **Absurdities of Special Education: The Best of Ants...Flying...and Logs**
Corwin Press
2455 Teller Rd
Thousand Oaks, CA 91320-2218 805-499-9734
800-233-9936
Fax: 805-499-5323
http://www.corwin.com
order@corwin.com
Kevin Ruelle, Editor
Michael F Giangreco, Author
Now available in this full color edition. Create beautiful transperances or use in PowerPoint presentations for staff development. Also a great gift for parents of educators. *$30.95*
114 pages Paperback
ISBN 1-890455-40-7

2449 **Access Aware: Extending Your Reach to People with Disabilities**
Alliance for Technology Access
1119 Old Humboldt Road
Jackson, TN 38305 731-554-5282
1-800-914-30
Fax: 731-554-5283
TTY: 731-554-5284
http://www.ataccess.org
atainfo@ataccess.org
Allegra Wilson, Administrative Assistant
Todd Plummer, Development Manager
This easy-to-use manual is designed to help any organization become more accessible for people with disabilities. *$45.00*
219 pages
ISBN 0-897933-00-1

2450 **Activities for a Diverse Classroom**
PEAK Parent Center
Ste 200
611 N Weber St
Colorado Springs, CO 80903-1072 719-531-9400
800-284-0251
Fax: 719-531-9452
http://www.peakparent.org
info@peakparent.org
Leah Katz, Author
Caren Sax, Co-Author
Douglas Fisher, Co-Author
A valuable resource for elementary teachers, this book helps begin the sometimes difficult conversation about diversity in the classroom. With the 18 fun, enriching, and do-it-tomorrow activities outlined in this text, teachers can help create a sense of community in the classroom as they introduce students to new ways of thinking about the need for friendships and the acceptance of others. *$11.00*
68 pages
ISBN 1-884720-07-2

2451 **Activity Schedules for Children with Autism: A Guide for Parents and Professionals**
Woodbine House
6510 Bells Mill Rd
Bethesda, MD 20817-1636 301-897-3570
800-843-7323
Fax: 301-897-5838
http://www.woodbinehouse.com
info@woodbinehouse.com
Lynn E McClannahan PhD, Author
Patricia J Krantz PhD, Author
Detailed instructions and examples help parents prepare their child's first activity schedule, then progress to more varied and sophisticated schedules. The goal of this system is for children with autism to make effective use of unstructured time, handle changes in routine, and help them choose among an established set of home, school, and leisure activities independently. *$14.95*
117 pages Paperback
ISBN 0-933149-93-X

2452 **Alternate Assessments for Students with Disabilities**
Corwin Press
2455 Teller Rd
Thousand Oaks, CA 91320-2218 805-499-9734
800-233-9936
Fax: 805-499-5323
http://www.corwin.com
order@corwin.com
Robb Clouse, Editorial Director
Sandra Thompson, Author
Martha Lurlow, Co-Author
Distinguished group of experts in a landmark book, co-published with the Council for Exceptional Children show you how to shift to high expectations for all learners, improve schooling for all. *$30.95*
168 pages Paperback
ISBN 0-761977-74-0

2453 **American Sign Language Concise Dictionary**
Harris Communications
15155 Technology Dr
Eden Prairie, MN 55344-2273 952-906-1180
800-825-6758
Fax: 866-870-7323
TDD: 952-906-1198
TTY: 800-825-9187
http://www.harriscomm.com
info@harriscomm.com
Martin Sternberg, Author
Darla Hudson, Customer Service
A portable version containing 2,000 of the most commonly used words and phrases in ASL. Illustrated with easy-to-follow hand, arm and facial movements. Part #B104. *$11.95*
737 pages Paperback

2454 **American Sign Language Dictionary: A Comprehensive Abridgement**
Harris Communications
15155 Technology Dr
Eden Prairie, MN 55344-2273
952-906-1180
800-825-6758
Fax: 866-870-7323
TDD: 952-906-1198
TTY: 800-825-9187
http://www.harriscomm.com
info@harriscomm.com
Martin Sternberg, Author
Darla Hudson, Customer Service
An abridged version of American Sign Language. A comprehensive dictionary with 4,400 illustrated signs. It has 500 new signs and 1,500 new illustrations. Third edition. Part #B103HC, and B103SC. *$24.00*
772 pages Paperback

2455 **Another Door to Learning**
Independent Publishers Group
814 N Franklin St
Chicago, IL 60610-3813
312-337-0747
800-888-4741
Fax: 312-337-5985
http://www.ipgbook.com
frontdesk@ipgbook.com
Judy Schwartz, Author
Stories of eleven atypical learners who got the help they needed to make a lasting difference in their lives.
ISBN 0-824513-85-1

2456 **Ants in His Pants: Absurdities and Realities of Special Education**
Corwin Press
2455 Teller Rd
Thousand Oaks, CA 91320-2218
805-499-9734
800-233-9936
Fax: 805-499-5323
http://www.corwin.com
order@corwin.com
Michael F Giangreco, Author
Kevin Ruelle, Editor
With wit, humor, and profound one liners, this book will transform your thinking as you take a lighter look at the often comical and occcasionally harsh truth in the field of special education. This carefully crafted collection of 101 cartoons can be made into transparencies for staff development and training. *$20.95*
128 pages
ISBN 1-890455-42-3

2457 **Attention-Deficit Hyperactivity Disorder**
slosson Educational Publications
PO Box 544
538 Buffalo Road
East Aurora, NY 14052
716-652-0930
888-756-7766
Fax: 800-655-3840
http://www.slosson.com
slosson@slosson.com
Steve Slosson, President
Sue Larson, Author
The book addresses issues of theory and practice quickly, with compassion and practicality and, most importantly, is very effective. Well-grounded answers and suggestions which would facilitate behavior, learning, social-emotional functioning, and other factors in preschool and adolescence are discussed.

2458 **Attention-Deficit Hyperactivity Disorder: A Handbook for Diagnosis and Treatment**
Guilford Publications
72 Spring St
New York, NY 10012-4019
212-431-9800
800-365-7006
Fax: 212-966-6708
http://www.guilford.com
info@guilford.com
Russell A Barkely, Author
Incorporates the latest findings on the nature, diagnosis, assessment, and treatment of ADHD. Clinicians, researchers, and students will find practical and richly referenced information on nearly every aspect of the disorder. *$ 55.00*
628 pages

2459 **Autism and the Family: Problems, Prospects and Coping with the Disorder**
Charles C Thomas Publisher
PO Box 19265
Springfield, IL 62794-9265
217-789-8980
800-258-8980
Fax: 217-789-9130
http://www.ccthomas.com
books@ccthomas.com
David E Gray, Author
Publisher of Education and Special Education books. *$52.95*
198 pages Hardcover
ISBN 0-398068-43-7

2460 **Backyards & Butterflies: Ways to Include Children with Disabilities**
Brookline Books
Suite B-001
8 Trumbull Rd
Northampton, MA 01060
413-584-0184
800-666-2665
Fax: 413-5846184
http://www.brooklinebooks.com
brbooks@yahoo.com
Doreen Greenstein PhD, Author
This colorful, profusely illustrated book shows parents and others who work with disabled children how to design and build simple, inexpensive assistive technology devices that open up the world of outdoor experiences for these children. *$14.95*
72 pages Paperback
ISBN 1-571290-11-7

2461 **Behavior Technology Guide Book**
The Eden Family of Services
2 Merwick Rd
Princeton, NJ 08540-5711
609-987-0099
Fax: 609-987-0243
http://www.edenautism.org
info@edenau.orgtism
Peter H. Bell, President
Jennifer Bizub, COO
John Inzilla, CFO
Techniques for increasing and decreasing behavior using the principles of applied behavior analysis and related teaching strategies — discrete trial, shaping, task analysis and chaining.

2462 **Children with Cerebral Palsy: A Parent's Guide**
Therapro
225 Arlington St
Framingham, MA 01702-8723
508-872-9494
800-257-5376
Fax: 508-875-2062
http://www.therapro.com
info@therapro.com
Elaine Geralis, Editor
This book explains what cerebral palsy is, and discusses its diagnosis and treatment. It also offers information and advice concerning daily care, early intervention, therapy, educational options and family life. *$18.95*
481 pages
ISBN 0-933149-82-4

2463 **Children with Special Needs: A Resource Guide for Parents, Educators, Social Worker**
Charles C Thomas
PO Box 19265
Springfield, IL 62794-9265
217-789-8980
800-258-8980
Fax: 217-789-9130
http://www.ccthomas.com
books@ccthomas.com
Michael P Thomas, President
Publisher of Education and Special Education books. *$57.95*
234 pages Cloth
ISBN 0-398069-33-6

2464 **Children with Tourette Syndrome**
Woodbine House
6510 Bells Mill Rd
Bethesda, MD 20817-1636
301-897-3570
800-843-7323
Fax: 301-897-5838
http://www.woodbinehouse.com
info@Woodbinehouse.com
Tracy Haerle, Editor
A guide for parents of children and teenagers with Tourette syndrome. Covers medical, educational, legal, family life, daily care, and emotional issues, as well as explanations of related conditions. *$14.95*
352 pages Paperback
ISBN 0-933149-39-5

2465 **Classroom Success for the LD and ADHD Child**
Therapro
225 Arlington St
Framingham, MA 01702-8723
508-872-9494
800-257-5376
Fax: 508-875-2062
http://www.therapro.com
info@therapro.com
Suzanne H Stevens, Author
Helpful book for parents and therapists who work with children with learning disabilities. It addresses specific issues such as organization, homework and concentration. Stevens offers practical suggestions on adjusting teaching techniques, adapting texts, adjusting classroom management procedures and testing and grading fairly. *$13.95*
342 pages Revised
ISBN 0-895871-59-9

2466 **Common Ground: Whole Language & Phonics Working Together**
Educators Publishing Service
PO Box 9031
Cambridge, MA 02139-9031
800-225-5750
Fax: 888-440-2665
http://eps.schoolspecialty.com
customer_service@epsbooks.com
Priscilla L Vail, Author
Offers guidelines for reading instruction in the primary grades that combines whole language with multisensory phonics instruction. *$8.95*
88 pages
ISBN 0-838852-11-4

2467 **Common Sense About Dyslexia**
Special Needs Project
Ste H
324 State St
Santa Barbara, CA 93101-2364
818-718-9900
800-333-6867
Fax: 818-349-2027
http://www.specialneeds.com
books@specialneeds.com
Ann Marshall Huston, Author
Offers important, need-to-know information about dyslexia. *$26.50*
284 pages Hardcover
ISBN 0-819163-23-6

2468 **Complete IEP Guide: How to Advocate for Your Special Ed Child**
NOLO
950 Parker St
Berkeley, CA 94710-2524
800-728-3555
Fax: 800-645-0895
http://www.nolo.com
Lawrence M Siegel, Author
This book has all the plain-English suggestions, strategies, resources and forms to develop an effective IEP. *$34.99*
402 pages paperback
ISBN 1-413305-10-5

2469 **Complete Learning Disabilities Resource Library**
Slosson Educational Publications
PO Box 544
538 Buffalo Road
East Aurora, NY 14052
716-652-0930
888-756-7766
Fax: 800-655-3840
http://www.slosson.com
slosson@slosson.com
Joan M Harwell, Author
These volumes provide easy-to-use tips, techniques, and activities to help students with learning disabilities at all grade levels. *$29.95*
320 pages Paperback
ISBN 0-787972-32-0

2470 **Computer & Web Resources for People with Disabilities: A Guide to...**
Alliance for Technology Access
1119 Old Humboldt Road
Jackson, TN 38305
731-554-5282
800-914-3017
Fax: 731-554-5283
TTY: 731-554-5284
http://www.ataccess.org
atainfo@ataccess.org
James Allison, President
Bob Van der Linde, VP
Mike Hewirr, Treasurer
This highly acclaimed book includes detailed descriptions of software, hardware and communication aids, plus a gold mine of published and online resources. *$20.75*
364 pages

2471 **Conducting Individualized Education Program Meetings that Withstand Due Process**
Charles C Thomas Publisher
PO Box 19265
Springfield, IL 62794-9265
217-789-8980
800-258-8980
Fax: 217-789-9130
http://www.ccthomas.com
books@ccthomas.com
James N Hollis, Author
Publisher of Education and Special Education books. *$41.95*
171 pages Hardcover
ISBN 0-398068-46-1

2472 **Connecting Students: A Guide to Thoughtful Friendship Facilitation**
PEAK Parent Center
Ste 200
611 N Weber St
Colorado Springs, CO 80903-1072
719-531-9400
800-284-0251
Fax: 719-531-9452
http://www.peakparent.org
info@peakparent.org
C Beth Schaffner, Author
Barbara Buswell, Co-Author

Offers real-life examples of how friendship facilitation can be implemented in natural ways in schools, neighborhoods, and communities. Perfect for anyone working to build classrooms and schools that ensure caring, acceptance and belonging for ALL students. *$11.00*
48 pages Paperback
ISBN 1-884720-01-3

2473 Contemporary Intellectual Assessment: Theories, Tests and Issues
Guilford Publications
72 Spring St
New York, NY 10012-4019
212-431-9800
800-365-7006
Fax: 212-966-6708
http://www.guilford.com
info@guilford.com
Patti L Harrison, Editor
Judy L Genshaft, Editor
This unique volume provides a comprehensive conceptual and practical overview of the current state of the art of intellectual assessment. The book covers major theories of intelligence, methods of assessing human cognitive abilities, and issues related to the validity of current intelligence test batteries. *$75.00*
667 pages Hardcover
ISBN 1-593851-25-1

2474 Deciding What to Teach and How to Teach It Connecting Students through Curriculum and Instruction
PEAK Parent Center
Ste 200
611 N Weber St
Colorado Springs, CO 80903-1072
719-531-9400
800-284-0251
Fax: 719-531-9452
http://www.peakparent.org
info@peakparent.org
Elizabeth Castagnera, Author
Douglas Fisher, Co-Author
Karen Rodifer, Co-Author
Provides exciting and practical resource tips to ensure that all students participate and learn successfully in secondary general education classrooms. Leads the reader through a step-by-step process for accessing general curriculum, making accommodations and modifications, and providing appropriate supports. Planning grids and concrete strategies make this an essential tool for both secondary educators and families. Support strategies are enhanced in this second edition *$ 14.00*
48 pages
ISBN 1-884720-19-6

2475 Defiant Children
Guilford Publications
72 Spring St
New York, NY 10012-4019
212-431-9800
800-365-7006
Fax: 212-966-6708
http://www.guilford.com
info@guilford.com
Russell A Barkley, Author
Christine M Benton, Co-Author
This book is written expressly for parents who are struggling with an unyielding or combative child, helping them understand what causes defiance, when it becomes a problem, and how it can be resolved. Its clear eight-step program stresses consistency and cooperation, promoting changes through a system of praise, rewards, and mild punishment. Filled with helpful sidebars, charts, and checklists. *$39.00*
264 pages Paperback
ISBN 1-572301-23-6

2476 Developing Fine and Gross Motor Skills
Therapro
225 Arlington St
Framingham, MA 01702-8723
508-872-9494
800-257-5376
Fax: 508-875-2062
http://www.therapro.com
info@therapro.com
Donna Staisiunas Hurley, Author
This new home exercise program has dozens of beautifully illustrated, reproducible handouts for the parent, therapists, health care and child care workers. Each interval of 3 to 6 months in the child's development is divided into a fine motor and a gross motor section. Each section has several exercise sheets that guide parents in ways to develop specific motor skills that typically occur at that age level. Also includes practical information on how to guide parents when doing the exerecises.
157 pages
ISBN 0-890799-43-1

2477 Diamonds in the Rough
Slosson Educational Publications
PO Box 544
538 Buffalo Road
East Aurora, NY 14052
716-652-0930
888-756-7766
Fax: 800-655-3840
http://www.slosson.com
slosson@slosson.com
Peggy Strass Dias, Author
An invaluable multidisciplinary reference guide to learning disabilities. It is an indispensable resource for educators, health specialists, parents and librarians. The author has printed a clear picture of the archetypical learner with a step-by-step view of the learning disabled child. *$53.00*
156 pages Spiral-Bound
ISBN 0-970379-90-0

2478 Dictionary of Special Education & Rehabilitation
Love Publishing Company
Ste 2200
9101 E Kenyon Ave
Denver, CO 80237-1854
303-221-7333
Fax: 303-221-7444
http://www.lovepublishing.com
lpc@lovepublishing.com
Glenn A Vergason, Author
M L Anderegg, Co-Author
This updated edition of one of the most valuable resources in the field is over six years in the making incorporates hundreds of additions. It provides clear, understandable definitions of more than 2,000 terms unique to special education and rehabilitation. *$34.95*
210 pages Paperback
ISBN 0-891082-43-3

2479 Early Childhood Special Education: Birth to Three
Connecticut Assoc for Children and Adults with LD
Ste 15-5
25 Van Zant St
Norwalk, CT 06855-1729
203-838-5010
Fax: 203-866-6108
http://www.cacld.org
cacld@optonline.net
J B Jordan, Author
Beryl Kaufman, Executive Director
Resources on early childhood education. *$34.00*
262 pages Paperback
ISBN 0-865861-79-X

2480 **Educating Deaf Children Bilingually**
Harris Communications
15155 Technology Dr
Eden Prairie, MN 55344-2273
952-906-1180
800-825-9187
Fax: 866-870-7323
TDD: 952-906-1198
TTY: 800-825-9187
http://www.harriscomm.com
info@harriscomm.com
Darla Hudson, Customer Service
Shawn Neal Mahshie, Author
Perspectives and practices in educating deaf children with the goal of grade-level achievement in fluency in the languages of the deaf community, general society and of the home are discussed in this book. Part #B442. *$16.95*
262 pages

2481 **Educating Students Who Have Visual Impairments with Other Disabilities**
Brookes Publishing Company
PO Box 10624
Baltimore, MD 21285
410-337-9580
800-638-3775
Fax: 410-337-8539
http://www.brookespublishing.com
custserv@brookespublishing.com
Sharon Z Sacks PhD, Editor
Rosanne K Silberman EdD, Editor
This text provides techniques for facilitating functional learning in students with a wide range of visual impairments and multiple disabilities. *$49.95*
552 pages Paperback
ISBN 1-557662-80-0

2482 **Effective Teaching Methods for Autistic Children**
Charles C Thomas
PO Box 19265
Springfield, IL 62794-9265
217-789-8980
800-258-8980
Fax: 217-789-9130
http://www.ccthomas.com
books@ccthomas.com
Rosalind C Oppenheim, Author
Publisher of Education and Special Education books. *$21.25*
116 pages Hardcover
ISBN 0-398028-58-3

2483 **Emergence: Labeled Autistic**
Academic Therapy Publications
20 Commercial Blvd
Novato, CA 94949-6120
415-883-3314
800-422-7249
Fax: 888-287-9975
http://www.academictherapy.com
books@ccthomas.com
Jim Arena, President
Joanne Urban, Manager
An autistic individual shares her history, and includes her own suggestions for parents and professionals. Technical Appendix, which overviews recent treatment methods and more.

2484 **Essential ASL: The Fun, Fast, and Simple Way to Learn American Sign Language**
Harris Communications
15155 Technology Dr
Eden Prairie, MN 55344-2273
952-906-1180
800-825-6758
Fax: 866-870-7323
TDD: 952-906-1198
TTY: 800-825-9187
http://www.harriscomm.com
info@harriscomm.com
Darla Hudson, Customer Service
This pocket version contains more than 700 frequently used signs with 2,000 easy-to-follow illustrations. Also, 50 common phrases. Part #B511. *$7.95*
322 pages Paperback

2485 **Family Guide to Assistive Technology**
Federation for Children with Special Needs
Suite 1102
529 Main Street
Boston, MA 02109
617-236-7210
800-331-0688
Fax: 617-241-0330
http://www.fcsn.org
fcsninfo@fcsn.org
Katherine A Kelker, Author
Roger Holt, Co-Author
John Sullivan, Co-Author
This guide is intended to help parents learn more about assistive technology and how it can help their children. Includes tips for getting started, ideas about how and where to look for funding and contact information for software and equipment. *$15.95*
160 pages Paperback
ISBN 1-571290-74-5

2486 **Family Place in Cyberspace**
Alliance for Technology Access
1119 Old Humboldt Road
Jackson, TN 38305
731-554-5282
800-914-3017
Fax: 731-554-5283
TTY: 731-554-5284
http://www.ataccess.org
atainfo@ataccess.org
Allegra Wilson, Administrative Assistant
Todd Plummer, Development Manager
Includes We Can Play, a variety of suggestions and ideas for making play activities accessible to all. Available in English and Spanish. Access in Transition. Information and resources for students with disabilities who are facing the transition from public school to the next stage in life. Includes links and resources. Assistive Technology in K-12 Schools gives a range of information about integrating assistive technology into schools.

2487 **Fine Motor Skills in Children with Downs Syndrome: A Guide for Parents and Professionals**
Therapro
225 Arlington St
Framingham, MA 01702-8773
508-872-9494
800-257-5376
Fax: 508-875-2062
http://www.theraproducts.com
info@theraproducts.com
Maryanne Bruni, Author
Fine motor skills are the hand skills that allow us to do the things like hold a pencil, cut with scissors, eat with a fork, and use a computer. This practical guide shows parents and professionals how to help children with Downs syndrome from infancy to 12 years improve fine motor functioning. Includes many age appropriate activities for home or school, with step by step instructions and photos. Invaluable for families and professionals. *$19.95*
241 pages Paperback
ISBN 1-890627-67-4

2488 **Fine Motor Skills in the Classroom: Screening & Remediation Strategies**
Therapro
225 Arlington St
Framingham, MA 01702-8773
508-620-0022
800-257-5376
Fax: 508-620-0023
http://www.theraproducts.com
info@theraproducts.com
Arthur Berry, Author

The Give Yourself a Hand program, revised. Developed as a tool to facilitate consultation in the classroom. The manual consists of training modules, a screening to administer to an entire class, report formats for teachers and parents, and classroom and home remediation activities. The program is designed to include everyone involved in the education process and to make them aware of the opportunites offered by occupational therapy in the classroom.
96 pages

2489 **Flying By the Seat of Your Pants: More Absurdities and Realities of Special Education**
Corwin Press
2455 Teller Rd
Thousand Oaks, CA 91320-2218
805-499-9734
800-233-9936
Fax: 805-499-5323
http://www.corwin.com
order@corwin.com
Michael F Giangreco, Author
Kevin Ruelle, Co-Author
In the sequel to Ants in His Pants, Giangreco continues to stimulate the reader to think differently about some of our current educational practices and raise questions about specific issues surrounding special education. Whether an educator, parent or advocate for persons with disabilities, you will smile, laugh aloud and ponder the hidden truths playfully captured in these carefully crafted cartoons. Transparencies may be created directly from the book. *$20.95*
112 pages Paperback
ISBN 1-890455-41-5

2490 **Gross Motor Skills Children with Down Syndrome: A Guide For Parents and Professionals**
Therapro
225 Arlington St
Framingham, MA 01702-8723
508-872-9494
800-257-5376
Fax: 508-875-2062
http://www.therapro.com
info@therapro.com
Patricia C Winders, Author
Children with Down syndrome master basic gross motor skills, everything from rolling over to running, just as their peers do, but may need additional help. This guide describes and illustrates more than 100 easy to follow activities for parents and professionals to practice with infants and children from birth to age six. Checklists and statistics allow readers to track, plan and maximize a child's progress. *$18.95*
236 pages
ISBN 0-933149-81-6

2491 **Guide for Parents on Hyperactivity in Children Fact Sheet**
Learning Disabilities Association of America
4156 Library Rd
Pittsburgh, PA 15234-1349
412-341-1515
Fax: 412-344-0224
http://www.ldanatl.org
ldanatl@usaor.net
Klaus K Minde, Author
Describes difficulties faced by a child with ADHD. Elaborates on types of management and ends with a section called 'A Day With a Hyperactive Child: Possible Problems'. *$2.00*
23 pages

2492 **Guide to Private Special Education**
Porter Sargent Handbooks
2 LAN Drive
Suite 100
Westford, MA 01886
978-692-9708
Fax: 978-692-2304
http://www.portersargent.com
info@portersargent.com
Daniel P. McKeever, Senior Editor
Leslie Weston, Manager
Lists and describes educational programs for families and consultants looking to place elementary and secondary students with special needs in the best possible learning environments. *$75.00*
1152 pages Triannual
ISBN 0-875581-50-1

2493 **Guidelines and Recommended Practices for Individualized Family Service Plan**
Education Resources Information Center
Suite 500
655 15th St. NW
Washington, DC 20005
800-538-3742
http://www.eric.ed.gov
Mary J McGonigel, Author
Presents a growing consensus about best practices for comprehensive family-centered early intervention services as required by Part H of the Individuals with Disabilities Education Act. *$15.00*
208 pages

2494 **Handbook for Implementing Workshops for Siblings of Special Needs Children**
Special Needs Project
Ste H
324 State St
Santa Barbara, CA 93101-2364
818-718-9900
800-333-6867
Fax: 818-349-2027
http://www.specialneeds.com
books@specialneeds.com
Donald Meyer, Author
Based on three years of professional experience working with siblings ages 8 through 13 and their parents, this handbook provides guidelines and technologies for those who wish to start and conduct workshops for siblings. *$40.00*
65 pages

2495 **Handbook of Research in Emotional and Behavioral Disorders**
Guilford Publications
72 Spring St
New York, NY 10012-4019
212-431-9800
800-365-7006
Fax: 212-966-6708
http://www.guilford.com
info@guilford.com
Robert B Rutherford Jr, Author
Mary Magee Quinn, Co-Author
Sarup R Mathur, Editor
Integrates current knowledge on emotional and behavioral disorders in the school setting. Also, emphasizes the importance of interdisciplinary collaboration in service provision and delineates best-practice guidelines for research. *$38.00*
622 pages Paperback
ISBN 1-593854-71-4

2496 **Handling the Young Child with Cerebral Palsy at Home**
Therapro
225 Arlington St
Framingham, MA 01702-8723
508-872-9494
800-257-5376
Fax: 508-875-2062
http://www.therapro.com
info@therapro.com
Nancie R Finnie, Author
This guide for parents remains a classic book on handling their cerebral palsied child during all activities of daily living. It has been said that its message is so important that it should be read by all those caring for such children including doctors, therapists, teachers and nurses. Many simple line drawings illustrate handling problems and solutions. *$55.95*
320 pages paperback
ISBN 0-750605-79-0

2497 **Help Build a Brighter Future: Children at Risk for LD in Child Care Centers**
Learning Disabilities Association of America
4156 Library Rd
Pittsburgh, PA 15234-1349
412-341-1515
Fax: 412-344-0224
http://www.ldanatl.org
ldanatl@usaor.net

Offers information for parents and professionals caring for the learning disabled child. *$3.00*

2498 **Help Me to Help My Child**
Hachette Book Group
3 Center Plz
Boston, MA 02108-2003
800-759-0190
Fax: 800-331-1664
http://www.hachettebookgroup.com
customer.service@hbgusa.com

Jill Bloom, Author

Contains nontechnical information on testing, advocacy, legal issues, instructional practices, and social-emotional development, as well as a resource list and bibliography.

324 pages Hardcover
ISBN 0-316099-81-3

2499 **Help for the Hyperactive Child: A Good Sense Guide for Parents**
Learning Disabilities Association of America
4156 Library Rd
Pittsburgh, PA 15234-1349
412-341-1515
Fax: 412-344-0224
http://www.ldanatl.org
ldanatl@usaor.net

William G Crook, Author

A practical guide; offering parents of ADHD children alternatives to Ritalin. *$16.95*

245 pages
ISBN 0-933478-18-6

2500 **Help for the Learning Disabled Child**
Slosson Educational Publications
PO Box 544
538 Buffalo Road
East Aurora, NY 14052
716-652-0930
888-756-7766
Fax: 800-655-3840
http://www.slosson.com
slosson@slosson.com

Lou Stewart, Author

An easy-to-read text describes observable behaviors, offers remediation techniques, materials, and specific test to assist in further diagnosis.

2501 **Helping Your Child with Attention-Deficit Hyperactivity Disorder**
Learning Disabilities Association of America
4156 Library Rd
Pittsburgh, PA 15234-1349
412-341-1515
Fax: 412-344-0224
http://www.ldanatl.org
ldanatl@usaor.net

M Fowler, Author

2502 **Helping Your Hyperactive Child**
Connecticut Assoc for Children and Adults with LD
Ste 15-5
25 Van Zant St
Norwalk, CT 06855-1729
203-838-5010
Fax: 203-866-6108
http://www.cacld.org
cacld@optonline.net

Beryl Kaufman, Executive Director
John Taylor, Author

A large, comprehensive book for parents, covering everything from techniques pertaining to sibling rivalry to coping with marital stresses. Contains thorough discussions of various treatments: nutritional, medical and educational. Also is an excellent source of advice and information for parents of kids with ADHD.

496 pages Hardcover
ISBN 1-559580-13-5

2503 **How the Special Needs Brain Learns**
Corwin Press
2455 Teller Rd
Thousand Oaks, CA 91320-2218
805-499-9734
800-233-9936
Fax: 805-499-5323
http://www.corwin.com
order@corwin.com

David A Sousa, Author

Research on the brain function of students with various learning challenges. Practical classroom activities and strategies, such as how to build self-esteem, how to work in groups, and strategies for engagement and retention. Focuses on the most commmon challenges to learning for many students. *$35.95*

248 pages Paperback
ISBN 1-412949-87-4

2504 **How to Get Services by Being Assertive**
Family Resource Center on Disabilities
Room 300
20 E Jackson Blvd
Chicago, IL 60604-2265
312-939-3513
800-952-4199
Fax: 312-854-8980
TDD: 312-939-3519
http://www.frcd.org
info@frcd.org

Charlotte Jardins, Executive Director
Myra Christian, Contact
Gloria Mikucki, Contact

A 100 page manual that demonstrates positive assertiveness techniques. Price includes postage and handling. *$12.00*

2505 **How to Organize Your Child and Save Your Sanity**
Learning Disabilities Association of America
4156 Library Rd
Pittsburgh, PA 15234-1349
412-341-1515
Fax: 412-344-0224
http://www.ldanatl.org
ldanatl@usaor.net

Ruth Brown, Author
13 pages $3.00

2506 **How to Organize an Effective Parent-Advocacy Group and Move Bureaucracies**
Family Resource Center on Disabilities
Room 300
20 E Jackson Blvd
Chicago, IL 60604-2265
312-939-3513
800-952-4199
Fax: 312-854-8980
TDD: 312-939-3519
http://www.frcd.org
info@frcd.org

Charlotte Jardins, Executive Director
Myra Christian, Contact
Gloria Mikucki, Contact

A 100-page handbook that gives step-by-step directions for organizing parent support groups from scratch. *$12.00*

2507 **How to Own and Operate an Attention Deficit Disorder**
Learning Disabilities Association of America
4156 Library Rd
Pittsburgh, PA 15234-1349
412-341-1515
Fax: 412-344-0224
http://www.ldanatl.org
ldanatl@usaor.net

Debra W Maxey, Author

Clear, informative and sensitive introduction to ADHD. Packed with practical things to do at home and school, the author offers her insight as a professional and mother of a son with ADHD. *$8.95*
43 pages

2508 **Hyperactive Children Grown Up**
Guilford Publications
72 Spring St
New York, NY 10012-4019
212-431-9800
800-365-7006
Fax: 212-966-6708
http://www.guilford.com
info@guilford.com
Gabrielle Weiss, Author
Long considered a standard in the field, this book explores what happens to hyperactive children when they grow into adulthood. Updated and expanded, this second edition describes new developments in ADHD, current psychological treatments of ADHD, contemporary perspectives on the use of medications, and assessment, diagnosis and treatment of ADHD adults. *$35.00*
473 pages Paperback
ISBN 0-898625-96-3

2509 **If it is to Be, It is Up to Me to Do it!**
AVKO Educational Research Foundation
Ste W
3084 Willard Rd
Birch Run, MI 48415-9404
810-686-9283
866-285-6612
Fax: 810-686-1101
http://www.avko.org
webmaster@avko.orgÿ
Don Mc Cabe, Research Director/Author
This is a tutors' book that can be used by anyone who can read this paragraph. It also contains the student's response pages. It is especially good to use to help an older child or adult. It uses the same basic format as Sequential Spelling I except it has the sentences to be read along with the word to be spelled. The students get to correct their own mistakes immediately. This way they quickly learn that mistakes are opportunities to learn. *$19.95*
96 pages
ISBN 1-564007-42-1

2510 **In Their Own Way: Discovering and Encouraging Your Child's Learning**
Special Needs Project
Ste H
324 State St
Santa Barbara, CA 93101-2364
818-718-9900
800-333-6867
Fax: 818-349-2027
http://www.specialneeds.com
books@specialneeds.com
Dr Thomas Armstrong, Author
An unconventional teacher has written a very popular book for a wide audience. It's customary to be categorical about youngsters who learn conventionally/are normal/are OK — and those who don't/who need special ed/are learning disabled. *$8.37*
224 pages Paperback
ISBN 0-791716-67-8

2511 **In Time and with Love**
Special Needs Project
Ste H
324 State St
Santa Barbara, CA 93101-2364
818-718-9900
800-333-6867
Fax: 818-349-2027
http://www.specialneeds.com
books@specialneeds.com
Marilyn Segal, Author
Wendy Masi, Co-Author
Roni Leiderman, Co-Author
Play and parenting techniques for children with disabilities. *$18.95*
256 pages Paperback

2512 **In the Mind's Eye**
Prometheus Books
59 John Glenn Drive
Amherst, NY 14228-2197
716-691-0133
800-421-0351
Fax: 716-691-0137
http://www.prometheusbooks.com
marketing@prometheusbooks.com
Thomas West, Author
The second edition will review a number of recent developments, which support and extend the ideas and perspectives originally set forth in the first edition. Among these will be brief profiles of two dyslexic scientists known for their ability to generate, in quite different fields, powerful but unexpected innovations and discoveries. *$25.98*
440 pages
ISBN 1-591027-00-3

2513 **Inclusion: A Practical Guide for Parents**
Corwin Press
2455 Teller Rd
Thousand Oaks, CA 91320-2218
805-499-9734
800-233-9936
Fax: 805-499-5323
http://www.corwin.com
order@corwin.com
Lorraine O Moore, Author
This comprehensive resource answers parent questions related to inclusive education and provides the tools to promote and enhance their child's learning. This publication includes practical strategies, exercises, questionnaires and do-it-yourself graphs to assist parents with their child's learning. Beneficial for parents, psychologists, social workers, and educators. *$28.95*
152 pages
ISBN 1-890455-44-6

2514 **Inclusion: Strategies for Working with Young Children**
Corwin Press
2455 Teller Rd
Thousand Oaks, CA 91320-2218
805-499-9734
800-233-9936
Fax: 805-499-5323
http://www.corwin.com
order@corwin.com
Lorraine O Moore, Author
Developed for early childhood through grade two educators and parents, this comprehensive developmentally focused publication focuses on the whole child. Hundreds of developmentally-based strategies help young children learn about feelings, empathy, resolving conflicts, communication, large/small motor development, prereading, writing and math strategies are included, plus much more. Excellent training tool. *$28.95*
146 pages
ISBN 1-890455-33-4

2515 **Inclusive Elementary Schools**
PEAK Parent Center
Ste 200
611 N Weber St
Colorado Springs, CO 80903-1072
719-531-9400
800-284-0251
Fax: 719-531-9452
http://www.peakparent.org
info@peakparent.org
Douglas Fisher, Author
Nancy Frey, Co-Author
Caren Sax, Co-Author

Walks readers through a state of the art, step-by-step process to determine what and how to teach elementary school students with disabilities in general education classrooms. Highlights strategies for accommodating and modifying assignments and activities by using core curriculum. Complete with user-friendly sample forms and creative support strategies, this is an essential text for elementary educators and parents. *$13.00*
45 pages Paperback
ISBN 1-884720-21-8

2516 **Innovations in Family Support for People with Learning Disabilities**
Brookes Publishing Company
PO Box 10624
Baltimore, MD 21285
410-337-9580
800-638-3775
Fax: 410-337-8539
http://www.brookespublishing.com
custserv@pbrookes.com
Barbara Coyne Cutler, Author
272 pages Paperback $22.00
ISBN 1-870335-15-5

2517 **Interventions for ADHD: Treatment in Developmental Context**
Guilford Publications
72 Spring St
New York, NY 10012-4019
212-431-9800
800-365-7006
Fax: 212-966-6708
http://www.guilford.com
info@guilford.com
Phyllis Anne Teeter, Author
This book takes a lifespan perspective on ADHD, dispelling the notion that it is only a disorder of childhood and enabling clinicians to develop effective and appropriate interventions for preschoolers, school-age children, adolescents, and adults. The author reviews empirically-and clinically-based treatment interventions including psychopharmacology, behavior management, parent/teacher training, and self-management techniques. *$40.00*
378 pages Hardcover
ISBN 1-572303-84-0

2518 **Invisible Disability: Understanding Learning Disabilities in the Context of Health & Edu.**
Learning Disabilities Association of America
4156 Library Rd
Pittsburgh, PA 15234-1349
412-341-1515
Fax: 412-344-0224
http://www.ldanatl.org
ldanatl@usaor.net
Pasquale Accardo, Author
50 pages Paperback $9.00
ISBN 0-937846-39-2

2519 **It's Your Turn Now**
Harris Communications
15155 Technology Dr
Eden Prairie, MN 55344-2273
952-906-1180
800-825-6758
Fax: 866-870-7323
TDD: 952-906-1198
TTY: 800-825-9187
http://www.harriscomm.com
info@harriscomm.com
Darla Hudson, Customer Service
Using dialogue journals with deaf students help the students learn to enjoy communicating ideas, information, and feelings through reading and writing. The book reviews teacher's questions and answers, frustrations and successes. Part #B584. *$14.95*
130 pages

2520 **Key Concepts in Personal Development**
Marsh Media
PO Box 8082
Shawnee Mission
Kansas City, MO 66208
800-821-3303
Fax: 866-333-7421
http://www.marshmedia.com
info@marshmedia.com
Puberty Education for Students with Special Needs. Comprehensive, gender-specific kits and supplemental parent packets address human sexuality education for children with mild to moderate developmental disabilities. *$19.95*

2521 **Ladders to Literacy: A Kindergarten Activity Book**
Brookes Publishing Company
PO Box 10624
Baltimore, MD 21285
410-337-9580
800-638-3775
Fax: 410-337-8539
http://www.brookespublishing.com
custserv@brookspublishing.com
Rollanda E O'Connor, Author
Angela Notari Syverson, Co-Author
Patricia F Vadasy, Co-Author
The kindergarten activities are designed for higher developmental levels, focusing on preacademic skills, early literacy development, and early reading development. Goals and scaffolding are more intense as children learn to recognize letters, match sounds with letters, and develop phonological awareness and the alphabetic principle. *$49.95*
337 pages Spiral bound
ISBN 1-557668-32-9

2522 **Ladders to Literacy: A Preschool Activity Book**
Brookes Publishing Company
PO Box 10624
Baltimore, MD 21285
410-337-9580
800-638-3775
Fax: 410-337-8539
http://www.brookespublishing.com
custserv@brookespublishing.com
Rollanda E O'Connor, Author
Angela Notari Syverson, Co-Author
The preschool activity book targets basic preliteracy skills such as orienting children toward printed materials and teaching letter sounds. It also provides professionals (and parents) with developmentally appropriate and ecologically valid assessment procedures — informal observation guidelines, structured performance samples, and a checklist — for measuring children's learning. *$49.95*
486 pages Spiral bound
ISBN 1-557669-13-9

2523 **Landmark School's Language-Based Teaching Guides**
Landmark School
429 Hale St
PO Box 227
Prides Crossing, MA 01965
978-236-3216
Fax: 978-927-7268
http://www.landmarkoutreach.org
outreach@landmarkschool.org
Robert Broudo, Author
Landmark School's Language-Based Teaching Guides provide research-based practical teaching strategies for teachers and parents working with students who have learning disabilities. Topics inlcude study skills, expressive langage skills, writing, mathematics. *$30.00*
104 pages Paperback
ISBN 0-962411-96-5

2524 **Language and Literacy Learning in Schools**
Guilford Publications
72 Spring St
New York, NY 10012-4019
212-431-9800
800-365-7006
Fax: 212-966-6708
http://www.guilford.com
info@guilford.com

Elaine R Stillman, Author
Louise C Wilkinson, Co-Author
Interweaves the voices of classroom teachers, speech-language pathologists whos children learning to become literate in English as a first or second language, and researchers from multiple disciplines. *$27.00*
366 pages Hardcover
ISBN 1-593854-69-2

2525 **Language-Related Learning Disabilities**
Brookes Publishing Company
PO Box 10624
Baltimore, MD 21285 410-337-9580
800-638-3775
Fax: 410-337-8539
http://www.brookespublishing.com
custserv@pbrookes.com
Adele Gerber, Author
416 pages Hardcover $47.00
ISBN 1-557660-53-0

2526 **Learning Disabilities & ADHD: A Family Guide to Living and Learning Together**
John Wiley & Sons Inc
111 River Street
Hoboken, NJ 07030-5774 201-748-6000
Fax: 201-748-6088
http://www.wiley.com
info@wiley.com
Betty Osman, Author
228 pages paperback $14.95
ISBN 0-471155-10-1

2527 **Learning Disabilities A to Z**
Simon and Schuster
1230 Avenue of the Americas
New York, NY 10020-1513 212-698-7000
800-233-2336
http://www.simonandschuster.biz
shop.feedback@simonsays.com
Corinne Smith, Author
Lisa Strick, Co-Author
Brings the best of recent research and educational experience to parents, teachers and caregivers who are responsible for children with information processing problems. Corinne Smith and Lisa Strick provide a comprehensive guide to the causes, indentification and treatment of learning disabilities. You will learn how these subtle neurological disorders can have a major impact on a child's development, both in and out of school. *$17.00*
416 pages Paperback
ISBN 0-684844-68-0

2528 **Learning Disabilities: Lifelong Issues**
Brookes Publishing Company
PO Box 10624
Baltimore, MD 21285 410-337-9580
800-638-3775
Fax: 410-337-8539
http://www.brookespublishing.com
custserv@brookespublishing.com
Shirley C Cramer, Author
William Ellis, Editor
Based on the diverse, representative viewpoints of educators, practitioners, policy makers, and adults with learning disabilities, this volume sets forth an agenda for improving the educational and ultimately, social and economic, futures of people with learning disabilities. *$36.00*
319 pages Paperback
ISBN 1-557662-40-1

2529 **Learning Disabilities: Literacy, and Adult Education**
Brookes Publishing Company
PO Box 10624
Baltimore, MD 21285 410-337-9580
800-638-3775
Fax: 410-337-8539
http://www.brookespublishing.com
custserv@pbrookes.com
Susan A Vogel PhD, Author
Stephen Reder PhD, Editor
This book focuses on adults with severe learning disabilities and the educators who work with them. *$49.95*
377 pages Paperback
ISBN 1-557663-47-5

2530 **Learning Disabilities: Theories, Diagnosis and Teaching Strategies**
Houghton Mifflin
222 Berkeley St
Boston, MA 02116-3748 617-351-5000
Fax: 617-351-1119
http://www.houghtonmifflinbooks.com
TradeCustomerService@hmhpub.com
J Lerner, Author
Theories on learning disabilities.
ISBN 0-395794-86-2

2531 **Learning Outside The Lines: Two Ivy League Students with Learning Disabilities and ADHD**
Fireside
1230 Avenue of the Americas
New York, NY 10020-1513 212-698-7000
800-233-2336
http://www.simonandschuster.biz
shop.feedback@simonsays.com
Edward M Hallowell, Author
Jonathan Mooney, Co-Author
David Cole, Co-Author
Takes you on a personal empowerment and profound educational change, proving once again that rules sometimes need to be broken. *$14.00*
288 pages
ISBN 0-684865-98-X

2532 **Legacy of the Blue Heron: Living with Learning Disabilities**
Oxton House Publishers
124 Main Street
Suite 203
Farmington, ME 04938 207-779-1923
800-539-7323
Fax: 207-779-0623
http://www.oxtonhouse.com
info@oxtonhouse.com
William Berlinghoff PhD, Managing Editor
Cheryl Martin, Marketing
Debra Richards, Office Manager
This book is available in soft cover or as a six-cassette audiobook. It is an engaging personal account by a severe dyslexic who became a successful engineer, business man, boat builder, and president of the Learning Disabilities Association of America. Drawing on his life experiences, the author presents a rich array of wise, common-sense advice for dealing with learning disabilities.
256 pages Paperback
ISBN 1-881929-20-5

2533 **Let's Learn About Deafness**
Harris Communications
15155 Technology Dr
Eden Prairie, MN 55344-2273 952-906-1180
800-825-6758
Fax: 866-870-7323
TDD: 952-906-1198
TTY: 800-825-9187
http://www.harriscomm.com
info@harriscomm.com
Darla Hudson, Customer Service
Hands-on activities, games, bulletin board displays, surveys, quizzes, craft projects, and skits used to help teachers and their students become more aware of deafness and its implications are included in this book. Part #B253. *$ 16.95*
82 pages

2534 **Life Beyond the Classroom: Transition Strategies for Young People with Disabilities**
Brookes Publishing Company
PO Box 10624
Baltimore, MD 21285
410-337-9580
800-638-3775
Fax: 410-337-8539
http://www.brookespublishing.com
custserv@brookespublishing.com
Paul Wehman, Author
Community living, leisure activities, personal relationships as well as employment. Planning with community, individualized, state and local governments, curriculum for transition, job development and placement, independent living plans for people with mild MR, severe disabilities, LD, physical and health impairments, and traumatic brain injury. *$74.95*
719 pages Hardcover
ISBN 1-557667-52-7

2535 **Living with a Learning Disability**
Southern Illinois University Press
1915 University Press Dr
Carbondale, IL 62901-4323
618-453-2281
800-621-2736
Fax: 800-453-1221
http://www.siupress.com
custserv@press.uchicago.edu
Barbara Martin, Director
Amy Etcheson, Marketing and Sales Manager
This book presents the kinds of adaptations needed for educating, communicating with, and parenting the child, the adolescent, and the young adult with learning disabilities. Deals with such issues as relationships, the legal process, implications for the professional, juvenile delinquency, and the future.
17.5 pages
ISBN 0-809316-68-4

2536 **Making the Writing Process Work: Strategies for Composition & Self-Regulation**
Brookline Books
Suite B-001
8 Trumbull Rd
Northampton, MA 01060
413-584-0184
800-666-2665
Fax: 413-5846184
http://www.brooklinebooks.com
brbooks@yahoo.com
Karen R Harris, Author
Steve Graham, Co-Author
Presents cognitive strategies for writing sequences of specific steps which make the writing process clearer and enable students to organize their thoughts about the writing task. *$24.95*
239 pages Paperback
ISBN 1-571290-10-9

2537 **McGraw Hill Companies**
PO Box 182604
Columbus, OH 43272-2604
877-833-5524
Fax: 614-759-3749
http://www.mcgraw-hill.com
customer.service@mcgraw-hill.com
Henry Hirschberg, President
Corrective reading program, helps students master the essential decoding and comprehension skills.

2538 **Me! A Curriculum for Teaching Self-Esteem Through an Interest Center**
Connecticut Assoc for Children and Adults with LD
Ste 15-5
25 Van Zant St
Norwalk, CT 06855-1729
203-838-5010
Fax: 203-866-6108
http://www.cacld.org
cacld@optonline.com
Beryl Kaufman, Executive Director
A curriculum for the professional. *$18.50*

2539 **Meeting the Needs of Students of ALL Abilities**
Corwin Press
2455 Teller Rd
Thousand Oaks, CA 91320-2218
805-499-9734
800-233-9936
Fax: 805-499-5323
http://www.corwin.com
order@corwin.com
Colleen Capper, Author
Elise Fattura, Co-Author
Maureen Keyes, Co-Author
Step-by-step handbook offers practical strategies for administrators, teachers, policymakers and parents who want to shift from costly special learning programs for a few students, to excellent educational services for all students and teachers, and adapting curriculum and instruction. *$75.95*
224 pages Hardcover
ISBN 0-761975-00-4

2540 **Misunderstood Child**
Connecticut Assoc for Children and Adults with LD
Ste 15-5
25 Van Zant St
Norwalk, CT 06855-1729
203-838-5010
Fax: 203-866-6108
http://www.cacld.org
cacld@optonline.net
Beryl Kaufman, Executive Director
A guide for parents of learning disabled children. *$14.95*
448 pages Paperback
ISBN 0-307338-63-0

2541 **Negotiating the Special Education Maze**
Woodbine House
6510 Bells Mill Rd
Bethesda, MD 20817-1636
301-897-3570
800-843-7323
Fax: 301-897-5838
http://www.woodbinehouse.com
info@woodbinehouse.com
Stephen Chitwood, Author
Deidre Hayden, Co-Author
Now in its fourth edition, Negotiating the Special Education Maze isone of the best tools available to parents and teachers for developing an effective special education program for their child or student. Every step is explained, from eligibility and evaluation to the Individualized Education Program and beyond. *$16.95*
264 pages Paperback
ISBN 0-933149-72-7

2542 **New Language of Toys**
Woodbine House
6510 Bells Mill Rd
Bethesda, MD 20817-1636
301-897-3570
800-843-7323
Fax: 301-897-5838
http://www.woodbinehouse.com
info@woodbinehouse.com
Sue Schwartz PhD, Author
This revised and updated edition presents a fun, hands-on approach to developing communication skills in children with disabilities using everyday toys. There's a fresh assortment of toys and books, as well as newe chapters on computer technology and language learning, videotapes and television. *$16.95*
289 pages Paperback 7x10
ISBN 0-933149-73-5

2543 **No One to Play with: The Social Side of Learning Disabilities**
Connecticut Assoc for Children and Adults with LD
Ste 15-5
25 Van Zant St
Norwalk, CT 06855-1729
203-838-4353
Fax: 203-866-6108
http://www.cacld.org
cacld@juno.com

Marie Armstrong, Information Specialist
Beryl Kaufman, Executive Director
Your child suffers from a learning disability and you have read reams on how to improve on her academic skills and now want to address his or her social needs. *$13.00*

2544 Nobody's Perfect: Living and Growing with Children who Have Special Needs
Brookes Publishing Company
PO Box 10624
Baltimore, MD 21285 410-337-9580
800-638-3775
Fax: 410-337-8539
http://www.brookespublishing.com
custserv@brookespublishing.com
Paul H Brookes, President
Melissa A Behm, VP
Study of four families with children who have special needs. How they all adapted in surviving, how they care for the child, family, parents and siblings. How families react and relate. What it is like in community and extended family? Basic issues dicussed: self-esteem, separating parent from the adult with special needs and other issues. *$23.00*
352 pages Paperback
ISBN 1-557661-43-X

2545 Opening Doors: Connecting Students to Curriculum, Classmate, and Learning, Second Edition
PEAK Parent Center
Ste 200
611 N Weber St
Colorado Springs, CO 80903-1072 719-531-9400
800-284-0251
Fax: 719-531-9452
http://www.peakparent.org
info@peakparent.org
Barbara Buswell, Author
Beth Schaffner, Co-Author
Alison B Seyler, Co-Author
This innovative text contains practical how-to's for inculding and supporting students with disabilities in the general education classroom. It explores the processes, thinking, and approaches that successful implementers of inclusion have used. Written for educators and parents of both elementary and secondary students, topics include instructional strategies, curriculum modifications, behavior, standards, literacy, and providing support. *$13.00*
ISBN 0-884720-12-9

2546 Optimizing Special Education: How Parents Can Make a Difference
Insight Books
233 Spring St
New York, NY 10013-1522 212-460-1500
800-221-9369
Fax: 212-647-1898
http://www.springer.com
info@springer.com
Rudiger Gebauer, Owner
The author shows families how to use education laws to increase services or change services to suit a child's needs. Book contains personal anecdotes and balanced viewpoint of parent and professional relationships. *$26.50*
300 pages
ISBN 0-306443-23-6

2547 Out of Sync Child: Recognizing and Coping with Sensory Integration Dysfunction
Therapro
225 Arlington St
Framingham, MA 01702-8723 508-872-9494
800-257-5376
Fax: 508-875-2062
http://www.therapro.com
info@therapro.com
Karen Conrad, Owner
Finally, a parent-friendly book about sensory integration (SI) clearly written to explain SI dysfunction from the perspective of a teacher who has worked extensively with an OT. Part I deals with recognizing SI dysfunction. Part II addresses coping with SI dysfunction.

2548 Out of the Mouths of Babes: Discovering the Developmental Significance of the Mouth
Therapro
225 Arlington St
Framingham, MA 01702-8723 508-872-9494
800-257-5376
Fax: 508-875-2062
http://www.therapro.com
info@therapro.com
Karen Conrad, Owner
Help children who have difficulty with focusing, staying alert, or being calm with these simple techniqes and activities. Learn how behavior is affected by suck/swallow/breathe (SSB) synchrony with suggestions for correcting specific problems. This informal writing style and many illustrations make it a great resource for parents, teachers and therapists.

2549 Parent Manual
Federation for Children with Special Needs
Suite 1102
529 Main Street
Boston, MA 02109 617-236-7210
800-331-0688
Fax: 617-241-0330
TDD: 617-236-7210
http://www.fcsn.org
fcsninfo@fcsn.org
Rich Robison, President
Outlines parents' and children's rights in special education as guaranteed by Chapter 766, the Massachusetts special education law, and the Individuals with Disabilities Education Act (IDEA), the federal special education law *$ 25.00*
75 pages

2550 Play Therapy
Books on Special Children
PO Box 3378
Amherst, MA 01004-3378 413-256-8164
Fax: 413-256-8896
http://www.boscbooks.com
irene@boscbooks.com
Irene Slovak, Founder
Kevin John O'Connor, Author
Leading authorities present various theoretical models of play therapy treatment and application. Case studies on how various treatments are applied. *$44.95*
350 pages Hardcover
ISBN 0-471106-38-0

2551 Positive Self-Talk for Children
PO Box 305
Congers, NY 10920 845-638-1236
Fax: 845-638-0847
http://www.boscbooks.com/
irene@boscbooks.com
D Bloch, Author
This book teaches positive talk and ideas to achieve positive self-esteem. Use this as a refererence in specific situations: ie: fears on 1st day of school, doctor's visit. Covers cases, includes specific dialogue.

2552 Practical Parent's Handbook on Teaching Children with Learning Disabilities
Charles C Thomas
PO Box 19265
Springfield, IL 62794-9265 217-789-8980
800-258-8980
Fax: 217-789-9130
http://www.ccthomas.com
books@ccthomas.com
Michael P Thomas, President

Publisher of Education and Special Education books. *$65.95*
308 pages Cloth
ISBN 0-398059-03-9

2553 Raising Your Child to be Gifted: Successful Parents
Brookline Books
Suite B-001
8 Trumbull Rd
Northampton, MA 01060
413-584-0184
800-666-2665
Fax: 413-5846184
http://www.brooklinebooks.com
brbooks@yahoo.com
James R Campbell PhD, Author
Moving beyond the usual genetic eplanations for giftedness, Dr. James Campbell presents powerful evidence that it is parental involvement- very specific methods of working with and nurturing a child which increases the child's chances of being gifted. *$21.95*
275 pages Paperback
ISBN 1-571290-94-X

2554 Right from the Start: Behavioral Intervention for Young Children with Autism: A Guide
Therapro
225 Arlington St
Framingham, MA 01702-8723
508-872-9494
800-257-5376
Fax: 508-875-2062
http://www.therapro.com
info@therapro.com
Karen Conrad, Owner
This informative and user-friendly guide helps parents and service providers explore programs that use early intensive behavioral intervention for young children with autism and related disorders. Within these programs, many children improve in intellectual, social and adaptive functioning, enabling them to move on to regular elementary and preschools. Benefits all children, but primarily useful for children age five and younger.
215 pages

2555 SMARTS: A Study Skills Resource Guide
Connecticut Assoc. for Children and Adults with LD
Ste 15-5
25 Van Zant St
Norwalk, CT 06855-1729
203-838-5010
Fax: 203-866-6108
http://www.cacld.org
cacld@juno.com
Marie Armstrong, Information Specialist
Beryl Kaufman, Executive Director
A comprehensive teachers handbook of activities to help students develop study skills. *$20.50*

2556 School-Based Home Developmental PE Program
Therapro
225 Arlington St
Framingham, MA 01702-8723
508-872-9494
800-257-5376
Fax: 508-875-2062
http://www.therapro.com
info@therapro.com
Karen Conrad, Owner
A wire bound flip book. Comprehensive developmental physical education program indentifies and improves motor ability right down to the specific sensory and perceptual motor areas for children. Has what you need: assessment; parent involvement; understandable directions; examples; and sample letters to parents. Includes fun sheets that parents/professionals can use with children. Activities are for vestibular integration, body awareness, eye-hand coordination, and fine motor manipulation.

2557 Seeing Clearly
Therapro
225 Arlington St
Framingham, MA 01702-8773
508-872-9494
800-257-5376
Fax: 508-875-2062
http://www.theraproducts.com
info@theraproducts.com
Karen Conrad, Owner
This booklet is chock-full of great information regarding vision andvisual perceptual problems and activities designed to improve visual skills of both adults and children. Begins with an overview of the development of vision with a checklist of warning signs of vision problems. 25 eye game activities are divided into those for Eye Movements, Suspended Ball, Chalkboard and Visualization (e.g. Pictures in your Mind, Spelling Comprehension, etc.)

2558 Self-Perception: Organizing Functional Information Workbook
Therapro
225 Arlington St
Framingham, MA 01702-8773
508-872-9494
800-257-5376
Fax: 508-875-2062
http://www.therapro.com
info@theraproducts.com
Karen Conrad, Owner
Kathleen Anderson MS CCC-SP, Author
Pamela Crow Miller, Co-Author
Recognizing human and animal body parts, discriminating between right and left, and exploring attitudes, emotions, humor and personal problem-solving.

2559 Sensory Integration and the Child: Understanding Hidden Sensory Challenges
Therapro
225 Arlington St
Framingham, MA 01702-8773
508-872-9494
800-257-5376
Fax: 508-875-2062
http://www.therapro.com
info@theraproducts.com
Karen Conrad, Owner
Designed to educate parents, students, and beginning therapists in sensory integration treatment.

2560 Sensory Integration: Theory and Practice
Therapro
225 Arlington St
Framingham, MA 01702-8773
508-872-9494
800-257-5376
Fax: 508-875-2062
http://www.therapro.com
info@theraproducts.com
Karen Conrad, Owner
This is the very latest in sensory integration theory and practice.The entire volume achieves an admirable balance between theory and practice, covering sensory integration theory, various kinds of sensory integrative dysfunction and comprehensive discussions of assessment, direct treatment, consultation and continuing research issues.

2561 Siblings of Children with Autism: A Guide for Families
Therapro
225 Arlington St
Framingham, MA 01702-8773
508-872-9494
800-257-5376
Fax: 508-875-2062
http://www.therapro.com
info@theraproducts.com
Karen Conrad, Owner
An invaluable guide to understanding sibling relationships, how they are affected by autism, and what families can do to support their other children while coping with the intensive needs of the child with autism.

2562 **Simple Steps: Developmental Activities for Infants, Toddlers & Two Year Olds**
Therapro
225 Arlington St
Framingham, MA 01702-8773 508-872-9494
800-257-5376
Fax: 508-875-2062
http://www.therapro.com
info@theraproducts.com
Karen Conrad, Owner
300 activites linked to the latest research in brain development. Outlines a typical developmental sequence in 10 domains: social/emotional, fine motor, gross motor, language, cognition, sensory, nature, music & movement, creativity and dramatic play. Chapters on curriculum development and learning environment also included.

2563 **Social Perception of People with Disabilities in History**
4156 Library Rd
Pittsburgh, PA 15234-1349 412-341-1515
Fax: 412-344-0224
http://www.ldanatl.org
ldanatl@usaor.net
Herbert C Covey, Author
Patrica H. Latham, President
Sharon Bloechle, Secretary
Shows how historical factors shape some of our current perceptions about disability. Of interest to special educators, historians, students of the humanities and social scientists.

2564 **Son Rise: The Miracle Continues**
Option Indigo Press
2080 S Undermountain Rd
Sheffield, MA 01257-9643 413-229-2100
800-562-7171
Fax: 413-229-8727
http://www.optionindio.com
indigo@bcn.net
Barry Neil Kaufman, Author
This book documents Raun Kaufman's astonishing develpment from a lifeless, autistic, retarded child into a highly verbal, lovable youngster with no traces of his former condition. It details Raun's extraordinary progress from the age of four into young adulthood. It also shares moving accounts of five families that successfully used the Son-Rise Program to reach their own special children. An awe-inspiring reminder that love moves mountains. A must for any parent, professional or teacher.-OUT OF *$14.95*
346 pages Bi-Annually
ISBN 0-915811-61-8

2565 **Study Skills: A Landmark School Teaching Guide**
Landmark School
429 Hale St
Prides Crossing, MA 01965 978-236-3216
Fax: 978-927-7268
http://www.landmarkoutreach.org
outreach@landmarkschool.org
Dan Ahearn, Program Director
Trish Newhall, Associate Director
Designed to help all students learn to comprehend and organize the information they must learn in school, Study Skills: A Landmark School Student Guide offers instruction in how to apply specific comprehension and study skills including multiple exercises to practice each skill. Intended for reading levels of middle school and beyond. *$25.00*
104 pages
ISBN 0-962411-96-5

2566 **Stuttering and Your Child: Questions and Answers**
Stuttering Foundation of America
PO Box 11749
Memphis, TN 38111 901-452-7343
800-992-9392
Fax: 901-761-0484
http://www.stutteringhelp.org
info@stutteringhelp.org
Jane Fraser, President
Provides help, information, and resources to those who stutter, their families, schools day care centers, and all others who need help for a stuttering problem. *$2.00*
64 pages
ISBN 0-933388-43-8

2567 **Substance Use Among Children and Adolescents**
John Wiley & Sons Inc
10475 Crosspoint Blvd
Indianapolis, IN 46256-3386 877-762-2974
Fax: 800-597-3299
http://www.wiley.com
Stephen M. Smith, President/CEO
Anne Marie Pagliaro, Author
Peter B. Wiley, Chairman
Exposure and use among infants, children and adolescents. Impact on mental and physical health. Ingestion of substances during pregnancy and effects on fetus and neonate. Drug abuse effects on learning, memory.. Preventing and treating children and adolescents. Available only as a print on demand title. *$132.00*
416 pages Hardcover
ISBN 0-471580-42-2

2568 **Success with Struggling Readers: The Benchmark School Approach**
Guilford Publications
72 Spring St
New York, NY 10012-4019 212-431-9800
800-365-7006
Fax: 212-966-6708
http://www.guilford.com
info@guilford.com
Irene West Gaskins, Author
Presents a proven approach for helping struggling students become fully engaged readers, learners, thinkers, and problem solvers. Demonstrates ways to teach effective strategies for decoding words and understanding concepts, and to give students the skills to apply these strategies across the curriculum based on their individual cognitive styles and the specific demands of the task at hand. *$30.00*
264 pages
ISBN 1-593851-69-3

2569 **Supporting Children with Communication Difficulties In Inclusive Settings**
Special Needs Project
Ste H
324 State St
Santa Barbara, CA 93101-2364 818-718-9900
800-333-6867
Fax: 818-349-2027
http://www.specialneeds.com
editor@specialneeds.com
Hod Gray, Founder/President
Linda McCormick, Author
Diane Frome Loeb, Co-Author
A collaboration of professionals and parents can achieve language communication competence in classroom and other settings. Essential background material, assessment and intervention and needs of special populations are discussed. Contains sectional headings and marginal comments, chapter summary. *$75.00*
530 pages Paperback
ISBN 0-023792-72-8

2570 **Tactics for Improving Parenting Skills (TIPS)**
Sopris West
4093 Specialty Pl
Longmont, CO 80504-5400 303-651-2829
800-547-6747
Fax: 303-776-5934
http://www.sprislearning.com.
Bob Algozzine, Author
Jim Ysseldyke, Author

Perhaps best described as a compliation of one-page parenting brochures, this helpful resource represents volumes of ideas and suggestions on topics of concern in today's families.OUT OF BUSINESS
202 pages
ISBN 1-570350-35-3

2571 **Teach Me Language**
Slosson Educational Publications
PO Box 280
East Aurora, NY 14052 716-652-0930
800-828-4800
Fax: 800-655-3840
http://www.slosson.com
slosson@slosson.com
Steven Slosson, President
Teach Me Language is designed for teachers, therapists, and parents, and includes a step-by-step how to manual with 400 pages of instructions, explanations, examples, and games and cards to attack language weaknesses common to children with peravasive developmental disorders. *$29.95*

2572 **Teaching Developmentally Disabled Children**
Slosson Educational Publications
PO Box 280
East Aurora, NY 14052 716-652-0930
800-828-4800
Fax: 800-655-3840
http://www.slosson.com
slosson@slosson.com
Steven Slosson, President
This instrructional program for teachers, nurses, and parents is clear and concisely shows how to help children who are developmentally disabled function more normally at home, in school, and in the community. *$34.00*
250 pages

2573 **Teaching Reading to Children with Down Syndrome**
Woodbine House
6510 Bells Mill Rd
Bethesda, MD 20817-1636 301-897-3570
800-843-7323
Fax: 301-897-5838
http://www.woodbinehouse.com
info@woodbinehouse.com
Patricia Logan Oelwin, Author
Teach your child with Down syndrome to read using the author's nationally recognized, proven method. From introducing the alphabet to writing and spelling, the lessons are easy to follow. The many pictures and flash cards included appeal to visual learners and are easy to photocopy! *$16.95*
392 pages Paperback
ISBN 0-933149-55-7

2574 **Teaching of Reading: A Continuum from Kindergarten through College**
AVKO Educational Research Foundation
Ste W
3084 Willard Rd
Birch Run, MI 48415-9404 810-686-9283
866-285-6612
Fax: 810-686-1101
http://www.avko.org
avkoemail@aol.com
Don Mc Cabe, Research Director/Author
Barry Chute, President
Gloria Goldsmith, Secretary
This book covers concepts, techniques, and practical diagnostic tests not normally taught in regular college courses on reading. It is designed to be used by teachers, parents, tutors, and college reading instructors willing to try new approaches to old problems. *$49.95*
364 pages
ISBN 1-564006-50-6

2575 **Teaching the Dyslexic Child**
Slosson Educational Publications
PO Box 280
East Aurora, NY 14052 716-652-0930
800-828-4800
Fax: 800-655-3840
http://www.slosson.com
slosson@slosson.com
Steven Slosson, President
Teaching the Dyslexic Child talks about the frustrations that the dyslexic youngsters and their parents encounter in the day to day collisions with life's demand. *$12.00*
128 pages

2576 **Understanding Learning Disabilities: A Parent Guide and Workbook, Third Edition**
York Press
P.O.Box 504
Timonium, MD 21094-0504 410-560-1557
800-962-2763
Fax: 410-560-6758
http://www.yorkpress.com
york@abs.net
Elinor Hartwig, President
An invaluable resource for parents who are new to the field of learning disabilities. Easy to read and overflowing with helpful information and advice. *$25.00*
380 pages
ISBN 0-912752-67-X

2577 **Understanding and Teaching Children with Autism**
John Wiley & Sons Inc
10475 Crosspoint Blvd
Indianapolis, IN 46256-3386 317-572-3000
Fax: 317-572-4000
http://www.wiley.com
Stephen M. Smith, President/CEO
Rita Jordan, Author
Stuart Powell, Co-Author
The triad of impairment: social, language and communication and thought behavior aspects of development discussed. Difficulties in interacting, transfer of learning and bizarre behaviors are syndome. Many LD are associated with autism. *$175.00*
188 pages Hardcover
ISBN 0-471958-88-3

2578 **What to Expect: The Toddler Years**
Workman Publishing
225 Varick St
New York, NY 10014-4304 212-254-5900
800-722-7202
Fax: 212-254-8098
http://www.workman.com
Info@workman.com
Peter Workman, President
Jenny Mandel, Special Markets Director
They guided you through pregnancy, they guided you through baby's first year, and now they'll guide you through the toddler years. In a direct continuation of What to Expect When You're Expecting and What to Expect the Frist Year, American's bestselling pregnancy and childcare authors turn their uniquely comprehensive, lively, and reassuring coverage to years two and three. *$15.95*
928 pages Paperback

Young Adults

2579 **Assertive Option: Your Rights and Responsibilities**
Research Press
PO Box 9177
Champaign, IL 61826-9177 217-352-3273
800-519-2707
Fax: 217-352-1221
http://www.researchpress.com
rp@researchpress.com
Russell Pence, President
Albert Ellis, Author

A self instructional assertiveness book, with many exercises and self tests. *$24.95*
348 pages
ISBN 0-878221-92-1

2580 **Behavior Survival Guide for Kids**
Free Spirit Publishing
Ste 200
217 5th Ave N
Minneapolis, MN 55401-1299 612-338-2068
866-703-7322
Fax: 612-337-5050
http://www.freespirit.com
help4kids@freespirit.com
Judy Galbraith, President
Offers up-to-date information, practical strategies, and sound advice for kids with diagnosed behavior problems (BD, ED, EBD) and those with general behavior problems so they can help themselves. *$14.95*
176 pages
ISBN 1-575421-32-1

2581 **Delivered form Distraction: Getting the Most out of Life with Attention Deficit Disorder**
Ballantine Books
1745 Broad way
New york, NY 10019 *Fax:* 212-572-6066
http://www.randomhouse.com
BBDPublicity@randomhouse.com
Edward M Hallowell, Author
John J Ratey, Co-Author
Random House has long been committed to publishing the best literature by writers both in the United States and abroad. In addition to their commercial success, books published by Random House, Inc. have won an unrivalled number of Nobel and Pulitzer Prizes. *$25.95*
416 pages
ISBN 0-345442-30-X

2582 **Education of Students with Disabilities: Where Do We Stand?**
National Council on Disability
Suite 1050
1331 F St NW
Washington, DC 20004 202-272-2004
Fax: 202-272-2022
TTY: 202-272-2074
http://www.ncd.gov
mquigley@ncd.ogv
Ethel D Briggs, Acting Executive Director
Brenda Bratton, Executive Secretary
The council reviews the education of students with disabilities as a critical priority. Success in education is a predictor of success in adult life. For students with disabilities, a good education can be the difference between a life of dependence and nonproductivity and a life of independence and productivity.

2583 **HEATH Resource Directory: Clearinghouseon Postsecondary Edu for Individuals with Disabilities**
George Washington University
2134 G St NW
Washington, DC 20052 202-973-0904
800-544-3284
Fax: 202-973-0908
http://www.heath.gwu.edu
askheath@gwu.edu
Donna Martinez, Director
Jessica Queener, Project Director
Reina Guartico, Principal Investigator
The HEATH Resource Center is an online clearinghouse on postsecondary education for individuals with disabilities. The HEATH Resource Center Clearinghouse has information for students with disabilities on educational disability support services, policies, procedures, adaptations, accessing college or university campuses, career-technical schools, and other postsecondary training entities.

2584 **Keeping Ahead in School: A Students Book About Learning Disabilities & Learning Disorders**
Educators Publishing Service
PO Box 9031
Cambridge, MA 02139-9031 617-547-6706
800-225-5750
Fax: 617-547-0412
http://www.epsbooks.com
eps@epsbooks.com
Gunnar Voltz, President
Alana Trisler, Author
Written for students 9 to 15 years of age with learning disorders. This book helps students gain important insights into their problems by combining realism with justifiable optimism. *$24.75*
ISBN 0-838820-09-7

2585 **Modern Consumer Education: You and the Law**
Triumph Learning
PO Box 1270
Northborough, MA 01460-4270 800-338-6519
Fax: 866-805-5723
http://www.triumphlearning.com
customerservice@triumphlearning.com
Buz Traugot, Sales Representative
An instructional program to teach independent living, with emphasis on legal resources and survival skills. *$59.00*

2586 **Phonemic Awareness: Lessons, Activities & Games**
Sage/Corwin Press
2455 Teller Rd
Thousand Oaks, CA 91320-2218 805-499-9734
Fax: 805-499-5323
http://www.corwinpress.com
order@corwin.com
Mike Soules, President
Lisa Shaw, Executive Director
Help struggling readers with Phonemic Awareness training. This all inclusive book iuncludes 48 scripted lessons. May be used as a prerequisite to reading or for stuggling students. Includes 49 reproductible masters. May be used with individual students or with groups. *$27.95*
176 pages

2587 **Reading Is Fun**
Teddy Bear Press
3703 S. Edmunds Street
Suite B-182
Seattle, WA 98118 858-560-8718
Fax: 866-870-7323
http://www.teddybearpress.net
fparker@teddybearpress.net
Fran Parker, President
Introduces 55 primer level words in six reading books and accompanting activity sheets. This easy to use reading program provides repition, visual motor, visual discrimination and word comprehension excersies. The manual and placement test. *$85.00*
ISBN 1-928876-01-3

2588 **Reading and Writing Workbook**
Therapro
225 Arlington St
Framingham, MA 01702-8773 508-872-9494
800-257-5376
Fax: 508-875-2062
http://www.theraproducts.com
info@theraproducts.com
Karen Conrad, Owner
Kathleen Anderson MS CCC-SP, Author
Pamela Crow Miller, Co-Author
Writing checks and balancing a checkbook, copying words and sentences, and writing messages and notes. Helps with recognition and understanding of calenders, phone books and much more.

2589 **Survival Guide for Kids with ADD or ADHD**
Free Spirit Publishing
Ste 200
217 5th Ave N
Minneapolis, MN 55401-1299 612-338-2068
866-703-7322
Fax: 612-337-5050
http://www.freespirit.com
help4kids@freespirit.com
Judy Galbraith, President
Explains how kids diagnosed with ADD and ADHD can help themselves succeed in school, get along better at home, and form healthy, enjoyable relationships with peers. In kid-friendly language and a format that welcomes reluctant and easily distracted readers, this book helps kids know they're not alone and offers practical strategies for taking care or oneself, modifying behavior, enjoying school, having fun, and dealing with doctos, counselors, and medication. Includes scenarios and quizzes. *$13.95*
128 pages
ISBN 1-575421-95-X

2590 **Survival Guide for Kids with LD Learning Differences**
Free Spirit Publishing
Ste 200
217 5th Ave N
Minneapolis, MN 55401-1299 612-338-2068
866-703-7322
Fax: 612-337-5050
http://www.freespirit.com
help4kids@freespirit.com
Judy Galbraith, President
Answers the many questions young people have, like 'Why is it hard for kids with LD to learn?' and 'What happens when you grow up?' It explains what LD means (and doesn't mean); defines different kinds of LD; describes what happens in LD programs; helps kids deal with sad, hurt, and angry feelings; suggests ways to get along better in school and at home; and inspires young people to set goals and plan for the future. Also includes resources for parents and teachers. *$10.95*
112 pages
ISBN 1-575421-19-4

2591 **Survival Guide for Teenagers with LD Learning Differences**
Free Spirit Publishing
Ste 200
217 5th Ave N
Minneapolis, MN 55401-1299 612-338-2068
866-703-7322
Fax: 612-337-5050
http://www.freespirit.com
help4kids@freespirit.com
Judy Galbraith, President
This guide helps young people with LD succeed in school and prepare for life as adults. It explains what LD is and how kids get into LD programs, clarifies readers' legal rights and responsibilities, and covers other vital topics including assertiveness, jobs, friends, dating, self-sufficiency, and responsible citizenship. *$12.95*
200 pages
ISBN 0-915793-51-2

2592 **Who I Can Be Is Up To Me: Lessons in Self-Exploration and Self-Determination**
Research Press
2612 N. Mattis Ave PO Box 9177
Champaign, IL 61822-9177 217-352-3273
800-519-2707
Fax: 217-352-1221
http://www.researchpress.com
rp@researchpress.com
Gloria D Campbell-Whatley, Author
Robert W. Parkinson, Founder
127 pages $24.95
ISBN 0-878224-84-X

2593 **Winning at Math: Your Guide to Learning Mathematics Through Successful Study Skills**
Academic Success Press
6023 26th St W
Bradenton, FL 34207-4402 941-746-1645
800-444-2524
Fax: 941-753-2882
http://www.academicsuccess.com
pnolting@ad.com
Paul Nolting, Owner
A guide that helps people with learning disabilities learn math easier. *$24.95*

2594 **Winning the Study Game**
Sage/Corwin Press
2455 Teller Rd
Thousand Oaks, CA 91320-2218 805-499-9734
Fax: 805-499-9734
http://www.corwinpress.com
order@corwin.com
Peggy Hammeken, President
Kevin Ruelle, Illustrator
A comprehensive study skills program for students with learning differences in grades 6-11. The student book has 16 units which will help students learn to study better, take notes, advance their thinking skills while stregthening their reading and writing. The student version is available in a reproducible or consumable format. Teachers guide sold separately. *$34.95*
2500 pages
ISBN 1-890455-48-2

General

2595 **A Student's Guide to Jobs**
NICHCY
1825 Connecticut Ave NW c/o FHI360
Suite 700
Washington, DC 20009
202-884-8200
800-695-0285
Fax: 202-884-8441
TDD: 800-695-0285
http://www.nichcy.org
nichcy@fhi360.org
Susan Ripley, Director
Young people with intellectual and developmental disabilities speak freely about their job-related experiences. *$2.00*
8 pages

2596 **A Student's Guide to the IEP**
NICHCY
1825 Connecticut Ave
Washington, DC 20009
202-884-8200
800-695-0285
Fax: 202-884-8441
http://www.nichcy.org
nichcy@fhi360.org
Susan Ripley, Director
A guide for students that features other students discussing their experiences as active members on their IEP team. *$2.00*
12 pages

2597 **Accessing Parent Groups**
NICHCY
1825 Connecticut Ave NW
Suite 700
Washington, DC 20009
202-884-8200
800-695-0285
Fax: 202-884-8441
http://www.nichcy.org
nichcy@fhi360.org
Susan Ripley, Director
Helps parents locate support groups where they can share information, give and receive emotional support, and address common concerns. *$2.00*
12 pages

2598 **Accessing Programs for Infants, Toddlers and Preschoolers**
NICHCY
1825 Connecticut Ave NW
Suite 700
Washington, DC 20009
202-884-8200
800-695-0285
Fax: 202-884-8441
http://www.nichcy.org
nichcy@fhi360.org
Susan Ripley, Director
This guide helps locate intervention services for infants and toddlers with disabilities. Also answers questions about educational programs for preschoolers. *$2.00*
20 pages

2599 **Advocacy Services for Families of Children in Special Education**
Arizona Department of Education
1535 W Jefferson St
Phoenix, AZ 85007-3209
1-800-352-45
800-352-4558
Fax: 602-542-5440
http://www.ade.state.az.us
ADE@ade.az.gov
Robert Plummer, Manager
Art Heikkila, Auditor
Information provided to families that have children in special education.

2600 **Assessing Children for the Presence of a Disability**
NICHCY
1825 Connecticut Ave NW
Suite 700
Washington, DC 20009
202-884-8200
800-695-0285
Fax: 202-884-8441
http://www.nichcy.org
nichcy@fhi360.org
Susan Ripley, Director
Describes the criteria and process preformed by school systems to determine if a child has a learning disabilty. *$4.00*
28 pages

2601 **Assessing the ERIC Resource Collection**
NICHCY
1825 Connecticut Ave NW
Suite 700
Washington, DC 20009
202-884-8200
800-695-0285
Fax: 202-884-8441
http://www.nichcy.org
nichcy@fhi360.org
Susan Ripley, Director
A nationwide network that gives access to education literature, this document explains how to search and retrieve documents from ERIC. Also explains how to find information about children with disabilites. *$2.00*
8 pages

2602 **Complete Set of State Resource Sheets**
NICHCY
1825 Connecticut Ave NW
Suite 700
Washington, DC 20009
202-884-8200
800-695-0285
Fax: 202-884-8441
http://www.nichcy.org
nichcy@fhi360.org
Susan Ripley, Director
Provides a sheet for every state and territory in the United States. *$10.00*
200 pages

2603 **Directory of Organizations**
NICHCY
1825 Connecticut Ave NW
Suite 700
Washington, DC 20009
202-884-8200
800-695-0285
Fax: 202-884-8441
http://www.nichcy.org
nichcy@fhi360.org
Susan Ripley, Director
Lists many organizations and services *$4.00*
28 pages

2604 **Education of Children and Youth with Special Needs: What do the Laws Say?**
NICHCY
1825 Connecticut Ave NW
Suite 700
Washington, DC 20009
202-884-8200
800-695-0285
Fax: 202-884-8441
http://www.nichcy.org
nichcy@fhi360.org
Susan Ripley, Director
Provides an overview of 3 laws that aid disabled children; 1. Section 504 of the Rehabilitation Act of 1973, 2. the Individuals with Disabilities Education Act, and 3. the Carl P. Perkins Vocational Educational Act. *$4.00*
16 pages

2605 **Ethical and Legal Issues in School Counseling**
American School Counselor Association
Ste 625
1101 King St
Alexandria, VA 22314-2957
703-683-2722
800-306-4722
Fax: 703-683-1619
http://www.schoolcounselor.org
asca@schoolcounselor.org
Richard Wong, Executive Director
Stephanie Will, Office Manager
Jill Cook, Assistant Director
Contains answers to many of the most controversial and challenging questions school counselors face every day. *$40.50*
ISBN 1-556200-55-2

2606 **Fact Sheet: Attention Deficit Hyperactivity Disorder**
Learning Disabilities Association of America
4156 Library Rd
Pittsburgh, PA 15234-1349
412-341-1515
Fax: 412-344-0224
http://www.ldanatl.org
ldanatl@usaor.net
Patrica H. Latham, President
Sharon Bloechle, Secretary
Ed Schlitt, Treasurer
A pamphlet offering factual information on ADHD.

2607 **Fundamentals of Autism**
Slosson Educational Publications
PO Box 280
East Aurora, NY 14052
716-652-0930
800-828-4800
Fax: 800-655-3840
http://www.slosson.com
slosson@slosson.com
Steven Slosson, President
John Slosson, Vice President
Provides a quick, user friendly effective and accurate approach to help in identifying and developing educationally related program objectives for children diagnosed as Autistic. These materials have been designed to be easily and functionally used by teachers, therapists, special education/learning disability resource specialists, psychologists, and others who work with children diagnosed with similar disabilites.

2608 **General Information about Autism**
NICHCY
1825 Connecticut Ave NW
Suite 700
Washington, DC 20009
202-884-8200
800-695-0285
Fax: 202-884-8441
http://www.nichcy.org
nichcy@fhi360.org
Susan Ripley, Director
Offers information about autism.

2609 **General Information about Disabilities**
NICHCY
1825 Connecticut Ave NW
Suite 700
Washington, DC 20009
202-884-8200
800-695-0285
Fax: 202-884-8441
http://www.nichcy.org
nichcy@fhi360.org
Susan Ripley, Director
A fact sheet offering information on the Education of the Handicapped Act.
2 pages

2610 **General Information about Speech and Language Disorders**
NICHCY
1825 Connecticut Ave NW
Suite 700
Washington, DC 20009
202-884-8200
800-695-0285
Fax: 202-884-8441
http://www.nichcy.org
nichcy@fhi360.org
Susan Ripley, Director
Offers characteristics, educational implications and associations in the area of speech and language disorders.

2611 **IDEA Amendments**
NICHCY
1825 Connecticut Ave NW
Suite 700
Washington, DC 20009
202-884-8200
800-695-0285
Fax: 202-884-8441
http://www.nichcy.org
nichcy@fhi360.org
Susan Ripley, Director
Examines the important changes that have occured in the Individuals Education Act, amended in June of 1997. *$4.00*
40 pages

2612 **If Your Child Stutters: A Guide for Parents**
Stuttering Foundation of America
PO Box 11749
Memphis, TN 38111
901-452-7343
800-992-9392
Fax: 901-452-3931
http://www.stutteringhelp.org
info@stutteringhelp.org
Jane Fraser, President
A guide that enables parents to provide appropriate help to children who stutter. *$1.00*

2613 **Individualized Education Programs**
NICHCY
1825 Connecticut Ave NW
Suite 700
Washington, DC 20009
202-884-8200
800-695-0285
Fax: 202-884-8441
http://www.nichcy.org
nichcy@fhi360.org
Susan Ripley, Director
Provides guidance regarding the legal requirement for beginning a student's IEP. *$2.00*
32 pages

2614 **Interventions for Students with Learning Disabilities**
NICHCY
1825 Connecticut Ave NW
Suite 700
Washington, DC 20009
202-884-8200
800-695-0285
Fax: 202-884-8441
http://www.nichcy.org
nichcy@fhi360.org
Susan Ripley, Director
A document that examines 2 different interventions for students who have learning disabilities; the first deals with strategies and the second with phonological awareness. *$4.00*
16 pages

2615 **National Resources**
NICHCY
1825 Connecticut Ave NW
Suite 700
Washington, DC 20009
202-884-8200
800-695-0285
Fax: 202-884-8441
http://www.nichcy.org
nichcy@fhi360.org

Susan Ripley, Director
Lists different organizations that provide information about different disabilities.
6 pages

2616 **National Toll-free Numbers**
NICHCY
1825 Connecticut Ave NW
Suite 700
Washington, DC 20009
202-884-8200
800-695-0285
Fax: 202-884-8441
http://www.nichcy.org
nichcy@fhi360.org
Susan Ripley, Director
Gives the names of organizations with toll-free numbers who specialize in different disabilities.
6 pages

2617 **Parenting a Child with Special Needs: A Guide to Reading and Resources**
NICHCY
1825 Connecticut Ave NW
Suite 700
Washington, DC 20009
202-884-8200
800-695-0285
Fax: 202-884-8441
http://www.nichcy.org
nichcy@fhi360.org
Susan Ripley, Director
Provides information to families whose child has been diagnosed with a disability. Also gives insight on how disabilities can in turn affect the family. *$4.00*
24 pages

2618 **Parents Guide**
NICHCY
1825 Connecticut Ave NW
Suite 700
Washington, DC 20009
202-884-8200
800-695-0285
Fax: 202-884-8441
http://www.nichcy.org
nichcy@fhi360.org
Lisa Kupper, Editor
Susan Ripley, Manager
Talks directly to parents about specific disability issues.

2619 **Planning a Move: Mapping Your Strategy**
NICHCY
1825 Connecticut Ave NW
Suite 700
Washington, DC 20009
202-884-8200
800-695-0285
Fax: 202-884-8441
http://www.nichcy.org
nichcy@fhi360.org
Susan Ripley, Director
This guide helps to make moving to a new place easier for parents and their children by listing available services in the new area and compiling educational and medical records. *$2.00*
12 pages

2620 **Planning for Inclusion: News Digest**
NICHCY
1825 Connecticut Ave NW
Suite 700
Washington, DC 20009
202-884-8200
800-695-0285
Fax: 202-884-8441
http://www.nichcy.org
nichcy@fhi360.org
Susan Ripley, Director
Provides a general guide to raising children with learning disabilities in an educational setting. *$4.00*
32 pages

2621 **Promising Practices and Future Directions for Special Education**
NICHCY
1825 Connecticut Ave NW
Suite 700
Washington, DC 20009
202-884-8200
800-695-0285
Fax: 202-884-8441
http://www.nichcy.org
nichcy@fhi360.org
Susan Ripley, Director
Examines different research regarding the educational methods for children with learning disabilities. *$4.00*
24 pages

2622 **Public Agencies Fact Sheet**
NICHCY
1825 Connecticut Ave NW
Suite 700
Washington, DC 20009
202-884-8200
800-695-0285
Fax: 202-884-8441
http://www.nichcy.org
nichcy@fhi360.org
Susan Ripley, Director
General information on public agencies that serve the disabled individual.
2 pages

2623 **Questions Often Asked about Special Education Services**
NICHCY
1825 Connecticut Ave NW
Suite 700
Washington, DC 20009
202-884-8200
800-695-0285
Fax: 202-884-8441
http://www.nichcy.org
nichcy@fhi360.org
Susan Ripley, Director
Offers information regarding special education.

2624 **Questions Often Asked by Parents About Special Education Services**
NICHCY
1825 Connecticut Ave NW
Suite 700
Washington, DC 20009
202-884-8200
800-695-0285
Fax: 202-884-8441
http://www.nichcy.org
nichcy@fhi360.org
Susan Ripley, Director
A publication to help parents learn about the Individuals with Disabilities Education Act. Also discusses how student access special education and other related services.
12 pages

2625 **Questions and Answers About the IDEA News Digest**
NICHCY
1825 Connecticut Ave NW
Suite 700
Washington, DC 20009
202-884-8200
800-695-0285
Fax: 202-884-8441
http://www.nichcy.org
nichcy@fhi360.org
Susan Ripley, Director
Covers the more commonly asked questions from families and professionals about the IDEA. *$4.00*
28 pages

2626 **Related Services for School-Aged Children with Disabilities**
NICHCY
1825 Connecticut Ave NW
Suite 700
Washington, DC 20009
202-884-8200
800-695-0285
Fax: 202-884-8441
http://www.nichcy.org
nichcy@fhi360.org
Susan Ripley, Director
Examines the different services offered to children with disabilities such as speech-language pathology, transportation, occupational and physical therapy and special health services. *$4.00*
24 pages

2627 **Resources for Adults with Disabilities**
NICHCY
1825 Connecticut Ave NW
Suite 700
Washington, DC 20009
202-884-8200
800-695-0285
Fax: 202-884-8441
http://www.nichcy.org
nichcy@fhi360.org
Susan Ripley, Director
Helps adults with disabilities find organizations that will help them find employment, education, recreation and independent living. *$2.00*
16 pages

2628 **Serving on Boards and Committees**
NICHCY
1825 Connecticut Ave NW
Suite 700
Washington, DC 20009
202-884-8200
800-695-0285
Fax: 202-884-8441
http://www.nichcy.org
nichcy@fhi360.org
Susan Ripley, Director
Part of the Parent's Guide series, this publication examines the different boards and committees on which parents of children with disabilities often serve. Also suggests ways to go about becoming involved with such organizations. *$2.00*
8 pages

2629 **Special Education and Related Services: Communicating Through Letterwriting**
NICHCY
1825 Connecticut Ave NW
Suite 700
Washington, DC 20009
202-884-8200
800-695-0285
Fax: 202-884-8441
http://www.nichcy.org
nichcy@fhi360.org
Susan Ripley, Director
Identifies the rights of parents and their children with disabilities and explains when and how to notify the school in writing about such conditions. *$2.00*
20 pages

2630 **State Resource Sheet**
NICHCY
1825 Connecticut Ave NW
Suite 700
Washington, DC 20009-1492
202-884-8200
800-695-0285
Fax: 202-884-8441
http://www.nichcy.org
nichcy@fhi360.org
Susan Ripley, Director
List numbers of different organizations that deal with disabilities by state.

2631 **Underachieving Gifted**
Council for Exceptional Children
2900 Crystal drive
Suite 1000
Arlington, VA 22202-3557
703-264-9454
888-232-7733
Fax: 703-264-9494
TTY: 866-915-5000
http://www.cec.sped.org/
service@cec.sped.org
Michael George, Director
A collection of annotated references from the ERIC and Exceptional Child Evaluation Resources (171 abstracts). Note: Abstracts only. Not the complete research. *$1.00*

2632 **What Every Parent Should Know about Learning Disabilities**
Connecticut Assoc. for Children and Adults with LD
Ste 15-5
25 Van Zant St
Norwalk, CT 06855-1729
203-838-5010
Fax: 203-866-6108
http://www.CACLD.org
Beryl Kaufman, Executive Director
What to do with a child with a learning disability.

2633 **Who's Teaching Our Children with Disabilities?**
NICHCY
1825 Connecticut Ave NW
Suite 700
Washington, DC 20009-1492
202-884-8200
800-695-0285
Fax: 202-884-8441
http://www.nichcy.org
nichcy@fhi360.org
Susan Ripley, Director
Takes a detailied look at the people who are teaching children with disabilities. *$4.00*
24 pages

2634 **Your Child's Evaluation**
NICHCY
1825 Connecticut Ave NW
Suite 700
Washington, DC 20009-1492
202-884-8200
800-695-0285
Fax: 202-884-8441
http://www.nichcy.org
nichcy@fhi360.org
Susan Ripley, Director
This document describes the steps that the school system will use to determine if you child has a learning disability. *$2.00*
4 pages

Adults

2635 International Dyslexia Association: Illinois Branch Newsletter
Bldg 7
751 Roosevelt Rd
Glen Ellyn, IL 60137-5904 630-469-6900
Fax: 630-469-6810
http://www.readibida.org
info@readibida.org.

Jo Ann Paldo, President
Kathleen L Wagner, Executive Director

2636 NICHCY News Digest
NICHCY
1825 Connecticut Ave NW
Suite 700
Washington, DC 20009-1492 202-884-8200
800-695-0285
Fax: 202-884-8441
http://www.nichcy.org
nichcy@fhi360.org

Lisa Kupper, Editor
Susan Ripley, Director
Addresses a single disability issue in depth.

2637 Volta Voices
Alexander Graham Bell Association
3417 Volta Pl NW
Washington, DC 20007-2737 202-337-5220
Fax: 202-337-8314
TTY: 202-337-5221
http://www.agbell.org
info@agbell.org

Melody Felzein, Production/Editing Manager
Harrison Judy, Director
Covers a wide variety of topics, including hearing aid and cochlear implants, early intervention and education, professional guidance, legislative updates and perspectives from individuals from across the United States and around the world.

Children

2638 Calliope
Cobblestone Publishing
Ste C
30 Grove St
Peterborough, NH 03458-1453 603-924-7209
800-821-0115
Fax: 603-924-7380
http://www.cobblestonepub.com
cobbfeedback@caruspub.com

Rosalie Baker, Editor
Kid's world history magazine, written for kids ages 9 to 14, goes beyond the facts to explore provoactive issues. *$29.95*
52 pages 9 times anually
ISSN 1050-7086

2639 KIND News
NAHEE
Washington, DC 02000 202-452-1100
Fax: 860-434-9579
http://www.kidsnews.org
membership@humanesociety.org

Wayne Pacelle, President
Laura Maloney, COO
Andrew Rowman, CIO
Four-page color newspaper with games, puzzles and entertaining, informative articles designed to install kindness to people, animals, and the enviroment and to make reading fun. *$30.00*
4 pages 9x school year
ISSN 1050-9542

2640 KIND News Jr: Kids in Nature's Defense
Kind News
2100 L St., NW
Washington, DC 02000 202-452-1101
Fax: 860-434-6282
http://www.kindnews.org
membership@humanesociety.org

Wayne Pacelle, President
Laura Maloney, COO
Andrew Rowman, CIO
Short, easy-to-read items on the environment and animal world with puzzles, contests and cartoons. Many illustrations, pictures.

2641 KIND News Primary: Kids in Nature's Defense
Kind News
2101 L St., NW
Washington, DC 02000 202-452-1102
Fax: 860-434-6282
http://www.kindnews.org
membership@humanesociety.org

Wayne Pacelle, President
Laura Maloney, COO
Andrew Rowman, CIO
Short, easy-to-read items on the environment and animal world with puzzles, pictures to color and cartoons. Many illustrations, pictures.

2642 KIND News Sr: Kids in Nature's Defense
NAHEE
2102 L St., NW
Washington, DC 02000 202-452-1103
Fax: 860-434-6282
http://www.kindnews.org
membership@humanesociety.org

Wayne Pacelle, President
Laura Maloney, COO
Lona Rowman, CIO
Publication put out by the National Association for Humane and Environmental Education, KIND News Sr. is intended for children between grades 5 through 6. The magazine covers different pet issues such as how to care for,feed and play with pets.

2643 Let's Find Out
Scholastic
555 Broadway
New York, NY 10012-3919 212-625-0778

Jamie Martillo, Editor
Richard Robinson, CEO
Get your PreK and K classes off to a great start with Free-trail copies of Let's Find Out, and bring all this to your teaching program: monthly seasonal themes in 32 colorful weekly issues, activity pages to develop early reading and math skills. *$4.25*

2644 National Association for Humane and Environmental Education
2100L St.,NW
Washington, DC 02000 202-452-1100
Fax: 860-434-6282
http://www.kidsnews.org
membership@humanesociety.org

Wayne Pacelle, President
Laura Maloney, COO
Andrew Rowman, CIO

2645 Ranger Rick
National Wildlife Foundation/Membership Services
989 Avenue of Americans
Suite 400
New York, NY 10018 212-730-1700
800-822-9919
Fax: 212-730-1823
http://www.nuf.org
info@nuf.com

Gerry Bishop, Editor
Mark Putten, CEO
Anthony Winn, Director,PSLDI

A magazine for children ages 6-12 that is dedicated to helping students gain a greater understanding and appreciation of nature. *$15.00*

2646 **Stone Soup, The Magazine by Young Writers& Artists**
Children's Art Foundation
PO Box 83
Santa Cruz, CA 95063
831-426-5557
800-447-4569
http://www.stonesoup.com
editor@stonesoup.com
Gerry Mandel, Editor
William Rubel, Editor
A literary magazine publishing fiction, poetry, book reviews and art by children through age 13. ISSN: 0094 579X. *$34.00*
48 pages 6x/year

Parents & Professionals

2647 **Association of Higher Education Facilities Officers Newsletter**
1643 Prince St
Alexandria, VA 22314-2818
703-684-1446
Fax: 703-549-2772
http://www.appa.org
webmaster@appa.org
Randolph Hare, President
Peter Strazdas, Vice President
Jerry Carlson, Secretary
A newsletter whose purpose is to promote excellence in the administration, care, operation, planning, and development of higher education facilities.

2648 **Children and Families**
National Head Start Association
1651 Prince St
Alexandria, VA 22314-2818
703-739-0875
Fax: 703-739-0878
http://www.nhsa.org
mmcgrady@nhsa.com
Vanessa Rich, Chairman
Alvin Jones, Vice Chairperson
Mary Cose Rox, Secretary
The magazine of the National Head Start Association.

2649 **Connections: A Journal of Adult Literacy**
Adult Literacy Resource Institute
100 William T Morrissey Blvd
Dorchester, MA 2125-3300
617-782-8956
Fax: 617-782-9011
TTY: 617-782-9011
http://www.alri.org
Connections is primarily intended to provide an opportunity for adult educators in the Boston area to communicate with colleagues.

2650 **Council for Exceptional Children**
2900 Crystal Dr.
Suite 100
Arlington, VA 22202-3557
888-232-7733
TTY: 866-915-5000
http://www.cec.sped.org
service@cec.sped.org
Laurie VanderPloeg, President
Mary Lynn Boscardin, President Elect
Jim McCormick, Treasurer
The Council for Exceptional Children (CEC) is the largest international professional organization dedicated to improving the educational success of individuals with disabilities and/or gifts and talents. CEC advocates for appropriate governmental policies, sets professional standards, provides professional development, advocates for individuals with exceptionalities, and helps professionals obtain conditions and resources necessary for effective professional practice.

2651 **Education Funding News**
Education Funding Research Council
1725 K St NW
Washington, DC 20006-1401
202-872-4000
800-876-0226
Fax: 800-926-2012
http://www.grantsandfunding.com
Emily Lechy, Editor
Phil Gabel, CEO
Provides the latest details on funding opportunities in education. *$298.00*
50 pages

2652 **Exceptional Children**
Council for Exceptional Children
2900 Crystal Drive
Ste 1000
Arlington, VA 22202
703-264-9454
888-232-7733
Fax: 703-264-9494
TTY: 703-264-9446
http://www.cec.sped.org
service@cec.sped.org
Robin D. Brewer, President
Mikki Garcia, Executive Director
John H. Hess, Consultant
Peer review journal publishing original research on the education and development of toddlers, infants, children and youth with exceptionality and articles on professional issues of concern to special educators. Published quarterly.

2653 **Exceptional Parent Magazine**
551 Main St
Johnstown, PA 15901-2032
877-372-7368
http://www.eparent.com
webmaster@eparent.com
Joseph M. Valenzano, President/CEO
Rick Rader, Editor in Chief
Ron Peterson, Webmaster
EP is the magazine for exceptional parents with exceptional children. Each month EP provides a forum to network with others who are providing a richer life for themselves and for their children. ISSN: 0046-9157. *$39.95*
92 pages Monthly

2654 **Federation for Children with Special Needs Newsletter**
529 Main St
Ste 1M3 Boston
Boston, MA 2129
617-236-7210
800-331-0688
Fax: 617-241-0330
http://www.fcsn.org
fcsninfo@fcsn.org
James F. Whalen, President/CEO
Michael Weiner, Treasurer
Miryam Wiley, Clerk
The mission of the Federation is to provide information, support, and assistance to parents of children with disabilities, their professional partners, and their communities. Major services are information and referrals and parent and professional training.

2655 **International Dyslexia Association Quarterly Newsletter: Perspectives**
4th Fl
40 York Rd
Baltimore, MD 21204-5243
410-296-0232
800-ABC-D123
Fax: 410-321-5069
http://www.interdys.org
jdallam@interdys.org
Hal Malchow, President
Ben Shifrin, Vice President
Suzzane Carreker, Secretary

Leading resource for individuals with dyslexia, their families, teachers, and educational professionals around the world. A non-profit organization dedicates to the study and treatment of dyslexia, we encourage you to join our mission and become a member. You will receive regular information about managing dyslexia, access to an international network of professionals in the field, discounts on conference fees and publications, quarterly and biannual publications
50-56 pages Free to Members

2656 **International Dyslexia Association: Illinois Branch Newsletter**
Bldg 7
751 Roosevelt Rd
Glen Ellyn, IL 60137-5904
630-469-6900
Fax: 630-469-6810
http://www.readibida.org
info@readibida.org
Dr.Suzzane O'Brien, President
Julia Nelson, Vice President
John Bloomfield, Treasurer
The Illinois Branch, serving the entire state of Illinois and founded in 1978, is dedicated to the study and remediation of dyslexia and to the support and encouragement of individuals with dyslexia and their families.

2657 **International Dyslexia Association: Philadelphia Branch Newsletter**
P.O.Box 251
Bryn Mawr, PA 19010-251
610-527-1548
Fax: 610-527-5011
Jann Glider, President
Amy Ress, Manager
An international 501 (c) (3) nonprofit, scientific and educational organization dedicated to the study and treatment of dyslexia. All branches hold at least one public meeting, workshop or conference per year.

2658 **International Reading Association Newspaper: Reading Today**
PO Box 8139
800 Barksdale Rd.
Newark, DE 19714-8139
302-731-1600
800-336-7323
Fax: 302-731-1057
http://www.reading.org
customerservice@reading.org
Jill Lewis-Spector, President
Diane Barone, Vice President
Marcie Craig Post, Executive Director
The International Reading Association is a professional membership organization dedicated to promoting high levels of literacy for all by improving the quality of reading instruction, disseminating research and information about reading, and encouraging the lifetime reading habit. Our members include classroom teachers, reading specialistsss, consultants, administrators, supervisors, university faculty, researchers, psychologists, librarians, media specialists, and parents.
Bi-monthly

2659 **Journal of Physical Education, Recreation and Dance**
1900 Association Dr
Reston, VA 20191-1502
703-476-3400
800-213-7193
Fax: 703-476-9527
http://www.shapeamerica.org
Dolly D. Lambdin, President
E.Paul Roetert, CEO
Gale Wiedow, Past President
Most frequently published, and most wide-ranging periodical reaching over 20,000 members and providing information on a greater variety of HPERD issues than any other publication. ISSN NUMBER: 0730-3084 *$9.00*
80 pages monthly

2660 **LDA Alabama Newsletter**
Learning Disabilities Association Alabama
PO Box 244023
Montgomery, AL 36124
334-277-9151
http://ldaalabama.org
Tamara Massey-Garrett, President
A non-profit grassroots organization whose members are individuals with learning disabilities, their families, and the professionals who work with them. LDAA is dedicated to identifying causes and promoting prevention of learning disabilities and to enhance the quality of life for all individuals with learning disabilities and their families by encouraging effective identification and intervention, fostering research, and protecting their rights under the law.

2661 **LDA Illinois Newsletter**
Learning Disabilities Association Illinois
Ste 106
10101 S Roberts Rd
Palos Hills, IL 60465-1556
708-430-7532
Fax: 708-430-7592
http://www.idanatl.org/illinois
Sharon Schussler, Manager
A non profit organization dedicated to the advancement of the education and general welfare of children and youth of normal or potentially normal intelligence who have perceptual, conceptual, coordinative or related learning disabilities.

2662 **Link Newsletter**
Parent Information Center of Delaware
5570 Kirkwood Hwy
Wilmington, DE 19808-5002
302-366-0152
888-547-4412
Fax: 302-999-7637
http://www.glrppr.org
l-barnes@illinois.edu
Laura Barnes, Executive Director
GLRPPR is a professional organization dedicated to promoting information exchange and networking to P2 professionals in the Great Lakes regions of the United States and Canada. *$12.00*
20 pages quarterly

2663 **OSERS Magazine**
Office of Special Education & Rehabilitative Svcs.
303 C St SW
Washington, DC 20202
202-727-6436
800-433-3243
TTY: 202-205-8241
http://www.ed.gov
Provides information, research and resources in the area of special learning needs.
Quarterly

2664 **Resources in Education**
US Government Printing Office
710 N Capitol St NW
Washington, DC 20401
202-512-0132
Fax: 202-512-1355
http://www.access.gpo.gov
Contactcenter@gpo.gov.in
Patricia Simmons, Manager
A monthly publication announcing education related documents.

2665 **TESOL Journal**
Teachers of English to Speakers of Other Languages
1925 Ballenger Avenue
Ste 500
Alexandria, VA 22314-4287
703-836-0774
888-547-3369
Fax: 703-836-7864
http://www.tesol.org
info@tesol.org
Rosa Aronson, Executive Director
Rita Gainer, Executive Assistant
Jim Trope, Director of Finance

TESOL Journal articles focus on teaching and classroom research for classroom practitioners. The journal includes articles about adult education and literacy in every volume year. Subscriptions available to members only.

2666 **TESOL Newsletter**
Teachers of English to Speakers of Other Languages
1925 Ballenger Avenue
Ste 500
Alexandria, VA 22314-4287
703-836-0774
888-547-3369
Fax: 703-836-7864
http://www.tesol.org
info@tesol.org

Rosa Aronson, Executive Director
Rita Gainer, Executive Assistant
Jim Trope, Director of Finance
TESOL produces the Adult Education Interest Section Newsletter and the Refugee Concerns Interest Section Newsletter. They provide news, ideas, and activities for ESL instructors. Subscriptions are available to members only.

2667 **TESOL Quarterly**
Teachers of English to Speakers of Other Languages
1925 Ballenger Avenue
Ste 500
Alexandria, VA 22314-4287
703-836-0774
888-547-3369
Fax: 703-836-7864
http://www.tesol.org
info@tesol.org

Rosa Aronson, Executive Director
Rita Gainer, Executive Assistant
Jim Trope, Director of Finance
TESOL Quarterly is a referred interdisciplinary journal teachers of English to speakers of other languages. Subscriptions available to members.

Young Adults

2668 **Get Ready to Read!**
National Center for Learning Disabilities
381 Park Ave S
New York, NY 10016-8806
212-545-7510
888-575-7373
Fax: 212-545-9665
http://www.ld.org
help@ncld.org

Frederic M. Poses, CEO
Mary Kalikow, Vice Chair
John R. Langeler, Treasurer
The National Center for Learning Disabilities (NCLD) works to ensure that the nation's 15 million children, adolescents, and adults with learning disabilities have every opportunity to succeed in school, work, and life.
Quarterly

2669 **LD Advocate**
National Center for Learning Disabilities
381 Park Ave S
New York, NY 10016-8806
212-545-7510
888-575-7373
Fax: 212-545-9665
http://www.ld.org
help@ncld.org

Frederic M. Poses, CEO
Mary Kalikow, Vice Chair
John R. Langeler, Treasurer
The National Center for Learning Disabilities (NCLD) works to ensure that the nation's 15 million children, adolescents, and adults with learning disabilities have every opportunity to succeed in school, work, and life.
Monthly

2670 **LD News**
National Center for Learning Disabilities
381 Park Ave S
New York, NY 10016-8806
212-545-7510
888-575-7373
Fax: 212-545-9665
http://www.ld.org
help@ncld.org

Frederic M. Poses, CEO
Mary Kalikow, Vice Chair
John R. Langeler, Treasurer
The National Center for Learning Disabilities (NCLD) works to ensure that the nation's 15 million children, adolescents, and adults with learning disabilities have every opportunity to succeed in school, work, and life.
Monthly

2671 **Our World**
National Center for Learning Disabilities
381 Park Ave S
New York, NY 10016-8806
212-545-7510
888-575-7373
Fax: 212-545-9665
http://www.ld.org
help@ncld.org

Frederic M. Poses, CEO
Mary Kalikow, Vice Chair
John R. Langeler, Treasurer
The National Center for Learning Disabilities (NCLD) works to ensure that the nation's 15 million children, adolescents, and adults with learning disabilities have every opportunity to succeed in school, work, and life.
Quarterly

General

2672 **Academic Communication Associates**
Educational Book Division
PO Box 4279
Oceanside, CA 92052-4279
760-758-9593
888-758-9558
Fax: 760-758-1604
http://www.acadcom.com
acom@acadcom.com

Larry Mattes, Founder/President
Publishes hundreds of speech and language products, educational books and assessment materials for children and adults with speech, language, and hearing disorders, learning disabilities, developmental disabilities, and special learning needs. Products include books, software programs, learning games, augmentative communication materials, bilingual/multicultural materials, and special education resources.

2673 **Academic Success Press**
6023 26th Street W
PO Box 132
Bradenton, FL 34206
888-822-6657
http://www.academicsuccess.com
info@academicsuccess.com

Paul D Nolting PhD, Learning Specialist
Kimberly Nolting, VP of Marketing & Research
Publishes books and materials in the interest of making the classroom learning experience less difficult, while improving student learning, to transform the classroom into a more successful environment where educators and students can use inventive learning techniques based on sound academic research.

2674 **Academic Therapy Publications/High Noon Books**
20 Leveroni Court
Novato, CA 94949-5746
415-883-3314
800-422-7249
Fax: 888-287-9975
http://www.academictherapy.com
sales@academictherapy.com

Academic Therapy Publications publishes assessments for speech-language pathologists, psychologists, occupational therapists and educators. High Noon Books publishes phonic-based and hi-lo chapter books for struggling readers of all ages. Audience also includes special education teachers, school psychologists, educational therapists, ESL teachers, parents, and specialists in all fields working with persons with reading, learning, and communication disabilities.

2675 **Active Parenting Publishers**
1220 Kennestone
Ste 130
Marietta, GA 30066-6022
770-429-0565
800-825-0060
Fax: 770-429-0334
http://www.activeparenting.com
cservice@activeparenting.com

Michael Popkin PhD, President
Melody Popkin, Manager of Christian Resources
Virginia Murray, Marketing Manager
Provides parenting education curricula, including one for parents of ADD/ADHD children.

2676 **Alexander Graham Bell Association for the Deaf and Hard of Hearing**
3417 Volta Pl NW
Washington, DC 20007-2737
202-337-5220
866-37-5226
Fax: 202-337-8314
TTY: 202-337-5221
http://www.agbell.org
info@agbell.org

Meredith K. Sugar, President
Emilio Alonso-Mendoza, CEO
Ted A. Meyer, Secretary
Publishes and distributes books, brochures, instructional materials, videos, CDs and audiocassettes relating to hearing loss. *$62.00*
64 pages Bimonthly

2677 **American Guidance Service**
PO Box 99
Circle Pines, MN 55014
651-287-7220
800-328-2560
Fax: 800-471-8457
http://www.agsnet.com
agsmail@agsnet.com

Produces assessments, textbooks, and instructional materials for people with a wide range of needs; publishes individually administered tests to measure cognitive ability, achievement, behavior, speech and language skills, and personal and social adjustment.

2678 **American Printing House for the Blind**
1839 Frankfort Avenue
PO Box 6085
Louisville, KY 40206-0085
502-895-2405
800-233-1839
Fax: 502-899-2284
http://www.aph.org
info@aph.org

Tuck Tinsley, President
Marsha Overstreet, Customer Service Manager
Tony Grantz, Business Development Manager
Promotes independence of blind and visually impaired persons by providing specialized materials, products, and services needed for education and life.

2679 **American Psychological Association**
750 First St. NE
Washington, DC 20002-4242
202-336-5500
800-374-2721
http://www.apa.org

Arthur C. Evans, Jr., CEO/Executive Vice President
Jessica Henderson Daniel, President
Jennifer F. Kelly, Secretary
Publishes periodicals, including PsycSCAN, a quarterly print abstract that provides citations to the journal literature on Learning Disorders and Mental Retardation, including theories, research, assessment, treatment, rehabilitation, and educational issues. Also publishes Psychological Abstracts, a monthly print reference tool containing summaries of journal articles, book chapters, and books in the field of psychology and related disciplines.

2680 **Associated Services for the Blind**
919 Walnut St
Philadelphia, PA 19107-5287
215-627-5930
Fax: 215-922-0692
http://www.asb.org
asbinfo@asb.org

Patricia C Johnson, CEO
Lauren Scarpa, Public Relations Officer
Linda Gaffney, Coordinator
Promotes self-esteem, independence, and self determination in people who are blind or visually impaired. ASB accomplishes this by providing support through education, training and resources, as well as through community action and public education, serving as a voice for the rights of all people who are blind or visually impaired.

2681 **Association on Higher Education and Disability (AHEAD)**
8015 West Kenton Circle
Suite 230
Huntersville, NC 28078
704-947-7779
Fax: 704-948-7779
http://www.ahead.org

Jamie Axelrod, President
Gaeir Dietrich, Treasurer
Stephen Smith, Executive Director

A professional membership organization for individuals involved in the development of policy and in the provision of quality services to meet the needs of persons with disabilities involved in all areas of higher education.
3,000 members 1977

2682 **At-Risk Youth Resources**
Sunburst Visual Media
PO Box 170
Farmingville, NY 11738
800-999-6884
Fax: 800-262-1886
http://www.at-risk.com
customerservice@guidance-group.com
Publisher of life-skills educational media for the K-12 market. In addition, we also produce science and social studies programs for students in grades K-8
78 pages

2683 **Bethany House Publishers**
6030 East Fulton Road
Ada, MI 49301
952-829-2500
800-877-2665
Fax: 952-829-2572
http://www.bethanyhouse.com
orders@bakerbooks.com
Gary Johnson, President
Teresa Fogarty, General Publicist
Publishes books in large-print format for the learning disabled.

2684 **Blackwell Publishing**
350 Main St
Malden, MA 2148-5020
781-870-1200
Fax: 781-388-8255
http://www.blackwellpublishing.com
dpeters@bos.blackwellpublishing.com
Lisa Bybee, President
Rene Olivieri, Chief Executive
Dawn Peters, Media Contact
Publishes books and journals for the higher education, research and professional markets, including several journals on topics relating to learning disabilities.

2685 **Brookes Publishing Company**
PO Box 10624
Baltimore, MD 21285
410-337-9580
800-638-3775
Fax: 410-337-8539
http://www.brookespublishing.com
custserv@brookespublishing.com
Paul Brooks, Owner
Melissa Behm, Vice President
Publishes books, texts, curricula, videos, tools and a newsletter based on research in disabilities, education and child development, including learning disabilities, ADHD, communication and language, reading and literacy, and special education.

2686 **Brookline Books/Lumen Editions**
34 University Rd
Brookline, MA 2445-4533
617-734-6772
800-666-2665
Fax: 617-734-3952
http://www.brooklinebooks.com
brbooks@yahoo.com
Milton Budoff, Executive Director
Publishes books on education, learning and topics relating to disabilities.

2687 **Charles C Thomas, Publisher, Ltd.**
2600 S 1st St
Springfield, IL 62704-4730
217-789-8980
800-258-8980
Fax: 217-789-9130
http://www.ccthomas.com
books@ccthomas.com
Michael P Thomas, President
Publisher of titles in Criminal Justice and Police Science, the Behavioral Sciences, Education and Special Education, Biomedical Sciences.

2688 **City Creek Press**
PO Box 8415
Minneapolis, MN 55408
612-823-2500
800-585-6059
Fax: 877-286-1163
http://www.citycreek.com
info@citycreek.com
Judy Liautaud, Owner
Publishes books and products offering a literature-based method of learning, such as books, clue cards, posters, magnetic math story boards, workbooks and audio tapes; the program is multisensory, interactive, and appeals to the visual, auditory and tactile learning styles.

2689 **Concept Phonics**
Oxton House Publishers
P.O.Box 209
Farmington, ME 4938-209
207-779-1923
800-539-7323
Fax: 207-779-0623
http://www.oxtonhouse.com
info@oxtonhouse.com
William Burlinghoff, Owner
Bobby Brown, Marketing Director
Publisher of effective, economical educational materials for early reading and math. We pay special attention to materials that work well for students with dyslexia and other learning disabilities.

2690 **Corwin Press**
Sage Publications
2455 Teller Rd
Woodbury
Thousand Oaks, CA 91320-2218
805-499-0721
800-818-7243
Fax: 805-499-9774
http://www.corwinpress.com
webmaster@sagepub.com
Mike Soules, President
Lisa Shaw, Executive Director
Kristin Anderson, Director of Learning
Publishes books and products for all learners of all ages and their educators, including subjects such as classroom management, early childhood education, guidance and counseling, higher/adult education, inclusive education, exceptional students, student assessment, as well as behavior, motivation and discipline.

2691 **Educators Publishing Service**
PO Box 9031
Cambridge, MA 2139-9031
617-547-6706
800-435-7728
Fax: 617-547-0285
http://www.epsbooks.com
epsbooks@epsbooks.com
Gunnar Voltz, President
Publishes vocabulary, grammar and language arts materials for students from kindergarten through high school, and specializes in phonics and reading comprehension as well as materials for students with learning differences.

2692 **Federation for Children with Special Needs**
529 Main St.
Suite 1M3
Boston, MA 02129
617-236-7210
800-331-0688
Fax: 617-241-0330
http://www.fcsn.org
fcsinfo@fcsn.org
Richard Robison, Executive Director
Tom Hamel, Director, Business/Finance
Jennetta Hyatt, Director, Human Resources

The mission of the Federation is to provide information, support, and assistance to parents of children with disabilities, their professional partners, and their communities. Major services are information and referrals and parent and professional training.

2693 **Free Spirit Publishing**

217 5th Ave N
Ste 200
Minneapolis, MN 55401-1299
612-338-2068
800-735-7323
Fax: 866-419-5199
http://www.freespirit.com
help4kids@freespirit.com

Judy Galbraith, Owner

Publishes non-fiction materials which empower young people and promote self-esteem through improved social and learning skills. Topics include self-awareness, stress management, school success, creativity, friends and family, and special needs such as gifted and talented learners and children with learning differences.

2694 **Gander Publishing**

450 Front St
Avila Beach, CA 93424
805-541-5523
800-554-1819
Fax: 805-782-0488
http://www.ganderpub.com

Wendy Cook, Sales Director

Publisher and distributor of Lindamood-Bell Programs; Seeing Stars, Visualizing and Verbalizing, On Cloud Nine and Talkies.

2695 **Gordon Systems & GSI Publications**

PO Box 746
Syracuse, NY 13214-746
315-446-4849
800-550-2343
Fax: 315-446-2012
http://www.gsi-add.com
info@gsi-add.com

Michael Gordon PhD, Founder

Books and videos for parents, teachers, children, siblings and adults re: ADHD and foster care. Gordon Diagnostic System is and FDA approved objective measure for use in evaluations of ADHD anf traumatic brain injury. Attention Training System is used in classroom with ADHD children.

2696 **Grey House Publishing**

4919 Route 22
Amenia, NY 12501
518-789-8700
800-562-2139
Fax: 845-373-6360
http://www.greyhouse.com
customerservice@greyhouse.com

Richard Gottlieb, President
Leslie Mackenzie, Publisher
Laura Mars, Vice President, Editorial

Publisher of reference materials, especially directories and encyclopedias. Other Health titles include: The Complete Directory for People with Disabilities; The Complete Directory of Pediatric Disorders; The Chronic Illness Directory; The Mental Health Directory; Older Americans Information Directory; The Directory of Hospital Personnel; The HMO/PPO Directory; and The Medical Device Register.

2697 **Guilford Publications**

72 Spring St
New York, NY 10012-4068
212-431-9800
800-365-7006
Fax: 212-966-6708
http://www.guilford.com
info@guilford.com

Bob Matloff, President
Chris Jennison, Senior Editor Education

Publishes books for education on the subjects of literacy, general education, school psychology and special education. Also offers books, videos, audio cassettes and software, as well as journals, newsletters, and AD/HD resources.

2698 **Hazelden Publishing**

PO Box 11
Center City, MN 55012
651-213-4200
800-257-7810
Fax: 651-213-4411
http://www.hazelden.org
info@hazelden.org

Sharon Birnbaum, Corporate Director
James A Blaha, CFO
Marvin D. Seppala, CMO

Hazelden a national nonprofit organization founded in 1949,helps people reclaim their lives from the disease of addiction.Built on decades of knowledge and exsperience,Hazelden offers a comprehensive approach to addiction that addresses the full range of patient,family, and professional needs, including treatment and continuing care for youth and adults,research,higher education, piblic education and advocacy,and publishing.

2699 **Heinemann-Boynton/Cook**

361 Hanover St
Portsmouth, NH 3802-6926
603-431-7894
800-225-5800
Fax: 603-431-7840
http://www.boyntoncook.com
custserv@heinemann.com

Lesa Scott, VP Human Resources

Publishes professional resources and provides educational services for teachers, and offers nearly 100 titles related to learning disabilities.

2700 **High Noon Books**

20 Commercial Blvd
Novato, CA 94949-6120
6
800-422-7249
Fax: 888-287-9975
http://www.academictherapy.com
sales@academictherapy.com

Jim Arena, President

Features over 35 sets of high-interest, low-level books written on a first through fourth grade reading level, for people with reading difficulties, ages nine and up.

2701 **JKL Communications**

Ste 707
2700 Virginia Ave NW
Washington, DC 20037-1909
202-333-1713
Fax: 202-333-1735
http://www.lathamlaw.org
lathamlaw@gmail.com

Peter S Latham JD, Director
Patricia Horan Latham JD, Director

Publishes books and videos on learning disabilities and ADD with a focus on legal issues in school, higher education and employment.

2702 **Jewish Braille Institute of America**

110 E 30th St
New York, NY 10016-7393
212-889-2525
800-433-1531
Fax: 212-689-3692
http://www.jewishbraille.org
eisler@jbilibrary.org

Dr. Ellen Isler, President
Israel Taub, Associate Director
Sandra Radinsky, Director of Development

Publishes magazines, a newsletter, and special resources available to the reading disabled who are themselves print-handicapped in varying degrees. Seeks the integration of Jews who are blind, visually impaired and reading disabled into the Jewish community and society.

2703 **Learning Disabilities Association of America (LDAA)**

4156 Library Rd.
Pittsburgh, PA 15234-1349
412-341-1515
Fax: 412-344-0224
http://www.ldaamerica.org
info@ldaamerica.org

Mary-Clare Reynolds, Executive Director
Stephanie Fedro-Byrom, Operations Manager
Myrna Mandlawitz, Policy Director
Maintains a large inventory of publications, videos, and other materials related to learning disabilities, and publishes two periodicals available by subscription as well as various books, booklets, brochures, papers, and pamphlets on topics related to learning disabilities.

2704 **Learning Disabilities Resources**
6 E Eagle Rd
Havertown, PA 19083-1424 610-446-6126
800-869-8336
Fax: 610-446-6129
http://www.learningdifferences.com
rcooper-ldr@comcast.net
Rich Cooper, Owner
Offers a variety of resources to help teach the learning disabled, including alternative ways to teach math, language, spelling, vocabulary, and also how to organize and study. Available in books, videos, and audio tapes.

2705 **Library Reproduction Service**
14214 S Figueroa St
Los Angeles, CA 90061-1034 310-354-2610
800-255-5002
Fax: 310-354-2601
http://www.lrs-largeprint.com
lrsprint@aol.com
Peter Jones, Owner
Offers large print reproductions to special needs students in first grade through post-secondary, as well as adult basic and continuing education programs; also produces an extensive collection of large print classics for all ages as well as children's literature.

2706 **LinguiSystems**
8700 Shoal Creek Blvd
Austin, TX 70757-6897 309-755-2300
800-897-3202
Fax: 800-397-7633
TDD: 800-933-8331
http://www.linguisystems.com
info@proedinc.com
Linda Bowers, CEO
Rosemary Huisingh, Co-Owner
Publishes a newsletter and speech-language materials for learning disabilities, ADD/ADHD, auditory processing and listening, language skills, fluency and voice, reading and comprehension, social skills and pragmatics, vocabulary and concepts, writing, spelling, punctuation and other specialized subjects.

2707 **Love Publishing Company**
Ste 2200
9101 E Kenyon Ave
Denver, CO 80237-1854 303-221-7333
Fax: 303-221-7444
http://www.lovepublishing.com
lpc@lovepublishing.com
Stan Love, Owner
Publishes titles for use in special education, counseling, social work, and individuals with learning differences.

2708 **Magination Press**
750 1st St NE
Washington, DC 20002-4241 202-336-5510
800-374-2721
Fax: 202-336-5500
http://www.apa.org
magination@apa.org
Norman B Anderson, CEO
L.Michael Honaker, Deputy CEO
Ellen G. Garrison, Senior Advisor
Publishes special books for children's special concerns, including starting school, learning disabilities, and other topics in psychology, development and mental health.

2709 **Marsh Media**
PO Box 8082
Kansas City, MO 66208-82 816-523-1059
800-821-3303
Fax: 866-333-7421
http://www.marshmedia.com
info@marshmedia.com
Joan Marsh, President
Puberty education for students with special needs curriculum. DVDs on personal safety and social skills.
1969

2710 **Mindworks Press**
4019 Westerly Pl
Ste 100
Newport Beach, CA 92660-2333 949-266-3700
Fax: 949-266-3770
http://amenclinics.com
contact@amenclinic.com
Daniel G Amen, Medical Director & CEO
Features books, audio, video, and CD-ROMs addressing a range of disorders, including anxiety, depression, obsessive-compulsiveness and ADD.

2711 **National Association for Visually Handicapped**
111 E 59th St
New York, NY 10022-1202 212-889-3141
Fax: 212-727-2931
http://www.lighthouse.org
staff@navh.org
Lorianie Marchi, CEO
Publishes information about sight and sight problems for adults and children. Offers a product line of low-vision aids, a collection of articles about eye conditions, causes and treatment modalities, and a newsletter issued four times a year with information to assist people in dealing with low vision.

2712 **National Bible Association**
488 Madison Ave
24 Floor
New York, NY 10022 917-371-0868
212-907-6427
Fax: 212-408-1360
http://www.nationalbible.org
nba@nationalbible.org
Richard Glickstein, President
Publishes Read it! A Journal for Bible Readers, which is issued three times a year. Also offers many versions of the Bible, including large-print editions and the easy-to-read Contemporary English Version.

2713 **Northwest Media**
326 W 12th Ave
Eugene, OR 97401-3449 541-343-6636
800-777-6636
Fax: 541-343-0177
http://www.sociallearning.com
nwm@northwestmedia.com
Lee White, President
Susan Larson, Marketing Director
Publishes material with a focus on independent living and foster care products. Training resources for parents: www.fosterparentcollege.com and for teens: www.vstreet.com.

2714 **PEAK Parent Center**
917 E Moreno Ave
Ste 140
Colorado Springs, CO 80903 719-531-9400
http://www.peakparent.org
info@peakparent.org
Barbara Buswell, Executive Director
David Meeks, President
Sid Inamdar, Vice President

A federally-designated Parent Traning and Information Center (PTI). As a PTI, PEAK supports and empowers parents, providing them with information and strategies to use when advocating for their children with disabilities by expanding knowledge of special education and offering new strategies for success.

2715 **Performance Resource Press**
Ste F
1270 Rankin Dr
Troy, MI 48083-2843
248-588-7733
800-453-7733
Fax: 248-588-6633
http://www.prponline.net
customerservice@prponline.net
George Watkins, President
Publishes over 600 products, including catalogs, journals, digests, newsletters, books, videos, posters and pamplets with a focus on behavioral health.

2716 **Peytral Publications**
PO Box 1162
Minnetonka, MN 55345
952-949-8707
877-739-8725
Fax: 952-906-9777
http://www.peytral.com
help@peytral.com
Peggy Hammeken, President
Publishes and distributes special education materials which promote success for all learners.

2717 **Phillip Roy Catalog**
Phillip Roy
PO Box 130
Largo, FL 33785
727-593-2700
800-255-9085
Fax: 727-595-2685
http://www.phillipro y.com
info@phillipro y.com
Phillip Roy, Owner
Ruth Bragman, President
Publishes educational materials written for students of any age with different learning abilities. Offers an alternative approach to traditional education. Free catalog upon request.

2718 **Reader's Digest Partners for Sight Foundation**
Reader's Digest Rd
Pleasantville, NY 10570
914-244-4900
800-877-5293
http://www.rd.com
partnersforsight@rd.com
Susan Olivo, VP/General Manager
Dianna Kelly-Naghizadeh, Program Manager
Thomas Ryder, CEO
Offers large type editions of select books and large print editions of Readers Digest Magazines, as well as a foundation newsletter, Sightlines, which is published in large format with large type.

2719 **Research Press Publisher**
PO Box 7886
Champaign, IL 61826-9177
217-352-3273
800-519-2707
Fax: 217-352-1221
http://www.researchpress.com
orders@researchpress.com
Gail ll Salyards, President
Dennis Wiziecki, Marketing
Research Press provides user-friendly research-based prevention and intervention materials.

2720 **Riggs Institute**
21106 479th Ave
White, SD 57276-6605
503-646-9459
800-200-4840
Fax: 503-644-5191
http://www.riggsinst.org
riggs@riggsinst.org
Myrna McCulloch, Founder/Director/Author
Publishes materials to help remedial students using the Orton method, a multisensory approach to learning. Offers a catalog of products, including teacher's editions, phonogram cards, audio CDs for students, student materials and classroom materials.

2721 **Scholastic**
557 Broadway
New York, NY 10012-3999
212-343-6100
800-246-2986
Fax: 212-343-6934
http://www.scholastic.com
Richard Robinson, CEO
Barbara A Marcus, VP/President Children's Books
Richard M Spaulding, Executive VP Marketing
Produces educational materials to assist and inspire students of all ages, including a range of special education books, software, and other products.

2722 **Schwab Learning**
201 Mission Strt
Ste 1960
San Francisco, CA 94105
415-795-4920
800-230-0988
Fax: 415-795-4921
http://www.schwabfoundation.org
info@schwabfoundation.org
Helen O. Schwab, President
Charles R. Schwab, Chairman
Nancy Bechtle, Director
Provides information, guidance, support and materials that address the emotional, social, practical and academic needs and concerns of children with learning difficulties, and their parents.

2723 **Slosson Educational Publications**
538 Buffalo Road
East Aurora, NY 14052-280
716-652-0930
888-756-7766
Fax: 716-655-3840
http://www.slosson.com
slossonprep@gmail.com
Steven Slosson, President
Publishes and distributes educational materials in the areas of intelligence, aptitude, developmental disabilities, school screening and achievement, speech-language and assessment therapy, emotional/behavior, and special needs. Offers a product line of testing and assessment materials, books, games, videos, cassettes and computer software intended for use by professionals, psychologists, teachers, counselors, students and parents.

2724 **Teddy Bear Press**
3703 S. Edmunds Street
Suite 67
Seattle, WA 98118
206-402-6947
Fax: 866-870-7323
http://www.teddybearpress.net
fparker@teddybearpress.net
Fran Parker, Author
Publishes books and reading materials designed with the beginning reader in mind, written and illustrated by a special education teacher specializing in elementary education, learning disabilities, and education for the emotionally and mentally challenged.

2725 **Therapro**
225 Arlington St
Framingham, MA 1702-8773
508-872-9494
800-257-5376
Fax: 508-875-2062
http://www.theraproducts.com
info@theraproducts.com
Karen Conrad, Owner

Offers specialty products and publications for all ages in the field of occupational therapy, including assistive technology, evaluations, handwriting programs, sensory-motor awareness and alerting products, oral motor products, early learning products, and perception, cognition and language resources.

2726 **Thomas Nelson Publishers**

PO Box 141000
Nashville, TN 37214-1000
615-248-2110
800-889-9000
Fax: 615-391-5225
http://www.thomasnelson.com
publicity@thomasnelson.com

Thomas Lewis Nelson, Owner
Michael S Hyatt, Executive VP/Group Publisher
Phil Stoner, Executive VP/Group Publisher

Publishes books and other resources for the learning disabled.

2727 **Thorndike Press**

295 Kennedy Memorial Dr
Waterville, ME 4901-4539
207-859-1000
800-223-1244
Fax: 207-859-1008
http://www.thorndike.gale.com
gale.printorders@cengage.com

Jamie Knobloch, Director Marketing
Jill Leckta, Publisher

Publishes and distributes over 900 new large-print editions per year, with an emphasis on bestsellers and genre fiction, as well as nonfiction titles.

2728 **Ulverscroft Large Print Books**

PO Box 1230
West Seneca, NY 14224-8230
716-674-4270
800-955-9659
Fax: 716-674-4195
http://www.ulverscroft.com
enquiries@ulverscroft.co.uk

Janice Gowan, Executive Director

Publishes large print books and audio products for people hard of seeing.

2729 **Wadsworth Publishing Company**

10 Davis Dr
Belmont, CA 94002-3002
650-598-9757
800-354-9706
Fax: 650-637-7544
http://www.wadworth.com
brian.joyner@cangage.com

Susan Badger, Acquisitions Editor

Publishes books on a wide range of topics in special education, including behavior modification, language disorders and development, and learning disabilities.

2730 **Woodbine House**

6510 Bells Mill Rd
Bethesda, MD 20817-1636
301-897-3570
800-843-7323
Fax: 301-897-5838
http://www.woodbinehouse.com
info@woodbinehouse.com

Irv Shapell, Owner

Specializes in books about children with special needs; publishes sixty-five titles within the Special Needs Collection, covering AD/HD, learning disabilities, special education, communication skills, and other disabilities, for use by parents, children, therapists, health care providers and teachers.

2731 **Xavier Society for the Blind**

154 E 23rd St
New York, NY 10010-4595
212-473-7800
http://www.xaviersocietyfortheblind.org
info@xaviersocietyfortheblind.org

Kathleen Lynch, Manager
Gina Ballero, Secretary to Director

Provides resources for the visually impaired, including large-print, braille, and audio products.

Classroom Resources

2732 **Collaboration in the Schools: The Problem-Solving Process**
Pro-Ed
8700 Shoal Creek Blvd
Austin, TX 78757-6897
512-451-3246
800-897-3202
Fax: 512-451-8542
http://www.proedinc.com
info@proedinc.com
Donald D Hammill, Owner
An inservice/preservice video that demonstrates the stages of the consultative/collaborative process, as well as many of the various communicative/interactive skills and collaborative problem solving skills. *$106.00*

2733 **Educational Evaluation**
Stern Center for Language and Learning
183 Talcott Road
Suite 101
Williston, VT 5495-9209
802-878-2332
800-544-4863
Fax: 802-878-0230
http://www.sterncenter.org
learning@sterncenter.org
Blanche Podhajski, President
Jane Nathan, Research Director
Michael Saphiro, CFO
The evaluation is an assessment of intelligence, academic achievement, language, and emotional and behavioral issues related to learning and includes pre- and post- evaluation conferences with parents and/ or students as well as an extensive written report detailing results and recommendations.

2734 **Fundamentals of Reading Success**
Educators Publishing Service
PO Box 9031
Cambridge, MA 2139-9031
617-547-6706
800-225-5750
Fax: 617-547-0412
http://www.epsbooks.com
eps@epsbooks.com
Arlene W Sonday, Author
This Orton-Gillingham-based video series teaches a phonic or code-emphasis approach to reading, spelling, and handwriting, and provides the foundation for a multisensory phonics curriculum. May be used by teachers and tutors. *$ 480.00*
ISBN 0-838872-52-2

2735 **Individual Instruction**
Stern Center for Language and Learning
135 Allen Brook Ln
Williston, VT 5495-9209
802-878-2332
800-544-4863
Fax: 802-878-0230
http://www.sterncenter.org
learning@sterncenter.org
Blanche Podhajski, President
Jane Nathan, Research Director
Michael Saphiro, CFO
Individualized instruction to help students develop literacy skills and achieve academic success, building on learning strengths and compensating for areas of difficulty.

2736 **Instructional Strategies for Learning Disabled Community College Students**
Graduate School and University Center
365 5th Ave
New York, NY 10016-4309
212-817-7000
Fax: 212-817-1503
http://www.gc.cuny.edu
Frances Degenhorowitz, President
For working with a cross-section of types of individuals with learning problems. *$47.50*

2737 **Key Concepts in Personal Development**
Marsh Media
PO Box 8082
Kansas City, MO 66208-82
816-523-1059
800-821-3303
Fax: 866-333-7421
http://www.marshmedia.com
info@marshmedia.com
Joan Marsh, President
Puberty Education for Children with Special Needs. Comprehensive, gender-specific kits and supplemental parent packets address human sexuality for children with miild to moderate developmental disabilities.

2738 **Living With Attention Deficit Disorder**
Aquarius Health Care Media
30 Forest Road
Millis, MA 20054
508-376-1244
888-440-2963
Fax: 508-376-1245
http://www.aquariusproductions.com
aquarius@aquariusproductions.com
Leslie Kussmann, President
Anne Baker, Billing and Accounting
This video presents tips for teachers and students how to deal with ADD, including how to adapt school structures and classes. *$125.00*
Video, 22 mins

2739 **New Room Arrangement as a Teaching Strategy**
Teaching Strategies
7101 Wisconsin Avenue
Suite 700
Bethesda, MD 20814
301-634-0818
800-637-3652
Fax: 301-657-0250
http://www.teachingstrategies.com
info@teachingstrategies.com
Andrea Valentine, President
Ron Davies, CEO
Amy Houser, CMO
A manual and video present the impact of the early childhood classroom environment on how children learn, how they relate to others and how teachers teach. *$35.00*

2740 **Now You're Talking: Extend Conversation**
Educational Productions
7101 Wisconsin Avenue
Suite 700
Bethesda, MD 20814
800-637-3652
Fax: 301-634-0826
http://www.teachingstrategies.com
info@teachingstrategies.com
Andrea Valentine, President
Ron Davies, CEO
Amy Houser, CMO
Video. Teachers in a language-based preschool and speech-language pathologists model effective techniques that focus and extend conversations of young children. *$295.00*

2741 **Phonemic Awareness: Lessons, Activities and Games**
Sage/Corwin Press
2455 Teller Rd
Thousand Oaks, CA 91320-2218
805-410-7408
Fax: 805-499-2692
http://www.corwinpress.com
Mike Soules, President
Lisa Shaw, Executive Director
Kristin Anderson, Director of Learning
Exceptional field tested guide to help educators who want to reach phonemic awareness as a prerequisite to reading, and/or to supplement the current curriculum. Special educators and speech clinicians will find this practical guide especially helpful as research indicates that deficits in phonemic awareness is often a major contributor to reading disabilities. This book or video contains fifty-eight scripted lessons, forty-nine reproducible blackline master and progress charts.

2742 **Professional Development**
Stern Center for Language and Learning
183 Talcott Road
Suite 101
Williston, VT 5495-9209
802-878-2332
800-544-4863
Fax: 802-878-0230
http://www.sterncenter.org
learning@sterncenter.org
Blanche Podhajski, President
Jane Nathan, Research Director
Michael Saphiro, CFO
Staff development programs for preschool through grade 12 designed in response to requests from teachers and administrators for cutting-edge information about different kinds of learners and the teaching strategies most successful for them.

2743 **Purdue University Speech-Language Clinic**
100 N University St
West Lafayette, IN 47907-2098
765-494-3663
800-359-2968
Fax: 765-494-3660
http://www.cla.purdue.edu
Irwin Weiser, Dean
The Speech-Language Clinic provides opportunities for individuals with communication problems to receive individual and group diagnostic evaluations, screenings and therapy services. The clinic provide services for children and adults with mild to severe speech sound problems and/or impaired oral-motor control, language problems associated with autism, language-learning disabilities, hearing impairment, stuttering, and voice problems. *$81.00*

2744 **Restructuring America's Schools**
Association for Supervision/Curriculum Development
1703 N Beauregard St
Alexandria, VA 22311-1746
703-578-9600
Fax: 703-549-3891
http://www.ascd.org
Nancy Gibson, President
Marie Adair, Executive Director
Jon Chapman, Chief Strategy Officer
A leader's guide and videotape designed for administrators, teachers, parents, school board members, and community leaders.

2745 **Skillstreaming Video: How to Teach Students Prosocial Skills**
Research Press
PO Box 9177
Champaign, IL 61826-9177
217-352-3273
800-519-2707
Fax: 217-352-1221
http://www.researchpress.com
rp@researchpress.com
Russell Pence, President
A video and two books providing an overview of a training procedure for teaching elementary and secondary level students the skills they need for coping with typical social and interpersonal problems. *$365.00*

2746 **Spelling Workbook Video**
Learning Disabilities Resources
PO Box 716
Arlington, VA 22206
610-525-8336
800-869-8336
Fax: 703-998-2060
http://www.ldonline.org
An instructional video which works through the spelling workbooks for teachers and students. *$16.00*

2747 **Strategic Planning and Leadership**
Association for Supervision/Curriculum Development
1703 N Beauregard St
Alexandria, VA 22311-1714
703-578-9600
800-933-2723
Fax: 703-575-5400
http://www.ascd.org
Nancy Gibson, President
Marie Adair, Executive Director
Jon Chapman, Chief Strategy Officer
Designed to explain and illustrate effective approaches to dealing with change through strategic planning.

2748 **Teaching Adults with Learning Disabilities**
Stern Center for Language and Learning
183 Talcott Road
Suite 101
Williston, VT 5495-9209
802-878-2332
800-544-4863
Fax: 802-878-0230
http://www.sterncenter.org
bpodhajski@sterncenter.org
Blanche Podhajski, President
Jane Nathan, Research Director
Michael Saphiro, CFO
A videotape training program and companion guide designed to help adult literacy teachers identify and instruct adults with learning disabilities. The focus of this five hour video series is on teaching basic reading and spelling skills. *$199.95*

2749 **Teaching Math**
Learning Disabilities Resources
2775 S. Quincy St
Arlington, VA 22206
610-525-8336
800-869-8336
Fax: 610-525-8337
http://www.ldonline.org
ldonline@weta.org
Neol Gunther, Executive Director
Susannah Harris, Senior Manager
A video for educational professionals teaching math to disabled children. *$12.00*

2750 **Teaching People with Developmental Disabilities**
Research Press
PO Box 9177
Champaign, IL 61826-9177
217-352-3273
800-519-2707
Fax: 217-352-1221
http://www.researchpress.com
rp@researchpress.com
Russell Pence, President
A set of four videotapes and accompanying participant workbooks designed to help teachers, staff, volunteers, or family members master task analysis, prompting, reinforcement and error correction. *$595.00*

2751 **Teaching Strategies Library: Research Based Strategies for Teachers**
Association for Supervision/Curriculum Development
1703 N Beauregard St
Alexandria, VA 22311-1714
703-548-9600
Fax: 703-575-5400
http://www.ascd.org
Nancy Gibson, President
Marie Adair, Executive Director
Jon Chapman, Chief Strategy Officer
A trainer's manual and five videotapes designed for inservice education of teachers K-12 focusing on four different types of learning expected of students: mastery, understanding, synthesis and involvement.

2752 **Teaching Students Through Their Individual Learning Styles**
St. John's University, Learning Styles Network
PO Box 417
Henrietta, NY 14467
888-887-7552
Fax: 256-740-0310
http://www.learningstyles.net
James Benson, Executive Director
A set of six videotapes introducing the Dunn and Dunn learning styles model. Explains the environmental, emotional, sociological, physical and psychological elements of style.

2753 **Telling Tales**
KET, The Kentucky Network Enterprise Division
600 Cooper Dr
Lexington, KY 40502-1669
859-258-7000
800-354-9067
Fax: 859-258-7396
http://www.tellingtales.org
info@tellingtales.org

Susan Jasper, Founder
Resource for teachers,librarians and drama departments at all levels of instruction. Telling Tales can be used to encourage creativity and self expression and help students understand their cultural and language arts skills, and develop openess to diverse cultures, build self confidence and leadership skills, improve communication and language arts skills and develop oral history projects. *$30.00*

2754 **Word Feathers**
KET, The Kentucky Network Enterprise Division
600 Cooper Dr
Lexington, KY 40502-1669
859-258-7000
800-354-9067
Fax: 859-258-7396
http://www.tellingtales.org
info@tellingtales.org

Susan Jasper, Founder
An activity-oriented language arts video series.

Parents & Professionals

2755 **3 R'S for Special Education: Rights, Resources, Results**
Brookes Publishing Company
PO Box 10624
Baltimore, MD 21285
410-337-9580
800-638-3775
Fax: 410-337-8539
http://www.pbrookes.com
custserv@pbrookes.com

Paul H Brooks, Owner
This video helps parents navigate the steps of the special education system and work towards securing the best education and services for their children. *$49.95*
Video

2756 **A Child's First Words**
Orange County Learning Disabilities Association
PO Box 25772
Santa Ana, CA 92799-5772
714-547-4206
http://www.oclda.org
info@oclda.org

Shows the importance of not waiting until your child is older to worry about their speech. *$20.00*
Catalog #7353

2757 **A Culture Undiscovered**
Fanlight Productions
32 Court St
21 Floor
Brooklyn, NY 11201
718-488-8900
800-876-1710
Fax: 718-488-8642
http://www.fanlight.com
info@fanlight.com

Miguel Gallardo, PsyD, Author
Ben Achtenberg, Owner
Explores the needs and experiences of college students, from diverse racial and/or ethnic backgrounds, who have learning disabilities. *$149.00*
Video, 36 min
ISBN 1-572959-22-3

2758 **A Mind of Your Own**
Fanlight Productions
32 Court St
21 Floor
Brooklyn, NY 11201
718-488-8900
800-876-1710
Fax: 718-488-8642
http://www.fanlight.com
info@fanlight.com

Gail Sweeney National Film Board of Canada, Author
Ben Achtenberg, Owner
New video on learning disabilities from the National Film Board of Canada, follows four learning disabled students through their struggles academically and socially as well as their successes in learning to cope with their disabilities and develop their own unique talents. Amtec Award of Merit. 37 minutes. *$199.00*
Video, 38 mins.
ISBN 1-572959-08-8

2759 **ABC's of Learning Disabilities**
American Federation of Teachers
555 New Jersey Ave NW
Washington, DC 20001-2029
202-879-4400
Fax: 202-879-4597
http://www.aft.org
online@aft.org

Sandra Feldman, President
This film illustrates the case histories of four learning disabled students with various learning disabilities.

2760 **ADHD**
Brookes Publishing Company
PO Box 10624
Baltimore, MD 21285
800-638-3775
Fax: 410-337-8539
http://www.pbrookes.com
custserv@pbrookes.com

Paul H Brooks, President
Melissa A Behm, Executive Vice President
George Stamathis, Vice President/Publisher
This video shows methods for helping students who have ADHD increase attention to tasks, improve listening skills, become better organized, and boost work production. *$99.00*
Video
ISBN 1-557661-15-4

2761 **ADHD in Adults**
Guilford Publications
72 Spring St
New York, NY 10012-4019
212-431-9800
800-365-7006
Fax: 212-966-6708
http://www.guilford.com
info@guilford.com

Bob Matloff, President
Jody Falco, Editor in Chief
This program integrates information on ADHD with the actual experiences of four adults who suffer from the disorder. Representing a range of professions, from a lawyer to a mother working at home, each candidly discusses the impact of ADHD on his or her daily life. These interviews are qugmented by comments from family members and other clinicians who treat adults with ADHD *$95.00*
36-min VHS

2762 **ADHD in the Classroom: Strategies for Teachers**
Guilford Publications
72 Spring St
New York, NY 10012-4019
212-431-9800
800-365-7006
Fax: 212-966-6708
http://www.guilford.com
info@guilford.com

Bob Matloff, President
Jody Falco, Editor in Chief

Viewers see the problems teachers encounter with children who suffer with ADHD, as well as instructive demonstrations of effective behavior management techbiques including color charts and signs, point system, token economy, and turtle-control technique. Also includes a Leader's Guide and a 42-page Manual. *$95.00*
36-min. VHS

2763 **ADHD: What Can We Do?**
Guilford Publications
72 Spring St
New York, NY 10012-4019
212-431-9800
800-365-7006
Fax: 212-966-6708
http://www.guilford.com
info@guilford.com
Bob Matloff, President
Jody Falco, Editor in Chief
A video program that introduces teachers and parents to a variety of the most effective techniques for managing ADHD in the classroom, at home, and on gamily outings. Includes Leader's Guide and 30-page Manual. *$95.00*
ISBN 0-898629-72-1

2764 **ADHD: What Do We Know?**
Guilford Publications
72 Spring St
New York, NY 10012-4019
212-431-9800
800-365-7006
Fax: 212-966-6708
http://www.guilford.com
info@guilford.com
Bob Matloff, President
Jody Falco, Editor in Chief
An introduction for teachers and special education practitioners, school psychologists and parents of ADHD children. Topics outlined in this videoinclude the causes and prevalence of ADHD, ways children with ADHD behave, otherconditions that may accompany ADHD and long-term prospects for children with ADHD. *$95.00*
Video

2765 **Adapting to Your Child's Personality**
Aquarius Health Media Care
30 Forest Road
Millis, MA 20054-1066
508-376-1244
888-440-2963
Fax: 508-376-1245
http://www.aquarisproductions.com
aquarius@aquarisproductions.com
Leslie Kussmann, President
Anne Baker, Billing and Accounting
Join a child behavioral specialist, two moms and their toddlers (with different personalities!) to find out how to mold your own responses so that you can more effectively influence your child. VHS: A-KIDSPERSONAL also on DVD. *$ 145.00*
Video, 30 mins

2766 **Adults with Learning Problems**
Learning Disabilities Resources
2775 S. Quincy St
Arlington, VA 22206
610-525-8336
800-869-8336
Fax: 703-998-2060
http://www.ldonline.org
ldonline@weta.org
Neol Gunther, Executive Director
Susannah Harris, Senior Manager
Educational materials for adults with a learning disability.

2767 **All Children Learn Differently**
Orange County Learning Disabilities Association
PO Box 25772
Santa Ana, CA 92799-5772
714-547-7206
http://www.oclda.org
info@oclda.org
Covers cognitive, perceptual, nutritional, optometric, speech and language motor aspects. *$29.95*
Catalog #6812

2768 **American Sign Language Phrase Book Videotape Series**
Harris Communications
15155 Technology Dr
Eden Prairie, MN 55344-2273
952-906-1180
800-825-6758
Fax: 952-906-1099
TDD: 952-906-1198
TTY: 800-825-9187
http://www.harriscomm.com
info@harriscomm.com
Darla Hudson, Customer Service
Includes book and three videotapes, each 60 minutes long. In Volume 1 you will find everyday expressions, signing and deafness, getting acquainted, health and water; in Volume 2 you will find family, school, food and drink, clothing, sports and recreation; and in Volume 3 you will find travel, animal, colors, civics, religion, numbers, time, dates and money. Set of books and videos. Part #BVT141. *$134.95*

2769 **Andreas: Outcomes of Inclusion**
Center on Disability and Community Inclusion
208 Colchester Avenue
3rd Floor
Burlington, VT 5405
802-656-3131
Fax: 802-656-1357
TTY: 802-656-4031
http://www.uvm.edu/zvapvt/timfox
syuan@uvm.edu
Tom Sullivan, President
Video portrays the academic, occupational, and social inclusion of a high school student with severe disabilities. Includes commentary of parents, administrators, teachers, support personnel, classmates.

2770 **Around the Clock: Parenting the Delayed ADHD Child**
Guilford Publications
72 Spring St
New York, NY 10012-4019
212-431-9800
800-365-7006
Fax: 212-966-6708
http://www.guilford.com
info@guilford.com
Bob Matloff, President
Jody Falco, Editor in Chief
This videotape provides both professionals and parents a helpful look at how the difficulties facing parents of ADHD children can be handled. *$150.00*
45-min. VHS

2771 **Art of Communication**
United Learning
Ste 100
1560 Sherman Ave
Evanston, IL 60201-4817
847-328-6700
800-424-0362
Fax: 847-328-6706
http://www.unitedlearning.com
info@unitedlearning.com
Ronald Reed, Vice President
Designed for parents and professionals, this video focuses on: effective parent-child communication; nonverbal communication in children; effective listening; effects of negative and critical messages; and deterrents limiting child/parent communication. *$99.00*

2772 **Attention Deficit Disorder**
Pro-Ed
8700 Shoal Creek Blvd
Austin, TX 78757-6816
512-451-3246
800-897-3202
Fax: 512-451-8542
http://www.proedinc.com
info@proedinc.com
Donald D Hammill, Owner
DR Jordan, Author

A video and book providing helpful suggestions for both home and classroom management of students with attention deficit disorder. *$60.00*
Yearly

2773 **Augmentative Communication Without Limitations**
Prentke Romich Company (PRC)
1022 Heyl Rd
Wooster, OH 44691-9786
330-262-1984
800-262-1984
Fax: 330-263-4829
http://www.prentrom.com
David L Moffatt, President
Cherie Weaver, Marketing Coordinator
Prentke Romich Company (PRC) is a worldwide leader in the development and manufacture of augmentative communication devices, computer access products, and other assistive technology for people with severe disabilities.

2774 **Autism**
Aquarius Health Media Care
30 Forest Road
Millis, MA 20054-1066
508-376-1244
888-440-2963
Fax: 508-376-1245
http://www.aquariusproductions.com
orders@aquariusproductions.com
Leslie Kussmann, President/Producer
Through therapeutic horseback riding a young boy emerges from his isolated world. He finds a connection with his horse when he isn't able to talk to adults. A teenage girl gains social confidence as she leads her llama at a local fair. This film explores the power animals can have on helping someone with autism to connect. This film is great for anyone working the autistic and their families. VHS: A-DISHWAA also on DVD. *$125.00*
Video, 30 mins

2775 **Beyond the ADD Myth**
Brookes Publishing Company
PO Box 10624
Baltimore, MD 21285
410-337-9580
800-638-3775
Fax: 410-337-8539
http://www.pbrookes.com
custerv@pbrookes.com
Paul H Brooks, President
Melissa A Behm, Executive VP
George Stamthis, VP/Publisher
This video builds on the theory that many of the behaviors associated with attention deficit disorder are not solely due to neurological dysfunction but actually result from a wide range of social, psychological, and educational causes. *$22.00*
Video
ISBN 1-557661-15-4

2776 **Child Who Appears Aloof: Module 5**
Educational Productions
7101 Wisconsin Avenue
Suite 700
Bethesda, MD 20814
503-297-6393
800-637-3652
Fax: 503-297-6395
http://www.teachingstrategies.com
info@teachingstrategies.com
Andrea Valentine, President
Ron Davies, CEO
Amy Houser, CMO
A 30 minute video and 60 page facilitation packet focusing on children who pull back, who avoid social contact. Teaches strategies to understand and support these children. Part of the Hand-in-Hand Series. *$295.00*

2777 **Child Who Appears Anxious: Module 4**
Educational Productions
7101 Wisconsin Avenue
Suite 700
Bethesda, MD 20814
503-297-6393
800-637-3652
Fax: 503-297-6395
http://www.teachingstrategies.com
info@teachingstrategies.com
Andrea Valentine, President
Ron Davies, CEO
Amy Houser, CMO
A 35 minute video and 60 page training facilitation packet examining the issues of anxious children and how a supporting adult can help bring them into play. Part of the Hand-in-Hand Series. *$295.00*

2778 **Child Who Dabbles: Module 3**
Educational Productions
7101 Wisconsin Avenue
Suite 700
Bethesda, MD 20814
503-297-6393
800-637-3652
Fax: 503-297-6395
http://www.teachingstrategies.com
info@teachingstrategies.com
Andrea Valentine, President
Ron Davies, CEO
Amy Houser, CMO
A 30-minute video and 60-page training facilitation guide that compares dabbling to quality, invested play and offers various strategies for adultsto help children build play skills. Part of Hand-in-Hand Series. *$295.00*

2779 **Child Who Wanders: Module 2**
Educational Productions
7101 Wisconsin Avenue
Suite 700
Bethesda, MD 20814
503-297-6393
800-637-3652
Fax: 503-297-6395
http://www.teachingstrategies.com
info@teachingstrategies.com
Andrea Valentine, President
Ron Davies, CEO
Amy Houser, CMO
A 30-minute video and 67-page training facilitation packet showing how to identify children who cannot engage in play so wander about the room. Shows creative interventions to help teach new skills. Part of Hand-in-Hand Series.

2780 **Child Who is Ignored: Module 6**
Educational Productions
7101 Wisconsin Avenue
Suite 700
Bethesda, MD 20814
503-644-7000
800-637-3652
Fax: 503-350-7000
http://www.teachingstrategies.com
info@teachingstrategies.com
Andrea Valentine, President
Ron Davies, CEO
Amy Houser, CMO
A 30 minute video and 60 page facilitation guide illustrating the children who are ignored by others and offering several interventions for them to learn social skills. Part of the Hand-in-Hand Series. *$295.00*

2781 **Child Who is Rejected: Module 7**
Educational Productions
7101 Wisconsin Avenue
Suite 700
Bethesda, MD 20814
503-297-6393
800-637-3652
Fax: 503-297-6395
http://www.teachingstrategies.com
info@teachingstrategies.com
Andrea Valentine, President
Ron Davies, CEO
Amy Houser, CMO

A 35-minute video and 60-page facilitation packet with strategies to help children whose behavior and/or appearance causes them to be rejected by other children. Part of Hand-in-Hand Series.

2782 **Concentration Video**
Center for Alternative Learning
6 E Eagle Rd
Havertown, PA 19083-1424
610-446-6126
800-204-7667
Fax: 610-446-6129
http://www.learningdifferences.com
rcooper-ldr@comcast.net
Rich Cooper, Director/Founder/Author
A 53 minute instructional video provides an optimistic perspective about attention problems ADD. Dr. Cooper discusses different types of attention problems causes and solutions. The second part of the video contains concentration exercises to help children and adults with attention problems. *$16.00*
53 Mins/Video

2783 **Degrees of Success: Conversations with College Students with LD**
4th Fl
240 Greene St
New York, NY 10003-6675
212-387-8205
Fax: 212-995-4114
http://www.nyu.edu/osl/csd
A new video which features college students with learning disabilities speaking in their own words about: making the decision to attend college, developing effective learning strategies, coping with frustrations and utilizing college support services. Includes resource packet with suggested discussion questions and list of other resources.

2784 **Developing Minds: Parent's Pack**
Learning Disabilities Resources
2775 S. Quincy St
Arlington, VA 22206
610-525-8336
800-869-8336
Fax: 703-998-2060
http://www.ldonline.org
ldonline@weta.com
Dr. Mel Levine, Author
Lia Salza, Editorial Associate
Created especially for parents, this video set provides an overview of why some children struggle with learning. The programs offer strategies for supporting kids' learning differences, based on the work of Dr. Mel Levin and his neurodevelopmental view on how to help children and adolescents become successful learners. *$59.90*
2 Videos

2785 **Developing Minds: Teacher's Pack**
Learning Disabilities Resources
2775 S. Quincy St
Arlington, VA 22206
610-525-8336
800-869-8336
Fax: 703-998-2060
http://www.ldonline.org
ldonline@weta.com
Dr. Mel Levine, Author
Lia Salza, Editorial Associate
Created especially for educators, this video set provides an overview of why some children struggle with learning. The programs offer strategies for supporting kids' learning differences, based on the work of Dr. Mel Levin and his neurodevelopmental view on how to help children and adolescents become successful learners. *$59.90*
2 Videos

2786 **Dyslexia: A Different Kind of Learning**
Aquarius Health Media Care
18 N Main St
Millis, MA 20054-1066
508-376-1244
888-440-2963
Fax: 508-376-1245
http://www.aquarisproductions.com
aquarius@aquarisproductions.com
Leslie Kussmann, President
Part of the Prescription for Learning Series. This programs shows us what it's like to grow up with dyslexia and the challenge people with dyslexia face in school. The video presents tips for teachers and students on how to deal with it, including how to adapt school structures and classes. VHS: A-TISDYSLEXIA *$125.00*
Video, 24 mins

2787 **FAT City**
Connecticut Assoc. for Children and Adults with LD
Ste 15-5
25 Van Zant St
Norwalk, CT 6855-1713
203-838-5010
Fax: 203-866-6108
http://www.CACLD.org
cacld@juno.com
Beryl Kaufman, Executive Director
Marie Armstrong, Information Specialist
Nationally acclaimed video designed to sensitize adults to the frustration, anxiety and tension that the learning disabled child experiences daily. Add $5.00 for shipping and handling. *$49.95*

2788 **First Steps Series: Supporting Early Language Development**
Educational Productions
7101 Wisconsin Avenue
Suite 700
Bethesda, MD 20814
503-297-6393
800-637-3652
Fax: 503-297-6395
http://www.teachingstrategies.com
info@teachingstrategies.com
Andrea Valentine, President
Ron Davies, CEO
Amy Houser, CMO
Four 20-minute videos used in early intervention efforts for training staff and parents. Teach how to support language acquisition and model responsive, connected adult-child relationships foundational for all development and learning

2789 **Getting Started With Facilitated Communication**
Syracuse Univ./Facilitated Communication Institute
370 Huntington Hall
Syracuse, NY 13244-2324
315-443-9379
Fax: 315-443-9218
http://www.soeweb.syr.edu/thefci
fcstaff@syr.edu
Annegret Schubert, Author
Douglas Biklen, Ph.D.ÿ, Director
Details on the getting started process, including discussion of candidacy, facilitator attitude, materials and equipment, and the components involved in a first session. Several first sessions are excerpted, showing a child, a teenager, a person with challenging behavior, and a child with significant but not fully functional speech.
14-min/Video

2790 **Getting Started with Facilitated Communication**
Syracuse University, Institute on Communication
370 Huntington Hall
Syracuse, NY 13244
315-443-9657
Fax: 315-443-2274
http://www.soeweb.syr.edu/thefci
fcstaff@syr.edu
Annegret Schubert, Author
Douglas Biklen, Ph.D.ÿ, Director

This videotape describes the details of the getting started process, including discussion of candidacy, facilitator attitude, materials and equipment, and the components involved in a first session.

2791 **Help! This Kid's Driving Me Crazy!**
Pro-Ed
8700 Shoal Creek Blvd
Austin, TX 78757-6816
512-451-3246
800-897-3202
Fax: 512-451-8542
http://www.proedinc.com
info@proedinc.com
Donald D Hammill, Owner
Designed for parents and professionals working with children up to five years old, this videotape and booklet offers information about the nature, special needs, and typical behavioral characteristics for young children with attention deficit disorder. *$5.00*

2792 **How Difficult Can This Be?**
Learning Disabilities Resources
2775 S. Quincy St
Arlington, VA 22206
610-525-8336
800-869-8336
Fax: 703-998-2060
http://www.ldonline.org
ldonline@weta.com
Richard Lavoie, Author
Lia Salza, Editorial Associate
This program looks at the world through the eyes of a child with learning disabilities by taking you to a unique workshop attended by parents, educators, psychologists, and social workers. There they join in a series of classroom activities that cause frustration, anxiety and tension - emotions all too familiar to the student with a learning disability. *$49.95*
70 mins/Video

2793 **I Want My Little Boy Back**
BBC - Autism Treatment Center of America
2080 S Undermountain Rd
Sheffield, MA 1257-9643
413-229-2100
877-766-7473
Fax: 413-229-8931
http://www.autismtreatment.com
autism@option.org
Tracy Baisden, Marketing Associate
This BBC documentary follows an English family with a child with autism before, during, and after their time at the Son-Rise Program. It uniquely captures the heart of the Son-Rise Program and is extremely useful in understanding its techniques. *$20.00*

2794 **I'm Not Stupid**
Learning Disabilities Association of America
4156 Library Rd
Pittsburgh, PA 15234-1349
412-341-1515
Fax: 412-344-0224
http://www.ldanatl.org
ldanatl@usaor.net
This video depicts the constant battle of the learning disabled child in school. *$22.00*

2795 **Identifying Learning Problems**
Center for Alternative Learning
6 E Eagle Rd
Havertown, PA 19083-1424
610-446-6126
800-204-7667
Fax: 610-446-6129
http://www.learningdifferences.com
rcooper-ldr@comcast.net
Rich Cooper, Director/Founder/Author
A presentation made to adult educators and volunteer tutors discusses what to look for in a student who has difficulty learning. The red flags (common behaviors and errors) are described. *$16.00*
1hr 40mins

2796 **Inclusion Series**
Comforty Mediaconcepts
2145 Pioneer Rd
Evanston, IL 60201-2564
847-475-0791
Fax: 847-475-0793
comforty@comforty.com
Jacky Comforty, Owner
A series of video programs on inclusive education and community life. Titles include: Choices, providing instruction for all audiences to the inclusion process; Inclusion: Issues for Educators, focusing on particular teachers and administrators in Illinois schools; Families, Friends, Futures, emphasizing the need for early inclusion; and Together We're Better, providing an overview of this comprehensive program. Videos available separately or as a set.

2797 **International Professional Development Training Catalog**
Center for Alternative Learning
6 E Eagle Rd
Havertown, PA 19083-1424
610-446-6126
800-204-7667
Fax: 610-446-6129
http://www.learningdifferences.com
scooper-ldr@comcast.net
Rich Cooper, Director
Training session details how individuals with learning differences, problems and disabilities think and learn.

2798 **Latest Technology for Young Children**
Western Illinois University: Macomb Projects
27 Horrabin Hall
Macomb, IL 61455
309-298-1955
Fax: 309-298-2305
http://www.mprojects.wiu.edu
PL-Hutinger@wiu.edu
Patricia Hutinger EdD, Director
Joyce Johanson, Coordinator
Amanda Silberer, Manager
This 25 minute videotape focuses on the Macintosh LC and adaptations for young children and includes a discussion of the features and advantages of the Macintosh LC, software demonstrations, footage of child applications, and ideas for off-computer activities. Videotape and written materials available.OUT OF BUSINESS *$40.00*
16-20 pages

2799 **Learning Disabilities and Discipline: Rick Lavoie's Guide to Improving Children's Behavior**
Connecticut Assoc. for Children and Adults with LD
Ste 15-5
25 Van Zant St
Norwalk, CT 6855-1713
203-838-5010
Fax: 203-866-6108
http://www.CACLD.org
cacld@juno.com
Beryl Kaufman, Executive Director
In this video, Richard Lavoie, a nationally known expert on learning disabilities, offers practical advice on dealing with behavioral problems quickly and effectively. Shows how preventive discipline can anticipate many problems before they start. Explains how teachers and parents can create stable, predictable environments in which children with learning disabilities can flourish. 62 minutes. *$49.95*

2800 **Learning Disabilities and Self-Esteem**
Connecticut Assoc. for Children and Adults with LD
Ste 15-5
25 Van Zant St
Norwalk, CT 6855-1713
203-838-5010
Fax: 203-866-6108
http://www.CACLD.org
cacld@juno.com
Beryl Kaufman, Executive Director

The 60 minute Teacher video contains program material for building self-esteem in the classroom. The 60 minute Parent video contains program material for building self-esteem in the home. A 16 page Program Guide accompanies each video. Dr. Robert Brooks, a clinical psychologist, renowned speaker and nationally known expert on learning disabilities, is on the faculty at Harvard Medical School and is the author of The Self-Esteem Teacher. *$49.95*

2801 **Learning Disabilities and Social Skills: Last One Picked..First One Picked On**
Connecticut Assoc. for Children and Adults with LD
Ste 15-5
25 Van Zant St
Norwalk, CT 6855-1713 203-838-5010
Fax: 203-866-6108
http://www.CACLD.org
cacld@juno.com
Beryl Kaufman, Executive Director
Nationally recognized expert on learning disabilities, Richard Lavoie, gives examples on how to help LD children succeed in everyday social situations. Lavoie helps students dissect their social errors to learn correct behavior. Mistakes are seen as opportunities for learning. Available in parent (62 min.) or teacher (68 min.) version. *$49.95*

2802 **Learning Disabilities: A Complex Journey**
Aquarius Health Media Care
18 N Main St
Millis, MA 20054-2324 508-376-1244
888-440-2963
Fax: 508-376-1245
http://www.aquariusproductions.com
orders@aquariusproductions.com
Leslie Kussmann, President/Producer
Does your child have trouble reading? Does your daughter seem to have more difficulty with schoolwork than you would expect, even though she's trying her hardest? Is your son avoiding school, claiming illness a little to often, insisitng that he's stupid when you know that's not really true? If so, your child may have a learning disability— a neurological problem processing information that he's actually smart enough to understand. How do you find out? VHS: A-KIDSLD also on DVD. *$125.00*
Video, 26 mins

2803 **Learning Problems in Language**
Center for Alternative
6 E Eagle Rd
Havertown, PA 19083-1424 610-446-6126
800-204-7667
Fax: 610-446-6129
http://www.learningdifferences.com
rcooper-ldr@comcast.net
Rich Cooper, Founder/Director/Author
This video was recorded at the National Laubach Conference in 1992 for reading tutors and teachers. In the video, Dr. Cooper discusses ideas for teaching reading and other academic skills to adults. *$16.00*
2hr, 50 mins

2804 **Legacy of the Blue Heron: Living with Learning Disabilities**
Oxton House Publishers
PO Box 209
Farmington, ME 4938 207-779-1923
800-539-7323
Fax: 207-779-0623
http://www.oxtonhouse.com
info@oxtonhouse.com
William Berlinghoff PhD, Managing Editor
Cheryl Martin, Marketing
Debra Richards, Office Manager
Thi book is available in soft cover or as a six-cassette audiobook. It is an engaging personal account by a servere dyslexic who became a successful engineer, business man, boat builder, and president of the Learning Disabilities Association of America. Drawing on his life experiences, the author presents a rich array of wise, common-sense advice for dealing with learning disabilities.

2805 **Letting Go: Views on Integration**
Iowa University Affiliated Programs
300 CMAB
Iowa City, IA 52242-1016 319-353-6390
800-272-7713
Fax: 319-356-8284
http://www.healthcare.uiowa.edu
disability-library@uiowa.edu
Three parents share their thoughts regarding the struggle between protecting their children with disabilities verses allowing the same freedom as other children. *$25.00*
19 mins/Video

2806 **Lily Videos : A Longitudinel View of Lily with Down Syndrome**
Davidson Films
Ste 210
735 Tank Farm Rd
San Luis Obispo, CA 93401-7073 805-594-0422
888-437-4200
Fax: 805-594-0532
http://www.davidsonfilms.com
dfi@davidsonfilms.com
Elaine Taunt, Manager
Fran Davidson, Owner
1. Lily: A Story About a Girl Like Me 2. Lily: A Sequal 3. Lily: At Thirty.

2807 **Making Sense of Sensory Integration**
Therapro
225 Arlington St
Framingham, MA 1702-8773 508-872-9494
800-257-5376
Fax: 508-875-2062
http://www.theraproducts.com
info@theraproducts.com
Karen Conrad, Owner
A discussion for parents and caregivers about sensory integration (SI), how it affects children throughout their lives, how diagnosis is made, appropriate treatment, recognizing red flags, and how SI difficulties affect child and family in their everyday lives. Informative 33 page book included. 75 minute CD. *$17.95*
31 pages Audio CD
ISBN 1-931615-14-4

2808 **Motivation to Learn: How Parents and Teachers Can Help**
Association for Supervision/Curriculum Development
1703 N Beauregard St
Alexandria, VA 22311-1746 703-578-9600
800-933-2723
Fax: 703-575-5400
http://www.ascd.org
Nancy Gibson, President
Marie Adair, Executive Director
Two videos intended for all those concerned about how educators and families can develop student motivation to learn, solve motivational problems, and effectively participate in parent-teacher conferences.

2809 **Normal Growth and Development: Performance Prediction**
Love Publishing Company
9101 East Kenyon Ave
Ste 2200
Denver, CO 80237 303-221-7333
Fax: 303-221-7444
http://www.lovepublishing.com
lovepublishing@compuserve.com
Dan Love, Director
Stan Love, Owner
Teaches the age at which skills are normally achieved by children ages 0 to 48 months. *$140.00*
Video

2810 **Oh Say What They See: Language Stimulation**
Educational Productions
9000 SW Gemini Dr
Beaverton, OR 97008-7151
503-644-7000
800-950-4949
Fax: 503-350-7000
http://www.edpro.com
custserv@edpro.com
Linda Freedman, Owner
Molly Krumm, Marketing Director
A complete video training program illustrating indirect language stimulation techniques to teachers, parents, students, child care staff, and other adult caregivers working with children.

2811 **Parent Teacher Meeting**
Learning Disabilities Resources
2775 S. Quincy St
Arlington, VA 22206
610-525-8336
800-869-8336
Fax: 703-998-2060
http://www.ldonline.org
ldonline@weta.org
Discusses learning differences and instructional techniques. *$12.00*

2812 **Phonemic Awareness: The Sounds of Reading**
Sage/Corwin Press
2455 Teller Rd
Thousand Oaks, CA 91320-2218
805-410-7408
Fax: 805-499-2692
http://www.corwinpress.com
order@corwin.com
Mike Soules, President
Lisa Shaw, Executive Director
Kristin Anderson, Director of Learning
This staff development video may be used with paraprofessionals and teachers to learn the techniques of teaching pnomemic awareness. *$59.95*
Video
ISBN 1-890455-29-6

2813 **Puberty Education for Students with Special Needs**
Marsh Media
PO Box 8082
Shawnee Mission, KS 66208
802-821-3303
Fax: 866-333-7421
http://www.marshmedia.com
info@marshmedia.com
Liz Smith, Author
Liz Sweeney, Co-Author
Two gender-specific kits include an instructional video, a comprehensive teaching guide and packets of 10 student booklets. These reassuring titles are clear, practical and positive and are intended for the following special populations: Students with developmental disabilities or delays, Intrusive behavior or mental illness, Down Syndrome, Autism Spectrum Disorder, Learning disabilities, Behavioral disabilities, Communicative disorders.
36 pages

2814 **Regular Lives**
WETA-TV, Department of Educational Activities
Ste 440
2775 S Quincy St
Arlington, VA 22206
610-525-8336
800-869-8336
Fax: 703-998-2060
http://www.weta.com
info@weta.com
Sharon P Rockefeller, President
Designed to show the successful integration of handicapped students in school, work and community settings. Demonstrates that sharing the ordinary routines of learning and living is essential for people with disabilities.

2815 **STEP/Teen: Systematic Training for Effective Parenting of Teens**
AGS
PO Box 99
Circle Pines, MN 55014
763-786-4343
800-328-2560
Fax: 763-786-9077
http://www.agsnet.com
agsmail@agsnet.com
Kevin Brueggeman, Manager
A parent training program designed to help parents of teenagers in the following areas: understanding misbehavior; improving communication and family relationships; understanding and expressing emotions and feelings and discipline. *$229.50*

2816 **Speech Therapy: Look Who's Not Talking**
Aquarius Health Media Care
18 N Main St
Sherborn, MA 1770-1066
508-650-1616
888-440-2963
Fax: 508-650-1665
http://www.aquariusproductions.com
aquarius@aquarisproductions.com
Leslie Kussmann, President
A Keeping Kids Healthy Series. Your child is old enough to be talking - other children are by this age - but for some reason, your child just can't put the words together. When should you step in to help? And what, exactly, can you do? VHS: A-KIDSSPEECH. Also available on DVD. *$125.00*
Video, 14 mins

2817 **Student Directed Learning: Teaching Self Determination Skills**
Beech Center on Disability, University of Kansas
1200 Sunnyside Ave
Lawrence, KS 0
785-864-7600
Fax: 785-864-7605
http://www.beachcenter.org
wehmeyer@ku.edu
Mike Wehmeyer, Associate Director
Written for educators and service providers who seek a comprehensive understanding of the process of helping students develop self-determination skills. The text follows academic principles and clearly is geared to professionals rather than to families. An educator seeking to understand technical self-determination concepts will find this organizational structure effective. *$73.00*
ISBN 0-534159-42-7

2818 **Study Skills: How to Manage Your Time**
Guidance Associates
31 Pine View Rd
Mount Kisco, NY 10549-3425
914-244-1055
800-431-1242
Fax: 914-244-1056
http://www.guidanceassociates.com
info@guidanceassociates.com
Fred Gaston Jr, Owner
Describes how to create a personal schedule that will help users get more accomplished each day and waste less time. *$61.00*
Video

2819 **The Power of Positive Communication**
Educational Productions
7101 Wisconsin Avenue
Suite 700
Bethesda, MD 20814
503-297-6393
800-637-3652
Fax: 503-297-6395
http://www.teachingstrategies.com
info@teachingstrategies.com
Andrea Valentine, President
Ron Davies, CEO
Amy Houser, CMO

A complete three-session training on CD-ROM teaches how and why to use clear, positive language to help children to follow expectations and learn. Emphasizes strategies that assist both children with special needs and English language learners.

2820 **Time Together: Adults Supporting Play**
Educational Productions
7101 Wisconsin Avenue
Suite 700
Bethesda, MD 20814
503-297-6393
800-637-3652
Fax: 503-297-6395
http://www.teachingstrategies.com
info@teachingstrategies.com
Andrea Valentine, President
Ron Davies, CEO
Amy Houser, CMO
A complete video training program for beginning childhood teachers,aides and parents illustrating when to join a child's play, how to enhance and extend the play, and when to step back.

2821 **Tools for Students**
Therapro
225 Arlington St
Framingham, MA 1702-8773
508-872-9494
800-257-5376
Fax: 508-875-2062
http://www.theraproducts.com
info@theraproducts.com
Karen Conrad, Owner
This is a 30 minute fun and participatory 'how-to' presentation which provides solutions to the problems indentified in the Tools for Teachers Video. It can be used by teachers in the classroom and by parents at home. There are 25 sensory tools for movement, proprioception, mouth and hand fidgets, calming and recess. Pencil-holding and hand games to develop hand manipulation skills are also demonstrated.
$25.95
Video

2822 **Tools for Teachers**
Therapro
225 Arlington St
Framingham, MA 1702-8773
508-872-9494
800-257-5376
Fax: 508-875-2062
http://www.theraproducts.com
info@theraproducts.com
Karen Conrad, Owner
Provides a logical approach to sensory integration and hand skill strategies for anyone to use, is ideal for in-services. Within 20 minutes, you'll learn how to help students calm down, focus, and increase their self-awareness. This is a great tool for teachers and therapists (it shows how to inplement sensory diet, into classroom), administrators and parents. *$25.95*
Video

2823 **TrainerVision: Inclusion, Focus on Toddlers and Pre-K**
Educational Productions
PO Box 957
Hillsboro, OR 97123
503-297-6393
800-950-4949
Fax: 503-297-6395
http://www.edpro.com
custserv@edpro.com
Linda Freedman, Owner
Instructive video clips focus on non-typically developing toddlers and pre-K children. Shows how to gently support skill building, independence and social competence. The clips are ideal to enrich training, classes and online courses.

2824 **Treatment of Children's Grammatical Impairments in Naturalistic Context**
Purdue University Continuing Education
1586 Stewart Ctr
West Lafayette, IN 47907
765-494-7231
800-830-0269
Fax: 765-494-0567
http://www.continuinged.purdue.edu/media/speech
Marc Fey, Presenter
The basic assumption is challenged that language intervention which takes place in naturalistic settings will be more effective than intervention that occurs in settings that are more heavily constrained by a clinician or other intervention agent. The concept of naturalness will be described as a continuum that is influenced by a number of factors that can be manipulated by clinicians. Several effective intervention approaches that reflect different levels of naturalness are presented. *$50.00*
1hr:42 mins

2825 **Understanding Attention Deficit Disorder**
Connecticut Assoc. for Children and Adults with LD
Ste 15-5
25 Van Zant St
Norwalk, CT 6855-1713
203-838-5010
Fax: 203-866-6108
http://www.CACLD.org
cacld@juno.com
Beryl Kaufman, Executive Director
A video in an interview format for parents and professionals providing the history, symptoms, methods of diagnosis and three approaches used to ease the effects of attention deficit disorder. A comprehensive general introduction to ADHD. 45 minutes. *$20.00*
Video

2826 **United Learning**
Ste 100
1560 Sherman Ave
Evanston, IL 60201-4817
847-328-6700
888-892-3494
Fax: 847-328-6706
http://www.unitedlearning.com
crechner@unitedlearning.com
Ronald Reed, President
Joel Altschul, Vice President
Coni Rechner, Vice President
United Learning is a provider of audio-visual materials that inform and educate people of all ages. It helps teachers teach more effectively and to help students learn more efficiently. Offering videos, cd's, dvd's, and now delivery of video clips and text via the internet.

2827 **What Every Teacher Should Know About ADD**
United Learning
Ste 100
1560 Sherman Ave
Evanston, IL 60201-4817
847-328-6700
888-892-3484
Fax: 847-328-6706
http://www.unitedlearning.com
info@unitedlearning.com
Ronald Reed, President
Mark Zinselmeier, Operations VP/General Manager
Coni Rechner, Marketing VP
This program is for teachers, paraprofessionals, administrators, and special educators because it separates clearly fact from fiction and is written specifically for and about educators who deal with disruptive, inattentive, and hyperactive pre-school and elementary age children on a daily basis.
$79.00
28-min. video

2828 **When a Child Doesn't Play: Module 1**
Educational Productions
PO Box 957
Hillsboro, OR 97123
800-950-4949
Fax: 503-297-6395
http://www.edpro.com
custserv@edpro.com
Linda Freedman, Owner
A 30 minute video with 100 pages of facilitation materials presentsdramatic footage of children with play problems and how they miss critical opportunities to learn. Illustrates supportive strategies for adults. Foundation program for Hand-in-Hand Series. *$350.00*

Vocational

2829 **Different Way of Learning**
Brookes Publishing Company
PO Box 10624
Baltimore, MD 21285
800-638-3775
Fax: 410-337-8539
http://www.pbrookes.com
custserv@pbrookes.com
Paul H Brooks, President
Melissa A Behn, Executive Vice President
George Stamthis, Vice President/Publisher
This video prepares students with learning disabilities for the transition from school to the workplace. *$49.00*
Video
ISBN 1-557663-49-1

2830 **Employment Initiatives Model: Job Coach Training Manual and Tape**
Young Adult Institute
460 W 34th St
New York, NY 10001-2320
212-273-6100
Fax: 212-268-1083
http://www.yai.org
ahorowitz@yai.org
Philip Levy, Manager
Thomas A Dern, Assoc. Executive Director
Aimee Horowitz, Project Specialist
Video and manual providing an overview and orientation for staff members involved in transition services to ensure that they are well-grounded inthe concepts, responsibilities, and activities that are required to provide quality supported employment services.

2831 **First Jobs: Entering the Job World**
Triumph Learning
PO Box 1270
Littleton, MA 1460-4270
800-338-6519
Fax: 212-675-8922
http://www.triumphlearning.com
customerservice@triumphlearning.com
Career/vocational education with emphasis on job search skills, job interviews and survival skills. *$139.00*

2832 **How Not to Contact Employers**
Nat'l Clearinghouse of Rehab. Training Materials
6524 Old Main Hil
Logan, UT 84322-6524
435-797-7537
Fax: 866-821-5355
http://https://ncrtm.org/
ncrtm@usu.edu
Sara P. Johnston, M.S, Director
Jennifer Robinson, Official Assistant
A single vignette of what not to do when visiting perspective employers to secure positions for clients. *$10.00*

2833 **KET Basic Skills Series**
KET, The Kentucky Network Enterprise Division
600 Cooper Dr
Lexington, KY 40502-2296
859-258-7000
800-354-9067
Fax: 859-258-7399
http://www.ket.org
feedback@ket.org
Barbra Ledford, President
Offers an independent learning system for workers who need retraining or help with basic skills

2834 **KET Foundation Series**
KET, The Kentucky Network Enterprise Division
600 Cooper Dr
Lexington, KY 40502-2296
859-258-7000
800-354-9067
Fax: 859-258-7399
http://www.ket.org
feedback@ket.org
Barbra Ledford, President
A highly effective basic skills series that is tailor-made for the needs of proprietary and vocational schools.

2835 **KET/GED Series**
KET, The Kentucky Network Enterprise Division
600 Cooper Dr
Lexington, KY 40502-1669
859-258-7000
800-354-9067
Fax: 859-258-7399
http://www.ket.org
feedback@ket.org
Barbra Ledford, President
This nationally acclaimed instructional series helps adults prepare for the GED test.

2836 **KET/GED Series Transitional Spanish Edition**
KET, The Kentucky Network Enterprise Division
600 Cooper Dr
Lexington, KY 40502-1669
859-258-7000
800-354-9067
Fax: 859-258-7399
http://www.ket.org
feedback@ket.org
Barbra Ledford, President
This award-winning series offers ESL students effective preparation for the GED test.

2837 **Life After High School for Students with Moderate and Severe Disabilities**
Beech Center on Disability, University of Kansas
3111 Haworth Hall
Lawrence, MA 0
785-864-7600
Fax: 785-864-7605
http://www.beachcenter.org
beachcenter@ku.edu
Shonda Anderson, Project Coordinator
A set of three videotapes and a participant handbook document, and a teleconference in which family members, people with disabilities, teachers, rehabilitation specialists, program administrators and policy makers focus on improving the quality of services in high school and supported employment programs.

2838 **On Our Own Transition Series**
Young Adult Institute
460 W 34th St
New York, NY 10001-2320
212-273-6100
Fax: 212-268-1083
http://www.yai.org
ahorowitz@yai.org
Philip Levy, Manager
Thomas A Dern, Assoc. Executive Director
Aimee Horowitz, Project Specialist
Designed for parents and professionals, this series of 15 videotapes examines innovative transitional approaches that help create marketable skills, instill self-esteem and facilitate successful transition for individuals with developmental disabilities.

General

2839 **www.HealthCentral.com**
Former Surgeon-General Dr. C Everett Koop
Information on health and conditions that affect learning, particularly heavy on the ADHD side.

2840 **www.ala.org**
American Library Association
Run by the American Library Association, this site works to raise public awareness about learning disabilities.

2841 **www.allaboutvision.com**
All About Vision
Vision information and resources, including articles on learning-related vision problems.

2842 **www.apa.org/psycinfo**
American Psychological Association
An online abstract database that provides access to citations to the international serial literature in psychology and related disciplines from 1887 to present. Available via PsycINFO Direct at www.psycinfo.com.

2843 **www.autismtreatment.com**
Autism Treatment Center of America
Since 1983, the Autism Treatment Center of America, has provided innovative training programs for parents and professionals caring for children challenged by Autism, Autism Spectrum Disorders, Pervasive Developmental Disorders (PDD) and other developmental difficulties. The Son-Rise Program teaches a specific yet comprehensive system of treatment and education designed to help families and caregivers enable their children to dramatically improve in all areas of learning.

2844 **www.childdevelopmentinfo.com**
Child Development Institute
Provides online information on child development, psychology, parenting, learning, health and safety as well as childhood disorders such as attention deficit disorder, dyslexia and autism. Provides comprehensive resources and practical suggestions for parents.

2845 **www.disabilityinfo.gov**
DisabilityInfo.gov
Provides one-stop online access to resources, services, and information available throughout the federal government to Americans with disabilities, their families, employers and service providers; also promotes awareness of disability issues to the general public.

2846 **www.disabilityresources.org**
Disability Resources
A guide to internet resources available with information and recommendations for disability assistance.

2847 **www.doleta.gov/programs/**
O'Net: Department of Labor's Occ. Information
Employment assistance, descriptions, and articles about learning disabled employees and government resources.

2848 **www.dyslexia.com**
Davis Dyslexia Association International
Links to internet resources for learning. Includes dyslexia, Autism and Asperger's Syndrome, ADD/ADHD and other learning disabilities.

2849 **www.familyvillage.wisc.edu**
University of Wisconsin-Madison
A global community that integrates information, resources and communication opportunities on the Internet for all those involved with cognitive and other disabilities.

2850 **www.funbrain.com**
Quiz Lab
Internet education site for teachers and kids. Access thousands of assessment quizzes online. Assign paperless quizzes that are graded automatically by email. Teaching tools are free and easy to use.

2851 **www.health.disovery.com**
Discovery Health
Information on conditions that impact learning.

2852 **www.healthanswers.com**
Health Answers Education
Health information, including learning disabilities, etc.

2853 **www.healthatoz.com**
Medical Network
Health information, including ADD, ADHD, etc.

2854 **www.healthcentral.com**
HealthCentral Network
Information and products for a healthier life. Includes conditions that impact learning.

2855 **www.healthymind.com**
HealthyMind.com
Information on ADD and learning disabilities.

2856 **www.hood.edu/seri/serihome.htm**
Special Education Resources on the Internet
Contains links to information about definitions, legal issues, and teaching and learning related to learning disabilities.

2857 **www.icpac.indiana.edu/infoseries/is-50.htm**
Finding Your Career: Holland Interest Inventory
Includes information on self-assessing one's skills and matching them to careers.

2858 **www.intelihealth.com**
Aetna InteliHealth
Includes information on learning disabilities.

2859 **www.irsc.org**
Internet Research for Special Children
Attention deficit and hyperactivity disorder help website, created so information, support and ADD coaching are available without having to pour over all 531,136 links that come up on a net search.

2860 **www.jobhunt.org/slocareers/resources.html**
Online Career Resources
Contains assessment tools, tutorials, labor market information, etc.

2861 **www.ld-add.com**
Attention Deficit Disorder (ADD or ADHD)
Do you think that you or your child has ADHD with or without learning disabilities? If the answer is yes, this webpage is for you.

2862 **www.ldonline.org**
Learning Project at WETA
Learning disabilities information and resources.

2863 **www.ldpride.net**
LD Pride Online
Inspired by Deaf Pride, a site developed as an interactive community resource for youth and adults with learning disabilities and ADD.

2864 **www.ldteens.org**
Study Skills Web Site
Run by the New York State Chapter of the International Dyslexia Association; a site for students, created by students; provides helpful tips and links.

2865 **www.marriottfoundation.org**
Marriott Foundation
Provides information on job opportunities for teenagers and young adults with disabilities.

2866 **www.my.webmd.com**
Web MD Health
Medical website with information which includes learning disabilities, ADD/ADHD, etc.

2867 **www.ntis.gov**
National Techinical Information Service
A worldwide database for research, development and engineering reports on a range of topics, including architectural barrier removal, employing individuals with disabilities, alternative testing formats, job accommodations, school-to-work transition for students with disabilities, rehabilitation engineering, disability law and transportation.

2868 **www.ocde.K12.ca.us/PAL/index2.html**
Peer Assistance Leadership (PAL)
A California-based outreach program for elementary, intermediate and high school students.

2869 **www.oneaddplace.com**
One A D D Place
A virtual neighborhood of information and resources relating to ADD, ADHD and learning disorders.

2870 **www.optimums.com**
JR Mills, MS, MEd
Information on learning disabilities.

2871 **www.pacer.org**
Does My Child Have An Emotional Disorder
Our mission is to expand opportunities and enhance the quality of life of children and young adults with disabilities and their families, based on the concept of parents helping parents.

2872 **www.parentpals.com**
Ameri-Corp Speech and Hearing
Offers parents and professionals special education support, teaching ideas and tips, special education continuing education, disability-specific information and more.

2873 **www.peer.ca/peer.html**
Peer Resources Network
A Canadian organization that offers training, educational resources, and consultation to those interested in peer helping and education. Their resources section has information on books, articles and videos.

2874 **www.petersons.com**
Peterson's Education and Career Center
Contains postings for full-and part-time jobs as well as summer job opportunities.

2875 **www.specialchild.com**
Resource Foundation for Children with Challenges
Variety of information for parents of children with disabilities, including actual stories, family and legal issues, diagnosis search, etc.

2876 **www.specialneeds.com**
Special Needs Project
A place to get books about disabilities.

2877 **www.wrightlaw.com**
Wrightslaw
Provides information about advocacy.

Counseling & Psychology

2878 **American Psychologist**
American Psychological Association
750 1st St NE
Washington, DC 20002-4242
202-336-5500
800-374-2721
Fax: 202-336-5518
TDD: 202-336-6123
TTY: 202-336-6123
http://www.apa.org
journals@apa.org

Norman B Anderson, Editor
Contains archivel documents and articles covering current issues in psychology, the science and practice of psychology, and psychology's contribution to public policy.
9 times x year
ISSN 0003-066X

2879 **Educational Therapist Journal**
Association of Educational Therapists
7044 S. 13th Street
Oak Creek, WI 53154
414-908-4949
Fax: 414-768-8001
http://www.aetonline.org
aet@aetonline.org

Jeanette Rivera, President
A multidisciplinary publication, that publishes articles and reviews on clinical practice, research, and theory. In addition, it serves to inform the reader of AET activities and business and presents issues relevant to the practice of educational therapy. *$40.00*
Quarterly

2880 **Journal of Social and Clinical Psychology**
Guilford Press
72 Spring Street
New York, NY 10012-4019
800-365-7006
Fax: 212-966-6708
http://www.guilford.com
info@guilford.com

Thomas E Joiner PhD, Editor
Discusses theory, research and research methodology from personality and social psychology toward the goal of enhancing the understanding of human well-being and adjustment. Also covers a wide range of areas, including intimate relationships, attributions, stereotyping, social skills, depression research, coping strategies, and more. It fosters interdisciplinary communication and scholarship among students and practitioners of social/personality and clinical/counseling/health psychology. *$165.00*
128 pages 10x a year
ISSN 0736-7236

2881 **Learning Disabilities Research & Practice**
Blackwell Publishing
350 Main St
Malden, MA 2148-5089
781-388-8200
Fax: 781-388-8210
http://www.blackwellpublishing.com

Charles Hughes, Editor
Because learning disabilities is a multidisciplinary field of study, this important journal publishes articles addressing the nature and characteristics of learning disabled students, promising research, program development, assessment practices, and teaching methodologies from different disciplines. In so doing, LDRP provides information of great value to professionals involved in a variety of different disciplines including school psychology, counseling, reading and medicine. *$68.00*
Quarterly
ISSN 0938-8982

2882 **School Psychology Quarterly**
American Psychological Association
750 1st St NE
Washington, DC 20002-4241
202-336-5500
800-374-2721
Fax: 202-336-5518
TDD: 202-336-6123
TTY: 202-336-6123
http://www.apa.org
journals@apa.org

Norman B Anderson, Editor
This journal advances the latest research, theory, and practice and features a new book review section. Strengthening the relationship between school psychology and broad-based psychological science. *$57.00*
Quarterly
ISSN 1045-3830

General

2883 **ASCD Express**
Association for Supervision/Curriculum Development
1703 N Beauregard St
Alexandria, VA 22311-1714
703-578-9600
800-933-2723
Fax: 703-575-5400
http://www.ascd.org
express@ascd.org

Rick Allen, Editor
Willona Sloan, Editor
This newsletter highlights articles on research-based teaching practices and provides you with quick links to these articles, relevant resources, and multimedia clips. *$29.00*
Bi-weekly

2884 **American Journal of Occupational Therapy**
American Occupational Therapy Association
4720 Montgomery Lane
Bethesda, MD 20814
301-652-2682
800-729-2682
Fax: 301-652-7711
TDD: 800-377-8555
http://www.aota.org
ajoteditor@cox.net

Mary A Corcoran PhD, Editor
An official publication of the American Occupational Therapy Association, inc. This peer reviewed journal focuses on research, practice, and health care issues in the field of occupational therapy. Also publishes articles that are theoretical and conceptual and that represent theory-based research, research reviews, and applied research realted to innovative program approaches, educational activities, and professional trends. *$50.00*
6x a year

2885 **American School Board Journal**
National School Boards Association
1680 Duke St
Alexandria, VA 22314-3474
703-838-6722
703-838-6722
Fax: 703-549-6719
http://www.asbj.com

Marilee C Rist, Publisher
Glenn Cook, Editor
American School Board Journal chronicles change, interprets issues, and offers readers — some 40,000 school board members and school administrators — practical advice on a broad range of topics pertinent to school go9vernance and management, policy making, student achievement, and the art of school leadership. In addition, regular departments cover education news, school law, research, and new books.
$54.00
Monthly

2886 **Annals of Otology, Rhinology and Laryngology**
Annals Publishing Company
4507 Laclede Ave
Saint Louis, MO 63108-2103 314-367-4987
Fax: 314-367-4988
http://www.annals.com
manager@annals.com
Ken Cooper, President
Richard J. H Smith, Managing Director
Offers original manuscripts of clinical and research importance in otolaryngology - head and neck surgery, audiology, speech pathology, head and neck oncology and surgery, and related specialties. All papers are peer-reviewed *$ 179.00*
112 pages Monthly
ISSN 0003-4894

2887 **Autism Research Review International**
Autism Research Institute
4182 Adams Ave
San Diego, CA 92116-2599 619-281-7165
Fax: 619-563-6840
http://www.autism.com
Steve Edelson, Editor
Janet Johnson, Managing Director
Covering biomedical and educational advances in autism research. *$18.00*
Quarterly

2888 **CABE Journal**
Connecticut Association of Boards of Education
81 Wolcott Hill Rd
Wethersfield, CT 6109-1286 860-571-7446
800-317-0033
Fax: 860-571-7452
http://www.cabe.org
bcarney@cabe.org
Robert Rader, Executive Director
Patrice McCarthy, Deputy Director
Reaches virtually all board members, superintendents and business managers in Connecticut. It's the only publication which does so on a regular basis. It is designed to encompass all material in an easy-to-read fashion. Readers if the journal find a wide range of topics covered in each issue.
11x a year

2889 **CEC Today**
Council for Exceptional Children
Ste 300
1110 N Glebe Rd
Arlington, VA 22201-5704 703-245-0600
888-232-7733
Fax: 703-264-9494
TTY: 866-915-5000
http://www.cec.sped.org
service@cec.sped.org
Lynda Voyles, Editor
Drew Albritten M.D., President
Bruce Ramirez, Manager
An online member newsletter that keeps you up-to-date on professional and legal developments.
4x per year

2890 **Disability Compliance for Higher Education**
LRP Publications
PO Box 24668
West Palm beach
Palm Beach Gardens, FL 33418-7106 561-622-6520
800-341-7874
Fax: 561-622-0757
http://www.lrp.com
webmaster@lrp.com
Kenneth Kahn, CEO
Virginia Charleston, Product Group Manager
Cynthia Gomez, Author
Combines insightful analyses of disability laws with details of innovative accomodations for your students and staff. *$198.00*
12 issues/yr

2891 **Education Digest**
Prakken Publications
PO Box 8623
Ann Arbor, MI 48107-8623 734-975-2800
Fax: 734-975-2787
http://www.eddigest.com
pam@eddigest.com
Pam Moore, Editor
The Education Digest reviews recent periodicals and reports on education to produce 12 or more condensations for quick, easy reading, along with the regular monthly columns and features. *$32.00*
9 Issues

2892 **Education Week**
Editorial Projects in Education
Ste 100
6935 Arlington Rd
Bethesda, MD 20814-5287 301-280-3100
800-346-1834
Fax: 301-280-3200
http://www.edweek.org
Virginia Edwards, Editor
Offers articles of interest to educators, teachers, professionals and special educators on the latest developments, laws, issues and more in the various fields of education. *$74.94*

2893 **Educational Leadership**
Association for Supervision/Curriculum Development
1703 N Beauregard St
Alexandria, VA 22311-1746 703-578-9600
800-933-2722
Fax: 703-575-5400
http://www.ascd.org
edleadership@ascd.org
Marge Scherer, Editor
RICHARD J. H. SMITH
8x a year

2894 **Educational Researcher**
American Educational Research Association
1430 K St., NW
Suite 1200
Washington, DC 20005 202-238-3200
Fax: 202-238-3250
http://www.aera.net
pubs@aera.net
Carolyn D. Herrington, Editor
Jason A. Grissom, Editor
Educational Researcher (ER) publishes scholarly articles that are of general significance to the education research community and that come from a wide range of areas of education research and related disciplines. ER aims to make major programmatic research and new findings of broad importance widely accessible. ER is one of AERA's flagship journals and is received by all members of the association.
9x a year
ISSN 0013-189X

2895 **Educational Technology**
Educational Technology Publications
700 E Palisade Ave
Englewood Cliffs, NJ 7632-3060 201-871-4007
800-952-BOOK
Fax: 201-871-4009
http://www.asianvu.com/bookstoread/etp
edtecpubs@aol.com
Lawrence Lipsitz, Editor
The world's leading periodical publication covering the entire field of educational technology, an area pioneered by the magazine's editors in the early 1960s. *$179.00*
6x annually

2896 **Gifted Child Today**
Prufrock Press
Ste 220
5926 Balcones Dr
Austin, TX 78731-4263
512-300-2220
Fax: 512-300-2221
http://www.prufrock.com
info@prufrock.com
Susan K Johnsen PhD, Editor
Sarah Morrison, Editor
Offers teachers information about teaching gifted children. Offers parents information about raising a gifted child, how to tell if your child is gofted, and effective strategies for parenting a gifted child. *$40.00*
Quarterly

2897 **Journal of Learning Disabilities**
Sage Publications
2455 Teller Rd
Thousand Oaks, CA 91320-2218
805-499-9774
800-818-7243
Fax: 805-499-0871
http://www.sagepub.com
journals@sagepub.com
H Lee Swanson, Editor
Recognized internationally as the oldest and most authoritative journal in the area of learning disabilities. The editorial board reflects the international, multidisciplinary nature of JLD, comprising researchers and practitioners in numerous fields, including education, psychology, neurology, medicine, law and counseling. *$69.00*
Bimonthly
ISSN 0022-2194

2898 **Journal of Postsecondary Education and Disability**
Association on Higher Education and Disability
Ste 204
107 Commerce Centre Dr
Huntersville, NC 28078-5870
704-947-7779
Fax: 704-948-7779
http://www.ahead.org
ahead@ahead.org
James Martin PhD, Editor
Serves as a resource to members and other professionals dedicated to the advancement of full participation in higher education for persons with disabilities. Is also the leading forum for scholarship in the field of postsecondary disability support services.

2899 **Journal of Rehabilitation**
National Rehabilitation Association
PO Box 150235
Alexandria, VA 22314-4109
703-836-0850
888-258-4295
Fax: 703-836-0848
http://www.nationalrehab.org
info@nationalrehab.org
Daniel C Lustig, Editor
David R Strauser, Editor
Sara Sundeen, President
The Journal of Rehabilitation publishes articles by leaders in the fields of rehabilitation. The articles are written for rehabilitation professionals and students studying in the fields of rehabilitation *$65.00*
Quarterly
ISSN 0022-4154

2900 **Journal of School Health**
Blackwell Publishing
350 Main St
Malden, MA 2148-5089
781-388-8200
Fax: 781-388-8210
http://www.blackwellpublishing.com
customerservices@blackwellpublishing.com
James H Price, Editor
Committed to communicating information regarding the role of schools and school personnel in facilitating the development and growth of healthy youth and healthy school environments.
Monthly
ISSN 0022-4391

2901 **Journal of Special Education Technology**
Council for Exceptional Children
2900 Crystal Drive
Ste 1000
Arlington, VA 22202-3557
703-245-0600
888-232-7733
Fax: 703-264-9494
http://www.cec.sped.org
service@cec.sped.org
J Emmett Gardner, Editor
The Journal of Special Education Technology (JSET) is a refereed professional journal that presents up-to-date information and opinions about issues, research, policy, and practice related to the use of technology in the field of special education. The publication is sent to subscribers and members of the Technology and Media Division of the Council for Exceptional Children. *$60.00*
Quarterly

2902 **LDA Alabama Newsletter**
Learning Disabilities Association of Alabama
PO Box 244023
Montgomery, AL 36124
334-277-9151
http://ldaalalabama.org
Tamara Massey-Garrett, President
A non-profit grassroots organization whose members are individuals with learning disabilities, their families, and the professionals who work with them. LDAA is dedicated to identifying causes and promoting prevention of learning disabilities and to enhance the quality of life for all individuals with learning disabilities and their families by encouraging effective identification and intervention, fostering research, and protecting their rights under the law.

2903 **LDA Rhode Island Newsletter**
Learning Disabilities Association of Rhode Island
4156 Library Road
Pittsburgh, PA 15234-1349
412-341-1515
Fax: 412-344-0224
TDD: 401-946-6968
http://www.ldanatl.org
info@ldaamerica.org
Mary Clare Reynolds, Interim Executive Director
Frank Kline PhD, Editor
A nonprofit, volunteer organization whose members give their time and support to children with learning disabilities as well as share information with other parents, professionals and individuals with learning disabilities.

2904 **Learning Disabilities Quarterly**
Council for Learning Disabilities
PO Box 405
Overland Park, KS 66201
913-491-1011
Fax: 913-941-1012
http://www.cldinternational.org
ldq@bc.edu
David Scanlon, Editor
Presents scientifically-based research, and includes articles by nationally known authors.
4x a year

2905 **Learning Disabilities: A Multidisciplinary Journal**
Learning Disabilities Association of America
4156 Library Rd
Pittsburgh, PA 15234-1349
412-341-1515
Fax: 412-344-0224
http://www.LDAAmerica.org
info@ldaamerica.org
Steve Russell, Editor
A technical publication oriented toward professionals in the field of learning disabilities. *$30.00*
Quarterly

2906 **Learning and Individual Differences**
Elsevier
6277 Sea Harbor Dr
Orlando, FL 32887
407-563-6022
877-839-7126
Fax: 407-363-1354
TDD: 301-657-4155
http://www.elsevier.com
journalcustomerservice-usa@elsevier.com
E L Grigorenko, Editor
A multidisciplinary journal in education.
ISSN 1041-6080

2907 **National Organization on Disability**
77 Water St.
Suite 204
New York, NY 10005
646-505-1191
Fax: 646-505-1184
http://www.nod.org
info@nod.org
Gov. Tom Ridge, Baord Chairman
Carol Glazer, President
Miranda Pax, Director, External Affairs
The mission of the National Organization on Disability is to expand the participataion and contribution of America's 57 million men, women, and children with disabilities in all aspects of life.

2908 **OT Practice**
American Occupational Therapy Association
PO Box 31220
Bethesda, MD 20824-1220
301-652-2682
800-SAY-AOTA
Fax: 301-652-7711
TDD: 800-377-8555
http://www.aota.org
otpractice@aota.org
Laura Collins, Editor
Frederick P Somers, Executive Director
The clinical and professional magazone of the AOTA. It serves as a comprehensive, authoritative source for practical information to help occupational therapists and occupational therapy assistants to succeed professionally. Provides professional news and information on all aspects of practice and encourages a dialogue among AOTA members on professional concerns and views.
64 pages

2909 **Occupational Outlook Quarterly**
US Department of Labor
200 Constitution Ave
Washington, DC 20212
202-693-5000
Fax: 202-693-6111
http://www.dol.gov
Olivia Crosby, Editor
Information on new educational and training opportunities, emerging jobs, prospects for change in the work world and the latest research findings.

2910 **Publications from HEATH**
HEATH Resource Center
2134 G St NW
Washington, DC 20052
202-973-0904
Fax: 202-994-3365
http://www.heath.gwu.edu
askheath@gwu.edu
Donna Martinez, Director
Dr. Lynda West, Principal Investigator
A newsletter offering information on postsecondary education for individuals with disabilities.

2911 **Teaching Exceptional Children**
Council for Exceptional Children
2900 Crystal Drive
Ste 1000
Arlington, VA 22202-3557
888-232-7733
Fax: 703-264-9494
TTY: 866-915-5000
http://www.cec.sped.org/
service@cec.sped.org
Drew Albritten MD, President
Bruce Ramirez, Manager
Published specifically for teachers and administrators of children who are gifted. Features practical articles that present methods and materials for classroom use as well as current issues in special education teaching and learning. Brings together its readers the latest data on technology, assistive technology, and procedures and techniques with applications to students with exceptionalities. The focus of its practical content is on immediate application.
6x per year

2912 **Texas Key**
Learning Disabilities Association of Texas
PO Box 831392
Richardson, TX 75083-1392
800-604-7500
Fax: 512-458-3826
http://www.ldat.org
contact@ldat.org
Ann Robinson, Editor
Jean Kueker, President
Quarterly newsletter providing information of intrest to parents and professionals in the field of learning.
16-24 pages

Language Arts

2913 **ASHA Leader**
American Speech-Language-Hearing Association
2200 Research Blvd
Rockville, MD 20850-3289
301-296-5700
800-498-2071
Fax: 301-296-8580
http://www.asha.org
leader@asha.org
Susan Boswell, Editor
Pertains to the professional and administrative activities in the fields of speech-language pathology, audiology and the American Speech-Language-Hearing Association.
16X/year

2914 **American Journal of Speech-Language Pathology: A Journal of Clinical Practice**
American Speech-Language-Hearing Association
2200 Research Blvd
Rockville, MD 20850-3289
301-296-5700
800-498-2071
Fax: 301-296-8580
http://www.asha.org
subscribe@asha.org
Laura Justice, Editor
The journal pertains to all aspects of clinical practice in speech-language pathology. Articles address screening, assessment, and treatment techniques; prevention; professional issues; supervision; and administration, and may appear in the form of clinical forums, clinical reviews, letters to the editor, or research reports that emphasize clinical practice.
Quarterly
ISSN 1058-0360

2915 **Communication Outlook**
Michigan State University Artificial Language Lab
405 Computer Ctr
East Lansing, MI 48824-1042
517-353-0870
Fax: 517-353-4766
http://www.msu.edu
artlang@pilot.msu.edu
Rebecca Ann Baird, Editor

Quarterly journal which focuses on communication aids and techniques. Provides information also for blind and visually impaired persons. *$18.00*
Quarterly

2916 **Journal of Speech, Language, and Hearing Research**
American Speech-Language-Hearing Association
2200 Research Blvd
Rockville, MD 20850-3289
301-296-5700
888-498-2071
Fax: 301-296-8580
http://www.asha.org
subscribe@asha.org

Katherine Verdolini, Editor
Karla K McGregor, Editor
Robert Slauch, Editor
Pertains broadly to the studies of the processes and disorders of hearing, language, and speech and to the diagnosis and treatment of such disorders. Articles may take any of the following forms: reports of original research, including single-study experiments; theoretical, tutorial, or review pieces; research notes; and letters to the editor.
Bi-Monthly
ISSN 1092-4388

2917 **Kaleidoscope, Exploring the Experience of Disability Through Literature and Fine Arts**
United Disability Services
701 S Main St
Akron, OH 44311-1019
330-762-9755
Fax: 330-762-0912
http://www.udsakron.org
kaleidoscope@udsakron.org

Gail Willmott, Editor
Creatively focuses on the experience of disability through diverse forms of literature and the fine arts. An award-winning magazine unique to the field of disability studies, it is open to writers with or without disabilities. KALEIDOSCOPE strives to express how disability does or does not affect society and individuals feelings and reactions to disability. Its portrayals of disability reflect a conscious effort to challenge and overcome stereotypical and patronizing attitudes. *$6.00*
64 pages $10.00/year

2918 **Language Arts**
National Council of Teachers of English
1111 W Kenyon Rd
Urbana, IL 61801
217-328-3870
877-369-6283
Fax: 217-328-9645
http://www.ncte.org

Wanda Brooks, Editor
Jonda McNair, Editor
Kelly Wissman, Editor
Language Arts provides a forum for discussions on all aspects of language arts learning and teaching, primarily as they relate to children in pre-kindergarten through the eighth grade. Articles discuss both theory and classroom practice, highlight current research, and review children's and young adolescent literature, as well as classroom and professional resources of interest to language arts educators. *$25.00*
Bi-monthly

College Guides

2919 **NACE Journal**
National Association of Colleges and Employers
62 Highland Ave
Bethlehem, PA 18017-9481
610-868-1421
800-544-5272
Fax: 610-868-0208
http://www.naceweb.org
callen@naceweb.org
Marilyn Mackes, Editor
Gives hard data on practitioners, budgets, the college relations and recruitment function, entry-level hiring, on-campus recruitment, new hires and much much more. *$70.00*
100+ pages Quarterly

Counseling & Psychology

2920 **Accommodations in Higher Education under the Americans with Disabilities Act (ADA)**
Guilford Press
72 Spring St
New York, NY 10012-4019
800-365-7006
Fax: 212-966-6708
http://www.guilford.com
info@guilford.com
Michael Gordon, Editor
Shelby Keiser, Editor
This practical manual offers essential information and guidance for anyone involved with ADA issues in higher education settings. Fundamental principals and actual clinical and administrative procedures are outlined for evaluating, documenting, and accommodating a wide range of mental and physical impairments. *$29.00*
245 pages
ISBN 1-572303-23-9

2921 **Affect and Creativity**
Routledge
7625 Empire Drive
Florence, KY 41042-2919
212-216-7800
800-634-7064
Fax: 212-563-2269
http://www.routledge.com
book.orders@tandf.co.uk
Sandra Walker Russ, Author
This volume offers information on the role of affect and play in the creative process. Designed as a required or supplemental text in graduate level courses in creativity, children's play, child development, affective/cognitive development and psychodynamic theory. *$39.95*
160 pages
ISBN 0-805809-86-4

2922 **Best Practice Occupational Therapy: In Community Service with Children and Families**
Therapro
225 Arlington St
Framingham, MA 1702-8773
508-872-9494
800-257-5376
Fax: 508-875-2062
http://www.theraproducts.com
info@theraproducts.com
Winnie Dunn PhD OTR FAOTA, Author
An invaluable resource for sudents and practitioners interested in working with children and families in early intervention programs and public schools. Includes screening, pre-assessment, the referral process, best practice assessments, designing best paractice services and examples of IEPs and IFSPs. Many of the forms (screenings, checklists for teachers, referral forms assessment planning guide, etc.) are reproducible. The case studies give good examples of reports. *$55.00*

2923 **Cognitive-Behavioral Therapy for Impulsive Children**
Guilford Press
72 Spring St
New York, NY 10012-4019
800-365-7006
Fax: 212-966-6708
http://www.guilford.com
info@guilford.com
Philip C Kendall, Author
Lauren Braswell, Co-Author
The first edition of this book has been used successfully by thousands of clinicians to help children reduce impulsivity and improve their self-control. Building on the procedures reviewers call powerful tools and of great value to professionals who work with children. This second edition includes treatments, assessment issues and procedures and information on working with parents, teachers and groups of children. *$39.00*
239 pages
ISBN 0-898620-13-9

2924 **Curriculum Based Activities in Occupational Therapy: An Inclusion Resource**
Therapro
225 Arlington St
Framingham, MA 1702-8773
508-872-9494
800-257-5376
Fax: 508-875-2062
http://www.theraproducts.com
info@theraproducts.com
Lisa Loiselle, Author
Susan Shea, Co-Author
This book is a comprehensive guide to classroom based occupational therapy. The authors have compiled over 162 classroom activities developed to provide a strong linkage between educational and therapeutic goals. Each structured activity is categorized into standard curriculum subsections (reading, math, written language, etc.). Designed for a 3rd and 4th grade classroom, it can be modified for use in lower grades. *$35.00*
225 pages

2925 **Emotional Disorders & Learning Disabilities in the Elementary Classroom**
Corwin Press
2455 Teller Rd
Thousand Oaks, CA 91320-2218
805-499-9734
800-233-9936
Fax: 805-499-5323
http://www.corwinpress.com
order@corwinpress.com
Jean Cheng Gorman, Author
This unique book focuses on the interaction between learning disabilities and emotional disorders, fostering an understanding of how learning problems affect emotional well-being and vice-versa. This resource and practical classroom guide for all elementary school teachers includes an overview of common learning disabilities and emotional problems and a classroom-tested, research-based list of classroom interactions and interventions. *$30.95*
160 pages
ISBN 0-761976-20-2

2926 **Emotionally Abused & Neglected Child: Identification, Assessment & Intervention**
John Wiley & Sons Inc
111 River St
Hoboken, NJ 7030-5773
201-748-6000
Fax: 201-748-6088
http://www.wiley.com
info@wiley.com
Dorota Iwaniec, Author
Describes emotional abuse and neglect and how it affects child's growth, development and well-being. Diagnosis, assessment and issues that should be addressed. *$60.00*
424 pages Paperback
ISBN 0-470011-01-7

2927 **Ethical Principles of Psychologists and Code of Conduct**
American Psychological Association
750 1st St NE
Washington, DC 20002-4241
202-336-5500
800-374-2722
Fax: 202-336-5633
TDD: 202-336-6123
http://www.apa.org
psycinfo@apa.org
Marion Harrell, Deport Manager
Norman Anderson, CEO
General ethical principles of psychologists and enforceable ethical standards.

2928 **General Guidelines for Providers of Psychological Services**
American Psychological Association
750 1st St NE
Washington, DC 20002-4241
202-336-5500
800-374-2722
Fax: 202-336-5633
TDD: 202-336-6123
http://www.apa.org
psycinfo@apa.org
Marion Harrell, Deport Manager
Norman Anderson, CEO
Offers information for the professional in the area of psychology.

2929 **HELP...at Home**
Therapro
225 Arlington St
Framingham, MA 1702-8773
508-872-9494
800-257-5376
Fax: 508-875-2062
http://www.theraproducts.com
info@theraproducts.com
Stephanie Parks MA, Author
Practical and convenient format covers the 650 assesment skills from the Hawaii Early Learning Profile, with each page formatted as a separate, reproducible activity sheet. Therapist annotates, copies and hands out directly to parents to facilitate their involvement. *$112.50*

2930 **Handbook of Psychological and Educational Assessment of Children**
Guilford Press
72 Spring St
New York, NY 10012-4019
800-365-7006
Fax: 212-966-6708
http://www.guilford.com
info@guilford.com
Cecil R Reynolds, Editor
Randy W Kamphaus, Editor
Provides practitioners, researchers, professors, and students with an invaluable resource, this unique volume covers assessment of intelligence, learning styles, learning strategies, academic skills, and special populations, and discusses special topics in mental testing. Chapter contributions are by eminent psychologists and educators in the field of assessment with special expertise in research or practice in their topic areas. *$89.00*
718 pages

2931 **Helping Students Become Strategic Learners: Guidelines for Teaching**
Brookline Books
8 Trumbull Rd
Suite B-001
Northampton, MA 1060
413 584 0184
Fax: 413-584-6184
http://www.brooklinebooks.com
brbooks@yahoo.com
Karen Schneid, Author
A practical book that helps the beginning or experienced teacher translate skill-specific strategy methods into their classroom teaching. The author demonstrates how teachers can implement cognitive strategy instruction in their own classrooms. Each chapter includes an introduction to the principles of a given teaching strategy and a review of the skill area in question—namely reading, writing and mathematics. *$27.95*
Paperback
ISBN 0-914797-85-9

2932 **Overcoming Dyslexia in Children, Adolescents and Adults**
Pro-Ed
8700 Shoal Creek Blvd
Austin, TX 78757-6897
512-451-3246
800-397-7633
Fax: 512-451-8542
http://www.proedinc.com
info@proedinc.com
Dale R Jordan, Author
This book describes some forms of dyslexia in detail and then relates those problems to the social, emotional and personal development of dyslexic individuals. *$42.00*
417 pages

2933 **Pathways to Change: Brief Therapy Solutions with Difficult Adolescents**
Guilford Press
72 Spring St
New York, NY 10012-4019
800-365-7006
Fax: 212-966-6708
http://www.guilford.com
info@guilford.com
Matthew D Selekman, Author
This innovative, practical guide presents an effective brief therapy model for working with challenging adolescents and their families. The solution-oriented techniques and strategies so skillfullly presented in the original volume are now augmented by ideas and findings from other therapeutics traditions, with a heightened focus on engagement and relationship building. *$44.00*
292 pages
ISBN 1-572309-59-8

2934 **Practitioner's Guide to Dynamic Assessment**
Guilford Press
72 Spring St
New York, NY 10012-4019
800-365-7006
Fax: 212-966-6708
http://www.guilford.com
info@guilford.com
Carol S Lidz, Author
A hands-on guide that is degined specifically for practitioners who engage in diagnostic assessment related to the functioning of children in school. It reviews and critiques current models of dynamic assessment and presents the research available on these existing models. *$25.00*
210 pages Paperback
ISBN 0-898622-42-5

2935 **Reading and Learning Disability: A Neuropsychological Approach to Evaluation & Instruction**
Charles C Thomas
2600 S 1st St
Springfield, IL 62704-4730
217-789-8980
800-258-8980
Fax: 217-789-9130
http://www.ccthomas.com
books@ccthomas.com
Estelle L Fryburg, Author
Publisher of Education and Special Education books. *$74.95*
398 pages Paper
ISBN 0-398067-45-8

2936 **Revels in Madness: Insanity in Medicine and Literature**
University of Michigan Press
839 Greene St
Ann Arbor, MI 48104-3209 734-764-4388
Fax: 734-615-1540
http://www.press.umich.edu
ump.webmaster@umich.edu
Allen Thiher, Author
Karen Hill, Interim Director
Kelly Sippell, Assistant Director
Revels in Madness offers a history of western culture's shifting understanding of insanity as evidenced in its literature and as influenced by medical knowledge. *$75.00*
368 pages Cloth
ISBN 0-472110-35-3

2937 **Teaching Students with Learning and Behavior Problems**
Pro-Ed
8700 Shoal Creek Blvd
Austin, TX 78757-6816 512-451-3246
800-897-3202
Fax: 512-451-8542
http://www.proedinc.com
info@proedinc.com
Donald D Hammill, Author
Nettie R Bartel, Co-Author
Provides teachers with a comprehensive overview of the best practices in informal assessment and adaptive instruction. With the current trend both regular and exceptional students will find this text a useful resource. *$63.00*

2938 **Treating Troubled Children and Their Families**
Guilford Press
72 Spring St
New York, NY 10012-4019 800-365-7006
Fax: 212-966-6708
http://www.guilford.com
info@guilford.com
Ellen F Wachtel, Author
Integrating systemic, psychodynamic, and cognitive-behavioral perspectives, this acclaimed book presents an innovative framework for therapeutic work. Shows how parents and children all too often get entangled in patterns that cause grief to both generations, and demonstrates ho to help being about change with a combinations of family-focused interventions. *$30.00*
320 pages Paperback
ISBN 1-593850-72-7

General

2939 **A History of Disability**
University of Michigan Press
839 Greene St
Ann Arbor, MI 48104-3209 734-764-4388
Fax: 734-615-1540
http://www.press.umich.edu
ump.webmaster@umich.edu
Henri Jacques Stiker, Author
A bold analysis of the evolution of western attitudes toward disability. The book traces the history of western cultural responses to disability, from ancient times to the present. *$23.95*
264 pages Paper
ISBN 0-472086-26-9

2940 **A Human Development View of Learning Disabilities: From Theory to Practice**
Charles C Thomas, 2nd Ed.
2600 S 1st St
Springfield, IL 62704-4730 217-789-8980
800-258-8980
Fax: 217-789-9130
http://www.ccthomas.com
books@ccthomas.com
Corraine E Kass, Author
Cleborne D Maddux, Co-Author
Publisher of Education and Special Education books. 252 pp (7x10), 5 tables, ISBN 978-0-398-07565-1 (paper) $39.95 Published 2005 *$35.95*
252 pages Paper
ISBN 0-398075-65-1

2941 **Academic Skills Problems Workbook**
Guilford Press
72 Spring St
New York, NY 10012-4019 800-365-7006
Fax: 212-966-6708
http://www.guilford.com
info@guilford.com
Edward S Shapiro, Author
This user-friendly workbook offers numerous opportunities for practicing and mastering direct assessment and intervention procedures. The workbook also includes teacher and student interview forms; a complete guide to using the Behavioral Observation of Students in Schools (BOSS) Observation code, exercises on administering assessments and scoring, interpreting, and graphing the results; and much more. *$30.00*
147 pages
ISBN 1-572309-68-7

2942 **Academic Skills Problems: Direct Assessment and Intervention**
Guilford Press
72 Spring St
New York, NY 10012-4019 800-365-7006
Fax: 212-966-6708
http://www.guilford.com
info@guilford.com
Edward S Shapiro, Author
Provides comprehensive framework for the direct assessment of academic skills. Presented is a readily applicable, four-step approach for working with students experiencing a range of difficulties with reading, spelling, written language, or math. *$45.00*
370 pages
ISBN 1-572309-77-6

2943 **Adapted Physical Education for Students with Autism**
Charles C Thomas, Publisher, Ltd.
2600 S 1st St
Springfield, IL 62704-4730 217-789-8980
800-258-8980
Fax: 217-789-9130
http://www.ccthomas.com
books@ccthomas.com
Kimberly Davis, Author
Publisher of Education and Special Education books. 142 pp. (7x10), 10 il. ISBN 978-0-398-06085-5 (paper) $29.95. Published 1990. *$27.95*
142 pages Paper
ISBN 0-398060-85-5

2944 **Adapting Curriculum & Instruction in Inclusive Early Childhood Settings**
Indiana Institute on Disability and Community
2853 E 10th St
Bloomington, IN 47408-2601 812-855-9396
Fax: 812-855-9630
TTY: 812-855-9396
http://www.iidc.indiana.edu
iidc@indiana.edu
David Mank, Director
Offers ideas and strategies that will be beneficial to all young children, including children with identified disabilities, children who are at risk, and students who need enriched curricular options. This is also an excellent resource for preservice training as well as inservice training for independent child care providers, center, and schools. *$11.00*

2945 **Annals of Dyslexia**
International Dyslexia Association
4th Fl
40 York Rd
Baltimore, MD 21204-5243 410-296-0232
Fax: 410-321-5069
http://www.interdys.org
subscriptions@springer.com
Rob Hott, Editor
Chris Schatschneider PhD, Editor
Lee Grossmanÿ, Executive Director
The Society's scholarly journal contains updates on current research and selected proceedings from talks given at each ODS international conference. Issues of Annals are available from 1982 through the present year. *$15.00*
2X / year

2946 **Art for All the Children: Approaches to Art Therapy for Children with Disabilities, 2nd Ed.**
Charles C Thomas, Publisher, Ltd.
2600 S 1st St
Springfield, IL 62704-4730 217-789-8980
800-258-8980
Fax: 217-789-9130
http://www.ccthomas.com
books@ccthomas.com
Frances E Anderson, Author
Publisher of Education and Special Education books. *$56.95*
398 pages Paper
ISBN 0-398060-07-7

2947 **Art-Centered Education & Therapy for Children with Disabilities**
Charles C Thomas, Publisher, Ltd.
2600 S 1st St
Springfield, IL 62704-4730 217-789-8980
800-258-8980
Fax: 217-789-9130
http://www.ccthomas.com
books@ccthomas.com
Frances E Anderson, Author
Publisher of Education and Special Education books. 284 pp (6-3/4x9), 100 il, 14 tables. ISBN 978-0-398-06006-0 (paper) $42.95. Published 1994. *$41.95*
284 pages Cloth
ISBN 0-398058-96-2

2948 **Atypical Cognitive Deficits in Developmental Disorders: Implications for Brain Function**
Routledge
7625 Empire Drive
Florence, KY 41042-2919 212-216-7800
Fax: 212-563-2269
http://www.routledge.com
book.orders@tandf.co.uk
Sarah H Broman, Editor
Jordan Grafman, Editor
This volume is based on a conference held to examine what was known about cognitive behaviors and brain structure and function in three syndromes. *$99.95*
360 pages
ISBN 0-805811-80-0

2949 **Auditory Processes**
Academic Therapy Publications
20 Commercial Blvd
Novato, CA 94949-6120 415-883-3314
800-422-7249
Fax: 888-287-9975
http://www.academictherapy.com
sales@academictherapy.com
Jim Arena, President
Joanne Urban, Manager
Pamela Gillet PhD, Author
Explains how teachers, educational consultants and parents can identify auditory processing problems, understand their impact and implement appropriate instructional strategies to enhance learning. *$15.00*
120 pages
ISBN 0-878790-94-2

2950 **Body and Physical Difference: Discourses of Disability**
University of Michigan Press
839 Greene St
Ann Arbor, MI 48104-3209 734-764-4388
Fax: 734-615-1540
http://www.press.umich.edu
ump.webmaster@umich.edu
David T Mitchell, Editor
Sharon L Synder, Editor
Karen Hill, Executive Director
For years the subject of human disability has engaged those in the biological, social and cognitive sciences, while at the same time, it has been curiously neglected within the humanitites. The Body and Physical Difference seeks to introduce the field of disability studies into the humanities by exploring the fantasies and fictons that have crystallized around conceptions of physical and cognitive difference. *$65.00*
320 pages cloth
ISBN 0-472066-59-9

2951 **Brief Intervention for School Problems: Outcome-Informed Strategies**
Guilford Press
72 Spring St
New York, NY 10012-4019 800-365-7006
Fax: 212-966-6708
http://www.guilford.com
info@guilford.com
John J Murphy, Author
Barry L Duncan, Co-Author
This practical guide provides innovative strategies for resolving academic and behavioral difficulties by enlisting the strengths and resources of students, parents, and teachers. *$30.00*
210 pages
ISBN 1-593854-92-7

2952 **Cognitive Strategy Instruction That Really Improves Children's Performance**
Brookline Books
PO Box 1209
Brookline, MA 2446 617-734-6772
800-666-2665
Fax: 413-584-6184
http://www.brooklinebooks.com
brbooks@yahoo.com
Michael Pressley, Author
A concise and focused work that summarily presents the few procedures for teaching strategies that aid academic subject matter learning that are empirically validated and fit well with the elementary school curriculum. *$27.95*
203 pages
ISBN 0-914797-66-2

2953 **Competencies for Teachers of Students with Learning Disabilities**
Council for Exceptional Children
Ste 300
1110 N Glebe Rd
Arlington, VA 22201-5704 703-245-0600
888-232-7733
Fax: 703-264-9494
TTY: 703-264-9446
http://www.cec.sped.org/
service@cec.sped.org
Amme Graves, Author
Mary Landers, Author
Bruce Ramirez, Manager

Lists 209 specific professional competencies needed by teachers of students with learning disabilities and provides a conceptual framework for the ten areas in which the competencies are organized. *$5.00*
25 pages

2954 Cooperative Learning and Strategies for Inclusion
Brookes Publishing Company
PO Box 10624
Baltimore, MD 21285 410-337-9580
800-638-3775
Fax: 410-337-8539
http://www.brookspublishing.com
custserv@brookespublishing.com
JoAnne Putnam PhD, Editor
This book supplies educators, classroom support personnel, and administrators with numerous tools for creating positive, inclusive classroom environments for students from preschool through high school. *$32.95*
288 pages Paperback
ISBN 1-557663-46-7

2955 Creative Curriculum for Preschool
Teaching Strategies
7101 Wisconsin Avenue
Suite 700
Bethesda, MD 20814 301-634-0818
800-637-3652
Fax: 301-657-0250
http://www.teachingstrategies.com
info@teachingstrategies.com
Andrea Valentine, President
Ron Davies, CEO
Amy Houser, CMO
Focuses on the developmentally appropriate program in early childhood education. Illustrates how preschool and kindergarten teachers set the stage for learning, and how children and teachers interact and learn in various interest areas. *$44.95*
540 pages
ISBN 1-879537-43-5

2956 Curriculum Development for Students with Mild Disabilities
Charles C Thomas, Publisher, Ltd.
2600 S 1st St
Springfield, IL 62704-4730 217-789-8980
800-258-8980
Fax: 217-789-9130
http://www.ccthomas.com
books@ccthomas.com
Carroll J Jones, Author
Publisher of Education and Special Education books. 454 pp. ISBN 978-0-398-079911-6, $69.95. Published 2010. *$38.95*
258 pages Spiral (paper)
ISBN 0-398707-18-2

2957 Curriculum-Based Assessment: A Primer, 3rd Ed.
Charles C Thomas
2600 S 1st St
Springfield, IL 62704-4730 217-789-8980
800-258-8980
Fax: 217-789-9130
http://www.ccthomas.com
books@ccthomas.com
Charles H Hargis, Author
Publisher of Education and Special Education books. 210 pp (8-1/2x11), 59 tables, ISBN 978-0-398-07815-7 (spiral) $39.95. Published 2008. *$33.95*
174 pages Paperback
ISBN 0-398075-52-1

2958 Curriculum-Based Assessment: The Easy Wayto Determine Response-to-Intervention, 2nd Ed.
Charles C Thomas
2600 S 1st St
Springfield, IL 62704-4730 217-789-8980
800-258-8980
Fax: 217-789-9130
http://www.ccthomas.com
books@ccthomas.com
Carroll J Jones, Author
Publisher of Education and Special Education books. 210 pp, (8-1/2x11), 59 tables, ISBN 978-0-398-07815-7 (spiral) $39.95. Published 2008. *$33.95*
174 pages Spiral (paper)

2959 Defects: Engendering the Modern Body
University of Michigan Press
839 Greene St
Ann Arbor, MI 48104-3209 734-764-4388
Fax: 734-615-1540
http://www.press.umich.edu
ump.webmaster@umich.edu
Charles Watkinson, Director
Aaron McCollough, Director of Editorial
Defects brings together essays on the emergence of the concept of monstrosity in the eighteenth century and the ways it paralleled the emergence of notions of sexual difference. *$27.95*
344 pages Paper
ISBN 0-472066-98-8

2960 Developmental Variation and Learning Disorders
Educators Publishing Service
PO Box 9031
Cambridge, MA 2139-9031 800-435-7228
Fax: 888-440-2665
http://www.epsbooks.com
eps@epsbooks.com
Melvin D Levine MD FAAP, Author
The Second Edition of this useful reference includes completely revised on attention, memory, and language, with significant modifications of the remaining chapters. Sections on educational skills have been expanded and updated; the chapter on causes and complications of learning disorders has been updated to include recent references and ongoing reseach efforts. *$61.80*
ISBN 0-838819-92-3

2961 Dictionary of Special Education and Rehabilitation
Love Publishing Company
Ste 2200
9101 E Kenyon Ave
Denver, CO 80237-1854 303-221-7333
Fax: 303-221-7444
http://www.lovepublishing.com
lpc@lovepublishing.com
Glenn A Vergason, Author
M L Anderegg, Co-Author
This updated edition of one of the most valuable resources in the field is over six years in the making and incorporates hundreds of additions. It provides clear, understandable definitions of more than 2,000 terms unique to special education and rehabilitation. It also provides listing of professional organizations and resources, includes latest terms, and is a critical reference for anyone in the special education field. *$34.95*
210 pages Paperback
ISBN 0-891802-43-3

2962 Directory for Exceptional Children
Porter Sargent Handbooks
2 Lan Drive Ste 100 Westford
Boston, MA 1886 978-842-2812
800-342-7870
Fax: 978-692-2304
http://www.portersargent.com
info@portersargent.com

Daniel McKeever, Editor
John Yonce, Director
Leslie Weston, Production Editor
A comprehensive survey of 3000 schools, facilities, and organizations across the USA. Serving children and yound adults with developmental, physical, medical, and emotional disabilities. Aide to parents, consultants, educators, and other professionals. *$75.00*
1152 pages
ISBN 0-875581-31-5

2963 **Eden Family of Services Curriculum Series:**
Eden Services
One Eden Way
Princeton, NJ 8540-5711 609-987-0099
Fax: 609-987-0243
http://www.edenservices.org
info@edenservices.org
Tom Mc Cool, President
This volume contains teaching programs for students ages three through adult in the area of cognitive skills; self-care and domestics; vocational skills; speech and languages and physcial education, recreation and leisure. Complete series $700; individual volumes $150-200

2964 **Educating All Students Together**
Corwin Press
2455 Teller Rd
Thousand Oaks, CA 91320-2218 805-499-9734
800-233-9936
Fax: 805-499-5323
http://www.corwinpress.com
order@corwinpress.com
Mike Soules, President
Lisa Shaw, Executive Director
Kristin Anderson, Director of Learning
A plan for unifying the separate and parallel systems of special and general education. Key concepts include: schools embracing special services personnel; the role of the community; program evaluation and incentives; brain and holographic design; collaboration between school administrators and teachers; and adapting curriculum; and instruction. *$33.95*
264 pages
ISBN 0-761976-98-1

2965 **Educating Children with Multiple Disabilities: A Collaborative Approach**
Brookes Publishing Company
PO Box 10624
Baltimore, MD 21285 410-337-9580
800-638-3775
Fax: 410-337-8539
http://www.brookespublishing.com
custserv@brookespublishing.com
Fred P Orelove PhD, Editor
Dick Sobsey EdD, Editor
Rosanne K Silberman EdD, Editor
Gives undergraduate and graduate students up-to-the-minute research and strategies for educating children with severe and multiple disabilities. *$49.00*
672 pages Paperback
ISBN 1-557667-10-1

2966 **Ending Discrimination in Special Education**
Charles C Thomas
2600 South 1st Street
Springfield, IL 62704-4730 217-789-8980
800-258-8980
Fax: 217-789-9130
http://www.ccthomas.com
books@ccthomas.com
Herbert Grossman, Author
Charles C. Thomas, Publisher
Publisher of Education and Special Education books. *$23.95*
142 pages Paper
ISBN 0-398073-04-6

2967 **Exceptional Teacher's Handbook: First Year Special Education Teacher's Guide for Success**
Corwin Press
2455 Teller Rd
Thousand Oaks, CA 91320-2218 805-499-9734
800-233-9936
Fax: 805-499-5323
http://www.corwinpress.com
order@corwinpress.com
Mike Soules, President
Lisa Shaw, Executive Director Editorial
Elena Nikitina, Executive Director, Marketing
Provides a step-by-step management approach complete with planning checklists and other ready-to-use forms. Arranged sequentially, the book guides new teachers through the entire school year, from preplanning to post planning. *$ 35.95*
240 pages
ISBN 0-761931-96-6

2968 **Focus on Exceptional Children**
Love Publishing Company
9101 E Kenyon Ave
Suite 2200
Denver, CO 80237-1854 303-221-7333
Fax: 303-221-7444
http://www.lovepublishing.com
lpc@lovepublishing.com
Edwin S Ellis, Editor
Timothy J Lewis, Editor
Chriss S Thomas, Editor
Published monthly except June, July, and August, get a constant flow of fresh teaching ideas-and keep up with the latest research- with this monthly newsletter that translates theory into strategies for action. Each issue focuses in depth on a single topic, such as assessment, cooperative learning, attention deficit disorders, inclusion, classroom management, discipline, and ohter timely issues. *$36.00*
ISSN 0015-511X

2969 **Frames of Reference for the Assessment of Learning Disabilities**
Brookes Publishing Company
PO Box 10624
Baltimore, MD 21285-0624 410-337-9580
800-638-3775
Fax: 410-337-8539
http://www.brookespublishing.com
custserv@brookespublishing.com
Lauren Rohe, Regional Sales Consultant
Cary Gold, Educational Sales Representative
Paul Kelly, College/University Sales Manager
This valuable reference offers an in-depth look at the fundamental concerns facing those who work with children with learning disabilities — assessment and identification. *$59.95*
672 pages Hardcover
ISBN 1-557661-38-3

2970 **HELP Activity Guide**
Therapro
225 Arlington Street
Framingham, MA 01702-8723 508-872-9494
800-257-5376
Fax: 508-875-2062
http://www.theraproducts.com
info@theraproducts.com
Karen Conrad, Owner
Setan Furuns PhD, Author
Takes you easily beyond assesment to offer the important next step, thousands of practical, task-analyzed curriculum activities and intervention strategies indexed by the 650 HELP skills. With up to ten activities and strategies per skill, this valuable resource includes definitions for each skill, illustrations, cross-references to skills in other developmental areas and a glossary. *$40.00*
190 pages

2971 **HELP for Preschoolers Assessment and Curriculum Guide**
Therapro
225 Arlington Street
Framingham, MA 01702-8723
508-872-9494
800-257-5376
Fax: 508-875-2062
http://www.theraproducts.com
info@theraproducts.com
Karen Conrad, Owner
Setan Furuns PhD, Author
Assessment procedure and instructional activities in one easy to use reference. Offers 6 sections of key information for each of the 622 skills: Definition, Materials, Assesment Procedures, Adaptions, Instructional Materials, and Instructional Activities.

2972 **Hidden Youth: Dropouts from Special Education**
Council for Exceptional Children
2900 Crystal Drive
Suite 1000
Arlington, VA 22202-3557
888-232-7733
Fax: 703-264-9494
TTY: 866-915-5000
http://www.cec.sped.org/
service@cec.sped.org
Donald L MacMillan, Author
Robin D. Brewer, President
James P. Heiden, President Elect
Christy A. Chambers, Immediate Past President
Examines the characteristics of students and schools that place students at risk for early school leaving. Discusses the accounting procedures used by different agencies for estimating graduation and dropout rates and cautions educators about using these rates as indicators of educational quality. *$8.90*
37 pages
ISBN 0-865862-11-7

2973 **How Difficult Can This Be?**
CT Association for Children and Adults with LD
Ste 15-5
25 Van Zant St
Norwalk, CT 06855-1713
203-838-5010
Fax: 203-866-6108
http://www.cacld.org
caccld@optonline.net
Richard Lavoie, Producer
FAT City Workshop video and discussion guide. Looks at the world through the eyes of a learning disabled child. Features a unique workshop attended by educators, psychologists, social workers, parents, siblings and a student with LD. They participate in a series of classroom activities which cause Frustration, Anxiety, and Tension-emotions all too familiar to the student with a learning disability. A discussion of topics ranging from school/home communication to social skills follows. *$49.95*

2974 **How Does Your Engine Run? A Leaders Guide to the Alert Program for Self Regulation**
Therapro
225 Arlington Street
Framingham, MA 01702-8723
508-872-9494
800-257-5376
Fax: 508-875-2062
http://www.theraproducts.com
info@theraproducts.com
Karen Conrad, Owner
Mary Sue Williams OTR, Author
Sherry Schellenberge OTR, Co-Author
Introduces the entire Alert Program. Explains how we regulate our arousal states and describes the use of sensorimotor strategies to manage levels of alertness. This program is fun for students and the adults working with them, and translates easily into real life.

2975 **How to Write an IEP**
Academic Therapy Publications
20 Leveroni Court
Novato, CA 94949-5746
415-883-3314
800-422-7249
Fax: 888-287-9975
http://www.academictherapy.com
sales@academictherapy.com
Jim Arena, President
Joanne Urban, Manager
This practical guide for teachers and parents contains the latest updates to the 2004 Individuals with Disabilities Education Act (IDEA). *$19.00*
168 pages
ISBN 1-571284-43-5

2976 **IEP Success Video**
Sopris West
17855 Dallas Parkway
Suite 400
Dallas, TX 75287-3520
303-651-2829
800-547-6747
http://www.voyagersopris.com
customerservice@sopriswest.com
Barbara D Baterman JD PhD, Author
Explains the five underlying principles of the individualized education program (IEP) process: evaluation and identification, IEPs and related services, placement, funding, and procedural safeguards. *$98.95*

2977 **Implementing Cognitive Strategy Instruction Across the School: The Benchmark Manual for Teachers**
Brookline Books
8 Trumbull Rd
Suite B-001
Northampton, MA 01060
413-584-0184
800-666-2665
Fax: 413-584-6184
http://www.brooklinebooks.com
brbooks@yahoo.com
Irene Gaskins, Author
Thorne Elliot, Author
Describes a classroom based program planned and executed by teachers to focus and guide students with serious reading problems to be goal oriented, planful, strategic and self-assessing. *$24.95*
Paperback
ISBN 0-914797-75-1

2978 **Improving Test Performance of Students with Disabilities in the Classroom**
Corwin Press
2455 Teller Rd
Thousand Oaks, CA 91320-2218
805-499-9734
800-233-9936
Fax: 805-499-5323
http://www.corwinpress.com
order@corwinpress.com
Mike Soules, President
Lisa Shaw, Executive Director Editorial
Elena Nikitina, Executive Director, Marketing
Elliott and Thurlow, long-time colleagues at the National Center on Educational Outcomes build on their highly respected work in accountability and assessment of students with disabilities to focus now on improving test performance — with an emphasis throughout on practical application. Common learning disabilities and emotional problems and a classroom-tested, research-based list of classroom interventions. *$35.95*
232 pages Paperback
ISBN 1-412917-28-X

2979 Including Students with Severe and Multiple Disabilities in Typical Classrooms

Brookes Publishing Company
PO Box 10624
Baltimore, MD 21285-0624 410-337-9580
800-638-3775
Fax: 410-337-8539
http://www.brookespublishing.com
custserv@brookespublishing.com
Lauren Rohe, Regional Sales Consultant
Cary Gold, Educational Sales Representative
Paul Kelly, College/University Sales Manager

This straightforward and jargon-free resource gives instructors the guidance needed to educate learners who have one or more sensory impairments in addition to cognitive and physical disabilities. *$44.95*

352 pages Paperback
ISBN 1-557669-08-2

2980 Inclusion: 450 Strategies for Success

Corwin Press
2455 Teller Rd
Thousand Oaks, CA 91320-2218 805-499-9734
800-233-9936
Fax: 805-499-5323
http://www.corwinpress.com
order@corwinpress.com
Mike Soules, President
Lisa Shaw, Executive Director Editorial
Elena Nikitina, Executive Director, Marketing

Commences with step-by-step guidelines to help develop, expand and improve the existing inclusive education setting. Hundreds of practical teacher tested ideas and accommodations are conveniently listed by topic and numbered for quick, easy reference. *$33.95*

192 pages Educators
ISBN 1-890455-25-3

2981 Inclusion: An Essential Guide for the Paraprofessional

Corwin Press
2455 Teller Rd
Thousand Oaks, CA 91320-2218 805-499-9734
800-233-9936
Fax: 805-499-5323
http://www.corwinpress.com
order@corwinpress.com
Mike Soules, President
Lisa Shaw, Executive Director Editorial
Elena Nikitina, Executive Director, Marketing

This best-selling publication is developed specifically for paraprofessionals and classroom assistants. The book commences with a simplified introduction to inclusive education, handicapping conditions, due process, communication, collaboration, confidentiality and types of adaptations. Used by many schools and universities as a training tool for staff development. *$35.95*

224 pages
ISBN 1-890455-34-2

2982 Inclusive Elementary Schools

PEAK Parent Center
611 North Weber Street
Suite 200
Colorado Springs, CO 80903-1072 719-531-9400
800-284-0251
Fax: 719-531-9452
http://www.peakparent.org
info@peakparent.org
Barbara Buswell, Executive Director
Kent Willis, President
Sarah Billerbeck, Vice President

Walks readers through a state of the art, step-by-step process to determine what and how to teach elementary school students with disabilities in general education classrooms. Highlights strategies for accommodating and modifying assignments and activities by using core curriculum. Complete with user-friendly sample forms and creative support strategies, this is an essential text for elementary educators and parents. *$13.00*

2983 Instructional Methods for Secondary Students with Learning & Behavior Problems

Allyn & Bacon
75 Arlington St
Suite 300
Boston, MA 02116-3988 800-848-9500
Fax: 877-260-2530
http://home.pearsonhighered.com
Patrick J Schloss, Author
Maureen A Schloss, Co-Author
Cynthia N Schloss, Co-Author

This book presents teaching principles useful to general high school educators and special educators working with students demonstrating a variety of academic, behavioral, and social needs in secondary schools. *$120.00*

432 pages
ISBN 0-205442-36-6

2984 Intervention in School and Clinic

Sage Publications
2455 Teller Rd
Thousand Oaks, CA 91320-2218 805-499-0721
800-818-7243
Fax: 805-583-2665
http://www.sagepub.com
journals@sagepub.com
Blaise R. Simqu, President
Tracey A. Ozmina, Executive VP/COO
Gretchen Bataille, Director

Equips teachers and clinicians with hands-on tips, techniques, methods and ideas for improving assessment, instruction, and management for individuals with learning disabilities or behavior disorders. Articles focus on curricular, instructional, social, behavioral, assessment, and vocational strategies and techniques that have a direct application to the classroom setting. This innovative and readable periodical provides educational information ready for immediate implementation

5 times a year
ISSN 1053-4512

2985 KDES Health Curriculum Guide

Harris Communications
15155 Technology Dr
Eden Prairie, MN 55344-2273 800-825-6758
800-825-9187
Fax: 952-906-1099
TTY: 800-825-9187
http://www.harriscomm.com
info@harriscomm.com
Sara Gillespie, Author
Doris Schwartz, Co-Author
Darla Hudson, Customer Service

This guide provides students with the information they need to make wise choices for healthy living. Divided into age-appropriate sections; preschool through middle school; the units cover four main areas: Health and Fitness, Safety and First Aid, Drugs, and Life. Asspendices provide resource lists and information on topics such as hygiene, street safety, teaching health. Part #B568. *$9.95*

125 pages

2986 Making School Inclusion Work: A Guide to Everyday Practices

Brookline Books
8 Trumbull Rd
Suite B-001
Northampton, MA 01060 413-584-0184
800-666-2665
Fax: 413-584-6184
http://www.brooklinebooks.com
brbooks@yahoo.com
Katie Blenk, Author
Doris Fine, Author

Tells the reader how to conduct a truly inclusive school program that educates a diverse student body together, regardless of ethnic or racial background, economic level, or physical or cognitive ability. Indication given on what is ment by true inclusion, what inclusion is not, and who should not be conducting an inclusive program. *$24.95*
264 pages Paperback
ISBN 0-914797-96-4

2987 **Mentoring Students at Risk: An Underutilized Alternative Education Strategy for K-12 Teachers**
Charles C Thomas
2600 South 1st Street
Springfield, IL 62704-4730
217-789-8980
800-258-8980
Fax: 217-789-9130
http://www.ccthomas.com
books@ccthomas.com
Gary Reglin, Author
Charles C. Thomas, Publisher
Publisher of Education and Special Education books. *$20.95*
110 pages Paper
ISBN 0-398068-33-2

2988 **Myofascial Release and Its Application to Neuro-Developmental Treatment**
Therapro
225 Arlington Street
Framingham, MA 01702-8723
508-872-9494
800-257-5376
Fax: 508-875-2062
http://www.theraproducts.com
info@theraproducts.com
Karen Conrad, Owner
Regi Boehme OTF, Author
This fully illustrated resource provides the therapist with techniques to approach myofascial restrictions which are secondary to tonal dysfunction in children and adults with neurological deficits. The Neuro-Developmental Treatment approach is included in the illustrated treatment rationale.

2989 **Narrative Prosthesis: Disability and the Dependencies of Discourse**
University of Michigan Press
839 Greene Street
Ann Arbor, MI 48104-3209
734-764-4388
Fax: 734-615-1540
http://www.press.umich.edu
dshafer@umich.edu
Charles Watkinson, Director
Ellen Bauerle, Executive Editor
Gabriela Beres, Business Manager
This book develops a narrative theory of the pervasive use of disability as a device of characterization in literature and film. It argues that, while other marginalized identities have suffered cultural exclusion due to dearth of images reflecting their experience, the marginality of disabled people has occurred in the midst of the perpetual circulation of images of disability in print and visual media. *$65.00*
264 pages Cloth
ISBN 0-472097-48-7

2990 **Points of Contact: Disability, Art, and Culture**
University of Michigan Press
839 Greene Street
Ann Arbor, MI 48104-3209
734-764-4388
Fax: 734-615-1540
http://www.press.umich.edu
dshafer@umich.edu
Charles Watkinson, Director
Ellen Bauerle, Executive Editor
Gabriela Beres, Business Manager
A richly diverse collection of essays, memoir, poetry and photography on aspects of disability and its representation in art. Brings together contributions by leading writers, artists, scholars, and critics to provide a remarkably broad and consistently engaging look at the intersection of disability and the arts. *$60.00*
312 pages Cloth
ISBN 0-472097-11-1

2991 **Prescriptions for Children with Learning and Adjustment Problems: A Consultant's Desk Reference**
Charles C Thomas
2600 South 1st Street
Springfield, IL 62704-4730
217-789-8980
800-258-8980
Fax: 217-789-9130
http://www.ccthomas.com
books@ccthomas.com
Ralph F Blanco, Author
Charles C. Thomas, Publisher
Publisher of Education and Special Education books. *$35.95*
264 pages Paper

2992 **Preventing Academic Failure**
Educators Publishing Service
PO Box 9031
Cambridge, MA 02139-9031
617-547-6706
800-225-5750
Fax: 888-440-2665
http://www.epsbooks.com
Feedback.EPS@schoolspecialty.com
Rick Holden, President
Phyllis Bertin, Author
Eileen Perlman, Co-Author
This multisensory curriculum meets the needs of children with learning disabilities in regular classrooms by providing a four-year sequence of written language skills (reading, writing and spelling). PAF has a handwriting and numerical program. *$42.00*
ISBN 0-838852-71-8

2993 **Resourcing: Handbook for Special Education RES Teachers**
Council for Exceptional Children
2900 Crystal Drive
Suite 1000
Arlington, VA 22202-3557
888-232-7733
888-232-7733
Fax: 703-264-9494
TTY: 866-915-5000
http://www.cec.sped.org
service@cec.sped.org
Mary Yeomans Jackson, Author
Robin D. Brewer, President
James P. Heiden, President Elect
Christy A. Chambers, Immediate Past President
Be prepared to function at your best as a member of a school-based team. Resourcing wil help you take a leadership role as you work in collaboration with general classroom teachers and other practitioners. Assess your personal readiness for being a resource professional within your school. Includes many useful forms and checklists for conducting meetings and organizing your workday. *$12.00*
64 pages
ISBN 0-865862-19-2

2994 **School-Home Notes: Promoting Children's Classroom Success**
Guilford Press
72 Spring Street
New York, NY 10012-4019
800-365-7006
Fax: 212-966-6708
http://www.guilford.com
info@guilford.com
Seymour Weingarten, Editor-in-Chief
Jim Nageotte, Senior Editor
Jody Falco, Managing Editor

Describes common obstacles to parent and teacher communication and clearly explicates how these obstacles can be overcome. It provides a critical appraisal of the relevant literature on parent-and-teacher managed contingency systems and factors influencing the efficacy of the procedure.
$28.00
198 pages Paperback
ISBN 0-898622-35-2

2995 **Segregated and Second-Rate: Special Education in New York**
Advocates for Children of New York
151 West 30th St
5th Floor
New York, NY 10001-4024 212-947-9779
866-427-6033
Fax: 212-947-9790
http://www.advocatesforchildren.org
info@advocatesforchildren.org
Eric F. Grossman, President
Harriet Chan King, Secretary
Paul D. Becker, Treasurer
Highlights the fact that New York rates last among all states in inclusive education.

2996 **Sensory Integration: Theory and Practice**
Therapro
225 Arlington Street
Framingham, MA 01702-8723 508-872-9494
800-257-5376
Fax: 508-875-2062
http://www.theraproducts.com
info@theraproducts.com
Karen Conrad, Owner
Anne Fisher, Author
Elizabeth Murray, Co-Author
The very latest in sensory integration theory and practice.
$60.00
481 pages

2997 **Strangest Song: One Father's Quest to Help His Daughter Find Her Voice**
Prometheus Books
59 John Glenn Drive
Amherst, NY 14228-2197 716-691-0133
800-421-0351
Fax: 716-691-0137
http://www.prometheusbooks.com
marketing@prometheusbooks.com
Jill Maxick, Vice President of Marketing
Lisa Michalski, Senior Publicist
Mary A Read, Permissions Manager
The first book to tell the story of Williams syndrome and the extraordinary musicality of many of the people who have it. An inspiring blend of human interest and breakthrough science, offers startling insights into the mysteries of the brain and hope that science can find new ways to help the handicapped. *$24.00*
296 pages
ISBN 1-591024-78-1

2998 **Take Part Art**
CT Association for Children and Adults with LD
Ste 15-5
25 Van Zant St
Norwalk, CT 06855-1713 203-838-5010
http://www.cacld.org
cacld@optonline.net
Bob Gregson, Author
Offers information on art therapies and their inclusion in learning disabled environments. *$19.50*

2999 **Teachers Ask About Sensory Integration**
Therapro
225 Arlington Street
Framingham, MA 01702-8723 508-872-9494
800-257-5376
Fax: 508-875-2062
http://www.theraproducts.com
info@theraproducts.com
Karen Conrad, Owner
Carol Kranowitz, Author
Stacey Szkult, Co-Author
A narration and discussion for teachers and school professionals about how to teach children with sensory integration problems. 60 page book included, filled with checklists, idea sheets, sensory profiles and resorces. 86 minute audio tape.
Audio Tape

3000 **Teaching Gifted Kids in the Regular Classroom CD-ROM**
Free Spirit Publishing
217 5th Ave North
Suite 200
Minneapolis, MN 55401-1299 612-338-2068
800-735-7323
Fax: 612-337-5050
http://www.freespirit.com
help4kids@freespirit.com
Judy Galbraith, President
Judy Galbrai
Includes all of the forms from the book, plus many additional extension menus, ready to customize and print for classroom use. Macintosh and Windows compatible. *$17.95*
ISBN 1-575421-01-4

3001 **Teaching Gifted Kids in the Regular Classroom**
Free Spirit Publishing
217 5th Ave North
Suite 200
Minneapolis, MN 55401-1299 612-338-2068
800-735-7323
Fax: 612-337-5050
http://www.freespirit.com
help4kids@freespirit.com
Judy Galbraith, President
The definitive guide to meeting the learning needs of gifted students, as well as those labeled slow, remedial, or LD, in the mixed-abilities classroom, without losing control, causing resentment, or spending hours preparing extra materials. The updated edition includes more than 50 reproducible forms and handouts for all grades. *$34.95*
256 pages
ISBN 1-575420-89-9

3002 **Teaching Students Ways to Remember: Strategies for Learning Mnemonically**
Brookline Books
8 Trumbull Rd
Suite B-001
Northampton, MA 01060 413-584-0184
800-666-2665
Fax: 413-584-6184
http://www.brooklinebooks.com
brbooks@yahoo.com
Margo Mastropieri MD, Author
This book was written in response to the enormous interest in mnemonic instruction by teachers and administrators, telling them how it can be used with their students. *$21.95*
ISBN 0-398074-77-7

3003 **Teaching Visually Impaired Children, 3rd Ed.**
Charles C Thomas
2600 South 1st Street
Springfield, IL 62704-4730 217-789-8980
800-258-8980
Fax: 217-789-9130
http://www.ccthomas.com
books@ccthomas.com
Virginia E Bishop, Author
Charles C. Thomas, Publisher

Publisher of Education and Special Education books. *$49.95*
352 pages Paper
ISBN 0-398065-95-0

3004 To Teach a Dyslexic
AVKO Educational Research Foundation
3084 Willard Rd
Birch Run, MI 48415-9404
810-686-9283
866-285-6612
Fax: 810-686-1101
http://www.avko.org
webmaster@avko.org

Don McCabe, President
Linda Heck, Vice President
Michael Lane, Treasurer
Just as it takes a thief to catch a thief, this is an autobiography of a dyslexic who discovered how to teach dyslexics. Common sense, logical approach, valuable to all who teach in our nation's classrooms. *$14.95*
288 pages
ISBN 1-564000-04-4

3005 Understanding & Management of Health Problems in Schools: Resource Manual
Temeron Books
PO Box 896
Bellingham, WA 98227
Fax: 360-738-4016
http://www.temerondetselig.com
temeron@telusplanet.net

H Moghadam, Author
Intended as a supplement to information given by parents and physicians, this book is a valuable aid to teachers and other school personnel in regards to some of the primary health issues that affect children and adolescents. *$ 13.95*
152 pages
ISBN 1-550591-21-5

3006 Understanding and Managing Vision Deficits
Therapro
225 Arlington Street
Framingham, MA 01702-8723
508-872-9494
800-257-5376
Fax: 508-875-2062
http://www.theraproducts.com
info@theraproducts.com

Mitchell Scheiman, OD, Author
Karen Conrad, Owner
This book is a unique and comprehensive collaboration from OT's and optometrists developed to increase the understanding of vision. Learn to screen for common visual deficits and effectively manage patients with vision disorders. Provides recommendations for direct intervention techniques for a variety of vision problems and supportive and compensatory stratagies for visual field deficits and visual neglect.

3007 Working with Visually Impaired Young Students: A Curriculum Guide for 3 to 5 Year-Olds
Charles C Thomas
2600 South 1st Street
Springfield, IL 62704-4730
217-789-8980
800-258-8980
Fax: 217-789-9130
http://www.ccthomas.com
books@ccthomas.com

Ellen Trief, Editor
Charles C Thomas, Publisher
Publisher of Education and Special Education books. *$42.95*
208 pages Spiral Paper
ISBN 0-398068-75-2

Language Arts

3008 Communication Skills for Visually Impaired Learners, 2nd Ed.
Charles C Thomas, Publisher, Ltd.
2600 South 1st Street
Springfield, IL 62704-4730
217-789-8980
800-258-8980
Fax: 217-789-9130
http://www.ccthomas.com
books@ccthomas.com

Randall K Harley, Author
Charles C Thomas, Publisher
LaRhea D Sanford, Co-Author
Publisher of Education and Special Education books. 322 pp. (7x10), 39 il, $59.95 (paper) ISBN 978-0-398-06693-2
$57.95
322 pages Paper
ISBN 0-398066-93-2

3009 First Start in Sign Language
Harris Communications
15155 Technology Dr
Eden Prairie, MN 55344-2273
800-825-6758
800-825-9187
Fax: 952-906-1099
TTY: 800-825-9187
http://www.harriscomm.com
info@harriscomm.com

Amy J Strommer, Author
Darla Hudson, Customer Service
Fun pictures, stories, and activities are all included in this introduction to American Sign Language. Students first learn to sign words for people, animals, objects and actions. Then they learn to produce simple sentences and to sign stories. Reproducible activity pages are included throughout the book. For students in kindergarten through sixth grade. Part #B469. *$32.00*
190 pages Paperback

3010 From Talking to Writing: Strategies for Scaffolding Expository Expression
Landmark School
429 Hale Street
P.O. Box 227
Prides Crossing, MA 01965
978-236-3216
Fax: 978-927-7268
http://www.landmarkoutreach.org
outreach@landmarkschool.org

Dan Ahearn, Director
Terrill M Jennings, Author
Charles W Haynes, Co-Author
Designed for teachers who work with students who have difficulty with writing and/or expressive language skills, this book provides practical strategies for teaching expository expression at the word, sentence, paragraph, and short essay levels. *$25.00*
191 pages

3011 Language Learning Everywhere We Go
Academic Communication Associates
PO Box 4279
Oceanside, CA 92052-4279
760-722-9593
888-758-9558
Fax: 760-722-1625
TDD: 952-906-1198
TTY: 800-825-9187
http://www.acadcom.com
acom@acadcom.com

Cecilia Casas, Author
Patricia Portillo, Co-Author
Students learn the vocabulary associated with each situation that they encounter on their travels with Bernardo Bear. Questions and vocabulary lists are included in English and Spanish for each picture. The 103 situational pictures may all be reproduced. *$34.00*
209 pages Paperback

3012 **Making the Writing Process Work: Strategies for Composition & Self-Regulation**

Brookline Books
8 Trumbull Rd
Suite B-001
Northampton, MA 01060
413-584-0184
800-666-2665
Fax: 413-584-6184
http://www.brooklinebooks.com
brbooks@yahoo.com
Karen R Harris, Author
Steve Graham, Co-Author

Presents cognitive strategies for writing sequences of specific steps which make the writing process clearer and enable students to organize their thoughts about the writing task. The strategies help students know how to turn thoughts into writing products. This is especially important for students having difficulty producing acceptable writing products, but all students benefit from learning these procedures. *$24.95*

ISBN 1-571290-10-9

3013 **Multisensory Teaching Approach**

MTS Publications
415 N McGraw St
Forney, TX 75126-8661
972-564-6960
877-552-1090
Fax: 972-552-9889
http://www.mtsedmar.com
msmith@mtsedmar.com
Margaret Smith, Author
Margaret T. Smith, Executive Director

MTA is a comprehensive, multisensory program in reading, spelling, cursive handwriting, and alphabet and dictionary skills for both regular and remedial instruction. Ungraded, MTA is based on the Orton-Gillingham techniques and Alphabetic Phonics. *$192.99*

3014 **Signs of the Times**

Harris Communications
15155 Technology Dr
Eden Prairie, MN 55344-2273
800-825-6758
800-825-9187
Fax: 952-906-1099
TTY: 800-825-9187
http://www.harriscomm.com
info@harriscomm.com
Edgar H Shroyer, Author
Darla Hudson, Customer Service

Containing 1,185 signs in 41 lessons, this classroom text is an excellent beginning Pidgin or Contact Sign English book that fills the gap between sign language dictionaries and American Sign Language texts. Each lesson contains clearly illustrated vocabulary, English glosses and synonyms, sample sentences to defice vocabulary context, and sentences for practice. Part #B202. *$34.95*

433 pages Softcover

3015 **Slingerland Multisensory Approach to Language Arts**

Slingerland Institute for Literacy
12729 Northup Way
Suite 1
Bellevue, WA 98005-1935
425-453-1190
Fax: 425-635-7762
http://www.slingerland.org
mail@slingerland.com
Bonnie Meyer, Author
Beth H. Slingerland, Founder

This adaptation of the Orton-Gillingham approach for classroom teachers provides a phonetically structured introduction to reading, writing and spelling. Books 1 and 2 are for first and second grade, Book 3 for primary classrooms and older students. Numerous supplementary materials are available.

3016 **Teaching Language Deficient Children: Theory and Application of the Association Method**

Pro-Ed
8700 Shoal Creek Blvd
Austin, TX 78757-6897
512-451-3246
800-897-3202
Fax: 512-451-8542
http://www.proedinc.com
general@proedinc.com
N Etoile DuBard, Author
Maureen K Martin, Co-Author

This revised and expanded edition of Teaching Aphasics and Other Language Deficient Children offers information on its theory, implementation of the method and sample curriculum. *$52.00*

360 pages

ISBN 0-838823-40-8

3017 **Visualizing and Verbalizing for Language Comprehension and Thinking**

Lindamood Bell
416 Higuera St
San Luis Obispo, CA 93401-3833
805-541-3836
800-233-1819
Fax: 805-541-8756
http://www.lindamoodbell.com
Nanci Bell, Author

This book identifies the important sensory connection that imagery provides and teaches specific techniques. Specific steps and sample dialog are presented. Summary pages after each step make it easy to implement the program in the classroom.

284 pages

ISBN 0-945856-01-6

3018 **Writing: A Landmark School Teaching Guide**

Landmark School
429 Hale Street
P.O. Box 227
Prides Crossing, MA 01965
978-236-3216
Fax: 978-927-7268
http://www.landmarkoutreach.org
outreach@landmarkschool.org
Dan Ahearn, Director
Deborah Blanchard, Academic Dean
Jean Gudaitis Tarricone, Author

This book offers strategies for teaching writing at the paragraph and short essay levels. It emphasizees the integration of language and critical thinking skills within a five-step writing process. Sample templates and graphic organizers as well as exercises that teachers can use in their classrooms are included. *$25.00*

92 pages

Math

3019 **Landmark Method for Teaching Arithmetic**

Landmark School
429 Hale Street
P.O. Box 227
Prides Crossing, MA 01965
978-236-3216
Fax: 978-927-7268
http://www.landmarkoutreach.org
outreach@landmarkschool.org
Dan Ahearn, Director
Deborah Blanchard, Academic Dean
Christopher Woodin, Author

This book is written for teachers who work with students having difficulty learning math. It includes practical strategies for teaching multiplication, division, word problems, and math facts. It also introduces the reader to two learning tools developed at Landmark — Woodin Ladders and Woodmark Icons. Sample templates and exercises are included. *$25.00*

145 pages

3020 **Math and the Learning Disabled Student: A Practical Guide for Accommodations**

Academic Success Press
3547 53rd Ave. W.
PMB 132
Bradenton, FL 34210-4402
941-746-1645
888-822-6657
Fax: 941-753-2882
http://www.academicsuccess.com
info@academicsuccess.com
Paul D Nolting PhD, Author
Kim Ruble, Editor
Kimberly Nolting, MAT, VP for Marketing and Research

More and more learning disabled students are experiencing difficulty passing mathematics. The book is especially written for counselors and mathematics instructors of learning disabled students, and provides information on accommodations for students with different types of learning disabilities. *$49.95*

256 pages

ISBN 0-940287-23-4

3021 **Teaching Mathematics to Students with Learning Disabilities**

Pro-Ed
8700 Shoal Creek Blvd
Austin, TX 78757-6897
512-451-3246
800-897-3202
Fax: 512-451-8542
http://www.proedinc.com
general@proedinc.com
Nancy S Bley, Author
Carol A Thornton, Co-Author

Offers information on problem-solving, estimation and the use of computers in teaching mathematics to the child with learning disabilities. *$49.00*

Preschool

3022 **Access for All: Integrating Deaf, Hard of Hearing, and Hearing Preschoolers**

Harris Communications
15155 Technology Dr
Eden Prairie, MN 55344-2273
800-825-6758
800-825-9187
Fax: 952-906-1099
TTY: 800-825-9187
http://www.harriscomm.com
info@harriscomm.com
Gail Solit, Author
Maral Taylor, Co-Author
Darla Hudson, Customer Service

Covers basic information needed to establish a successful preschool program for deaf and hearing children; interagency cooperation, staff training, and parental involvement. Part #BUT103. *$29.95*

169 pages Video-90 min.

3023 **When Slow Is Fast Enough: Educating the Delayed Preschool Child**

Guilford Press
72 Spring Street
New York, NY 10012-4019
800-365-7006
Fax: 212-966-6708
http://www.guilford.com
info@guilford.com
Seymour Weingarten, Editor-in-Chief
Jim Nageotte, Senior Editor
Jody Falco, Managing Editor

This bold and controversial book asks what we are accomplishing in early intervention programs that attempt to accelerate development in delayed young children. She questions the value of such programs on educational, psychological, and moral grounds, suggesting that in pressuring these children to perform more, and sooner, we undermine their capacity for independent development and deprive them of the freedom we insist upon for the nondelayed. *$29.00*

306 pages Paperback

ISBN 0-898624-91-6

Reading

3024 **Gillingham Manual**

Educators Publishing Service
PO Box 9031
Cambridge, MA 02139-9031
617-547-6706
800-225-5750
Fax: 617-547-0412
http://www.epsbooks.com
Feedback.EPS@schoolspecialty.com
Rick Holden, President
Anna Gillingham, Author
Bessie W Stillman, Co-Author

This classic in the field of specific language disability has now been completely revised and updated. The manual covers reading, spelling, writing and dictionary technique. It may be used with individuals or small groups. *$74.15*

352 pages

ISBN 0-838802-00-1

3025 **Phonology and Reading Disability**

University of Michigan Press
839 Greene Street
Ann Arbor, MI 48104-3209
734-764-4388
Fax: 734-615-1540
http://www.press.umich.edu
dshafer@umich.edu
Charles Watkinson, Director
Ellen Bauerle, Executive Editor
Gabriela Beres, Business Manager

Discusses the importance to the learning process of the phonological structures of words. *$52.50*

184 pages Cloth

ISBN 0-472101-33-7

3026 **Preventing Reading Difficulties in Young Children**

National Academies Press
500 Fifth St NW
Washington, DC 20001
202-334-3313
888-624-8373
Fax: 202-334-2451
http://www.nap.edu
customer_service@nap.edu
Barbara Kline Pope, Director
Ann Merchant, Deputy Executive Director
Stephen Mautner, Executive Editor

Explores how to prevent reading difficulties in the context of social, historical, cultural, and biological factors. *$34.16*

448 pages Hardback

ISBN 0-309064-18-X

3027 **Readability Revisited: The New Dale-Chall Readability Formula**

Brookline Books
8 Trumbull Rd
Suite B-001
Northampton, MA 01060
413-584-0184
800-666-2665
Fax: 413-584-6184
http://www.brooklinebooks.com
brbooks@yahoo.com
Jeanne Chall, Author
Edgar Dale, Co-Author

Information is given on reading difficulties in children with learning disabilities and how to overcome them. *$29.95*

168 pages

ISBN 1-571290-08-7

3028 **Reading Problems: Consultation and Remediation**
Guilford Press
72 Spring Street
New York, NY 10012-4019 800-365-7006
Fax: 212-966-6708
http://www.guilford.com
info@guilford.com
Seymour Weingarten, Editor-in-Chief
Jim Nageotte, Senior Editor
Jody Falco, Managing Editor
Designed to both help school psychologists and reading specialists effectively assume the consultation role, this volume provides an overview of reading problems while serving as a guide to effective practice. *$42.00*
285 pages

3029 **Reading Programs that Work: A Review of Programs from Pre-K to 4th Grade**
Milken Family Foundation
1250 4th St
Santa Monica, CA 90401-1353 310-570-4800
Fax: 310-570-4801
http://www.mff.org
media@mff.org
Lowell Milken, Chairman & Co Founder
Richard Sandler, Executive Vice President
Ralph Finerman, Senior Vice President
This publication tackles two questions, joining the research behind why children fail to read with research on effective solutions to reverse this failure. Included in the reading report are analyses of 35 different reading programs and their impact on student achievement.
72 pages

3030 **Reading and Learning Disabilities: A Resource Guide**
NICHCY
1825 Connecticut Ave NW
Suite 700
Washington, DC 20009 202-884-8200
800-695-0285
Fax: 202-884-8441
TDD: 800-695-0285
http://www.nichcy.org
emulligan@fhi360.org
Lisa Kupper, Editor
This publication describes some of the most common learning disabilities that can cause reading problems and provides information on organizations that can provide needed assistance.

3031 **Reading and Learning Disability: A Neuropsychological Approach to Evaluation & Instruction**
Charles C Thomas
2600 South 1st Street
Springfield, IL 62704-4730 217-789-8980
800-258-8980
Fax: 217-789-9130
http://www.ccthomas.com
books@ccthomas.com
Estelle L Fryburg, Author
Charles C. Thomas, Publisher
Publisher of Education and Special Education books. *$74.95*
398 pages Paper
ISBN 0-398067-45-8

3032 **Starting Out Right: A Guide to Promoting Children's Reading Success**
National Academies Press
500 Fifth St NW
Washington, DC 20001 202-334-3313
888-624-8373
Fax: 202-334-2451
http://www.nap.edu
customer_service@nap.edu
Barbara Kline Pope, Director
Ann Merchant, Deputy Executive Director
Stephen Mautner, Executive Editor
This book discusses how best to help children succeed in reading. This book also includes 55 activities yo do with children to help them become successful readers, a list of recommended children's books, and a guide to CD-ROMs and websites. A must read for specialists in primary education as well as pediatricians, childcare providers, tutors, literacy advocates, and parents. *$13.46*
192 pages
ISBN 0-309064-10-4

3033 **Teaching Reading to Disabled and Handicapped Learners**
Charles C Thomas
2600 South 1st Street
Springfield, IL 62704-4730 217-789-8980
800-258-8980
Fax: 217-789-9130
http://www.ccthomas.com
books@ccthomas.com
Harold D Love, Author
Charles C. Thomas, Publisher
Publisher of Education and Special Education books. *$43.95*
260 pages Paperback
ISBN 0-398062-48-4

3034 **Textbooks and the Students Who Can't Read Them**
Brookline Books
8 Trumbull Rd
Suite B-001
Northampton, MA 01060 413-584-0184
800-666-2665
Fax: 413-584-6184
http://www.brooklinebooks.com
brbooks@yahoo.com
Jean Ciborowski, Author
This book proposes how to involve low readers more effectively in textbook learning. It presents instructional techniques to improve students' willingness to work in mainstream textbooks. *$21.95*
Paperback
ISBN 0-914797-57-3

Social Skills

3035 **ADHD in the Schools: Assessment and Intervention Strategies**
Guilford Press
72 Spring Street
New York, NY 10012-4019 800-365-7006
Fax: 212-966-6708
http://www.guilford.com
info@guilford.com
Seymour Weingarten, Editor-in-Chief
Jim Nageotte, Senior Editor
Jody Falco, Managing Editor
This popular reference and text provides essential guidance for school-based professionals meeting the challenges of ADHD at any grade level. Comprehensive and practical, the book includes several reproducible assessment tools and handouts. *$30.00*
330 pages
ISBN 1-593850-89-1

3036 **Behavior Change in the Classroom: Self-Management Interventions**
Guilford Press
72 Spring Street
New York, NY 10012-4019 800-365-7006
Fax: 212-966-6708
http://www.guilford.com
info@guilford.com
Seymour Weingarten, Editor-in-Chief
Jim Nageotte, Senior Editor
Jody Falco, Managing Editor

This book presents practical approaches for designing and implementing self-management interventions in school settings. Rich with detailed instruction, the volume covers the conceptual foundation for the development of self-management from both contingency management and cognitive-behavioral perspectives. *$35.00*
204 pages
ISBN 0-898623-66-9

3037 **Group Activities to Include Students with Special Needs**

Corwin Press
2455 Teller Road
Thousand Oaks, CA 91320-2218
805-499-9734
800-233-9936
Fax: 805-499-5323
http://www.corwin.com
order@corwin.com

Mike Soules, President
Lisa Shaw, Executive Director
Elena Nikitina, Executive Director

This hands-on resource offers 120 group activities emphasizing participation, cooperation, teamwork, mutual support, and improved self-esteem. This practical guide provides instant activities that can be used without preparation and incorporated into the daily routine with ease and confidence. Classroom games, gym and outdoor games, and ball games are designed to help your students gain the valuable skills they need to interact appropriately within the school setting. *$35.95*
240 pages
ISBN 0-761977-26-1

Publications

3038 **Beyond Transition: An Interative Workbook for College-Bound Students with LD & ADHD**
Association on Higher Education & Disability
8015 W Kenton Circle
Ste 230
Huntersville, NC 28078
704-947-7779
Fax: 704-948-7779
http://www.ahead.org
Mary Barrows, Jennifer Newton, Emily Collins, Author
Kristie Orr, President
Stephan Smith, Executive Director
An interactive guide to assistant students with a learning disability or ADHD through their studies. Designed to facilitate communication between students and their parents as they transition to college. *$45.00*

3039 **Essentional Six: A Parent's Guide: How to Pace the Road to Self-Advocacy for College Students**
Association on Higher Education & Disability
8015 W Kenton Circle
Ste 230
Huntersville, NC 28078
704-947-7779
Fax: 704-948-7779
http://www.ahead.org
Lorri Comeau, Mickey Cronin, Author
Kristie Orr, President
Stephan Smith, Executive Director
The Essentional Six series focuses on the development of self-advocacy skills for students with learning disabilities and how parents can help encourage their children throughout the course of their education. *$35.00*

3040 **ISS Directory of International Schools**
International Schools Services
15 Roszel Rd
PO Box 5910
Princeton, NJ 08543
609-452-0990
Fax: 609-452-2690
http://www.iss.edu
iss@iss.edu
Liz Duffy, President
Bruce McWilliams, Senior Leadership Executive
Kristin Evins, Chief Financial Officer
Comprehensive guide to over 550 American and international schools worldwide. Annually published since 1981.

3041 **Interpreting Diagnostic Assessments for Adolescents and Adults with Learning Disabilities**
Association on Higher Education & Disability
8015 W Kenton Circle
Ste 230
Huntersville, NC 28078
704-947-7779
Fax: 704-948-7779
http://www.ahead.org
Janet Medina, Author
Kristie Orr, President
Stephan Smith, Executive Director
A guide to diagnostic assesment examines the current proceess for learning disability evaluations, including tools and tests. *$45.00*

3042 **Member Directory**
NAPSEC
601 Pennsylvania Ave
Ste 900, South Bldng
Washington, DC 20004
202-434-8225
http://www.napsec.org
napsec@napsec.org
Tom Dempsey, President
Dr. Tom McCool, Vice President
Tom Celli, Treasurer
A membership directory listing NAPSEC'S members, disabilities served, program descriptions, school profiles, admissions procedures and funding approval.

3043 **Testing Accommodations Reference Manual**
Association on Higher Education & Disability
8015 W Kenton Circle
Ste 230
Huntersville, NC 28078
704-947-7779
Fax: 704-948-7779
http://www.ahead.org
Trisha Tonge Barefield, Sarah Kesler, Author
Kristie Orr, President
Stephan Smith, Executive Director
This manual is an updated version of previous publication, Exam Accommodations. This edition reflects the most up-to-date practices in disability services and provides detailed information regarding accommodations at the postsecondary level, including: assistive technology and online exams. *$30.00*

3044 **The Guide to Assisting Students with Disabilities Equal Access in Health Science & Prof Education**
Association on Higher Education & Disability
8015 W Kenton Circle
Ste 230
Huntersville, NC 28078
704-947-7779
Fax: 704-948-7779
http://www.ahead.org
Lisa M. Meeks, Neera R. Jain, Author
Kristie Orr, President
Stephan Smith, Executive Director
This textbook is aimed towards administrators and faculty in health science programs. Addresses accommodation policies, disability law, and civil rights. *$65.00*

3045 **Veterans with Disabilities: Promoting Success in Higher Education**
Association on Higher Education & Disability
8015 W Kenton Circle
Ste 230
Huntersville, NC 28078
704-947-7779
Fax: 704-948-7779
http://www.ahead.org
Tom Church, Author
Kristie Orr, President
Stephan Smith, Executive Director
This publication provides information for veterans with disabilities in regards to legal accommodations, employement opportunities, and a variety of support organizations. *$25.00*

3046 **Winning at Math: Your Guide to Learning Mathematics Through Successful Study Skills**
Association on Higher Education & Disability
8015 W Kenton Circle
Ste 230
Huntersville, NC 28078
704-947-7779
Fax: 704-948-7779
http://www.ahead.org
Paul Nolting, PhD, Author
Kristie Orr, President
Stephan Smith, Executive Director
A guidebook for students designed for use inside and outside of the classroom. Includes trational math courses, study guides, and math labs.] *$29.95*

Alabama

3047 **Auburn University**
EAGLES Program
100 Ramsay Hall
Auburn, AL 36849
334-844-5927
Fax: 337-844-5950
http://web.auburn.edu
atliweb@auburn.edu
Courtney K. Dotson, PhD, Director
The EAGLES Program stands for Education to Accomplish Growth in Life Experiences for Success. A two-year or four-year on-campus non-degree program experience. Students learn to increase independence, improve leadership and advocacy skills, prepare to enter the workforce, and develop life skills.

3048 **Auburn University at Montgomery**
Center for Disability Services
PO Box 244023
Montgomery, AL 36124-4023 334-244-3631
Fax: 334-244-3907
http://www.aum.edu
cds@aum.edu

Carl A. Stockton, Chancellor
Carolyn Campbell-Golden, Chancellor of Advancement
Scott Parsons, Vice Chancellor, Finance/Admin
Offers a variety of services to students with disabilities including equipment, extended testing time, interpreting services, counseling services, and special accommodations.

3049 **Birmingham-Southern College**
900 Arkadelphia Rd
Birmingham, AL 35254 800-523-5793
http://www.bsc.edu

Katie Hatch, Associate Director, HR
Offers a variety of services to students with disabilities including notetakers, extended testing time, counseling services, and special accommodations.

3050 **Chattahoochee Valley State Community College**
2602 College Dr
Phenix City, AL 36869 334-291-4900
http://www.cv.edu
terrah.long@cv.edu

Jacqueline Screws, President
Vickie Williams, Director, Student Development
Terrah Long, Administrative Assistant
Offers a variety of services to students with disabilities including note takers, extended testing time, counseling services and special accommodations.

3051 **Churchill Academy**
395 Ray Thorington Rd
Montgomery, AL 36117 334-270-4225
Fax: 334-270-7805
http://www.churchillacademy.net
A one-of-a-kind school for bright children with unique learning differences.

3052 **Enterprise State Community College**
600 Plaza Dr
PO Box 1300
Enterprise, AL 36331 334-347-2623
Fax: 334-347-5569
http://www.escc.edu
admissions@escc.edu

Matt Rodgers, President
A public two-year college with 15 special education students out of a total of 600. Certified by the Federal Aviation Administration, and offers the only comprehensive aviation maintenance training program in the state of Alabama, with instruction in airframe, powerplant and avionics.

3053 **Horizons School**
2018 15th Ave S
Birmingham, AL 35205 205-322-6606
Fax: 205-322-6605
http://www.horizonsschool.org

Dr. Brian Geiger, Executive Director
Dr. Karen Dixon, Assistant Director
Don Lutomski, President
Offers a non-degree transition program specifically designed to facilitate personal, social and career independence for students with specific learning disabilities and other handicapping conditions.

3054 **Jacksonville State University**
Disability Support Services
700 Pelham Rd N
Jacksonville, AL 36265 256-782-5781
800-231-5291
http://www.jsu.edu
info@jsu.edu

John M. Beehler, PhD, President
Ronald William Smith, Chair
Thomas W. Dedrick, Sr., Vice Chair
Offers a variety of services to students with disabilities including notetakers, extended testing time, counseling services, and special accommodations.

3055 **Troy State University Dothan**
Student Disability Services
500 University Dr
Alabama, AL 36303 334-983-6556
886-291-0371
Fax: 334-983-4580
http://www.troy.edu
afarver@troy.edu

Amy Farver, Coordinator
Offers a variety of services to students with disabilities including notetakers, extended testing time, counseling services, and special accommodations.

3056 **University of Alabama**
Office of Disability Services
1000 Houser Hall
PO Box 870185
Tuscaloosa, AL 35487-0185 205-348-4285
Fax: 205-348-0804
http://ods.ua.edu/contact
ods@ua.edu

Stuart R. Bell, President
Kevin Whitaker, Executive Vice President
David Grady, VP, Student Affairs
A public four-year college with approximately 650 students identified with disabilities out of a total of 19,200.

3057 **University of Montevallo**
Office of Disability Services
Station 6250
Montevallo, AL 35115 205-665-6250
http://www.montevallo.edu
dss@montevallo.edu

Dr. John W. Stewart III, President
Deborah S. Braswell, Disability Compliance Officer
Offers a variety of services to students with disabilities including notetakers, extended testing time, counseling services, and special accommodations.

3058 **University of North Alabama**
Office of Disability Support Services
Guillot University Center
Room 111
Florence, AL 35632 256-765-4214
http://www.una.edu
dss@una.edu

Jeremy Martin, MEd, Director
Stacy C. Lee, Coordinator
R. Darlene Crowden, Administrative Assistant
Offers a variety of services to students with disabilities including notetakers, extended testing time, counseling services, and special accommodations.

3059 **University of South Alabama**
Student Disability Services
320 Alumni Circle
Educational Services Bldng, Ste 19
Mobile, AL 36688 251-460-7212
Fax: 251-414-8176
http://www.southalabama.edu/departments/sds
disabilityservices@southalabama.edu
Dr. Andrea Agnew, Assistant Dean of Students
Laventrice Ridgeway, Coordinator
Greta Washington, Secretary
Offers a variety of services to students with disabilities including note takers, extended testing time, counseling services, and special accommodations.

3060 **Wallace Community College Selma**
3000 Earl Goodwin Parkway
PO Box 2530
Selma, AL 36702-2530
334-876-9227
http://www.wccs.edu
info@wccs.edu
James Mitchell, President
Tammie Briggs, Associate Dean, Student Learning
Offers a variety of services to students with disabilities including note takers, extended testing time, counseling services and special accommodations.

Alaska

3061 **Alaska Pacific University**
Disabled Student Services
4101 University Drive
Anchorage, AK 99508
http://www.alaskapacific.edu
admissions@alaskapacific.edu
Bob Onders, President
Laura See, Development Specialist
Four-year college offering special services to students that are learning disabled.

3062 **Juneau Campus: University of Alaska Southeast**
11066 Auke Lake Way
Juneau, AK 99801
907-796-6100
http://www.uas.alaska.edu
uas.info@uas.alaska.edu
Richard Caulfield, PhD, Chancellor
Eric Scott, Dean of Students & Campus Life
Offers a variety of services to students with disabilities including notetakers, extended testing time, counseling services, and special accommodations.

3063 **Ketchikan Campus: University of Alaska Southeast**
2600 7th Ave
Ketchikan, AK 99901
228-4511
888-550-6177
Fax: 225-3624
TTY: 888-550-6177
http://www.uas.alaska.edu/ketchikan
ketch.info@uas.alaska.edu
Richard Caulfield, PhD, Chancellor
Eric Scott, Dean of Students & Campus Life
Offers a variety of services to students with disabilities including note takers, extended testing time, counseling services and special accommodations.

3064 **University of Alaska Anchorage**
Disability Support Services
3211 Providence Dr
Anchorage, AK 99508
907-786-1800
http://www.uaa.alaska.edu
Sam Gingerich, Chancellor
Bruce R. Schultz, Vice Chancellor, Student Affairs
Provides equal opportunites for students who experience disabilities.

Arizona

3065 **New Way Learning Academy**
5048 E Oak St
Phoenix, AZ 85008
602-389-8600
Fax: 602-389-8601
http://www.newwayacademy.org
Bill Jacoby, Chairman
Stephanie La Loggia, Vice Chairman
Todd Brown, Treasurer
Non-profit, private K-12 day school specializing in children with learning differences, including students with dyslexia and AD/HD.

3066 **SALT Center**
University of Arizona
1010 North Highland Ave
PO Box 210136
Tucson, AZ 85721
520-621-1242
Fax: 520-626-3260
http://www.salt.arizona.edu
uasaltcenter@email.arizona.edu
Gabrielle Miller, Director
Laurel Grigg Mason, Senior Associate Director
Deb Evano, Administrative Associate
An academic support program that provides a comprehensive range of fee-based services to University of Arizona students with learning and attention challenges.

3067 **Upward Foundation**
Special Education Program
6306 N 7th St
Phoenix, AZ 85014
602-279-5801
Fax: 602-279-0033
http://www.upwardaz.org
info@upwardaz.org
Jos Anshell, President
Daniel G. Perez, Vice President
James L. Kieffer, Secretary
Improving the lives of children with severe disabilities and other special needs.

Arkansas

3068 **Jones Learning Center**
University of the Ozarks
415 N College Ave
Clarksville, AR 72830
479-979-1403
http://www.ozarks.edu
jlc@ozarks.edu
Julia Frost, Director
Dodi Pelts, Assistant Director
Richard L. Dunsworth, JD, President
Offers enhanced services to students who show potential for success in a competitive academic environment.

3069 **Philander Smith College**
Disability & Support Services
900 West Daisy Bates Drive
Little Rock, AR 72202-3717
501-370-5356
http://www.philander.edu
bmartin@philander.edu
Brenda Martin, Coodinator
Roderick L. Smothers, Sr., President
Offers a variety of services to students with disabilities including notetakers, extended testing time, counseling services, and special accommodations.

3070 **Southern Arkansas University**
Disabled Student Programs and Services
100 E University
Magnolia, AR 71753-5000
870-235-5113
Fax: 870-235-4133
http://web.saumag.edu/support
eewalker@saumag.edu
Eunice Walker, Director
Dr. Trey Berry, President
Offers a variety of services to students with disabilities including notetakers, extended testing time, counseling services, and special accommodations.

3071 **University of Arkansas**
Center for Educational Access
209 ARKU
Fayetteville, AR 72701
479-575-3104
Fax: 479-575-7445
http://www.uark.edu
ada@uark.edu
Joseph E. Steinmetz, Chancellor
Jim Coleman, Vice Chancellor,Academic Affairs

Offers a variety of services to students with disabilities including note takers, extended testing time, counseling services, and special accommodations.

California

3072 **ACCESS Program**
Moorpark College
7075 Campus Rd
Moorpark, CA 93021 805-378-1461
Fax: 805-378-1594
TDD: 805-378-1461
http://www.moorparkcollege.edu
Silva Arzunyan, Coordinator
Bonnie Lara, Student Services Assistant
Marc Lazar, Disabilities Services Technician
A public two-year college with 154 special education students out of a total of 12,414.

3073 **Allan Hancock College**
800 S College Dr
Santa Maria, CA 93454 805-922-6966
http://www.hancockcollege.edu
Kevin G. Walthers, PhD, President
Melinda Martinez, Executive Secretary
Students with mobility, visual, hearing and speech impairments, learning disabilities, acquired brain injury, developmental disabilities, psychological and other disabilities are eligible to receive special services which enable them to fully participate in the community college experience at Allan Hancock College.

3074 **Antelope Valley College**
Office for Students with Disabilities
3041 W Ave K
Lancaster, CA 93536 661-722-6300
http://www.avc.edu
Edward Knudson, President
Provides support services, specialized instruction, and educational accommodations to students with disabilities so that they can participate as fully and benefit as equitably from the college experience as their non-disabled peers.

3075 **Aspen Education Group**
20400 Stevens Creek Blvd
6th Fl
Cupertino, CA 95014 855-259-2288
888-972-7736
http://aspeneducation.crchealth.com
Susan Cambria, President
Joel Rosenhaus, Vice President
Provider of education programs for the struggling or underachieving young people. Offers professionals and families the opportunity to choose a setting that best meets a student's unique academic and emotional needs.

3076 **Bakersfield College**
Disabled Student Programs and Services
1801 Panorama Dr
Bakersfield, CA 93305 661-395-4334
Fax: 661-395-4079
TTY: 661-395-4334
http://www.bakersfieldcollege.edu
terri.goldstein@bakersfieldcollege.edu
Terri Goldstein, Director
Offers a variety of services to students with disabilities including equipment, extended testing time, interpreting services, counseling services, and special accommodations.

3077 **Barstow Community College**
ACCESS Program
2700 Barstow Rd
Barstow, CA 92311 760-252-2411
Fax: 760-252-1875
TTY: 760-252-6759
http://www.barstow.edu
mhenderson@barstow.edu
Eva Bagg, PhD, Superintendent/President
Michelle Henderson, Executive Assistant
Educational support program for disabled students including special classes and support services for all disabled students.

3078 **Bridge School**
Educational Program
545 Eucalyptus Ave
Hillsborough, CA 94010-6404 650-696-7295
http://www.bridgeschool.org
Dr. Vicki Casella, Executive Director
Pegi Young, President
Based on the principle of providing access to and participation in an age-appropriate curriculum adapted to the special needs of children with motor, sensory and speech impairments.

3079 **Butte College**
Disabled Student Programs and Services
3536 Butte Campus Dr
Oroville, CA 95965 530-895-2455
Fax: 530-895-2235
TTY: 530-895-2599
http://www.butte.edu
dsps@butte.edu
Offers a variety of services to students with disabilities including equipment, extended testing time, interpreting services, counseling services, and special accommodations.

3080 **Cabrillo College**
Accessibility Support Center
6500 Soquel Dr
Aptos, CA 95003 831-479-6100
Fax: 831-479-6393
TTY: 831-479-6421
http://www.cabrillo.edu
jonapoli@cabrillo.edu
M. Beth McKinnon, ASC Director
Nikki A. Oneto, Program Director
Peggy Church, ASC Conselor
Offers a variety of services to students with disabilities including equipment, extended testing time, interpreting services, counseling services, and special accommodations.

3081 **California State University: East Bay**
25800 Carlos Bee Blvd
Library Complex 2400
Hayward, CA 94542 510-885-3868
Fax: 510-885-4775
http://www.csueastbay.edu/accessibility
as@csueastbay.edu
Dr. Leroy Morishita, President
Debbie Chaw, VP, Admin/Finance & CFO
Derek Atiken, Chief of Staff
Students with documented disabilities and functional limitations are eligible for accomodations designed to provide equivalent access to general campus and classroom programs and activities. The campus provides an SDRC - Student Disability Resource Center - with assistive technology and testing accomodations. They also offer Project Impact and the EXCEL Program, both of which serve their disabled student body.

3082 **California State University: Fullerton**
Disability Support Services
800 N State College Blvd
Fullerton, CA 92831 657-278-3112
http://www.fullerton.edu
Lori Palmerton, Director
Jacquelyn Gerali, Disability Management Specialist
Douglas Liverpool, Learning Disability Specialist
Offers a variety of services to students with disabilities including equipment, extended testing time, interpreting services, counseling services, and special accommodations.

3083 **California State University: Long Beach-Stephen Benson Program**
Disabled Student Services
Brotman Hall
Room BH 270
Long Beach, CA 90840 562-985-4430
Fax: 562-985-4529
http://www.csulb.edu/sbp
Brian.Carey@csulb.edu
Brian Carey, Assistant Director
Tina Sutera, Learning Disability Specialist
Dominique Somoano, Office Coordinator
Four-year college offers a program for students with learning disabilities and attention deficits.

3084 **Chaffey Community College District**
Disability Programs and Services
5885 Haven Avenue
Rancho Cucamonga, CA 91737-3002 909-652-6379
Fax: 909-652-6385
TTY: 909-652-6393
http://www.chaffey.edu/dps
dps.staff@chaffey.edu
Janet Trenier, Program Assistant
Jean Oh, Learning Disability Specialist
Melissa Johannsen, Counselor
Chaffey College's Disabled Student Programs and Services (DSP&S) offer instruction and support services to students with developmental, learning, physical, psychological disabilities or aquired brain injury. Students can recieve a variety of services such as: test facilitation, note taking, tutoring, adaptive physical education, pre-vocational training, career preparation, and job placement.

3085 **Charles Armstrong School**
1405 Solana Dr
Belmont, CA 94002 650-592-7570
Fax: 650-591-3114
http://www.charlesarmstrong.org
information@charlesarmstrong.org
Audrey Fox, President
Sydney Bernier, Vice President
Clint Oram, Treasurer
Serves students with language-based learning differences, such as dyslexia, by providing an appropriate educational experience which enables the students to acquire language skills, while instilling a joy of learning, enhancing self-worth, and allowing each student the right to identify, understand and fulfill personal potential.

3086 **Chartwell School: Seaside**
2511 Numa Watson Rd
Seaside, CA 93955 831-394-3468
Fax: 831-394-6809
http://www.chartwell.org
info@chartwell.org
Katrina Maestri, President
Robert Egnew, Vice President
Hunter Lowder, Treasurer
To educate children with a wide range of language-related visual and auditory learning challenges in a way that provides them with the learning skills and self-esteem necessary to return successfully to mainstream education. Chartwell also helps individuals with specific learning challenges access their full potential by providing leading-edge education, research and community outreach.

3087 **College of Alameda**
Programs & Services for Students with Disabilities
555 Ralph Appezzato Memorial Pkwy
Alameda, CA 94501 510-748-2328
Fax: 510-748-2339
http://alameda.peralta.edu/dsps
Timothy Karas, President
Tina Vasconcellos, PhD, VP, Student Services
William Bruce, Dean of Special Programs
Accommodations, assessment and special classes are provided for learning disabled students enrolled at College Alameda, a 2 year college located by San Francisco Bay.

3088 **College of Marin**
ADA Accessibility
835 College Ave
Kentfield, CA 94904 415-457-8811
http://www1.marin.edu/ada-accessibility
David Wain Coon, Ed.D., Superintendent/President
Philip Kranenburg, Vice President
Stuart Tanenberg, Clerk
Offers a variety of services to students with disabilities including notetakers, extended testing time, counseling services, and special accommodations. Also offers diagnostic testing and remedial classes for learning disabled students.

3089 **College of the Canyons**
Disabled Student Programs and Services
26455 Rockwell Canyon Rd
Santa Clarita, CA 91355 661-362-3341
http://www.canyons.edu
jane.feuerhelm@canyons.edu
Jane A. Feuerhelm, PhD, Director
Offers a variety of services to students with disabilities including equipment, extended testing time, interpreting services, counseling services, and special accommodations.

3090 **College of the Redwoods**
Disabled Student Programs and Services
7351 Tompkins Hill Rd
Eureka, CA 95501 707-476-4280
Fax: 707-476-4418
TTY: 707-476-4284
http://www.redwoods.edu/dsps
cheryl-krueger@redwoods.edu
Dr. Keith Snow-Flamer, President
Cynthia Petrusha, Assistant to the President
Cheryl Krueger, Director
Mission is to assist individual students in the development of a realistic self-concept, assist in the development of educational interests and employment goals, provide the advice, counseling, and equipment necessary to facilitate success, starting with specialized assistance in the registration process.

3091 **College of the Sequoias**
Disability Resource Center
915 S. Mooney Blvd
Visalia, CA 93277 559-730-3805
Fax: 559-730-3803
TDD: 559-302-9976
http://www.cos.edu
AAC@cos.edu
Sandra Calderon, Director
Kyle Campbell, Support Services Coordinator
Neal Powell, Assistive Technology Manager
The Access & Ability Center provides academic and disability-related counseling on an appointment or walk-in basis.

3092 **College of the Siskiyous**
800 College Ave
Weed, CA 96094 530-938-5297
888-397-4339
Fax: 530-938-5378
http://www.siskiyous.edu/dsps
dsps@siskiyous.edu
Sunny Greene, DSPS Director
Offers services to learning and physically disabled students throught the DSPS - Disabled Students Programs & Services.

3093 **Columbia College**
11600 Columbia College Dr
Sonora, CA 95370 209-588-5100
Fax: 209-588-5104
http://www.gocolumbia.edu
osborns@yosemite.edu
Sean Osborn, MSW, DSPS Coordinator/Counselor
Santanu Bandyopadhyay, President
Cari Craven, Exec. Assistant to the President

Offers a variety of services to students with disabilities including note takers, extended testing time, counseling services and special accommodations.

3094 **Cuesta College**
PO Box 8106
Highway 1
San Luis Obispo, CA 93403-8106
805-546-3148
Fax: 805-546-3930
http://www.cuesta.edu
Jennifer Donaldson, Director
Judy Rittmiller, Program Assistant
Loren Buckingham, Testing Coordinator
A public, two-year community college, offering instruction and services to students with learning disabilities since 1973. A comprehensive set of services and special classes are available. Contact the program for further information.

3095 **East Los Angeles College**
1301 Avenida Cesar Chavez
Monterey Park, CA 91754
323-265-8787
Fax: 323-265-8714
http://www.elac.edu
dspstests@elac.edu
Marvin Martinez, President
Hao Xie, Financial Administrator
Danielle Fallert, Dean of Student Services
Offers a variety of services to students with disabilities including equipment, extended testing time, interpreting services, counseling services, and special accommodations.

3096 **Excelsior Academy**
Disabled Student Programs
7200 Parkway Dr
LaMesa, CA 91942
619-583-6762
Fax: 619-583-6764
http://www.excelsior-academy.com
kwilson@excelsioracademy.com
Nance Maguire, Ed.D, Executive Director
Shirley Willadsen, EdS, Director, Educational Operations
Provide a safe and nurturing environment wherein students become literate, thinking, independent, and productive citizens. Serving students in Grade 3-12 with unique learning profiles.

3097 **Fresno City College**
Disabled Student Programs and Services
1101 E University Ave
Fresno, CA 93741
559-442-8237
Fax: 559-499-6038
TDD: 599-442-8237
http://www.fresnocitycollege.edu
Thom Gaxiola-Rowles, Dir., Student Learning Support
Offers a variety of services to students with disabilities including equipment, extended testing time, interpreting services, counseling services, and special accommodations.

3098 **Frostig Center**
Marianne Frostig Center of Educational Therapy
971 N Altadena Dr
Pasadena, CA 91107
626-791-1255
Fax: 626-798-1801
http://www.frostig.org
center@frostig.org
Nancy Hogg, EdD, Chair
Debbie Baroi, PhD, Vice Chair
Vicki Seamons, Secretary
Dedicated to providing children with learning disabilities a quality academic program that also promotes their language, motor, social-emotional, and creative growth.

3099 **Gavilan College**
Disabled Student Programs and Services
5055 Santa Teresa Blvd
Gilroy, CA 95020
408-848-4865
Fax: 408-848-4914
TTY: 408-848-4924
http://www.gavilan.edu
drc@gavilan.edu
Kathleen Moberg, Vice President, Student Services
Kathleen A. Rose, President
Offers a variety of services to students with disabilities including note takers, extended testing time, counseling services and special accommodations.

3100 **Hartnell College**
Disabled Student Programs and Services
411 Central Ave
Salinas, CA 93901
831-755-6706
http://www.hartnell.edu
lserrano@hartnell.edu
Lucille Serrano, Executive Assistant
Willard Lewallen, PhD, Superintendent/President
Offers a variety of services to students with disabilities including equipment, extended testing time, interpreting services, counseling services, and special accommodations.

3101 **Institute for the Redesign of Learning**
Transition and Adult Services
625 Fair Oaks Ave
Ste 300
South Pasadena, CA 91030
323-341-5632
877-837-4332
Fax: 323-341-5644
http://www.redesignlearning.org
Nancy J. Lavelle, PhD, President
Edward Amey, Managing Diredtor
Nita Davis, MPA, Program Director
A full day school serving 100 boys and girls, at-risk infants and children. Vocational Program serves adults and includes Supported Employment Services and an Independent Living Program.

3102 **Irvine Valley College**
Disabled Student Programs and Services
5500 Irvine Center Dr
Irvine, CA 92618
949-541-5630
Fax: 949-451-5386
TDD: 949-333-0595
http://students.ivc.edu/dsps
ivcdsps@ivc.edu
Glenn R. Roquemore, PhD, President
Deejay Santiago, EdD, Dir., Student Success & Support
Dr. Linda Fontanilla, EdD, Vice President, Student Services
The goal is to effectivly provide assistance to all students with disabilities to achieve academic success while at Irvine Valley. The primary function is to accommodate a student's disability, whether it is a physical, communication, learning or psychological disability.

3103 **Kayne Eras Center**
Exceptional Children's Foundation
5359 Machado Rd
Culver City, CA 90232
310-204-3300
http://www.ecf.net
gwoods@ecf.net
Scott D. Bowling, President & CEO
Leslie B. Abell, Esq., Chairperson
George Woods, Director, School Programs
Operates a state certified, non-public school for youth ages 5 to 22 who are having difficulty functioning in the public school system due to developmental delays, learning disabilities, emotional or behavior challenges, and/or health impairments.

3104 **Laney College**
Disabled Student Programs & Services
900 Fallon St
Bldng E, Room 251
Oakland, CA 94607
510-464-3428
TTY: 510-464-3400
http://www.laney.peralta.edu
Tammeil Y. Gilkerson, EdD, President
Provides services and instructional programs for students with disabilities.

3105 **Long Beach City College: Liberal Arts Campus**
Disabled Student Programs and Services
4901 E Carson St
Long Beach, CA 90808 562-938-4111
http://www.lbcc.edu
Reagan F. Romali, President
DSPS provides many support services that enable students with disability related limitations to participate in the college's programs and activities. DSPS offers a wide range of services that compensate for a students limitations, like note taking assistance, interpretive services, alternative media, etc.

3106 **Los Angeles Mission College**
Disabled Student Programs and Services
13356 Eldridge Ave
Sylmar, CA 91342 818-364-7732
http://www.lamission.edu/dsps
DSPSinfo@lamission.edu
Monte E. Perez, PhD, President
A support system that enables students to fully participate in the college's regular programs and activities. Provides a variety of services from academic and vocational support to assistance with finacial aid. All services are individulalized according to specific needs. They do not replace regular programs, but rather, accommodate students special requirements.

3107 **Los Angeles Pierce College**
Disabled Student Programs and Services
6201 Winnetka Ave
Woodland Hills, CA 91371 818-719-6430
TDD: 818-436-0467
http://www.piercecollege.edu
special_services@piercecollege.edu
Dr. Genice Sarcedo-Magruder, Dean, Student Services & Equity
Miriam Gottlieb, Disabilities Specialist
John James, Counselor
Offers a variety of services to students with disabilities including equipment, extended testing time, interpreting services, counseling services, and special accommodations.

3108 **Los Angeles Valley College**
Services for Students with Disabilities (SSD)
5800 Fulton Ave
Student Services Annex, Room 175
Valley Glen, CA 91401 818-947-2681
Fax: 818-778-5775
TDD: 818-947-2680
TTY: 818-947-2680
http://www.lavc.edu
ssd@lavc.edu
David Green, Associate Dean
Katherine Tejeda-May, Counselors
Armenuhi Juharyan, Student Services Assistant
Provides specialized support services to students with disabilities which are in addition to the regular services provided to all students. Special accommodations and services are determined by the nature and extent of the disability related educational limitations of the student and are provided based upon the recommendation of DSPS.

3109 **Monterey Peninsula College**
Access Resource Center
980 Fremont St
STS 115
Monterey, CA 93940 831-646-4070
Fax: 831-646-4171
http://www.mpc.edu
arcinfo@mpc.edu
Dr. Walter Tribley, President
Charles Brown, Chair
Jaque Evans, Coordinator & Counselor
Supportive Services & Instruction program provides services and specialized instruction for enrolled students with disabilities.

3110 **Mount San Antonio Community College**
Accesibility Resource Centers for Students
1100 N Grand Ave
Walnut, CA 91789 909-274-4290
Fax: 909-274-2943
http://www.mtsac.edu/access
access@mtsac.edu
William T. Scroggins, President & CEO
Dr. Audrey Yamagata-Noji, Vice President, Student Services
Abe Ali, Vice President, Human Resources
Offers a variety of services to students with disabilities including equipment, extended testing time, interpreting services, counseling services, and special accommodations.

3111 **Napa Valley College**
Disabled Student Programs and Services
2277 Napa Valley Highway
Room 1769D
Napa, CA 94558 707-256-7453
http://www.napavalley.edu
sbarros@napavalley.edu
Sheryl Fernandez, Coordinator & Counselor
Farrel Dobbins, Secretary
Sandy Barros, Student Services Specialist
Offers a variety of services to students with disabilities including note takers, extended testing time, counseling services and special accommodations.

3112 **Ohlone College**
Student Accessibility Services (SAS)
43600 Mission Blvd
Bldng 7, 2nd Fl, Room 7217
Fremont, CA 94539 510-659-6079
Fax: 510-979-7401
http://www.ohlone.edu
sas@ohlone.edu
Ann Burdett, Director
Diane Cheney, Learning Specialist
Marcie Avina, Special Programs Assistant
Special services are provided to meet the unique needs of Deaf, Hard of Hearing, and Disabled students and help them achieve a successful college career.

3113 **Orange Coast College**
Disabled Students Program & Services
2701 Fairview Rd
Costa Mesa, CA 92626-5561 714-432-5807
http://www.orangecoastcollege.edu
occdisabledstudents@occ.cccd.edu
Vanessa Dominguez, Director
Thomas Stephenson, Disability Services Associate
Michael Ravellette, Disability Services Associate
Offers a variety of services to students with disabilities including equipment, extended testing time, interpreting services, counseling services, and special accommodations.

3114 **Park Century School**
3939 Landmark St
Culver City, CA 90232 310-840-0500
Fax: 310-840-0590
http://www.parkcenturyschool.org
Hilary Garland, President
Judith Fuller, Head of School
Jennifer Palmer, Chief Operating Officer
A non-profit independent co-educational day school designed to meet the specific educational needs of bright children, ages 7-14 years, who have learning disabilities.

3115 **Prentice School**
18341 Lassen Dr
North Tustin, CA 92705 714-538-4511
http://www.prentice.org
Mark Gaines, President
Devon Green, MS, Head Of School
Sabrina Clark, Director of Program
The Prentice School is an independent, nonprofit, coeducational day school for children ages Pre-K through 8th grade with language learning differences.

3116 **Raskob Learning Institute and Day School**
3520 Mountain Blvd
Oakland, CA 94619 510-436-1275
Fax: 510-436-1106
http://www.raskobinstitute.org
raskobinstitute@hnu.edu
Edith Ben Ari, Executive Director
Jessica Baiocchi, Director of Admission
Stefani Wulkan, Assistant Director/Lead Teacher
A co-educational school for students from diverse cultural and economic backgrounds with language-based learning disabilities. Raskob seeks to recognize and nurture the talents and strengths of each student while remediating areas of academic weakness.

3117 **San Diego City College**
Disabled Student Programs and Services
1313 Park Blvd
L-206
San Diego, CA 92101 619-388-3513
Fax: 619-388-3801
http://www.sdcity.edu/dsps
citydsps@sdccd.edu
Brianne Kennedy, Coordinator
Ricky Shabazz, EdD, President
Offers a variety of services to students with disabilities including note takers, extended testing time, counseling services, and special accommodations.

3118 **San Diego Miramar College**
Disability Support Programs and Services
10440 Black Mountain Rd
San Diego, CA 92126-2999 616-388-7312
Fax: 619-388-7917
http://www.sdmiramar.edu
miradsps@sdccd.edu
Patricia Hsieh, EdD, President
Offers a variety of services to students with disabilities including equipment, extended testing time, interpreting services, counseling services, and special accommodations.

3119 **San Diego State University**
Student Disability Services
5500 Campanile Dr
San Diego, CA 92182 619-594-5200
http://go.sdsu.edu
Adela de la Torre, President
Thomas McCarron, Vice President & CFO
Eric Rivera, Vice President, Student Affairs
Program and Support services are available to students with certified visual limitations, hearing and communication impairments, learning disabilities, mobility, and other functional limitations.

3120 **Santa Monica College**
Center for Students with Disabilities
1900 Pico Blvd
Santa Monica, CA 90405 310-434-4265
Fax: 310-434-4272
http://www.smc.edu
Barry Snell, Chair
Margaret Quinones-Perez, Vice Chair
Kathryn E. Jeffery, Superintendent/President
Offers guidance and counseling on admissions requirements and procedures, as well as a number of special programs to help students with their academic, vocational, and career planning goals. In addition, the Center offers services such as tutoring, specialized equipment, test proctoring, among many other accommodations for students who are eligible.

3121 **Santa Rosa Junior College**
Adapted Physical Education
1501 Mendocino Ave
Santa Rosa, CA 95401-4395 707-527-4470
Fax: 707-522-2780
http://www.santarosa.edu
kbell@santarosa.edu
Frank Chong, Ed.D, President
Kathy Bell, Coordinator
Offers a variety of regular classes each semester for people with disabilities.

3122 **Stanbridge Academy**
515 E Poplar Ave
San Mateo, CA 94401 650-375-5860
Fax: 650-375-5861
http://www.stanbridgeacademy.org
mainoffice@stanbridgeacademy.org
Julie Smith, Head of School
Susan Coyne, Director of Admissions
Ward Quincey, Director of Finance & Operations
A private, non-profit school for students with mild to moderate learning differences, primary grades through high school.

3123 **Stellar Academy for Dyslexics**
38325 Cedar Blvd
Newark, CA 94560 510-797-2227
Fax: 510-797-2207
http://www.stellaracademy.org
Beth Mattsson-Boze, Director
Karen Taylor, Dyslexia Tutor Center
Michele Muhamedcani, Office Administrator
To serve the needs of children with dyslexia using the Slingerlandr approach.

3124 **Sterne School**
838 Kearny St
San Francisco, CA 94108 415-922-6081
http://www.sterneschool.org
Ed McManis, Head of School
Susan Cain, Communications
Jaime Tollas, Director of Development
A private school serving students in 6-12 grade who have specific learning disabilities.

3125 **Summit View School**
6455 Coldwater Canyon Ave
Valley Glen, CA 91606 818-623-6300
Fax: 818-623-6390
http://www.summitview.org
Keri Borzello, Head of School
Catherine Lee, Clinical Director
Carol Cao, Director of Curriculum
Serving students with specific learning disabilities.

3126 **Summit View School: Los Angeles**
12101 W Washington Blvd
Los Angeles, CA 90066 310-751-1100
Fax: 310-397-4417
http://www.summitview.org
Keri Borzello, Head of School
Trudy Barker, Principal
Carol Cao, Director of Curriculum
Serving students with specific learning disabilities.

3127 **Tobinworld School: Glendale**
920 E Broadway
Glendale, CA 91205 818-247-7474
Fax: 818-247-6516
http://www.tobinworld.org
A non-profit school for children and young adults with behavior problems. Typically students have been classified as severely emotionally disabled, autistic or developmentally disabled.

3128 **Turning Point School**
8780 National Blvd
Culver City, CA 90232 310-841-2505
Fax: 310-841-5420
http://www.turningpointschool.org
info@turningpointschool.org
Dr. Laura Konigsberg, Head of School
Robert Friedman, President
Dana Kitaj, Vice President
A private, nonprofit school providing education for those with specific learning disabilities, including Dyslexia.

3129 **University of California: Irvine**
Office for Disability Services
100 Disability Services Center
Bldng 313
Irvine, CA 92697-5250
949-824-7494
Fax: 949-824-3083
TDD: 949-824-6272
http://www.dsc.uci.edu
dsc@uci.edu
Karen Andrews, Director
Jenna Roberts, Accommodations Coordinator
Rosezetta Henderson, Senior Disability Specialist
To provide effective and reasonable academic accommodations and related disability services to UCI students, Extension and Summer Session students, and other program participants. Consults with and educates faculty about reasonable academic accommodations. Strives to improve access to UCI programs, activities, and facilities for students with disabilities. Advises and educates academic and administrative departments about access issues to programs or facilities.

3130 **University of Redlands**
1200 E Colton Ave
PO Box 3080
Redlands, CA 92373
909-793-2121
Fax: 909-793-2029
http://www.redlands.edu
Ralph W. Kuncl, President
Michelle L. Rogers, Chief of Staff
Lisa Caldera, Executive Secretary
Small, private 4-year, residential, liberal arts university.

3131 **Ventura College**
Assitive Technology Training Center
4667 Telegraph Rd
Ventura, CA 93003
805-289-6000
http://www.venturacollege.edu
khoffmans@vcccd.edu
Kimberly Hoffmans, VP, Student Learning
Sebastian Szczebiot, Senior Administrative Assistant
Provides instruction in computer access to students with a broad range of disabilities, using the latest assistive technology available.

3132 **Westmark School**
5461 Louise Ave
Encino, CA 91316
818-986-5045
Fax: 818-986-2605
http://www.westmarkschool.org
cgoodman@westmarkschool.org
Claudia Koocheck, Head of School
Cindy Goodman, Director of Admissions
Steve Taylor, Director of Finance/Operations
Provides a caring environment where motivated students with learning differences discover their unique paths to personal and academic excellence in preparation for a successful college experience.

3133 **Westview School**
12101 W Washington Blvd
Los Angeles, CA 90066
310-478-5544
Fax: 310-397-4417
http://www.westviewschool.com
info@westviewschool.com
Alicia M. Jennings, Director of Education
Cheryl Myers, Administrative Principal
A private, non-profit day school in Los Angeles for students with learning, attentional and/or mild emotional concerns in grades 6-12.

Colorado

3134 **Denver Academy**
4400 E Iliff Ave
Denver, CO 80222
303-777-5870
Fax: 303-777-5893
http://www.denveracademy.org
info@denveracademy.org
Ed Callahan, Chair
Lisa Patterson, Vice Chair
Mark Twarogowski, Headmaster
The only co-ed 1st-12th grade independent school in the Denver-metro area dedicated to teaching students with learning differences and unique learning profiles.

3135 **Havern School**
4000 S Wadsworth Blvd
Littleton, CO 80123
303-986-4587
http://www.havernschool.org
info@havernschool.org
Christopher Koupal, Chair
Scott Stone, Secretary
Cathleen Pasquariello, Head of School
Provides a specialized education program for elementary and middle school students with learning disabilities.

3136 **Lamar Community College**
2401 S Main Street
Lamar, CO 81052
719-336-2248
http://www.lamarcc.edu
information@lamarcc.edu
Linda Lujan, PhD, President
Offers a variety of services to students with disabilities including notetakers, extended testing time, counseling services, and special accommodations.

3137 **Regis University**
Disability Services
3333 Regis Blvd
Clarke Hall, Room 225
Denver, CO 80221
303-458-4941
303-964-6595
Fax: 303-964-5498
http://www.regis.edu
disability@regis.edu
Father John P. Fitzgibbons, SJ, President
Barbara J. Wilcots, PhD, VP, Student Affairs
Salvador D. Aceves, EdD, SVP & CFO
Offers a variety of services to students with disabilities including equipment, extended testing time, interpreting services, counseling services, and special accommodations.

3138 **University of Colorado: Boulder**
Academic Resource Team (ART)
107 CU-Boulder
Boulder, CO 80309-0107
303-492-8671
TDD: 303-492-8671
http://disabilityservices.colorado.edu
dsinfo@colorado.edu
Joe Andenmatten, Ast. Dir., Access Services
Anirban Banerjee, Project Manager
Shanti Devasagayam, Program Administrator
Provides a variety of services to individuals with nonvisible disabilities, including individualized strategy sessions with a disability specialist, an assistive technology lab, and a career program for students with disabilities. Disability specialists also assist with obtaining reasonable accommodations if documentation meets disability services requirements and supports the need for them.

3139 **University of Denver**
Learning Effectiveness Program
1999 E Evens Ave
Ruffatto Hall, 4th Fl
Denver, CO 80208
303-871-2372
Fax: 303-871-3939
http://www.du.edu
lep-info@du.edu

Jimmie Smith, Director
Julie Law, Assistant Director
Jane Parks, Enrollment & Office Manager
A fee for service program offering comprehensive, individualized services to University of Denver Students with learning disabilities and or ADHD. The LEP is part of a larger organization called University Disability Services.

Connecticut

3140 **Ben Bronz Academy**
Learning Incentive
11 Wampanoag Dr
West Hartford, CT 06117 860-236-5807
Fax: 860-233-9945
http://www.learningincentive.org
Cynthia Cordes, Program Director
Ben Bronz Acadamy is a day school for bright disabled students. Guides 60 students through an intensive school day that includes writing, mathematics, literature, science and social studies. Oral language is developed and stressed in all classes.

3141 **Connecticut College**
Student Accessibility Services
270 Mohegan Ave
New London, CT 06320 860-447-1911
http://www.conncoll.edu
info@conncoll.edu
Katherine Bergeron, President
Melissa Shafner, Director
Offers a variety of services to students with disabilities including notetakers, extended testing time, counseling services, and special accommodations.

3142 **Eagle Hill School**
45 Glenville Rd
Greenwich, CT 06831 203-622-9240
http://www.eaglehillschool.org
Marjorie E. Castro, Head of School
Jeremy Henderson, Co-Chair
Patricia Murphy, Co-Chair
A language based remedial program committed to educating children with learning disabilities.

3143 **Forman School**
12 Norfolk Rd
PO Box 80
Litchfield, CT 06759 860-567-8712
Fax: 860-567-8317
http://www.formanschool.org
admissions@formanschool.org
Scott Sutherland, President
David Walter, Vice President
Michael L. Cook, Secretary
Forman offers students with learning differences the opportunity to achieve academic excellence in a traditional college preparatory setting. Daily remedial instruction balanced with course offerings rich in content provide each student with a flexible program that is tailored to his or her unique learning style and needs.

3144 **Marvelwood School**
476 Skiff Mountain Rd
Kent, CT 06757 860-927-0047
http://www.marvelwood.org
Blythe Everett, Head of School
William Dennett, Director of Enrollment
A coeducational boarding and day school enrolling 150 students in grades 9-12. Provides an environment in which young people of varying abilities and learning needs can prepare for success in college and in life. In a nurturing, structured community, students who have not thrived academically in traditional settings are guided and motivated to reach and exceed their personal potential.

3145 **Mitchell College**
Bentsen Learning Center
437 Pequot Ave
3rd Fl
New London, CT 06320 860-629-6214
http://www.mitchell.edu/academic-support/blc
murallo_a@mitchell.edu
Alice Murallo, Assistant Director
Kristina Smith, Office Manager
Kelby Chappelle, Director of Admissions
Small private college with comprehensive subject program for student with Learning Disabilities and/or ADHD.

3146 **The Glenholme School Devereux Connecticut**
81 Sabbaday Lane
Washington, CT 06793 860-868-7377
Fax: 860-868-7894
http://www.theglenholmeschool.org
Courtney Hoefer-Delaney, Director of Development
David Dunleavy, Director of Admissions
Julie Smallwood, Director of External Affairs
The Glenholme School is a therapeutic boarding school for students, ages 10-21, with high-functioning autism spectrum disorders, ADHD, OCD, Tourette's, depression, anxiety and various learning differences.

3147 **University of Hartford**
Learning Plus Program
200 Bloomfield Ave
West Hartford, CT 06117 860-768-4100
http://www.hartford.edu
E. Lynne Golden, Director
Patty O'Donovan, Administrative Secretary
Provides academic support to students with specific learning disabilities and/or attention deficit disorder. The support consists of one 45 minute appointment a week with an adult Learning Plus specialist presenting applicable learning strategies.

3148 **Vista Life Innovation**
1356 Old Clinton Rd
Westbrook, CT 06498 860-399-8080
http://www.vistalifeinnovations.org
Andi Barouh, Chair
Steven Seigelaub, Esq., Vice Chair
Helen K. Bosch, MS, Executive Director
Formerly known as the Vocational & Life Skills Center, Vista focuses on building self-esteem and confidence in the lives of adults with disabilities through work, independence and friendship. Offers a post-secondary program for young adults with learning disabilities providing individualized training and support in career development, independent living skills, social skills development and community involvement.

3149 **Woodhall School**
58 Harrison Ln
PO Box 550
Bethlehem, CT 06751 203-266-7788
http://www.woodhallschool.org
woodhallschool@woodhallschool.org
Matthew C. Woodhall, Head of School
Vince B Vincent, Associate Head of School
Julie Bohan, President
Offers an opportunity to experience success for young men of above average intellectual ability in grades 9-12 who have not achieved at a level commensurate with their ability in traditional school programs.

Delaware

3150 **Centreville Layton School**
6201 Kennett Pike
Centreville, DE 19807 302-571-0230
Fax: 302-571-0270
http://centrevillelayton.org
Barton Reese, Head of School

Provides an educational program that produces academic success and social development for children with learning disabilities.

District of Columbia

3151 **American University**
Learning Services Program
4400 Massachusetts Ave NW
Washington, DC 20016 202-885-1000
http://www.american.edu
Nancy Sydnor-Greenberg, Coordinator
Focuses on assisting students with their transition from high school to college during their freshman year. It is a small, mainstream program offering weekly individual meetings with the coordinator of the Learning Services Program throughout the student's first year.

3152 **Catholic University of America**
Disability Support Services
620 Michigan Ave NE
Washington, DC 20064 202-319-5211
Fax: 202-319-5126
TTY: 202-319-5211
http://dss.cua.edu
cua-dss@cua.edu
Philip V. Magalong, Director
Caitlin Rothwell, DSS Coordinator
Justin McPherson, Administrative Assistant
Four-year college that has support services for students with learning disabilities.

3153 **Georgetown University**
Disability Support Services
600 New Jersey Ave NW
Washington, DC 20001 202-662-4042
http://www.georgetown.edu
disabilityservices@georgetown.edu
Angela Tingler, Special Programs Coordinator
A four-year private university with a total enrollment of 6,418.

3154 **Saint Coletta: Greater Washington**
1901 Independence Ave SE
Washington, DC 20003 202-350-8680
Fax: 202-350-8699
TTY: 202-350-8695
http://www.stcoletta.org
Sue Goodhart, President
Joseph Watkins, Vice President
Delmas Johnson, Secretary
A non-sectarian, non-profit organization that operates school and adult day programs for children and adults with developmental disabilities and Autism.

3155 **The Lab School of Washington**
4759 Reservoir Rd NW
Washington, DC 20007-1921 202-965-6600
http://www.labschool.org
katherine.schantz@labschool.org
Katherine Schantz, Head of School
Diana Meltzer, Associate Head
Robert Lane, Director of Admissions
An innovative, rigorous, arts-based program for intelligent students with moderate to severe learning disabilities.

Florida

3156 **Barry University**
Center for Advanced Learning
11300 NE 2nd Ave
Miami Shores, FL 33161-6695 305-899-3687
800-756-6000
http://www.barry.edu
admissions@barry.edu
Linda Bevilacqua, President
John M. Bussel, Chair
Gerald W. Moore, Esq., Vice Chair
A comprehensive support program for students with learning disabilities and attention deficit disorders.

3157 **Beacon College**
105 E Main St
Leesburg, FL 34748 855-220-5374
Fax: 352-787-0721
http://www.beaconcollege.edu
admissions@beaconcollege.edu
George Hagerty, President
Brian T. Cobb, Chair
Sarah Flanagan, Vice Chair
Offer academic degree programs to students with learning disabilities.

3158 **Center Academy**
6710 86th Ave N
Pinellas Park, FL 33782 727-541-5716
http://www.centeracademy.com
NickiMaddalena@centeracademy.com
Mack R. Hicks, Founder and Chairman
Andrew P. Hicks, Chief Executive Officer
Eric V. Larson, President & COO
Private school, college prep, AD/HD, SLD, small classes, SACS & NIPSA accredited.

3159 **DePaul School for Dyslexia**
2747 Sunset Point Rd
Clearwater, FL 33759 727-796-7679
Fax: 727-796-7927
http://www.thedepaulschool.org
admin@thedepaulschool.org
Provides an alternative educational experience for students K-8th grade with dyslexia, ADHD, ADD and other learning disabilities and attention deficits.
1983

3160 **Dyslexia Research Institute**
5746 Centerville Rd
Tallahassee, FL 32309 850-893-2216
Fax: 850-893-2440
http://www.dyslexia-add.org
dri@dyslexia-add.org
Patricia K. Hardman, Founder, CEO
Robyn Rennick, Program Director
Addresses academic, social and self-concept issues for dyslexic and ADD children and adults. College prep courses, study skills, advocacy, diagnostic testing, seminars, teacher training, day school, tutoring and an adult literacy and life skills program is available using an accredited MSLE approach.

3161 **Florida Community College: Jacksonville**
Independent Living for Adult Blind
101 W State St
Jacksonville, FL 32202 904-633-8100
http://www.fscj.edu
An instructional program for adults who have vision loss to a degree that they experience some difficulty in their daily activities. Through guidance and specialized training offered through the ILAB program, individuals learn necessary skills for work and independence in their home and community.

3162 **Jericho School for Children with Autism and Other Developmental Delays**
1351 Sprinkle Dr
Jacksonville, FL 32211 904-744-5110
Fax: 904-744-3443
http://www.thejerichoschool.org
jerichoschool@yahoo.com
Angelo Martinez, Executive Director
Amie Austria, Education Director
Johann Schnell, Treasurer

Provides comprehensive, individualized science-based education not otherwise available in the community. Believes that those children with autism and other developmental delays deserve the opportunity to reach their full potential.

3163 **Lynn University**
Institute for Achievement and Learning
3601 N Military Trl
Boca Raton, FL 33431
561-237-7000
800-994-LYNN
Fax: 561-237-7100
http://www.lynn.edu
admission@lynn.edu
Shaun Exsteen, Executive Director
Kevin M. Ross, President
Anthony Altieri, VP, Student Affairs
Provides a series of support services to students with learning differences through a series of programs designed to help the students to succeed in their academic endeavors.

3164 **Morning Star School of Pinellas Park**
4661 80th Ave N
Pinellas Park, FL 33781
727-544-6036
Fax: 727-546-9058
http://www.morningstarschool.org
info@morningstarschool.org
Sue Conza, Principal
Students with special educational requirements need more care and attention than is offered in a traditional school setting.

3165 **PACE-Brantley School**
3221 Sand Lake Rd
Longwood, FL 32779
407-869-8882
http://pacebrantley.org
eshaffer@pacebrantley.org
Pam Tapley, Head of School
Dr. Rick Dunn, Chairman
Adam Haba, Vice Chairman
Specializes in teaching learning disabled children. Children that have been diagnosed with ADD, ADHD, and Dyslexia attend PACE.

3166 **Paladin Academy**
14900 NW 20th St
Pembroke Pines, FL 33028
954-431-4224
http://www.paladinacademy.com
jody.miller@nlcinc.com
Offers a college-prep curriculum for students with mild learning disabilities from grades K-12.

3167 **Tampa Bay Academy of Hope**
5118 N 56th St
Ste 230
Tampa, FL 33610-5400
813-620-4029
Fax: 813-620-4225
http://www.tampahope.org
info@tampahope.org
Titania Lamb, Executive Director
Christopher Shaver, Board Member
Amy Munroe, Board Member
The curriculum is designed with academic goals that encompass both special and vocational education. The mission of Tampa Bay Academy of Hope is to keep children on the path to success.
1996

3168 **Tampa Day School**
12606 Henderson Rd
Tampa, FL 33625
813-269-2100
http://www.tampadayschool.com
Lois Delaney, Head of School
Patricia Soloski, Learning Solutions Director
Pat Missak, Business Manager
To provide a learning environment that promotes that individual feeling of success for each child, and to find the unique key that opens the door to optimize his/her learning potential.

3169 **The Vanguard School**
22000 Hwy 27
Lake Wales, FL 33859
863-676-6091
Fax: 863-676-8297
http://www.vanguardschool.org
info@vanguardschool.org
Harold Maready, Head of School
Marya Marcum-Jones, Principal
Candi Medeiros, Director of Admissions
The Vanguard School is a fully accredited (SCAS and FCIS) coeducational boarding school and day school educating students in grades 5-12 with learning differences such as attention issues, challenging reading disorder, dyslexia, and Asperger's Syndrome.

3170 **The Victory Center**
18900 NE 25th Ave
North Miami Beach, FL 33180
305-466-1142
Fax: 305-466-1143
http://www.thevictoryschool.org
office@thevictoryschool.org
Raquel Pancer, Chief Executive Officer
David Barnett, Chairman
Michael Yavner, Vice Chairman
A Florida, non-secretarian, not-for-profit corporation that provides children with autism and smiliar disorders comprehensive individualized treatment with a 1:1 student/teacher ratio, in a classroom setting that is unique in Southeast Florida.

Georgia

3171 **Andrew College**
FOCUS Program
501 College St
Cuthbert, GA 39840-5599
229-732-5908
800-664-9250
http://www.andrewcollege.edu
benniemattox@andrewcollege.edu
Bennie Mattox, Director
Donna Manry, Academic Support Facilitator
The FOCUS program offers an intensive level of academic support designed for and limited to documented learning disabilities or attention deficit disorder. While FOCUS supplements and complements the tutorial and advising to all students, the program also provides an additional level of professional assistance and mentoring. Those accepted into FOCUS are charged regular tuition andd fees, plus a FOCUS laboratory fee.

3172 **Atlanta Speech School**
3160 Northside Pkwy NW
Atlanta, GA 30327
404-233-5332
Fax: 404-266-2175
http://www.atlantaspeechschool.org
Billy Levine, Chairman
Nancy Brumley Robitaille, Vice Chairman
Kathryn B. Miller, Secretary
For children ages 5 to 12 years old with average to very superior intelligence and mild to moderate language-based learning disabilities. The types of learning disabilities that are served include written language disorders, mathematical disabilities, ADD, dyslexia, and difficulty understanding and/or using spoken language.

3173 **Brandon Hall School**
1701 Brandon Hall Dr
Atlanta, GA 30350
770-394-8177
http://www.brandonhall.org
Dean J. Fusto, President/Head of School
Terry D. Lufkin, Associate Head & CFO
Andrew Smith, Director, Business Development
College preparatory, co-ed day and boys' boarding school for students in grades 4-12. Designed for academic underachievers and students with minor learning disabilities, attention deficit disorders and dyslexia.

3174 **Cottage School**
700 Grimes Bridge Rd
Roswell, GA 30075
770-641-8688
Fax: 770-641-9026
http://www.cottageschool.org
Steven T. Palmer, Executive Director
Bob Crenshaw, Chief Financial Officer
Kim Weber, Director of Advancement
Building a sense of self for students with special learning needs through academic and experiential programming, The Cottage School prepares individuals for fulfillment of their true potential as confident, productive, and independent adults.

3175 **Fort Valley State University**
Differently Abled Services Center
1005 State University Dr
Fort Valley, GA 31030
478-825-6744
877-462-3878
http://www.fvsu.edu/differently-abled-services
brownj02@fvsu.edu
Joyce Brown, Director
To increase retention for students with learning disorders by ensuring equal treatment, opportunity, and access for persons with impairments and/or disorders.

3176 **Georgia State University**
Margaret A Staton Office of Disability Services
Student Center E, Ste 205
55 Gilmer St
Atlanta, GA 30303
404-413-1560
http://disability.gsu.edu
dismail@gsu.edu
Mark P. Becker, President
Works with any student who has a disability to ensure meaningful access to the goods and services offered by GSU. To achieve this goal, academic accommodations are often made on behalf of the student.

3177 **Howard School**
1192 Foster St NW
Atlanta, GA 30318
404-377-7436
Fax: 404-377-0884
http://www.howardschool.org
info@howardschool.org
Marifred Cilella, Head of School
Anne Beisel, Admissions Director
Marci Mitchell, Director of Communications
Educates students with language learning disabilities and differences. Instruction is personalized to complement individual learning styles, to address student needs and to help each student understand his or her learning process. The curriculum focuses on depth of understanding in order to make learning meaningful and therefore, maximize educational success.

3178 **Mill Springs Academy**
13660 New Providence Rd
Alpharetta, GA 30004
770-360-1336
Fax: 770-360-1341
http://www.millsprings.org
rmoore@millsprings.org
Bruce Clayton, Chair
Robert W. Moore, Headmaster
Committed to a comprehensive, holistic program design that is multifaceted to meet the needs of the 'total child'.

3179 **Schenck School**
282 Mount Paran Rd NW
Atlanta, GA 30327
404-252-2591
Fax: 404-252-7615
http://www.schenck.org
office@schenck.org
Josh J. Clark, Head of School
Cathy Coleman, Director of Development
Terry Sherali, Director of Student Services
Offers a unique learning environment for children with dyslexia, as well as several auxiliary programs

3180 **St. Francis School**
9375 Willeo Rd
Roswell, GA 30075
770-641-8257
Fax: 770-641-0283
http://www.saintfrancisschools.com
dbuccellato@sfschools.net
Drew Buccellato, Headmaster
Linda Crawford, Associate Headmaster
Karen Harrison, Principal
Providing an educational program of the highest quality that can meet the needs of students with diverse abilities who would profit from a smaller teacher-pupil ratio than is available in most public or private schools.

3181 **Toccoa Falls College**
107 Kincaid Dr
Toccoa Falls, GA 30598
706-886-7299
http://www.tfc.edu
admissions@tfc.edu
Robert M. Myers, President
Abigail Davis, VP, Student Affairs
Emily Kerr, VP, Enrollment Management
Four-year college that provides services to the learning disabled.

Hawaii

3182 **University of Hawaii: Manoa**
Center on Disability Services
1410 Lower Campus Rd
Ste 171F
Honolulu, HI 96826
808-956-2065
http://www.cds.hawaii.edu
pmorriss@hawaii.edu
Patricia Morrissey, Director
JoAnn Yuen, Associate Director
Marla Arquero, Student Support Specialist
Dedicated to supporting the quality of life, inclusion, and empowerment of all persons with disabilities and their families through partnerships in training, service, evaluation, research, dissemination, and technical assistance. Nurtures, sustains, and expands promising practices for people with disabilities.

Idaho

3183 **Community High School**
1 Community School Dr
Sun Valley, ID 83353
208-622-3955
Fax: 208-622-3962
http://www.communityschool.org
info@communityschool.org
Brent Stevens, Chair
Will Hovey, Treasurer
Steve Shafran, Secretary
Offers a complete school prep curriculum for students with learning disabilities and ADD from grades 9 to 12.

3184 **University of Idaho**
Center on Disabilities and Human Development
1187 Alturas Dr
Moscow, ID 83843-8331
208-885-6000
800-393-7290
Fax: 208-885-6145
http://www.idahocdhd.org
idahocdhd@uidaho.edu
Chuck Staben, President
Currently operates a variety of independent grant programs and carries out training, services, technical assistance, research and dissemination activities across the state and nation.

Illinois

3185 **Acacia Academy**
6425 Willow Springs Rd
LaGrange, IL 60525
708-579-9040
Fax: 708-579-5872
http://www.acaciaacademy.com
info@acaciaacademy.com

Kathryn Fouks, Principal
Eileen Petzold, Asst. Principal
Jim Shoemaker-Saif, Head of High School
A school for grades 1-12 for children with learning disabilities. NCA accrediated and approved for out of district students in special education in the state of Illinois. Acacia Academy also offers a transition program for students ages 18-22, to help them achieve independence.

3186 **Brehm Preparatory School**
950 S Brehm Ln
Carbondale, IL 62901
618-457-0371
http://www.brehm.org
admissionsinfo@brehm.org

Stacy Brehm Tate, President
Daniel Maher, Vice President
Rita Dodd, Secretary
A coeducational boarding school for students with learning differences. Services are provided for students in grades 6-12. A post-secondary program, OPTIONS, is also available.

3187 **College of Dupage**
Vocational Skills Program
425 Fawell Blvd
Glen Ellyn, IL 60137
630-942-2176
Fax: 630-942-3785
http://www.cod.edu

Deanne Mazzochi, Chair
Frank Napolitano, Vice Chair
Christine M. Fenne, Secretary
Offers courses to students challenged with mild to moderate cognitive impairment. The courses are developmental-level, non-transferable credit courses designed to develop vocational skills that can lead to competitive, entry-level employment and enhance everyday living skills.

3188 **Cove School**
350 Lee Rd
Northbrook, IL 60062
847-562-2100
Fax: 847-562-2112
http://www.coveschool.org
ssover@coveschool.org

Sally Sover, Executive Director
John Stieper, III, Director of Education
Robin S. Johnstone, Clinical Director
For children and young adults in grades K-12 who are coping with a wide range of learning disabilities. The Cove School creates an exceptional environment for the children where they develop the emotional and social skills needed to reach their fullest potential.

3189 **DePaul University**
Center for Students with Disabilities
25 E Jackson Blvd
Lewis 1400
Chicago, IL 60604
312-362-5680
http://www.depaul.edu
studentaffairs@depaul.edu

Patricia O'Donoghue, Interim President
Robert L. Kozoman, CPA, Executive Vice President
Edward R. Udovic, Secretary
Offers a variety of services to students with disabilities including equipment, extended testing time, interpreting services, counseling services, and special accommodations.

3190 **Hamel Elementary School**
Edwardsville Community Unit District 7
400 W State St
Hamel, IL 62046
618-692-7444
Fax: 618-633-1702
http://www.ecusd7.org/schools

Matthew Sidarous, Principal
Offer programs for students with learning disabilities, ADD and/or emotional difficulties.

3191 **Kaskaskia College**
27210 College Rd
Centralia, IL 62801
618-545-3040
Fax: 618-545-3393
http://www.kaskaskia.edu
kcadmissions@kaskaskia.edu

George Evans, President
Cathy Quick, Administration
Offers a variety of services to students with disabilities including note takers, extended testing time, counseling services, and special accommodations.

3192 **Lewis and Clark Community College**
College Life Program
5800 Godfrey Rd
Godfrey, IL 62035
618-468-7000
800-YES-LCCC
http://www.lc.edu/disability
rellington@lc.edu

Roselyn Ellington, Program Coordinator
Kathy Haberer, Director
Emily DeGrand, Special Learning Needs Counselor
For those students with disabilities who have had few inclusive experiences in high school, the College for Life Program provides courses that continue the educational experience and also provides social growth opportunities on a college campus.

3193 **Roosevelt University**
Learning and Support Services Program
430 S Michigan Ave
Chicago, IL 60605-1394
312-341-3811
http://www.roosevelt.edu
academicsuccess@roosevelt.edu

Ali Malekzadeh, President
Andrew Harris, VP & CFO
The Disabled Student Services office serves all students with special needs. The use of services is voluntary and confidential. This office is a resource for students and faculty. The goal of this office is to ensure educational opportunity for all students with special needs by providing access to full participation in all aspects of campus life and increase awareness of disability issues on campus.

3194 **Saint Xavier University**
Student Success Program
3700 W 103rd St
Chicago, IL 60655
773-298-3330
Fax: 773-298-3331
http://www.sxu.edu
flynn@sxu.edu

Kristel Flynn, Director
James Alford, Student Support Specialist
Ann Ornelas, Office Manager
Offers a variety of services to students with disabilities including notetakers, extended testing time, counseling services, and special accommodations.

3195 **Southern Illinois University: Carbondale**
Clinical Center Achieve Program
625 Wham Dr
Mailcode 4602, Wham Bldng, Room 141
Carbondale, IL 62901
618-453-2361
Fax: 618-453-6130
http://clinicalcenter.siu.edu
jmeuth@siu.edu

Carlo Montemagno, Chancellor
Matt Baughman, Chief of Staff
Lori Stettler, Vice Chancellor, Student Affairs

Clinical Center Achieve Program is a comprehensive academic support service for students with LD and/or ADHD. Students must apply to both Achieve and the University.

3196 **University of Illinois: Chicago**
Institute on Disability and Human Development
1640 W Roosevelt Rd
Chicago, IL 60608 312-413-1647
Fax: 312-413-1630
http://ahs.uic.edu/disability-human-development
cherylj@uic.edu
Cheryl Johnson, Director
Dedicated to promoting the independence, productivity and inclusion of people with disabilities into all aspects of society.

3197 **University of Illinois: Urbana**
Disability Resources and Educational Services
1207 S Oak St
Champaign, IL 61820 217-333-1970
Fax: 217-244-0014
http://www.disability.illinois.edu
disability@illinois.edu
Pat Malik, Director
Maureen Gilbert, Coordinator
Marlene Hedrick, Clerk
Provides comprehensive disability services to University of Illinois students with disabilities, including disabilities.

Indiana

3198 **Ball State University**
Disabled Student Development
2000 W University Ave
Muncie, IN 47306 765-289-1241
800-382-8540
Fax: 765-285-5295
TTY: 765-285-2206
http://www.bsu.edu
dsd@bsu.edu
Courtney Jarrett, Director
Sharon Harper, Administrative Coordinator
Offers a variety of services to students with disabilities including note takers, extended testing time, counseling services, and special accommodations.

3199 **Cathedral High School**
5225 E 56th St
Indianapolis, IN 46226 317-542-1481
Fax: 317-542-1484
http://www.gocathedral.com
Robert Bridges, President
David Worland, Principal
Colleen O'Brien-Teasley, Chief Financial Officer
Provides, to a diverse group of students, opportunities for spiritual, intellectual, social, emotional and physical growth through service and academic excellence.

3200 **Indiana Wesleyan University**
TRIO Scholars Program
4201 S Washington St
Ste 220
Marion, IN 46953 765-677-2257
Fax: 765-677-2140
http://www.indwes.edu
karen.newhard@indwes.edu
Karen Newhard, Coordinator
David Wright, President
To help students realize their full potential in relation to their academic pursuits at Indiana Wesleyan University. Benefits to TRIO Scholars include academic and cultural enrichment, disability services, mentoring, personal counseling, tutorial support, and the opportunity to apply for grant aid.

3201 **Ivy Tech Community College**
3501 N 1st Ave
Evansville, IN 47710 888-IVY-LINE
http://www.ivytech.edu
Dr. Sue Ellspermann, President
Andy Bowne, SVP & COO
Anne Brinson, Chief Information Officer
Provides reasonable and effective accommodations to qualified students with learning disabilities.

3202 **Manchester College**
Services for Students with Disabilities
604 E College Ave
North Manchester, IN 46962 260-982-5000
http://www.manchester.edu
Laura Turner-Reed, Director
Mia Miller, Academic Coach
Diana Nettleton, Academic Coach
Offers a variety of services to students with disabilities including equipment, extended testing time, interpreting services, counseling services, and special accommodations.

3203 **Saint Mary-of-the-Woods College**
1 St Mary of Woods Coll
Saint Mary of the Woods, IN 47876 812-535-5151
http://www.smwc.edu
smwc@smwc.edu
Dottie L. King, PhD, President
Janet Clark, PhD, VP, Academic & Student Affairs
Brennan Randolph, VP, Enrollment Management
Offers a variety of services to students with disabilities including note takers, extended testing time, counseling services, and special accommodations.

3204 **University of Indianapolis**
BUILD Program
1400 E Hanna Ave
Indianapolis, IN 46227 317-788-3536
800-232-8634
http://www.uindy.edu/ssd/build
foutse@uindy.edu
Betsy Fouts, Director
Mary Catherine Davis, Administrative Assistant
A full support program at the University of Indianapolis designed to help the college students with specific learning disability earn an associate or baccalureate degree.

3205 **Worthmore Academy**
4601 N Emerson Ave
Indianapolis, IN 46226 877-700-6516
Fax: 317-251-6516
http://www.worthmoreacademy.org
bjackson@worthmoreacademy.org
Brenda Jackson, Founder & Director
A place where children with learning differences may come and receive individualized instruction to help remediate his or her learning differences.

Iowa

3206 **Clinton High School**
1401 12th Ave N
Clinton, IA 52732 563-243-9600
Fax: 563-243-5405
http://www.clinton.k12.ia.us
dbloom@clintonia.org
David Bloom, Student Services Director
Julie Matzen, Student Enrollment Secretary
Gary DeLacy, Superintendent
Provide services for individuals with special needs to achieve high levels of learning through equitable access to quality education for each student in an environment of mutual respect, trust, enthusiasm and cooperation.

3207 **Des Moines Area Community College**
2006 S Ankeny Blvd
Ankeny, IA 50023
515-964-6200
800-362-2127
http://www.dmacc.edu
rjdenson@dmacc.edu

Robert J. Denson, President
Joe Pugel, Chair
Kevin Halterman, Vice Chair
DMACC is committed to providing an accessible environment that supports students with disabilities in reaching their full potential. Support services are available for students with disabilities to ensure equal access to educational opportunities.

3208 **Iowa Central Community College**
One Triton Circle
Fort Dodge, IA 50501
515-576-7201
800-362-2793
http://www.iowacentral.edu

Dr. Dan Kinney, President
Mark R. Crimmins, Board Member
Darrell Determann, Board Member
Offers a variety of services to students with disabilities including equipment, extended testing time, interpreting services, counseling services, and special accommodations.

3209 **Iowa Lakes Community College: Emmetsburg**
3200 College Dr
Emmetsburg, IA 50536
712-852-5219
800-242-5108
Fax: 712-582-2152
http://www.iowalakes.edu
info@iowalakes.edu

Jody Condon, Educational Counselor
Thomas Brotherton, Executive Dean
Offers a variety of services to students with disabilities including equipment, extended testing time, interpreting services, counseling services, and special accommodations.

3210 **Iowa Western Community College**
2700 College Rd
Council Bluffs, IA 51503
712-325-3299
Fax: 712-388-6850
http://www.iwcc.edu
disabilityservices@iwcc.edu

Dan Kinney, President
Tori Christie, VP, Student Services
Offers a variety of services to students with disabilities including equipment, extended testing time, interpreting services, counseling services, and special accommodations.

3211 **Loras College**
Loras Lynch Learning Center
1450 Alta Vista St
Dubuque, IA 52001
563-588-7134
800-245-6727
http://www.loras.edu
lynch.learningcenter@loras.edu

James E. Collins, President
Mary Ellen Carroll, PhD, Senior Vice President
Arthur Sunleaf, VP, Student Development
Offers a variety of services to students with disabilities including equipment, extended testing time, interpreting services, counseling services, and special accommodations.

3212 **North Iowa Area Community College**
On Track: Time Management Program
500 College Dr
Mason City, IA 50401
641-422-4296
888-GO-NIACC
http://www.niacc.edu
vancelis@niacc.edu

Lisa Vance, Counselor
Dr. Steven Schulz, President
On Track Program is meant for students with disabilities who have realized they need a little extra help keeping track of assignments, due dates, and a busy schedule of activities.

3213 **SAVE Program**
Iowa Lakes Community College: Emmetsburg
3200 College Dr
Emmetsburg, IA 50536-1055
712-852-5274
800-242-5108
Fax: 712-852-2152
http://www.iowalakes.edu
mkogel@iowalakes.edu

Michelle Kogel, Program Coordinator
Provide special education secondary students with an option where they will receive, based on their IEP goals, further education in the areas of life skills training, vocational/employability skills training, and transitional/self advocacy skills training.

3214 **Simpson College**
The Center for Academic Resources
701 N C St
Indianola, IA 50125
515-961-1682
http://www.simpson.edu/hawley
car@simpson.edu

Drew Van Winkle, Director, Student Accessibility
Sarah Davitt, Academic Coach
Ron Warnet, Academic Coach
Offers a variety of services to students with disabilities including equipment, extended testing time, interpreting services, counseling services, and special accommodations.

3215 **University of Iowa**
Realizing Educational and Career Hopes Program
240 S Madison St
Iowa City, IA 52242
319-384-2127
http://education.uiowa.edu/services/reach
reach@uiowa.edu

Bruce Harreld, President
Specifically designed to meet the needs of young adults with multiple learning and cognitive disabilities.

3216 **Wartburg College**
Pathways Center
100 Wartburg Blvd
Waverly, IA 50677
319-352-8230
800-772-2085
Fax: 319-352-8365
http://www.wartburg.edu
nicole.willis@wartburg.edu

Nicole Willis, Academic Success Associate
Offers a variety of services to students with disabilities including equipment, extended testing time, interpreting services, counseling services, and special accommodations.

Kansas

3217 **Baker University**
Student Academic Success
PO Box 65
Baldwin City, KS 66006
785-597-8352
http://www.bakeru.edu
robin.liston@bakerU.edu

Dr. Robin Liston, Coordinator, Academic Advising
Samantha Cheek, Academic Success Assistant
Kathy Wilson, Academic Achievement
Offers a variety of services to students with disabilities including equipment, extended testing time, interpreting services, counseling services, tutoring and special accommodations.

3218 **Fort Scott Community College**
2108 S Horton St
Fort Scott, KS 66701
800-874-3722
http://www.fortscott.edu

John Bartelsmeyer, Chair
Alysia Johston, President
Robert Nelson, Vice Chair
A public two-year college with 34 special education students out of a total of 1,928.

3219 **Horizon Academy**
4901 Reinhardt Dr
Ste A
Roeland Park, KS 66205 913-789-9443
Fax: 913-789-8180
http://www.horizon-academy.org
info@horizon-academy.com
Julie Altman, Principal
Vicki Asher, Head of School
Trish Arnold, Development Director
Private school for children with learning disabilities. Students learn word decoding skills in reading, oral and written language comprehension and/or expression, math skills, organizational and social skills.

3220 **Newman University**
3100 McCormick St
Wichita, KS 67213-2097 316-942-4291
http://www.newmanu.edu
Noreen Carrocci, President
Victor Trilli, VP, Student Affairs
Norm Jones, VP, Enrollment Management
Offers a variety of services to students with disabilities including notetakers, extended testing time, counseling services, and special accommodations.

Kentucky

3221 **Brescia University**
717 Frederica St
Owensboro, KY 42301 270-685-3131
http://www.brescia.edu
chris.houk@brescia.edu
Father Larry Hostetter, President
Provides the following for students with learning disabilities: developmental courses (English, mathematics and study skills); individual tutoring for all areas; and academic and career counseling.

3222 **DePaul School**
1925 Duker Ave
Louisville, KY 40205 502-459-6131
http://www.depaulschool.org
dpinfo@depaulschool.org
Tony Kemper, Head of School
Lisa Stepp, Principal
Phil Howell, Dean of Students
The dePaul School embraces all sorts of learning differences and accommidate learning disabilities.

3223 **Eastern Kentucky University**
Project SUCCESS
521 Lancaster Ave
Whitlock Bldng, Room 361
Richmond, KY 40475 859-622-2933
Fax: 859-622-6794
http://accessibility.eku.edu/project-success
accessibility@eku.edu
Joslyn Glover, JD, Director
Lee Ann Griesheimer, Academic Success Coordinator
Jessica Denise Harris Hunt, Accessibility Coordinator
Offers a comprehensive support program for college students with learning disabilities, attention deficit disorder and other cognitive disorders. Upon admittance, Project SUCCESS develops an individualized program of services which serve to enhance the academic success of each student.

Louisiana

3224 **Louisiana College**
Student Success Center
1140 College Dr
PO Box 545
Pineville, LA 71359-0001 318-487-7629
http://www.lacollege.edu
JoLynn McConley, Director
Offers a variety of services to students with disabilities including equipment, extended testing time, interpreting services, counseling services, tutoring and special accommodations.

3225 **Louisiana State University: Alexandria**
8100 Highway 71 S
Alexandria, LA 71302 318-445-3672
888-473-6417
http://www.lsua.edu
advising@lsua.edu
Dr. Guiyou Huang, Chancellor
Offers a variety of services to students with disabilities including extended testing time, counseling services, and special accommodations.

3226 **Louisiana State University: Eunice**
Office of Disability Services
2048 Johnson Hwy
PO Box 1129
Eunice, LA 70535 337-550-1204
Fax: 337-550-1268
http://www.lsue.edu
ods@lsue.edu
F. King Alexander, President
Jason Droddy, Chief of Staff
Hannah Rovira, Coordinator
Offers a variety of services to students with disabilities including equipment, extended testing time, interpreting services, counseling services, tutoring and special accommodations.

3227 **Nicholls State University**
Student Access Center
PO Box 2087
Thibodaux, LA 70310 985-448-4430
Fax: 985-449-7009
http://www.nicholls.edu/disability
Lizetta M. Frederick, Director
The Center provides assessments and remediation to students with Dyslexia and related learning disabilities. Programs are offered for college students as well as K-12 students.

3228 **Northwestern State University**
Office of Disability Support
309 Student Union
Rm234
Natchitoches, LA 71497 318-357-4460
Fax: 318-357-6502
http://studentaffairs.nsula.edu
faucheauxc@nsula.edu
Catherine C. Faucheaux, Director
Holley Shivers, Counselor
Northwestern State University's Office of Disability Support (ODS) offers services and accommodations for students with disabilities. ODS is also available to provide information pertaining to disability-related issues.

3229 **Southeastern Louisiana University**
Disability Services
War Memorial Student Union 1304
SLU Box 10496
Hammond, LA 70402 985-549-2247
Fax: 985-549-3482
http://www.southeastern.edu/admin/ds
disabilityservices@southeastern.edu
Angela James, Director
Facilitates academic accommodations for students with disabilities and collaborate with other University departments to ensure full access and participation in all activities, programs, and services offered by the University.

Maine

3230 **University of Maine**
Student Accessibility Services
121 East Annex
Orono, ME 04469
207-581-2319
Fax: 207-581-9420
http://www.umaine.edu
um.sas@maine.edu

Sarah Henry, Director
Amy Sturgeon, Assistant Director
Merlin Littlefield, Administrative Specialist
The primary goal of the Student Accessibility Services is to create educational access for students with disabilities at UMaine by providing a point of coordination, information and education for those students and the campus community.campus community.

3231 **University of New England: University Campus**
Student Access Center
Student Academic Success Building
Biddeford, ME 04005
207-602-2815
Fax: 207-602-5971
http://www.une.edu/student-access-center
bcstudentaccess@une.edu

Hahna Patterson, Director
Laura Cutter, Coordinator
Dawn M. Jewett, Test Center Supervisor
The Student Access Center seeks to promote respect for individual differences and to ensure that students with disabilities have equal opportunities to succeed and take an active role in their education.

Maryland

3232 **Chelsea School**
2970 Belcrest Center Dr
Ste 300
Hyattsville, MD 20782
240-467-2100
http://www.chelseaschool.edu
information@chelseaschool.edu

Mindelyn Anderson, Program Director
Kristal Weems-Bradner, Principal, Middle School
Frank Mills, Principal, Upper School
To prepare students with language based learning disabilities for higher education by providing a world-class school which embeds literacy remediation and technology into all aspects of the curriculum.
1976

3233 **Greenwood School**
6525 Belcrest Rd.
Suites G-80 & G-90
Hyattsville, MD 20782
301-458-4860
Fax: 301-458-4863
http://www.greenwoodschoolmd.org
greenwoodschoolmd@verizon.net

Laurie Klinovski, Director
Greenwood School is a private pre-school that serves infants through kindergarten. If a student requires special educational needs, the school works with the parents and teacher in order to develop a program catered to the child.

3234 **Harbour School**
1277 Green Holly Dr
Annapolis, MD 21409
410-974-4248
Fax: 410-757-3722
http://www.harbourschool.org
info@harbourschool.org

Linda J. Jacobs, EdD, Executive Director
Bryon Fracchia, Program Director
Noel Butler, Curriculum Coordinator
To provide a supportive, caring and individualized education to students with learning disabilities, autism, speech language impairments, and other disabilities like ADD/ADHD in grades one through twelve by assisting each child to attain academic and personal achievement and success commensurate with the child's abilities.

3235 **Highlands School**
2409 Creswell Rd
Bel Air, MD 21015
410-836-1415
Fax: 410-412-1098
http://www.highlandsschool.net
info@highlandsschool.net

Phil Piercy, Head of School
Suzanna Lippa, Director of Admissions
Paula Carmody, Educational Director
Offering a full academic program for students in grades k-8 with dyslexia, ADHD, and laguage based learning differences.

3236 **Ivymont School**
Autism Program
11614 Seven Locks Rd
Rockville, MD 20854
301-469-0223
Fax: 301-469-0778
http://www.ivymount.org
sholt@ivymount.org

Susan Holt, CEO & Director
Amy Alvord, Education Director
M. Kimball Clark, Autism Program Director
Provides a non-diploma functional life skills program for students ages 6-21 diagnosed with autism and offers a proactive generalization program which ensures student progress is generalized to their community and home.

3237 **James E Duckworth School**
11201 Evans Trl
Beltsville, MD 20705
301-572-0620
http://www1.pgcps.org/jameseduckworth
Yolanda G. Cosby, Principal
Tracey Johnson, Administrative Assistant
A public school in the Prince George's County Public School System., And serves students with moderate to severe disabilities ages 5 through 21.

3238 **Jemicy School**
11 Celadon Rd
Owings Mills, MD 21117
410-653-2700
Fax: 410-653-1972
http://www.jemicyschool.org
mmcgowan@jemicyschool.org

Megan McGowan, Head of School
Empowers students with dyslexia and language-based learning differences to realize their intellectual and social potential through a proven, multisensory curriculum.

3239 **Margaret Brent School**
100 E 26th St
Baltimore, MD 21218
401-396-6509
http://www.baltimorecityschools.org/53
PSmith01@bcps.k12.md.us

Pamela Smith, Principal
Offers a language-based curriculum which infuses both language and literacy skills throughout the curriculum, utilizing picture communication symbols.

3240 **McDaniel College**
Student Academic Support & Disability Services
2 College Hill
Ste 117
Westminster, MD 21157
410-857-2504
Fax: 410-386-4617
http://www.mcdaniel.edu
sass@mcdaniel.edu

Melanie Conley, Director
Lisa Breslin, SASS Consultant
Dana Neville, Associate Director

SASS offers basic accommodations (free) as well as more intensive levels of support (fee-based). In addition, each fall they offer Step Ahead, a week-long workshop, to a limited number of incoming first year and transfer students. This intensive experience works to equip students with the necessary academic, independence, and social skills to assist with a smooth transition to college. Step Ahead peer mentors provide outreach throughout the semester.

3241 **Odyssey School**
3257 Bridle Rdg
Stevenson, MD 21153 410-580-5551
Fax: 410-580-5352
http://www.theodysseyschool.org
acusick@theodysseyschool.org
Martha H. Sweeney, Head of School
Provides a warm and creative environment that balances a stimulating hands-on curriculum with a personalized approach to meet the needs of the individual child. Early intervention program, daily tutoring, visual arts/music/dance, leading edge technology, sports, character education and clubs.

3242 **Summit School**
Academic Program
664 Central Ave E
Edgewater, MD 21037 410-798-0005
Fax: 410-798-0008
http://www.thesummitschool.org
info@thesummitschool.org
Joan A. Mele-McCarthy, Executive Director
Elizabeth A. Crabtree, Chair
Chris Lamon, Vice Chair
Committed to providing a mainstream academic program that challenges intelligent young minds while addressing students with dyslexia and other learning differences.

3243 **The Forbush School at Hunt Valley**
Sheppard Pratt Health System
11201 Pepper Rd
Hunt Valley, MD 21031 410-527-9505
Fax: 410-527-0329
http://www.sheppardpratt.org
tyearick@sheppardpratt.org
Tim Yearick, Principal
Harsh K. Trivedi, President & CEO
Armando Colombo, Executive VP & COO
Special education classes for children and young adults ages 5-21 with autism, developmental delays, pervasive developmental disorder and multiple learning problems. Programs include motor skill development and sensory integration strategies, natural aided language stimulation, positive behavioral support and vocational programming.

3244 **Towson University**
Disability Support Services
8000 York Rd.
Towson, MD 21252 410-704-2638
Fax: 410-704-4247
http://www.towson.edu/dss
tudss@towson.edu
Kim Schatzel, President
Debra Moriarty, VP, Student Affairs
David Vanko, Acting Provost/VP
With more than 23,000 students, Towson University is the second largest public university in Maryland. Founded in 1866, the University offers more than 100 bachelor's, master's and doctoral degree programs in the liberal arts, STEM programs, fine arts, business and applied professional fields. Approximately 1,800 students are registered with the Disability Support Services office on campus.

Massachusetts

3245 **American International College**
Supportive Learning Services Program
1000 State St
Springfield, MA 01109 800-242-3142
http://www.aic.edu
inquiry@www.aic.edu
Frank Colaccino, Chair
A. Craig Brown, Treasurer
Vincent Maniaci, President
An independent four-year college with 95 special education students out of a total of 1,433. There is an additional fee for the special education program.

3246 **Berkshire Center**
40 Main St
Ste 3
Lee, MA 01238 413-243-2576
Fax: 413-243-3351
http://cipworldwide.org/cip-berkshire/berkshire
admissions@cipworldwide.org
Miral Kruh, Program Director
Matthew Kosiorek, Director, Student Life Services
Judy Gerich, Academic Coordinator
Provides individualized social, academic, career & life skills instruction to young adults 18-26 with Aspergers, ADD and other learning differences. With our support and direction, students learn to realize & develop their potential.

3247 **Berkshire Meadows**
249 N Plain Rd
Housatonic, MA 01236 413-528-2523
http://www.jri.org/berkshiremeadows
lkelly@jri.org
Liisa Kelly, Senior Program Director
A residential school for children with intellectual physical disabilities. Nursing and medical services available. Programs based on the philosophy that all people, no matter how severe their disabilities, should be given the opportunity to achieve their maximum potential.

3248 **Boston College**
140 Commonwealth Ave
Chestnut Hill, MA 02467 617-552-8000
http://www.bc.edu
William P. Leahy, SJ, President
Peter K. Markell, Chair
Joseph L. Hooley III, Vice Chair
An independent four-year college with 195 special education students out of a total of 14,230. There is an additional fee for the special education program in addition to the regular tuition.

3249 **Boston University**
Office of Disability Services
One Silber Way
Boston, MA 02215 617-353-3658
Fax: 617-353-9646
http://www.bu.edu
access@bu.edu
Lorre Wolf, Program Director
Grace Daley, Student Services Coordinator
Christopher S. Robinson, Outreach/Training Coordinator
Provides basic support services such as test taking accommodations, note taking assistance, etc. Provides comprehensive services that include learning strategies instruction for an additional fee. LDSS offers a six-week summer program, The Summer Transition Program, for high school graduates.

3250 **Bristol Community College**
Office of Disability Services
777 Elsbree St
L109
Fall River, MA 02720 774-357-2955
http://www.bristolcc.edu
ODSaccess@bristolcc.edu

Laura L. Douglas, President
Joan M. Medeiros, Chair
Steven A. Torres, Esq., Vice Chair
Provides an integrated program of early academic and career guidance for students with physical and/or learning disabilities.

3251 **Carroll School**
25 Baker Bridge Rd
Lincoln, MA 01773 781-314-9731
http://www.carrollschool.org
admissions@carrollschool.org
Richard Waters, Chair
Charles Brizius, Vice Chair
Steve Wilkins, Head of School
A dynamic independent day school for elementary and middle school students who have been diagnosed with specific learning disabilities in reading and writing, such as dyslexia.

3252 **Cotting School**
453 Concord Ave
Lexington, MA 02421 781-862-7323
Fax: 781-861-1179
http://www.cotting.org
info@cotting.org
David W. Manzo, Executive Director/President
Bridget Irish, Chief Operating Officer
Michael Pembroke, Chief Financial Officer
Day school for children with a broad spectrum of learning and communication disabilities, physical challenges, and complex medical conditions.

3253 **Curry College**
Program for Advancement of Learning
1071 Blue Hill Ave
Milton, MA 02186 617-333-0500
Fax: 617-333-2114
http://www.curry.edu
pal@curry.edu
Dr. Laura Vanderberg, PAL Director
Kathy Wilmot, Admissions Coordinator
Dr. Janis Peters, Student & Parent Concerns
PAL is a program within Curry College, a co-educational, four-year liberal arts institution serving 2,000 students and located in the Boston suburb of Milton, Massachusetts. For over 25 years, PAL has both shaped and been shaped by Curry's distinctive philosophy of education. Serves college age students with specific learning disabilities.

3254 **Dearborn Academy**
575 Washington St
Newton, MA 02458 781-641-5992
Fax: 781-641-5997
http://www.dearbornacademy.org
raltepeter@dearbornacademy.org
Rebecca Altepeter, Head of School
Pam Sweeney, Director
Sheilah Gauch, Director
A program of psycho-educational day schools serving children in elementary, middle, and high school with emotional, behavioral, and learning difficulties. Students struggling to learn find a secure environment in which to thrive.

3255 **Eagle Hill School**
242 Old Petersham Rd
PO Box 116
Hardwick, MA 01037 413-477-6000
Fax: 413-477-6837
http://www.eaglehill.school
Jim Richardson, Chair
Marilyn Waller, President
Alden Bianchi, Vice President
Co-educational, college preparatory boarding and day school for students in grades 8-12 diagnosed with learning disabilities and ADD.

3256 **Evergreen Center**
Educational Programs and Services
345 Fortune Blvd
Milford, MA 01757 508-478-2631
Fax: 508-634-3251
http://www.evergreenctr.org
services@evergreenctr.org
A residential school serving children and adolescents with severe developmental disabilities.

3257 **Harvard School of Public Health**
Harvard University
677 Huntington Ave
Boston, MA 02115 617-495-1000
http://www.hsph.harvard.edu
Stacey Herman, Associate Dean, Student Services
Leah Kane, Director of Student Affairs
An independent four-year college with 45 special education students out of a total of 6,621. Disabled students are encouraged to take advantage of opportunities available to help them achieve their educational goals.

3258 **Hillside School**
404 Robin Hill Rd
Marlborough, MA 01752 508-485-2824
Fax: 508-485-4420
http://www.hillsideschool.net
admission@hillsideschool.net
Ed Chase, Headmaster
Tanner Church, Learning Specialist
Hillside School is an independent boarding and day school for boys, grades 4-9. Hillside provides educational and residential services to boys needing to develop their academic and social skills while building self-confidence and maturity. The 200-acre school is located in a rural section of Marlborough and includes a working farm. Hillside accommodates both traditional learners who want a more personalized education, and those boys with learning difficulties and/or attention problems.

3259 **Landmark Elementary and Middle School Program**
Landmark School
429 Hale St
PO Box 227
Prides Crossing, MA 01965 978-236-3010
Fax: 978-927-7268
http://www.landmarkschool.org
admission@landmarkschool.org
Moira McNamara James, Chair
Martin P. Slark, Vice Chair
Rob Kahn, Head of School
Landmark School's mission is to enable and empower students with language-based learning disabilities to realize their educational and social potential through an exemplary school program complemented by outreach and training, diagnosis, and research.

3260 **Landmark High School Program**
Landmark School
429 Hale St
PO Box 227
Prides Crossing, MA 01965 978-236-3010
http://www.landmarkschool.org
admission@landmarkschool.org
Moira McNamara James, Chair
Martin P. Slark, Vice Chair
Robert J. Broudo, President and Headmaster
Landmark School's mission is to enable and empower students with language-based learning disabilities to realize their educational and social potential through an exemplary school program complemented by outreach and training, diagnosis, and research.

3261 **Landmark School Outreach Program**
Landmark School
429 Hale St.
P.O. Box 227
Prides Crossing, MA 01965 978-236-3216
Fax: 978-927-7268
http://www.landmarkoutreach.org
outreach@landmarkschool.org
Dan Ahearn, Director
Keryn Kwedor, Associate Director
Jenna Lanoue, Operations Manager
Seeks to empower children with language-based learning disabilities by offering their teachers an exemplary program of applied research and professional development.
1971Grade Range: 2-8

3262 **Lesley University**
Threshold Program
29 Everett St
Cambridge, MA 02138-2790 617-349-8181
800-999-1959
http://www.lesley.edu
threshold@lesley.edu
Hans D. Strauch, Chair
Juanita James, Vice Chair
Jeff A. Weiss, President
The Threshold Program is a comprehensive, nondegree campus-based program at Lesley University for highly motivated young adults with diverse learning disabilities and other special needs.

3263 **Middlesex Community College**
Transition Program
591 Springs Rd
Bedford, MA 01730-1197 781-280-3630
Fax: 781-275-7126
http://www.middlesex.mass.edu
darceyd@middlesex.mass.edu
Nancy Sleger, Program Coordinator
Pat Bruno, Associate Dean, Student Support
Dyan Darcey, Administrative Assistant
Designed expressly for students with significant learning disabilities. This two-year certificate program teaches consumer and business skills, independent living, and personal and social development.

3264 **Northeastern University**
Learning Disabilities Program
135 Forsyth Building
360 Huntington Ave
Boston, MA 02115 617-373-4526
Fax: 617-373-4142
http://www.northeastern.edu/ldp
j.newton@northeastern.edu
Jennifer Newton, Director
Offers a variety of services to students with disabilities including note takers, extended testing time, counseling services, and special accommodations.

3265 **Pre-College Workshop for Students with Disabilities**
Bridgewater State University
10 Shaw Rd
Bridgewater, MA 02325 508-531-2194
Fax: 508-531-4194
http://www.bridgew.edu
disability_resources@bridgew.edu
Timothy Pure, Assistant Director
Pamela Spillane, Learning Disabilities Specialist
A two-day program for new students with disabilities. Gives new students with disabilities an opportunity to talk about what BSC offers with upper-class students with disabilities.

3266 **Riverview School**
551 Route 6A
East Sandwich, MA 02537 508-888-0489
Fax: 508-833-7001
http://www.riverviewschool.org
admissions@riverviewschool.org
Stewart Miller, Head of School
Nancy Hopkins, Director of Admissions
Richard Dalrymple, Director of Finance
An independent, residential school of international reputation and service enrolling 183 male and female students in its secondary and post-secondary programs. Students share a common history of lifelong difficulty with academic achievement and the development of friendships. On measures of intellectual ability, most students score within the 70-100 range and have a primary diagnosis of learning disability and/or complex language or learning disorder.

3267 **Smith College**
Disability Services
College Hall 104
Northampton, MA 01063-0001 413-585-2071
TDD: 413-585-2071
TTY: 413-585-2071
http://www.smith.edu
ods@smith.edu
Laura Rauscher, Director
Lisa Roberge, Administrative Assistant
Jeanette Landrie, Coordinator, Academic Access
Support services office for students, staff and faculty with disabilities.

3268 **Springfield Technical Community College**
One Armory Square, Ste 1
PO Box 9000
Springfield, MA 01102-9000 413-781-7822
Fax: 413-755-6344
http://www.stcc.edu
John B. Cook, PhD, President
Christopher C. Johnson, Chair
Franklin D. Qingley, Jr., Vice Chair
Springfield Technical Community College, a leader in technology and instructional innovation, transforms lives through educational opportunities that promote personal and professional success.

3269 **White Oake School**
533 North Rd
Westfield, MA 01085 413-562-9500
Fax: 413-562-9010
http://www.whiteoakschool.org
admissions@whiteoakschool.org
David Drake, Headmaster
Jody Michalski, Dean of Academics
Gerard McGovern, Dean of Students
Offer programs for students with learning disabilities, ADD and/or emotional difficulties.

3270 **Willow Hill School**
98 Haynes Rd
Sudbury, MA 01776 978-443-2581
Fax: 978-443-7560
http://www.willowhillschool.org
mgreid@willowhillschool.org
Marilyn G. Reid, Head of School
Mark Hall, Director of Education
Tom Rimer, Director of Admissions
Offers secondary level students with learning challenges opportunities to acquire academic and social skills needed to shape their own future.

Michigan

3271 **Andrews University**
8975 US 31
Berrien Springs, MI 49104 269-471-7771
http://www.andrews.edu
enroll@andrews.edu
Dr. Andrea Luxton, President
Dr. Christon Arthur, Provost
Artur Stele, Chair

Offers a variety of services to students with disabilities including notetakers, extended testing time, counseling services, and special accommodations.

3272 **Aquinas College**
1700 Fulton St E
Grand Rapids, MI 49506-1801 616-632-8900
http://www.aquinas.edu
admissions@aquinas.edu

Kevin Quinn, PhD, President
An independent four-year college with 32 special education students out of a total of 2,300 students.

3273 **Calvin College**
Center for Student Success
3201 Burton St SE
Spoelhof College Center 360
Grand Rapids, MI 49546-4402 616-526-6155
http://calvin.edu
successcenter@calvin.edu

Lisa Kooy, Disability Coordinator
Kyle Heys, Access Program Director
Javonna Allen, Academic Conselor
Provides the coaching program for students with learning disabilities, attention deficit disorders and other students who benefit from help with time management and study skills.

3274 **Eastern Michigan University**
Disability Resource Center
246 Student Center
Ypsilanti, MI 48197 734-487-2470
Fax: 734-483-6515
http://www.emich.edu
drc@emich.edu

James M. Smith, President
Rhonda Longworth, PhD, Provost/EVP
Mike Valdes, Chief Financial Officer
Four year college that offers students with learning disabilities support and services.

3275 **Eton Academy**
Academic Program
1755 E Melton Rd
Birmingham, MI 48009 248-642-1150
http://www.etonacademy.org
contact@etonacademy.org

Pete Pullen, Head of School
To help students who learn differently achieve their fullest potential for academic excellence. Eton Academy offers a comprehensive curriculum that integrates the best available multi-sensory, hands-on and experiential learning methods to meet the individual needs of its students.

3276 **Lake Michigan Academy**
2428 Burton St SE
Grand Rapids, MI 49546 616-464-3330
Fax: 616-285-1935
http://www.mylma.org
info@mylma.org

Nanette Clatterbuck, CEO
Veronica Beitner, Director of Operations
Amy Barto, Academic Consultant
Lake Michigan academy provides academic excellence for students with specific learning disabilities and/or attention deficit disorder in grades 1-12.

3277 **Michigan Technological University**
1400 Townsend Dr
Houghton, MI 49931-1295 906-487-1885
888-688-1885
http://www.mtu.edu
mtu4u@mtu.edu

Richard Koubek, President
Jacqueline Huntoon, Provost/VP for Academic Affairs
David Reed, Chief Financial Officer
Offers services for students with physical or learning disabilities, including extended testing time, audio textbooks, and counseling.

3278 **Montcalm Community College**
2800 College Dr
Sidney, MI 48885 989-328-2111
http://www.montcalm.edu
info@montcalm.edu

Karen Carbonelli, Chair
Robert Marston, Vice Chair
Robert C. Ferrentino, J.D., President
Offers a variety of services to students with disabilities including note takers, extended testing time, counseling services, and special accommodations.

3279 **Northwestern Michigan College**
Disability Support Services
1701 E Front St
Osterlin Bldng O115 ML
Traverse City, MI 49686 231-995-1000
800-748-0566
http://www.nmc.edu
lbaumeler@nmc.edu

Leanne Baumeler, Disability Support Specialist
Kennard R. Weaver, Chair
Chris M. Bott, Vice Chair
Offers a variety of services to students with disabilities including note takers, extended testing time, counseling services, and special accommodations.

Minnesota

3280 **Alexandria Technical and Community College**
1601 Jefferson St
Alexandria, MN 56308 320-762-0221
http://www.alextech.edu
info@alextech.edu

Educational Institution

3281 **Augsburg College**
Center for Learning and Adaptive Student Services
2211 Riverside Ave
Minneapolis, MN 55454 612-330-1000
Fax: 612-330-1590
http://www.augsburg.edu
admissions@augsburg.edu

Paul C. Pribbenow, PhD, President
Karen L. Kaivola, Provost & Chief Academic Officer
Leif Anderson, VP & Chief Strategy Officer
The Center for Learning and Adaptive Student Services coordinates academics accommodations and services for students with learning, attentional and psychiatric disabilities.

3282 **College of Saint Scholastica**
1200 Kenwood Ave
Duluth, MN 55811-4199 800-447-5444
http://www.css.edu
admissions@css.edu

Colette McCarrick, PhD, President
Steve Lyons, VP, Student Affairs
Offers a variety of services to students with disabilities including note takers, extended testing time, counseling services, and special accommodations.

3283 **Groves Academy**
3200 Highway 100 S
St Louis Park, MN 55416 952-920-6377
Fax: 952-920-2068
http://www.grovesacademy.org
alexanderj@grovesacademy.org

Thomas Schnack, Chair
Megan Prindiville, Vice Chair
John Alexander, Executive Director
A private, independent, day school for adults with langauge, learning and attentional disabilities.

3284 **Institute on Community Integration**
University of Minnesota
109 Pattee Hall
150 Pillsbury Dr SE
Minneapolis, MN 55455
612-624-6300
Fax: 612-624-9344
http://ici.umn.edu
ici@umn.edu

Amy S. Hewitt, PhD, Director
A federally designated University Center for Excellence in Developmental Disabilities, has over 400 print and electronic resources on topics relating to community living for persons with intellectual and developmental disabilities across the lifespan.

3285 **Minnesota Life College**
7501 Logan Ave S
STE 2A
Richfield, MN 55423
612-869-4008
Fax: 612-869-0443
http://www.miccommunity.org
agudmestad@miccommunity.org

Mark Ziegler, Chair
Rob Bass, Vice Chair
Amy Gudmestad, Executive Director
Minnesota Life College is a not-for-profit, vocational and life skills training program for young adults with learning disabilities.

3286 **Minnesota State Community and Technical College: Moorhead**
1900 28th Ave S
Moorhead, MN 56560
218-299-6500
877-450-3322
Fax: 218-299-6810
TTY: 800-627-2539
http://www.minnesota.edu
jerome.migler@minnesota.edu

Dr. Peggy D. Kennedy, President
Pat Nordick, CFO
Kathleen Brock, Chief Academic Officer
Offers a variety of services to students with disabilities including notetakers, extended testing time, counseling services, and special accommodations.

3287 **Northwest Technical College**
1900 28th Ave S
Moorhead, MN 56560-4899
218-299-6500
877-450-3322
Fax: 218-299-6810
TTY: 800-627-3529
http://www.minnesota.edu
jerome.migler@minnesota.edu

Tom Julsrud, President
Marlis Ziegler, Secretary
Richard Smestad, Vice President
Offers a variety of services to students with disabilities including notetakers, extended testing time, counseling services, and special accommodations.

3288 **Student Accessibility Services**
St. Cloud State University
720 4th Ave S
St Cloud, MN 56301-4498
320-308-4080
http://www.stcloudstate.edu/sas
sas@stcloudstate.edu

Andria Belisle, Director
Jane Eckhoff, Office Manager
A public comprehensive university that provides services for students with learning disabilities and other needs: alternative testing, note taking, referrals to campus resources and advocacy/support.

3289 **University of Minnesota: Morris**
Disability Resource Center
600 E 4th St
240 Briggs Library
Morris, MN 56267
320-589-6178
Fax: 320-589-6473
TTY: 800-627-3529
http://www.morris.umn.edu

Matthew Hoekstra, Coordinator
Offers a variety of services to students with disabilities including note takers, extended testing time, counseling services, and special accommodations.

Mississippi

3290 **Mississippi State University**
Adaptive Driving Program
PO Box 9736
326 Hardy Rd
Mississippi State, MS 39762
662-325-1028
Fax: 662-325-0896
TTY: 662-325-0520
http://www.msstate.edu
ek77@msstate.edu

Eric Knox, Director
Specializes in the evaluation and training of persons with disabilities who wish to consider driving. Services may result in a recommendation for driving or further training, and when appropriate, will include specific recommendations regarding vehicle modifications and adaptive driving equipment. Also offers evaluation and training services for driving candidates using bioptic lenses.

3291 **University of Southern Mississippi**
118 College Dr
Hattiesburg, MS 39406-0001
601-266-1000
http://home.usm.edu

Rodney D. Bennett, President
Steven R. Moser, PhD, Provost & SVP, Academic Affairs
Allyson Easterwood, VP, Finance & Administration
Four year college that provides students with support and resources whom are disabled.

Missouri

3292 **Central Missouri State University**
Office of Accessibility Services
Elliott Union 224
Warrensburg, MO 64093
660-543-4421
Fax: 660-543-4724
http://www.ucmo.edu
access@ucmo.edu

John A. Collier, President
Mary Dandurand, Secretary
Provider of equal opportunity to education for students with disabilities through notetakers, extended testing time, interpreters and other accommodations.

3293 **Churchill Center and School for Learning Disabilities**
1021 Municipal Center Dr.
Town & Country, MO 63131
314-997-4343
Fax: 314-997-2760
http://www.churchillstl.org
info@churchillstl.org

Sandra Gilligan, Director
Anne Evers, Director, Admissions
Deborah Warden, Assistant Director
The Churchill School is a private, not-for-profit, co-educational day school. It is designed to serve children between the ages of 8-16 with diagnosed learning disabilities. The goal is to help each child reach his or her full potential and prepare them for a successful return to a traditional classroom in as short a period of time as possible.

3294 **Metropolitan Community College: Longview**
Disability Support Services
500 SW Longview Rd
Lee's Summit, MO 64081-2015 816-604-2254
Fax: 816-672-2025
http://www.mcckc.edu/disability-services
Dr. Utpal Goswami, President
Dr. Bill Dial], Chief HR Officer
Sandra Garcia, Chief Legal Officer
The program teaches students with neurological disabilities including, but not limited to: learning disabilities or brain injuries how to become independent learners.

3295 **Missouri State University**
Learning Diagnostic Clinic
300 S Jefferson
Ste 502
Springfield, MO 65806 417-836-4787
Fax: 417-836-5475
http://www.psychology.missouristate.edu/ldc
LearningDiagnosticClinic@missouristate.edu
Steven C. Capps, Director
Hannah Jayne Harris, Assistant Director
Provides services and support to all students. The clinic ensures all students with learning disabilities have access and actively participate in the services provided by the university.

3296 **North Central Missouri College**
1301 Main St
Trenton, MO 64683 660-359-3948
http://www.ncmissouri.edu
Dr. Lenny Klaver, President
Offers a variety of services to students with disabilities including note takers, extended testing time, counseling services, and special accommodations.

3297 **St Louis Community College: Forest Park**
5600 Oakland Ave
St Louis, MO 63110 314-644-9100
http://www.stlcc.edu
Julie Fickas, Interim Provost
Franklyn Taylor, Dean, Student Development
St. Louis Community College creates accessible, dynamic learning environments focused on the needs of their diverse students.

3298 **St Louis Community College: Meramec**
11333 Big Bend Rd
Kirkwood, MO 63122 314-984-7500
http://www.stlcc.edu
Carol Lupardus, Provost
Kim Fitzgerald, Dean, Student Development
St. Louis Community College creates accessible, dynamic learning environments focused on the needs of their diverse students.

3299 **University of Missouri: Kansas City**
Student Disability Services
5110 Oak St
Ste 225
Kansas City, MO 64110 816-235-5612
http://info.umkc.edu/disability-services
disability@umkc.edu
Scott Laurent, Director
Offers a variety of services to students with disabilities including note takers, extended testing time, counseling services, and special accommodations.

Montana

3300 **Western Montana College**
710 S Atlantic St
Dillon, MT 59725 406-683-7331
http://w.umwestern.edu
Dr. Beth Weatherby, Chancellor
Michael Reid, Vice Chancellor
A public four-year college with 6 special education students out of a total of 1,100.

Nebraska

3301 **Midland Lutheran College**
Academic Program Support
900 N Clarkson
Fremont, NE 68025 402-941-6027
800-642-8382
http://www.midlandu.edu
info@midlandu.edu
Leaha Hammer, ADA Coordinator
Four-year college that provides academic support for students who have a learning disability.

3302 **Southeast Community College: Beatrice Campus**
Academic Advising & Support
4771 W Scott Rd
Beatrice, NE 68310 402-228-3468
http://www.southeast.edu
Nancy A. Seim, Chair
James J. Garver, Vice Chair
Robert J. Feit, Treasurer
Offers academic counselling to students regarding admissions, courses, academic requirements, credit transfers, etc.

3303 **University of Nebraska: Omaha**
Accessibility Services Center (ASC)
6001 Dodge St
Milo Bail Student Center 126
Omaha, NE 68182 402-554-2872
800-858-8648
Fax: 402-554-6015
http://www.unomaha.edu
rjacobs@unomaha.edu
Jeffrey P. Gold, Chancellor
Hank M. Bounds, President
Becky Jacobs, Interim Director
Offers a variety of services to students with disabilities including notetakers, extended testing time, counseling services, and special accommodations.

New Hampshire

3304 **Dartmouth College**
Student Accessibility Services
6174 Carson Hall
Ste 125
Hanover, NH 03755 603-646-9900
http://dartmouth.edu
Student.Accessibility.Services@Dartmouth.edu
Ward Newmeyer, Direcror
Alicia Brandon, Associate Director
Megan Nemeroff, Auxiliary Service Coordinator
The Student Accessibility Services (SAS) Office works with students, faculty and staff to ensure that the programs and activities of Dartmouth College are accessible, and students with disabilities receive reasonable accommodations.in their curricular and co-curricular pursuits. Services include note takers, extended testing time, and counseling services.

3305 **Hampshire Country School**
28 Patey Circle
Rindge, NH 03461 603-899-3325
Fax: 603-899-6521
http://www.hampshirecountryschool.org
office@hampshirecountryschool.net
Bernd Foecking, Headmaster
Thomas Ciglar, Director of Operations
William Dickerman, Director of Admissions
Hampshire Country School is a boarding school for middle school boys with very high ability who need an unusual amount of adult attention and support, including boys with Asperger's, nonverbal learning disabilities and ADHD.
1948Grade Range: Ages 8-18

3306 **Hunter School**
PO Box 600
768 Doetown Rd
Rumney, NH 03266
603-786-9427
Fax: 603-786-2221
http://www.hunterschool.org
info@hunterschool.org
A small, non-profit school where young boys and girls with Attention Deficit Disorder (ADD), Attention Deficit/Hyperactivity Disorder (ADHD) or Asperger's Syndrome are nurtured, educated and celebrated. Offers both a residential program and a day school.

3307 **Keene State College**
Office of Disability Services
229 Main St
Keene, NH 03435
603-358-2353
800-KSC-1909
Fax: 603-358-2313
http://www.keene.edu
Jane Warner, Director
Lisa David, Associate Director
Melanie Morel, Assistive Tech Coordinator
Offers a variety of services to students with disabilities including note takers, extended testing time, counseling services, and special accommodations.

3308 **Learning Skills Academy**
1247 Washington Rd
Rye, NH 03870
603-964-4903
http://www.learningskillsacademy.org
lsa@learningskillsacademy.org
Karen Elrod Staines, Executive Director
Sean Kotkowski, Program Administrator
Mary Anker, Chair
Learning Skills Academic strives to help students reach their full potential both academically and socially. The program prepares them for success in life by helping them to understand their learning profile: advocate for their needs; interact appropriately in scholastic and social situations; and bring their academic work to a level that matches their potential.
1985

3309 **Manchester Community College**
1066 Front St
Manchester, NH 03102
603-206-8000
Fax: 603-668-5354
http://www.mccnh.edu
Dr. Susan Huard, President
Offers a variety of services to students with disabilities including notetakers, extended testing time, counseling services, and special accommodations.

3310 **New England College**
Disability Services Office
98 Bridge St
Henniker, NH 03242
603-428-2302
Fax: 603-428-2433
http://www.nec.edu
disabilityservices@nec.edu
Michelle D. Perkins, President
Megan Hotaling, Director of Student Engagement
Kim Bolton, Asst., Student Development
The Disability Services Office works with students, faculty and staff in order to ensure all students have access and are capabale of fully participating in both the social and academic communities at the college.

3311 **Rivier College**
Office Disability Services
420 S Main St
The Learning Commons, 1st Fl
Nashua, NH 03060
603-897-8497
800-44-RIVIE
Fax: 603-897-8816
http://www.rivier.edu
damurphy@rivier.edu
Darcy Murphy, Director
Sr. Paula Marie Buley, President
Kurt Stimeling, VP, Student Affairs
Offers a variety of services to students with disabilities including note takers, extended testing time, counseling services, and special accommodations.

3312 **Southern New Hampshire University**
Campus Accessibility Center (CAC)
2500 N River Rd
Manchester, NH 03106
603-644-3118
http://www.snhu.edu
cac@snhu.edu
Paul Leblanc, President
R. Yvette Clark, SVP & General Counsel
Amelia Manning, Chief Operating Officer
Offers services to students with disabilities based on recommendations from documentaion supporting a disability. Accommodations are made for specific needs.

3313 **University of New Hampshire**
Student Accessibility Services (SAS)
201 Smith Hall
3 Garrison Ave
Durham, NH 03824-3594
603-862-2607
Fax: 603-862-4043
TTY: 800-735-2964
http://www.unh.edu/studentaccessibility
michael.shuttic@unh.edu
Michael Shuttic, Director
Janice Carlson, Disability Specialist
Maureen Bourdeau, Assistive Technology Specialist
Student Accessibility Services provides services to students with documented disabilities to ensure that University activities and programs are accessible. It also promotes the development of student self-reliance and the personal independence necessary to succeed in a university climate.

New Jersey

3314 **Banyan School**
12 Hollywood Ave
Fairfield, NJ 07004
973-439-1919
http://www.banyanschool.com
wmcneill@banyanschool.com
Wendy McNeill, Executive Director
A private, nonprofit elementary and high school for students with significant language-based learning disabilities. Banyan School works to identify each student's strengths and abilities and adapts the curriculum accordingly.
1993

3315 **Caldwell College**
Office of Disability Services
120 Bloomfield Ave
Caldwell, NJ 07006
973-618-3488
Fax: 973-618-3488
http://www.caldwell.edu
bmoran@caldwell.edu
Barbara Moran, Coordinator
Offers a variety of services to students with disabilities including note takers, extended testing time, counseling services, and special accommodations.

3316 **Camden County College**
Office of Disability Services
200 N Broadway
Blackwood, NJ 08012-118
856-227-7200
http://www.camdencc.edu
jkinzy@camdencc.edu
Joanne Kinzy, Director
Donald A. Borden, President
Offers a variety of services to students with disabilities including note takers, extended testing time, counseling services, and special accommodations.

3317 **Catapult Learning**
Two Aquarium Dr
Camden, NJ 08103 800-841-8739
http://catapultlearning.com
info@catapultlearning.com
Jeffrey Cohen, Chief Executive Officer
Stephen Freeman, Vice Chairman
Chris Catalano, Chief Financial Officer
Catapult Learning works with students and tachers from both public and nonpublic schools to provide education solutions to any barriers the system may face. Offers family support services, professional development assistance, special education and alternative education programs.

3318 **Centenary University**
Office of Disabilities Services
400 Jefferson St
Hackettstown, NJ 07840 908-852-1400
http://www.centenaryuniversity.edu
dso@centenaryuniversity.edu
Michelle Meyer, Director
Marcella Lamura, Learning Support Specialist
Laura Rhodes, Learning Support Specialist
Offers two programs specifically designed to support students with mild emotional and learning disabilities: Project Able and Step Ahead. The goals of these programs are to provide a bridge between the structured and sometimes modified secondary-school setting to the predominantly self-directed college environment.

3319 **Children's Center of Monmouth County**
1115 Green Grove Rd
Neptune, NJ 07753 732-922-0228
Fax: 732-922-8133
http://www.ccprograms.com
Offers educational services, training in adaptive living and pre-vocational skills for students, ages 3 to 21, with multiple disabilities or a diagnosis of autism and pervasive developmental delays.

3320 **College of New Jersey**
Disability Support Services
121 Roscoe W 2000 Pennington Rd
Ewing, NJ 08628-0718 609-771-3199
Fax: 609-637-5121
http://differingabilities.tcnj.edu
dss@tcnj.edu
Meghan L. Sooy, Director
Kathryn A. Foster, President
Offers a variety of services to students with disabilities including note takers, extended testing time, counseling services, and special accommodations.

3321 **College of Saint Elizabeth**
Accessibility Services
2 Convent Rd
Morristown, NJ 07960-6989 973-290-4261
http://www.cse.edu
lseneca@cse.edu
Lisa Seneca, Coordinator
Offers a variety of services to students with disabilities including notetakers, extended testing time, counseling services, and special accommodations.

3322 **Craig School**
10 Tower Hill Rd
Mountain Lakes, NJ 07046 973-334-1295
Fax: 973-334-1299
http://www.craigschool.org
admissions@craigschool.org
Frank Velocci, Chair
Gary Levinson, Vice Chair
Grant L. Jacks, Head of School
A school for children with learning differences such as dyslexia, auditory processing issues and ADD.

3323 **Cumberland County College**
Physical & Learning Disabilities
3322 College Dr
Vineland, NJ 08360 856-691-8600
http://www.cccnj.edu
mvicente@cccnj.edu
Meredith Vicente, Senior Director
Offers a variety of services to students with disabilities including note takers, extended testing time, counseling services, and special accommodations.

3324 **Fairleigh Dickinson University: Metropolitan Campus**
1000 River Rd
Teaneck, NJ 07666-1914 201-692-7100
800-338-8803
Fax: 201-692-7100
http://www.fdu.edu
Christopher A. Capuano, PhD, President
Comprehensive support services to students with language based LD.

3325 **Forum School**
107 Wyckoff Ave
Waldwick, NJ 07463 201-444-5882
Fax: 201-444-4003
http://www.theforumschool.com
info@theforumschool.com
Steven Krapes, Executive Director
Linda Oliver, Office Manager
Day school for children through age 16 who have neurologically based developmental disabilities, including autism, ADHD, LD, and asperger syndrome. Services include extended year, speech, adaptive physical education, music, art therapy, and parent program.

3326 **Georgian Court University**
The Learning Connection (TLC)
900 Lakewood Ave
Lakewood, NJ 08701 732-987-2650
800-458-8422
Fax: 732-987-2000
http://www.georgian.edu
fahrl@georgian.edu
Luana E. Fahr, Director
The Learning Connection is an assistance program that provides an environment for students with mild to moderate learning disabilities who desire a college education. An individualized support program to assist candidates in becoming successful college students. Emphasis is placed on developing self-help strategies, study techniques, content tutoring, time management, organization skills, and social skills all taught by a certified professional.

3327 **Hudson County Community College**
70 Sip Ave
Jersey City, NJ 07306 201-714-7100
http://www.hccc.edu
Chris Reber, President
Offers a variety of services to students with disabilities including note takers, extended testing time, counseling services, and special accommodations.

3328 **Kean University**
Counselling & Disabilities Services
1000 Morris Ave
Union, NJ 07083 908-737-4850
Fax: 908-737-4855
http://www.kean.edu
counselling@kean.edu
Dawood Farahi, PhD, President
Ada Morell, Chair
Michael D'Agostino, Vice Chair
Offers a variety of services to students with disabilities including note takers, extended testing time, counseling services, and special accommodations.

3329 **Middlesex County College**
Project Connections
2600 Woodbridge Avenue
Johnson Learning Center, Rm 230
Edison, NJ 08818-3050 732-906-2507
Fax: 732-906-7767
http://www.middlesexcc.edu
CKolber@middlesexcc.edu

Cheryl Kolber, Director
Diane Manatch, Project Associate
Project Connections is a comprehensive academic and counseling service for students with learning disabilities who are enrolled in mainstream programs at Middlesex County College.

3330 **Morristown-Beard School**
70 Whippany Rd
Morristown, NJ 07960 973-539-3032
Fax: 973-539-1590
http://www.mbs.net
admission@mbs.net

John Fey, President
Gail Kurz, Vice President
David Gately, Vice President
Offer programs for students with learning disabilities, ADD and/or emotional difficulties.

3331 **New Jersey City University**
Office of Specialized Services
2039 Kennedy Blvd
Karnoustsos Hall, Rm 105
Jersey City, NJ 07305 201-200-2091
http://www.njcu.edu

Jennifer Aitken, Director
Jazmin Zegarra, Coordinator, Specialized Service
Joan Serafin, Coor. Supplemental Instruction
Offers a variety of services to students with disabilities including notetakers, extended testing time, counseling services, and special accommodations.

3332 **Ocean County College**
College Dr
Toms River, NJ 08754 732-255-0400
http://www.ocean.edu

Carl V. Thulin, Jr., Chair
Linda L. Novak, Vice Chair
Jon H. Larson, PhD, President
A regional resource center and comprehensive support center for college students with learning disabilities, offering a range of services including psycho-educational assessments, faculty/staff in-service training, program development assistance and consultation, and technical support. Individual and/or small group counseling is available, and vocational/career counseling on transition issues is also offered.

3333 **Princeton University**
Office of Disability Services
241 First Campus Center
Princeton, NJ 08544 609-258-8840
Fax: 609-258-1621
http://ods.princeton.edu
eerickso@princeton.edu

Liz Erickson, Director
Asha Nambiar, Assistant Director
Siobhan Strickhart, Accommodations Coordinator
Offers a variety of services to students with disabilities including note takers, extended testing time, counseling services, and special accommodations.

3334 **Ramapo College of New Jersey**
Office of Specialized Services
505 Ramapo Valley Rd
Mahwah, NJ 07430 201-684-7514
Fax: 201-684-7004
TTY: 201-684-7092
http://www.ramapo.edu
oss@ramapo.edu

David C. Nast, Director
Barbara Stienstra, Specialized Services Coordinator
Ramona Kopacz, Learning Disabilities Specialist
Offers a variety of services to students with disabilities including note takers, extended testing time, counseling services, and special accommodations.

3335 **Raritan Valley Community College**
118 Lamington Rd
Branchburg, NJ 08876 908-526-1200
http://www.raritanval.edu

Michael J. McDonough, President
Deborah E. Preston, Provost/VP, Academic Affairs
Cheryl Wallace, Executive Director, HR
A public two-year college with 250 students with disabilities of a total of 6,000 per semster.

3336 **Rider University**
2083 Lawrenceville Rd
Lawrenceville, NJ 08648 609-896-5000
800-257-9026
http://www.rider.edu
accessibility@rider.edu

Robert Schimek, Chair
John Guarino, Vice Chair
Gregory G. Dell'Omo, President
Four-year college that provides resources, programs and support for students with learning disabilities through their SASS (Student Accessibility and Support Services) program.

3337 **Robert Wood Johnson Medical School**
The Boggs Center on Developmental Disabilities
335 George St
3rd Fl
New Brunswick, NJ 08901 732-235-9300
http://rwjms.rutgers.edu/boggscenter

Deborah M. Spitalnik, PhD, Executive Director
Robert L. Barchi, President
The Elizabeth M. Boggs Center, as a University Center for Excellence in Developmental Disabilities, values uniqueness and individuality and promotes the self-determination and full participation of people with disabilities and their families in all aspects of community life. The Boggs Center prepares students through interdisciplinary programs, provides community training and technical assistance, conducts research, and disseminates information and educational materials.

3338 **Rowan College at Gloucester County**
1400 Tanyard Rd
Sewell, NJ 08080 856-415-2265
http://www.rcgc.edu
dcook@gccnj.edu

Dennis M. Cook, Director, Special Services
Almarie J. Jones, Executive Dir., Diversity/Equity
Frederick Keating, President
The Office of Special Needs Services addresses supportive needs toward academic achievement for those students with documented disabilties such as having a learning disability, a visual, hearing or mobility impairment.

3339 **Salem Community College**
460 Hollywood Ave
Carneys Point, NJ 08069 856-299-2100
http://www.salemcc.edu
info@salemcc.edu

Michael R. Gorman, President
Dorothy D. Hall, Chair
Scott T. Kramme, Vice Chair
Offers a variety of services to students with disabilities including extended testing time, counseling services, and special accommodations.

3340 **Seton Hall University**
Disability Support Services
400 S Orange Ave
Duffy Hall, Rm 67
South Orange, NJ 07079
973-761-9000
http://www.shu.edu

Angela Millman, Director
Dana Giroux, Assistant Director
Diane Delorenzo, Secretary
Student Support Services is an academic program that addresses the needs of students with disabilities.

3341 **Stockton University**
Learning Access Program
101 Vera King Farris Dr
Galloway, NJ 08205-9441
609-652-4988
http://www2.stockton.edu
lap@stockton.edu

Stephen Davis, Dean of Students
Roseann Stollenwerk, Assistant Supervisor
Offers a variety of services to students with disabilities including note takers, extended testing time, counseling services, and special accommodations.

3342 **Sun Valley Community School**
1 Community School Dr
PO Box 2118
Sun Valley, ID 83353
208-622-3955
Fax: 208-622-3962
http://www.communityschool.org
info@communityschool.org

Ben Pettit, Head of School
Becca Hemingway, Director of Development
Katie Robins, Admissions Director
Comprehensive academic program for LD/ADD children grades K-8; NY and NJ funding available.

3343 **William Paterson University**
Accessibility Resource Center
300 Pompton Rd
Speert Hall, Rm 134
Wayne, NJ 07470
973-720-2853
Fax: 973-720-3293
http://www.wpunj.edu

Joy Durham, Director
Elsie Baires, Accessibility Specialist
Kelly Farrell, Program Assistant
Offers a variety of services to students with disabilities including notetakers, extended testing time, counseling services, and special accommodations.

New Mexico

3344 **Central New Mexico Community College**
Disability Resource Center
525 Buena Vista Dr SE
Albuquerque, NM 87106-4096
505-224-3259
888-453-1304
Fax: 505-224-3261
http://www.cnm.edu

Pauline J. Garcia, Chair
Thomas E. Swisstack, Vice Chair
Nancy Baca, Board Member
Provides or coordinates services for students with all disabilities. For students with learning disabilities can arrange for special testing situations, notetaker/scribes, tape recorders, use of wordprocessors or other accommodations based on individual needs.

3345 **College of Santa Fe**
6401 Richards Ave
Santa Fe, NM 87508
505-428-1000
http://www.sfcc.edu

Linda Siegle, Chair
Jack Sullivan, Vice Chair
George Gamble, Secretary
Offers a variety of services to students with disabilities including note takers, extended testing time, counseling services, and special accommodations.

3346 **Eastern New Mexico University**
Disability and Testing Services
1500 S Ave K
Student Academic Services (SAS), Rm 186
Portales, NM 88130
575-562-2280
http://www.enmu.edu

Vee Lucas, Coordinator
Offers a variety of services to students with disabilities including note takers, extended testing time, counseling services, and special accommodations.

3347 **Eastern New Mexico University: Roswell**
Disability Services Office
PO Box 6000
Roswell, NM 88202-6000
575-624-7286
800-243-6687
http://www.roswell.enmu.edu

Dr. Shawn Powell, President
Dr. Jeff Elwell, Chancellor
Offers a variety of services to students with disabilities including note takers, extended testing time, counseling services, and special accommodations.

3348 **Institute of American Indian Arts**
83 Avan Nu Po Rd
Santa Fe, NM 87508
505-424-2325
http://www.iaia.edu
adaoffice@iaia.edu

Jeminie Shell, Rention Director
Nena Martinez Anaya, Chief Enrollment Officer
Dr. Robert Martin, President
Offers a variety of services to students with disabilities including note takers, extended testing time, counseling services, and special accommodations.

3349 **New Mexico Institute of Mining and Technology**
801 Leroy Pl
Socorro, NM 87801
575-835-5620
http://www.nmt.edu
thomas.guenerich@nmt.edu

Stphen G. Wells, President
Melissa Jaramillo-Fleming, Dean of Students
Offers a variety of services to students with disabilities including note takers, extended testing time, counseling services, and special accommodations.

3350 **New Mexico Junior College**
1 Thunderbird Circle
Hobbs, NM 88240
575-392-4510
800-657-6260
http://www.nmjc.edu

Kelvin W. Sharp, President
Pat Chappelle, Chair
Ron Black, Secretary
A public two-year college with 170 special education students out of a total of 2,438.

3351 **New Mexico State University**
Student Accessibility Services
PO Box 30001
MSC 4149
Las Cruces, NM 88003
575-646-6840
Fax: 575-646-5222
http://www.nmsu.edu
sas@nmsu.edu

Trudy Luken, Director
Dan E. Arvizu, Chancellor
John Floros, President
Offers a variety of services to students with disabilities including note takers, extended testing time, counseling services, and special accommodations.

3352 **Northern New Mexico Community College**
Accessibility Resource Center
921 N. Paseo de O¤ate
Espanola, NM 87532 505-747-2152
http://www.nnmc.edu
accessibility@nnmc.edu
Verna A. Trujillo, Director
Richard J. Bailey, Jr., President
Ivan Lopez, Provost/VP for Academic Affairs
Offers a variety of services to students with disabilities including note takers, extended testing time, counseling services, and special accommodations.

3353 **San Juan College**
Advising and Counseling Center
4601 College Blvd
Farmington, NM 87402 505-566-3271
Fax: 505-566-4408
http://www.sanjuancollege.edu
disabilityservices@sanjuancollege.edu
Toni Hopper Pendergrass, President
Edward DesPlas, Executive Vice President
Adrienne Forgette, VP, Learning
Offers a variety of services to students with disabilities including note takers, extended testing time, counseling services, and special accommodations.

3354 **University of New Mexico**
Accessibility Resource Center
302 Cornell Dr NE
Rm 2021
Albuquerque, NM 87131 505-277-3506
Fax: 505-277-3750
http://www.unm.edu
arcsrvs@unm.edu
Joan Green, Director
Christina Chavez, Senior Program Manager
Rhiannon Doyle, Program Coordinator
Offers a variety of services to students with disabilities including notetakers, extended testing time, counseling services, and special accommodations.

3355 **University of New Mexico/School of Medicine**
Center for Development and Disability
2300 Menaul Blvd NE
Albuquerque, NM 87107 505-272-3000
800-552-8195
Fax: 505-272-2014
http://www.cdd.unm.edu
cdd@unm.edu
Chaouki Abdallah, Provost/VP of Academic Affairs
The mission of the CDD is the full inclusion of people with disabilities and their families in their community by: enganging individuals in making life choices; partnering with communities to build resources; and improving systems of care.

3356 **University of New Mexico: Los Alamos Branch**
Accessibility Resource Center
4000 University Dr
Los Alamos, NM 87544 505-662-5919
Fax: 505-662-0344
http://losalamos.unm.edu
arcsrvs@unm.edu
Joan Green, Director
Christina Chavez, Senior Program Manager
Rhiannon Doyle, Program Coordinator
Offers a variety of services to students with disabilities including notetakers, extended testing time, counseling services, and special accommodations.

3357 **University of New Mexico: Valencia Campus**
Accessibility Resource Center
280 La Entrada Rd
Los Lunas, NM 87131 505-925-8500
http://valencia.unm.edu
arcsrvs@unm.edu
Joan Green, Director
Christina Chavez, Senior Program Manager
Rhiannon Doyle, Program Coordinator
Offers a variety of services to students with disabilities including note takers, extended testing time, counseling services, and special accommodations.

3358 **Western New Mexico University**
Office of Disability Support Services
PO Box 680
Silver City, NM 88062 575-538-6138
800-872-9668
Fax: 575-538-6017
http://www.wnmu.edu
erlingj@wnmu.edu
JoBeth Erling, Coordinator
Offers a variety of services to students with disabilities including notetakers, extended testing time, counseling services, and special accommodations.

New York

3359 **Adelphi University**
Student Access Office
PO Box 701
1 South Ave
Garden City, NY 11530 516-877-3806
Fax: 516-877-3138
http://access-office.adelphi.edu
sao@adelphi.edu
Rosemary Garabedian, Director
Brian Flatley, Assistant Director
Melissa Dean, Administrative Assistant
Offers a variety of services to students with disabilities including note takers, extended testing time, counseling services, and special accommodations.

3360 **Albert Einstein College of Medicine**
1300 Morris Park Ave
Bronx, NY 10461 718-430-2000
http://www.einstein.yu.edu
supservices@einstein.yu.edu
Edward R. Burns, Executive Dean
Stephen G. Baum, Senior Advisor for Students
Claudia Gomez, Executive Assistant
Provides evaluation and psychoeducational treatment to children and adults of normal intelligence, 21 years or older, who have serious reading difficulties.

3361 **Bank Street College: Graduate School of Education**
610 W 112th St
New York, NY 10025 212-875-4400
http://graduate.bankstreet.edu
graduateschool@bankstreet.edu
Cecelia Traugh, Dean
Valentine Burr, Chair, Dept. Teaching/Learning
Anthony C. Conelli, Chair, Leadership Department
For college students with learning disabilities who are highly motivated to become teachers of children and youth with learning problems and who wish to earn a masters degree in Special Education.

3362 **Binghamton University**
Services for Students with Disabilities
4400 Vestal Pkwy E
Binghamton, NY 13902 607-777-2000
http://www.binghamton.edu
ssd@binghamton.edu
Harvey G. Stenger, President
Dianne Gray, Director
Anne Lewis, Learning Disabilities Specialist
Offers a variety of services to students with disabilities including note takers, extended testing time, counseling services, and special accommodations.

3363 **Bramson ORT College**
69-30 Austin St
Forest Hills, NY 11375 718-261-5800
http://www.bramsonort.edu
hpolynsky@bramsonort.edu
David Kanani, PhD, EECS, President
Helen Polynsky, Academic Dean
Angela Nasimova, Director, Student Services
Offers a variety of services to students with disabilities including notetakers, extended testing time, counseling services, and special accommodations.

3364 **CUNY Queensborough Community College**
222-05 56th Ave
Bayside, NY 11364 718-631-6257
http://www.qcc.cuny.edu
Bfreier@qcc.cuny.edu
Ben-Ami Freier, Director
Andrew Muller, Learning Disabilities Specialist
Amy Flannery, Administrative Assistant
The Office of Services for Students with Disabilities (Science Building, Room 132) offers special assistance and couseling to students with specific needs. The services offered include academic, vocational, psychological and rehabilitation counseling, as well as liasion with community social agencies.

3365 **Canisius College**
Accessibility Support Services
2001 Main St
Buffalo, NY 14208-1517 716-883-7000
Fax: 716-888-2525
http://www.canisius.edu
info@canisius.edu
Anne-Marie Dobies, Director
Eileen Abbatoy, Associate Director
Sierra Bonerb, Assistant Director
Offers a variety of services to students with disabilities including note takers, extended testing time, counseling services, and special accommodations.

3366 **Cazenovia College**
Center for Teaching and Learning
22 Sullivan St
Cazenovia, NY 13035 315-655-7208
800-654-3210
http://www.cazenovia.edu
admissions@cazenovia.edu
Ron Chesbrough, President
An independent college with a significant number of special education students.

3367 **Center for Spectrum Services: Ellenville**
4 Yankee Pl.
Ellenville, NY 12428 845-647-6464
Fax: 845-647-3456
http://www.centerforspectrumservices.org
info@centerforspectrumservices.org
Crystal C. Jacob, President
Brain Schug, Jr., Vice President
Samuel Kandel, Treasurer
This center-based program is a school for preschool and school-age children who are 3 through 8 eight years old and have the educational classification of preschooler with a disability, autism, emotional disability, or multiple disabilities.

3368 **Center for the Advancement of Post Secondary Studies**
Maplebrook School
5142 Route 22
Amenia, NY 12501 845-373-8191
Fax: 845-373-7029
http://www.maplebrookschool.org
admissions@maplebookshool.org
Mark J. Metzger, Chairman
Robert S. Audia, Vice Chair
Donna Konkolics, Head of School
A program based on students successfully completing the goals and objectives designed to prepare them for integration into today's world. Through small group and individualized instruction, the student will be assisted in reaching his/her academic, social, vocational, and physical potential.

3369 **Churchill School and Center**
Programs for Children
301 E 29th St
New York, NY 10016 212-722-0610
http://www.churchillschoolnyc.org
Timothy P. Madigan, PhD, Head of School
Cynthia Wainwright, President
Maryl Hosking, Secretary
Offers educational programs, professional development in the field of learning disabilities, and advisory and referral services to students, parents, teachers of general and special education, and related service provides.

3370 **Colgate University**
Academic Support and Disability Services
13 Oak Dr
Hamilton, NY 13346 315-228-7000
http://www.colgate.edu
admission@mail.colgate.edu
Lynn Waldman, Director
Brian W. Casey, President
Daniel B. Hurwitz, Chair
Offers a variety of services to students with disabilities including note takers, extended testing time, counseling services, and special accommodations.

3371 **College of Saint Rose**
Office of Services for Students with Disabilities
432 Western Ave
Albany, NY 12203 518-337-2335
800-637-8556
http://www.strose.edu
cantwell@strose.edu
Lynn Cantwell, Director
Carolyn J. Stefanco, President
Offers a variety of services to students with disabilities including note takers, extended testing time, counseling services, and special accommodations.

3372 **College of Staten Island of the City University of New York**
Center for Student Accessibility
2800 Victory Blvd
Staten Island, NY 10314 718-982-2510
Fax: 718-982-2117
http://www.csi.cuny.edu
CSA@csi.cuny.edu
Stefan Charles-Pierre, Director
Joanne D'Onofrio, Associate Director
Steven Sullam, Ast. Dir., Assistive Technology
Offers a variety of services to students with disabilities including note takers, extended testing time, counseling services, and special accommodations.

3373 **Columbia College**
Disability Services
105 Bard Hall
50 Haven Ave
New York, NY 10032 212-304-7029
http://health.columbia.edu
disability@columbia.edu
Lee C. Bollinger, President
Gerald M. Rosberg, Senior Executive Vice President
Jerome Davis, Secretary
Offers a variety of services to students with disabilities including note takers, extended testing time, counseling services, and special accommodations.

3374 **Columbia-Greene Community College**
4400 Route 23
Hudson, NY 12534 518-828-4181
http://www.sunycgcc.edu

Edward Schneier, Jr., Chair
Peter O'Hara, Vice Chair
James R. Campion, President
Services available to students with a documented learning disability include various academic accommodations, peer tutoring and academic counselling. Six developmental courses are offered in reading, math, English, and study skills.

3375 **Concordia College: New York**
Center for Student Success
171 White Plains Rd
Bronxville, NY 10708 914-337-9300
http://www.concordia-ny.edu
ghg@concordia-ny.edu
Rev. John Arthur Nunes. PhD, President
Offers a variety of services to students with disabilities including note takers, extended testing time, counseling services, tutoring, writing center, and special accommodations.

3376 **Cornell University**
Student Disability Services
110 Ho Plz
Ithaca, NY 14853-3102 607-245-4545
Fax: 607-255-1562
http://sds.cornell.edu
sds_cu@cornell.edu
Katherine Fahey, Director/Disability Counselor
Joshua Smith, Accommodations Specialist
Andrea Dietrich, Accommodations Specialist
Cornell University is committed to ensuring that students with disabilities have equal access to all university programs and activities. Policy and procedures have been developed to provide students with as much independence as possible, to preserve confidentiality, and to provide students with disabilities the same exceptional opportunities available to all Cornell students.

3377 **Corning Community College**
Accessibility Services
1 Academic Dr
Corning, NY 14830 607-962-9262
Fax: 607-962-9249
http://www.corning-cc.edu
accessibility@corning-cc.edu
Deborah Joseph, Coordinator
Cindy Drake, Program Assistant
A variety of services are available to students with LD, including specialized advising and registration, individualized tutoring, academic advisoring, and accommodations. Also on campus: Kurzweil reading machines, voice activated word processing, etc.

3378 **Dutchess Community College**
53 Pendell Rd
Poughkeepsie, NY 12601 845-431-8000
http://www.sunydutchess.edu
admissions@sunydutchess.edu
Thomas E. LeGrand, Chair
Michael Francis Dupree, Vice Chair
Pamela E. Edington, President
A public two-year college with 45 special education students out of a total of 7,511.

3379 **Erie Community College: South Campus**
Special Education Department
4041 Southwestern Blvd
Orchard Park, NY 14127 716-851-1003
Fax: 716-851-1629
TDD: 716-851-1831
http://www.ecc.edu
adamsjm@ecc.edu
Jack Quinn, Counselor
William Reuter, CEO
A public two-year college with 200 special education students out of a total of 3,455.

3380 **Farmingdale State University**
2350 Broadhollow Rd
Farmingdale, NY 11735-1021 631-420-2000
http://www.farmingdale.edu
malka.edelman@farmingdale.edu
Malka Edelman, Director
Melissa Aziz, Disability Counseling Specialist
John S. Nader, PhD, President
Designed to meet the unique educational needs of currently enrolled students with documented permanent or temporary disabilities. The Office of Support Services is dedicated to the principle that equal opportunity be afforded each student to realize his/her fullest potential.

3381 **Finger Lakes Community College**
3325 Marvin Sands Dr
Canandaigua, NY 14424 585-394-FLCC
http://www.flcc.edu
admissions@flcc.edu
Geoffrey Astles, Chair
Stephen R. Martin, Vice Chair
Robert K. Nye, President
Provides services such as pre-admission counseling, academic advisement, tutorials, computer assistance, workshops, peer counseling and support groups. The college does not offer a formal program, but aids students in arranging appropriate accommodations.

3382 **Fordham University**
Disability Services
441 E Fordham Rd
O'Hare Hall, Lower Level
Bronx, NY 10458 718-817-0655
Fax: 718-817-0888
http://www.fordham.edu
disabilityservices@fordham.edu
Joseph M. McShane, SJ, President
Jonathan Crystal, Interim Provost
Jeffrey Gray, SVP, Student Affairs
The Office of Disability Services collaborates with students, faculty and staff to ensure appropriate services for students with disabilities. The University will make reasonable acccommodations, and provide appropriate aids.

3383 **Fulton-Montgomery Community College**
2805 State Hwy 67
Johnstown, NY 12095 518-736-3622
http://www.fmcc.suny.edu
Ryan B. Weitz, Chair
Geoffrey Peck, Vice Chair
Dustin Swanger, Ed.D, President
Offers a variety of services to students with disabilities including note takers, extended testing time, counseling services, and special accommodations.

3384 **Gateway School of New York**
211 W 61st St
6th Fl
New York, NY 10023 212-777-5966
Fax: 212-777-5794
http://www.gatewayschool.org
info@gatewayschool.org
Carolyn Salzman, Head of School
Jodi Schwartz, Chair
Benson Kutrieb, Secretary
An ungraded lower school dedicated to helping children with learning disabilities develop the academic skills, learning strategies, social competence and self-confidence necessary to succeed.

3385 **Genesee Community College**
SUNY (State University of New York) Systems
1 College Rd
Batavia, NY 14020 585-343-0055
866-CALL-GCC
http://www.genesee.edu
admissions@genesee.suny.edu

Donna M. Ferry, Chair
Peter R. Call, Vice Chair
James M. Sunser, President
Offers a variety of services to students with disabilities including note takers, extended testing time, counseling services, and special accommodations.

3386 **Hamilton College**
198 College Hill Rd
Clinton, NY 13323 315-859-4011
Fax: 315-859-4457
http://www.hamilton.edu
David Wippman, President
Irene Cornish, Director, Auxiliary Services
Jan Risel, Secretary to the VP
Four year college that offfers services for learning disabled students.

3387 **Harmony Heights**
PO Box 569
Oyster Bay, NY 11771 516-922-4060
Fax: 516-922-4133
http://www.harmonyheights.org
kathy.nastri@harmonyheights.org
Kathryn Nastri, Executive Director
Lori Neazer, Clinical Director, Admissions
Denis Garbo, President
A therapeutic residential and day school serving girls with emotional needs that cannot be adequately served in the standard high school setting.

3388 **Herkimer County Community College**
Academic Support Center
100 Reservoir Rd
Herkimer, NY 13350 315-866-0300
844-464-4375
http://www.herkimer.edu
Cathleen McColgin, President
Shari Hunt, Secretary
Leslie Cornish, Coordinator, Disability Services
Offers a variety of services to students with disabilities including note takers, extended testing time, counseling services, tutoring and special accommodations.

3389 **Hofstra University**
Program for Academic Learning Skills
212 Memorial Hall
Hempstead, NY 11549-1000 516-463-7075
http://www.hofstra.edu
sas@hofstra.edu
W. Houston Dougharty, VP, Student Affairs
Gail M. Simmons, Provost/SVP, Academic Affairs
Stuart Rabinowitz, President
Provides auxillary aids and compensatory services to certified learning disabled students who have been accepted to the University through regular admissions. These services are provided free of charge.

3390 **Houghton College**
Center for Academic Success & Advising (CASA)
1 Willard Ave
Houghton, NY 14744 800-777-2556
http://www.houghton.edu
admission@houghton.edu
Sharon Mulligan, Director
Karen Wise, Digital Text Coordinator
Deborah Young, Office Manager
Offers a variety of services to students with disabilities including note takers, extended testing time, counseling services, and special accommodations.

3391 **Hudson Valley Community College**
Center for Access & Assistive Technology
80 Vandenburgh Ave
Troy, NY 12180 518-629-7154
877-325-4822
Fax: 518-629-4831
TDD: 518-629-7596
http://www.hvcc.edu/caat
d.martocci@hvcc.edu
DeAnne Martocci, Director
Donna Totaro, Ast. Director/LD Specialist
Ann Peterson, Coordinator of Accessibility
Offers a variety of services to students with disabilities including note takers, extended testing time, counseling services, and special accommodations.

3392 **Hunter College of the City University of New York**
Office of AccessABILITY
695 Park Ave
New York, NY 10065 212-772-4857
http://www.hunter.cuny.edu
sshayest@hunter.cuny.edu
Sudi Shayesteh, Director
Jennifer J. Raab, President
Dr. Lon Kaufman, Provost/VP of Academic Affairs
Provides services to over 250 students with learning disabilities. A learning disability is a disorder in one or more of the basic psychological processes involved in understanding or in using spoken or written language.

3393 **Iona College**
College Assistance Program
715 North Ave
New Rochelle, NY 10801 914-633-2077
800-231-IONA
Fax: 914-633-2642
http://www.iona.edu
lrobertello@iona.edu
Daneshea Palmer, Director
J. Kevin Delvin, Sr. Director, Student Success
Darrell P. Wheeler, Provost/VP, Academic Affairs
Offers a comprehensive support program for students with learning disabilities. CAP is designed to encourage success by providing instruction tailored to individual strenghts and needs.

3394 **Ithaca College**
Student Accessibility Services
100 Rothschild Pl
953 Danby Road
Ithaca, NY 14850 607-274-1005
Fax: 607-274-3957
http://www.ithaca.edu/sas
sas@ithaca.edu
Leslie Reid, Manager
Jean Celeste-Astorina, Student Accessibility Specialist
Valerie Ober, Adaptive Technology Specialist
Offers a variety of services to students with disabilities including note takers, extended testing time, counseling services, and special accommodations.

3395 **Ithaca College: Speech and Hearing Clinic**
953 Danby Road
202 Smiddy Hall
Ithaca, NY 14850 607-274-3714
http://www.ithaca.edu
Shirley M. Collado, President
La Jerne Terry Cornish, Provost/SVP, Academic Affairs
Rosanna Ferro, VP, Student Affairs/Campus Life
Offers a variety of services to students with disabilities including notetakers, extended testing time, counseling services, and special accommodations.

3396 **Jamestown Community College**
State University of New York Systems
525 Falconer St
PO Box 20
Jamestown, NY 14702
716-665-1000
800-388-8557
http://www.sunyjcc.edu
admissions@mail.sunyjcc.edu
Wally Huckno, Chair
Carole Faulk, Secretary
Daniel DeMarte, President
Offers a variety of services to students with disabilities including note takers, extended testing time, counseling services, and special accommodations.

3397 **Jefferson Community College**
1220 Coffeen St
Watertown, NY 13601
315-786-2200
888-435-6522
http://www.sunyjefferson.edu
webmaster@sunyjefferson.edu
Nathan P. Hunter, Chair
Judith L. Gentner, Vice Chair
Ty A. Stone, President
Offers a variety of services to students with disabilities including note takers, extended testing time, counseling services, and special accommodations.

3398 **John Jay College of Criminal Justice of the City University of New York**
524 W 59th St
New York, NY 10019
212-237-8000
http://jjay.cuny.edu/accessibility
Benno C. Schmidt, Chair
Philip Alfonso Berry, Vice Chair
Karol V. Mason, President
Offers a variety of services to students with disabilities including note takers, extended testing time, counseling services, and special accommodations.

3399 **Kildonan School**
425 Morse Hill Rd.
Amenia, NY 12501
845-373-8111
Fax: 845-373-9793
http://www.kildonan.org
admissions@kildonan.org
C. Wilson Anderson, Jr., Chair
Richard S. Berg, Vice Chair
Bruce Karsk, Treasurer
Offers a fully accredited College Preparatory curriculum. The school is co-educational, enrolling boarding students in Grades 6-Postgraduate and day students in Grade 2-Postgraduate. Provides daily one-on-one Orton-Gillingham tutoring to build skills in reading, writing, and spelling. Daily independent reading and writing work reinforces skills and improves study habits. Interscholastic sports, horseback riding, clubs, and community service enhance self-confidence.

3400 **Long Island University Post**
Academic Resource Program
720 Northern Blvd
Brookville, NY 11548-1300
516-299-3057
Fax: 516-299-2126
http://www.liu.edu/CWPost/Campus-Life
marie.fatscher@liu.edu
Marie Fatscher, Director, Leaning Support Center
A comprehensive, structured, fee-for-service, support program designed to teach undergraduate students with learning disabilities and/or ADHD skill and strategies that will help then achiece their academic potential in a university setting.

3401 **Manhattan College: Specialized Resource Center**
4513 Manhattan College Pkwy
Thomas Hall 3.15
Riverdale, NY 10471
718-862-7409
Fax: 718-862-7808
TTY: 718-862-7885
http://www.manhattan.edu
srcdirector@manhattan.edu
Brennan O'Donnell, PhD, President
The Specialized Resource Center serves all students with special needs including individuals with temporary disabilities, such as those resulting from injury or surgery. The mission of the center is to ensure educational opportunity for all students with special needs by providing access to full participation in all aspects of the campus life.

3402 **Maplebrook School**
Academic Program
5142 Route 22
Amenia, NY 12501
845-373-8191
Fax: 845-373-7029
http://www.maplebrookschool.org
admissions@maplebrookschool.org
Mark J. Metzger, Chairman
Robert S. Audia, Vice Chair
George T. Whalen, Jr., Treasurer
The school offers several levels of academic achievement toward which a student may strive. Their curriculum follows the New York State guidelines, the teachers are trained in a multi-sensory approach and provide a small, nurturing classroom in which each student can reach their full potential.

3403 **Maria College**
700 New Scotland Ave
Albany, NY 12208
518-438-3111
Fax: 518-438-7170
http://www.mariacollege.edu
accessibilityservices@mariacollege.edu
Thomas J. Gamble, President
Kim Noakes, Director, Accessibility Services
Offers a variety of services to students with disabilities including note takers, extended testing time, counseling services, and special accommodations.

3404 **Marist College**
Learning Disabilities Support Program
3399 North Rd
Donnelly Hall, Rm 226
Poughkeepsie, NY 12601
845-575-3274
Fax: 845-575-3011
http://www.marist.edu
accommodations@marist.edu
Ross A. Mauri, Chair
Thomas J. Ward, Treasurer
David Yellen, President
Provides a comprehensive range of academic support services and accommodations which promote the full integration of students with disabilities into the mainstream college environment.

3405 **Marymount Manhattan College**
Academic Access Program
221 E 71st St
Carson Hall, Ste 500
New York, NY 10021
212-774-0724
http://www.mmm.edu
dnash@mmm.edu
Diana Nash, Director
Kerry Walk, President
Carol L. Jackson, VP, Student Affairs
The College's program for students with learning disabilities is designed to provide a structure that fosters academic success.

3406 **Medaille College**
Academic Support Center: Accessibility Resources
18 Agassiz Cir
Buffalo, NY 14214
716-880-2000
800-292-1582
http://www.medaille.edu
Genevieve.M.Kruly@medaille.edu
Genevieve M. Kruly, Coordinator
Kenneth M. Macur, President
Howard K. Hitzel, Secretary
Offers a variety of services to students with disabilities including notetakers, extended testing time, counseling services, and special accommodations.

3407 **Mercy College**
Star Program
555 Broadway
Dobbs Ferry, NY 10522
914-674-7600
877-MERCY-GO
http://www.mercy.edu
Bruce J. Haber, Chair
Joseph P. Carlucci, Vice Chair
Timothy L. Hall, President
Designed by the Division of Student Affairs to highlight and distinguish students' achievements throughout their academic career.

3408 **Mohawk Valley Community College**
Office of Accessibility Resources
1101 Sherman Dr
Utica, NY 13501
315-731-5813
http://www.mvcc.edu
jdaoreuang@mvcc.edu
Jimsak Daoreuang, Director
Katelyn Ouderkirk, Transition Support Specialist
Tamara Mariotti, Coordinator
Service provided to students with learning disabilities include advocacy, information and referral to on and off campus services, testing accommodations, taped materials, loaner tape recorders and note takers.

3409 **Molloy College**
1000 Hempstead Avenue
PO Box 5002
Rockville Centre, NY 11571-5002
888-4-MOLLOY
http://www.molloy.edu
info@molloy.edu
John P. McEntee, Chair
Diane Fornieri, Secretary
Drew Bogner, President
STEEP (Success Through Expanded Education), is a program specifically designed to assist students with learning disabilities and enable them to become successful students. The program offers the student the opportunities to learn techniques which alleviate some of their problems. Special emphasis is directed toward the development of positive self-esteem.

3410 **Nassau Community College**
Disability Services
1 Education Dr
Garden City, NY 11530-6793
516-572-7241
Fax: 516-572-9874
http://www.ncc.edu
CSDoffice@ncc.edu
Molly Ludmar, Chair, Student Personel Services
Orval Jewett, Disability Services Coordinator
Gina Esposito-Sales, Disability Counselor
Offers a variety of services to students with disabilities including note takers, extended testing time, counseling services, and special accommodations.

3411 **Nazareth College of Rochester**
Student Accessibility Services
4245 East Ave
Rochester, NY 14618
585-389-2498
Fax: 585-389-2499
http://www.naz.edu
SASoffice@naz.edu
Erika M. Hess, Program Director
Suzanne Marie Welker, Program Coordinator
Daan Braveman, President
Four-year college that offers students with a learning disablility support and services.

3412 **New York City College of Technology**
Center for Student Accesibility
300 Jay St
Atrium 237
Brooklyn, NY 11201
718-260-5143
Fax: 718-254-8539
http://www.citytech.cuny.edu/accessibility
jcurrie@citytech.cuny.edu
John R. Currie, Director
Lewanda Miller, Coor., Disability Services
Carrie N. Baram, Literacy Specialist
The Center for Student Accessibility provides comprehensive services to students with disabilities. The array of interventions includes counseling, tutorials, workshops, use of computer lab with adaptive software, testing accommodations, sign-language interpreters, captioning, and implementation of accommodations as per documentation.

3413 **New York University**
Henry and Lucy Moses Center
726 Broadway
3rd Fl
New York, NY 10003
212-998-4980
http://www.nyu.edu/csd
mosescsd@nyu.edu
William R. Berkley, Chair
Daniel R. Tisch, Vice Chair
Andrew Hamilton, President
The Henry and Lucy Moses Center for Students with Disabilities (CSD) functions to determine qualified disability status and to assist students in obtaining appropriate accommodations and services. CSD operates according to the Independent Living Philosophy, and thus strives in its policies and practices to empower each student to become an independent as possible. Services are designed to encourage independence, backed by a strong system of supports.

3414 **New York University Medical Center**
Learning Diagnostic Program
550 First Avenue
New York, NY 10016
212-263-7300
Fax: 212-263-7721
http://www.med.nyu.edu
Kenneth G. Langone, Chair
Laurence D. Fink, Vice Chair
John Sexton, President
Assessment team, neurology, neuro-psychology, psychiatry services are offered.

3415 **Niagara County Community College**
3111 Saunders Settlement Rd
Sanborn, NY 14132
716-614-6222
Fax: 716-614-6700
http://www.niagaracc.suny.edu
Dr. William Murabito, Interim President
The College provides reasonable accommodations for students with disabilties, including those with specific learning disabilities. Students with learning disabilities must provide documentation by a qualified professional that proves thry are eligible for accommodations.

3416 **Niagara University**
Accessibility Services
Seton Hall
1st Fl
Niagara University, NY 14109
716-286-8541
http://www.niagara.edu/accessibility-services
kadams@niagara.edu
Kelly Enger, Program Coordinator
Timothy O. Ireland, Provost/VP, Academic Affairs
James J. Maher, President

Reasonable accommodations are provided to students with disabilities based on documentation of disability. Depending on how the disability impacts the individual, reasonable accommodations may include extended time on tests taken in a separate location with appropriate assistance, notetakes or use of a tape recorder in class, interpreter, textbooks and course materials in alternative format, as well as other academic and non-academic accommodations.

3417 **Norman Howard School**
275 Pinnacle Rd
Rochester, NY 14623 585-334-8010
http://www.normanhoward.org
info@normanhoward.org
Joseph M. Martino, Executive Director
Jennifer Baker, Director of Students
Rosemary Hodges, Director of Education
An independent co-educational day school for students with learning disabilities. An approved special education program by the New York State Education Department and accredited by the New York Association of Independent Schools. Program supports many youngsters with various types of learning disabilities, including dyslexia, non-verbal LD, Asperger's Syndrome, anxiety and ADHD.

3418 **North Country Community College**
State University of New York
23 Santanoni Ave
PO Box 89
Saranac Lake, NY 12983 518-891-2915
888-879-6222
Fax: 518-891-2915
http://www.nccc.edu
admissions@nccc.edu
Fred Smith, Learning Lab/Malone
Scott Lambert, Enrollment/Financial Aid Counsel
Dr. Steve Tyrell, President
Located in the Adirondack Olympic Region of northern New York, NCCC is committed to providing a challenging and supportive environment where the aspirations of all can be realized. The college provides a variety of services for students with special needs which includes: specialized advisement, tutors and supplemental instruction, specialized accommodations, technology and equipment to accommodate learning disabilities and other resources.

3419 **Office of Resources, Equity, Accessibility and Learning (REAL)**
College of New Rochelle
29 Castle Pl
New Rochelle, NY 10805 914-654-5556
http://www.cnr.edu
REALsupport@cnr.edu
William Latimer, President
Gwen Adolph, Esq., Chair
Elizabeth Spadaccini, Director
Offers a variety of services to students with disabilities including notetakers, extended testing time, counseling services, and special accommodations.

3420 **Onondaga Community College**
Disability Services Office
4585 W Seneca Turnpike
Syracuse, NY 13215 315-498-2622
Fax: 315-498-2977
http://www.sunyocc.edu
occinfo@sunyocc.edu
Margaret M. O'Connell, Chair
Allen J. Naples, Vice Chair
Casey Crabill, President
A public two-year college with 650 students with disabilities.

3421 **Orange County Community College**
115 South St
Middletown, NY 10940-6437 845-341-4444
Fax: 845-341-4998
http://www.sunyorange.edu
Joan H. Wolfe, Chair
Helen G. Ullrich, Vice Chair
Dr. William Richards, President
The Office of Special Services for the Disabled provides support services to meet the individual needs of students with disabilities. Such accommodations include oral testing, extended time testing, tape recorded textbooks, writing lab, note-takers and others. Pre-admission counseling ensures accessibility for the qualified student.

3422 **Purchase College State University of New York**
Special Services Office
735 Anderson Hill Rd
Purchase, NY 10577 914-251-6020
Fax: 914-251-6019
http://www.purchase.edu
Thomas J. Schwarz, President
Donna Siegmann, Coordinator Supported Education
Offers a variety of services to students with disabilities including note takers, extended testing time, counseling services, and special accommodations.

3423 **Queens College City University of New York**
Special Services Office
65-30 Kissena Blvd
Flushing, NY 11367 718-997-5000
Fax: 718-997-5895
TDD: 718-997-5870
http://www.qc.cuny.edu/
christopher_rosa@qc.edu
Evangelos Gizis, Interim President
Elizabeth Hendrey, Provost/VP for Academic Affairs
William Keller, VP for Finance & Administration
Services include tutoring and notetaking, accommodating testing alternatives, counseling, academic and vocational advisement, as well as diagnostic assessments in order to pinpoint specific deficits.

3424 **Readiness Program**
New York Institute for Special Education
999 Pelham Pkwy
Bronx, NY 10469 718-519-7000
Fax: 718-231-9314
http://www.nyise.org
bkappen@nyise.org
Bernadette M Kappen PhD, Executive Director
A pre-school that helps children who are developmentally delayed from ages 3 to 5. They have disabilities that include speech impairment, mild orthopedic impairment, or a learning or emotional disability. By providing specialized instruction, intensive therapies and early intervention many are able to be mainstreamed or are placed in a least restrictive educational environment when they reach the age of five.

3425 **Rensselaer Polytechnic Institute**
110 8th St
Troy, NY 12180-3590 518-276-6000
800-448-6562
Fax: 518-276-4072
http://www.rpi.edu
hamild@rpi.edu
Shirley Ann Jackson, Disabled Student Services
Claude Rounds, VP, Administration Division
An independent four-year college with 53 learning disabled students out of a total of 6,000.

3426 **Rochester Business Institute**
1630 Portland Ave
Rochester, NY 14621 585-266-0430
888-741-4271
Fax: 585-266-8243
http://www.rochester-institute.com
dpfluke@cci.edu
Carl Silvio, President
Jim Rodriguez, Admissions Representative
An independent two-year college with 12 special education students out of a total of 528.

3427 **Rochester Institute of Technology**
Structured Monitoring Program
1 Lomb Memorial Drive
Rochester, NY 14623-5603 585-475-2411
Fax: 585-475-2215
http://www.rit.edu
smacst@rit.edu

Lisa Fraser, Chair Leraning Support Services
Pamela Lloyd, Disability Services Coordinator
Albert Simone, President
An independent four-year college offers a wide variety of accommodations and support services to students with documented disabilities.

3428 **Rockland Community College**
145 College Rd
Suffern, NY 10901 845-574-4000
Fax: 845-574-4424
http://www.sunyrockland.edu

Dr. Cliff L. Wood, President
Joseph Marra, Assoc. VP, Finance/Controller
Dr. Nayyer Hussain, VP for Admin & Finance
A public two-year college with 300 special education students out of a total of 5,500. The office of Disability Services provides a variety of support services tailored to meet the individual needs and learning styles of students with documented learning disabilities.

3429 **Rose F Kennedy Center**
Albert Einstein College of Medicine
1410 Pelham Pkwy S
Bronx, NY 10461-1116 718-430-8522
Fax: 718-904-1162
http://www.einstein.yu.edu.com

Robert Marion, Director
Mission is to help children with disabilities reach their full potential and to support parents in their efforts to get the best care, education, and treatment for their children.

3430 **Ryken Educational Center**
Xaverian High School
7100 Shore Rd
Brooklyn, NY 11209 718-836-7100
http://www.xaverian.org
ctrasborg@xaverian.org

Lawrence Harvey, Chair
Daniel E. Skala, Vice chair
Robert B. Alesi, President
Provides programs and services for high school students of average, or above-average intelligence who have specific learning disabilities. Its mission is to challenge and support learning disabled young men so that they achieve academically at their intellectual level. Our goal is to turn them into effective life-long learners who will go on to college.

3431 **SUNY Adirondack**
640 Bay Rd
Queensbury, NY 12804 518-743-2200
888-SUNY-ADK
Fax: 518-745-1433
http://www.sunyacc.edu
access@sunyacc.edu

John Jablonski, VP, Academic Affairs
Jason Enser, Dean for Student Affairs
Marcell Mallette, Executive Director, Development
Offers a variety of services to students with disabilities including note takers, extended testing time, counseling services, and special accommodations.

3432 **SUNY Canton**
34 Cornell Dr
Campus Center 233
Canton, NY 13617-1098 315-386-7011
800-388-7123
Fax: 315-379-3877
TDD: 315-386-7943
http://www.canton.edu
leev@canton.edu

Zvi Szafran, President
Karen Spellacy, Provost/VP Academic Affairs
Courtney Bish, Dean of Students
Four year state college that provides resources and services to learning disabled students.

3433 **SUNY Cobleskill**
142 Schenectady Ave
State Route 7
Cobleskill, NY 12043 518-255-5011
800-295-8988
Fax: 518-255-6430
TDD: 518-255-5454
TTY: 518-255-6500
http://www.cobleskill.edu/
dss@cobleskill.edu

Dr. Debra H. Thatcher, President
Carol Bishop, VP for Business& Finance
Bonnie Martin, VP for Operations
A public two-year college with a Bachelor of Technology component in agriculture. Approximately 170 students identify themselves as having a learning disability out of the 2,000 total population. Tuition $3,500 in state/$8,300 out of state. Academic support services and accommodations for documented LD students.

3434 **SUNY Institute of Technology: Utica/Rome**
100 Seymour Road
Utica, NY 13502 315-792-7500
866-278-6948
Fax: 315-792-7837
http://www.sunyit.edu
admissions@sunyit.edu

Robert E. Geer, President
William W. Durgin, Provost
Upper division bachelor's degree in a variety of professional and technical majors; masters degree and continuing educational coursework is also available.

3435 **Sage College**
140 New Scotland Ave
Albany, NY 12208 518-244-2000
Fax: 578-292-1910
http://www.sage.edu
chowed@sage.edu

Dr. Susan Scrimshaw, President
Terry S. Weiner, Provost
Kevin R. Stoner, Associate Provost
Four year college that offers services to students with a learning disability.

3436 **Schenectady County Community College**
Disability Services Department
78 Washington Ave
Schenectady, NY 12305 518-381-1200
Fax: 518-346-0379
http://www.sunysccc.edu

Ann Fleming Brown, Chair
Dr. William Levering, Vice Chair
Martha Asselin, Ph.D., President
Access for All program is designed to make programs and facilities accessible to all students in pursuit of their academic goals. Disabled Student Services seeks to ensure accessible educational opportunities in accordance with individual needs. Offers general support services and program services such as: exam assistance, special scheduling, adaptive equipment, readers, taping assistance and more.

3437 **Schermerhorn Program**
New York Institute for Special Education
999 Pelham Pkwy N
Bronx, NY 10469-4905 718-519-7000
Fax: 718-231-9314
http://www.nyise.org
bkappen@nyise.org

Bernadette M Kappen PhD, Executive Director

It offers diverse educational services to meet the needs of children who are legally blind, from the ages of 5 to 21. Students participate in individually designed academic and modified academic programs that emphasize independence.

3438 **Siena College**
515 Loudon Rd
Loudonville, NY 12211
518-785-6537
888-AT-SIENA
Fax: 518-783-4293
http://www.siena.edu
jpellegrini@siena.edu

Howard S. Foote, Chair
John F. Murray, Vice Chair
Fr. Kevin Mullen, President
Four year college that offers programs for the learning disabled.

3439 **St. Bonaventure University**
Teaching & Learning Center
3261 West State Road
St Bonaventure, NY 14778
716-375-2000
800-462-5050
Fax: 716-375-2072
http://www.sbu.edu
nmatthew@sbu.edu

Raymond C. Dee, Chair
Robert J. Daughtery, Vice Chair
Margaret Carney, President
Catholic University in the Franciscan tradition. Independent coeducational institution offering programs through its schools of arts and sciences, business administration, education and journalism and mass communication. 2500 students, tuition $16,210, room and board $6,190.

3440 **St. Lawrence University**
23 Romoda Dr
Canton, NY 13617
800-285-1856
Fax: 315-229-5502
http://www.stlawu.edu
jmeagher@mail.stlawu.edu

William L. Fox, President
Liv Regosin, Director of Advising
The Office of Special Needs is here to ensure that all students with disabilities can freely and actively participate in all facets of University life, to coordinate support services and programs that enable students with disabilities to reach their educational potential, and to increase the level of awareness among all members of the University so that students with disabilites are able to perform at a level limited only by their abilities, not their disabilities.

3441 **St. Thomas Aquinas College**
Pathways
125 Route 340
Sparkill, NY 10976
845-398-4000
Fax: 845-359-8136
http://www.stac.edu
pathways@stac.edu

Lanny S. Cohen, Chair
Joseph McSweeny, Vice Chair
Margaret Fitzpatrick, President
Comprehensive support program for selected college students with learning disabilites and/or ADHD. Services include individual professional mentoring, study groups, academic counseling, priority registration, assistive technology, and a specialized summer program prior to the first semester.

3442 **State University of New York College Technology at Delhi**
2 Main St
Delhi, NY 13753
607-746-4000
800-96-DELHI
Fax: 607-746-4004
http://www.delhi.edu
weinbell@delhi.edu

Dr. Candace Vancko, President
Carol Bishop, VP Business and Finance
Dr. John Nader, Provost
Provide services for students with disabilities. Alternate test-taking arrangements, adapted equipment, assistive technology, accessibility information, note taking services, reading services, tutorial assistance, interpreting services, accessble parking and elevators, sounseling, guidance and support, refferral information and advocacy services, workshops and support groups.

3443 **State University of New York College at Brockport**
State University of New York
350 New Campus Dr
Brockport, NY 14420
585-395-5409
800-382-8447
Fax: 585-395-5291
TDD: 585-395-5409
http://www.brockport.edu
osdoffic@brockport.edu

John R. Halstead, PhDÿ, President
Mary Ellen Zuckerman, Provost/VP Academic Affairs
James Willis, VP Administration and Finance
Provides support and assistance to students with medical, physical, emotional or learning disabilities, specially those experiencing problems in areas such as academic environment.

3444 **State University of New York College of Agriculture and Technology**
State Route 7
Cobleskill, NY 12043
518-255-5011
800-295-8988
Fax: 518-255-6430
TDD: 518-255-5454
TTY: 518-255-5454
http://www.cobleskill.edu
labarno@cobleskill.edu

Dr. Debra H. Thatcher, President
Carol Bishop, VP for Business& Finance
Bonnie Martin, VP for Operations
The primary objective is to develop and maintain a supportive campus environment that promotes academic achievement and personal growth for students with disabilities. Services provide by the office are based on each student's documentation and are tailored to each student's unique individual needs.

3445 **State University of New York: Albany**
1400 Washington Ave
Albany, NY 12222
518-442-3300
Fax: 518-442-5400
TDD: 518-442-3366
http://www.albany.edu

Robert Jones, President
Susan D. Phillips, Provost/VP Academic Affairs
Leanne Wirkkula, Chief of Staff
4-year public University.

3446 **State University of New York: Buffalo**
Special Services Department
1300 Elmwood Ave
Buffalo, NY 14222
716-878-4000
Fax: 716-645-3473
TTY: 716-645-2616
http://www.buffalostate.edu
savinomr@buffalostate.edu

Katherine Conway-Turner, President
Denise K. Ponton, Provost
Bonita R. Durand, Chief of Staff
The Office of Disability Services (ODS) is the University at Buffalo's center for coordinating services and accommodations to ensure accessiblity and usability of all programs, services and activities of UB by people with disabilities, and is a resource for information and advocacy toward their full participation in all aspects of campus life.

3447 **State University of New York: Geneseo College**

1 College Cir
Geneseo, NY 14454 585-245-5000
Fax: 585-245-5032
http://disability.geneseo.edu
web@geneseo.edu

Carol S. Long, President
Dr. Savi Iyer, Dean of Curriculum

To provide qualified students with disabilities, whether temporary or permanent, equal and comprehensive access to college-wide programs, services, and campus facilities by offering academic support, advisement, and removal of architectural and attitudinal barriers.

3448 **State University of New York: Oswego**

Disability Services Office
7060 Route 104
Oswego, NY 13126-3599 315-312-2500
Fax: 315-312-2943
http://www.oswego.edu
dss@oswego.edu

Deborah F. Stanley, President
Lorrie Clemo, VP for Academic Affairs/Provost
Nicholas Lyons, VP for Administration & Finance

A public four-year college of arts and sciences currently serving 140 students identified with disabling conditions. Total enrollment is approximately 8,000. Full time coordinator of academic support services for students with disabilities works with students on an individual basis.

3449 **State University of New York: Plattsburgh**

Student Support Services
101 Broad St
Plattsburgh, NY 12901 518-564-2000
Fax: 518-564-2807
http://www.plattsburgh.edu
michele.carpentier@plattsburgh.edu

John Ettling, President
Keith Tyo, Executive Assistant
Dawn Short, Secretary

Academic support program funded by the United States Department of Education. Staffed by caring and commited professional whose mission is to provide services for students with disabilities.

3450 **State University of New York: Potsdam**

44 Pierrepont Avenue
Potsdam, NY 13676 315-267-2000
Fax: 315-267-3268
TDD: 315-267-2071
TTY: 315-267-2071
http://www.potsdam.edu
housese@potsdam.edu

H.Carl McCall, Chair
Samuel L. Stanley, President
Nancy L. Zimpher, Chancellor

A public four-year college with approximately 200 students with disabilities out of a total of 4,000.

3451 **Stony Brook University**

Disability Support Services
128 Educational Communications Ctr
Stony Brook, NY 11794 631-632-6000
Fax: 631-632-6747
TTY: 631-632-6748
http://www.sunysb.edu
dss@notes.cc.sunysb.edu

H.Carl McCall, Chair
Samuel L. Stanley, President
Nancy L. Zimpher, Chancellor

The Office of Disability Support Services provides assistance for both students and employees. It coordinates advocacy and support services for students with disabilities in their academic and student life activities. Assuring campus accessibility, assisting with academic accommodations and providing assistive devices are important components of the programs.

3452 **Suffolk County Community College: Ammerman**

Special Services
533 College Rd
Selden, NY 11784-2899 631-451-4045
Fax: 631-451-4473
TTY: 631-451-4041
http://www.sunysuffolk.edu

Dafny Irizarry, Chair
Dr. Shaun L. McKay, President
Bryan Lilly, Secretary

Office of services for students with disabilities.

3453 **Suffolk County Community College: Eastern Campus**

Speonk-Riverhead Rd
Riverhead, NY 11901 631-548-2500
Fax: 631-369-2641
http://www.sunysuffolk.edu

Dafny Irizarry, Chair
Dr. Shaun L. McKay, President
Bryan Lilly, Secretary

The Eastern Campus is an accessible, open admissions institution. Services are provided to learning disabled students to allow them the same or equivalent educational experiences as nondisabled students.

3454 **Suffolk County Community College: Western Campus**

Crooked Hill Rd
Brentwood, NY 11717 631-851-6700
Fax: 631-851-6509
http://www.sunysuffolk.edu

Dafny Irizarry, Chair
Dr. Shaun L. McKay, President
Bryan Lilly, Secretary

The goal of Suffolk Community College with regard to students with disabilities is to equalize educational opportunities by minimizing physical, psychological and learning barriers. We attempt to provide as typical a college experience as is possible, encouraging students to achieve academically through the provision of special services, auxillary aids, or reasonable program modifications.

3455 **Sullivan County Community College**

Learning & Student Development Services
112 College Rd
Loch Sheldrake, NY 12759 845-434-5750
800-577-5243
Fax: 845-434-4806
http://www.sullivan.suny.edu

Russ Heyman, Chair
Lyman Holmes, Vice Chair
Patricia Adams, Trustee

SCCC is fully committed to institutions accessability for individuals with disabilities. Students who wish to obtain particular services or accommodations should communicate their needs and concerns as early as possible. These may include, but are not limited to, extended time for tests, oral examinations,reader and notetaker services, campus maps, and elevator privileges. Books on tape may be ordered through recordings for the blind. Appropriate documentation needed.

3456 **Syracuse University**

Services For Students with Disabilities
900 South Crouse Ave
Syracuse, NY 13244 315-443-1870
Fax: 315-443-4410
TDD: 315-443-1312
http://www.syracuse.edu
dtwillia@syr.edu

Richard L. Thompson, Chair
Joanne F. Alper, Vice Chair
James D. Kuhn, Vice Chair

The office of disability services provides and coordinates services for students with documented disabilities. Students must provide current documentation of their disability in order to receive disability services and reasonable accommodations.

3457 **The Gow School**
2491 Emery Rd.
South Wales, NY 14139 716-652-3450
http://www.gow.org
admissions@gow.org
M. Bradley Rogers, Jr., Headmaster
Boarding school for boys, grades 7-12, with dyslexia and other language based learning disabilities.

3458 **Trocaire College**
360 Choate Ave
Buffalo, NY 14220-2094 716-826-1200
Fax: 716-828-6107
http://www.trocaire.edu
Paul Hurley, President
An independent two-year college with 3 special education students out of a total of 1,056.

3459 **Ulster County Community College**
Student Support Services
491 Cottekill Rd
Stone Ridge, NY 12484 845-687-5000
800-724-0833
Fax: 845-687-5292
http://www.sunyulster.edu
William L. Spearman, Chair
Timothy J. Sweeney, Vice Chair
Dr. Donald C Katt, President
The Student Support Services program promotes student success for students who are academically disadvantaged, economically disadvantaged, first-generation college students, and or students with disabilities. The goals of the program are to increase the retention, graduation, and transfer rates of those enrolled.

3460 **University of Albany**
1400 Washington Ave.
Albany, NY 12222 518-442-3300
Fax: 518-442-3583
TDD: 518-442-3366
http://www.albany.edu
cmalloch@uamail.albany.edu
Robert J. Jones, President
Leanne Wirkkula, Chief of Staff
Susan Supple, Senior Assistant to President
Offers a full time Learning Disability Specialist to work with students that have learning disabilities and or attention deficit disorder. The specialist offers individual appointments to develop study and advocacy skills.

3461 **Utica College**
1600 Burrstone Rd
Utica, NY 13502 315-792-3111
Fax: 315-223-2504
http://www.utica.edu
admiss@utica.edu
Kateri Henkel, Learning Services Director
Provides students with disabilities individualized learning accommodations designed to meet the academic needs of the student. Counseling support and the development of new strategies for the learning challenges posed by college level work are an integral part of the services offered through Academic Support Services.

3462 **Van Cleve Program**
The New York Institute for Special Education
999 Pelham Pkwy
Bronx, NY 10469 718-519-7000
Fax: 718-231-9314
http://www.nyise.org
Bernadette M Kappen PhD, Executive Director
Thomas Bergett, Ph.D, Assistant Executive Director
The children of this program have emotional or learning difficulties. Our goal is to reduce the behavioral and learning deficits of students by providing academic and social skills necessary to enter less restrictive programs.

3463 **Vassar College**
124 Raymond Ave
Box 9
Poughkeepsie, NY 12604-9 845-437-7400
Fax: 845-437-7187
TTY: 845-437-5458
http://www.vassar.edu
info@vassar.edu
Frances D Fergusson, Director
Milbrey Rennie Taylor, President
Matthew Vassar, Founder
Offers a variety of services to students with disabilities including note takers, extended testing time, counseling services, and special accommodations.

3464 **Wagner College**
1 Campus Rd
Staten Island, NY 10301 718-390-3100
800-221-1010
Fax: 718-390-3467
http://www.wagner.edu
Dr. Richard Guarasci, President
Pat Fitzpatrick, Assistant to the President
An independent four-year college with 25 special education students out of a total of 1,272. There is an additional fee for the special education program in addition to the regular tuition.

3465 **Westchester Community College**
75 Grasslands Rd
Valhalla, NY 10595 914-606-6600
Fax: 914-785-6540
http://www.sunywcc.edu
Joseph N. Hankin, President
Gloria Leon, Director
Students with Disabilities parallels the mission of WCC to be accessable, community centered, comprehensive, adaptable and dedicated to lifelong learning for all students. Full participation for students with disabilities is encouraged.

3466 **Xaverian High School**
Legacy Program
7100 Shore Rd
Brooklyn, NY 11209 718-836-7100
http://www.xaverian.org
ctrasborg@xaverian.org
Lawrence Harvey, Chair
Daniel E. Skala, Vice Chair
Robert B. Alesi, President
Our mission is to challenge and support learning disabled young men so that they achieve academically at their intellectual level. Our goal is to turn them into effective life-long learners who will go on to college.

North Carolina

3467 **Appalachian State University**
Learning Disability Program
ASU Box 32158
Boone, NC 28608 828-262-3056
Fax: 828-262-7904
http://www.ods.appstate.edu
ods@appstate.edu
Maranda R. Maxey, Director Disability Services
Courtney K. McWhorter, Assistant Director
The Office of Disability Services (ODS) assists students with indentified disabilities by providing the support they need to become successful college graduates. ODS provides academic advising, alternative testing, assistance with technology, tutoring, practical solutions to learning problems, counseling, self-concept building and career exploration.

3468 **Bennett College**
900 E Washington St
Greensboro, NC 27401
336-571-2100
800-413-5323
Fax: 336-517-2228
http://www.bennett.edu

Charles Barrentine, Chair
Deborah W. Foster, Vice Chair
Dr. Rosalind Fuse-Hall, President
An independent four-year college with 10 special education students out of a total of 568.

3469 **Brevard College**
Office for Students with Special Needs & Disab
1 Brevard College Dr
Brevard, NC 28712
828-883-8292
800-527-9090
Fax: 828-884-3790
http://www.brevard.edu
admissions@brevard.edu

David C. Joyce, President
Four year college provides services to special needs students.

3470 **Caldwell Community College and Technical Institute**
Basic Skills Department
2855 Hickory Blvd
Hudson, NC 28638
828-726-2200
Fax: 828-726-2216
http://www.cccti.edu
ccrump@cccti.edu

Kenneth A. Boham, President
Cindy Richards, Administrative Assistant
A public two-year college with 18 special education students out of a total of 2,744.

3471 **Catawba College**
Learning Disability Department
2300 W Innes St
Salisbury, NC 28144
704-637-4259
800-CATAWBA
Fax: 704-637-4401
http://www.catawba.edu
ekgross@catawba.edu

Brien Lewis, President
Jim Stringfield, Dean
Steve McKinzie, Director
An independent four-year liberal arts college with an enrollment of 1,400.

3472 **Catawba Valley Community College**
Student Services Office
2550 Us Highway 70 SE
Hickory, NC 28602-8302
828-327-7000
Fax: 828-327-7276
http://www.cvcc.edu
dulin@cvcc.edu

Charles R. Preston, Chair
Larry Aiello, Vice Chair
Garrett D. Hinshaw, President
The following is a partial list of accommodations provided by the college: counseling services, tutors, note-takers and carbonless duplication paper, recorded textbooks, tape recorders for taping lecture classes, interpeters, computer with voice software, and extended time for texts. Catawba Valley Community College provides services for students with disabilities.

3473 **Central Carolina Community College**
1105 Kelly Dr
Sanford, NC 27330-9840
919-775-5401
Fax: 919-718-7380
http://www.ccc.edu

Paula Wolff, Chair
Ellen Alberding, Vice Chair
Larry R. Rogers, Secretary
Adopted to guide its delivery of services to students with disabilities that states that no otherwise qualified individual shall by reason of disability be excluded from the participation in, be denied benefits of, or be subjected to discrimination under any program at Central Carolina Community College. The college will make program modification adjustments in instructional delivery and provide supplemental services.

3474 **Central Piedmont Community College**
Learning Disability Department
PO Box 35009
Charlotte, NC 28235-5009
704-542-0470
Fax: 704-330-4020
TDD: 704-330-5000
TTY: 704-330-4223
http://www.cpcc.edu/
patricia.adams@cpcc.edu

Edwin A. Dalrymple, Chair
Judith A. Allison, Vice Chair
P. Anthony Zeiss, President
A public two-year college with 300 special education students out of a total of 60,000.

3475 **Davidson County Community College**
PO Box 1287
Lexington, NC 27293-1287
336-249-8186
Fax: 336-249-0088
http://www.davidsonccc.edu
emorse@davidsonccc.edu

Ed Morse MD, Dean
Mary Rittling, President
Offers a variety of services to students with disabilities including notetakers, extended testing time, counseling services, and special accommodations.

3476 **Dore Academy**
5146 Parkway Plaza Blvd.
Charlotte, NC 28217
704-365-5490
Fax: 704-365-3240
http://johncroslandschool.org/
info@johncroslandschool.org

Sean Preston, Head of School
Portia Eley, Admissions Director
Faye Lakey, Director of Finance & Operations
Dore Academy is Charlotte's oldest college-prep school for students with learning differences. A private, non-profit, independent day school for students in grades 1-12, it is approved by the state of North Carolina, Division of Exceptional children. All teachers are certified by the state and trained in the theory and treatment of dyslexia and attention disorders. With a maximum of 10 students per class (5 in reading classes), the teacher student ratio is 1 to 7.

3477 **East Carolina University**
Project STEPP
E 5th Street
Greenville, NC 27858-4353
252-328-6131
http://www.ecu.edu
williamssar@ecu.edu

Dr. Marilyn Sheerer, Provost
Chris Locklear, Chief of Staff
The program offers comprehensive academic, social, and life-skills support to a select number of students with identified Specific Learning Disabilities who have shown the potential to succeed in college.

3478 **Evergreen Valley College**
Disabilities Support Programs
East Fifth Street
Greenville, NC 27858-4353
252-328-6131
Fax: 408-223-6341
TDD: 408-238-8722
http://www.euc.edu
bonnie.clark@euc.edu

David W Coon, LD Specialist
John D. Messick, President
A public two-year college with 82 learning disabled students out of a total of 9,000.

3479 **Fletcher Academy**
400 Cedarview Ct
Raleigh, NC 27609
919-782-5082
Fax: 919-782-5980
http://www.thefletcheracademy.com
info@thefletcheracademy.com
Paul Atkinson, Headmaster
Tiffany Gregory, Dean of Admissions
Nancy Steinauer, Business Manager/ IT Specialist
A coeducational, independent day school serving students from grades 1-12 with learning differences.

3480 **Gardner-Webb University**
Noel Program
PO Box 997
110 South Main Street
Boiling Springs, NC 28017
704-406-4000
Fax: 704-406-3524
http://www.gardner-webb.edu
cpotter@gardner-webb.edu
Dr. A Frank Bonner, President
Dr. Ben Leslie, Provost
Four year college that provides a program for disabled students.

3481 **Guilford Technical Community College**
PO Box 309
601 E. Main Street
Jamestown, NC 27282
336-334-4822
Fax: 336-841-2158
TTY: 336-841-2158
http://www.gtcc.cc.nc.us
dcameron@gtcc.cc.nc.us
Dr. Randy Parker, President
Sonny White, Vice President
The purpose of disability access services is to provide equal access and comprehensive, quality services to all students who experience barriers toacademic, personal and social success.

3482 **Hill Center**
3200 Pickett Rd.
Durham, NC 27705
919-489-7464
Fax: 919-489-7466
http://www.hillcenter.org
info@hillcenter.org
Beth Anderson, Executive Director
Bryan Brander, Head of School
Beth Hawkins, Director, Finance/Operations
Half day school and teacher training facility, established for students with LD/ADHD.
1977

3483 **Isothermal Community College**
Department of Disability Services
PO Box 804
286 ICC Loop Road
Spindale, NC 28160
828-286-3636
Fax: 828-286-8109
TDD: 828-286-3636
TTY: 828-288-9844
http://www.isothermal.edu/
kharris@isothermal.cc.nc.us
John Condrey, Chair
Bobby England, Vice Chair
Buck Petty, Trustee
Isothermal Community College, in compliance with the Americans with Disabilities Act, makes every effort to provide accommodations for students with disabilities. It is our goal to integrate students with disabilities into the college and help them participate and benefit from programs and activities enjoyed by all students. We at Isothermal are committed to improving life through learning.

3484 **Johnson C Smith University**
Disability Support Services Department
100 Beatties Ford Rd
Charlotte, NC 28216
704-378-1010
Fax: 704-372-1242
http://www.jcsu.edu
admissions@jcsu.edu
Ronald L. Carter, President
James Saunders, Director
Four year college that provides support to those who are disabled.

3485 **Key Learning Center**
Carolina Day School
1345 Hendersonville Rd
Asheville, NC 28803
828-274-0757
Fax: 828-274-0116
http://www.cdschool.org
bsgro@cdschool.org
Jeff Baker, Chair
Marie-Louise Murphy, President
Kirk Duncan, Head of School
Provides students with learning differences the educational opportunity to overcome their differences and to achieve their maximum potential in school and life.

3486 **Lenoir-Rhyne College**
PO Box 7470
Hickory, NC 28603-7470
828-328-7315
Fax: 828-328-7329
http://www.lr.edu
kirbydr@lrc.edu
Donavon Kirby, Coordinator
Wayne Powell, President
Four year college that provides services for those students that are learning disabled.

3487 **Mariposa School for Children with Autism**
203 Gregson Dr
Cary, NC 27511-6495
919-461-0600
Fax: 919-461-0566
http://www.mariposaschool.org
info@mariposaschool.org
Dane Shears, Chairman
Palma Fouratt, Vice Chair
Jacinta Johnson, Executive Director
Provides year round one-on-one instruction to children with autism, using innovative teaching techniques targeting multiple developmental areas in a single integrated setting. A school of excellence choice for children with autism to maximize developemtn of their communication, social and academic skills.

3488 **Mars Hill College**
100 Atletic Street
PO Box 370
Mars Hill, NC 28754
866-642-4968
800-543-1514
Fax: 828-689-1478
http://www.mhu.edu/
ccain@mhc.edu
J. Dixon Free, Chairman
Cheryl B. Pappas, Vice Chair
Dan Lunsford, President
An independent four-year college with 15 special education students out of a total of 1,321.

3489 **Mayland Community College**
Support Options for Achievement and Retention
PO Box 547
Spruce Pine, NC 28777
828-766-1200
800-462-9526
http://www.mayland.edu
dcagle@mayland.edu
Charles Ronald Kates, Chairman
Edwina Sluder, Vice Chair
Dr. John C. Boyd, President

Offers a variety of services to students with disabilities including notetakers, extended testing time, counseling services, and special accommodations.

3490 McDowell Technical Community College
Student Enrichment Center
54 College Dr
Marion, NC 28752
828-652-6021
Fax: 828-652-1014
http://www.mcdowelltech.edu
donnashort@cc.nc.us

Darren Waugh, Chairman
Joy Shuford, Vice Chair
Dr. Bryan W Wilson, President
A public two-year college with 15 special education students out of a total of 857. Free auxiliary services for LD students include: tutors, books on tape, unlimited testing, oral testing, notetakers and counseling. All faculty are trained in working with the LD student.

3491 Montgomery Community College: North Carolina
1011 Page St
Troy, NC 27371-8387
910-576-6222
Fax: 910-576-2176
http://www.montgomery.edu

Mary Kirk, President
Offers a variety of services to students with disabilities including note takers, extended testing time, counseling services, and special accommodations.

3492 North Carolina State University
Campus Box 7509
Raleigh, NC 27695
919-515-2011
Fax: 919-513-2840
TDD: 919-515-8830
TTY: 919-515-8830
http://www.ncsu.edu/dso
cheryl_branker@ncsu.edu

Cheryl Branker, Director
Academic accommodations and services are provided for students at the university who have documented learning disabilities. Admission to the university is based on academic qualifications and learning disabled students are considered in the same manner as any other student. Special assistance is available to accommodate the needs of these students, including courses in accessible locations when appropiate.

3493 North Carolina Wesleyan College
3400 N Wesleyan Blvd
Rocky Mount, NC 27804
252-985-5100
800-488-6292
Fax: 252-985-5284
http://www.ncwc.edu
albunn.infowc@edu

Will H. Lassiter III, Chairman
Michael Hancock, Vice Chair
Dr. Dewey G. Clark, President
The Center provides support to students interested in achieving academic success. The staff works to provide you with information about academic matters and serves as an advocate for you. Services focus on pre-major advising, tutoring, mentoring, skills enrichment, disabilities assistance, self-assessment and retention.

3494 Piedmont International University
420 S Broad St
Winston Salem, NC 27101-5025
336-725-8344
800-937-5097
Fax: 336-725-5522
http://www.pbc.edu

Dr. Charles Petitt, President
Dr. Beth Ashburn, Provost
Dr. Barkev Trachian, VP Graduate Studies
Prepares men and women for Christian ministries, both lay and professional, through a rigorous program of biblical, general and professional studies.

3495 Randolph Community College
629 Industrial Park Ave
Asheboro, NC 27205
336-626-0200
Fax: 336-629-4695
http://www.randolph.edu/
jbranch@randolf.edu

F. Mac Sherrill, Chairman
Fred E. Meredith, Vice Chair
Robert S. Shackleford Jr, President
A public two-year college with 23 special education students out of a total of 1,487. Applicants with disabilities who wish to request accommodations in compliance with the ADA must identify themselves to the admissions counselor before placement testing.

3496 Rockingham Community College
215 Wrenn Memorial Road
Hwy. 65
Wentworth, NC 27375
336-342-4261
Fax: 336-349-9986
TDD: 336-634-0132
http://www.rockinghamcc.edu
rkeys@rcc.cc.nc.us

William C Aiken, President
Suzanne Rohrbaugh, Vice President, Academic Affairs
Steve Woodruff, VP Administrative Services
Offers a variety of services to students with disabilities including notetakers, extended testing time, counseling services, and special accommodations.

3497 Salem College
S Church Street
Winston-Salem, NC 27108
336-721-2600
Fax: 336-917-5339
http://www.salem.edu
smith@salem.edu

Stephen G. Jennings, Chair
Leigh Flippin Krause, Vice Chair
Lorraine Sterritt, President
Offers a variety of services to students with disabilities including notetakers, extended testing time, counseling services, and special accommodations.

3498 Sandhills Community College
3395 Airport Rd
Pinehurst, NC 28374
910-692-6185
800-338-3944
Fax: 910-695-1823
http://www.sandhills.edu

George Little, Chair
Robert Hayter, Vice Chair
John R Dempsey, President
Offers a variety of services to students with disabilities including notetakers, extended testing time, counseling services, and special accommodations.

3499 Southwestern Community College: North Carolina
447 College Dr
Sylva, NC 28779
828-339-4000
800-447-4091
Fax: 828-339-4613
http://www.southwesterncc.edu
cheryl@southwest.cc.nc.us

Terry Bell, Chair
W. Paul Holt, Vice Chair
Don Tomas, Ed.D., President
Southwestern Community College provides equal access to education for persons with disabilities. It is the responsibility of the student to make their disability known and to request academic adjustments. Requests should be made in a timely manner and submitted to the Director of Student Support Services. Every reasonable effort will be made to provide service, however, not requesting services prior to registration may delay implementation.

3500 **St Andrews Presbyterian College**
1700 Dogwood Mile
Laurinburg, NC 28352
910-277-5555
800-763-0198
Fax: 910-277-5020
http://www.sapc.edu
info@sapc.edu
Paul Baldasare, President
Glenn Batten, VP Administration
Erin Cooper Balduf, Admissions Counselor
Four year college that supports and provides services to the learning disabled students.

3501 **Stone Mountain School**
126 Camp Elliott Rd
Black Mountain, NC 28711-9003
888-631-5994
Fax: 828-669-2521
http://www.stonemountainschool.org
smoore@stonemountainschool.com
Sam Moore, Executive Director
Paige Thomas, Admissions Director

3502 **Surry Community College**
630 S Main St
Dobson, NC 27017
336-386-8121
Fax: 336-386-8951
http://www.surry.edu
riggsj@surry.edu
Dr. Ann Vaughn, Chair
George L. Anderson, Vice Chair
Tony Martin, Vice President, Finance
Offers a variety of services to students with disabilities including notetakers, extended testing time, counseling services, and special accommodations.

3503 **University of North Carolina Wilmington**
Disability Resource Center
601 S College Rd
Wilmington, NC 28403
910-962-3000
Fax: 910-962-7556
TDD: 800-735-2962
TTY: 800-735-2962
http://www.uncw.edu/disability
waybrantj@uncw.edu
Wendy F. Murphy, Chair
Britt A. Preyer, Vice Chair
Bill Sederburg, Chancellor
Offer accommodative services, consultation, counseling and advocacy for students with disabilities enrolled at UNCW.

3504 **University of North Carolina: Chapel Hill**
450 Ridge Rd
Ste 2109
Chapel Hill, NC 27599-5135
919-962-3782
Fax: 919-962-7797
http://learningcenter.unc.edu
learning_center@unc.edu
Kim Abels, Director
Robin Blanton, Academic Coach
Billie Shambley, Program Manager
Promotes learning by providing academic support to meet the individual needs of students diagnosed with specific learning disabilities. Strives to ensure the independence of participating students so that they may succeed during and beyond their university years.

3505 **University of North Carolina: Charlotte**
Special Education Department
9201 University Blvd
Charlotte, NC 28223-1
704-687-8622
Fax: 704-547-3239
http://www.uncc.edu
abennett@email.uncc.edu
Karen A. Popp, Chair
Joe L. Price, Vice Chair
Philip L. Dubois, Chancellor
Introduction to Students with Special Needs. Characteristics of students with special learning needs, including those who are gifted and those who experience academic, social, emotional, physical and developmental disabilities. Legal, historical and philosophical foudations of special education and current issues in providing appropriate educational services to students with special needs.

3506 **University of North Carolina: Greensboro**
Disability Services
910 Raleigh Rd.
PO Box 2688
Chapel Hill, NC 27514
919-962-1000
Fax: 336-334-4412
http://www.uncg.edu
ods@uncg.edu
John C. Fennebresque, Chair
W. Louis Bissette, Vice Chair
Thomas W. Ross, President
A public four-year university with over 300 students with disabilities out of a total of 12,000.

3507 **Wake Forest University**
1834 Wake Forest Road
Winston Salem, NC 27106
336-758-5000
Fax: 336-758-6074
http://www.wfu.edu
Donald E. Flow, Chair
Donna A. Boswell, Vice Chair
Bobby R. Burchfield, Vice Chair
Offers a variety of services to students with disabilities including notetakers, extended testing time, counseling services, and special accommodations.

3508 **Wake Technical Community College**
Disabilities Support Department
9101 Fayetteville Rd
Raleigh, NC 27603
919-866-5000
Fax: 919-779-3360
TDD: 919-779-0668
http://www.waketech.edu
jtkillen@waketech.edu
Stephen C Scott, Director
Elaine Sardi, Coordinator
If you are a person with a documented disability who requires accommodations to achieve equal access to Wake Tech facilities, academic programs or other activities, you may request reasonable accommodations.

3509 **Western Carolina University**
Student Support Services
137 Killian Anx
Cullowhee, NC 28723
828-227-7211
Fax: 828-227-7078
http://www.wcu.edu
mellen@wcu.edu
Teresa Wiiliams, Chair
F. Edward Broadwell, Vice Chair
David O. Belcher, Chancellor
Students with a documented disability may be provided with appropriate academic accommodations such as, note takers, testing accomadations, books on tape, readers/scribes, use of adaptive equipment and priority registration.

3510 **Wilkes Community College**
Student Support Services
PO Box 120
1328 S.Collegiate Dr.
Wilkesboro, NC 28697
336-838-6100
Fax: 336-838-6277
http://www.wilkescc.edu
nancy.sizemore@wilkescc.edu
Kim Faw, Director
Nancy Sizemore, Disability Coordinator
A public two-year community college. Special services include: testing and individualized education plans; oral and extended time testing; individual and small group tutoring; study skills; readers and proctors and specialized equipment.

3511 **Wilson County Technical College**
North Carolina Community College
PO Box 4305
902 Herring Avenue
Wilson, NC 27893
252-291-1195
Fax: 252-243-7148
TDD: 252-246-1362
http://www.wilsoncc.edu

Dr. Rusty Stephens, President
Lynn Moore, Director
Jane S. Elliott, Grant Assistant
Offers a variety of services to students with disabilities including notetakers, extended testing time, counseling services, and special accommodations.

3512 **Wingate University**
Disability Services Department
220 N. Camden St.
Wingate, NC 28174
704-233-8000
800-755-5550
Fax: 704-233-8014
http://www.wingate.edu
admit@wingate.edu

Dr. Jerry McGee, President
Peter Frank, Associate Professor of Economics
Joe Graham, Professor of Accounting
An independent four-year college with 50 special education students out of a total of 1,372. There is an additional fee for the special education program in addition to the regular tuition.

3513 **Winston-Salem State University**
601 S. Martin Luther King Jr. Drive
Winston Salem, NC 27110
336-750-2000
Fax: 336-750-2392
http://www.wssu.edu/

Brenda A. Allen, Provost
Donald J. Reaves, Ph.D, Chancellor
Dr. Carolyn Berry, Associate Provost
Offers a variety of services to students with disabilities including notetakers, extended testing time, counseling services, and special accommodations.

North Dakota

3514 **Anne Carlsen Center for Children**
701 3rd St., NW.
P.O. Box 8000
Jamestown, ND 58402
800-568-5175
http://www.annecenter.org

Tim Eissinger, Chief Executive Officer
Stephanie Nelson, Chief Operations Officer
Daniel Johnson, Chief Financial Officer
Provides students a safe, secure, and loving atmosphere to learn and grow. The program is filled with an array of sensory and literary enriched experiences and materials that allow each student to become an independent, freethinking being.

3515 **Bismarck State College**
1500 Edwards Ave
PO Box 5587
Bismarck, ND 58506
701-224-5400
800-445-5073
Fax: 701-224-5550
http://www.bsc.nodak.edu
Ischlafm@gwmail.nodak.edu

Patrick J. Bjork, Web Manager
Zachery Allen, Project Manager
Dusty Anderson, Production Coordiator
Offers a variety of services to students with disabilities including notetakers, extended testing time, counseling services, and special accommodations.

3516 **Dakota College at Bottineau**
105 Simrall Blvd
Bottineau, ND 58318
701-228-5488
800-542-6866
Fax: 701-228-5499
http://www.dakotacollege.edu
jan.nahinurk@dakotacollege.edu

David Fuller, President
Dr. Ken Grosz, Dean
Karen Bowen, Director of Business Affairs
Dakota College at Bottineau offers a variety of services to students with disabilities including note takers, extended testing time, academic advising, and special accommodations.

3517 **Dickinson State University**
Student Support Services
291 Campus Dr
Dickinson, ND 58601
701-483-2507
800-279-HAWK
Fax: 701-483-2006
http://www.dickinsonstate.edu/
dsu.hawk@dickinsonstate.edu

D. C. Coston, President
Dr. Cynthia Pemberton, Provost/ VP for Academic Afairs
Mark Lowe, VP for Finance & Administration
Four year college offers support services to learning disabled students.

3518 **Fort Berthold Community College**
PO Box 490
280 8th Ave. N.
New Town, ND 58763
701-627-4378
Fax: 701-627-3609
http://www.fortbertholdcc.edu/
lgwin@spcc.bia.edu

Patrick J. Packineau, President
Phillip Lewis, CFO/ VP, Support Services
Keith Smith, Faciltíes Manager
An independent two-year college with 3 special education students out of a total of 279.

3519 **Mayville State University**
Learning Disabilities Department
330 3rd St NE
Mayville, ND 58257
701-788-2301
800-437-4104
Fax: 701-788-4748
http://www.mayvillestate.edu
kyllo@mayvillestate.edu

Charlotte Anderson, Office Manager
Karen A. Amundson, Business Office
Jessica P. Amb, Administrative Coordinator
Offers a variety of services to students with disabilities including notetakers, extended testing time, counseling services, and special accommodations.

3520 **Minot State University**
North Dakota Center for Persons with Disabilities
500 University Ave W
Minot, ND 58707
701-858-3371
800-777-0750
Fax: 701-858-3686
TDD: 701-858-3580
http://www.minotstateu.edu
ndcpd@minotstateu.edu

Leslie Coughlin, Chair
Steven W. Shirley, President
Brian Foisy, VP for Finance & Administration
NDCPD works with the disability community, university, faculty and researchers, policy makers and service providers to identify emerging needs in the disability community and how to obtain resources to address them.

3521 **North Dakota State College of Science**
Disability Support Services (DSS) Office
800 6th St N
Wahpeton, ND 58076
701-671-2401
800-342-4325
Fax: 701-671-2499
http://www.ndscs.nodak.edu
joy.eichhorn@ndscs.nodak.edu

Gregory Anderson, Chair
John Richman, President
Christine Ahlsten, Director
A public two-year comprehensive college with a student population of 2400. Students with disabilites comprise seven percent of the population. Tuition $2025.

3522 **North Dakota State University**
Disability Services
Post Office Box 6050
Fargo, ND 58108-6050
701-231-8011
Fax: 701-231-6318
TDD: 800-366-6888
http://www.ndsu.edu
bunnie.johnson-messelt@ndsu.edu

Dean L. Brescian, President
Bruce Bollinger, VP for Finance & Administration
Timothy Alvarez, VP for Student Affairs
Students with permanent physical, psychological or learning disabilities may obtain accommodations. The Disability Services (DS) staff meet with the student to determine eligibility and identify reasonable accomodations. Accomodations are based on the functional limitations of the disability. DS staff assist in the implementation of approved accommodations. Referrals for disability diagnosis and for other support services such as tutoring are also provided by staff.

3523 **Standing Rock College**
9299 Hwy 24
Fort Yates, ND 58538
701-854-8000
Fax: 701-854-3403
http://www.sittingbull.edu
info@sbci.edu

Sharon Two Bears, Chair
Joe L. McNeil, Vice Chair
Dr.Laurel Vermillion, President
Offers a variety of services to students with disabilities including notetakers, extended testing time, counseling services, and special accommodations.

Ohio

3524 **Art Academy of Cincinnati**
1212 Jackson St
Cincinnati, OH 45202
513-562-6262
800-323-5692
Fax: 513-562-8778
http://www.artacademy.edu/

Mark Grote, Chair
Susan Crabtree, Vice Chair
John M. Sullivan, President
Offers a variety of services to students with disabilities including notetakers, extended testing time, counseling services, and special accommodations.

3525 **Baldwin-Wallace College**
275 Eastland Rd
Berea, OH 44017-2088
440-826-2900
Fax: 440-826-3777
http://www.bw.edu
info@bw.edu

Paul H. Carleton, Chair
Robert C. Helmer, President
Stephen D. Stahl, Provost
Offers a variety of services to students with disabilities including notetakers, extended testing time, counseling services, and special accommodations.

3526 **Bluffton College**
Special Student Services
1 University Dr.
Bluffton, OH 45817-2104
419-358-3000
800-488-3257
Fax: 419-358-3323
http://www.bluffton.edu
bergerd@bluffton.edu

James H. Harder, President
Four year college offers special programs to learninig disabled students.

3527 **Bowling Green State University**
413 S Hall
Bowling Green, OH 43403-1
419-372-2531
Fax: 419-372-8496
http://www.bgsu.edu
dss@bgsu.edu

Mary Ellen Mazey, President
Dr. Rodney Rogers, SVP for Academic Affairs/Provost
Jill Carr, VP for Student Affairs
The Disability Services Office is evidence of Bowling Green State University's commitment to provide a support system which assists in conquering obstacles that persons with disabilities may encounter as they pursue their educational goals and activities. Our hope is to facilitate mainstream mobility and recognize the diverse talents that persons with disabilities have to offer to our university and our community.

3528 **Brown Mackie College: Akron**
2791 Mogadore Rd
Akron, OH 44320
330-896-3600
Fax: 330-733-5853
http://www.brownmackie.edu

Jannette Mason, Administrative Assistant
Fred Baldwin, Dean of Academic Services
Offers a variety of services to students with disabilities including notetakers, extended testing time, counseling services, and special accommodations.

3529 **Case Western Reserve University**
10900 Euclid Ave
Cleveland, OH 44106
216-368-2000
Fax: 216-368-8826
http://www.cwru.edu

Barbara R. Snyder, President
W.A. Bud Baeslack III, EVP & Provost
Robert Clark Brown, Treasurer
While all students will have preferences for learning, students with physical or learning disabilities have different actual needs as well. Students with physical disabilities such as visual impairments, hearing impairments, or temporary or permanent motor impairments may need guide dogs, interpeters, note-takers, wheelchair accessible rooms, or other types of assistance to help them attend and participate in class. Also available, extra time or a separate room for exams, tutoring and more.

3530 **Central Ohio Technical College**
Developmental Education
1179 University Dr
Newark, OH 43055
740-366-9494
800-963-9275
Fax: 740-366-5047
http://www.cotc.edu

Cheryl Snyder, Chair
John Hinderer, Vice Chair
Bonnie Coe, President
Learning Assitance Center and Disability Services (LAC/DS) is the academic support unit in Student Support Services. LAC/DS provides FREE programs and services designed to help students sharpen skills necessary to succeed in college.

3531 **Central State University**
Office of Disability Services
1400 Brush Row Rd
PO Box 1004
Wilberforce, OH 45384
937-376-6011
800-388-2781
Fax: 937-376-6245
http://www.centralstate.edu
publicrelations@centralstate.edu
Curtis Pettis, Executive Director
Daarel E. Burnette, VP for Adminstration & CFO
Charles Wesley Ford, Provost
Four year college that provides services for the learning disabled students.

3532 **Cincinnati State Technical and Community College**
3520 Central Pkwy
Cincinnati, OH 45223
513-569-1500
Fax: 513-569-1719
TDD: 877-569-0115
http://www.cincinnatistate.edu
dcover@cinstate.cc.oh.us
Cathy T. Crain, Chair
Mark D. Walton, Vice Chair
O'Dell M. Owens, M.D., M.P.H, President
Services include assistance and support services for students with permanent and temporary disabilities, test proctoring, readers/scribes, taping, tape recording loan, reading machines, assistance with locating interpeters, mediating between student and faculty to overcome specific disability issues; also offers braille access.

3533 **Clark State Community College**
Disability Retention Center
570 East Leffel Lane
Springfield, OH 45505-4795
937-325-0691
Fax: 937-328-6133
http://www.clarkstate.edu
Jo Alice Blondin, Ph.D., President
James N. Doyle, Chair
Peggy Noonan, Vice Chair
In accordance with the Americans with Disabilities Act, it is the policy of Clark State Community College to provide reasonable accommodations to persons with disabilities. The office of disability services offers a variety of services to Clark State students who have documented physical, mental or learning disabilities.

3534 **Cleveland Institute of Art**
Academic Services
11141 East Boulevard
Cleveland, OH 44106-1700
216-421-7450
800-223-4700
Fax: 216-421-7438
http://www.cia.edu
cinema@cia.edu
Michael Schwartz, Board Chair
Grafton Nunes, President and CEO
Almut Zvosec, VP Business AffairS/CFO
No student should be discouraged from attending CIA because of a learning disability. A student working on their BFA degree at the Institute of Art can get academic support from the tutoring director in the Office of Academic Services. Services include books-on-tape, one-on-one tutoring, alternative curriculum advising, notetaking services, alternative test taking and assignment arrangements. Services outside the scope of the program can be arranged at the student's expense.

3535 **Cleveland State University**
2121 Euclid Avenue
Cleveland, OH 44115-2214
216-687-2000
888-278-6446
Fax: 216-687-9366
http://www.csuohio.edu
m.zuccaro@csuohio.edu
Ronald ÿM. Berkman, President
Michael Artbauer, Chief of Staff
Barbara E. Smith, Director Special Events
CSU aims to provide equal opportunity to all of its students. Services are available to those who might need some extra help because of a physical disability, communication impairment or learning disability. This program is designed to address the personal and academic issues of the physically handicapped students as they become oriented to campus. A full range of services is offered.

3536 **College of Mount Saint Joseph**
Project EXCEL
5701 Delhi Road
Cincinnati, OH 45233-1670
513-244-4200
800-654-9314
Fax: 513-244-4601
http://www.msj.edu
debra_mato@mail.msj.edu
Tony Aretz, Ph.D., President
Kenneth W. Stecher, Chairperson
Jason P. Niehaus, Vice Chairperson
Project EXCEL is a nationally recognized, comprehensive academic support system for students with specific learning disabilities and/or Attention Deficit/Attention Deficit Hyperactivity Disorder. Project EXCEL is a fee-for-service program. Students must be admitted to the College of Mount St. Joseph before applying for Project EXCEL.

3537 **College of Wooster**
1189 Beall Ave
Wooster, OH 44691-2363
330-263-2000
Fax: 330-263-2427
http://www.wooster.edu
Grant H. Cornwell, President
David H. Gunning, Chairman
Douglas F. Brush, Vice Chairman
Offers a variety of services to students with disabilities including notetakers, extended testing time, counseling services, and special accommodations.

3538 **Columbus State Community College Disability Services**
550 East Spring St
Columbus, OH 43215-1722
614-287-5353
800-621-6407
Fax: 614-287-3645
TDD: 614-287-2570
TTY: 614-287-2570
http://www.cscc.edu
information@cscc.edu
David T. Harrison, Ph.D., President
Richard D. Rosen, Chair
Michael E. Flowers, Vice-Chair
A public two-year college serving qualified students with disabilities, including learning disabilities. Support services are provided based on disability documentation and can include, books, tapes, alternative testing, notetaking, counseling, equipment use, reader, scribe, and peer tutoring.

3539 **Cuyahoga Community College: Eastern Campus**
4250 Richmond Road
Highland Hills, OH 44122-6195
800-954-8742
866-933-5175
Fax: 216-987-2054
TDD: 866-933-5175
http://www.tri-c.edu
Maryann.Syarto@tri-c.cc.oh.us
Jerry L. Kelsheimer, Chairman
Nadine H. Feighan, Vice Chairperson
Alex Johnson, Ph.D., President
The ACCESS Programs strive to assist Tri-C students with disabilities to realize their learning potential, bring them into the mainstream of the College community, enhance their self-sufficiency, and enable them to achieve academic success. Services include tuoring, test proctoring, interpreters, adaptive equipment, readers and/or scribes for exams, alternative test taking arrangements, alternative format for printed materials and textbooks on tape.

3540 **Cuyahoga Community College: Western Campus**
1000 West Pleasant Valley Rd
Parma, OH 44130
216-987-5077
800-954-8742
Fax: 516-987-5050
TDD: 216-987-5117
http://www.tri-c.edu
rose.kolovrat@tri-c.edu

Jerry L. Kelsheimer, Chairman
Nadine H. Feighan, Vice Chairperson
Alex Johnson, Ph.D., President
The ACCESS programs strive to assist Tri-C students with disabilities to realize their learning potential, bring them into the mainstream of the College community, enhance their self-suffciency and enable them to achieve academic success. Services provided include tutoring, test proctoring, interpeters, adaptive equipment, readers/scribes for exams, alternative testing arrangements, alternative format for printed material and textbooks on tape.

3541 **Defiance College**
701 N Clinton St
Defiance, OH 43512-1695
419-784-4010
800-520-4632
Fax: 419-784-0426
http://www.defiance.edu
admissions@defiance.edu

Mark C. Gordon, President
Lois McCullough, VP for Finance and Management
Michael Suzo, VP for Enrollment Management
Offers a variety of services to students with disabilities including notetakers, extended testing time, counseling services, and special accommodations.

3542 **Denison University**
100 West College St.
Granville, OH 43023
740-587-6666
800-336-4766
Fax: 740-868-1168
http://www.denison.edu
arc@denison.edu

Adam Weinberg, President
Jennifer Grube Vestal, Associate Dean/ARC Director
The Academic Resource Center (ARC) offers a wide range of services for students with disabilities. In supporting students as they move forward toward graduation and the world of work beyond, the ARC strongly encourages and promotes self advocacy regarding disability related issues.

3543 **FOCUS Program**
Program for Students with Learning Disabilities
2550 Lander Road
Pepper Pike, OH 44124-4318
440-449-4200
888 URSULINE
Fax: 440-684-6138
http://www.ursuline.edu
info@ursuline.edu

Eileen Delaney Kohut, Director
John M. Newman, Jr., Chair
Sister Diana Stano, President
A voluntary, comprehensive, fee-paid program for students with learning disabilities and ADHD. The goals of the FOCUS Program include providing a smooth transition for college life, helping students learn to apply the most appropriate learning strategies in college courses, and teaching students self-advocacy skills.

3544 **Franklin University**
201 S Grant Ave
Columbus, OH 43215-5399
614-797-4700
877-341-6300
Fax: 614-224-8027
http://www.franklin.edu
admissions@franklin.edu

Dr. David Decker, President
Gary L. Flynn, Chairman of the Board
Mary Laird Duchi, Vice Chairman
Students who have disabilities may notify the University of their status by checking the appropriate space on the registration form each trimester.Then the Coordinator of Disability Services will help them file proper documentation so that accommodations can be made for their learning needs.

3545 **Hiram College**
11715 Garfield Road
Hiram, OH 44234-67
330-569-3211
800-705-5050
Fax: 330-569-5398
http://www.hiram.edu
alumnirel@hiram.edu

Lori E. Varlotta, President
Brittney Braydich, Director of Major Gifts
Patrick Roberts, VP Dev & Alumni Relations
Offers a variety of services to students with disabilities including notetakers, extended testing time, counseling services, and special accommodations.

3546 **Hocking College**
3301 Hocking Parkway
Nelsonville, OH 45764-9588
740-753-3591
877-462-5464
Fax: 740-753-7065
http://www.hocking.edu
admissions@hocking.edu

John Light, President
Rosie Smith, Director
The Access Center Office of Disability Support Services is dedicated to serving the various needs of individuals with disabilities and promoting their participation in college life.

3547 **ITT Technical Institute**
1030 North Meridian Road
Youngstown, OH 44509-4098
330-270-1600
800-832-5001
Fax: 330-270-8333
http://www.itt-tech.edu

Frank Quartini, Manager
Offers a variety of services to students with disabilities including note takers, extended testing time, counseling services, and special accommodations.

3548 **Julie Billiart School**
4982 Clubside Rd
Lyndhurst, OH 44124
216-381-1191
Fax: 216-381-2216
http://www.juliebilliartschool.org
jjohnston@jbschool.org

Lannie Davi-Frecker, MEd, President & CEO
Jodi Johnston MEd, Principal
Rooted in the educational vision of the Sisters of Notre Dame, Julie Billiart School is a Catholic, alternative K-8 school, which educates children of all faith traditions who experience special learning needs.

3549 **Julie Billiart School - Akron**
380 Mineola Ave
Akron, OH 44320
234-206-0941
http://www.juliebilliartschool.org
akron@jbschool.org

Lannie Davi-Frecker, MEd, President & CEO
Jason Wojnicz, MEd, Principal
Rooted in the educational vision of the Sisters of Notre Dame, Julie Billiart School is a Catholic, alternative K-8 school, which educates children of all faith traditions who experience special learning needs.

3550 **Lorain County Community College**
1005 N Abbe Road
Elyria, OH 44035-1691
440-366-4100
800-955-5222
Fax: 440-365-6519
http://www.lorainccc.edu
info@lorainccc.edu

Roy Church, President
Lawrence Goodmanÿ, Chairman
Benjamin Fligner, Vice Chairman
LCCC serves over 80 learning disabled students per year out of a total student population of about 7,000. Services include readers/testers, scribes, notetaking accommodations, assistive technology, advocacy training and personal counseling. Free tutoring is available to all students at the college. No diagnostic testing is available.

3551 **Malone University**
2600 Cleveland Ave NW
Canton, OH 44709-3308
330-471-8100
800-521-1146
Fax: 330-471-8149
TDD: 330-471-8496
http://www.malone.edu
ameadows@malone.edu
Anna Meadows, Student Access Services Director
Dr Wil Friesen, President
David P. Murray, Chair?
An independent four-year college with about 40 special education students out of a total of almost 2,000.

3552 **Marburn Academy**
1860 Walden Drive
Columbus, OH 43229-3627
614-433-0822
Fax: 614-433-0812
http://www.marburnacademy.org
marburnadmission@marburnacademy.org
Earl B Oremus, Headmaster
A not-for-profit, independent, day school devoted to serving the educational needs of bright students with learning differences such as dyslexia and ADHD. The school programs are designed to help the student's learn strong work habits, teach values of persistance and courage in overcoming challenges and to build effective social interaction and problem solving patterns.

3553 **Marietta College**
Marietta College
215 Fifth Street
Marietta, OH 45750-4047
740-376-4786
800-331-7896
Fax: 740-376-4530
http://www.marietta.edu
higgisd@marietta.edu
Walter Miller, Director
Jean Scott, President
An Independent four-year college that offers a variety of servies to students with disabilities including note takers, extended testing time, counseling services, and special accommodations. There is no separate fee for these services.

3554 **Marion Technical College**
1467 Mount Vernon Ave
Marion, OH 43302-5694
740-389-4636
Fax: 740-389-6136
http://www.mtc.edu
enroll@mtc.edu
J Richard Bryson,Ph.D., President
Jeff Nutter, VP/CFO
Brenda Feasel, Director of Human Resources
The Student Resource Center also houses the Office of Disabilities. The SRC director will advocate on student's behalf for resonable accommodations for those with physical, mental and or emotional disabilities.

3555 **Miami University Rinella Learning Center**
Room 14
501 E. High St.
Oxford, OH 45056-2481
513-529-1809
http://www.muohio.edu
David C. Hodge, President
Ray Gorman, Interim Provost and EVP
J. Peter Natale, VP Information Technology
A public four-year college.

3556 **Miami University: Middletown Campus**
4200 N University Blvd
Middletown, OH 45042-3458
513-727-3200
86-MIAMI-MID
Fax: 513-727-3451
TDD: 513-727-3308
TTY: 513-727-3431
http://www.mid.muohio.edu
nferguson@mid.muohio.edu
Kelly Cowan, Executive Director
Margir Perkins, Academic Services
Offers a variety of services to students with disabilities including notetakers, extended testing time, counseling services, and special accommodations.

3557 **Mount Vernon Nazarene College**
800 Martinsburg Rd
Mount Vernon, OH 43050-9500
740-392-6868
866-462-6868
Fax: 740-393-0511
http://www.mvnu.edu
admissions@mvnu.edu
Dr. Henry Spaulding, II, President
Dr. Robert Hamill, VP for Finances & CFO
Dr. Lanette Sessink, VP for Student Life
Four year college that provides programs for learning diabled students.

3558 **Muskingum College**
Center for Advancement of Learning
163 Stormont Street
New Concord, OH 43762
740-826-8137
800-752-6082
Fax: 740-826-8100
http://www.muskingum.edu
adminfo@muskingum.edu
Beth DaLonzo, Senior Director of Admission
Jake Burnett, Associate Director of Admission
Gary Atkins, Assistant Director of Admission
The PLUS Program provides students identified as learning-disabled with individual and group learning strategies instruction embedded within course content.

3559 **Oberlin College**
Academic Support for Students with Disabilities
101 N. Professor St.
Oberlin, OH 44074
440-775-8411
800-622-6243
Fax: 440-775-6905
http://www.oberlin.edu
college.admissions@oberlin.edu
Marvin Krislov, President
Debra Chermonte, VP/Dean of Admissions
Tom Abeyta, Senior Associate Director
An independent four-year college with small percentage of education students.

3560 **Ohio State University Agricultural Technical Institute**
1328 Dover Road
Wooster, OH 44691-4000
330-287-1330
800-647-8283
Fax: 330-287-1333
http://ati.osu.edu
ati@osu.edu
Rhonda Billman, Assistant Director
Jim Kinder, Ph.D., Interim Director
Gail Miller, Director - Upward Bound
A public two-year college with nearly 10% special education students. There is no fee for the special education program in addition to the regular tuition.

3561 **Ohio State University: Lima Campus**
Disability Services
4240 Campus Dr
Lima, OH 45804
567-242-7510
Fax: 419-995-8483
http://www.lima.ohio-state.edu
meyer.193@osu.edu

Deborah Ellis, Chair
Susan Hubbell, Vice Chair
Lori Schleeter, Secretary
A public four-year college providing services to learning disabled students including extended test time, counseling, notetakers and other special accommodations.

3562 **Ohio State University: Mansfield Campus**
Disability Services
1760 University Drive
Mansfield, OH 44906-1547
419-755-4011
Fax: 419-755-4241
http://mansfield.osu.edu
abedon.1@osu.edu
Stephen M. Gavazzi, Ph.D., Dean and Director
Christ J. Ticoras, Chair
Patrick A. Heydinger, Vice-Chair
A public four-year college providing services to learning disabled students including peer tutoring, extended test time, quiet rooms and other special accommodations.

3563 **Ohio State University: Marion Campus**
1465 Mount Vernon Avenue
Marion, OH 43302-5628
740-389-6786
Fax: 740-725-6258
http://www.osumarion.osu.edu
Matt Moreau, Director
Kathleen Clemons, Counselor
Holly Jacobson, Coordinator of Admission
A public four-year college providing a full range of services for students with disabilities.

3564 **Ohio State University: Newark Campus**
1179 University Drive
Founders Hall
Newark, OH 43055-1797
740-366-9333
800-963-9275
Fax: 740-364-9645
http://www.newark.osu.edu
William L. Mac Donald, Dean/Director
Anne Federlein, President
Ann Donahue, Director of Admissions
A public four-year college providing services to learning disabled students including peer tutoring, extended test time, quiet rooms and other special accommodations. There is no separate fee for these services.

3565 **Ohio State University: Nisonger Center**
1581 Dodd Drive
Columbus, OH 43210-1257
614-685-3192
855-983-9955
Fax: 614-366-6373
TDD: 614-688-8040
http://www.nisonger.osu.edu
nisongeradmin@osumc.edu
Marc J. Tasse, Director
Jane Case-Smith, President
Paula Rabidoux, Associate Director
The Ohio State University Nisonger Center for Mental Retardation and Developmental Disabilities provides interdisciplinary training, research and exemplary services pertaining to people with developmental disabilities. The center, which is a part of a national network of activities called University Afffiliated Programs, was founded in 1968. Training is provided in medicine (pediatrics and psychiatry), dentistry, education, physical therapy, psychology and other relevant disciplines.

3566 **Ohio University**
Ohio University
101 University Drive
P.O. Box 629
Chillicothe, OH 45601
740-774-7200
Fax: 740-593-2708
http://www.ohiou.edu
chillicothe@ohio.edu
David Brightbill, Chairÿ
David A. Wolfort, Vice Chair
Rodrick J. McDavis, President
A public four-year college with a small percentage of special education students.

3567 **Ohio University Chillicothe**
101 University Drive
Chillicothe, OH 45601-629
740-774-7200
877-462-6824
Fax: 740-774-7290
http://www.ohiou.edu/~childept
diekroge@ohio.edu
Diane Diekroger MD, Student Support Coordinator
Richard Bebee, Manager
Offers a variety of services to students with disabilities including note takers, extended testing time, counseling services, and special accommodations.

3568 **Otterbein College**
1 S. Grove St.
Westerville, OH 43081-2006
614-823-1618
800-488-8144
Fax: 614-823-1983
http://www.otterbein.edu
lmonaghan@otterbein.edu
Rebecca D. Vazquez-Skillings, VP for Business Affairs
Kathy Krendl, President
Alec Wightman, Secretary
An independent four-year college with a small percentage of special education students.

3569 **Owens Community College**
Disability Resources Department
PO Box 10000
Toledo, OH 43699-1947
567-661-7000
800-466-9367
Fax: 419-661-7607
http://www.owens.edu
bscheffert@owens.cc.oh.us
Thomas P Perin, Associate Vice President
Dr. Mike Bower, Ph.D., President
Renay M Scott, Vice President/Provost
A comprehensive Community College that offers educational programs in over 50 technical areas of study leading to the Associate of Applied Science, Associate of Applied Business or Associate of Technical Studies degree. Provides programs designed for college transfer and leads to the Associate of Arts or Associate of Science degree. Finally, a number of certificate programs as well as short term credit and non-credit programs are available.

3570 **Shawnee State University**
940 Second Street
Portsmouth, OH 45662-4347
740-351-4778
800-959-2778
Fax: 740-351-3470
TTY: 740-351-3159
http://www.shawnee.edu
jmoore@shawnee.edu
Rita Rice-Morris, President
Elinda C. Boyles, Ph.D, VP of Finance & Administration
Elizabeth Blevins, M.S., Director of Communications
Offers a variety of services to students with disabilities including notetakers, extended testing time, counseling services, and special accommodations.

3571 **Sinclair Community College**
Learning Disability Support Services
Rm 11342
444 West Third Street
Dayton, OH 45402-1453
937-512-2855
800-315-3000
Fax: 937-512-4564
TDD: 937-512-3096
http://www.sinclair.edu
Jeff Boudouris, Vice President
Dr. Dave Collins, Provost
Steven L. Johnson, Ph.D., President and CEO

Funded by the Federal Department of Education, Student Support Services is an organization devoted to helping students meet the challenges of college life. Our goals are to help students stay in school, then eventually graduate and/or transfer to a four-year college or university. We strive to develop new ways of helping students achieve their educational, career and professional goals.

3572 **Southern State Community College**
100 Hobart Drive
Hillsboro, OH 45133-9406
937-393-3431
Fax: 937-393-9831
http://www.sscc.edu
Robin Lashley, Exe Assistant to the President
Dr Kevin Boys, President
James Bland, Vice President
Offers a variety of services to students with disabilities including notetakers, extended testing time, counseling services, and special accommodations.

3573 **Terra State Community College**
Special Education Services
2830 Napoleon Road
Fremont, OH 43420-9600
419-559-2349
866-288-3772
Fax: 419-334-3667
http://www.terra.cc.us/terra2.html
admissions@terra.eduÿ
Jerome Webster, President ÿ
Jack Fatica, VP, Academic Affairsÿ
Jeffery Huffman, Director
Provides quality learning experiences which are accessible and affordable. Terra is actively committed to excellence in learning and offers associate degrees in various technologies as well as in arts and sciences, applied business, and applied science. Our office of student support services works with students with learning disabilities and other disabilities.

3574 **University of Cincinnati: Raymond Walters General and Technical College**
9555 Plainfield Road
Blue Ash, OH 45236-1007
513-745-5600
Fax: 513-745-5780
TDD: 513-745-8300
http://www.ucblueash.edu
questions@ucblueash.edu
Cady Short-Thompson, Dean
Raymond Waltersÿ, President
Meredith Delaney, Director of Development
Offers a variety of services to students with disabilities including notetakers, extended testing time, counseling services, and special accommodations.

3575 **University of Findlay**
Disability Services Office
1000 N. Main St.
Findlay, OH 45840-3653
419-422-8313
800-472-9502
Fax: 419-434-4822
TDD: 419-434-5532
http://www.findlay.edu
campuscompact@findlay.edu
Debow Freed, Ph.D., President Emeritus
Katherine Fell, President
William D. Miller, Director of Christian Ministry
An independent four-year college with a small percentage of special needs students.

3576 **University of Toledo**
Libbey Hall
Mail Stop 524
Toledo, OH 43606-3390
419-530-8888
Fax: 419-530-4505
http://www.utoledo.edu
enroll@utoledo.edu
Patricia M. Mowery, B.A., Interim Director
Julianne Bonitati, Administrative Assistant
Nagi Naganathan, PhD, President
A public four-year college whose mission is to provide the support services and accommodations necessary for all students to succeed.

3577 **Urbana University**
Student Affairs Office
597 College Way
Urbana, OH 43078
937-772-9200
Fax: 937-484-1322
http://www.urbana.edu
webmaster@urbana.edu
Dr. David Decker, Presidentÿ
J. Steven Polsley, Chairman
Jim Wehrman, Vice Chair
An independent four-year college with a small percentage of special education students.

3578 **Walsh University**
2020 East Maple Street
North Canton, OH 44720-3336
330-490-7090
800-362-9846
Fax: 330-499-7165
http://www.walsh.edu
bfreshour@walsh.edu
Richard Jusseaume, President
Nancy Blackford, Vice President
Derrick Wyman, Director
An independent four-year college. The Office of Student Support Services maintains an early warning system for students in academic, financial, social and/or emtional difficulty. The Office proudly communicates regularly with students regarding their general well being, and assists in the students' academic and financial concerns with referals to appropriate offices.

3579 **Washington State Community College**
710 Colegate Drive
Marietta, OH 45750-9225
740-374-8716
Fax: 740-376-0257
http://www.wscc.com
Bradley J. Ebersole, Ph.D, President
Gary Williams, Executive Director
Jess N. Raines, CPA, CFO/Treasurer
A public two-year college with a small percentage of special education students.

3580 **Wilmington College of Ohio**
1870 Quaker Way
Wilmington, OH 45177-2499
937-382-6661
800-341-9318
Fax: 937-382-7077
http://www.wilmington.edu
Jim Renoylds, President
Robert Touchton, Chair
Sandra W. Neville, Vice Chair
Offers a variety of services to students with disabilities including notetakers, extended testing time, counseling services, and special accommodations.

Oklahoma

3581 **Bacone College**
2299 Old Bacone Rd
Muskogee, OK 74403-1568
918-683-4581
888-682-5514
Fax: 918-682-5514
http://www.bacone.edu
stewarta@bacone.edu
Dr. Robert K Brown, Executive Vice President
Ann Stewart, Coordinator
Frank K. Willis, President
Offers a variety of services to students with disabilities including notetakers, extended testing time, counseling services, and special accommodations.

3582 **Cascade College**
PO Box 11000
2501 E.Memorial Road
Edmond, OK 73013-1100
405-425-5000
800-877-5010
Fax: 503-257-1222
http://www.cascade.edu
info@oc.edu
John DeSteiguer, President
Dr. Bill Goad, Executive Vice President
Scott LaMascus, VP Academic Affairs
Offers a variety of services to students with disabilities including note takers, extended testing time, counseling services, and special accommodations.

3583 **East Central University**
1100 E 14th St
Ada, OK 74820-6999
580-332-8000
Fax: 580-310-5654
http://www.ecok.edu/
Duane C. Anderson, Provost and Vice President
Jessica A. Boles, VP, Administration and Finance
John R. Hargrave, President
A public four-year college with a small percentage of special education of students.

3584 **Moore-Norman Technology Center**
PO Box 4701
Norman, OK 73070-4701
405-364-5763
Fax: 405-360-9989
http://www.mntechnology.com
sjohnson@mntechnology.com
Jane Bowen, Superintendent
Barbara Rice, Disability Coordinator
Roger Adair, Director, Finance
Offers a variety of services to students with disabilities including notetakers, extended testing time, counseling services, and special accommodations.

3585 **Northeastern State University**
600 N Grand Ave
Tahlequah, OK 74464-2301
918-456-5511
800-722-9614
Fax: 918-458-2363
http://www.nsuok.edu
offices.nsuok.edu/publicsafety
Dr. Laura D Boren, Vice President Student Affairs
Ben Hardcastle, Executive Director
Dr. Steve Turner, President
Four year college that offers programs and services to disabled students.

3586 **Oklahoma City Community College**
Department of Student Support Services
7777 South May Avenue
Oklahoma City, OK 73159-4444
405-682-1611
Fax: 405-682-7585
TDD: 405-682-7520
TTY: 405-682-7529
http://www.occc.edu
webmaster@occc.edu
Teresa Moisant, Chair
Devery Youngblood, Vice-Chair
Dr. Paul W. Sechrist, President
Comprehensive community college with individualized services and accommodations for students with disabilities arranged by the Office of Student Support Services. Services include Deaf Program, and accommodations as described by section 504 & ADA. Five tutoring labs are available on campus and assistive technology including voice synthesizers and voice recognition for computer based word processing.

3587 **Oklahoma Panhandle State University**
PO Box 430
Goodwell, OK 73939-430
580-349-2611
800-664-OPSU
Fax: 580-349-2302
TDD: 580-349-1559
http://www.opsu.edu
opsu@opsu.edu
David A. Bryan, President
Lynna Brakhage, Director
Apryl Burleson, Financial Aid Conselor
Four year college that offers programs to the learning disabled.

3588 **Oklahoma State University: Oklahoma City Technical School**
900 N Portland Ave
Oklahoma City, OK 73107-6195
405-947-4421
800-580-4099
Fax: 405-945-3289
http://www.osuokc.edu
emilytc@osuokc.edu
Natalie Shirley, President
Shane Crawford, Assoc. Vice President
Rachel Rittenhouse, Secretary
Offers access to students with disabilities based upon the diagnostic documentation which is provided by the student and the functional impact of the disability.

3589 **Oklahoma State University: Okmulgee Technical School**
1801 E 4th Street
Okmulgee, OK 74447-3901
918-293-4678
800-722-4447
Fax: 918-293-4643
http://www.osuit.edu
osuit.admissions@okstate.edu
Claudette Butcher, Exe Assistant to the President
Bill R. Path, President
Dr. Linda Avant, Executive Vice President
Offers a variety of services to students with disabilities including notetakers, extended testing time, counseling services, and special accommodations.

3590 **Oral Roberts University**
7777 South Lewis Avenue
Tulsa, OK 74171
918-495-6161
Fax: 918-495-7229
http://www.oru.edu
droberson@oru.edu
William M. Wilson, President
Reverend Robert Hoskins, Board Chair
Mart Green, Vice Chair
Four year college that offers resources to students with a learning disability.

3591 **Rogers State University**
1701 W Will Rogers Blvd
Claremore, OK 74017-3259
918-343-7777
800-256-7511
Fax: 918-343-7712
http://www.rsu.edu
msith@rsu.edu
Misty Smith, Acting VP for Student Affairs
Richard A. Beck, VP for Academic Affairs
Thomas M. Volturo, EVP Administration and Finance
A public four-year university with several special education students out of a total of approximately 3,300.

3592 **Rose State College**
Academic Support Department
6420 SE 15th Street
Midwest City, OK 73110-2704
405-733-7673
866-621-0987
Fax: 405-733-7399
TDD: 405-736-7308
http://www.rose.edu
rjones@rose.edu

Dr. Jeanie Webb, President
Dr. Jeff Caldwell, Vice President
Betty J.C Wright, Chairman
Services and facilities include academic advisement, referal and liaison with other community agencies, recorded textbooks and individual testing for qualified students.

3593 **Southeastern Oklahoma State University**
1405 North 4th Ave
Durant, OK 74701-609
580-745-2000
800-435-1327
Fax: 580-745-2515
TDD: 580-745-2704
http://www.se.edu
sdodson@sosu.edu
Dr. Doug McMillan, VP for Academic Affairs
Sean Burrage, President
Michele Campbell, Executive Assistant
Four year college that provides services to the learning disabled students.

3594 **Southwestern Oklahoma State University**
100 Campus Drive
Weatherford, OK 73096-3098
580-774-3063
Fax: 580-774-3795
http://www.swosu.edu
cindy.dougherty@swosu.edu
John Hays, President
Offers a variety of services to students with disabilities including notetakers, extended testing time, counseling services, and special accommodations.

3595 **St. Gregory's University**
Partners in Learning
1900 W. MacArthur St.
Shawnee, OK 74804-2403
405-878-5100
Fax: 405-878-5198
TDD: 405-878-5103
http://www.stgregorys.edu
info@stgregorys.edu
D. Gregory Main, President
Donald Wolf, Board Chair
Michael Scaperlanda, Vice Chair
Four-year college offering assistive programs for students with learning disabilities.

3596 **Tulsa Community College**
Disabled Student Resource Center
909 South Boston Avenue
Tulsa, OK 74119-2095
918-595-7000
800-331-3050
Fax: 918-595-7179
TDD: 918-595-7287
http://www.tulsacc.edu
admission@utulsa.edu
Roger N. Blais, Provost/VP for Academic Affairs
Kevan C. Buck, EVP/Treasurer
Dr. Steadman Upham, President
Offers a variety of services to students with disabilities including note takers, extended testing time, counseling services, and special accommodations.

3597 **Tulsa University**
Center for Student Academic Support
800 South Tucker Drive
Tulsa, OK 74104-9700
918-631-2000
Fax: 918-631-5003
TDD: 918-631-3329
http://www.utulsa.edu
jcorso@utulsa.edu
Jane Corso PhD, Director
Ruby Wile, Assistant Director
Dr. Steadman Upham, President
The Center offers a comprehensive range of support services and accommodations for students with disabilities.

3598 **University of Oklahoma**
660 Parrington Oval
Norman, OK 73019-0390
405-325-0311
800-522-0772
Fax: 405-325-7605
TDD: 405-325-4173
http://www.ou.edu/
sdyer@ou.edu
Suzette Dyer, Disability Services Director
Caryn Pacheco, Director, Financial Aid
David L. Boren, President
A public doctoral degree-granting research university. The University of Oklahoma is an equal opportunity institution.

Oregon

3599 **Central Oregon Community College**
2600 NW College Way
Bend, OR 97701-5933
541-383-7700
Fax: 541-383-7506
http://www.cocc.edu
James E. Middleton, President
Julie Smith, Executive Assistant
Jeff Stuermer, Board Chair
Central Oregon Community College will be a leader in regionally and globally responsive adult, lifelong, postsecondary education for Central Oregon.

3600 **Clackamas Community College**
Disability Resource Center
19600 Molalla Avenue
Oregon City, OR 97045
503-594-6100
Fax: 503-722-5865
TDD: 503-650-6649
http://www.clackamas.edu
admissions@clackamas.edu
Joanne Truesdell, President
Lisabeth Pacheco, Disability Coordinator
A public two-year college. Special education services are designed to support student success by creating full access and providing appropriate accommodations for all students with disabilities.

3601 **Corban College**
5000 Deer Park Drive SE
Salem, OR 97317-9392
503-581-8600
Fax: 503-585-4316
http://www.corban.edu
visit@corban.edu
Heidi Stowman, Director of Admissions
Reno Hoff, President
Chris Vetter, Associate Provost
Private four year Christian college offering assistance for learning disabled students.

3602 **George Fox University**
Disability Services Office
414 N Meridian St
Newberg, OR 97132-2697
503-538-8383
800-765-4369
Fax: 503-554-3880
http://ds.georgefox.edu
webmaster@georgefox.edu
Rick Muthiah, Associate Director
Missy Terry, Executive Assistant
Robin Baker, President
An independent faith-based four-year college with a small percentagge of students with disabilities.

3603 **Lane Community College**
4000 East 30th Ave.
Eugene, OR 97405-640
541-463-3100
Fax: 541-463-5201
TDD: 541-463-3079
http://www.lanecc.edu
webmaster@lanecc.edu

Mary Spilde, President
Sonya Christian, Vice-President
Anna Kate Malliris, Assistant to the Vice President
We provide accommodations, technology, advising, support systems, training and education.

3604 Linfield College
900 SE Baker St
McMinnville, OR 97128-6894 503-883-2200
Fax: 503-883-2472
TDD: 503-883-2396
TTY: 503-883-2396
http://www.linfield.edu
admission@linfield.edu
Susan Agre-Kippenhan, VP for Academic Affairs
Thomas L. Hellie, President
Susan Hopp, Vice President
An independent four-year college. Services include tutoring, extended time for testing, assistance with advising and counseling. Student needs are considered in customizing individual programs of support for documented special needs.

3605 Linn-Benton Community College Office of Disability Services
6500 Pacific Blvd. SW
Albany, OR 97321 541-917-4999
Fax: 541-917-4328
TDD: 541-917-4703
http://www.linnbenton.edu/go/ds
ods@linnbenton.edu
Carol Raymundo, Coordinator
Greg Hamann, President
Dave Henderson, Vice President
A public two-year college. LBCC provides a number of services and programs for students with disabilities including classes, supportive services and aids.

3606 Mount Bachelor Academy
33051 NE Ochoco Hwy
Prineville, OR 97754-7990 541-462-3404
800-462-3404
Fax: 541-462-3430
http://www.mtba.com/
Sharon Bitz, Executive Director
Matthew Lovell, Program Director
Kelli Hoffman, Admissions Director
Aspen Education Group is recognized nationwide as the leading provider of education programs for struggling or underachieving young people. As the largest and most comprehensive network of therapeutic schools and programs, Aspen offers professionals and families the opportunity to choose a setting that best meets a student's unique academic and emotional needs.

3607 Mt. Hood Community College Disability Services Department
Learning Disabilities Department
26000 SE Stark St
Gresham, OR 97030-3300 503-491-6422
Fax: 503-491-7670
http://www.mhcc.edu
dsoweb@mhcc.edu
Richard Doughty, VP Administrative Services
Pam Benjamin, Executive Assistant
Debbie Derr, Ed.D, President
A commitment to providing educational opportunities for all students forms the foundation of the disability services program. If you are a student with a disability, disability services will help you overcome potential obstacles so that you may be successful in your area of study. Disability services gives you the needed support to help you meet your goals without separating you and other students with disabilities from existing programs.

3608 Oregon Institute of Technology
Oregon State University Systems
3201 Campus Drive
Klamath Falls, OR 97601-8801 541-885-1000
800-422-2017
Fax: 541-885-1777
TDD: 541-885-1072
TTY: 541-885-1072
http://www.oit.edu
access@oit.edu
Christopher Maples, President
MaryAnn Zemke, VP Finance & Administration
Bradley Burda, Provost/VP For Academic Affairs
A public four-year college enrolling about 3,000 students. Accommodations are tailored to the needs of individual students on a case-by-case basis for those self-identified as having learning disabilities.

3609 Oregon State University
Services for Students with Disabilities
A202 Kerr Administration Building
1500 SW Jefferson Avenue
Corvallis, OR 97331-2133 541-737-4098
Fax: 541-737-7354
TDD: 541-737-3666
http://www.oregonstate.edu
disabilty.services@oregonstate.edu
Martha Smith, Director
Dr. Edward Ray, President
Elizabeth Grubb, Executive Secretary
A public four-year college with a small percentage of students.

3610 Portland Community College
PO Box 19000
Portland, OR 97280-990 503-244-6111
866-922-1010
Fax: 503-977-4882
TTY: 503-246-4072
http://www.pcc.edu
Deanna Palm, Vice Chair
Dr. Jeremy Brown, President
Denise Frisbee, Chair
Our team includes rehabilitation guidance counselors, learning disability specialists, sign language interpreters, a technology specialist, vocational progarm and special needs coordinatiors.

3611 Reed College
3203 SE Woodstock Blvd
Portland, OR 97202 503-777-7511
800-547-4750
Fax: 503-777-7553
http://www.reed.edu
admissions@reed.edu
Hugh Porter, President
Lorraine Arvin, Vice President & Treasurer
Mike Brody, VP, Student Affairs
Offers a variety of services to students with disabilities including notetakers, extended testing time, counseling services, and special accommodations.

3612 Southwestern Oregon Community College
1988 Newmark Ave
Coos Bay, OR 97420-2911 541-888-2525
800-962-2838
Fax: 541-888-7285
http://www.socc.edu
Patty M. Scott,Ed. D., President
Marcia Jensen, Chair
David Bridgham, Vice-Chair
The college will provide reasonable accommodation for students with learning disabilities. Some instructors in academic skills have special training in working with learning disabled students.

3613 **Treasure Valley Community College**
650 College Blvd
Ontario, OR 97914-3423
541-881-8822
Fax: 541-881-2717
http://www.tvcc.cc.or.us

Dana M. Young, President
Randy Griffin, VP Administrative Services
Dr. Rachel Anderson, VP Academic Affairs
Offers a variety of services to students with disabilities including notetakers, extended testing time, counseling services, and special accommodations.

3614 **Umpqua Community College**
PO Box 967
1140 Umpqua College Rd
Roseburg, OR 97470-226
541-440-4622
Fax: 541-440-4666
http://www.umpqua.edu

Elin Miller, Board Chair
David Beyer, Administrator
Dr. Joe Olson, UCC President
A public two-year college with a small percentage of special education students.

3615 **University of Oregon**
5278 University of Oregon
164 Oregon Hall
Eugene, OR 97403-5278
541-346-1155
Fax: 541-346-6013
TTY: 541-346-1155
http://www.ds.uoregon.edu
uoaec@uoregon.edu

Michele Gottfredson, President
Yvette Marie Alex-Assensoh, VP Equity and Inclusion
Scott Coltrane, SVP/Provost
A public four-year college with about 5% of students with disabilities.

3616 **Warner Pacific College**
2219 SE 68th Ave
Portland, OR 97215-4099
503-517-1142
800-582-7885
Fax: 503-517-1350
http://www.warnerpacific.edu
webmaster@warnerpacific.edu

Andrea P. Cook, Ph.D., President
Steve Anderson, Chair
Steve Robertson, Vice-Chair
Offers a variety of services to students with disabilities including notetakers, extended testing time, counseling services, and special accommodations.

3617 **Western Oregon University**
345 N. Monmouth Avenue
Monmouth, OR 97361-1371
503-838-8000
877-877-1593
Fax: 503-838-8399
http://www.wou.edu
webmaster@wou.edu

Louann Brant, Program Assistant
Mark D. Weiss, President
Malissa Larson, Director
A public four-year college. Strives to provide and promote a supportive, accessible, non-discriminatory learning and working environment for students, faculty, staff and community members with disabilities. These goals are realized through the provision of individualized support services, advocacy and the identification of current technology and information.

3618 **Willamette University**
Learning Disabilities Department
900 State Street
Salem, OR 97301-3930
503-370-6300
Fax: 503-370-6148
TDD: 503-375-5383
http://www.willamette.edu/dept/disability/main.
jhill@willamette.edu

Kristen Grainger, VP
Marlene Moore, VP Academic Affairs
Stephen E. Thorsett, President
Offers a variety of services to students with disabilities including notetakers, extended testing time, counseling services, and special accommodations. Provides services for all students on campus, including graduate schools.

Pennsylvania

3619 **Albright College**
13th & Bern Streets
P.O. Box 15234
Reading, PA 19612-5234
610-921-2381
Fax: 610-921-7530
http://www.albright.edu
albright@alb.edu

Kathleen C. Hittner, M.D, Vice Chair
Lex O. McMillan III, Ph.D., President
Jeffrey J. Joyce, Chair
An independent four-year college with a small percentage of special education students. There is an additional fee for the education program in addition to the regular tuition.

3620 **Bloomsburg University**
400 E. Second St.
Bloomsburg, PA 17815-1301
570-389-4000
Fax: 570-389-3700
http://www.bloomu.edu
buadmiss@bloomu.edu

MAry Vasta, Vice Chairperson
David L. Soltz, President
Patrick Wilson, Chairperson
Offers a variety of services to students with disabilities including notetakers, extended testing time, counseling services, and special accommodations.

3621 **Bryn Mawr College**
Educational Support Services
101 North Merion Avenue
Bryn Mawr, PA 19010-2899
610-526-5000
Fax: 610-526-6525
http://www.brynmawr.edu
info@brynmawr.edu

Kim Cassidy, President
Marge Garber, Vice President
Jerry Berenson, Chief Administrative Officer
Bryn Mawr is a private liberal arts college located in Bryn Mawr, Pennsylvania not far from Philadelphia. The College provides support services for qualified students with documented learning, physical, and psychological disabilities. For additional information visit www.brynmawr.edu/access_services .

3622 **Cabrini College**
Disability Support Services
610 King of Prussia Rd
Radnor, PA 19087-3698
610-902-8100
Fax: 610-902-8204
TDD: 610-902-8582
http://www.cabrini.edu
ama722@cabrini.edu

Thomas P. Nerney, Chair
Frank R. Emmerich Jr., Vice Chair
Donald B. Taylor, Ph.D., President
Offers support services and appropriate accommodations to students with documented learning disabilities.

3623 **Carnegie Mellon University**
Equal Opportunity Services, Disability Resources
143 North Craig Street
Whitfield Hall
Pittsburgh, PA 15213
412-268-3386
Fax: 412-268-1524
http://www.cmu.edu/hr/eos/disability/index.html
hrhelp@andrew.cmu.edu

Larry Powell, Manager, Disability Resources
Daniel McNulty, Interim Associate Vice President
Haley Lantz, Senior Administrative
Four year college that offers its students services for the learning disabled.

3624 **College Misericordia**
Alternative Learners Project
301 Lake St
Dallas, PA 18612-1090
570-674-6400
800-262-6363
Fax: 570-675-2441
http://www.misericordia.edu
info@misericordia.edu
Thomas J. Botzman, Ph.D, President
John Metz, Chair
Christopher Borton, Vice Chair
An independent four-year college with about 5% special education students.

3625 **Community College of Allegheny County: College Center, North Campus**
Learning Disabilities Services
8701 Perry Highway
Pittsburgh, PA 15237-5353
412-366-7000
Fax: 412-366-7000
TDD: 412-369-4110
TTY: 412-369-4110
http://www.ccac.edu
kwhite@ccac.edu
Amy M. Kuntz, Chair
Quintin B. Bullock, President
Mary Frances Archey, VP Student Success & Completion
Support services for students with disabilities are provided according to individual needs. Services include assistance with testing, advisement, registration, classroom accommodations, professor and agency contact.

3626 **Community College of Allegheny County: Boyce Campus**
595 Beatty Road
Monroeville, PA 15146-1396
724-327-1327
Fax: 724-325-6733
TTY: 724-325-6733
http://www.ccac.edu
mailto:Pflorent@ccac.edu
Amy M. Kuntz, Chair
Quintin B. Bullock, President
Mary Frances Archey, VP Student Success & Completion
A 2 year community college campus in a suburban setting. Offers a variety of services to students with disabilities including notetakers, extended testing time, counseling services, and special accommodations.

3627 **Community College of Philadelphia**
Center on Disability
1700 Spring Garden Street
Philadelphia, PA 19130-3991
215-751-8010
Fax: 215-751-8762
http://www.ccp.edu
fdirosa@ccp.edu
Dr. Donald Generals, President
Matthew Bergheiser, Chair
Suzanne Biemiller, Vice Chair
ÿWith more than 70 associate's degree, certification and continuing education programs, a lively campus near Center City, and a supportive, top-flight faculty,ÿCommunity College of Philadelphia is your path to possibilities.

3628 **Delaware County Community College**
901 S. Media Line Road
Media, PA 19063-1027
610-359-5000
Fax: 610-359-5055
TDD: 610-359-5020
TTY: 610-359-5020
http://www.dccc.edu
abinder@dccc.edu
Donald L. Heller, Vice-Chair
Jerome S. Parker, President
Michael L. Ranck, Chair
Delaware County Community College, the ninth largest college in the Philadelphia metropolitan area, is a public, two year institution offering more than 60 programs of study. Its open-door policy, and affordable tuition make it accessible to all. Services to physically and learning disabled students include counseling services, tutoring, extended testing, tape recorded lectures, spelling allowances, assistive equipment, notes copied and study skills workshops.

3629 **Delaware Valley College of Science and Agriculture**
700 East Butler Ave
Doylestown, PA 18901-2698
215-345-1500
Fax: 215-230-2968
http://www.delval.edu
Admitme@delval.edu
Frances Flood, Transfer Coordinator
Bashar W. Hanna, VP Academic Affairs
Thomas O'Connor, Associate Director of Admission
Offers a variety of services to students with disabilities including notetakers, extended testing time, counseling services, and special accommodations.

3630 **Delaware Valley Friends School**
19 E Central Avenue
Paoli, PA 19301-1345
610-640-4150
Fax: 610-296-9970
http://www.dvfs.org
Pritchard Garrett, Head of School
Rick Mosenkis, President and CEO
Robert Turner, Chairman
Our mission is to prepare students with learning differences for future work and study.

3631 **Dickinson College**
Services for Students with Disabilities
Post Office Box 1773
Carlisle, PA 17013-2896
717-243-5121
800-644-1773
Fax: 717-245-1080
TTY: 717-245-1134
http://www.dickenson.edu
admissions@dickinson.edu
Bronte Jones, VP Finance and Administration
Nancy A. Roseman, President
Joyce Bylander, VP, Student Development
The Office of Counseling and Disability Services is dedicated to the enhancement of healthy student development. Professional and paraprofessional staff offer confidential individual and group counseling sessions and outreach services which help students with both general developmental issues and with specific personal or interpersonal difficulties.

3632 **Drexel University**
Office of Disability Services
3141 Chestnut Street
Main Building, Room 212, 2nd Floor
Philadelphia, PA 19104-2875
215-895-2000
Fax: 215-895-1414
http://www.drexel.edu
John A. Fry, President
Mark L. Greenberg, PhD, Provost and SVP
Susan C. Aldridge, PhD, Senior Vice President
Drexel University's mission is to serve their students and society through comprehensive integrated academic offerings enhanced by technology, co-operative education, and clinical practice in an urban setting, with global outreach embracing research, scholarly activities, and community initiatives.

3633 **East Stroudsburg University of Pennsylvania**
200 Prospect St
East Stroudsburg, PA 18301-2999
570-422-3211
877-230-5547
Fax: 570-422-3777
TDD: 570-422-3543
http://www.esu.edu
emiller@po-box.esu.edu

Marcia G. Welsh, Ph.D., President
L. Patrick Ross, Chair
Nancy V. Perretta, Vice Chair
Four year college that offers services to disabled students.

3634 **Gannon University**
Program for Students with Learning Disabilities
109 University Square
Erie, PA 16541
814-871-7000
814-426-6668
Fax: 814-871-7338
http://www.gannon.edu
theisen001@gannon.edu

Thomas C. Guelcher, Vice Chairperson
Keith Taylor, Ph.D., President
Lawrence T. Persico, Chairperson
Special Support Services are provided for students who have a diagnosed learning disability and choose to enroll in PSLO. Charge of $300.00 per semester special services include individual sessions with Educational Specialists, Kurzweil Reader, Copying Services, Advocacy Seminar Courses I and II, Reading Efficiency sessions, testing accommodations, etc.

3635 **Gettysburg College**
300 N Washington Street
Gettysburg, PA 17325-1483
717-337-6100
800-431-0803
Fax: 717-337-6145
http://www.gettysburg.edu
admiss@gettysburg.edu

Janet Morgan Riggs, President
Gail Sweezey, Director of Admissions
Darryl Jones, Senior Associate Director
Offers a variety of services to students with disabilities including notetakers, extended testing time, counseling services, and special accommodations.

3636 **Gwynedd: Mercy College**
PO Box 901
1325 Sumneytown Pike
Gwynedd Valley, PA 19437-901
215-646-7300
800-342-5462
Fax: 215-641-5598
http://www.gmc.edu
guido.r@gmc.edu

Dr. Frank E. Scully, Jr., VP for Academic Affairs
Kathleen Owens, PhD, President
Kevin O'Flaherty, VP Finance and Administration
Recognizing the diversity of our student population and the challenges and needs this brings to the educational enterprise, Gwynedd-Mercy College, within the bounds of its resources, intends to provide reasonable accommodations for students with disabilities so that all students accepted into a program of study have equal access and subsequent opportunity to reach their academic and personal goals. Requests for specific accommodations are processed on an individual basis.

3637 **Harcum Junior College**
750 Montgomery Ave
Bryn Mawr, PA 19010-3476
610-525-4100
Fax: 610-526-6086
http://www.harcum.edu

Denise Beauchamp, Executive Director
Susan E. Barrett, Ed.D., Vice President
Jon Jay DeTemple, PhDÿ, President
An independent two-year college. There is an additional fee for the special education program in addition to the regular tuition.

3638 **Harrisburg Area Community College**
Disability Services Office
One Hacc Drive
Harrisburg, PA 17110-2999
717-780-2538
800-222-4222
Fax: 717-780-2551
http://www.hacc.edu
bookstor@hacc.edu

Edna V Baehre, Affairs/Enrollment Management
Carol Keeper, Director
John J. Sygielski, President
A public two-year college with a small percentage of special needs students.

3639 **Hill Top Preparatory School**
737 S. Ithan Ave.
Rosemont, PA 19010
610-527-3230
Fax: 610-527-7683
http://www.hilltopprep.org

Tom Needham, Headmaster
Lex Nugent, Business Manager
Prepares students in grades 5-12 with diagnosed learning differences for higher education and successful futures. The school is a co-educational day school that offers an individually structured, rigorous curriculum that is complemented by a counseling support and menotoring program.

3640 **Indiana University of Pennsylvania**
1011 South Dr ive
Indiana, PA 15705-1098
724-357-2100
800-442-6830
Fax: 724-357-6281
TDD: 724-357-4067
http://www.iup.edu/advisingtesting
admissions_inquiry@iup.edu

Michael A. Driscoll, President
Susan S. Delaney, Chair
Jonathan B. Mack, Vice Chair
Disability Support Services is a component of the Advising and Testing Center. The mission of DSS is to ensure that students with disabilities who attend Indiana University of Pennsylvainia receive an integrated, quality education.

3641 **Keystone Junior College**
P.O .Box 50
One College Green
La Plume, PA 18440-0200
570-945-8000
877-4college
Fax: 570-945-8962
http://www.keystone.edu
admissions@keystone.edu

Dr. David Coppola, President
Cheryl Guse, Executive Assistant
Nancy Allan, Secretary to the President
Offers a variety of services to students with disabilities including notetakers, extended testing time, counseling services, and special accommodations.

3642 **King's College**
Academic Skills Center
133 N River Street
Wilkes Barre, PA 18711-801
570-208-5900
Fax: 570-208-5967
http://www.kings.edu
admissions@kings.edu

John Ryan, C.S.C., Ph.D., President
Thomas R. Smith, Chairman
Mark DeCesaris, Vice Chairman
First Year Academic Studies Program (FASP) - A proactive program to facilitate transition to college with intensive first-year programming with indivdual support in subsequent years. Students are enrolled as full-time students completing general education and major course requirements. Support includes regular meetings with a learning disability specialist, faculty tutorials/study groups, priority advisement, and development of self-advocacy skills. A fee charged for the first year.

3643 **Kutztown University of Pennsylvania**
15200 Kutztown Road
Kutztown, PA 19530
610-683-4000
Fax: 610-683-1520
TDD: 610-683-4499
http://www.kutztown.edu
sutherla@kutztown.edu
Jesus Pena, Esq, Associate Vice President
Dr. Carlos Vargas-Aburto, Acting President
Gerald Silberman, VP Administration and Finance
Kutztown University of Pennsylvania, a member of the Pennsylvania State System of Higher Education, was founded in 1856 as Keystone Normal School, and achieved University status in 1983. Today Kutztown University is a modern, comprehensive University. There are approximately 7,900 full and part time undergraduate and graduate students.

3644 **Lebanon Valley College**
101 N College Avenue
Annville, PA 17003-1400
717-867-6275
Fax: 717-867-6124
http://www.lvc.edu
perry@lvc.edu
Dr. Lewis Evitts Thayne, President
Shawn P. Curtin, VP Finance and Administration
Karen M. Feather, Executive Assistantt
Four year college that offers learning disabled students support and services.

3645 **Lehigh Carbon Community College**
4525 Education Park Drive
Schnecksville, PA 18078-2598
610-799-2121
Fax: 610-799-1527
TTY: 610-799-1792
http://www.lccc.edu
mmitchell@lccc.edu or lkelly@lccc.edu
Thomas C. Leamer, President
Brian Kahler, VP Finance and Facilities
Audrey L. Larvey, Chair
Disability Support Services provides learning support to qualified students with disabilities in compliance with section 504 of the Rehabilitation Act and Americans with Disabilities Act, 1990. Requests for access and/or academic accommodations are reviewed on a case by case basis. Additional learning support is available through Educational Support Services.

3646 **Lock Haven University of Pennsylvania**
Learning Disabilities Office
401 N Fairview St
Lock Haven, PA 17745-2390
570-893-2011
800-332-8900
Fax: 570-893-2432
http://www.lhup.edu
admissions@lhup.edu
Dr. Michael Fiorentino, Jr., President
Dr. Donna Wilson, Provost/SVP
William Hanelly, VP Finance and Administration
A public four-year college with a small percentage of students with disabilities.

3647 **Lycoming College**
700 College Place
Williamsport, PA 17701
570-321-4000
800-345-3920
Fax: 570-321-4337
http://www.lycoming.edu
webmaster@lycoming.edu
Peter R. Lynn, Chair of the Board
Kent Trachte, Ph.D., President
Jeff Bennett, VP Finance and Administration
An independent four-year college with a small percentage of special education students.

3648 **Manor Junior College**
700 Fox Chase Road
Jenkintown, PA 19046-3399
215-885-2360
Fax: 215-576-6564
http://www.manor.edu
ftadmiss@manor.edu
Sister Mary Cecilia Jurasinski, President
Sally Mydlowec, Executive Vice President
Jeffrey Levine, M.Ed., Director of Admissions
Offers a variety of services to students with disabilities including notetakers, extended testing time, counseling services, and special accommodations.

3649 **Mansfield University of Pennsylvania**
Services for Students with Learning Disabilities
31 South Academy St.
Ste. 1
Mansfield, PA 16933
570-662-4000
800-577-6826
Fax: 570-662-4995
http://www.mansfield.edu
wchabala@mansfield.edu
Steven M. Crawford, Vice Chairman
Francis L. Hendricks, President
Ralph H. Meyer, Chairman
Offers a variety of services to students with disabilities including, extended testing time, counseling services, and special accommodations.

3650 **Marywood University**
Special Education Department
2300 Adams Avenue
Scranton, PA 18509-1598
570-348-6211
866-279-9663
Fax: 570-961-4739
http://www.marywood.edu
Anne Munley, I.H.M., Ph.D., President
Alan M. Levine, Ph.D., Vice President
Marion Munley, Chair
Marywood challenges students to broaden their understanding of globale issues and to make decisions based on spiritual, ethical, and religious values.

3651 **Mercyhurst College**
Learning Differences Program
501 East 38th Street
Erie, PA 16546
814-824-2000
800-825-1926
Fax: 814-824-2438
http://www.mercyhurst.edu
drogers@mercyhurst.edu
Thomas J. Gamble, Ph.D., President
Marlene D Mosco, Chair of the Board
Richard A. Lanzillo, Vice Chair
Mercyhurst provides a comprehensive program of academic accommodations and support services to students with documented learning disabilities. Accommodations may include audiotaped textbooks, extended time for tests, a test reader and use of a computer to complete essay tests.

3652 **Messiah College**
One College Avenue
Suite 3059
Mechanicsburg, PA 17055-9800
717-796-5382
800-233-4220
Fax: 717-796-5217
http://www.messiah.edu
disabilityservices@messiah.edu
Kim S. Phipps, Ph.D., President
Anne Barnes, Executive Assistant
Carol Wickey, Special Assistant
Private Christian college.

3653 **Millersville University of Pennsylvania**
Disability and Learning Services
1 South George St
P.O. Box 1002
Millersville, PA 17551-302 717-872-3011
Fax: 717-871-2129
http://www.millersv.edu
admissions@millersville.edu
John M. Anderson, Ph.D., President
Dr. Aminta Hawkins Breaux, Vice President
Michael G. Warfel, Chairman
Four year college that provides services to learning disabled students.

3654 **Moravian College**
1200 Main Street
Bethlehem, PA 18018 610-861-1320
800-441-3191
Fax: 610-861-1577
http://www.moravian.edu
memld02@moravian.edu
Robert J. Schoenen, Jr., Vice Chair
Bryon L. Grigsby, President
Kenneth J. Rampolla, Chair
Four year college that offers programs for the learning disabled.

3655 **Northampton Community College**
Disability Support Services
3835 Green Pond Rd
Bethlehem, PA 18020-7599 610-861-5300
Fax: 610-861-5373
TDD: 610-861-5351
http://www.northampton.edu/disabilityservices
LDemshock@northampton.edu
Robert R. Fehnel, Vice Chairman
Dr. Mark H. Erickson, President
Karl A. Stackhouse, Chairman
Encourages academically qualified students with disabilities to take advantage of educational programs. Services and accommodations are offered to facilitate accessiblity to both college programs and facilities. Services provided to students with disabilities are based upon each student individual needs.

3656 **Pace School**
2432 Greensburg Pike
Pittsburgh, PA 15221-3611 412-244-1900
Fax: 412-244-0100
http://www.paceschool.org
pace@paceschool.org
Gerri L. Sperling, President
Robert Gold, Vice President
Brian P. Fagan, Secretary
A placement option for school districts in Allegheny and surrounding counties that serves kids, K-9, with emotional challenges or Autism.

3657 **Pathway School**
162 Egypt Rd.
Jeffersonville, PA 19403 610-277-0660
http://www.pathwayschool.org
info@pathwayschool.org
William S. Harrigan, Chair
Edmond A. Watters III, Vice Chair
Brad Kerr, Treasurer
Provides a comprehensive program of services for children between the ages of 9 and 21 for whom mainstream public and private school education is insufficient to meet their needs. These youngsters display severe neuropsychiatric disorders and complex learning issues necessitating focused learning environments.

3658 **Pennsylvania Institute of Technology**
800 Manchester Ave
Media, PA 19063-4089 610-892-1000
800-422-0025
Fax: 610-892-1510
http://www.pit.edu
info@pit.edu
Walter R. Garrison, President
Gerard C. Gambs Jr., Program Manager
Raymond P. Altieri, Chair
Offers a variety of services to students with disabilities including notetakers, extended testing time, counseling services, and special accommodations.

3659 **Pennsylvania State University**
Support Services for Students with Learning Disab
116 Boucke Building
University Park, PA 16802-5902 814-863-1807
Fax: 814-863-3217
TDD: 814-863-1807
http://www.equity.psu.edu/ods
william.welsh@equity.psu.edu/ods
Eric J. Barron, President
Keith Masser, Chairman
Janine S. Andrews, Director
Penn State provides academic accommodations and support services to students with documented learning disabilities. Accommodations may include audiotaped textbooks, extended time for tests, a test reader and use of a computer to complete essay tests.

3660 **Pennsylvania State University: Mont Alto**
1 Campus Dr
Mont Alto, PA 17237-9799 717-749-6000
Fax: 717-749-6116
http://www.ma.psu.edu
nmhz@psu.edu
Derk S. Barnett, Assistant Director of Admissions
Dr. Francis Achampong, Chancellor
Dr. Michael Doncheski, Director of Academic Affairs
It is the intention of Penn State University to provide equal access to students with disabilities as mandated by the Americans with Disabilities Act, and the Rehabilitiation Act. Students with disabilities are encouraged to take advantage of the support services provided to help them successfully meet the high academic standards of the university.

3661 **Pennsylvania State University: Schuylkill Campus**
Disability Services
200 University Drive
Schuylkill Haven, PA 17972-2202 570-385-6000
Fax: 570-385-3672
http://www.sl.psu.edu
Allen E. Kiefer, President
Charles M. Miller, 1st Vice President
Dr. Jack T. Dolbin, 2nd Vice President
Offers a variety of services to students with disabilities including notetakers, extended testing time, counseling services, and special accommodations.

3662 **Pennsylvania State University: Shenango Valley Campus**
Office for Disability Services
147 Shenango Avenue
Sharon Hall 207
Sharon, PA 16146-5902 724-983-2803
Fax: 724-983-2820
TDD: 814-863-1807
TTY: 814-863-1807
http://www.equity.psu.edu/ods
william.welsh@equity.psu.edu/ods
Thomas Burich, President
Sam Bernstine, Vice President
Fredric M. Leeds, Secretary

Penn State encourages academically qualified students with disabilities to take advantage of its educational programs. To be eligible for disability related accommodations, individuals must have a documented disability as defined by the Americans with Disabilities Act. A disability is defined by the physical or mental impairment that substantially limits a major life function. Individuals seeking accommodations are required to provided documentation.

3663 **Pennsylvania State University: Worthington Scranton Campus**
120 Ridgeview Drive
Dunmore, PA 18512-1699
570-963-2500
Fax: 570-963-2535
http://www.sn.psu.edu

Dean L. Butler, Chair
Darlene Dunay D.O., Vice Chair
Dr. Alan Peslak, President
Penn State encourages academically qualified students with disabilities to take advantage of its educational programs. It is the policy of the university not to discriminate against persons with disabilities in its admissions policies or procedures or its educational programs, services and activities.

3664 **Point Park College**
Program for Academic Success
201 Wood Street
Pittsburgh, PA 15222-1984
412-391-4100
800-321-0129
Fax: 412-392-3998
http://www.pointpark.edu
pboykin@pointpark.edu

Dr. Karen S. McIntyre, SVP, Academics
Dr. Paul Hennigan, President
Anne Lewis, Chair
Provides appropriate, reasonable accommodations for students who are disabled in accordance with the Americans with Disabilities Act. All campus accommodations are coordinated through the Program for Academic Success (PAS).

3665 **Reading Area Community College**
10 South Second Street
Reading, PA 19603-1706
610-372-4721
800-626-1665
Fax: 610-607-6264
http://www.racc.edu

Dr. Anna Weitz, President
Edwin L. Stock, Chair
Zylkia R. Rivera, Vice Chair
A public two-year college with a small percentage of special education students.

3666 **Seton Hill University**
One Seton Hill Drive
Greensburg, PA 15601
724-834-2200
800-826-6234
Fax: 724-834-2752
TTY: 724-830-1151
http://www.setonhill.edu
bassi@setonhill.edu

Michele Ridgeÿ, Chair
David Myron, Vice President for Finance, CFO
Mary C. Finger, President
Offers programs to those who are eligible and learning disabled.

3667 **Shippensburg University of Pennsylvania**
1871 Old Main Drive
Shippensburg, PA 17257-2299
717-477-1301
Fax: 717-477-1273
http://www.ship.edu
lawate@wharf.ship.edu

Dr. Jody Harpster, President
Robin Maun, Executive Assistant
Joy Arnold, Secretary to the President
Four year college that offers services to the learning disabled students.

3668 **Solebury School**
Learning Skills Program
6832 Phillips Mill Road
New Hope, PA 18938-9682
215-862-5261
Fax: 215-862-3366
http://www.solebury.org
admissions@solebury.org

Tom Wilschutz, Head of School
Scott Eckstein, Director of Admission
Janice Poinsett, Associate Director of Admission
A special program for bright students who are hampered by specific learning differences. It is ideally suited for students who require specialized instruction to assist them in unlocking their potential.

3669 **Stratford Friends School**
2 Bishop Hollow Rd.
Newtown Square, PA 19073
610-355-9580
Fax: 610-355-9585
http://www.stratfordfriends.org
info@stratfordfriends.org

Jill Dougherty, Head of School
Bethann Lynch, Director, Advancement
Corinne News, Associate Head of School
Offer programs for students with language-based learning disabilities who have had difficulty learning in a traditional classroom.

3670 **Summer Matters**
1777 North Valley Rd
PO Box 730
Paoli, PA 19301
610-296-6725
Fax: 610-640-0132
http://www.summermatters.org
info@summermatters.org

James Kirkpatrick, Chief Financial Officer
Scott Wheeler, Chair
Mark Oebbecke, Vice-Chair
Represents a continuum of innovative summer enrichment and remedial experiences for youth and young adults. Offers 3 separate and unique programs for learning and fun.

3671 **Temple University**
1301 Cecil B Moore Avenue
100 Ritter Annex
Philadelphia, PA 19122
215-204-1280
Fax: 215-204-6794
TTY: 215-204-1786
http://www.temple.edu/disability
drs@temple.edu

Vanessa Dash, Student Services Coordinator
Reene Kirby, Assistant Director
Aaron Spector, Associate Director
Offers a variety of services to students with disabilities including proctoring, interpreting and academic accommodations.

3672 **Thaddeus Stevens College of Technology**
750 East King Street
Lancaster, PA 17602-3198
717-299-7701
800-842-3832
Fax: 717-391-6929
http://www.stevenscollege.edu
admissions@stevenscollege.edu

Ronald E. Ford, Vice Chair
William E. Griscom, ED.D., President
Donna Kreiser, Chairperson
A 2-year trade and technical college primarily serving socially and economically under-resourced students.

3673 **Thiel College**
Office of Special Needs
75 College Ave
Greenville, PA 16125-2181
724-589-2000
800-248-4435
Fax: 724-589-2850
http://www.thiel.edu
scowan@thiel.edu

Mark Benninghoff, Chair
Lynn Franken, Ph.D., VP Academic Affairs
Troy D. VanAken, Ph.D., President
Four year college that provides an Office of Special Needs for those students with disabilities.

3674 **University of Pennsylvania**
3101 Walnut Street
Philadelphia, PA 19104 215-898-5000
Fax: 215-898-5756
http://www.upenn.edu
lrcmail@pobox.upenn.edu
Valerie Dorsey Allen, Director
Gregory S. Rost, Vice President/Chief of Staff
Dr. Amy Gutmann, President
Services for People with Disabilities coordinates academic support services for students with disabilities; services include readers, notetakers, library research assistants, tutors or transcribers.

3675 **University of Pittsburgh: Bradford**
Learning Development Department
300 Campus Drive
Bradford, PA 16701-2898 814-362-7500
800-872-1787
Fax: 814-362-7684
http://www.upb.pitt.edu
William C. Conrad, Executive Director
Thomas R. Bromeley, Chairman and CEO
Dr. Livingst Alexander, President
Offers a variety of services to students with disabilities including extended testing time, counseling services, and special accommodations.

3676 **University of Pittsburgh: Greensburg**
Disabilities Services Office
150 Finoli Drive
Greensburg, PA 15601 724-837-7040
Fax: 724-836-7134
http://www.pitt.edu/~upg
upgadmit@pitt.edu
Rick A. Fogle, Dean of Student Services
J. Wesley Jamison, VP Academic Affairs
Sharon P. Smith, PhDÿ, President
The Learning Resources Center is an important place for students with disabilities at Pitt Greensburg. Students are encouraged to register with Lou Ann Sears to recieve any accommodations they are entitled to.

3677 **University of Scranton**
Memorial Hall
800 Linden Street
Scranton, PA 18510-4699 570-941-7400
Fax: 570-941-7899
http://http://matrix.scranton.edu
addmissions@scranton.edu
Donald R. Boomgaarden, Ph.D., Provost/Senior Vice President
Kevin P. Quinn, S.J., President
Gary R. Olsen, Vice President
Four year college that offers programs for learning disabled students.

3678 **University of the Arts**
320 S Broad St
Philadelphia, PA 19102-4994 215-717-6030
800-616-2787
Fax: 215-717-6045
http://www.uarts.edu
Sean T. Buffington, President
Thomas H. Carnwath, VP
Megan Storti, Executive Assistant
Within this community of artists, the process of learning engages, refines, and articulates all of our creative capabilities; the Office of Educational Accessibility is here to assist students with disabilities in the pursuit of their personal, creative, artisitic and educational objectives.

3679 **Ursinus College**
PO Box 1000
Collegeville, PA 19426-1000 610-409-3000
Fax: 610-489-0627
http://www.ursinus.edu
admissions@ursinus.edu
Jonathan Ivec, VP for Finance & Administration
Bobby Fong, President
Terry Winegar, Dean of the College
Offers a variety of services to students with disabilities including notetakers, extended testing time, counseling services, and special accommodations.

3680 **Valley Forge Educational Services**
1777 North Valley Road
PO Box 730
Paoli, PA 19301 610-296-6725
Fax: 610-640-0132
http://www.vfes.net
info@vfes.net
Tim Krushinski, Director of The Vanguard School
Janet McDwell, Admin Assistant for Director
Lynne Sansone, Administrative Assistant
Offers a wide variety of educational services focused on guiding 21st century learners to independence. Provides premier educational optoins for young children, adolescents and pre-21 adults ranging from school-based and summer programs to career planning to clinical and consulting services.

3681 **Vanguard School**
1777 North Valley Rd.
Malvern, PA 19355 610-296-6700
Fax: 610-296-6530
http://www.vfes.net/vanguard
Dr. Grace Fornicola, Executive Director
Dr. Darren Levin, Director, Clinical Services
Lisa Wood, Director, Education
Serves students whose exceptionalities include austism spectrum disorders, mild emotional disturbance, and cognitive disabilities.

3682 **Washington and Jefferson College**
60 South Lincoln Street
Washington, PA 15301-4801 724-229-5139
888-926-3529
Fax: 724-503-1049
http://www.washjeff.edu
SAIL@washjeff.edu
Tori Haring-Smith, President
Denny Trelka, Dean
John Zimmerman, VP Academic Affairsÿ
An independent four-year college with a small percentage of special education students.

3683 **Westmoreland County Community College**
145 Pavilion Lane
Youngwood, PA 15697 724-925-4000
800-262-2103
Fax: 724-925-3823
TDD: 724-925-4297
http://www.wccc.edu
beresm@wccc-pa.edu
Kevin Pahach, Vice Chairman
Larry J. Larese, Chairman
Tuesday Stanley, President
Offers a variety of services to students with disabilities including notetakers, extended testing time, counseling services, and special accommodations. All services are based on a review of a current evaluation presented by the student. Appropriate services are then arranged by the student support service counselor.

3684 **Widener University**
Disabilities Services
One University Place
Chester, PA 19013-5792
610-499-4000
Fax: 610-499-4386
http://www.widener.edu
csimonds@mail.widener.edu
James T Harris III, President
Linda S. Durant, MEd, SVP for University Advancement
Nicholas P. Trainer, Chairÿ
An independent four-year college with comprehensive support services, including disabilities services, academic coaching, tutoring services, a math center and writing center.

Rhode Island

3685 **Brown University, Disability Support Services**
20 Benevolent St
Box 1876
Providence, RI 02912-9012
401-863-2378
Fax: 401-863-9300
TDD: 401-863-9588
http://www.brown.edu
dss@brown.edu
Kimberly Roskiewicz, Assistant To The President
Christina H. Paxson, President
Elizabeth Huidekoper, EVP Administration and Finance
Brown University has as its primary aim the education of a highly qualified and diverse student body and respects each student's dignity, capacity to contribute, and desire for personal growth and accomplishment. Brown's commitment to students with disabilities is based on awareness of what students require for success. The University desires to foster both intellectual and physical independence to the greatest extent possible in all of its students.

3686 **Bryant College**
Academic Services
1150 Douglas Pike
Smithfield, RI 02917-1287
401-232-6000
Fax: 401-232-6319
http://www.bryant.edu
lhazard@bryant.edu
Ronald K. Machtley, President
James Damron, VP for University Advancement
James Patti, M.B.A., Executive Assistant
An independent four-year Business and Liberal Arts College. A learning specialist is on campus to provide services for students with learning disabilities.

3687 **Community College of Rhode Island: Knight Campus**
400 East Ave
Warwick, RI 02886-1807
401-825-1000
Fax: 401-825-2365
http://www.ccri.edu
webservices@ccri.edu
Deb Zielinski, Assistant to the President
Ray M. Di Pasquale, President
Greg Lamontagne, VP Academic Affairs
Academic accommodations are available to students with disabilities who demonstrate a documented need for the requested accommodation. Accommodations include but are not limited to adapted equipment, alternative testing, course accommodations, sign language interpreters, reader/audio taping services, scribes and peer note-takers.

3688 **Disability Services for Students**
University of Rhode Island
302 Memorial Union
Kingston, RI 02881
401-874-2098
Fax: 401-874-5574
TTY: 800-745-5555
http://www.uri.edu
dss@etal.uri.edu
Dr. David M. Dooley, President
Dr. Gerald Sonnendeld, VP Research & Economic Dev
Naomi R. Thompson, AVP Community
Disability Service for Students fosters a barrier free environment to individuals with disabilities through education that focuses on inclusion, awareness, and knowledge of ADA/504 compliance. Our mission is two fold: 1. To encourage a sense of empowerment for students with disabilities by providing a process that involves the student. 2. To be an information resource to the University faculty and staff regarding disability awareness and academic services.

3689 **Johnson & Wales University**
8 Abbott Park Place
Providence, RI 02903-3775
401-598-1000
800-343-2565
Fax: 401-598-2880
http://www.jwc.edu
mberstein@jwu.edu
Mim Runey, President
Marie Bernardo-Sousa, SVP Administration
Diane H. D'Ambra, VP Human Resources
An independent four-year university servicing about 5% special education students. Accommodations are individualized to students presenting documentation and may include extended time testing, tape recorders in class, notetaking assistance, reduced course load, preferential scheduling and tutorial assistance.

3690 **Providence College**
Disability Support Services
1 Cunningham Square
Providence, RI 02918
401-865-1000
Fax: 401-865-2057
TDD: 401-865-2494
http://www.providence.edu/oas
oas@providence.edu
Nancy Kelley, Executive Assis to the President
Brian J. Shanley, President
Kenneth Sicard, O.P., Executive Vice President
Offers a variety of services to students with disabilities including note takers, extended testing time, counseling services, and special accommodations.

3691 **Rhode Island College**
Paul V Sherlock Center on Disabilities
600 Mount Pleasant Ave
Providence, RI 02908-1991
401-456-8072
Fax: 401-456-8150
TDD: 401-456-8773
http://www.sherlockcenter.org
aantosh@ric.edu
Michael Ducharme, Director
Patricia Nolin, Special Assistant
Nancy Carriuolo, President
The University Affiliated Program (UAP) of Rhode Island is a member of a national network of UAPs. The UAP is charged with four core functions: 1. Providing pre-service training to prepare quality service providers. 2. Providing community outreach training and technical assistance. 3. Disseminating information about research and exemplary practice. 4. Research.

3692 **Roger Williams University**
One Old Ferry Road
Bristol, RI 02809
401-253-1040
800-458-7144
Fax: 401-254-3185
http://www.rwu.edu
admit@rwu.edu
Donald J. Farish, Ph.D., J.D., President
Robert H. Avery, Esq., General Counsel/SVP
Catherine C. Capolupo, VP Enrollment Management
An independent comprehensive four-year university with about 5% special education students.

South Carolina

3693 **Aiken Technical College**
Student Services
PO Drawer 696
2276 J. Davis Highway
Graniteville, SC 29829
803-593-9231
Fax: 803-593-9231
http://www.atc.edu
weldon@atc.edu

Richard Weldon, Counselor
Jennifer Pinckney, Manager
Winsor Susan, President
A public two-year college offering services to the learning disabled.

3694 **Camperdown Academy**
501 Howell Rd
Greenville, SC 29615-2028
864-244-8899
Fax: 864-244-8936
http://www.camperdown.org

Dan Blanch, Head of School
Our mission is to enable students with average to above average intelligence, who also experience learning difficulties in the areas of reading, organization, language processing, and written expression, to reach their maximum academic potential.

3695 **Citadel-Military College of South Carolina**
171 Moultrie St
Charleston, SC 29409
843-953-5230
Fax: 843-953-7036
http://www.citadel.edu
admissions@citadel.edu

John W. Rosa, President
Thomas J. Elzey, Vice President
John W. Powell Jr., Director
Offers a variety of services to students with disabilities including notetakers, extended testing time, counseling services, and special accommodations.

3696 **Clemson University**
Student Development Services
707 University Under
Clemson, SC 29634
864-656-3311
Fax: 864-656-0514
http://www.clemson.edu
bmartin@clemson.edu

David H. Wilkins, Chairman
James P. Clements, President
Nadim M. Aziz, Vice President
Four-year college offers services to learning disabled students.

3697 **Coastal Carolina University**
Disability Services Department
PO Box 261954
Conway, SC 29528-6054
843-347-3161
Fax: 843-349-2990
http://www.coastal.edu

D. Wyatt Henderson, Chairman
William S. Biggs, Vice Chair
David A. DeCenzo, President
Coastal Carolina University provides a program of assistance to students with disabilities. Upon acceptance to the University, students will become eligible for support services by providing documentation of their disability. Accommodations include academic labs, tutorial referral, study skills, counseling, auxillary aids, coordination with other agencies and classroom accommodations.

3698 **Erskine College**
2 Washington St
P.O. Box 338
Due West, SC 29639
864-359-4358
888-359-4358
Fax: 864-379-2167
http://www.erskine.edu

Dr. Paul D. Kooistra, President
W.S. Cain, Chairman
N. Bradley Christie, SVP Academic Affairs
Offers a variety of services to students with disabilities including notetakers, extended testing time, counseling services, and special accommodations.

3699 **Francis Marion University**
PO Box 100547
Florence, SC 29502-547
843-661-1310
800-368-7551
Fax: 843-661-1202
http://www.fmarion.edu

Luther F Carter, President
George C. McIntyre, Chair
L. Franklin Elmore, Vice Chair
A public four-year college with services for special education students.

3700 **Glenforest School**
1041 Harbor Drive
West Columbia, SC 29169-3609
803-796-7622
Fax: 803-796-1603
http://www.glenforest.org
info@glenforest.org

Cheri Riddell, Principal
Daphne Perugini, Vice-Principal
Ina Fournier, Superintendent
A K-12 independent, SACS accredited, non-profit day school dedicated to educationg students who learn differently. Dedicated to serving children with learning differences and attention issues including: ADD/ADHD, Dyslexia, Dysgraphia and Autism Spectrum Disorders.

3701 **Greenville Technical College**
PO Box 5616
506 S. Pleasantburg Drive
Greenville, SC 29606-5616
864-250-8000
800-922-1183
Fax: 864-250-8580
http://www.greenvilletech.com
Susan M. Jones, Associate VP of Human Resources
Jacqueline DiMaggio, Vice President for Finance
Dr. Keith Miller, President
Committed to providing equal access for all students and assisting students in making their college experience successful in accordance with ADA/504 and the Rehabilitation Act. The Office of Special Needs for Students with Disabilities has counselors available to assist in the planning and implementation of appropriate accommodations.

3702 **Limestone College**
Program for Alternative Learning Styles
1115 College Dr
Gaffney, SC 29340-3799
864-489-7151
800-795-7151
Fax: 864-487-8706
http://www.limestone.edu
kkearse@limestone.edu

Dr. Walt Griffin, President
Dr. Karen Gainey, VP Academic Affairs & Exe. VP
Dr. William Baker, Special Assistant
Independent four-year college with a program designed to serve students with learning disabilities. There is an additional fee for the first year in the program in addition to the regular tuition. However, that additional cost is reduced by 50% after the freshman year depending on the grade point average.

3703 **Midlands Technical College**
PO Box 2408
Columbia, SC 29202-2408
803-738-8324
800-922-8038
Fax: 803-790-7524
TDD: 803-822-3401
http://www.midlandstech.edu
askmtc@midlandstech.edu

Dr. Marshall White, Jr., President
Gina Mounsield, Vice President
Derrah Cassidy, Director of Admissions
Services to Students with Disabilities counselors support and assist students with disabilities in meeting their personal, educational and career goals. Services include academic and career planning, faculty/student liasion, assistive technology, readers, writers, interpeters, closed circuit television in libraries, TDD, testing services, orientation sessions and a support group.

3704 **North Greenville College**
Learning Disabilities Services
7801 N. Tigerville Rd
P. O. Box 1892
Tigerville, SC 29688-1892
864-977-7000
800-468-6642
Fax: 864-977-7021
http://www.ngc.edu
nisgett@ngc.edu
Nancy Isgett, Learning Disabilities Liaison
Dr. James B. Epting, President
Offers a variety of services to students with disabilities including notetakers, extended testing time, counseling services, and special accommodations.

3705 **South Carolina State University**
300 College Street NE
Orangeburg, SC 29117
864-587-4000
800-772-7286
Fax: 864-587-4355
http://www.scsu.edu
gouveia@scsu.edu
W. Franklin Evans, VP for Academic Affairs
Andrew Hugine, President
Dr. William Small, Jr., Chair
Four-year college that provides information and resources for the learning disabled.

3706 **Spartanburg Methodist College**
1000 Powell Mill Road
Spartanburg, SC 29301
864-587-4000
800-772-7286
Fax: 864-587-4355
http://www.smcsc.edu
admiss@smcsc.edu
Dr. Phinnize Fisher, Chair
Dr. Colleen Perry Keith, President
James Fletcher Thompson, Vice Chair
2-year educational institution, Junior College

3707 **Technical College of Lowcountry: Beaufort**
921 Ribaut Road
Beaufort, SC 29901-1288
843-525-8211
Fax: 843-525-8285
http://www.tcl.edu
Rodney Adams, Dean of Students
Richard J. Gough, President
Offers a variety of services to students with disabilities including note takers, extended testing time, counseling services, and special accommodations.

3708 **Trident Academy**
1455 Wakendaw Rd.
Mount Pleasant, SC 29464
843-884-7046
Fax: 843-881-8320
http://www.tridentacademy.com
admissions@tridentacademy.com
Mike Jeresaty, President
Chad Anderson, Vice President
Andrea Martin, Secretary
An independent learning disabilities school for students in grades K-12 who have Dyslexia, Dysgraphia, Dyscalculia, Non-verbal Learning Disabilities, ADHD, CAPD, and other learning differences.

3709 **Trident Technical College**
PO Box 118067
Charleston, SC 29423-8067
843-574-6111
877-349-7184
Fax: 843-574-6682
http://www.tridenttec.edu
Mary Thornley, President
Patricia J. Robertson, Vice President For Academic Aff
Patrice Mitchell, Vice President For Student Ser
Recognizes its responsibility to identify and maintain the standards (academic, admissions, scores, etc.) that are necessary to provide quality academic programs while ensuring the rights of students with disabilities.

3710 **University of South Carolina**
Disability Services
902 Sumter Street Access/Lieber Col
Columbia, SC 29208
803-777-7000
800-868-5872
Fax: 803-777-0101
TDD: 803-777-6744
http://www.sc.edu
kpettus@sc.edu
Harris Pastides, President
Eugene P Warr, Jr., Chairman
John C. von Lehe, Jr., Vice Chairman
The Office of Disability Services provides accommodations for students with documented physical, emotional, and learning disabilities. The professionally trained staff works toward accessiblity for all university programs, services, and activities in compliance with ADA/504. Services include orientation,priority registration, library access, classroom adaptions, interpeters, and access to adapted housing.

3711 **University of South Carolina: Aiken**
471 University Parkway
Aiken, SC 29801
803-648-6851
Fax: 803-641-3362
http://www.usca.edu
kayb@aiken.sc.edu
Ernest R. Allen, Chairman
Teresa Haas, Vice Chairman
Sandra Jordan, Chancellor
The mission of Disability Services (DS) is to facilitate the transition of students with disabilities into the University eniviroment and to provide appropriate accommodations for each student's special needs in order to ensure equal access to all programs, activities and services at USCA.

3712 **University of South Carolina: Beaufort**
801 Carteret Street
Beaufort, SC 29902-4601
843-521-4100
Fax: 843-521-4194
http://www.sc.edu/beaufort
Joan Lemoine MD, Associate Dean
Jane T. Upshaw, Chancellor
A public two-year college with services for special education students.

3713 **University of South Carolina: Lancaster**
Admissions Office
PO Box 889
101 N. Main Street
Lancaster, SC 29721-889
803-285-1565
Fax: 803-313-7106
http://www.lancaster.sc.edu
ksaile@gwm.sc.edu
Debbie Horne, Administrator
Hal Hiott, Director
Carrie W. Helms, Treasurer
Offers a variety of services to students with disabilities including notetakers, extended testing time, counseling services, and special accommodations.

3714 **Voorhees College**
PO Box 678
Denmark, SC 29042-678
803-780-1234
866-685-9904
Fax: 866-685-9904
http://www.voorhees.edu
info@voorhees.edu
Cleveland L. Dr. Cleveland L., President and CEO
Dr. Lugenia Rochelle, Interim EVP, Academic Affairs
St. Clair P. Guess, III, Chair
Four-year college that offers programs to learning disabled students.

3715 **Winthrop University**
Student Disabilities Department
701 Oakland Ave
Rock Hill, SC 29733-7001
803-323-2211
Fax: 803-323-4861
TDD: 803-323-2233
http://www.winthrop.edu
smithg@winthrop.edu
Anthony Digiorio, Director
Rosanne Wallace, Administrator
DebraÿC. Boyd, Ph.D., Provost/VP Academic Affairs
Since each student has a unique set of special needs, the Counselor for Students with Disabilities makes every effort to provide the student with full access to programs and services. Reasonable accommodations are provided based on needs assessed through proper documentation and an intake interview with the couselor. The majority of buildings on campus are accessible.

South Dakota

3716 **Black Hills State College**
1200 University St
Unit 9502
Spearfish, SD 57799-9502
605-642-6343
800-255-2478
Fax: 605-642-6099
http://www.bhsu.edu
admissions@bhsu.edu
Beth Oaks, Director of Admissions
Tom Jackson Jr., President
Joe Rainboth, Assistant Director of Admissions
Provide the comprehensive supports necessary in meeting the individual needs of students with disabilities.

3717 **Children's Care Hospital and School**
Educational Program
2501 West 26th Street
Sioux Falls, SD 57105-2498
605-444-9500
800-584-9294
Fax: 605-336-0277
http://www.cchs.org
Jessica Wells, Foundation President
Dave Timpe, Interim CEO
Angie Brown, V.P. Strategic Initiatives
Provides a variety of innovative educational services based on the individual learning, medical, and therapeutic needs of the child.

3718 **Northern State University**
1200 S Jay St
Aberdeen, SD 57401-7198
605-626-3011
800-678-5330
Fax: 605-626-2587
http://www.northern.edu
admissions@northern.edu
Laurie Nichols, Director
James Smith, President
Four-year college that provides services to students with a learning disability.

3719 **South Dakota School of Mines & Technology**
501 East Saint Joseph Street
Rapid City, SD 57701-3995
605-394-2511
800-544-8162
Fax: 605-394-6131
http://www.sdsmt.edu
fcampone@sdsmt.edu
Heather Wilson,Dphil, President
Duane C Hrncir, Provost/VP, Academic Affairs
Patricia G Mahon, VP, Student Affairs
Four-year college that offers support services to those students whom are disabled.

3720 **South Dakota State University**
PO Box 2201
Brookings, SD 57007
605-688-4121
800-952-3541
Fax: 605-688-6891
TDD: 605-688-4394
http://www.sdstate.edu
SDSU_Admissions@sdstate.edu
Robert Otterson, Executive Assis to the President
David L. Chicoine, Ph.D., President
Laurie Nichols, Provost/VP Academic Affairs
Committed to providing equal opportunities for higher education for learning disabled students.

3721 **Yankton College**
PO Box 133
Yankton, SD 57078-133
605-665-3661
866-665-3661
Fax: 605-665-3662
http://www.yanktoncollege.org
nfo@yanktoncollege.org
Charles Kaufman, President
Joan Neubauer, Chairÿ
Joseph Ward, Vice-Chair
Offers a variety of services to students with disabilities including note takers, extended testing time, counseling services, and special accommodations.

Tennessee

3722 **Austin Peay State University**
Office of Disability Services
PO Box 4578
Clarksville, TN 37044
931-221-6230
Fax: 931-221-7102
TDD: 931-221-6278
TTY: 931-221-6278
http://www.apsu.edu/disability
acadaffairs@apsu.edu
Amy Deaton, Director of Admissions
Tracy Comer, Assistant Director
Megan Mitchell, Associate Director
The Office of Disability Services is dedicated to providing academic assistance for students with disabilities enrolled at Austin Peay State University. We provide information to students, faculty, staff and administrators about the needs of students with disabilities. We ensure the accessiblity of programs, services, and activities to students having a disability. We are a resource of information pertaining to disability issues and advocate participation in campus life.

3723 **Bryan College: Dayton**
721 Bryan Drive
Dayton, TN 37321-7000
423-775-2041
800-277-9522
Fax: 423-775-7300
http://www.bryan.edu
info@bryan.edu
John Haynes, Chairman
Kevin Clauson, J.D., Vice President of Academics
Stephen D. Livesay , Ph.D., President

Committed to providing quality education for those who meet admission standards but learn differently from others. Modifications are made in the learning environment to enable LD students to succeed. Some of the modifications made require documentation of the specific disability while other adaptations do not. In addition to modifications the small teacher-student ratio allows the school to provide much individual attention to those with learning difficulties.

3724 **Carson-Newman College**
2130 Branner Ave.ÿ
Jefferson City, TN 37760-2232
865-471-2000
800-678-9061
Fax: 865-471-3502
http://www.cn.edu
ckey@cn.edu

J Randall O'Brien, President
Tom Harmon, Chairman
Janet Hayes, Vice Chairman
An independent four-year college with support services for special education students.

3725 **East Tennessee State University**
1276 Gilbreath Dr.
Box 70300
Johnson City, TN 37614-1700
423-439-1000
Fax: 903-886-5702
http://www.etsu.edu
go2etsu@etsu.edu

Cecilia McIntosh, PhD, Dean of Graduate Studies
Scott Kirkby, PhD, Assistant Dean
Karin Bartoszuk, PhD, Associate Dean of Grad. Studies
Offers a variety of services to students with disabilities including note takers, extended testing time, counseling services, and special accommodations.

3726 **Knoxville Business College**
1000 Volunteer Boulevard
Knoxville, TN 37996-4160
865-974-5001
Fax: 865-974-4989
http://www.kbcollege.edu
execed@utk.edu

Stephen L. Mangum, Dean
Kate Atchley, Executive Director
Tom Cervone, Managing Director
Offers a variety of services to students with disabilities including notetakers, extended testing time, counseling services, and special accommodations.

3727 **Middle Tennessee State University**
1301 East Main Street
Murfreesboro, TN 37132-1
615-898-2300
Fax: 615-898-5444
http://www.mtsu.edu
dssemail@mtsu.edu

Sidney McPhee, President
John Morgan, Chancellor
Dale Sims, Vice Chancellor
We offer a wide variety of services to students with disabilities including testing accommodations, providing access to adaptive computer technologies and acting as a liaison to University departments.

3728 **Motlow State Community College**
PO Box 8500
Lynchburg, TN 37352-8500
931-393-1500
800-654-4877
Fax: 931-393-1764
http://www.mscc.edu
asimmons@mscc.cc.tn.us

A. Simmons, Dean Student Development
Billy Soloman, Owner
MaryLou Apple, President
A public two-year college with support services for special education students.

3729 **Northeast State Community College**
PO Box 246
2425 Highway 75
Blountville, TN 37617-0246
423-323-3191
800-836-7822
Fax: 423-279-7649
TDD: 423-279-7640
TTY: 423-279-4649
http://www.northeaststate.edu
memask@northeaststate.edu

A. Lee Shillito, Chair
Dr. Allana Hamilton, VP, Academic Affairs
Matt DeLozier, Interim VP of Student Affairsÿ
To assure equal educational opportunities for individuals with disabilities.

3730 **Pellissippi State Technical Community College**
PO Box 22990
10915 Hardin Valley Road
Knoxville, TN 37933-990
865-694-6400
Fax: 865-539-7217
http://www.pstcc.edu
admissions@pstcc.edu

Joanne Monhollen, Executive Secretary
Rebecca Ashford, Vice President
Dr.Anthony Wise, President
Services for Students with Disabilities develops individual educational support plans, provides prioriy registration and advisement, furnishes volunteer notetakers, provides readers, scribes, tutor bank, provides interpeter services and publishes a newsletter. The office acts as a liaison, and assists students in location of resources appropriate to their needs.

3731 **Shelby State Community College**
P.O. Box 780
Memphis, TN 38101-0780
901-333-5000
877-717-7822
Fax: 901-333-5711
http://www.sscc.cc.tn.us

Sherman Greer, Executive Assis to the President
Ron Parr, VP Fnancial & Admin Services
Dr. Nathan Essex, President
A two-year college providing information and resources to disabled students.

3732 **Southern Adventist University**
Academic Support
5010 University Driveÿ
P.O. Box 370ÿ
Collegedale, TN 37315-370
423-236-2000
800-768-8437
Fax: 423-236-1000
http://www.ldpsych.southern.edu
adossant@southern.edu

Ron Smith, Chairman
Marc Grundy, Vice President
Gordon Bietz, President
A private university offering undergraduate degrees in education designed for K-8, 1-8, 7-12, and K-12 certification plus graduate degrees designed for inclusion (special needs in the regular classroom), multiage/multigrade teaching, outdoor education, and psychology and counseling of exceptional individuals. College age students with special needs and those desiring to teach students with special needs are welcome to apply.

3733 **Southwest Tennessee Community College**
5983 Macon Cove
P.O. Box 780
Memphis, TN 38101-780
901-333-5000
877-717-7822
Fax: 901-333-4788
http://www.southwest.tn.edu
vesails@southwest.tn.edu

Dr.Anthony Wise, President
Sherman Greer, Executive Assistant
Ron Parr, VP Fnancial & Admin Services

Offers a variety of services to students with disabilities including note takers, extended testing time, counseling services, and special accommodations.

3734 **Tennessee State University**
Office of Disabled Student Services
3500 John a Merritt Blvd
P. O. Box 9609
Nashville, TN 37209-1561
615-963-5000
888-463-6878
Fax: 615-963-2930
TDD: 615-963-7440
http://www.tnstate.edu
pscudder@tnstate.edu
Dr. Glenda Baskin Glover, President
Monique Mitchell, Administrative Assistant ll
Steven McCrary, Coordinator
Four year college offers services for learning disabled students.

3735 **University of Memphis**
110 Wilder Tower N
Memphis, TN 38152
901-678-2911
Fax: 901-678-5023
TDD: 901-678-2880
http://www.saweb.memphis.edu
sds@memphis.edu
Susan TePaske, Director
Jennifer Murchison, Asst Director
Phil Minyard, Coordinator
Emphasizes individual responsibility for learning by offering a developmentally oriented program of college survival skills, learning strategies, and individualized planning and counseling based on the student's strengths and weaknesses. The program also coordinates comprehensive support services, including test accommodations, tutoring and learning strategies, alternate format tests and assistive technology. The program serves 400 to 500 students with learning disabilities and ADHD per year.

3736 **University of Tennessee**
Boling Center for Developmental Disabilities
711 Jefferson Ave
Memphis, TN 38105-5003
901-448-6512
888-572-2249
Fax: 901-448-7097
TDD: 901-448-4677
http://www.utmem.edu
Jimmy G. Cheek, Chancellor
Susan Martin, Provost
Kennard Brown, Executive Vice Chancellor/COO
Interdisciplinary or focused evaluation of learning, behavioral and developmental problems in infants, toddlers, children and young adults. Treatment of some conditions offered.

3737 **University of Tennessee: Knoxville**
Disability Services Office
2227 Dunford Hall
915 Volunteer Blvd
Knoxville, TN 37996-0001
865-974-6087
Fax: 865-974-9552
TDD: 865-974-6087
http://www.ods.utk.edu
ods@utk.edu
Jimmy G. Cheek, Chancellor
Susan Martin, Provost
Kennard Brown, Executive Vice Chancellor/COO
The mission of the Office of Disability Services is to provide each individual an equal opportunity to participate in the University of Tennessee's programs and activities.

3738 **University of Tennessee: Martin**
554 University Street
Martin, TN 38238-0001
731-881-7000
Fax: 731-881-1886
http://www.utm.edu
success@utm.edu
Edie B. Gibson, Executive Assis to Chancellor
Dr. Margaret Toston, Vice Chancellor
Tom Rakes, Chancellor
A four-year independent college that offers a program called Program Access for College Enhancement for students with learning disabilities.

3739 **Vanderbilt University**
Vanderbilt University
2301 Vanderbilt Place
Nashville, TN 37235
615-322-7311
Fax: 615-322-3762
TDD: 615-322-4705
http://www.vanderbilt.edu
melissa.a.smith@vanderbilt.edu
Jackson W. Moore, Vice Chairman
Nicholas S. Zeppos, Chancellor
Mark Dalton, Chairman
An independent four-year college with support services for special education students.

3740 **William Jennings Bryan College**
HEATH Resource Center
721 Bryan Drive
2121 K St NW
Dayton, TN 20202-2524
423-775-2041
800-544-3284
Fax: 202-973-0908
http://www.heath.gwu.edu
nfo@bryan.edu
Stephen D. Livesay , Ph.D., President
Kevin Clauson, J.D., Interim Vice President
John Haynes, Chairman
A public four-year college. The HEALTH Resource Center operates the national clearinghouse on postsecondary education for individuals with disabilities.

Texas

3741 **Alvin Community College**
Alvin Community College
3110 Mustang Road
Alvin, TX 77511-4807
281-756-3500
Fax: 281-756-3858
http://www.alvincollege.edu
info@alvincollege.edu
Christal M. Albrecht, President
Alyssa Reeves, Admission Specialist
Jim Crumm, Vice President
A public two-year college with support services for special education students.

3742 **Angelina College**
Student Services Office
PO Box 1768
3500 S 1st St
Lufkin, TX 75901-1768
936-639-1301
Fax: 936-639-4299
http://www.angelina.edu
jtwohig@angelina.edu
Patricia M. McKenzie, Ed.D., VP/Dean of Instruction
Larry M. Phillips, President
Tim Stacy, Secretary
A public community college that offers two-year degrees in the arts and sciences designed to transfer to four-year colleges and universities as well as one and two year programs in technical and occupational fields.

3743 **Brookhaven College**
Special Services Office
3939 Valley View Ln
Farmers Branch, TX 75244-4997
972-860-4700
Fax: 972-860-4897
http://www.dcccd.edu.bhc
bhcInfo@dcccd.edu
Sharon Blackman, Grants Manager
Thom D. Chesney, Ph.D., President
Rodger Bennett, Vice President

Physically challenged and learning disabled special services office offers advisement, additional diagnostic evaluations, mobility assistance, note taking, textbook taping, interpreters for the deaf and assistance in test taking.

3744 **Cedar Valley College**
3030 N Dallas Ave
Lancaster, TX 75134-3799 972-860-8201
http://www.cedarvalleycollege.edu
Dr Jennifer Wimbish, President
Dr. Nancy Cure, Vice President of Instruction
Dr. Mickey Best, Executive Dean of Liberal Arts
The mission of Cedar Valley College is to provide quality learning that prepares students for success in a dynamic world.

3745 **Central Texas College**
PO Box 1800
Killeen, TX 76540-1800 254-526-7161
800-792-3348
Fax: 254-526-1700
TDD: 254-526-1378
http://www.ctcd.edu
Thomas Klincar, Chancellor
Rex Weaver, Chair
Jimmy Towers, Vice Chair
Offers a variety of services to students with disabilities including extended testing time, counseling services, and assistive technology.

3746 **Cisco College**
101 College Heights
Cisco, TX 76437 254-442-5000
Fax: 254-442-5100
http://www.cisco.edu
Bobby Smith, President
Jerry Dodson, Ed.D., VP Student Services
Carol Dupree, Ph.D., Provost
Provides affordable, accessible education to more than 4,200 students through its two locations in Cisco and Abilene. Offers a variety of career and technical education programs and academic transfer options as well as many student support services like tutoring, academic intervention and counseling to ensure student success.

3747 **College of the Mainland**
Student Support Services
1200 Amburn Rd
Texas City, TX 77591-2499 409-938-1211
888-258-8859
Fax: 409-938-1306
http://www.com.edu
kkimbark@com.edu
Dr. Beth Lewis, President
Roney G. McCrary, Chair
Wayne H. Miles, Vice Chair
Offers a variety of services to students with disabilities including notetakers, extended testing time, counseling services, and special accommodations. The mission of services for students with disabilities is to provide each student with the resources needed to register, enroll and complete their course work and/or degree plan.

3748 **Collin County Community College**
2200 W University Drive
McKinney, TX 75071-2999 972-548-6790
Fax: 972-548-6716
http://www.collin.edu
Cary A. Israel, President
Mac Hendricks, Chair
Dr. Sherry Schumann, VP/Provost
A public two-year college. ACCESS provides resonable accommodations, individual attention and support for students with disabilities who need assistance with any aspect of their campus experience such as accessibility, academics and testing.

3749 **Dallas Academy**
950 Tiffany Way
Dallas, TX 75218-2743 214-324-1481
Fax: 214-327-8537
http://www.dallas-academy.com
mail@dallas-academy.com
Jim Richardson, Headmaster
Troy Sturrock, Chair
Terrence S. Welch, Vice Chair
Offers a variety of services to students with disabilities including notetakers, extended testing time, counseling services, and special accommodations.

3750 **Dallas Academy: Coed High School**
950 Tiffany Way
Dallas, TX 75218-2743 214-324-1481
Fax: 214-327-8537
http://www.dallas-academy.com
mail@dallas-academy.com
Troy Sturrock, Chair
Terrence S. Welch, Vice Chair
Jim Richardson, Headmaster
Coed Day School for bright children grades 7-12 with diagnosed learning differences. Curriculum includes sports, art, music, and photography programs.

3751 **Dallas County Community College**
701 Elm St.
Dallas, TX 75202-2033 214-860-2283
Fax: 972-860-7227
http://www.dcccd.edu/
5HCRC@dcccd.edu
Charletta Rogers Compton, Chair
Dr. Joe May, Chancellor
Susan Hall, Executive Director
Offers a variety of services to students with disabilities including note takers, extended testing time, counseling services, and special accommodations.

3752 **East Texas Baptist University**
One Tiger Drive
Marshall, TX 75670-1498 903-935-7963
800-804-3828
Fax: 903-938-7798
http://www.etbu.edu
Admissions@etbu.edu
Dr. Lawrence Ressler, Interim President
Offers a variety of services to students with disabilities including notetakers, extended testing time, counseling services, and special accommodations.

3753 **Eastfield College**
3737 Motley Drive
Mesquite, TX 75150-2099 972-860-7100
Fax: 972-860-7622
http://www.eastfieldcollege.edu
efcdso@dcccd.edu
Dr Jean Conway, President
Sharon Cook, Assistant to the President
Dr. Adrian Douglas, VP Business Services
Offers a variety of support services for students with disabilities and/or special requirements. Services are coordinated to fit the individual needs of the student and may include sign language interpreters, computer aided real-time translation services, notetaking services, tutoring referral, textbook taping, testing accomodations, and use of adaptive technology. Academic counseling, priority registration, and referral information are also available.

3754 **El Centro College**
801 Main Street
Dallas, TX 75202 214-860-2000
Fax: 214-860-2440
http://www.elcentrocollege.edu
Norman Howden, Executive Dean
Karin Reed, Disability Services Coordinator
Paul McCarthy, President

A public two-year college with support services for special education students.

3755 **Fairhill School**
16150 Preston Road
Dallas, TX 75248-3558
972-233-1026
Fax: 972-233-8205
http://www.fairhill.org
Carla Stanford, Executive Director
Deborah Atchley, Head of Lower School
Carla Hilts, Administrative Assistant
A private, non-profit college preparatory school serving students in grades one through twelve. Fairhill's primary purpose is to provide a superior education for students of average and above intelligence who have been diagnosed with a learning difference such as Dyslexia, Dysgraphia, Dyscalculia, Auditory Processing Disorder, or Attention Deficit/Hyperactivity Disorder.

3756 **Frank Phillips College**
Special Populations Department
PO Box 5118
1301 W. Roosevelt St.
Borger, TX 79008-5118
806-457-4200
800-687-2056
Fax: 806-457-4225
http://www.fpctx.edu
Jarel Whitehead, Chairperson
Charlotte Hale, Vice Chairperson
Lew K Hunnicutt, Ph.D., VP Extended Services
Offers a variety of services to students with disabilities including notetakers, extended testing time, counseling services, and special accommodations.

3757 **Galveston College**
4015 Avenue Q
Galveston, TX 77550-7496
409-944-4242
Fax: 409-944-1500
TDD: 866-483-4242
http://www.gc.edu
W. Myles Shelton EdD, President
Armin Cantini, Chairperson
Raymond Lewis, Jr., Vice Chairperson
A public two-year college. A variety of services and programs are available to assist students with disabilities, those who are academically and/or economically disadvantaged and those with limited English proficiency.

3758 **Great Lakes Academy**
6000 Custer Road
Building 7
Plano, TX 75023-5100
972-517-7498
Fax: 972-517-0133
http://www.greatlakesacademy.com
admissions@greatlakesacademy.com
Marjolein J. Borsten, Executive Director
Jolene Wofford, Director
Jason Campbell, Assistant Director
A full day non-profit private school that provides 1st-12th grade students with average to above-average intelligence, diagnosed with various Learning Differences, Asperger's Syndrome, ADD or AD/HD a stimulating environment and favorable atmosphere which affords each student opportunities to develop both socially and academically.

3759 **Hill School**
4817 Odessa Ave
Fort Worth, TX 76133-1640
817-923-9482
Fax: 817-923-4894
http://www.hillschool.org
hillschool@hillschool.org
Whit Perryman, President
David G. Bucher, Senior Vice President
Tim Carter, Chairman of the Board
Hill School is a college preparatory, full-service school for bright students who learn differently. Our exceptional faculty emphasize intensive small-group instruction in core subject areas to ensure that all students have an opportunity to reach their full academic potential. Our students explore interests and affinities through athletics, fine arts (drama, visual arts, music, band) and a wide variety of community involvement activities. Also located in SW Ft. Worth and Grapevine.

3760 **Jarvis Christian College**
PO Box 1470
Hawkins, TX 75765-1470
903-769-5700
800-292-9517
Fax: 903-769-5005
http://www.jarvis.edu
florine_white@jarvis.edu
Florine White MD, Student Support Services Dir.
Lester C. Newman, President
Stephanie Brown, Administrative Staff
Student Support Services is a federally funded program whose purpose is to improve the retention and graduate rate of program participants. Eligible program participants include low income, first generation college students and students with learning and physical disabilities. A variety of support services are provided.

3761 **Lamar State College - Port Arthur**
PO Box 310
1500 Procter Street
Port Arthur, TX 77640-0310
409-983-4921
800-477-5872
Fax: 409-984-6056
TDD: 409-984-6242
http://www.pa.lamar.edu
andrea.munoz@lamarpa.edu
Mary Wickland, Vice President for Finance
Dr. Charles Gongre, Dean of Academic Programs
W. Sam Monroe, President
A public two-year college with support services for special education students.

3762 **Laredo Community College**
Special Populations Office
West End Washington Street
Laredo, TX 78040
956-721-5109
Fax: 956-721-5367
http://www.laredo.edu
sylviat@laredo.cc.tx.us
Eleazar Gonzalez, Chief Administrative Officer/CFO
Dr. Juan L. Maldonado, President
Vincent R. Solis, VP
Offers a variety of services to students with disabilities including notetakers, extended testing time, counseling services, and special accommodations.

3763 **Lon Morris College**
Disability Services: Cole Learning Enrichment Ctr
600 College Avenue
Jacksonville, TX 75766
903-589-4000
800-259-5733
Fax: 903-589-4001
http://www.beabearcat.com
Sandra White, Director, Enrichment Center
Angela Jones, Assistant
Dasvid Russ, Advisor
A two-year liberal arts college that offers a learning support program (the Cole Learning Enrichment Center) for students with learning disabilities. Students work collaboratively with the director of the center to develop and achieve realistic career and education goals, determine educational needs based on testing data, and foster independence while developing and demonstrating their full potential and abilities.

3764 **Lubbock Christian University**
5601 19th Street
Lubbock, TX 79407-2099
806-796-8800
800-933-7601
Fax: 806-720-7255
http://www.lcu.edu
admissions@lcu.edu
L. Timothy Perrin, President
Dr. Brian Starr, Vice President
Monica Lopez Barnard, General Counsel
Offers a variety of services to students with disabilities including notetakers, extended testing time, counseling services, and special accommodations.

3765 **McLennen Community College**
1400 College Drive
Waco, TX 76708-1499
254-299-8622
Fax: 254-299-8654
http://www.mclennan.edu
helpdesk@mclennan.edu
Dr. Johnette McKown, President
Mickey Reyes, Desktop Publishing Technician
Harry Harelik, Executive Director
A public two-year college with support services for special education students.

3766 **Midwestern State University**
Disability Counseling Office
3410 Taft Boulevard
Wichita Falls, TX 76308-2096
940-397-4352
800-842-1922
Fax: 940-397-4780
TDD: 940-397-4515
http://www.mwsu.edu
counselling@mwsu.edu
Jesse W Rogers, President
Dr. Marilyn Fowle, Vice President
Dr. Keith Lamb, VP
A public four-year college with support services for special education students.

3767 **North Lake College**
Disabilities Services Office
Rm A438
5001 N Macarthur Blvd
Irving, TX 75038-3899
972-273-3000
Fax: 972-273-3431
TDD: 972-273-3169
http://www.dcccd.edu
Debbie Eberla, Assistant to the President
Martha Hughes, VP Academic Affairs
Christa Slejko, President
A public two-year college. Our mission is to provide a variety of support services to empower students, foster independence, promote achievement of realistic career and educational goals and assist students in discovering, developing and demonstrating full potential and abilities.

3768 **Notre Dame School**
2018 Allen Street
Dallas, TX 75204-2604
214-720-3911
Fax: 214-720-3913
http://www.notredameschool.org
tfrancis@notredameschool.org
Theresa Francis, Principal
Bruce Newsome, Vice President
Randy Bacon, President
Providing a quality education to children with developmental disabilities ages 6 to 21 and facilitating their intergration into society.

3769 **Odyssey School**
4407 Red River St
Austin, TX 78751-4039
512-472-2262
Fax: 512-236-9385
http://www.odysseyschool.com
info@odysseyschool.com
Nancy Wolf, Head of School
Paul R. Teich, Vice President
F. Scott McCown, President
Committed to the development of academic excellence and self-acceptance for students with learning and attentional differences. We believe all children can be successful in their intellectual, creative and social development. Our goal is to help each student discover his or her individual potential for greatness.

3770 **Pan American University**
Office of Disability Services
1201 W University Drive
Edinburg, TX 78539-2999
956-381-3306
Fax: 956-381-5196
TDD: 956-316-7092
http://www.panam.edu
Brinda V. Torres, Assistant toÿVP
Maqdalena Hinojosa, Senior Associate VP
Robert S. Nelsen, President
Offers a variety of services to students with disabilities including note takers, extended testing time, counseling services, and special accommodations.

3771 **Rawson-Saunders School**
Soaring Eagles Program
2614-A Exposition Boulevard
Austin, TX 78703-1702
512-476-8382
Fax: 512-476-1132
http://www.rawson-saunders.org
info@rawson-saunders.org
Laura Steinbach, Head of School
Samer Zabaneh, Legal Counsel
Kaye Knox, Chair
Developed to help learning disabled students, grades 1 to 8, maintain their language arts and math skills while increasing their self-esteem. Students participate in small group, hands-on activities in math, language arts, organized games/movement, keyboarding, sign language, and science or creative problem solving.

3772 **Richland College**
12800 Abrams Rd
Dallas, TX 75243-2199
972-238-6100
Fax: 972-238-6346
http://www.rlc.dcccd.edu
Steve Mittelstet, President
Finney Varghese, Associate Vice President
Richland College's mission is teaching, learning, and community building.

3773 **Sam Houston State University**
1806 Avenue J
Huntsville, TX 77340
936-294-1111
Fax: 936-294-3794
TDD: 936-294-3786
http://www.shsu.edu
disability@shsu.edu
Dana G. Hoyt, President
Jaimie Hebert, Provost and Vice President
Al Hooten, VP Finance and Operation
Offers a variety of services to students with disabilities including note takers, extended testing time, counseling services, and special accommodations.

3774 **San Jacinto College: Central Campus**
P.O.Box 2007
8060 Spencer Hwy.
Pasadena, TX 77505-2007
281-998-6150
Fax: 281-476-1892
http://www.sjcd.cc.tx.us
Van Wigginton, Provost
Laurel Williamson, Deputy Chancellor/SJCD President
Joanna Zimmermann, Interim VP, Student Services
Offers a variety of services to students with disabilities including notetakers, extended testing time, counseling services, and special accommodations such as test readers and writers.

3775 **San Jacinto College: South Campus**
San Jacinto College: South Campus
13735 Beamer Rd
Houston, TX 77089-6099
281-998-6150
Fax: 281-922-3401
http://www.sjcd.edu
eeverett@sjcd.edu
Laurel Williamson, Deputy Chancellor/SJCD President
Joanna Zimmermann, Interim VP of Student Services
Brenda Jones, Provost
A public two-year college with support services for special education students.

3776 **Schreiner University**
2100 Memorial Blvd
Kerrville, TX 78028-5697
830-792-7217
800-343-4919
Fax: 830-282-4638
http://www.schreiner.edu
jgallik@schreiner.edu
Tim Summerlin, President
Bill Muse, VP for Administration & Finance
Mike Pate, Chairman of the Board
Comprehensive support program for students with diagnosed specific learning disabilities with demonstrated potential for success at the college level.

3777 **Shelton School**
15720 Hillcrest Road
Dallas, TX 75248-4161
972-774-1772
Fax: 972-991-3977
http://www.shelton.org
Suzanne Stell, Executive Director
Gary Webb, Chairman
Paul Neubach, M.D., Vice Chairman
Primary emphasis is providing learning-different children (average or above intelligence) with full, effective curriculum through individualized, structured multisensory programs. Learning differences include dyslexia, attention deficit disorder (ADD), attention deficit hyperactivity disorder (ADHD), speech and language disorders.

3778 **South Plains College**
1401 College Ave
Levelland, TX 79336-6595
806-894-9611
Fax: 806-897-2800
http://www.spc.cc.tx.us
Kelvin W. Sharp, Ed.D., President
Jim Walker, M.P.A., Vice President for Academic Aff
Cathy Mitchell, M.Ed., Vice President for Student Aff
Offers a variety of services to students with disabilities including notetakers, extended testing time, counseling services, and special accommodations.

3779 **Southern Methodist University**
Disability Accommodations & Success Strategies
PO Box 750201
Dallas, TX 75275-100
214-768-2000
Fax: 214-768-1225
http://www.smu.edu/alec/dass.asp
ugadmission@smu.edu
Michael M. Boone, Chair
R. Gerald Turner, President
Thomas E. Barry, Vice President
Provides access and accomodations to all SMU students with a disability. Also offers academic waching to undergraduates with learning and attention disorders.

3780 **Southwestern Assemblies of God University**
1200 Sycamore St
Waxahachie, TX 75165-2397
972-937-4010
888-YES-SAGU
Fax: 972-923-0488
http://www.sagu.edu
sagu@sagu.edu
Kermit S Bridges, President
Paul Brooks, Vice President for Academics
Katie White, Administrative Academic
Offers a variety of services to students with disabilities including notetakers, extended testing time, counseling services, and special accommodations.

3781 **St. Edwards University**
Learning Disabilities Services
3001 South Congress Avenue
Austin, TX 78704-6489
512-448-8400
855-468-6738
Fax: 512-448-8492
http://www.stedwards.edu
seu.admit@stedwards.edu
George E. Martin, President
Donna Jurick, SND, Executive Vice President
Christie Campbell, Associate Vice President
An independent four-year college. Students with disabilities meet with a counselor from academic planning and support and they work together to ensure equal access to all academic services.

3782 **St. Mary's University of San Antonio**
1 Camino Santa Maria St
San Antonio, TX 78228-8500
210-436-3011
Fax: 210-436-3782
http://www.stmarytx.edu
Thomas Mengler, J.D., President
Charles T. Barrett Jr., Chairman of the Board
Andre Hampton, Provost and VP
Offers a variety of services to students with disabilities including tutoring, extended testing time, and academic counseling services.

3783 **Stephen F Austin State University**
Office of Disability Services
2008 Alumni Drive
Rusk Building, Room 206
Nacogdoches, TX 75962-3940
936-468-2504
Fax: 936-468-3849
http://www.sfasu.edu
admissions@sfasu.edu
Richard Berry, Provost/VP for Academic Affairs
Tito Guerrero, President
Mr. James H. Dickerson, Secretary
Offers a variety of services to students with disabilities including note takers, extended testing time, counseling services, and special accommodations.

3784 **Tarleton State University**
Box T-0001
1333 W. Washington
Stephenville, TX 76402
254-968-9000
Fax: 254-968-9703
http://www.tarleton.edu
Joe Standridge, Jr. P.E., Associate Vice President
Angie Brown, Assistant Vice President
F Dominic Dottavid, President
Four year college that provides students with learning disabilities support and services.

3785 **Tarrant County College**
Disability Support Services
1500 Houston Street
Fort Worth, TX 76102
817-515-5100
Fax: 817-515-6112
TDD: 817-515-6812
http://www.tccd.edu
judy.kelly@tccd.edu
Larry Darlage, President, Northeast Campus
O.K. Carter, Secretary
Gary Smith, M.S., VP Academic Affairs
Offers a variety of support services to students with disabilities including notetakers, testing accommodations, as well as special accommodations, tutoring.

3786 **Texas A&M University**
0200 TAMU
750 Agronomy Road, Suite 1601
College Station, TX 77843-200 979-845-3313
Fax: 979-845-2647
http://www.tamu.edu
anne@stulife2.tamu.edu
Dr. Brett Giroir, Executive Vice President and CEO
Dr. Karan L. Watson, Provost/EVP for Academic Affairs
Mark A. Hussey, President
A public four-year college with support services for special education students.

3787 **Texas A&M University: Commerce**
PO Box 3011
Commerce, TX 75429-3011 903-886-5835
888-868-2682
Fax: 903-468-3220
http://www.tamu-commerce.edu
frank_perez@tamu-commerce.edu
Linda King, Executive Asst. to the President
Dan R. Jones, Ph.D., President & CEO
Sharon Johnson, Vice President
Four-year college that provides student support services and programs to those students who are learning disabled.

3788 **Texas A&M University: Kingsville**
1210 Retama Dr
Kingsville, TX 78363 361-592-4762
Fax: 361-593-2006
http://www.tamuk.edu
kacjaol@tamuk.edu
Jeanie Alexander, Coordinator Disability Svcs
Dr. Steven Tallant, President
Four-year college that provides an academic support center for students who are disabled.

3789 **Texas Southern University**
3100 Cleburne St
Houston, TX 77004-4597 713-313-7011
Fax: 713-313-7851
http://www.tsu.edu
Janis J. Newman, Chief of Staf
Dr. John M. Rudley, President
Wendy H. Adair, VP, University Advancement
A public four-year college with support services for special education students.

3790 **Texas State Technical Institute: Sweetwater Campus**
300 Homer K Taylor Drive
Sweetwater, TX 79556-4108 325-235-7300
http://www.sweetwater.tstc.edu
Kyle Smith, Interim President
Mike Reeser, MBA, Chancellor
Dixon Bailey, Vice President
Offers a variety of services to students with disabilities including notetakers, extended testing time, counseling services, and special accommodations.

3791 **Texas Tech University**
AccessTECH & TECHniques Center
2500 Broadway
Lubbock, TX 79409 806-742-2011
Fax: 806-742-4837
TDD: 806-742-2092
TTY: 806-742-4837
http://www.accesstech.dsa.ttu.edu
webmaster@ttu.edu
M. Duane Nellis, Ph.D., President
Lawrence Schovanec, Provost/Senior Vice President
Robert V. Duncan, Vice President for Research
AccessTECH & TECHniques Center offer TTU students every opportunity to succeed in independence and education.

3792 **Texas Woman's University**
Disability Support Services
PO Box 425966
Denton, TX 76204-5966 940-898-3835
Fax: 940-898-3965
TDD: 940-898-3830
http://www.twu.edu
dss@twu.edu
A public four-year college with support services for special education students.

3793 **Tri-County Community College**
1500 Houston Street
Fort Worth, TX 76102 817-515-8223
Fax: 828-837-3266
TDD: 724-228-4028
http://www.tccd.edu
Louise Appleman, President
Kristin Vandergriff, Vice President
Erma Johnson Hadley, Chancellor
Offers a variety of services to students with disabilities including notetakers, extended testing time, counseling services, and special accommodations.

3794 **Tyler Junior College**
PO Box 9020
Tyler, TX 75711-9020 903-510-2200
800-687-5680
Fax: 903-510-2434
http://www.tyler.cc.tx.us
Vickie Geisel, Special Services
Aubry Sharp, Manager
L. Michael Metke, President
Offers a variety of services to students with disabilities including note takers, extended testing time, counseling services, and special accommodations.

3795 **University of Austin Texas**
Texas Center for Disability Studies
1 University Station C1200
Austin, TX 78712 512-471-3434
800-828-7839
Fax: 512-232-0761
http://www.utexas.edu
txcds@uttcds.org
Patricia L. Clubb, VP for University Operations
Brad Englert, AVP/CIO
William Powers Jr, President
The mission of the Texas Center for Disability Studies (TCDS) is to serve as a catalyst so that people with developmental and other disabilities are fully included in all levels of their communities and in control of their lives.

3796 **University of Houston**
Disability Support Services
4800 Calhoun Road
Houston, TX 77004 713-743-2255
Fax: 713-743-5396
TDD: 713-749-1527
TTY: 713-749-1527
http://www.uh.edu
wscrain@mail.uhe.edu
Eli D. Cipriano, Associate Vice President
Lisa Holdeman, Assistant Vice President
Renu Khator, President
A public four-year college with support services for students with disabilities.

3797 **University of North Texas**
Office of Disability Accommodation
PO Box 310770
1155 Union Circle #311277
Denton, TX 76203-5017 940-565-4323
Fax: 940-369-7969
TDD: 940-369-8652
http://www.unt.edu/oda
branding@unt.edu

Dr. Warren Burggren, Provost/VP for Academic Affairs
Neal J. Smatresk, President
Elizabeth With, VP Student Affairs
The mission of the ODA is to provide reasonable accommodations to students and to apply appropriate adjustments to the classroom and associated learning environments. In order to facilitate this process, the ODA maintains all student diability-related medical and psychological documentation and the corresponding accommodation request records.

3798 **University of Texas at Dallas**
PO Box 830688
800 West Campbell Road
Richardson, TX 75083-3021 972-883-2111
Fax: 972-883-2098
http://www.utdallas.edu
Kerry Tate, Asst Director Disability Service
David E. Daniel, President
Judy Snellings, Executive Associate
Offers a variety of services to students with disabilities including notetakers, extended testing time, counseling services, and special accommodations.

3799 **University of Texas: Pan American**
1201 W University Drive
Edinburg, TX 78539-2999 956-381-2011
866-441-UTPA
Fax: 956-381-2150
http://www.panam.edu
Dr. Havidan Rodriguez, Provost/VP for Academic Affairs
Martin V. Baylor, VP, Business Affairs
Robert S. Nelsen, President
Offers a variety of services to students with disabilities including notetakers, extended testing time, counseling services, and special accommodations.

3800 **University of the Incarnate Word**
4301 Broadway St
CPO #285
San Antonio, TX 78209-6318 210-829-6000
800-749-WORD
Fax: 210-829-3847
http://www.uiw.edu
uiwhr@universe.uiwtx.edu
Louis J Agnese Jr, President
Kathleen Coughlin, VP, Institutional Adv.
Dr. Denise Doyle, Chancellor
Four year college that provides services to learning disabled students.

3801 **Wharton County Junior College**
911 E Boling Hwy
Wharton, TX 77488-3298 781-583-7561
800-561-9252
Fax: 888- 898-620
http://www.wcjc.cc.tx.us/
Gary P. Trochta, Vice Chair
Betty A. McCrohan, President
P. D. Gertson, III, Chair
Offers a variety of services to students with disabilities including note takers, extended testing time, counseling services, and special accommodations.

3802 **Wiley College**
711 Wiley Ave
Marshall, TX 75670-5151 903-927-3300
800-658-6889
Fax: 903-938-8100
http://www.wilec.edu
vdavis@wileyc.edu
Haywood L Strickland, President and CEO
Dr. Glenda Carter, Executive Vice President
Dr. Ernest Plata, VP for Academic Affairs
Offers a variety of services to students with disabilities including notetakers, extended testing time, counseling services, and special accommodations.

3803 **Winston School**
5707 Royal Lane
Dallas, TX 75229-5500 214-691-6950
Fax: 214-691-1509
http://www.winston-school.org
info@winston-school.org
Pamela K. Murfin, Head of School
Paula Tuffin, President
Scott Becchi, 1st Vice President
Our mission is to realize the extraordinary potential of bright students who learn differently through individualized learning strategies, and to aid in preparing graduates for college level work.

Utah

3804 **College of Eastern Utah**
451 East 400 North
Price, UT 84501-2699 435-613-5000
888-202-8783
Fax: 435-613-5112
http://www.ceu.edu
Michael King, DRC Director
John Shattuck, President
The DRC at CEU provides academic accommodations for the learning disabled.

3805 **Latter-Day Saints Business College**
95 North 300 West
Salt Lake City, UT 84101-1302 801-524-8100
Fax: 801-524-1900
http://www.ldsbc.edu
Thomas S Monson, Chairman
J. Lawrence Richards, President
Bob H. Wiser, VP Finance and Controller
Offers a variety of services to students with disabilities including notetakers, extended testing time, counseling services, and special accommodations.

3806 **Salt Lake Community College**
Disability Resource Center
4600 South Redwood Road
Salt Lake City, UT 84123-3197 801-957-4111
Fax: 801-957-4440
TDD: 801-957-4646
TTY: 801-957-4646
http://www.slcc.edu
linda.bennett@slcc.edu
Deneece Huftalin, Ph.D., President
Gail Miller, Chair
Nancy Singer, Ph.D., Vice President
A program to assist students with disabilities in obtaining equal access to college facilities and programs. The resource center serves all disabilities and provides services and accommodations such as testing, adaptive equipment, text on tape, readers, scribes, note takers, and interpreters for the deaf.

3807 **Snow College**
150 College Ave
Ephraim, UT 84627-1299 435-283-7000
800-848-3399
Fax: 435-283-5259
http://www.snow.edu
Gary Carlston, President
Theressa Alder, Chair
Spencer Hill, Vice President of Finance
A public two-year college with support services for special education students.

3808 **Southern Utah University**
351 West University Boulevard
Cedar City, UT 84720-2470 435-586-7700
Fax: 435-865-8223
http://www.suu.edu
thompson@suu.edu

Michael T Benson, Executive Director
Scott Wyatt, President
Stuart Jones, Vice President
A public four-year University with support services for special education students.

3809 **University Accessibility Center**
Brigham Young University
800 West, University Parkway
MS 190
Orem, UT 84058-5999
801-863-8747
Fax: 801-863-8377
TTY: 801-221-0908
http://www.uac.byu.edu
uac@byu.edu
Sandy Parsons, Chair
Gretchen Tousey, President
Dani Anguiano, VP University Affairs
REACH was established to assist students with disabilities to reach their full potential. It is our goal to provide an environment where the pursuit of excellence is expected, and students are strongly encouraged to make a contribution toward their own success.

3810 **University of Utah**
201 Presidents Cir
Room 201
Salt Lake City, UT 84112-9049
801-581-7200
800-444-8638
Fax: 801-585-5257
TDD: 801-581-5020
http://www.utah.edu
onadeau@saun.saff.utah.edu
Bryon Buchmiller, Chair
Patti Carpenter, Secretary / Treasurer
Paul Larsen, President
A public four-year college. Services include admissions requirements modification, testing accommodations, priority registration, advisement on course selection and number, adaptive technology, support group. Documentation of learning disability is required.

3811 **Utah State University**
0160 Old Main Hill
Rm 102
Logan, UT 84322-0160
435-797-1079
800-488-8108
Fax: 435-797-0130
TDD: 435-797-0740
http://www.usu.edu
diane.baum@usu.edu
Katie Nielsen, Director of Admissions
Tagg Archibald, Assistant Director
Jeff Sorensen, Associate Director of Admissions
A public four-year college with support services for students with learning disabilities.

3812 **Utah Valley State College**
Accessibility Services Department
800 W University Pkwy
Orem, UT 84058
801-863-8105
Fax: 801-863-7265
http://www.uvu.edu
info@uvsc.edu
Jono Andrews, Associate VP, Academic Programs
Brian Brich, VP, Development & Alumni
Matthew Holland, President
The mission for Accessibility Services at Utah Valley State College is to ensure, in compliance with federal and state laws, that no qualified individual with a disability be excluded from participation in or be denied the benefits of a quality education at UVSC or be subjected to discrimination by the college or its personnel. UVSC offers a large variety of support services, accommodative services and assistive technology for individuals with learning disabilities.

3813 **Weber State University**
Disabilities Support Office
3848 Harrison Blvd.
Ogden, UT 84408
801-626-6000
Fax: 801-626-6744
TDD: 801-626-7283
http://www.weber.edu
recruit1@weber.edu
Charles A. Wight, President
Bret R. Ellis, VP Information Technology
Alan E. Hall, Chair
Offers a variety of services to students with disabilities including notetakers, extended testing time, counseling services, and special accommodations.

3814 **Westminster College of Salt Lake City**
Learning Disability Program
1840 South 1300 East
Salt Lake City, UT 84105-3697
801-484-7651
800-748-4753
Fax: 801-468-0916
TDD: 801-832-2286
http://www.westminstercollege.edu
gdewitt@westminstercollege.edu
Thomas A. Ellison, ESQ, Chair
William Orchow, Vice Chair
Dr.Brian Levin-Stankevich, President
Offers a variety of services to students with disabilities including notetakers, extended testing time, counseling services, and special accommodations.

Vermont

3815 **Burlington College**
351 North Avenue
Burlington, VT 05401-2998
802-862-9616
800-862-9616
Fax: 802-660-4331
http://www.burlington.edu
jsanders@burlcol.edu
Christine Plunkett, President
Yves Bradley, Chair
Stephen St. Onge, Vice President for Academic
Education process vs test and grades. Small classes. Learning specialist available.

3816 **Champlain College**
Support Services
251 South Willard St.
Burlington, VT 05401-3950
802-860-2700
800-570-5858
Fax: 802-860-2750
http://www.champlain.edu
peterson@champlain.edu
Robert D. Botjer, Chairman
Donald J. Laackman, President
RJ Sweeney, Vice President
Four year college that supports students with a learning disability.

3817 **College of St. Joseph**
71 Clement Rd
Rutland, VT 05701-3899
802-773-5900
877-270-9998
Fax: 802-773-5900
http://www.csj.edu
admissions@csj.edu
Richard Lloyd, President
Judy Morgan, Assistant to the President
James Lambert, Director of Communications
Offers a variety of services to students with disabilities including note takers, extended testing time, counseling services, and special accommodations.

3818 **Community College of Vermont**
Student Services Office
PO Box 489
660 Elm Street
Montpelier, VT 05602-489
802-828-2800
800-228-6686
Fax: 802-828-2805
http://www.ccv.vsc.edu
ccvinfo@ccv.vsc.edu
Joyce Judy, President
Lisa Yaeger, Director of Human Resources
Tapp Barnhill, Executive Director
A public two-year college offering courses, certificates and associate degrees.

3819 **Green Mountain College**
Calhoun Learning Center
1 Brennan Cir
Poultney, VT 05764-1078
800-776-6675
Fax: 802-287-8099
http://www.greenmtn.edu
admiss@greenmtn.edu
Robert C. Allen, Chair
Matthew Menner, SVP Sales and Alliance
Paul J. Fonteyn, President
Four-year college that offers support through the school's Calhoun Learning center to students with disabilities.

3820 **Landmark College**
19 River Road South
Putney, VT 05346
802-387-4767
Fax: 802-387-6880
http://www.landmark.edu
institute@landmark.edu
Peter Eden, President
Gregory Matthews, VP Enrollment Management
Carroll Pare, Senior Director
Our programs are specially designed for a particular audience. designed exclusively for students with dyslexia, attention deficit hyperactivity disorder (AD/HD), or other specific learning disabilities.

3821 **Norwich University**
Learning Support Center
158 Harmon Dr
Northfield, VT 05663-1035
802-485-2000
800-468-6679
Fax: 802-485-2032
http://www.norwich.edu
gills@norwich.edu
Richard W Schneider, President
Dr. Guiyou Huang, Senior Vice President
Gordon R. Sullivan, Chairman
The Learning Center offers an opportunity for individualized assistance with many aspects of academic life in a supportive, personalized atmosphere. Students may voluntarily choose from a wide variety of service options.

3822 **Pine Ridge School**
101 Thorpe circle
Pine Ridge, SD 57770-9598
802-434-2161
Fax: 802-434-5512
http://www.pineridgeschool.com
dkb3131@yahoo.com
Dana Blackhurst, Head of School
Mona Miyasato, Principal
Dora Gwein, Assistant Principal
An educational community that is committed to empowering students with dyslexia and other language based learning disabilities, to define and achieve success throughout their lives.

3823 **The Greenwood School**
14 Greenwood Ln.
Putney, VT 05346
802-387-4545
http://www.greenwood.org
frontdesk@greenwood.org
Caryl Frankenberger, Head of School
Anne Swayze, Assistant Head of School
Jim Kane, Director, Finance/Operations
A boarding and day school dedicated to taking bright and talented boys with learning differences and learning disabilities (LD) such as dyslexia, attentional difficulties (ADD/ADHD), or executive functioning deficits and empowering them with the skills and strategies necessary to bridge the gap between their outstanding promise and present abilities.

3824 **University of Vermont**
ACCESS
A170 Living Learning Center
Burlington, VT 05405
802-656-7753
Fax: 802-656-0739
TDD: 802-656-3865
TTY: 802-656-7753
http://www.uvm.edu/access
access@uvm.edu
Jean Haverstick, Learning Specialist
Nick Ogrizovich, Information Specialist
Diana Williams, M.A., M.S., Learning Specialist
Provides accommodation, consultation, collaboration and educational support services as a means to foster opportunities for students with disabilities to participate in a barrier free learning environment.

3825 **Vermont Technical College**
PO Box 500
124 Admin Drive
Randolph Center, VT 05061
802-728-1000
800-442-8821
Fax: 802-728-1321
TDD: 802-728-1278
http://www.vtc.vsc.edu
rgoodall@vtc.edu
Pamela Ankuda, Director of Human Resources
Jim Smith, Chief Technology Officer
Dan Smith, Interim President
Offers a variety of services to students with disabilities including individualized accommodations, counseling services, academic counseling.

Virginia

3826 **Averett College**
Support Services for Students
420 West Main St.
Danville, VA 24541
434-791-5600
Fax: 804-791-4392
http://www.averett.edu
priedel@averett.edu
Pamela Riedel MD, Support Services Coordinator
Bill Bradford, Assistant Professor of Aviation
Dr. Tiffany McKillip Franks, President
Four-year college that offers services for the learning disabled.

3827 **College of William and Mary**
PO Box 8795
Williamsburg, VA 23187-8795
757-221-4000
TDD: 757-221-1154
http://www.wm.edu
Terry Driscoll, Director
Taylor Reveley, President
Anna Martin, VP Administration
Offers a variety of services to students with disabilities including notetakers, extended testing time, counseling services, and special accommodations.

3828 **Eastern Mennonite University**
Academic Support Center - Student Disability Svcs.
1200 Park Rd
Harrisonburg, VA 22802-2462
540-432-4000
800-368-2665
Fax: 540-432-4444
TDD: 540-432-4631
TTY: 540-432-4599
http://www.emu.edu
hedrickj@emu.edu
Loren E Swartzendruber, Coordinator
Dr. Loren Swartzendruber, President
EMU is committed to working out reasonable accommodations for students with documented disabilities to ensure equal access to the University and its related programs.

3829 **Emory & Henry College**
PO Box 947
Emory, VA 24327-0947
276-944-4121
800-848-5493
Fax: 276-944-6180
http://www.ehc.edu
helpdesk@ehc.edu
Jake Schrum, President
David Haney, Vice President/Dean of Faculty
Pam Gourley, Vice President/Dean of Students
A private four-year liberal arts college located in the foothills of southwest Virginia. Student enrollment of appox. 1,000, almost equally divided between men and women. The Paul Adrian Powell III resource center offers a variety of services to students with disabilities including extended testing time, counseling services, and special accommodations, as well as tutorial services.

3830 **Ferrum College**
PO Box 1000
Ferrum, VA 24088-9001
540-365-2121
800-868-9797
Fax: 540-365-4203
TDD: 540-365-4614
http://www.ferrum.edu
Jennifer L Braaten, President
Dr. Gail Summer, VP Academic Affairs
Samuel L. Lionberger, Jr.m, Chairman
An independent four-year college with support services for special education students.

3831 **GW Community School**
9001 Braddock Road
Suite 111
Springfield, VA 22151-1002
703-978-7208
Fax: 703-978-7226
http://www.gwcommunityschool.com
SchoolInfo@GWCommunitySchool.com
Alexa Warden, Director
Richard Goldie, Assistant Director
Cassie Sinichko, Administrative Director
The GW Community School is owned and operated by teachers who understand the learning process and the students' needs, and who genuinely enjoy teaching adolesents. They work closely with students and their families to maximize learning. The GW School for Divergent Learners embodies a vision shared by teachers, parents, and students. A school committed to developing and optimizing the giftedness and intellegence of each student and fostering a sense of social awareness and civic responsibility

3832 **Hampden-Sydney College**
1 College Road
Hampden Sydney, VA 23943-685
434-223-6000
Fax: 434-223-6346
http://www.hsc.edu
Keary Mariannino, Executive Secretary to President
DR. Christop Howard, President
Dale Jones,Ph.D., VP Administration
Offers a variety of services to students with disabilities including note takers, extended testing time, counseling services, and special accommodations.

3833 **James Madison University**
Office of Disabilities Services
738 S Mason St
Student Success Center, Suite 1202
Harrisonburg, VA 22807
540-568-6705
Fax: 540-568-7099
TDD: 540-568-6705
TTY: 540-568-6705
http://www.jmu.edu/ods
disability-svcs@jmu.edu
Jonathan R. Alger, President
Dr. A. Jerry Benson, Provost/Senior Vice President
Maggie Burkhart Evans, Executive Assistant
Offers Learning Strategies Instruction and Strategic Learning Course. Learning Resource Centers in writing, communication, math, science, and critical thinking. Assistive technology lab with various software and hardware include scanners, Kurzweil, etc. High speed scanner support alternate text accommodations. Students with learning disabilities of ADHD may participate in Learning Leaders program.

3834 **John Tyler Community College**
Office of Disability Services
13101 Jefferson Davis Hwy
Chester, VA 23831-5316
804-796-4000
800-552-3490
Fax: 804-796-4362
TDD: 804-796-4197
http://www.jtcc.edu
Mara Hilliar, Executive Secretary to President
Dr. Edward Raspiller, President
Dr. L. Ray Drinkwater, VP Student Affairs
A public two-year college with support services for special education students.

3835 **Liberty University**
Office of Academic Disability Support
1971 University Boulevard
Lynchburg, VA 24515-2213
434-582-2000
Fax: 434-582-2976
TDD: 434-522-0420
http://www.liberty.edu
wdmchane@liberty.edu
Lee Beaumont, SVP for Auxiliary Service
Jerry Falwell, President
Neal A. Askew, SVP Special Project
Religiously oriented, private, coeducational, comprehensive four year institution. Students who have documented learning disabilities are eligible to receive support services. These would include academic advising, priority class registration, tutoring and testing accommodations.

3836 **Little Keswick School**
P.O. Box 24
Keswick, VA 22947-0024
434-295-0457
Fax: 434-977-1892
http://www.littlekeswickschool.net
Terry Columbus, M.Ed., Director, Admissions
Marc J. Columbus. M.Ed., Headmaster
Jody Berkey, M.Ed., Assistant Head of School
A therapeutic boarding school for 33 boys who have learning, emotional, and behavioral difficulties.
1963

3837 **Longwood College**
201 High Street
Graham Hall
Farmville, VA 23909
434-395-2391
800-281-4677
Fax: 434-395-2434
http://www.longwood.edu/disability
disabilityresources@longwood.edu
Lindsay F. Farrar M.S., CRC, Director
Dana Kieran M.S., Assistant Director
Cameron D. Patterson, Program Coordinator
A public four-year college with support services for special education students.

3838 **Lord Fairfax Community College**
173 Skirmisher Lane
Middletown, VA 22645-1745
540-868-7000
800-906-5322
Fax: 540-868-7100
TDD: 540-868-7218
http://www.lfcc.edu

Mary E. Greene, Chair
Dr. Cheryl Thompson-Stacy, President
Chris Boies, Vice President
A public two-year college. Students are encouraged to identify special needs during the admissions process and to request support services, such as individualized placement testing, developmental studies, learning assistance programs, and study skills. A 504 faculty team recommends accommodations to academic programs, and communicates with area service providers.

3839 **Mary Washington College**
University of Mary Washington Disability Services
1301 College Ave
Fredericksburg, VA 22401-5300
540-654-1000
Fax: 540-654-1073
TDD: 540-654-1102
http://www.umw.edu
jhample@umw.edu

Jeffrey W. Rountree, Executive Director and CEO
Salvatore M. Meringolo, Vice President
Richard V. Hurley, President
A public four-year college with support services for special education students.

3840 **New River Community College**
PO Box 1127
5251 College Drive
Dublin, VA 24084-1127
540-674-3600
866-462-6722
Fax: 540-674-3644
TDD: 540-674-3619
http://www.nr.edu
nrdixoj@nr.ca.cc.va.us

Pat Huber, Vice President for Instruction
F. Brad Denardo, Chair
Jack Lewis, President
A public two-year college with support services for special education students.

3841 **Norfolk State University**
700 Park Avenue
Norfolk, VA 23504-8090
757-823-8396
800-274-1821
Fax: 757-823-2078
http://www.nsu.edu
admissions@nsu.edu

Paula Paula, Assistant to the President
Eddie N. Moore Jr., President
Clementine Cone, Executive Assistant
Four year university that offers programs for the students with learning disabilities.

3842 **Northern Virginia Community College**
Disability Support Department
8333 Little River Turnpike
Annandale, VA 22003-3796
703-323-7000
Fax: 703-323-3559
http://www.nvcc.edu

Robert G Templon Jr, President
John T Denver, Executive Vice President
Pat Gary, Chair
A public two-year college.

3843 **Oakwood School**
7210 Braddock Rd.
Annandale, VA 22003
703-941-5788
Fax: 703-941-4186
http://www.oakwoodschool.com
oakwood@oakwoodschool.com

Robert McIntyre, Chairman
A private, non-profit, co-educational day school for elementary and middle school students with mild to moderate learning differences.

3844 **Old Dominion University**
5115 Hampton Boulevard
Norfolk, VA 23529-0001
757-683-4655
Fax: 757-683-3000
TDD: 757-683-5356
http://www.studentaffairs.odu.edu/disability
disabilityservices@odu.edu

Velvet Grant, Assistant to the President/CEO
John R Broderick, President
Bob Fenning, VP Administration & Finance
Providing accomodations for students admitted to Old Dominion University that have a documented disability.

3845 **Patrick Henry Community College**
Patrick Henry Community College
645 Patriot Avenue
Martinsville, VA 24112-5311
276-638-8777
800-232-7997
Fax: 276-656-0327
TDD: 276-638-2433
http://www.ph.vccs.edu
klandrum@patrickhenry.edu

Angeline D. Godwin, Ph.D., J.D., President
Christopher Parker, PhD., VP Institutional Advancement
Debbie Bryant, Financial Assistant
Offers a variety of services to students with disabilities including note takers, adaptive testing, counseling services, peer tutoring and adaptive equipment, and accessible transportation.

3846 **Paul D Camp Community College**
PO Box 737
100 North College Drive
Franklin, VA 23851-737
757-569-6700
Fax: 757-569-6773
TDD: 757-569-7946
http://www.pdc.edu/
info@pdc.edu

Richard Brooks, Chair
Paul W. Conco, President
Randy Betz, VP Workforce Development
A public two-year institution with two campuses. Students with learning disabilities are eligible for special services provided by the Student Support Service Program. Learning-disabled students may take advantage of tutors (outside of class time and during class labs), notetakers, and taped textbooks. A counselor serves as student advocate and helps students arrange for classroom accommodations with instructors.

3847 **Piedmont Virginia Community College**
501 College Dr
Charlottesville, VA 22902-7589
434-977-3900
Fax: 434-971-8232
http://www.pvcc.edu
admissions@pvcc.edu

Frank Friedman, President
John R. Donnelly, Vice President
Corinne Lauer, Administrative Assistant
A two-year comprehensive community college dedicated to the belief that individuals should have equal opportunity to develop and extend their skills and knowledge. Consistent with this philosophy and in compliance with the Americans with Disabilities Act, we encourage persons with disabilities to apply.

3848 **Randolph-Macon Woman's College**
2500 Rivermont Ave
Lynchburg, VA 24503-1526
434-947-8000
800-745-RMWC
Fax: 434-947-8139
TDD: 434-947-8608
http://http://www.randolphcollege.edu
admissions@randolphcollege.edu

Bradley W. Bateman, Ph.D., President
Rebecca Morrison Dunn, Chair
Wesley R. Fugate, Ph. D., Vice President
An independent four-year college with support services for students with disabilities.

3849 **Rappahannock Community College**
12745 College Drive
Glenns, VA 23149-2616
804-758-6700
800-836-9381
Fax: 804-758-3852
http://www.rcc.vccs.edu
mcralle@rappahannock.edu
Elizabeth Hinton Crowther, President
D. Kim McManus, Vice President, Finance & Admin
Cherie N. Carl, Director of College Advancement
Offers a variety of services to students with disabilities including notetakers, extended testing time, counseling services, and special accommodations.

3850 **Riverside School**
2110 McRae Rd.
North Chesterfield, VA 23235
804-320-3465
Fax: 804-320-6146
http://www.riversideschool.org
info@riversideschool.org
William J. Longan, Jr., President
Richard W. Fowlkes, Vice President
Juliette Sykes, Treasurer
Provides remediation of language skills of at-risk students with dyslexia in grades 1-8, so that they can return to mainstream education fully prepared to realize their highest potential.

3851 **Saint Coletta: Alexandria**
Adult Programs
207 S Peyton Street
Alexandria, VA 22314-2812
571-438-6940
Fax: 571-438-6949
TTY: 202-350-8695
http://www.stcoletta.org
Sharon B. Raimo, Chief Executive Officer
John Shank, VP Federal Legislative Affairs
David Pryor, Jr., President
Offer adults age 18 and older opportunities to participate in vocational and pre-vocational training, life skills training, and community integration in order to achieve greater independence.

3852 **Southern Virginia College**
One University Hill Drive
Buena Vista, VA 24416-3038
540-261-8400
800-229-8420
Fax: 540-266-3806
http://http://svu.edu/
student.finances@svu.edu
Paul K. Sybrowsky, President
Robert E. Huch, Vice President of Finance
Glade M. Knight, Chair
Offers a variety of services to students with disabilities including note takers, extended testing time, counseling services, and special accommodations.

3853 **Southside Virginia Community College**
109 Campus Drive
Alberta, VA 23821-2930
434-949-1000
http://www.sv.vccs.edu
rhina.jones@southside.edu
John J Cavan, President
Dorcas Helfant-Browning, Chair
Idalia Fernandez, Vice Chair
Offers a variety of services to students with disabilities including notetakers, extended testing time, counseling services, and special accommodations.

3854 **Southwest Virginia Community College**
PO Box SVCC
Richlands, VA 24641
276-964-2555
Fax: 276-964-9307
TDD: 276-964-7235
http://www.sw.edu
admissions@sw.edu
Dr. J. Mark Estepp, President
Michael Bales, Business Manager
Peggy Barber, Director
Offers a variety of services to students with disabilities including note takers, extended testing time, counseling services, and special accommodations.

3855 **The New Community School**
4211 Hermitage Rd
Richmond, VA 23227
804-266-2494
Fax: 804-264-3281
http://www.tncs.org
info@tncs.org
Nancy L. Foy, Head of School
The New Community School is an independent day school specializing in college preparatory instruction and intensive remediation for students in grades 5-12 with dyslexia and related learning differences.

3856 **Thomas Nelson Community College**
99 Thomas Nelson Dr
Hampton, VA 23666
757-825-2700
Fax: 757-825-2763
http://www.tncc.edu
info@TNCC.edu
Thomas Kellen, Admissions Advisor
Dr. John.T Dever, President
Howard Taylor, Administrator
A public two-year college with support services for students with disabilities.

3857 **Tidewater Community College**
350 Granby Street
Norfolk, VA 23510
757-822-1110
TTY: 757-822-1248
http://www.tcc.edu
tcharro@tcc.edu
Edna Baehre-Kolovani, Ph.D., President
Mr. Franklin Dunn, Executive Vice President
Valary Lejman, Administrative Assistant
This public two-year college offers transfer and occupational/technical degrees on four campuses and a visual arts center in the Hampton Roads area of Virginia. TCC offers students evaluations, all reasonable accommodations, and a wide array of assistive technology.

3858 **University of Virginia**
Learning Needs & Evaluation Cetner
400 Brandon Avenue
PO Box 800760
Charlottesville, VA 22908-760
434-924-5362
Fax: 434-982-3956
http://www.virginia.edu/studenthealth/
studenthealth@virginia.edu
Chris P. Holstege, M.D., Executive Director
James.C Turner, Director
Full range of support services for students admitted to any of the ten schools of the university, including graduate/professional schools. Including, but not limited to, alternate texts, exam accommodations, peer-notetakers, TTY and interpreters, assistive devices and housing and transportation accommodations.

3859 **Virginia Commonwealth University**
Services for Students with Disabilities
901 W Franklin St
Richmond, VA 23284-9066
804-828-0100
800-841-3638
Fax: 804-828-1899
http://www.vcu.edu
vcuhsinternet@mcvh-vcu.edu

Michael Rao, Ph.D., President
Marti K. S. Heil, Vice president for Development
Mark E. Rubin, Executive Director
Offers a variety of services to students with disabilities including note takers, extended testing time, counseling services, and special accommodations.

3860 **Virginia Highlands Community College**
PO Box 828
100 VHCC Drive
Abingdon, VA 24212-828
276-739-2400
877-739-6115
Fax: 276-739-2590
http://http://www.vhcc.edu
helpdesk@vhcc.edu
James F. Rector, Jr., Chair
Virgil C. Wimmer, Vice-Chair
Gene C. Couch, Jr., President
A public two-year college. Strives to assist students with disabilities in successfully responding to challenges of academic study and job training.

3861 **Virginia Intermont College**
1013 Moore Street
Bristol, VA 24201-4298
276-669-6101
800-451-1842
Fax: 276-466-7963
http://www.vic.edu
bholbroo@vic.edu
E. Clorisa Phillips, Ph.D., President
Kathleen W. O'Brien, Chair
Linda C. Morgan, SVP for Administration
Virginia Intermont College is a private, four-year Baptist affiliated liberal arts college located near the Appalachian Mountains of Southwest Virginia. Intermont has an enrollment of 850 men and women students. Accommodations, such as notetakers, extended time on tests, transcribers, oral testing, tutors and other services, are provided based on documentiation of disabilities.

3862 **Virginia Polytechnic Institute and State University**
430 Old Turner Street
Blacksburg, VA 24061
540-231-3788
Fax: 540-231-3232
TTY: 540-231-0853
http://www.ssd.vt.edu
ssd@vt.edu
Susan Angle MD, Director For Disability Services
Charles Steger, President
Robyn Hudson, Assistant Director
A public four-year college with support services for special education students.

3863 **Virginia Wesleyan College**
Disabilities Services Office
1584 Wesleyan Dr
Norfolk, VA 23502-5599
757-455-3200
800-737-8684
Fax: 757-466-8526
http://www.vwc.edu
fpearson@vwc.edu
William T Greer Jr, President
Mr. Bruce Vaughan, Vice President of Operations
Gary D. Bonnewell, Chairman
Four year college that offers support to students with a learning disability.

3864 **Virginia Western Community College**
PO Box 14007
Roanoke, VA 24038-4007
540-857-7231
Fax: 540-857-6102
TDD: 540-857-6351
http://www.virginiawestern.edu
helpdesk@virginiawestern.edu
Michael Henderson, Special Services
Dana Asciolla, Admissions Staff
Robert Sandel, President
A public two-year college with support services for special education students.

Washington

3865 **Bellevue Community College**
3000 Landerholm Cir SE
Bellevue, WA 98007-6484
425-564-1000
Fax: 425-649-3173
TTY: 425-564-4110
http://www.bcc.ctc.edu
admissions@bellevuecollege.edu
Dave Rule, President
Carol Jones-Watkins, Coordinator
Disability Support Services provides accommodations for people with disabilities to make their academic careers a success. There is no separate fee for these services.

3866 **Center for Disability Services**
Central Washington University
400 E University Way
Ellensburg, WA 98926-7431
509-963-2171
Fax: 509-963-3235
http://www.cwu.edu
DS@cwu.edu
James L. Gaudino, President
Rob Harden, Director
Pamela Wilson, Associate Director
A public four-year college with disability support services for students with disabilities.

3867 **Centralia College**
600 Centralia College Blvd
Centralia, WA 98531-4099
360-736-9391
Fax: 360-330-7501
TTY: 360-807-6227
http://www.centralia.edu
demerson@centralia.ctc.edu
Robert A. Frost, President
Donna Emerson, Secretary Lead
Michael Grubiak, Vice President
The Special Services Office offers a variety of services to students with disabilities including notetakers, extended testing time, counseling services, and special accommodations.

3868 **Children's Institute for Learning Differences**
2640 Benson Rd. South
Renton, WA 98055
425-336-3260
866-492-4902
Fax: 425-277-7726
http://www.childnow.org
Carrie Fannin, Executive Director
Cathy DeLeon, Director, Clinical Services
Linda Foley, Director, Development
A full-day academic and therapeutic program for children ages 3 to 17. Provides social, emotional, developmental, and neurological strategies for children with challenging learning differences and behavior disorders.

3869 **Clark College**
1933 Fort Vancouver Way
Vancouver, WA 98663-3598
360-992-2314
Fax: 360-992-2879
http://www.clark.edu/dss
tjacobs@clark.edu
Robert K. Knight, President
Bob Williamson, Vice President
Dr. Tim Cook, Vice President
Offers a variety of services to students with disabilities including note takers, extended testing time, counseling services, and special accommodations.

3870 **Columbia Basin College, Resource Center Program**
2600 N 20th Ave
Pasco, WA 99301-4108
509-547-0511
Fax: 509-546-0401
TDD: 509-547-0400
http://www.columbiabasin.edu
pbuchmiller@columbiabasin.edu

Richard W. Cummins PhD, President
Peggy Buchmiller, Assistant Dean & Director
Pat Wright, Associate Director
Provides advocacy and Auxillary aids and services to students with a disability.

3871 Cornish College of the Arts
1000 Lenora St
Seattle, WA 98121-2718 800-726-ARTS
http://www.cornish.edu
hello@cornish.edu
Dr. Nancy Uscher, President
Lois Harris, Ph.D., Provost and Vice President
Virginia Anderson, Chair
Through the Student Affairs Office, appropriate accommodations are provided for students with learning disabilities.

3872 Dartmoor School
2340 130th Avenue NE
Suite 110
Bellevue, WA 98005-2322 425-649-8976
Fax: 425-603-0038
http://www.dartmoorschool.org
Doris.J Bower, Founder and Executive Director
Andrew Wahl, President
Denise Leiby, Director of Special Education
A school where intellectual development and interest creates a mentorship between teacher and student, where students call teachers by their first name, and where staff invest actively in student achievement.

3873 Eastern Washington University
124 Tawanka
Cheney, WA 99004 509-359-6871
Fax: 509-359-7458
http://www.ewu.edu
dsss@ewu.edu
Dr. Mary Cullinan, President
Paul Tanaka, Chair
Michael Finley, Trustee
Although the University does not offer a specialized program specifically for learning disabled students, the disability support services office works with students on a case by case basis.

3874 Edmonds Community College
20000 68th Ave W
Lynnwood, WA 98036-5999 425-640-1459
Fax: 425-640-1622
TDD: 425-354-3113
TTY: 425-774-8669
http://www.edcc.edu/ssd
ssdmail@edcc.edu
Dee Olson, Director
Kaleb Cameron, Assistant Director
Ruben Alatorre, Coordinator-Sign Language
Offers a variety of services to students with disabilities including notetakers, extended testing time, and special accommodations.

3875 Epiphany School
3611 East Denny Way
Seattle, WA 98122-3471 206-323-9011
Fax: 206-324-2127
http://www.epiphanyschool.org
office@epiphanyschool.orgÿ
Laurie Lootens Chyz, President
Hunter Wessells, VP
Belinda Buscher, Secretary
Now, with 233 students served by 43 faculty and staff, Epiphany School and the Board of Trustees turn their attention to a new educational vision, examining the student needs in a changing world, while staying true to the strengths that have served them well for over 53 years. Epiphany has proudly served more than 1,000 students, many of whom return to the School and increasingly bring their own children to be educated here.

3876 Everett Community College
Center for Disabilities Services
2000 Tower St
Everett, WA 98201-1390 425-388-9100
Fax: 425-388-9129
TDD: 425-388-9438
http://www.everettcc.edu
cds@everettcc.edu
Jerod Grant, Director
Esther Moss, Program Coordinator
Abraham Rodriguez-Hernandez, Program Manager
Offers a variety of services to students with disabilities including notetakers, extended testing time, adaptive software and individual accommodations.

3877 Evergreen State College
2700 Evergreen Pkwy NW
Olympia, WA 98505-5 360-867-6000
Fax: 360-867-6577
http://www.evergreen.edu
Thomas L Purce, President
Evergreen's mission is to sustain a vibrant academic community and to offer students an education that will help them excel in their intellectual, creative, professional and community service goals.

3878 Green River Community College
12401 SE 320th St
Room 126
Auburn, WA 98092-3622 253-833-9111
TDD: 253-288-3359
http://www.greenriver.edu
rblosser@greenriver.edu
Dr. Eileen Ely, President
Jennifer Nelson, Program Assistant
Tom Campbell, Chair
Support services for students with disabilities to ensure that our programs and facilities are accessible. Our campus is organized to provide reasonable accommodations, including core services, to qualified students with dissabilities.

3879 Heritage Christian Academy
19527 104thÿAvenue NE
Bothell, WA 98011-2930 425-485-2585
Fax: 425-486-2895
http://www.hcabothell.org
Info@hcabothell.org
Jack Middlebrooks, Chair
Cindy Bushnell, Parent Representative
Wendy Chappell, Preschool Director
Heritage Christian Academy has had the opportunity to educate thousands of children in the Puget Sound region. The school is well known throughout the region for its quality academic program and it is becoming known for its unwavering dedication in equipping students with a Kingdom Education that enables them to stand against a world view in opposition to Christian values.

3880 Highline Community College
PO Box 98000
Des Moines, WA 98198-9800 206-878-3710
Fax: 206-870-3773
TTY: 206-870-4853
http://www.highline.edu
cjones@highline.edu
Jini Allen, Human Resources Staff
Jack Bermingham, President
Debrena Jackson Gandy, Chair
Offers a variety of services to students with disabilities including note takers, extended testing time, counseling services, and special accommodations.

3881 Morningside Academy
901 Lenora Street
Seattle, WA 98121 206-709-9500
Fax: 206-709-4611
http://www.morningsideacademy.org
info@morningsideacademy.org

Aine O'Connor, Director of Operations
Dr. Kent Johnson, Executive Director
Tim Smith, Director
Morningside Academy's school helps both elementary and middle school students to catch up and get ahead. Its students have not previously reached their potential; many have learning disabilities or ADD/ADHD diagnoses; all have average to well above average intelligence. Morningside is not a school for children with significant emotional problems, behavioral problems, or developmental delays.

3882 **New Heights School**
Children's Institute for Learning Differences
4030 86th Ave SE
Mercer Island, WA 98040-4198 206-232-8680
Fax: 206-232-9377
http://www.childrensinstitute.com
micheleg@childrensinstitute.com
Carrie Fannin, Executive Director
Cathy DeLeon, OTR/L, Director of Clinical Services
Dominic Jimenezÿ, Director of Education
A Pre k-12 school based program serving children ages 3-18.

3883 **North Seattle Community College**
Educational Access Center
9600 College Way N
Seattle, WA 98103-3599 206-527-3600
Fax: 206-527-3606
http://northseattle.edu
Mary Ellen O'Keeffe, Interim President
Orestes Monterecy, Administrative Services
Jennie Dulas, Office of Advancement
The Educational Access Center offers a variety of services to students with disabilities including notetakers, extended testing time, counseling services, and special accommodations.

3884 **Northwest School**
1415 Summit Ave
Seattle, WA 98122-3619 206-682-7309
Fax: 206-467-7353
http://www.northwestschool.org
admissions@northwestschool.org
Cory Carlson, President
Lisa Anderson, Vice President
Mike McGill, Head of School
The Northwest School is set in an urban campus that is housed in a historic landmark cared for by our students, we provide a curriculum for grades 6-12 that offers an international perspective and encourages independent and creative thinking in every class. They educate and shape their students into global citizens who will one day shape the community, nation, and world.

3885 **Pacific Learning Solutions**
314 N Olympic Ave
Arlington, WA 98223-9541 360-403-8885
Fax: 360-403-7607
http://pacificlearningsolutions.com
pacificlearningsolutions@gmail.com
Nola Smith, President
Leslie Platt, Tutor
Rebecca Wesson, Tutor
Tutoring for dyslexia; therapy for processing, memory recall and learning difficulties; LiFT (Listening is Fitness Training), Teacher consultant with Academy Northwest Private school helping home school families.

3886 **Pierce Community College**
9401 Farwest Dr SW
Lakewood, WA 98498-1999 253-964-6500
Fax: 253-964-6599
http://www.pierce.ctc.edu
mharris@pierce.ctc.edu
Angie Roarty, Chair
Steve Smith, Vice Chair
Brett Willis, Trustee
A federally funded TRIO progrm providing academic support services to low income students, first generation college students and students with disabilities in order to improve their retention, academic proformance, graduation and transfer to four-year institutions.

3887 **Seattle Academy of Arts and Sciences**
1201 E Union St
Seattle, WA 98122-3925 206-323-6600
Fax: 206-323-6618
http://seattleacademy.org
admissions@seattleacademy.org
Jean Orvis, Administrator
Barbara Burk, Administrative Assistant
Joe Puggelli, Head of School
Seattle Academy prepares students to participate effectively in modern society. They seek a diversified student body and faculty.

3888 **Seattle Central Community College**
Seattle Community College District
1701 Broadway
Seattle, WA 98122-2400 206-587-3800
Fax: 206-344-4390
TDD: 206-934-5450
http://www.seattlecentral.org
SCCCWCC@sccd.ctc.edu
Paul T. Killpatrick, Ph.D., President
Warren Brown, EVP
Adam Nance, Executive Director
Offers a variety of services to students with disabilities including notetakers, extended testing time, counseling services, and special accommodations.

3889 **Seattle Christian Schools**
18301 Military Rd S
Seatac, WA 98188-4684 206-246-8241
Fax: 206-246-9066
http://www.seattlechristian.com
ghunter@seattlechristian.org
Gloria Hunter, Superintendent
Bryan Peterson, Principal
Dave Steele, Administrator
Independent, interdenominational Christian Day School established in 1946, serving 750+ students.

3890 **Seattle Pacific University**
3307 3rd Ave W
Ste 214
Seattle, WA 98119-1997 206-281-2000
Fax: 206-286-7348
TDD: 206-281-2475
TTY: 206-281-2224
http://www.spu.edu
centerforlearning3@spu.edu
Daniel J. Martin, President
Don Mortenson, VP
Jeff Jordan, VP
Offers a variety of services to students with disabilities including notetakers, extended testing time, books on tape, interpreters and special accommodations.

3891 **Shoreline Christian School**
2400 NE 147th St
Shoreline, WA 98155-7395 206-364-7777
Fax: 206-364-0349
http://www.shorelinechristian.org
admin@shorelinechristian.org
Michael C. Smith, Head of School
Tassie DeMoney, Dir., Development/Marketing
Shoreline Christian School educates students in preschool through grade 12, challenging them to grow academically, socially and spiritually.

3892 **Snohomish County Christian**
17931 64th Ave W
Lynnwood, WA 98037-7106 425-742-9518
Fax: 425-745-9306
http://www.cpcsschools.com/lynnwood

Dr. Clinton Behrends, District Superintendent
Jan Isakson, School Administrator
Mary Riley, Preschool/Childcare Director
The Lynnwood Campus is focused on a Christ-centered education that prepares their students to authentically live for God while serving Him and others.

3893 **South Puget Sound Community College**
2011 Mottman Rd SW
Olympia, WA 98512-6292 360-754-7711
Fax: 360-664-0780
http://www.spscc.ctc.edu
advising@spscc.ctc.edu
Gerald Pumphrey, Disability Support Coordinator
Kenneth Minnaert, President
Marilyn Adair, Nursing/Director
Offers a variety of services to students with disabilities including notetakers, extended testing time, books on tape, readers, scribes, interpreters, assistance with registration.

3894 **South Seattle Community College**
6000 16th Ave SW
Seattle, WA 98106-1499 206-764-5300
Fax: 206-764-5393
TDD: 800-833-6388
http://www.southseattle.edu
rtillman@sccd.ctc.edu
Jill Wakefield, President
Albert Shen, Chair
Courtney Gregoire, Vice Chair
Offers a variety of services to students with disabilities including notetakers, extended testing time, counseling services and special accommodations.

3895 **Spokane Community College**
1810 N Greene St
Spokane, WA 99217-5399 509-533-7000
800-248-5644
TDD: 509-533-7482
http://www.scc.spokane.edu
shanson@scc.spokane.edu
Christine Johnson, Chancellor
Scott Morgan, President
Ben Wolfe, Director
Offers a variety of services to students with disabilities including notetakers, extended testing time, counseling services, and special accommodations.

3896 **Spokane Falls Community College**
3410 W Fort George Wright Dr
Spokane, WA 99224-5288 509-533-3500
888-509-7944
Fax: 509-533-3237
TDD: 509-533-3838
TTY: 509-533-3838
http://www.spokanefalls.edu
Christine Johnson, Chancellor
Scott Morgan, President
Ben Wolfe, Director
Offers a variety of services to students with disabilities including notetakers, extended testing time, counseling services, and special accommodations.

3897 **St. Alphonsus**
5816 15th Ave NW
Seattle, WA 98107-3096 206-782-4563
Fax: 206-789-5709
http://www.stalphonsus-sea.org
Fr. Shane McKee, SOLT, Pastor
Matt Eisenhauer, Principal
Charleen Sweet, Administrative Assistant
The Society has assigned priests to serve the local Seattle area out of the parish rectory.The excellent relationship between the Archdiocese and the SOLT community has also afforded the assignment of dozens of SOLT sisters and novices to the convent located on St. Alphonsus parish grounds.

3898 **St. Matthew's**
1240 NE 127th St
Seattle, WA 98125-4021 206-363-6767
Fax: 206-362-4863
http://stmatthewseattle.org
parishoffice@stmatthewseattle.org
Fr. Jerry Burns, Priest
Jean Cooney, Administrative Assistant
Jon Rowley, Facilities Manager
St. Matthews believe in Jesus Christ and welcome all who seek God's Grace. Their compassionate community embraces many cultures. Through prayer, liturgy, our ministries and service to others, they cultivate a lifelong journey of faith.

3899 **St. Thomas School**
8300 NE 12th Street
Medina, WA 98039-124 425-454-5880
Fax: 425-454-1921
http://www.stthomasschool.org
info@stthomasschool.org
Kirk Wheeler, Ed.D., Head of School
Lyn-Felice Calvin, Director
Bill Palmer, Acting Director
St Thomas School aims to develop responsible citizens of a global society. In partnership with parents, they inspire and motivate intellectually curious students. Their small, nurturing environment supports the acquisition of a broad academic foundation with an emphasis on critical thinking, leadership skills, and the development of strong character and spiritual awareness.

3900 **University Preparatory Academy**
8000 25th Ave NE
Seattle, WA 98115-4600 206-525-2714
Fax: 206-525-9659
http://www.universityprep.org
Matt Levinson, Head of School
Susan Lansverk, CFO
Lora Kolmer, Director of Communications
An independent school serving grades six through twelve, they offer an outstanding academic program guided by our mission statement:ÿUniversity Prep is committed to developing each student's potential to become an intellectually courageous, socially responsible citizen of the world. Their innovative teachers offer a collaborative journey of learning in a diverse community of talented students and involved families.ÿ

3901 **University of Puget Sound**
University of Puget Sound
1500 N Warner St
Tacoma, WA 98416-5 253-879-3211
Fax: 253-879-3500
TDD: 253-879-3399
TTY: 800-833-6388
http://www.pugetsound.edu
admission@pugetsound.edu
Ronald R. Thomas, President
Linda Norwell King, Executive Assistant
Patti Turner, Residence Manager
Support services and accommodations are individually tailored depending upon a student's disability, its severity, the students academic environment and courses, housing situation, activities, etc. Accommodations include instruction in study strategies, free tutoring, assistance in note taking, sign language and additional academic advising.

3902 **University of Washington Disability Resources for Students**
011 Mary Gates
Box 352808
Seattle, WA 98195-2808 206-543-8924
Fax: 206-616-8379
TDD: 206-543-8925
http://depts.washington.edu/uwdrs
uwdss@u.washington.edu

Provides services and academic accommodations to students with documented permanent and temporary disabilities to ensure equal access to the university's educational programs and facilities. Services may include but are not limited to exam accommodations, notetaking, audio-taped class texts/materials, sign language interpreters, auxilary aids (assistive listening devices, and accessible furniture).

3903 **University of Washington: Center on Human Development and Disability**
PO Box 357920
Seattle, WA 98195-7920 206-543-7701
Fax: 206-543-3417
http://www.depts.washington.edu/chdd
chdd@uw.edu

Michael Guralnick, Director
Richard Masse, M.P.H., Director of Administration
Elizabeth Aylward, Ph.D., Associate Director
The Center on Human Development and Disability (CHDD) at the University of Washington makes important contributions to the lives of people with developmental disabilities and their families, through a comprehensive array of research, clinical services, training, community outreach and dissemination activities.

3904 **Walla Walla Community College**
500 Tausick Way
Walla Walla, WA 99362-9267 509-522-2500
877-992-9922
Fax: 509-527-4480
TDD: 509-527-4412
http://www.wwcc.edu

Darcey Fugman-Small, Chair
Don McQuary, Vice Chair
Kris Klaveano, Trustee
The Special Services Office offers a variety of services to students with disabilities including notetakers, extended testing time, counseling services, and special accommodations.

3905 **Washington State University**
Disability Resource Center
217 Washington Building
PO Box 642
Pullman, WA 99164-2322 509-335-3417
Fax: 509-335-8511
http://www.drc.wsu.edu
drc.frontdesk@ad.wsu.edu

Meredyth Goodwin, Director
Juli Anderson, Access Advisor
Kay Smith, Proctoring Coordinator
Provide leadership in the development of an inclusive environment at WSU by eliminating barriers, whether they are physical, attitudinal, informational, or programmatic.

3906 **Western Washington University**
516 High St
Old Main 120
Bellingham, WA 98225-9019 360-650-3083
Fax: 360-650-3715
http://www.wwu.edu/depts/drs
drs@wwu.edu

David Brunnemer, Director
Anna Talvi-Blick, Assistant Director
Kim Thiessen, Coordinator
disAbility Resources for Students (DRS) offers a variety of services to students with disabilities including note takers, extended testing time, counseling services and special accommodations.

3907 **Whatcom Community College**
237 W Kellogg Rd
Bellingham, WA 98226-8003 360-383-3000
Fax: 360-676-2171
http://www.whatcom.ctc.edu
advise@whatcom.ctc.edu

Dr. Kathi Hiyane-Brown, President
Anne Bowen, Executive Director
Patricia Onion, Vice President
A public two-year college with support services for special education students.

3908 **Whitworth College**
300 W Hawthorne Rd
Spokane, WA 99251 509-777-1000
Fax: 509-777-3725
http://www.whitworth.edu
mhansen@whitworth.edu

Marianne Hanson, Director of Admissions
Aaron McMurray, Director
Garrett Riddle, Associate Director
Offers a variety of services to students with disabilities including note takers, extended testing time, counseling services, and special accommodations.

3909 **Yakima Valley Community College**
S.16th Ave & Nob Hill Blvd.
Yakima, WA 98907-2520 509-574-4600
TDD: 509-574-4600
http://www.yvcc.edu

Robert Ozuna, Vice Chair
Paul McDonald, Trustee
Rosalinda Mendoza, Trustee
Offers a variety of services to students with disabilities including notetakers, extended testing time, counseling services, and special accommodations.

3910 **Yellow Wood Academy**
9655 SE 36th St
Suite 101
Mercer Island, WA 98040-3798 206-236-1095
Fax: 206-236-0998
http://www.yellowwoodacademy.org
info@ywacademy.org

Ruth Hayes-Short, Executive Director
Tina Kennedy, CFO
Susan Small, Director of Student Services
Assessment, referral, tutorial, courses for credit, advocacy, dissertation, adults and students that are school age.

West Virginia

3911 **Bethany College West Virginia**
Special Advising Program
Room 4
Morlan Hall
Bethany, WV 26032 304-829-7000
Fax: 304-829-7580
http://www.bethanywv.edu
alumni@bethanywv.edu

Dr. Scott D. Miller, President
Dr. Darin E. Fields, Vice President
William R. Kiefer, Executive Vice President
Bethany College is an academic community founded on the close interaction between students and faculty in the educational process. Bethany College values intellectual rigor and freedom, diversity of thought and lifestyle, personal growth within a community context, and responsible engagement with public issues.

3912 **Davis & Elkins College**
Learning Disability Program
100 Campus Dr
Elkins, WV 26241-3996 304-637-1900
800-624-3157
Fax: 304-637-1413
http://www.dewv.edu
mccaulj@dne.wvnet.edu

Dr. Michael P. Mihalyo, Jr., President
June B. Myles, Chair
Richard C. Seybolt, Vice Chair
Offers a program to provide individual support to college students with specific learning disabilities. This comprehensive program includes regular sessions with one of the three full-time learning disabilities instructors and specialized assistance and technology not available elsewhere on campus.

3913 **Fairmont State University**
Student Disabilities Services
1201 Locust Ave
Fairmont, WV 26554-2470
304-367-4892
800-641-5678
Fax: 304-367-1803
TDD: 304-367-4200
http://www.fairmontstate.edu
admit@FairmontState.edu

Maria C. Bennett Rose, President
Ron Tucker, Chairman
Dixie Yann, Vice Chair
Four year college provides services to learning disabled students.

3914 **Glenville State College**
Student Disability Services
200 High St
Glenville, WV 26351-1200
304-462-7361
800-924-2010
Fax: 304-462-4407
TDD: 304-462-4136
http://www.glenville.edu
cottrill@GLENVILLE.WVNET.EDU

Peter B Barr, President
Rich Heffelfinger, Chair
Greg Smith, Vice Chair
Glenville State College, often referred to as the Lighthouse on the Hill, is West Virginia's only centrally located public college.With an enrollment of approximately 1,400 students, the college has a student to faculty ratio of 19 to 1. The college's enrollment is made up of many first generation students with approximately 90% of the students coming from West Virginia counties.

3915 **Higher Education for Learning Problems (HELP)**
Marshall University
Myers Hall
520 18th St.
Huntington, WV 25755
304-696-6252
Fax: 304-696-3231
http://www.marshall.edu/help
help@marshall.edu

Debbie Painter, Director
Missi Fisher, Assistant Director
Renna Moore, Administrative Assistant
An organization that provides education support for individuals diagnosed with a learning disability and/or ADD/ADHD. Offers the following services: individual tutoring to assist with coursework; studying for tests; administration of oral tests when appropriate; assistance with improvement of memory; assistance with note taking; assistance to determine presence of learning problems.

3916 **Salem International University**
233 W Main St
Salem, WV 26426-1226
888-235-5024
Fax: 304-326-1246
TDD: 304-782-5011
http://www.salemu.edu
admissions@salemiu.edu

John Reynolds, President
Student Support Services grant program funded by the US Dept of Education for 125 college students who are identified as disadvantaged and/or disabled. On staff are a counselor, a learning disabled specialist in math and science and a learning specialist in reading and writing.

3917 **Southern West Virginia Community and Technical College**
PO Box 2900
Mount Gay, WV 25637-2900
304-896-7432
Fax: 304-792-7113
TTY: 304-792-7054
http://www.southernwv.edu
darrellt@southernwvnet.edu

Darrell Taylor, Dean of Student Development
Higher education

3918 **West Virginia Northern Community College**
1704 Market St
Wheeling, WV 26003-3643
304-233-5900
Fax: 304-233-0272
http://www.wvncc.edu

Martin Olshinsky, President
Dr. Darrell Cummings, Chair
Mary K. DeGarmo, Vice Chair
A public two-year college with support services for special education students.

3919 **West Virginia State College**
PO Box 1000
Institute, WV 25112-1000
304-766-3000
800-987-2112
Fax: 304-766-4100
http://www.wvstateu.edu

Kellie Dunlap, Disability Services
Dr.Brian.O Hemphill, President
Melvin Jones, Vice President
A public four-year college. Accommodations are individualized to meet student's needs.

3920 **West Virginia University**
Speech Pathology and Audiology
802 Allen Hall
PO Box 6122
Morgantown, WV 26506-6122
304-293-4241
Fax: 304-293-2905
http://www.wvu.edu/~speechpa
jack.aylor@mail.wvu.edu

Lynn Schrum, Dean
Cheryl Ridgway, Administrative Assistant
Jack Aylor, Director of Development
Provides high-quality programs of instruction at the undergraduate, graduate, and prefessional level; to stimulate and foster both basic and applied research and scholarship; to engage in and encourage other creative and artistic work; and to bring the resources of the University to all segments of society through continuing education, extension, and public activities.

3921 **West Virginia University at Parkersburg**
300 Campus Dr
Parkersburg, WV 26104-8647
304-424-8378
Fax: 304-424-8372
TDD: 304-424-8337
http://www.wvup.edu
wvup_disabilitysv@mail.wvu.edu

Christine Post, Dean Enrollment Management
John Gorrell, Assistant Dean/Director
Alice Harris, VP of Finance and Administration
Provides disability accomodations to qualified students based on appropriate documentation.

3922 **West Virginia Wesleyan College**
Mentor Advantage Program
59 College Ave
Buckhannon, WV 26201-2699
304-473-8000
800-722-9933
Fax: 304-472-2571
http://www.wvwc.edu
kuba_s@wvwc.edu

Pamela Balch, President
The mentoring program, developed from research on the transition and persistence of postsecondary students with learning disabilities and from self-regulated learning theory, is designed to create a bridge to academic regulation in the college environment.

Wisconsin

3923 **Alverno College**
3400 S 43rd St
Milwaukee, WI 53234-3922
414-382-6026
800-933-3401
Fax: 414-382-6354
http://www.alverno.edu
colleen.barnett@alverno.edu
Mary J Meehan, Ph.D., President
Mary Beth Berkes, Chair
Howard Jacob, Ph.D., Vice Chair
An independent liberal arts college with 2,000 students in its weekday and weekend degree programs. Support services for students with learning disabilities include appropriate classroom accommodations, assistance in developing self advocacy skills, instructor assistance, peer tutoring, study groups, study strategies workshops, a communication resource center and math resource center.

3924 **Beloit College**
700 College St
Beloit, WI 53511-5595
608-363-2000
Fax: 608-363-2717
http://www.beloit.edu
Scott Bierman, President
Dan Schooff, Chief of Staff and Secretary
Louise Denk, Executive Secretary
Offers a variety of services to students with disabilities such as self advocacy training, study skills and time management guidance, couseling services, and special accommodations.

3925 **Blackhawk Technical College**
6004 S County Road G
Janesville, WI 53546-9458
608-758-6900
800-498-1282
Fax: 608-757-7740
TDD: 608-743-4422
http://www.blackhawk.edu
OfficeofthePresident@blackhawk.edu
Dr Thomas Eckert, President
Dr. Diane Nyhammer, Vice President
Brian Gohlke, Vice President
A public two-year college with support services for special education students.

3926 **Cardinal Stritch University**
Academic Support
6801 N Yates Rd
Milwaukee, WI 53217-3985
414-410-4166
800-347-8822
Fax: 414-410-4239
http://www.stritch.edu
James P. Loftus, President
Robert J. Buckla, Ed.D, Vice President
Allan D Mitchler, M.A., Vice President
An independent four-year college with support services for special education students.

3927 **Carthage College**
Academic Support Program
2001 Alford Park Dr
Kenosha, WI 53140-1994
262-551-8500
Fax: 262-551-6208
http://www.carthage.edu
Gregory Woodward, President
William Abt, Senior Vice President
Dean Clark, Vice President
An independent four-year college with support services for special education students.

3928 **Chippewa Valley Technical College**
Chippewa Valley Technical College
620 W Clairemont Ave
Eau Claire, WI 54701-6162
715-833-6200
800-547-2882
Fax: 715-833-6470
http://www.cvtc.edu
infocenter@cvtc.edu
Bruce Barker, President
Joe Hegge, Vice President
Ronald Edwards, Manager
A public two-year college with support services for special education students.

3929 **Edgewood College**
1000 Edgewood College Dr
Madison, WI 53711-1997
608-663-4861
800-444-4861
Fax: 608-663-3291
http://www.edgewood.edu
admissions@edgewood.edu
Scott Flanagan, Ed.D., President
Michael Guns, VP Business and Finance
Christine Benedict, VP Enrollment Management
An independent four-year college with support services for students with learning disabilities.

3930 **Fox Valley Technical College**
1825 N. Bluemound Drive
PO Box 227
Appleton, WI 54912-2277
920-735-5600
800-735-3882
Fax: 920-831-4396
http://www.fvtc.edu
helpdesk@fvtc.eduÿ
Dr. Patricia Robinson, Executive Dean
Dr. Susan A. May, President
Jill McEwen, V.P. Administrative Services
A public two-year college with support services for special education students.

3931 **Gateway Technical College**
3520 30th Ave
Kenosha, WI 53144-1690
262-564-2200
Fax: 262-564-2201
TTY: 262-564-2206
http://www.gtc.edu
Bryan D Albrecht, President
In accordance with Section 504 of the Vocational Rehabilitation Act, Gateway provides a wide range of services that assist special needs students in developing independence and sel-reliance within the Gateway campus community. Reasonable accommodations will be made for students with learning disabilities or physical limitations.

3932 **Lakeshore Technical College**
Office For Special Needs
1290 North Ave
Cleveland, WI 53015-1414
920-693-1000
888-GOT-OLTC
Fax: 920-693-1363
TTY: 920-693-8956
http://www.gotoltc.edu
rivi.hatt@qotoltc.edu
Michael A. Lanser, Ed.D., President
Allison Weber, Executive Assistant
Rivi Hatt, Director Student Central
A two-year college that provides comprehensive programs to students with learning disablities.

3933 **Lawrence University**
711 E. Boldt Way
Appleton, WI 54911
920-832-7000
Fax: 920-832-6884
http://www.lawrence.edu
excel@lawrence.edu
Rudi Pakendorf, Associate Director, Development
Laura Zuege, Director, Off-Campus Programs
Sandy Isselmann, Director, Human Resources

Four year college that offers services to the learning disabled.

3934 **Maranatha Baptist Bible College**
745 W Main St
Watertown, WI 53094-7600
920-261-9300
800-622-2947
Fax: 920-261-9109
http://www.mbbc.edu
cmidcalf@mbbc.edu

Larry R Oats, Director
S. Marty Marriott, President
Matthew J Davis, Chair
Four year college that offers programs for the learning disabled.

3935 **Marian College of Fond Du Lac**
45 S National Ave
Fond Du Lac, WI 54935-4699
920-923-7600
800-2-MARIAN
Fax: 920-923-7154
http://www.marianuniversity.edu
admission@marianuniversity.eduÿ

Eric P. Stone, Chairperson
Terri L. Emanuel, Vice Chairperson
Anthony J. Ahern, Treasurer
Offers a variety of services to students with disabilities including note takers, extended testing time, counseling services, and special accommodations.

3936 **Marquette University**
Disability Services Department
1250 W. Wisconsin Ave.
Milwaukee, WI 53233
414-288-7250
800-222-6544
Fax: 414-288-3764
http://www.marquette.edu
patriciaalmon@marquette.edu

Michael R. Lovell, President
Arthur F. Scheuber, Vice President
Dr. Mary DiStanislaoÿ, Executive Vice President
An independent four-year university with support services for students with learning disabilities.

3937 **Mid-State Technical College**
500 32nd St N
Wisconsin Rapids, WI 54494-5512
715-422-5300
888-575-MSTC
Fax: 715-422-5345
http://www.mstc.edu
webmaster@midstate.tec.wi.us

Robert Beaver, Director
Patrick Costello, Director
Terry Reynolds, Director
Offers a variety of services to students with disabilities including notetakers, extended testing time, counseling services, and special accommodations.

3938 **Milwaukee Area Technical College**
700 W State St
Milwaukee, WI 53233-1419
414-297-MATC
Fax: 414-297-7990
http://www.matc.edu
info@matc.edu

Dr. Vicki J. Martin, President
A public two-year college with support services for disabled students.

3939 **Nicolet Area Technical College**
Disability Support Service
5364 College Dr
Rhinelander, WI 54501-0518
715-365-4410
800-544-3039
Fax: 715-365-4445
http://www.nicoletcollege.edu
inquire@nicoletcollege.edu

Ron Zimmerman, Chair
Thomas Umlauf, Treasurer
Robert Martini, Vice Chair
In support of the Nicolet Area Technical College Student services mission, the Special Needs Support Program provides appropriate accommodations empowering students with disabilities to identify and develop abilities for successful educational and life experiences.

3940 **Northcentral Technical College**
1000 W Campus Dr
Wausau, WI 54401-1899
715-675-3331
888-682-7144
Fax: 715-675-9776
http://www.ntc.edu
admissions@ntc.edu

Tom Felch, Trustee
Paul C. Proulx, Trustee
Kristine Gilmore, Trustee
Offers a variety of services to students with disabilities including notetakers, extended testing time, counseling services, and special accommodations.

3941 **Northeast Wisconsin Technical College**
Special Services Program
2740 W Mason St
PO Box 19042
Green Bay, WI 54307-9042
920-498-5400
800-422-6982
Fax: 920-498-6260
TTY: 920-498-6901
http://www.nwtc.edu
more.info@nwtc.edu

H. Jeffrey Rafn, Ph.D., President
Jim Blumreich, CFO
Jennifer Canavera, Procurement Manager
The Special Needs Office of NWTC offers assistance to individuals with disabilities when choosing educational and vocational goals, building self-steem and increasing their occupational potential. We offer a wide range of support services and accommodations which increases the potential of individuals with exceptional education needs to successfully complete Associate Degree and Technical Diploma programs.

3942 **Northland College**
Northland College
1411 Ellis Ave
Ashland, WI 54806-3999
715-682-1699
Fax: 715-682-1308
http://www.northland.edu
admit@northland.edu

Michael A. Miller, President
Margot Carroll Zelenz, Vice President
Robert Jackson, Vice President
Four year college that provides students with learning disabilities with support and services.

3943 **Oconomowoc Developmental Training Center**
36100 Genesee Lake Rd
Oconomowoc, WI 53066-9202
262-569-5515
Fax: 262-569-6337
http://www.odtc-wi.com

Christie Ducklow, Director
Our mission is to provide comprehensive residential treatment, educational and vocational services to children, adolescents, and young adults with dually-diagnosed emotional disturbances and developmental disabilities.

3944 **Ripon College**
Student Support Services
300 Seward Streetÿ
PO Box 248
Ripon, WI 54971-248
920-748-8107
800-947-4766
http://www.ripon.edu
adminfo@ripon.edu

Zach Messitte, President

Student Support Services (SSS) is a federally funded United States Department of Education TRIO program and provides a network of academic, personal and career services to hundreds of students on the Ripon campus who are first generation, lower income or physically or learning disabled.

3945 **St. Norbert College**
Academic Support Services
100 Grant St
De Pere, WI 54115-2099
920-337-3181
800-236-4878
Fax: 920-403-4008
http://www.snc.edu
karen.goode-bartholomew@snc.edu
Thomas Kunkel, President
Raechelle Clemmons, Chief Information Officer & VP
Dr. Jeffrey Frick, Dean of the College, Academic VP
Provides reasonable accommodations for documented disabilities.

3946 **University of Wisconsin Center: Marshfield Wood County**
2000 W 5th St
Marshfield, WI 54449-3310
715-389-6530
http://www.marshfield.uwc.edu
kimberly.kolstad@uwc.edu
Michelle Boernke, Assistant Dean Admin & Finance
Kimberly Kolstad, Academic Advisor
Matthew Lemmerman, Program Associate
A public two-year college with support services for special education students.

3947 **University of Wisconsin-Madison**
Waisman Center
1500 Highland Ave
Madison, WI 53705-2280
608-263-1656
Fax: 608-263-0529
TDD: 608-263-0802
http://www.waisman.wisc.edu
webmaster@waisman.wisc.edu
Marsha Mailick Seltzer, PhD, Director
Qiang Chang, PhDÿ, Faculty Core Co-Director
Joe Egan, MPA, Associate Director
To advance knowledge about human development, developmental disabilities, and neurodegenerative diseases.

3948 **University of Wisconsin: Eau Claire**
105 Garfield Ave
P.O Box 4004
Eau Claire, WI 54702-4004
715-836-4636
Fax: 715-836-3712
http://www.uwec.edu
hansonbj@uwec.eduÿ
James C. Schmidt, Chancellor
Martin Hanifin, Vice Chancellor
Dorothy Nelson, Associate Budget Director
Offers a variety of services to students with disabilities including note takers, extended testing time, counseling services, and special accommodations.

3949 **University of Wisconsin: La Crosse**
1725 State St
La Crosse, WI 54601-3742
608-785-8000
Fax: 608-785-6868
TDD: 608-785-6900
http://www.uwlax.edu
reinert.june@uwlax.edu
Joe Gow, Chancellor
Bob Hetzel, Vice Chancellor
Paula Knudson, Vice Chancellor
Offers a variety of services to students with disabilities including note takers, extended testing time, counseling services, and special accommodations.

3950 **University of Wisconsin: Madison**
McBurney Disability Resource Center
702 W. Johnson Street
Suite 2104
Madison, WI 53715
608-263-2741
Fax: 608-265-2998
TDD: 608-263-6393
TTY: 608-263-6393
http://www.mcburney.wisc.edu
mcburney@studentlife.wisc.edu
Cathleen Trueba, Director
B.A. Scheuers, Assistant Director
Barbara Lafferty, Office Manager
Offers a variety of services to students with disabilities including notetakers, extended testing time, counseling services, and special accommodations.

3951 **University of Wisconsin: Milwaukee**
Exceptional Education Department
PO Box 413
Milwaukee, WI 53201-413
414-229-4721
Fax: 414-229-4705
http://www.exed.soe.uwm.edu
oas@uwm.edu
Amy Otis Wilborn, Chairperson
Paul Ross, Director
Carol L. Colbeck, Dean
A public four-year college with support services for special education students.

3952 **University of Wisconsin: Oshkosh**
Project SUCCESS
800 Algoma Blvd
Oshkosh, WI 54901-8610
920-424-1234
TTY: 920-424-1319
http://www.uwosh.edu
wegner@uwosh.edu
Tim Merrill, Facilities Manager
Richard H. Wells, Chancellor
A remedial program for students with language-based learning disabilities attending the University of Wisconsin Oshkosh.

3953 **University of Wisconsin: Platteville**
1 University Plaza
Platteville, WI 53818-3099
608-342-1491
800-362-5515
Fax: 608-342-1122
http://www.uwplatte.edu
wilsonj@uwplatt.edu
Dennis J. Shields, Chancellor
Mittie N. Den Herder, Provost and Vice Chancellor
Robert Cramer, Vice Chancellor
Coordinates academic accommodations, provides an advocacy resource center for students with disabilities.

3954 **University of Wisconsin: River Falls**
410 S. 3rd Street
River Falls, WI 54022
715-425-3911
Fax: 715-425-3277
http://www.uwrf.edu
dots@uwrf.edu
Dean Van Galen, Chancellor
Fernando Delgado, Provost and Vice Chancellor
Elizabeth Frueh, Assistant Chancellor
Offers a variety of services to students with disabilities including note takers, extended testing time, counseling services, and special accommodations.

3955 **University of Wisconsin: Whitewater**
Project ASSIST
800 W. Main Street
Whitewater, WI 53190-1790
262-472-1234
Fax: 262-472-1518
http://www.uww.edu
amachern@uww.edu
Richard J. Telfer, Chancellor
Rebecca Reichert, Assistant to the Chancellor
Elizabeth Woolever, Program Assistant Confidential

The program is based on the philosophy that students with learning disabilities can learn specific strategies that will enable them to become independent learners who can be successful in a college setting.

3956 **Viterbo University**
900 Viterbo Dr
La Crosse, WI 54601-8804
608-796-3000
800-VITERBO
Fax: 608-796-3050
http://www.viterbo.edu
communication@Viterbo.edu
Dr. Richard Artman, President
Barbara Gayle, Vice President
Todd Ericson, Vice President
An independent four-year college with special services for special education students.

3957 **Walbridge School**
7035 Old Sauk Rd
Madison, WI 53717-1010
608-833-1338
Fax: 608-833-1338
http://www.walbridgeschool.com
info@walbridgeschool.com
Steve Lien, Interim Head of School
Nancy Donahue, Director
Kristina Jasmine, Office Manager
Offers an alternative and comprehensive full day elementary through middle school program emphasizing multi-sensory teaching and individualization to address the learning differences of children. Specialized and personalized instruction is geared to children with learning disabilities including dyslexia and ADHD.

3958 **Waukesha County Technical College**
Special Services Department
800 Main St
Pewaukee, WI 53072-4696
262-691-5566
877-892-9282
Fax: 262-691-5593
http://www.wctc.edu
djilbert@wctc.edu
Barbara A. Prindiville, Ph.D., President
Caroline Tindall, Executive Assistant to President
Karen Krause, Office Assistant
Offers technical and associate degree programs. Services for students with a documented disability may include academic support services, transition services, assistance with the admissions process, testing accommodations, interpreting services, note taking and assistance with RFB&D.

3959 **Western Wisconsin Technical College**
400 Seventh Street North
La Crosse, WI 54601
608-785-9200
800-322-9982
http://www.westerntc.edu
Daniel P. Hanson, Chair
David Laehn, Vice Chair
Edward J. Lukasek, Secretary
Offers a variety of services to students with disabilities including notetakers, extended testing time, counseling services, and special accommodations.

3960 **Wisconsin Indianhead Tech College: Ashland Campus**
505 Pine Ridge Driveÿ
Shell Lake, WI 54871-8727
715-468-2815
800-243-WITC
Fax: 715-468-2819
http://www.witc.edu
Bob Meyer, President
Morrie Veilleux, Chair
James Beistle, Treasurer
A public two-year college with support services for special education students.

3961 **Wisconsin Indianhead Technical College: Rice Lake Campus**
1900 College Drive
Rice Lake, WI 54868
715-234-7082
800-243-WITC
Fax: 715-234-5172
TTY: 888-261-8578
http://www.witc.edu
Bob Meyer, President
Morrie Veilleux, Chair
James Beistle, Treasurer
A public two-year college with support services for students with disabilities.

Wyoming

3962 **Child Development Services of Wyoming (CDSWY)**
PO Box 62
Story, WY 82842
307-752-0687
http://www.cdswy.org
sue@mediationwest.com
Sue Sharp, Executive Director
An organization of the Developmental Preschools Programs serving the state, CDSWY provides therapeutic and educational services to preschool children with developmental disabilities.
1972

3963 **Laramie County Community College: Disability Support Services**
1400 E. College Drive
Education & Enrichment Cntr, Room 222
Cheyenne, WY 82007-3295
307-778-1359
800-522-2993
Fax: 307-778-1262
TTY: 307-778-1266
http://lccc.wy.edu/services/disability
tkeney@lccc.wy.edu
Dr. Joe Schaffer, President
Vicki Boreing, Assistant to the President
Bill Dubois, Trustee
Disability Support Services provides comprehensive, confidential services for LCCC students with documented disabilities. Services and adaptive equipment to reduce mobility, sensory and perceptual problems are available through the DRC, and all services are provided free of charge to LCCC students.

3964 **University of Wyoming**
1000 E. University Avenue
Laramie, WY 82071
307-766-1121
http://www.uwyo.edu
An independent four-year college with support services for special education students.

3965 **Wyoming Institute For Disabilities**
University Of Wyoming
1000 E University Ave.
Department 4298
Laramie, WY 82071
307-766-2761
888-898-9463
http://www.uwyo.edu
wind.uw@uwyo.edu
Karen Williams, Executive Director WIND
Assists individuals with developmental disabilities and their families through early intervention, education, training and community services.

Alabama

3966 **Easterseals Alabama**
5960 E. Shirley Ln.
Montgomery, AL 36117 334-395-4489
Fax: 334-395-4492
http://www.easterseals.com/alabama/
info@al.easterseals.com
Lynne Stokley, CEO
A non-profit organization that provides services to individuals with autism, developmental disabilities, physical or mental disabilities, and other special needs.

3967 **Goodwill Easterseals**
2448 Gordon Smith Dr.
Mobile, AL 36617 251-471-1581
800-411-0068
http://www.gesgc.org
Frank Harkins, Administrator/CEO
Cindy Larry, Chief Financial Officer
Michael DeMattei, Chief Compliance Officer
Children and adults with disabilities and special needs find the highest-quality services designed to meet their individual needs.

3968 **Sequel TSI**
Sequel Youth And Family Services
1329 Browns Ferry Rd.
Madison, AL 35758 256-895-0710
http://www.threesprings.com
Jay Ripleyÿ, Co-Founder/Chairman
John Stupak, Chief Executive Officer
Mandy Moses, Executive VP/COO
Formally known as Three Springs, Sequel TSI is a nationally recognized leader in youth services, founded in 1999 to provide therapy and education to adolescents experiencing emotional, behavioral, and learning problems.

3969 **Wiregrass Rehabilitation Center**
WRC, Inc.
795 Ross Clark Circle
Suite 1
Dothan, AL 36303 334-792-0022
Fax: 334-712-7632
http://www.wrcjobs.com
cgreen@wrcjobs.com
Jeff Coleman, Chairman
Gloria Daughtry, Vice Chairman
Blaine Stewart, Treasurer
Trains individuals to become employable and helps in assisting them to find jobs within their communities.

3970 **Workshops, Inc.**
4244 3rd Ave. South
Birmingham, AL 35222 205-592-9683
Fax: 205-592-9687
http://www.workshopsinc.org
email@workshopsinc.org
Susan Crow, Executive Director
Dana Chang, Director of Programs
Kathy Dunn, Director of Operations
Work adjustment and job development services for people with disabilities.

Alaska

3971 **Center for Community**
700 Katlian
Suite B
Sitka, AK 99835 907-747-6960
800-478-6970
Fax: 907-747-4868
http://cfc.org/
Bryan O'Callaghan, Executive Director
Patrick Hughes, President
Barbara Stocker, Vice President
A state-wide provider of home and community-based services for people with disabilities, the elderly, and others who experience barriers to community living in Alaska.

3972 **Gateway School and Learning Center**
900 W. Fireweed Ln.
Anchorage, AK 99511 907-522-2240
Beverly Lau, Principal
Provides specialized educational services for students grades 1-12 with dyslexia and other language-processing disorders.

Arizona

3973 **Arizona Center Comprehensive Education and Lifeskills**
10251 N. 35th Ave.
Phoenix, AZ 85051 602-995-7366
http://www.accel.org
Cheryl Marvin, Vice President, Operations
Raymond Damm, Chief Development Officer/CFO
Connie Laird, Executive Director
A private, non-profit, special education school providing therapeutic, educational, and behavioral services to over 200 students, ages 3-21, with cognitive, emotional, orthopedic, and/or behavioral disabilities.

3974 **Devereux Arizona Treatment Network**
2025 N. 3rd St.
Suite 250
Phoenix, AZ 85004 602-283-1573
Fax: 480-443-5587
http://www.devereux.org
Lane Barker, Executive Director
Dr. Yvette Jackson, Assistant Executive Director
Janelle Westfall, Clinical Director
Provides a wide array of behavioral health and social welfare services for persons with emotional and behavioral disorders or who are victims of physical or sexual abuse and neglect.

3975 **Life Development Institute (LDI)**
18001 N. 79th Ave.
Suite B-42
Glendale, AZ 85308 866-736-7811
http://discoverldi.com
Robert Crawford, CEO
Veronica Lieb, President
Justin Coller, Director, Operations
Provides a supportive residential community that gives individuals the education, skills, and training they need to live independently. By offering these programs in a residential environment, the students are given a chance to learn independence, and instill in them a desire to succeed.

3976 **Raising Special Kids**
5025 E. Washington St.
Suite 204
Phoenix, AZ 85034 602-242-4366
800-237-3007
Fax: 602-242-4306
http://www.raisingspecialkids.org
info@raisingspecialkids.org
Christopher Tiffany, Executive Director
Janna Murrell, Assistant Executive Director
Maureen Mills, Communications Coordinator
A parent training and information center providing information, resources, and support to families of children with disabilities and special needs in Arizona. Services are offered free of charge.

Arkansas

3977 **Arkansas Disability Coalition**
1501 N. University Ave.
Suite 221
Little Rock, AR 72207 501-614-7020
http://www.adcpti.org
Lynne McAllester, Executive Director
Arkansas Disability Coalition's mission is to work for equal rights and opportunities for Arkansans with disabilities through public policy change, cross-disability collaboration, and empowerment of people with disabilities and their families.

California

3978 **Adaptive Learning Center**
3227 Clayton Rd.
Concord, CA 94519 925-827-3863
http://alc-ca.org
info@alc-ca.org
Donna Feingold, Executive Director
Jordane Tofighi, Associate Director
Barbara J. Simpson, Community Living Coordinator
The center provides a comprehsive program that is designed to address many needs; physical, social, emotional, and vocational. To empower adults with a developmental neurological disability to realize their own potential.

3979 **Almansor Transition & Adult Services**
The Institute for the Redesign of Learning
211 Pasadena Ave.
South Pasadena, CA 91030 323-341-5632
877-837-4332
Fax: 323-341-5644
http://www.redesignlearning.org
info@resdesignlearning.org
Nancy J. Lavelle, Executive Director
Nita Davis, Program Director
A multi-service, community-based education and training facility for at-risk youth. Offering a range of professional services and support to the students and their parents.

3980 **Ann Martin Children's Center**
1375 55th St.
Emeryville, CA 94608 510-655-7880
Fax: 510-655-3379
http://www.annmartin.org
Mojgan Vijeh, Chief Financial Officer
Hasse Leonard-Pagel, Interim Executive Director
Emily Cha, Development Coordinator
A non-profit community agency, providing psychotherapy, educational therapy, and diagnostic testing for children, adults, and families. Also offers a monthly lecture series for educators and child mental health professionals.

3981 **Center For Educational Therapy**
12301 Wilshire Blvd.
Los Angeles, CA 90025 310-979-7860
http://www.educational-therapy.org
cet.adrian@gmail.com
Adrian S. Whitchelo-Scott, Owner
Provides individuals with Autism Spectrum Disorders, Asperger's syndrome, severe ADHD and other learning disabilities with remedial programs and asssistive technology. Works with parents, school administrators, doctors, social workers, and psychologists.

3982 **Charles Armstrong School**
1405 Solana Dr.
Belmont, CA 94002 650-592-7570
Fax: 650-591-3114
http://www.charlesarmstrong.org
information@charlesarmstrong.org
Beth Springer, President
Sydney Bernier, Vice President
Clint Oram, Treasurer
The mission of the school is to serve the dyslexic learner by providing an appropriate educational experience which not only enables the students to acquire language skills, but also instills a joy of learning, enhances self-worth, and allows each student the right to identify, understand, and fulfill their personal potential.

3983 **Devereux California**
P.O. Box 6784
Santa Barbara, CA 93160 805-968-2525
Fax: 805-879-0398
http://www.devereux.org
info@devereux.org
Jennifer Pascoe, Direcore, Finance/Support
Veronica Arenas-Soto, Human Resources Director
Amy Evans, Executive Director
A treatment facility offering residential, educational, and adult vocational or day activity programs to individuals ages 8-85 with multiple diagnoses such as; autistic spectrum disorders, emotional and/or behavioral disorders, mental retardation, developmental disabilities, and medical conditions.

3984 **EDU-Therapeutics**
14401 Roland Canyon Rd.
Salinas, CA 93908 831-484-0994
Fax: 831-484-0998
http://www.edu-therapeutics.com
terry@EDU-Therapeutics.com
Terry McHenry, President
Dr. Joan Smith, Program Director
EDU-Therapeutics is a unique learning system that offers effective solutions for overcoming dyslexia, attention deficit, learning disabilities, and reading challenges.

3985 **Frostig Center**
971 N. Altadena Dr.
Pasadena, CA 91107 626-791-1255
Fax: 626-798-1801
http://www.frostig.org
center@frostig.org
Nancy Hogg, Chair
Debbie Baroi, Vice Chair
Dean Conklin, Executive Director
A non-profit organization that specializes in helping children who have learning disabilities. Offers parent training, consulting, school, and tutoring services to learning disabled children.

3986 **Help for Brain Injured Children**
Cleta Harder Developmental School
981 N. Euclid St.
La Habra, CA 90631 562-694-5655
Fax: 562-694-5657
http://www.hbic.org
Jason Cecil, Executive Director
Paula Frontroy, Human Resources Manager
Christopher W. Beswick, Education Program Specialist
Offers help for brain-injured children through long-term, low cost home rehabilitation programs. School programs, rehabilitation, academic, speech, and physical therapy, as needed. Offers an after-school program for youngsters in regular school who are experiencing difficulties.

3987 **Institute for the Redesign of Learning**
625 Fair Oaks Ave.
Suite 300
South Pasadena, CA 91030 323-341-5580
http://www.redesignlearning.org
Nancy J. Lavelle, President
Edward Amey, Managing Director
A multi-service, community-based education and training facility for at-risk youth. Offering a range of professional services and support to the students and their parents.

3988 **Kayne Eras Center**
Exceptional Children's Foundation
5350 Machado Rd.
Culver City, CA 90230 310-204-3300
http://www.ecf.net/programs/kayne-eras-center
Scott D. Bowling, President/CEO
Debbi Winter, Chief Development Officer
Denise Orme, Chief Financial Officer
Kayne-Eras accomplishes its mission by offering educational resources, direct service, and a professional training center. Kayne-Eras provides personalized programming to children and young adults from at risk conditions and those challenged by emotional, learning, developmental, chronic neurological, and/or medical disabilities.

3989 **Marina Psychological Services**
4560 Admiralty Way
Suite 255
Marina Del Rey, CA 90292 310-822-0109
http://wendyjsalz.com
wendy@wendyjsalz.com
Wendy J. Shalz, Psychologist
Comprehensive psychological services for children and adults with learning disabilities and attention deficit disorders. Private, individualized assessment and treatment.

3990 **Park Century School**
3939 Landmark St.
Culver City, CA 90232 310-840-0500
Fax: 310-840-0590
http://www.parkcenturyschool.org
Hilary Garland, President
Justin Hunt, Board Member
Paul Jennings, Board Member
An independent school for average and above average intellect children with learning disabilities. The program emphasizes developing the skills and strategies necessary to return to a traditional program. With a 2:1 student-staff ratio.

3991 **Pine Hill School**
Second Start, Inc.
1325 Bouret Dr.
San Jose, CA 95118 408-979-8210
http://www.secondstart.org/programs/
Tara Bevington, Executive Director
Ray Johnson, Pine Hill Site Manager
Greg Zieman, Director of Educational Programs
A private school that provides special education and alternative services to students with a wide range of learning and behavior disabilities.

3992 **Prentice School**
18341 Lassen Dr.
North Tustin, CA 92705 714-538-4511
http://www.prentice.org
Mark Gaines, Board President
Devon Green, Head of School
Laurie McKinley, Director, Operations/Finance
The Prentice School is an independent, non-profit, coeducational day school for children pre-k through 8th grade with language learning differences.

3993 **Providence Speech and Hearing Center**
1301 Providence Ave.
Orange, CA 92868 714-923-1521
855-901-7742
Fax: 714-639-2593
http://www.pshc.org
pshc@pshc.org
Kevin Timone, President
Kashif Khan, Director, Finance/Administration
Andrew Simone, Chief Executive Officer
Comprehensive services for testing and treatment of all speech, language, and hearing problems. Individual and group therapy beginning with parent/infant programs.

3994 **Raskob Learning Institute and Day School**
3520 Mountain Blvd.
Oakland, CA 94619 510-436-1275
Fax: 510-436-1106
http://www.raskobinstitute.org
raskobinstitute@hnu.edu
Edith Ben Ari, Executive Director
Jessica Baiocchiÿ, Director, Admissions
Polly Mayer, Clinic Director
A co-educational school for students from diverse cultural and economic backgrounds with language-based learning disabilities. Raskob seeks to recognize and nurture the talents and strengths of each student while remediating areas of academic weakness.

3995 **Sandhills School**
650 Clark Way
Palo Alto, CA 94304 650-688-3605
http://sandhillschool.org
info@sandhillschool.org
Jeff Kozlowski, Head of School
Heather Whitlock, Assistant Head of School
Ramsey Khasho, Chief Clinical Officer
A private, non-profit school for children with learning disabilities. Serves students from grades 1-8 and also offers diagnostic evaluations, summer school, and educational therapy for all ages. Boarding with local families is also available.

3996 **Santa Cruz Learning Center**
2560 Soquel Ave.
Suite 200
Santa Cruz, CA 95062 831-331-5611
http://www.santacruzlearningcenter.com
malika@santacruzlearningcenter.com
Malika Bell, Owner
Individualized one-to-one tutoring for individuals aged 5 to adult. Specializes in dyslexia, learning difficulties, and gifted persons. Includes test preparation, math, reading, self confidence, study skills, time organization, and related services.

3997 **Special Education Day School Program**
Inst. for the Redesign of Learning/Almansor Center
1955 Fremont Ave.
South Pasadena, CA 91030 323-257-3006
Fax: 323-341-5642
http://www.redesignlearning.org
info@resdesignlearning.org
Nancy J. Lavelle, Ph.D., President
Erik Quillen, Education Director
Lori Andrews, Education Director
Providing basic education and related services to children with language, learning, behavioral, developmental, and emotional needs.

3998 **Speech and Language Development Center**
8699 Holder St.
Buena Park, CA 90620 714-821-3620
TDD: 714-821-3628
http://www.sldc.net
info@sldc.net
Adrienne Kessler, Chief Executive Officer
Martin Pugno, Director, Finance
April Barnes, Director, Development
A school and therapy center for children and young adults with language, learning, and behavior disorders (many have multiple handicapping conditions), resulting in complex educational needs.

3999 **Stockdale Learning Center**
1701 Westwind Dr.
Suite 110
Bakersfield, CA 93301 661-326-8084
http://www.stockdalelearning.com
slc@igalaxy.net
Andrew J. Barling, Executive Director

A professional State Certified Educational Therapy clinic designed to collaboratively diagnose and assess individuals 5 years of age through adult who have learning disabilities. Offering extensive services for dyslexia, ADD/HD, and other specific learning disabilities.

4000 Stowell Learning Center
15192 Central Ave.
Chino, CA 91710
909-598-2482
Fax: 909-598-3442
http://www.learningdisability.com
info@learningdisability.com
Jill Stowell, President
Lorena Ghale, Director
A diagnostic and teaching center for learning and attention disorders. Specializes in instruction for dyslexic or learning disabled children and adults. Our services include diagnostic evaluation, developmental evaluation, cognitive and educational therapy which is provided on a one-to-one basis, and a full day class for elementary age students with reading disabilities.

4001 Stowell Learning Center: Irvine
1150 Main St
Ste C
Irvine, CA 92614
949-477-4133
Fax: 949-477-4082
http://www.learningdisability.com
info@learningdisability.com
Jill Stowell, President
Lauren Ma, Director
A diagnostic and teaching center for learning and attention disorders. Specializes in instruction for dyslexic or learning disabled children and adults. Our services include diagnostic evaluation, developmental evaluation, cognitive and educational therapy which is provided on a one-to-one basis, and a full day class for elementary age students with reading disabilities.

4002 Switzer Learning Center
2201 Amapola Court
Torrance, CA 90501-1431
310-328-3611
Fax: 310-328-5648
http://www.switzercenter.org
Rebecca Foo, Ph.D., Executive Director
Len Hernandez, Principal
Wendy White, Psy.D., Programs Manager
Provides a personalized academic program in a therapeutic environment. Has one elementary, one middle school and six high school classrooms, plus two classrooms for middle and high school students with a moderate to severe autistic spectrum disorder.

4003 Team of Advocates for Special Kids (TASK)
100 W. Cerritos Ave.
Anaheim, CA 92805
714-533-8275
Fax: 714-533-2533
http://www.taskca.org
Mario Haug, Executive Director
Dr. John Hess, President
Katherine Patel, Vice President
A parent training and information center that parents and professionals can turn to for assistance in seeking and obtaining needed early intervention and educational, medical, or therapeutic support service for children.

4004 Turning Point School
8780 National Blvd.
Culver City, CA 90232
310-841-2505
Fax: 310-841-5420
http://www.turningpointschool.org
info@turningpointschool.org
Dr. Laura Konigsberg, Head of School
Robert Friedman, President
Dana Kitaj, Vice President
A private, non-profit school for children with dyslexia, attention deficit disorder, and learning disabilities who have difficulties in reading, writing, spelling, and math. Also offers camping, after-school classes, and daycare.

4005 Vision Care Clinic
General, Preventive and Developmental Optometry
2730 Union Ave.
Suite A
San Jose, CA 95124
408-377-1150
http://www.visiondiva.com
Dr. V. Liane Rice, Director
Diagnostic and training for those with visual disabilities.

4006 Westmoreland Academy
Institute for the Redesign of Learning
5 & 6 Westmoreland Place
Pasadena, CA 91103
626-356-1500
Fax: 626-356-1501
http://www.redesignlearning.org
info@resdesignlearning.org
Nancy J. Lavelle, President
Paul Bailey, Director of Education
Nicholas Pinto, Director of Education
Speciality, non-public day school program for students with Autism Disorders. Offers a specialized curriculum that is scientifically-proven and evidence-based.

Colorado

4007 Developmental Disabilities Resource Center
11177 West 8th Ave.
Lakewood, CO 80215
303-233-3363
http://www.ddrcco.com
contact@ddrcco.com
Beverly Winters, Executive Director
Rob DeHerrera, Deputy Director/CFO
Jane Byron, Director, Human Resources
The mission is to provide leading-edge services that create opportunities for people with developmental disabilities and their families to participate fully in the community.

4008 Havern School
4000 S. Wadsworth Blvd.
Littleton, CO 80123
303-986-4587
http://www.havernschool.org
info@havernschool.org
Cathleen Pasquariello, Head of School
Christopher P. Koupal, Chairman
Don Wendell, Treasurer
School for children with learning disabilities. Educational programs, special language programs, and occupational therapy is available.

Connecticut

4009 American School for the Deaf
139 North Main St.
West Hartford, CT 06107
860-570-2300
TTY: 860-899-1217
http://www.asd-1817.org
information@asd-1817.org
Jeffery S. Bravin, Executive Director
Jennifer DelConte, Director, Education
Jennifer Pizzoferrato, Director, Finance/Operations
A residential/day program operating as a state-aided private school and governed by a board of directors. It is the oldest permanent school for the deaf in America, offering a comprehensive educational program for the deaf and hard of hearing students, infants, preschoolers, primary, elementary, junior high school, high school, and post-secondary students.

4010 Boys and Girls Village, Inc.
528 Wheelers Farms Rd.
Milford, CT 06461
203-877-0300
Fax: 203-876-0076
http://www.bgvillage.org/
Steven M. Kant, President/CEO
Kimberly Shaunesey, Chief Operating Officer
Maria Giaimo, Chief Financial Officer

The clients of Boys & Girls Village are children in crisis or children with learning difficulties who have experienced rejection, failure, or abuse. Through the years, the agency has evolved into a leading therapeutic and learning facility offering residential shelter, clinical, after-school, counseling, special educational, foster & adoptive recruitment, and training, family support services, and day programs for children and their families.

4011 **Child Care Programs**
Easterseals Connecticut/Oak Hill
733 Summer St.
Suite 104
Stamford, CT 06901 203-388-2192
Fax: 203-388-2196
http://www.easterseals.com/cfc/
Barry M. Simon, President/CEO, Oak Hill
Bruce Stovall, Chief Operating Officer
Meeting a growing need for high-quality child care for more than 20 million young children and their working parents, Easterseals offers child care for children ages 6 months to 5 years. Young children are welcomed to a unique environment where children of all abilities learn together.

4012 **Connecticut Transition Academy**
135 Kirtland St.
Deep River, CT 06417 860-343-1300
Fax: 860-239-0753
http://cttransitionacademy.org
Dr. Pamela L. Potemri, Chief Administrator
Michael R. Cote, Board President
Leszek T. Janik, 1st Vice President
A private, co-educational special education school service children with learning disabilities in grades 1 through 12+. They also offer jobs skills training, language based education, and extended day programming.

4013 **Eagle Hill School**
45 Glenville Rd.
Greenwich, CT 06831 203-622-9240
http://www.eaglehillschool.org
Marjorie E. Castro, Head of School
Robert M. Breakell, Assistant Head of School
Lisa Ferraro, Director, Development
Eagle Hill is a languaged-based, remedial program committed to educating children with learning disabilities. The curriculum is individualized, interdisciplinary, and transitional in nature.

4014 **FOCUS Center For Autism**
126 Dowd Ave.
P.O. Box 452
Canton, CT 06019-0452 860-693-8809
Fax: 860-693-0141
http://focuscenterforautism.org
info@focuscenterforautism.org
Donna Swanson, Executive Director
Fred Evans, Associate Director
Jenee Hepp, Finance Manager
FOCUS Center for Autism is a private, licensed, non-profit, year-round clinical program committed to the treatment of children ages 6-18 diagnosed with Autism Spectrum disorders, attention and anxiety disorders, or who have processing and/or learning problems.

4015 **Forman School**
12 Norfolk Rd.
P.O. Box 80
Litchfield, CT 06759 860-567-8712
Fax: 860-567-8317
http://www.formanschool.org
Scott Sutherland, President of the Board
David Walter, Vice President
Thomas G. Sorell, Treasurer
Forman offers students with learning differences the opportunity to achieve academic excellence in a traditional college preparatory setting. A coeducational boarding school of 180 students with daily remedial instruction balanced with course offerings rich in content that provides each student with a flexible program that is tailored to his or her unique learning style and needs.

4016 **Gengras Center**
University of Saint Joseph
1678 Asylum Ave.
West Hartford, CT 06117 860-232-5616
Fax: 860-231-6795
http://www.gengrascenter.org
GCinfo@usj.edu
This state approved, private special education facility, provides a highly structured, intensive, self-contained special education program for elementary, middle, and high school students. The program focuses on skill development in the core academic areas, functional application of skills, community life skills, work readiness skills, job training, social development, and independent living skills. Special attention is given to the behavioral challenges of individual students.

4017 **Intensive Education Academy**
840 North Main St.
West Hartford, CT 06117 860-236-2049
Fax: 860-231-2843
http://www.ie-academy.org/
info@ie-academy.org
Jeffrey L. Forman, Executive Director
Jillian Slater, Director, Education
Tracy Barbour, Assistant Director, Education
A state approved, non-profit, non sectarian special education facility for children 6 to 21 years with different learning styles. Individualized program with a 5:1 student teacher ratio. Program strives to help each student reach their potential by gaining confidence, recognizing their strengths and limitations, setting realistic goals, and attaining satisfaction by achieving these goals. State approved. Full-day curriculum is offered.

4018 **Klingberg Family Centers**
370 Linwood St.
New Britain, CT 06052 860-832-5503
http://www.klingberg.org
krystal.crockett@klingberg.org
Steven A. Girelli, President/CEO
Joseph Milke, Vice President
Mark Johnson, Vice President
Provides structured programs for residential, day treatment, and day school students in a therapeutic environment. A private, non-profit organization serving children and families from across Connecticut.

4019 **Learning Center**
Adelbrook
60 Hicksville Rd.
Cromwell, CT 06416 860-635-6010
http://www.adelbrook.org
info@adelbrook.org
Garrell Mullaney, President/CEO
Pat Clark, Chief Compliance Officer
David Maibaum, CFO/Facilities Manager
A private special education facility serving adolescents between the ages of 9 and 21. The flexibility of the program provides students with an opportunity to meet their academic needs. Technology is an important component of the program in addition to academics and an opportunity to participate in a vocational component.

4020 **Lorraine D. Foster Day School**
1861 Whitney Ave.
Hamden, CT 06517 203-230-4877
http://www.ldfds.com
ldfds@snet.net
Dominique S. Fontaine, Executive Director
Christine Kirschenbaum, Assistant Director

Teaches elementary grade children with special needs who have experienced difficulty learning in typical school settings.

4021 **Natchaug Hospital School Program**
189 Storrs Rd.
Mansfield Center, CT 06250-0260 860-456-1311
Fax: 860-423-5922
http://www.natchaug.org
Patricia Rehmer, President
Tom King, VP, Clinical Operations
Deborah Weidner, Medical Director
Natchaug Hospital operates three state approved K-12 special education programs for socially, emotionally disturbed youth. Natchaug Hospital also provides in patient and partial hospital programs at 9 Eastern Connecticut locations.

4022 **Natchaug's Network of Care**
Natchaug Hospital
189 Storrs Rd.
Mansfield Center, CT 06250 860-456-1311
Fax: 860-423-5922
http://www.natchaug.org
Patricia Rehmer, President
Tom King, VP, Clinical Operations
Deborah Weidner, Medical Director
The hospital's 54-bed facility in Mansfield Center, provides inpatient care for seriously emotionally disturbed children and adolescents as well as adults in crisis each year.

4023 **Oak Hill**
120 Holcomb St.
Hartford, CT 06112 860-242-2274
TTY: 860-286-3113
http://oakhillct.org
info@OakHillCT.org
Barry M. Simon, President/CEO
James T. Jones, Vice Presient, Finance
Bruce Stovall, Chief Operating Officer
A private non-profit community provider of services for people with disabilities in Connecticut. Oak Hill provides help to all ages and all intellectual, development, and physical disabilities.

4024 **STAR, Inc.**
182 Wolfpit Ave.
Norwalk, CT 06851 203-846-9581
Fax: 203-847-0545
http://www.starct.org
Katie Banzhaf, Executive Director
Bill Casale, Director of Operations
Denise Oakley, Director of Financial Services
A non-profit organization that serves individuals of all ages who have developmental disabilities. STAR provides a variety of educational, residential, and vocational services.

4025 **St. Vincent's Special Needs Services**
St. Vincent's Medical Center
95 Merritt Blvd.
Trumbull, CT 06611 203-375-6400
Fax: 203-380-1190
http://www.stvincentsspecialneeds.org
svsns@stvincents.org
Raymond G. Baldwin, Jr., President/CEO
Christina Longden, Senior Director, Operations
Beth Jezierny, Director, Adult Services
Began as therapy treatment program for children with cerebral palsy, and has evolved into a provider of specialized lifelong education and therapeutic programs for children and adults with multiple developmental disabilities and special health care needs.

4026 **The Children's Program**
Connecticut College
75 Nameaug Ave.
New London, CT 06320 860-439-2922
Fax: 860-439-5317
http://www.conncoll.edu/childrens-program/
info@conncoll.edu
Kathryn M. O'Connor, Director
Beatrice DeMitte, Associate Director
The mission of the Connecticut College Children's Program is to provide a child and family-focused early childhood program for infants and young children of diverse backgroungs and abilities.

4027 **The Foundation School**
719 Derby Milford Rd.ÿ
Orange, CT 06477 203-795-6075
Fax: 203-799-4797
http://www.foundationschool.org/Site/Home.html
Michael Nicholson, Education Director
For students ages 3-21 with developmental needs, learning deficits, behavioral challenges, and autism spectrum disorder. Basic developmental skills address speech/language and perceptual/motor areas. Academic skills are reading, writing, and arithmetic with social studies, science, and career studies.

4028 **The Glenholme School - Devereux Connecticut**
81 Sabbaday Ln.
Washington, CT 06793 860-868-7377
Fax: 860-868-7894
http://www.theglenholmeschool.org
info@theglenholmeschool.org
Julie Smallwood, Director, External Affairs
David Dunleavy, Director, Admissions
Rebecca Nieb, Admissions Associate
The Glenholme School is a therapeutic boarding school that provides a supportive program and exceptional learning environment to address varying levels of academic, social, and emotional development in boys and girls, ages 10-21, with high functioning autism spectrum disorders, ADHD, OCD, Tourette's, depression, anxiety and various learning differences. The goal of the program is to prepare graduates for post-secondary college and career opportunities.

4029 **The Learning Clinic**
P.O. Box 324
Brooklyn, CT 06234-0324 860-774-5619
Fax: 860-774-1037
http://www.thelearningclinic.org
admissions@thelearningclinic.org
Raymond W. DuCharme, Ph.D., Executive Director
A private, non-profit educational program that provides day and residential school focused on ADHD and learning and emotional issues. The program is coeducational and serves seventy students. The aim is to assist students in meeting their academic goals and preparing them for future experiences in educational, vocational, and community settings.

4030 **VISTA Life Innovations**
1356 Old Clinton Rd.
Westbrook, CT 06498 860-399-8080
http://www.vistalifeinnovations.org/
Helen Bosch, Chief Executive Officer
Tracey Celentano, Vice President, Operations
Kathy Townsend, Director, Finance
Educational and support services for young adults with Autism Spectrum Disorders, ADD, learning disabilities, traumatic brain injuries, and developmental delays.

4031 **Villa Maria Education Center**
Villa Maria School
161 Sky Meadow Dr.
Stamford, CT 06903 203-322-5886
Fax: 203-322-0228
http://www.villamariaedu.org
info@villamariaedu.org
Diane McManus, Head of School
Antoinette Keiser, Finance Director
Dedicated to developing the full potential of students who are learning disabled, and does this by providing an education that will help children who learn differently acquire knowledge, develop skills, and increase the self-acceptance and self-esteem necessary to become responsible adults.

4032 **Vocational Center for People who are Blind or Visually Impaired**
Oak Hill Center
120 Holcomb St.
Hartford, CT 06112
860-242-2274
TTY: 860-286-3113
http://www.ciboakhill.org
info@OakHillCT.org
Barry M. Simon, President/CEO
James T. Jones, Vice President, Finance
Bruce Stovall, Chief Operating Officer
Oak Hill provides children and adults with disabilities the opportunity to live, learn, and work in the community. The Vocational Center aids visually impaired adults with job searching and offers specialized training.

4033 **Waterford Country Schools**
78 Hunts Brook Rd.
Quaker Hill, CT 06375
860-442-9454
Fax: 860-442-2228
http://www.waterfordcountryschool.org
info@waterfordcs.org
William R. Martin, Executive Director
Chris Lacey, Assistant Executive Director
Sharon Butcher, Director, Education
The school offers academic, prevocational, behavior management, and life skills programs for children and young adults ages 8-18.

4034 **Wheeler Clinic, Inc.**
91 Northwest Dr.
Plainville, CT 06062
888-793-3500
http://www.wheelerclinic.org
Susan Walkama, President/CEO
Athena Dellas, Chief Financial Officer
Nicolangelo Scibelli, Chief Information Officer
A provider of behavioral health services for children, adolescents, adults, and families that include mental health, substance abuse, special education, early childhood development, prevention, an employee assistance program, and community education.

4035 **Wilderness School**
State of Connecticut Dept of Children & Families
240 N. Hollow Rd.
East Hartland, CT 06027
860-653-8059
800-273-2293
http://www.ct.gov
Wildernessjourney@ct.gov
Aaron Wiebe, Director
Scott Basile, Field Program Supervisor
Bonnie Sterpka, Field Program Supervisor
A prevention, intervention, and transition program for troubled youth from Connecticut. The school offers high impact wilderness programs intended to foster positive youth development.

Delaware

4036 **Bellweather Behavioral Health**
4185 Kirkwood-St. Georges Rd.
Bear, DE 19701
302-834-7018
http://www.bellbh.com
Mike Martin, Chief Executive Officer
Thomas Papa, SVP, Governmental Affairs
Provides services to individuals whose challenges have defied all previous attempts at treatment. Through proven, positive, and comprehensive strategies that teach individuals how to live problem-free, Bellweather can help overcome the burdens and barriers associated with severe and intractable problems.

4037 **Centreville Layton School**
6201 Kennett Pike
Centreville, DE 19807
302-571-0230
Fax: 302-571-0270
http://www.centrevillelayton.org
Edward Rosenthal, Ppresident
Paul M. McConnell, Vice President
Douglas Quaintance, Treasurer
Motivated by two fundamental goals; to provide learning disabled children a vibrant and challenging curriculum comparable to those found at any primary or intermediate level school, and to offer each student the specialized and focused support he or she needs.

4038 **Parent Information Center of Delaware**
404 Larch Cir
Wilmington, DE 19804
302-999-7394
888-547-4412
Fax: 302-999-7637
http://www.picofdel.org
Tika Hartsock, Chair
Jazmone Taylor, Executive Director
Meedra Surratte, Special Programs Manager
Assists individuals with disabilities and special needs and those who serve them; also provides information and referral to other agencies.

4039 **Pilot School**
208 Woodlawn Rd.
Wilmington, DE 19803
302-478-1740
Fax: 302-478-1746
http://www.pilotschool.org
info@pilotschool.org
Alexandra Kokkoris, Director
John Harrison, Finance Director
Colleen Shivone, Development Director
Pilot School provides a creative, nurturing environment for children with special learning needs. The schools works with each child to give them the specific developmental tools, guidance, and attention needed to learn and achieve in order to feel comfortable and successful.

District of Columbia

4040 **Kingsbury Center**
5000 14th St., N.W.
Washington, DC 20011
202-722-5555
Fax: 202-723-2082
http://www.kingsbury.org
center@kingsbury.org
Dr. Dennis Campbell, CEO/Head of School
Angie Harris, Chief Operating Officer
Jen Henderson, Director, Marketing/Comm.
DC's oldest non public school for children with learning disabilities.

4041 **The Lab School of Washington**
4759 Reservoir Rd., NW
Washington, DC 20007-1921
202-965-6600
http://www.labschool.org
Bill Tennis, Chair
John Jonas, Vice Chair
Susan Hutton, Treasurer
The Lab School is internationally recognized for its innovative programs for children and adults with learning disabilities. The Lab School offers individualized instruction to students in kindergarten through 12th grade.

Florida

4042 **Academic Achievement Center**
313 Pruett Rd.
Seffner, FL 33584
813-654-4198
Fax: 813-871-7468
http://www.iser.com/AAC-FL.html
ALSofAAC@aol.com
Lillian M Stark, Ph.D., Educational Administrator
Arnold L. Stark, Ph.D., Educational Director

A private program for bright and gifted children with LD and/or ADD, offering multisensory-based instruction; remediation of basic skills; academic challenge in science, social science, and literature; award-winning art and drama; and curriculum-enhancing field trips and travel. Maximum student body is 22 and it is coeducational. After school tutoring and phonelogical awareness training are also available.

4043 **Achievement Academy**
716 E. Bella Vista St.
Lakeland, FL 33805
863-683-6504
Fax: 863-688-9292
http://www.achievementacademy.com
information@achievementacademy.com
John Burton, Executive Director
Sam Houghton, President
Chandra Frederick, 1st Vice President
Serves children up to age 6 with autism, cerebral palsy, speech delays, and down syndrome. The Birth to Three program offers services to children up to three years of age who may be at risk for developmental delays.

4044 **Atlantis Academy**
Educational Services of America
1950 Prairie Rd.
West Palm Beach, FL 33406
561-220-4757
Fax: 561-969-1950
http://www.atlantisacademy.com
Donna Bussiere, Director
Jennifer Mandat, Assistant Director
A small, private, highly individualized program, Pre K-12, for children with attention disorders, dyslexia, and other academic learning problems. Day students only.

4045 **Baudhuin Preschool**
Nova SE University's Mailman Segal Institute
7600 SW 36th St.
Davie, FL 33328
954-262-6918
http://www.nova.edu
baudhuin@nova.edu
Roni Leiderman, Dean
Jamie Mayersohn, Director, Operations
Donna Hillier, Director, Academics
For autistic children, the program supports the qualities and capabilities of each child. This therapeutic program focuses on cognitive, social-emotional, adaptive, behavioral, motor, and communication skill development within a relationship-based environment. Providing each child with choices, challenges, and opportunities that nurture feelings of competence, promote intellectual growth, and enable each child to achieve his or her potential.

4046 **Children's Center for Development and Behavior**
440 Sawgrass Corporate Pkwy.
Suite 106
Sunrise, FL 33325
954-745-1112
866-290-6468
Fax: 954-745-1120
http://www.childpsych.org
administrative@childpsych.org
Shana Williams, Psy.D., Director, Psychological Services
David Lubin, Ph.D., Vice President, Clinical Affairs
Debbie White-Maynes, Ms. Ed, Director, Academic Services
Dedicated to supporting the social, physical, emotional, intellectual, and creative development in children with speech delays, general developmental disorders, Autism, and Down's Syndrome. Some of the programs include speech language pathology, behavior management, music therapy, occupational therapy, and sibling support groups.

4047 **Exceptional Student Education: Assistive Technology**
Orange County Public School
445 W. Amelia St.
Orlando, FL 32801
407-317-3229
Fax: 407-317-3310
http://www.ocps.net
ian.gesundheit@ocps.net
Ian Gesundheit, Senior Director
Services are provided for students who are mentally handicapped, emotionally handicapped, specific learning disabled, sensory impaired, speech and language impaired, physically impaired, hospital/homebound, Autistic, gifted, and developmentally delayed. Services such as occupational/physical therapy, assistive technology, and assistance for ESE bilingual students are also available.

4048 **Kurtz Center**
1201 Louisiana Ave.
Suite C
Winter Park, FL 32789
407-740-5678
Fax: 407-629-6886
http://www.learningdisabilities.com
dkurtz@learningdisabilities.com
Gail E. Kurtz, Co-Founder
Denton M. Kurtz, Co-Founder/Executive Director
A treatment facility and professional development provider, using scientifically based researched approaches in the treatment of those in need and in training other professionals, paraprofessionals, and parents to use these approaches. Develops individualized programs for all ages that conquer all forms of learning disabilities/difficulties, including the various dyslexias and attention focus problems.

4049 **McGlannan School**
10770 S.W. 84 St.
Miami, FL 33173
305-274-2208
http://www.mcglannanschool.com
Frances K. McGlannan, Founder/Director
A school that provides one-to-one learning for children with dyslexia and other learning disabilities. Diagnostic, multidisciplinary, prescriptive, research-based, and individualized to reach the whole child.

4050 **Morning Star School**
210 E. Linebaugh Ave.
Tampa, FL 33612
813-935-0232
Fax: 813-932-2321
http://www.morningstartampa.org
Eileen Odom, Principal
Alina Lopez, Assistant Principal
Denise Dwyer, Administrative Assistant
A non-profit school for elementary and junior-high age children with learning disabilities and related learning differences.

4051 **Pace Brantley School**
3221 Sand Lake Rd.
Longwood, FL 32779
407-869-8882
http://pacebrantley.org
eshaffer@pacebrantley.org
Pamela Tapley, Head of School
Dr. Rick Dunn, Chairman
Adam Haba, Vice Chairman
An independent, non-profit school for children with learning differences. The PACE program has been specifically designed for students who have been diagnosed with learning disabilities, attention deficit disorder, dyslexia, and similar challenges.

4052 **Summer Camp Program**
Tampa Day School
12606 Henderson Road
Tampa, FL 33625
813-269-2100
Fax: 813-490-2554
http://www.tampadayschool.com
Lois Delaney, Head of School
Andrea Mowatt, Head of Lower School
Crystal Haralambou, Director, Performing Arts
Summer camp program for children in grades K-8. Camp is held in the Citrus Park area and children are encouraged to learn, play and grow while enjoying such activies as arts and crafts, sports, field trips and more.

4053 **Susan Maynard Counseling**
7096 SW 48 Lane
Miami, FL 33155 305-667-5011
http://www.susanmaynardphd.com
info@susanmaynardphd.com
Susan Maynard, Ph.D., School Psychologist
Serices include testing, evaluations and consultations for children who are exhibiting learning/behavior problems or physical and motor difficulties.

4054 **Tampa Bay Day School**
12606 Henderson Rd.
Tampa, FL 33625 813-269-2100
Fax: 813-490-2554
http://www.tampadayschool.com
Lois Delaney, Head of School
T.J. Mullarkey, Associate Head of School
Paula Pennington, Director, Admissions
A school for children with learning differences in grades 2-8. The Tampa Bay Day School seeks to understand each child's unique strengths and needs in order to maximize their learning potential.

4055 **The Learning Academy**
The Els Center of Excellence
18370 Limestone Creek Rd.
Jupiter, FL 33458 561-296-1776
http://tlacad.org
info@tlacad.org
Dr. Toby Honsberger, Executive Director
Danielle Doherty, Director, Behavioral Services
Kathryn Steele, Assistant Principal
A charter high school that serves students ages 14-21 with Autism Spectrum Disorder. Shares it's campus with the Learning Center, a charter school for kids ages 3-14 with Autism.

4056 **The Learning Center**
The Els Center of Excellence
18370 Limestone Creek Rd.
Jupiter, FL 33458 561-320-9500
http://thelearningcenter.org
Stacie Routt, Executive Director
Lelis Rossique, Assistant Principal
Melisa Scott, Officer Manager
A charter school that develops and provides effective education and treatment programs for children ages 3-14 with autism.

4057 **Vanguard School**
22000 US Highway 27ÿ
Lake Wales, FL 33859 863-676-6091
Fax: 863-676-8297
http://www.vanguardschool.org
Harold Maready, Head of School
Marya Marcum-Jones, Principal
Candi Medeiros, Director, Admissions
The Vanguard School program is designed for students age 10 through high school who are experiencing academic difficulties due to learning disability such as dyslexia, dyscalculia, or an attention deficit.

Georgia

4058 **Atlanta Speech School**
3160 Northside Pkwy., NWÿ
Atlanta, GA 30327 404-233-5332
Fax: 404-266-2175
http://www.atlantaspeechschool.org
Jack Zimmermann, Chief Financial Officer
Comer Yates, Executive Director
Iris Goodson, Director, Human Resources
The Atlanta Speech School is one of the Southeast's oldest therapeutic educational centers for children and adults with hearing, speech, language, or learning disabilities. They help children and adults with communication disorders realize their full potential.

4059 **Bedford School**
5665 Milam Rd.
Fairburn, GA 30213 770-774-8001
Fax: 770-774-8005
http://www.thebedfordschool.org
Kris Kennedy, Finance Director
Jeff James, Head of School
Allison Day, Associate Head of School
Serves children in grades 1-9 with learning disabilities. Students are grouped by skill levels in classes of 8-12. Students receive the proper academic remediation, as well as specific remedial help with physical skills, peer interaction, and self-esteem.

4060 **Brandon Hall School**
1701 Brandon Hall Dr.
Atlanta, GA 30350 770-394-8177
http://www.brandonhall.org
Dean J. . Fusto, President/Head of School
Terry D. Lufkin, Assistant Head of School/CFO
Kirsten Perdue, Director, Enrollment Management
Provides both one-on-one and small group college preparatory classes for students who, for a variety of reasons, have not been achieving their potential or who otherwise need a more intensive educational setting.

4061 **Chatham Academy**
4 Oglethorpe Professional Blvd.
Savannah, GA 31406 912-354-4047
Fax: 912-354-4633
http://www.chathamacademy.com
info@chathamacademy.com
Carolyn Hannaford, Principal/Associate Director
Adelle Burnsed-Geffen, President
Jeff O'Connor, Treasurer
Providing a specialized curriculum and individualized instruction for students with diagnosed learning disabilities and/or attention deficit disorder. Chatham's goal is to improve students' functioning to levels commensurate with their potential in all areas so that they may return to and succeed in regular educational programs.

4062 **Creative Community Services**
1650 Oakbrook Dr.
Suite 445
Norcross, GA 30093 770-469-6226
Fax: 770-469-6210
http://www.ccsgeorgia.org
info@ccsgeorgia.org
Dave Collier, Board President
Dr. Dionne Poulton, Secretary
Sally Buchanan, Executive Director
Therapeutic foster care services for children and home-based support for developmentally disabled adults. CCS gives both kids and adults hope by encouraging independent living resulting in involved, engaged citizens and community members.

4063 **Horizons School**
1900 DeKalb Ave., NE
Atlanta, GA 30307 404-378-2219
Fax: 404-378-8946
http://www.horizonsschool.com
Les Garber, Head of School
An independent boarding and day school for grades k-12 that serves students with learning challenges. Horizons offers college prepatory classes, as well as classes in visual and performing arts.

4064 **Jacob's Ladder Neurodevelopmental School & Therapy Center**
407 Hardscrabble Rd.
Roswell, GA 30075 770-998-1017
http://www.jacobsladdercenter.com
Amy O'Dell, M.Ed., Founder/Executive Director
Jaclyn Rhodes, Director, HR/Admissions
Molly Parish, Director, Client Programming

A neurodevelopmental school and therapy center established to provide the child with Autism, PDD, ADD/ADHD, Asperger's, learning differences, Down Syndrome or any other neurological delay, the services they need in order to realize their full potential.

4065 **Mill Springs Academy**
13660 New Providence Rd.
Alpharetta, GA 30004 770-360-1336
Fax: 770-360-1341
http://www.millsprings.org
Robert W. Moore, Headmaster
Bruce Clayton, Chairperson
Ed Coco, Board Member
A value-based educational community dedicated to the academic, physical, and social growth of those students who have not realized their full potential in traditional classroom settings. Learning strategies are generated from psycho-educational evaluations, previous school records, diagnostic skills assessment, observations and communication with other professionals involved with the student.

4066 **The Howard School**
1192 Foster St., NW
Atlanta, GA 30318 404-377-7436
Fax: 404-377-0884
http://www.howardschool.org
Marifred Cilella, Head of School
Anne Beisel, Director, Admissions
Nancy Davis, Director, Advancement
The Howard School is an independent school for children in grades K-12 who have learning differences and language learning disabilities. Instruction is personalized to complement individual learning styles, to address student needs and to help each student understand his or her learning process. The curriculum focuses on depth of understanding in order to make learning meaningful and therefore, maximize educational success.

4067 **Wardlaw School**
Atlanta Speech School
3160 Northside Pkwy., NW
Atlanta, GA 30327 404-233-5332
Fax: 404-266-2175
http://www.atlantaspeechschool.org
Jack Zimmermann, Chief Financial Officer
Comer Yates, Executive Director
Iris Goodson, Director, Human Resources
Dedicated to serving children with average to very superior intelligence and mild to moderate learning disabilities. Children served in the Wardlaw School typically exhibit underlying auditory and/or visual processing problems that make it difficult for them to learn in their present educational setting.

Hawaii

4068 **Center on Disability Studies**
University of Hawaii at Manoa
1410 Lower Campus Rd.
Suite 171F
Honolulu, HI 96826 http://www.cds.hawaii.edu
Patricia Morrissey, Director
JoAnn Yuen, Associate Director
Jennifer Tarnay, Chair
The Center for Disability Studies is a Hawaii University Affiliated Program at the University of Hawaii at Manoa. The mission of the CDS is to support the quality of life, community inclusion, and self-determination of all persons with disabilities and their families.

4069 **Learning Disabilities Association of Hawaii**
245 N. Kukui St.
Suite 205
Honolulu, HI 96817 808-536-9684
Fax: 808-537-6780
http://www.ldahawaii.org
ldah@ldahawaiii.org
Rosie Rowe, Executive Director
Bev Reidy, Education & Training Manager
Stephanie Tim Sing, Administrative Assistant
Serving families with children with learning disabilities and other special needs that interfere with learning by providing education advocacy, training, and support in order to remove barriers and promote awareness and full educational opportunity. LDAH has several special projects that helps fulfill the mission of removing barriers and promoting awareness and full educational opportunity. The Parent Training and Information Center is one of these special projects that is offered.

4070 **Variety School of Hawaii**
710 Palekaua St.
Honolulu, HI 96816 808-732-2835
Fax: 808-732-4334
http://www.varietyschool.org
info@varietyschool.org
Duane Yee, Executive Director
To identify and educate children with learning disabilities and to assist in achieving their maximum potential through a multi-disciplinary approach.

Idaho

4071 **Brain Balance of Eagle**
3210 E. Chinden Blvd.
Suite 113
Eagle, ID 83616 208-337-3559
http://www.brainbalancecenters.com
Dr. Ray Booth, Owner
Dawna Booth, Owner/Executive Director
Using a holistic and integrated approach, Brain Balance helps children with behavioral, social, and academic learning problems.

4072 **Idaho Parents Unlimited, Inc.**
4619 W. Emerald St.
Suite E
Boise, ID 83706 208-342-5884
800-242-4785
Fax: 208-342-1408
http://www.ipulidaho.org
Angela Lindig, Executive Director
Sarah Tueller, Parent Education Coordinator
Amy Ireland, Parent Education Coordinatorÿ
A statewide organization founded to provide support, information, and technical assistance to parents of children and youth with disabilities.

4073 **Joshua Institute**
2150 W. Cherry Ln.
Meridian, ID 83642 208-893-5130
http://joshuainstitute.org
info@cvcs.com
Connie Risser, Executive Director
Debbie Cedergren, Educational Coach
Carmen Classen, Educational Coach
A non-profit organization that helps students with learning disabilities of all types, such as dyslexia, dysgraphia, and auditory processing issues.

4074 **Lee Pesky Learning Center**
3324 Elder St.
Boise, IS 83705 208-333-0008
http://www.lplearningcenter.org
info@lplearningcenter.org

Michael Shaughnessy, Jr., Board Chair
Greg Pesky, Vice Chair
Gregory Byron, Secretary
Founded in 1997, the Lee Pesky Learning Center helps children, families, and schools understand and overcome obstacles to learning.

Illinois

4075 **Acacia Academy**
6425 Willow Springs Rd.
LaGrange Highlands, IL 60525 708-579-9040
Fax: 708-579-5872
http://www.acaciaacademy.com
info@acaciaacademy.com
Kathryn Fouks, Principal/Director
Eileen Petzold, Assistant Principal & Director
Jim Shoemaker-Saif, Head of High School
Offering personalized and exceptional educational instruction to each individual student in the development of his/her intellectual and academic potential.

4076 **Allendale Association**
P.O. Box 1088
Lake Villa, IL 60046 847-356-2351
http://www.allendale4kids.org
Jason Keeler, President/CEO
Connie Borucki, COO/SVP, Human Resources
Chris Schrantz, CFO/SVP, Finance & Business
A private, not-for-profit organization serving children and adolescents with moderate to profound emotional and behavioral disabilities. Allendale is dedicated to excellence and innovation in the care, education, treatment, and advocacy for troubled children, youth, and their families.

4077 **Associated Talmud Torahs of Chicago**
3531 Madison St.
Skokie, IL 60076 773-973-2828
Fax: 773-973-6666
http://www.att.org
webmaster@att.org
Rabbi Mordechai Raizman, Executive Director, Operations
Rabbi Avrohom Moller, Superintendent of Education
Rabbi Yehuda Polstein, Principal of MIE Torah High
An organization that serves the Jewish community by offering mainstreaming, independent skills, therapeutic swim classes, and psychological services.

4078 **Brehm Preparatory School**
950 South Brehm Ln.
Carbondale, IL 62901 618-457-0371
http://www.brehm.org
admissionsinfo@brehm.org
Stacey Brehm Tate, President
Daniel Maher, Vice President
Rita Dodd, Secretary
A boarding school specifically designed to meet the needs of students with complex learning disabilities and attention deficit disorder issues.

4079 **Center for Audiology, Speech, Language, and Learning**
Northwestern University
2315 Campus Dr.
Evanston, IL 60208 847-491-3165
Fax: 847-467-7141
http://nucasll.northwestern.edu
nucasll@northwestern.edu
Francis K. Block, Clinical Instructor
Diane Novak, Assistant Director
Denise Boggs, Director
A teaching clinic that provides diagnostic evaluations for children and adults, remediation for children, and theory-based coursework for graduate students interested in teaching people with learning disabilities.

4080 **Center for Speech and Language Disorders**
310-D S. Main St.
Lombard, IL 60148 630-652-0200
Fax: 630-652-0300
http://www.csld.org
info@csld.org
Karine Faden, Executive Director
Sara Belczak, Director, Clinical Services
Ciara Nally, Clinical Supervisor
The mission is to help children with speech and language disorders reach their full potential. CSLD is an internationally recognized leader in the diagnosis and treatment of hyperlexia and other language disorders.

4081 **Children's Center for Behavioral Development**
353 N. 88th St.
East Saint Louis, IL 62203 618-398-1152
Special education programs for children and adults who are learning disabled, emotionally distubed, or have behavioral disorders. Some of the programs include vocational education classes, computer classes, art, and physical education.

4082 **Cove School**
350 Lee Rd.
Northbrook, IL 60062 847-562-2100
Fax: 847-562-2112
http://www.coveschool.org
Dr. Sally L. Sover, Executive Director
John Stieper, III, Director, Education
Robin S. Johnstone, Clinical Director
The Cove School was established in 1947, to educate students with learning disabilities and to facilitate their return to their neighborhood schools in the shortest possible time. The heart of Cove's educational philosophy is to design a program that pulls out the child's skills.

4083 **Educational Services of Glen Ellyn**
364 Pennsylvania Ave.
Glen Ellyn, IL 60137 630-469-1479
http://www.esgetutoring.com
Megan Burke, Owner
Tutoring for all ages in all subject areas. Diagnostic testing, specializing in learning disabilities and career counseling for learning disabled adults.

4084 **Elim Christian Services**
13020 S. Central Ave.
Crestwood, IL 60418 708-389-0555
877-9-ELIMCS
http://www.elimcs.org
info@elimcs.org
Frederick Wezeman, Chairman
Dr. Mackenzi Huyser, Vice Chairman
William Lodewyk, President
Elim Christian Services is a non-profit corporation that seeks to equip persons with special needs to achieve to their highest God-given potential.

4085 **Esperanza Community Services**
520 N. Marshfield Ave.
Chicago, IL 60622 312-243-6097
http://www.esperanzacommunity.org
info@esperanzacommunity.org
Joy Decker, Executive Director
Jeff Fenwick, Director, Development
Terrell Wilson, Finance Administrator
Accredited by the Rehabilitation Accreditation Commission; Esperanza School is a private, therapeutic school serving students ages 5 to 21 with Autism, mild/moderate/severe cognitive disabilites, traumatic brain injuries, and other health impairements.

4086 **Family Resource Center on Disabilities**
11 E. Adams St.
Suite 1002
Chicago, IL 60603
312-939-3513
Fax: 312-854-8980
http://www.frcd.org
info@frcd.org
Charlotte Des Jardins, Executive Director
FRCD was organized by parents, professionals, and volunteers who seek to improve services for all children with disabilities.

4087 **Illinois Center for Autism**
548 S. Ruby Ln.
Fairview Heights, IL 62208
618-398-7500
Fax: 618-394-9869
http://www.illinoiscenterforautism.org
info@illinoiscenterforautism.org
Joy Rick, Chairperson
Gary Guthrie, Vice Chairperson
Troy Metheny, Executive Director
A not-for-profit, mental health treatment, and educational agency dedicated to serving people with autism. Referrals for possible student placement are made through local school districts, hospitals, regional special education centers, and doctors.

4088 **Joseph Academy**
1101 Gregory St.
Des Plaines, IL 60016
847-803-1930
Fax: 847-803-8669
http://www.josephacademy.org
Mike Schack, Executive Director
Sandy Schillinger, Business Manager
Ken Cozzi, Administrative Consultant
Founded in 1983, Joseph Academy provides a nurturing and challenging environment for young people. Their mission is to serve children and adolescents with behavioral, emotional, and learning disorders by helping them develop the social, academic, and vocational skills they need to function in society.

4089 **Path to Academics, Community and Employment (P.A.C.E.)**
National-Louis University
122 S. Michigan Ave.
Chicago, IL 60603
312-261-3770
http://www.nl.edu/pace
paceprogram@nl.edu
Iva Kolarov, Executive Director
T.C. Schneck, Program Operations Manager
Angie Wanek, Student Life Manager
PACE is a three-year, certificate program located on the campus of National-Louis University. The PACE program is designed especially to meet the transitional needs of young adults with multiple learning disabilities in a university setting.

4090 **South Central Community Services**
8316 South Ellis Ave.
Chicago, IL 60619
773-483-0900
Fax: 773-483-8090
http://www.sccsinc.org
Malcom Weems, Chairperson
Willie DeShong, 1st Vice Chairperson
Gene A. Linton, 2nd Vice Chairperson
A comprehensive human service agency committed to improving the quality of life for individuals and families by providing mental health, educational, socio-economic, and recreational programs and services throughout the State of Illinois.

4091 **Special Education Day School**
Catholic Children's Home
1400 State St.
Alton, IL 62002
618-465-3594
Fax: 618-465-4023
http://www.catholicchildrenshome.com
info@catholicchildrenshome.com
Michael Shelton-Montez, Administrator
Steven Roach, Executive Director
Kimberly Speidel, Educational Director
For children with learning disabilities, developmental, and behavioral disorders and through its comprehensive residential services for children in crisis. Providing year-round educational and therapuetic services to students who, due to a variety of social, emotional and/or educational difficulties, have been unsuccessful in public school programs.

4092 **Summit School, Inc.**
333 West River Rd.
Elgin, IL 60123
847-468-0490
http://www.summitinc.org
jwhite@summitelgin.org
Leo Flanagan, Jr., Chair
Mike Polchopek, Vice Chair
Michael Brown, Treasurer
The Summit School offers an array of services to children and young adults with learning difficulties. The school provides the necessary academic and interpersonal skills needed so that the students can live productive and meaningful lives.

4093 **The Achievement Centers**
Acacia Academy
6425 Willow Springs Rd.
LaGrange Highlands, IL 60525
708-579-9040
Fax: 708-579-5872
http://www.acaciaacademy.com
info@acaciaacademy.com
Kathryn Fouks, Principal/Director
Eileen Petzold, Assistant Principal & Director
Jim Shoemaker-Saif, Head of High School
The Achievement Centers offers programs for students with various learning disabilities, including dyslexia, dysgraphia, ADD/ADHD, anxiety, and more. Programs include testing/diagnostic services, private tutoring, speech theraphy, and more.

4094 **The Baby Fold**
Hammit School
108 E. Willow St.
Normal, IL 61761
309-452-1170
Fax: 309-862-2902
http://www.thebabyfold.org
publicrelations@thebabyfold.org
Dianne Schultz, President/CEO
Kathy Kujawa, VP, Business Operations
Dr. Rob Lusk, Clinical Director
A multi-service agency that provides Residential, Special Education, Child Welfare, and Family Support Services to children and families in central Illinois. Educational services are held at the Hammitt Elementary school and the Hammitt Junior-Senior High School for children and adolescents with behavioral, learning, emotional, and pervasive developmental disabilities.

4095 **The Hope Learning Academy**
The Hope Institute for Children and Families
15 E. Hazel Dell Ln.
Springfield, IL 62712
217-585-5437
TTY: 217-529-5766
http://www.thehopeschool.org
info@thehopeschool.org
Clint Paul, President/CEO
Amanda Brott, Chief Operating Officer
Kristi Kramp, Chief Human Resources Officer
The Hope School is a private, not-for-profit eduational and residential center that has been serving children with multiple disabilities and their families since 1957.

Indiana

4096 **Brain Balance of Indianapolis**
Brain Balance Achievement Centers
9510 N. Meridian St.
Suite D
Indianapolis, IN 46260 317-843-9200
http://www.brainbalancecenters.com
Dirk Bryce Lindley, Executive Director
Using a holistic and integrated approach, Brain Balance helps children with behavioral, social, and academic problems.

4097 **Dyslexia Institute of Indiana**
8359 Keystone Crossing
Suite 110
Indianapolis, IN 46240 317-222-6635
http://www.diin.org
Bill Herman, CEO
Lynn Leonard, Director, Programs
Deniese Hofmeister, Associate Director, Operations
Services children, teens, and adults with dyslexia and other learning disabilities through one-on-one tutoring, psycho-educational evaluations, and parent and educator training.

4098 **IN*SOURCE**
Indiana Resource Cntr-Families with Special Needs
1703 South Ironwood Dr.
South Bend, IN 46613 800-332-4433
Fax: 574-234-7279
http://www.insource.org
insource@insource.org
Joel Boehner, Executive Director
Scott Carson, Assistant Director
Rhett Lehman, Business Manager
The mission of IN*SOURCE is to provide parents, families, and service providers in Indiana the information and training necessary to assure effective educational programs and appropriate services for children and young adults with disabilities.

4099 **Learning Disabilities Association of Indiana**
P.O. Box 2452
West Lafayette, IN 47996 http://www.ldaofindiana.net
Patty Useem, President
Dr. Tammy Mahon, Vice President
Josh Tolbert, Treasurer
A non-profit affiliate of the LDA Association of America, that assists individuals affected by learning disabilities.

4100 **LearningRx Indianapolis Northeast**
9767 Fall Creek Rd.
Indianapolis, IN 46256 317-845-1999
http://www.learningrx.com
indianapolisne.in@learningrx.net
Heather Koenig, Owner/Director
LearningRx helps children and adults with improving their cognitive skills relating to learning, reading, memory, and attention. LearningRx has helped people with ADD/ADHD, Dyslexia, Autism Spectrum Disorders, and more.

Iowa

4101 **Access for Special Kids Resource Center (ASK)**
5665 Greendale Rd.
Suite D
Johnston, IA 50131 515-243-1713
800-450-8667
Fax: 515-243-1902
http://askresource.org
info@askresource.org
Karen Thompson, Executive Director
Ashley Gill, Operations Coordinator
A parent training, information, and advocacy center that helps parents and families with special needs children.

4102 **Center for Disability and Development**
University of Iowa Health Care
100 Hawkins Dr.
Iowa City, IA 52242 888-573-5437
http://uihc.org/ucedd
julie-christensen@uiowa.edu
Julie Christensen, Director
Lane Strathearn, Co-Director
Derrick Willis, Associate Director
The Center for Disability and Development is a University Center for Excellence in Developmental Disabilities (UCEDD), and aims to help Iowans with disabilities and their families through employment, health and wellness, education, and community living.

4103 **LearningRx Ankeny**
1205 N. Ankeny Blvd.
Suite 201
Ankeny, IA 50023 515-224-4819
http://www.learningrx.com
ankeny.ia@learningrx.net
Nancy Pim, Executive Director
LearningRx helps children and adults, ages 4-104, with improving their cognitive skills relating to learning, reading, memory, and attention. LearningRx has helped people with ADD/ADHD, Dyslexia, Autism Spectrum Disorders, and more.

Kansas

4104 **Families Together**
5611 SW Barrington Court S
Suite 120
Topeka, KS 66614-2489 785-233-4777
800-264-6343
Fax: 785-233-4787
http://www.familiestogetherinc.org
topeka@familiestogetherinc.org
Dee Steinbach, Board Member
Sheryl Davenport, Board Member
Melanie Jacobs, Board Member
Families Together is a statewide non-profit organization assisting Kansas families which include sons and/or daughters who have any form of disability.

4105 **Heartspring School**
8700 East 29th St. North
Wichita, KS 67226 316-634-8700
800-835-1043
http://www.heartspring.org
David Stupay, President/CEO
Stacie Williamson, Director, Development
Carolyn Wilhelm, Chief Financial Officer
Heartspring School has earned an international reputation for improving the lives of children. Heartspring is a not-for-profit private residential school that serves children 5-21. They serve children with disabilities such as Autism, Asperger's, communication disorders, developmental disabilities, dual diagnosed, behavior disorders, and hearing or vision impairments.

Kentucky

4106 **KY-SPIN, Inc.**
Kentucky Special Parent Involvement Network, Inc.
10301-B Deering Rd.
Louisville, KY 40272 502-937-6894
800-525-7746
Fax: 502-937-6464
http://www.kyspin.com
spininc@kyspin.com
Paulette Logsdon, Executive Director
Rhonda Logsdon, Assistant Director
Provides training, information, and support to people with disabilities, their parents and families, and information on all types of disabilities and topics for all age groups.

4107 Meredith-Dunn School
3023 Melbourne Ave.
Louisville, KY 40220 502-456-5819
http://meredithdunnschool.org
info@meredithdunnschool.org
Kathy Beam, Head of School
Meredith-Dunn School's instruction is designed to empower students with average or above-average abilities who learn differently in becoming accomplished learners and resilient indiviiduals. Grades 1-8.

4108 Shedd Academy
401 S. 7th St.
Mayfield, KY 42066 270-247-8007
Paul Thompson, Executive Director
The mission of the Shedd Academy is to prepare students with dyslexia/ADD for college or vocational training and for their future by helping them to understand their unique learning styles; fulfill their intellectual, academic, physical, artistic, creative, social, spiritual, and emotional potential; develop a sense of self responsibility; assume a value system so that they can become contributing members of society; and increase their skills to ensure they are armed with a variety of abilities.

4109 The de Paul School
1925 Duker Ave.
Louisville, KY 40205 502-459-6131
Fax: 502-805-0505
http://www.depaulschool.org
Tony Kemper, Head of School
Lisa Stepp, Principal
Elea Fox, Chief Development Officer
Teaches students with specific learning differences how to: learn, be independent, and be successful. Co-ed, grades 1-8.

Louisiana

4110 Families Helping Families
700 Hickory Ave.
Harahan, LA 70123 504-888-9111
800-766-7736
http://fhfofgno.org
Mary Jacob, Executive Director
Greg Brenan, Chairman
Lisa Ledet, Vice Chairwoman
A resource center for individuals with disabilities and their families serving all of Louisiana. They provide peer to peer support, information, resources, and training on disability, health care needs, and special education.

4111 Lanier Evaluation & Learning Center
332 Farrel Rd.
Suite B
Lafayette, LA 70508 337-988-5758
http://www.cynthialanier.com
info@cynthialanier.com
Cynthia D. Lanier, Owner/Director
A private practice that offers educational therapy, tutoring, evaluations, and consultations for individuals with learning disabilities.

4112 LearningRx Shreveport-Bossier
8856 Youree Dr.
Suite D
Shreveport, LA 71115 318-797-8523
http://www.learningrx.com/shreveport-bossier/
shreveport.la@learningrx.net
Donesa Walker, Director
LearningRx helps children and adults with improving their cognitive skills relating to learning, reading, memory, and attention. LearningRx has helped people with ADD/ADHD, Dyslexia, Autism Spectrum Disorders, and more.

4113 Louisiana Center for Dyslexia and Related Learning Disorders
Nicholls State University
FACS Building, Room 6
P.O. Box 2050
Thibodaux, LA 70310 985-448-4214
Fax: 985-448-4423
http://www.nicholls.edu/dyslexia/
karen.chauvin@nicholls.edu
Karen Chauvin, Director
Rachel Hebert, Program Coordinator
Octave Hymel, Program Coordinator
Serves NSU students and the community who have been diagnosed with dyslexia and/or a related disorder. The Center provides support services for college students, and also training for teachers through in-service workshops.

Maine

4114 ACCESS Unity
Unity College
90 Quaker Hill Rd.
Unity, ME 04988 833-UnityGo
http://www.unity.edu
admissions@unity.edu
Dr. Melik Khoury, University President
Dr. John Zavodney, Chief of Staff
Bert Audette, Chief Information Officer
ACESS Unity provides support services to students with learning disabilities, such as alternate testing environment, extended exam time, note-taking assistance, and more.

4115 Aucocisco School
126 Spurwink Ave.
Cape Elizabeth, ME 04107 207-773-7323
http://www.aucociscoschool.org
information@aucociscoschool.org
A school and learning center that provides remedial education for sudents with Dyslexia, reading differences, Dyscalculia, Dysgraphia, ADHD, and language and auditory processing issues.

4116 Children's Center
1 Alden Ave.
Augusta, ME 04330 207-626-3497
800-894-6264
Fax: 207-621-6211
http://www.childrensctr.org
Jeffrey Johnson, Executive Director
Heather Dubord, Director, Finance/Human Resource
Shelley Roy, Intake Coordinator
Provides specialized programs to young children with disabilities, ages birth-5, including early education, pediatric therapies, specialized programs for children with Autism Spectrum Disorderders, family support, and more.

4117 Maine Parent Federation
484 Maine Ave. 2D
Farmingdale, ME 04344 207-588-1933
800-870-7746
Fax: 207-588-1938
http://www.mpf.org
parentconnect@mpf.org
Carrie Woodcock, Executive Director
Jane K. Morse, Chair
Anne Osolinski, Vice Chair
A non-profit organization that provides information, referral, support, and training to parents of children with disabilities. Services are provided at no cost.

Maryland

4118 Chelsea School
2970 Belcrest Center Dr.
Suite 300
Hyattsville, MD 20782 240-467-2100
http://www.chelseaschool.edu
Paul Hagens, Chair
Mindelyn Anderson, Vice Chair
Kevin Claggett, Treasurer
Committed to providing superior education to children with language-based learning disabilities. Grades 5-12.

4119 Children's Developmental Clinic
Prince George's Community College
301 Largo Rd.
Largo, MD 20774-2199 301-546-0519
http://www.pgcc.edu
Charlene M. Dukes, President
Howard W. Stone, Chair
Sidney L. Gibson, Vice Chair
The Children's Development Clinic is a continuing education program conducted by the Workforce Development and Continuing Education Division at Prince George's Community College. The clinic provides special services to children, birth and up, who are experiencing various development difficulties such as learning problems, developmental delays, physical fitness and coordination problems, brain injury, emotional problems, or orthopedic challenges.

4120 Frost School
4915 Aspen Hill Rd.
Rockville, MD 20853-3700 301-933-3451
Fax: 301-933-0350
http://www.sheppardpratt.org
Chip Maust, Education Director
Claire Cohen, Program Director
Part of the Sheppard Pratt Health System, The Frost school's programs and therapeutic day programs serve emotionally troubled and autistic children and adolescents and their families.

4121 High Road School Of Baltimore County
11685 Crossroads Circle
Suites S-U
White Marsh, MD 21220 410-282-8500
Fax: 410-282-1047
http://catapultlearning.com/schools/
Danielle Peck, Director
Caitlin Rosing, Associate Director
Kelly Mlynski, Associate Director
Offers programs serving the educational, social, and emotional needs of children with specific learning disabilities, communication disorders, and/or behavioral difficulties.

4122 Kennedy Krieger Institute
University Affiliated Program
707 North Broadway
Baltimore, MD 21205 443-923-9200
800-873-3377
http://www.kennedykrieger.org
info@kennedykrieger.org
Gary W. Goldstein, President/CEO
Internationally recognized for improving the lives of children and young adults with disorders of the brain, spinal cord, and musculoskeletal system. Serves more than 14,000 individuals each year through inpatient and oupatient clinics; homes and community services; and school-based programs.

4123 Nora School
955 Sligo Ave.
Silver Spring, MD 20910 301-495-6672
Fax: 301-495-7829
http://www.nora-school.org
Marcia Miller, Director, Admissions
A small, progressive, college preparatory high school that nurtures and empowers bright students who have been frustrated in larger, more traditional school settings.

4124 Phillips Programs for Children and Families
8920 Whiskey Bottom Rd.
Laurel, MD 20723 301-470-1620
Fax: 301-470-1624
http://www.phillipsprograms.org
Piper Phillips Caswell, President/CEO
Trixie Herbert, Chief Operating Officer
Marbeth Ingle Levy, Director, HR
Phillips is a non-profit, private organization serving the needs of individuals with emotional and behavioral problems and their families through education, family support services, community education, and advocacy.

4125 Ridge School of Montgomery County
Adventis Behavioral Health
14915 Broschart Rd.
Rockville, MD 20850 301-217-5412
http://www.adventisthealthcare.com
Terry Forde, President/CEO
Susan L. Glover, SVP/Chief Quality Officer
James G. Lee, EVP/Chief Financial Officer
The school provides both a special education program and a general education program to meet the needs of the students who have difficulty learning in a traditional school environment.

4126 The Forbush School at Glyndon
Sheppard Pratt Health System
407 Central Ave.
Reisterstown, MD 21136 410-517-5400
Fax: 410-517-5600
http://www.sheppardpratt.org
Andy Parsley ÿ, Director, Education
Kathy Ourand, Middle School Principal
Scott Derby, High School Principal
Provides educational and therapeutic services for children and young adults through 12th grade who have learning disabilities. Curriculum is designed to help the growth of each student in emotional and cognitive areas, and each student follows a program that is designed to meet their needs.

4127 The Parents' Place of Maryland
801 Cromwell Park Dr.
Suite 103
Glen Burnie, MD 21061 410-768-9100
800-394-5694
Fax: 410-768-0830
http://www.ppmd.org
info@ppmd.org
Rene Averitt-Sanzone, Executive Director
Suzie Shannon, Director, Operations
Val Englert, Communications Coordinator
Serving the parents of children with disabilities throughout Maryland, regardless of the nature of their child's disability or the age of their child. The staff helps families obtain the appropriate information on education, health care, and services for their child's disabilities.

Massachusetts

4128 Adult Center at PAL: Program for Advancement of Learning
1071 Blue Hill Ave.
Milton, MA 02186 617-333-0500
Fax: 617-333-2114
http://www.curry.edu/pal
Dr. Laura Hubbard, Adult Center Coordinator
The Adult Center at PAL (Program for Advancement of Learning) is the first program to offer academic and socio-emotional services to adults with LD/ADHD/Dyslexia in a college setting in the New England area. The ACD offers one-to-one academic tutorials; small support groups that meet weekly; and Saturday Seminars that explore issues that impact the lives of adults with LD/ADHD.

4129 **Berkshire Meadows**
249 North Plain Rd.
Housatonic, MA 01236 413-528-2523
Fax: 413-528-0293
http://jri.org/services/
lkelly@jri.org
Liisa Kelly, Senior Program Director
Berkshire Meadows is a year-round residential school that helps children and young adults with severe cognitive disabilities, autism, and challenging behaviors.

4130 **CAST**
40 Harvard Mills Square
Suite 3
Wakefield, MA 01880-3233 781-245-2212
http://www.cast.org
cast@cast.org
Linda Gerstle, Chief Executive Officer
Wendy Scott Keeney, Chief Development Officer
Carole Lacy, CFO/Director, Human Resources
A non-profit organization that works to expand learning opportunities for all individuals, especially those with disabilities, through the research and development of innovative, technology-based educational resources and strategies.

4131 **College Internship Program**
The Berkshire Center
199 South St.
Pittsfield, MA 01201 413-344-4109
Fax: 617-238-2122
http://cipworldwide.org
Michael McManmon, Founder
Dan McManmon, President
Sharona Sommer, Director, Family Services
The College Internship Program provides individualized, post-secondary academic, internship, and independent living experiences for young adults with learning differences. With the support and direction, students learn to realize and develop their potential.

4132 **Commonwealth Learning Center**
220 Reservoir St.
Suite 6
Needham, MA 02494-3133 781-444-5193
Fax: 781-444-6916
http://www.commlearn.com
info@commlearn.com
Beth Dinelli, Director
Offers individualized one-to-one instruction specializing in multisensory methodologies such as Orton-Gillingham. Works with students of all ages in academic support, organizational and study skills, and test preparation.

4133 **Cotting School**
453 Concord Ave.
Lexington, MA 02421 781-862-7323
Fax: 781-861-1179
http://www.cotting.org
info@cotting.org
David W. Manzo, M.Ed., President/Executive Director
Krista Macari, M.S., Chief Academic Officer
Bridget Irish, Chief Operating Officer
Cotting School is for students with moderate to severe learning disabilities requiring assessment of learning style, remediation techniques, and one-to-one instruction.

4134 **Devereux Massachusetts**
60 Miles Rd.
P.O. Box 219
Rutland, MA 01543-0219 508-886-4746
Fax: 508-886-4773
http://www.devereux.org
Kerry Ann Goldsmith, Executive Director
Nadyia Abbas, Assistant Executive Director
Patricia Susen, Director, Education
A residential program for children, adolescents, and young adults who have emotional, behavioral, and substance abuse problems with developmental and learning disabilities.

4135 **Educational Options**
5 Suburban Rd.
Apt. 603
Worcester, MA 01602 508-459-9158
Fax: 617-864-8864
http://www.optionsined.com
rgoldberg227@gmail.com
Renee Goldberg, Director
Neil Kalt, Ph.D., Staff
Full-service educational consulting practice dedicated to assisting students plan their future. Works with students to identify their strengths and match these qualities with an academic setting that meets their educational, cultural, and social aspirations.

4136 **Evergreen Center**
345 Fortune Blvd.
Milford, MA 01757 508-478-2631
Fax: 508-634-3251
http://www.evergreenctr.org
Robert Littleton, Jr., Executive Director
The Evergreen Center is a residential school serving children and adolescents with severe developmental disabilities.

4137 **F.L. Chamberlain School**
Frederick L. Chamberlain Center, Inc.
1 Pleasant St.
P.O. Box 778
Middleboro, MA 02346 508-947-7825
Fax: 508-947-1593
http://www.chamberlainschool.org
William Schulpen Doherty, Co-Founder/Executive Director
Jeanne Edwards, Co-Founder/COO
The F. L. Chamberlain School offers a highly structured program for students ages 11-22 who have difficulties that influence learning and behavior. Students may either live on campus or attend day classes, and academic programming is tailored to meet the specific needs of each student.

4138 **John Dewey Academy**
389 Main St.
Great Barrington, MA 01230 413-528-9800
Fax: 413-528-5662
http://www.jda.org
info@jda.org
Andrea E. Leln, Head of School
Andrea Nathans, Executive Director, Admissions
Lisa Sinsheimer, Clinical Consultant
Provides an individualized and comprehensive education in a non-traditional therapeutic boarding school setting. Students are bright, troubled adolescents with a history of self-defeating or self-destructive choices. The peer-based approach leads students to high levels of achievement and inspires them to develop in ways that promote self-respect, maturity, and respect for others.

4139 **Landmark School Outreach Program**
Landmark School
429 Hale St.
P.O. Box 227
Prides Crossing, MA 01965 978-236-3216
Fax: 978-927-7268
http://www.landmarkoutreach.org
outreach@landmarkschool.org
Dan Ahearn, Director
Keryn Kwedor, Associate Director
Jenna Lanoue, Operations Manager
The Outreach Program provides professional development programs and publications that offer practical and effective strategies to help children learn. These strategies are based on Landmark's Six Teaching Principles and reflect Landmark's innovative instruction of students with language-based learning disabilites.
1971

4140 Landmark School and Summer Programs
Landmark School
429 Hale St.
P.O. Box 227
Prides Crossing, MA 01965 978-236-3010
Fax: 978-927-7268
http://www.landmarkschool.org
admission@landmarkschool.org
Robert Broudo, Headmaster/President
Dan Ahearn, Director, Outreach
Mark Brislin, CFO/Business Manager
Landmark is a co-educational boarding and day school for emotionally healthy students who have been diagnosed with a language based learning disability. Landmark individualizes instruction for each student, providing an intensive program emphasizing the development of language and learning skills within a highly structured environment. They also offer an intensive six-week summer program for students who wish to explore the benefits of short-term, skill-based learning.

4141 League School of Greater Boston
300 Boston-Providence Turnpike
Walpole, MA 02032 508-850-3900
Fax: 508-660-2442
http://www.leagueschool.com
info@leagueschool.com
Kimberly Driskell, Chief Financial Officer
Patrick Fuller, Principal
Frank Gagliardi, Executive Director
Providing social, academic, and vocational programs for children with Autism/Asperger Spectrum Disorders who need a specialized alternative to public school, preparing them to transfer into an environment offering greater independence.

4142 Living Independently Forever, Inc.
550 Lincoln Road Extension
Hyannis, MA 02601 508-790-3600
http://www.lifecapecod.org
info@lifecapecod.org
Jo Ann Simons, Chairperson
Peter Barrett, Vice Chairperson
Diane Enochs, Executive Director
Living Independently Forever, Inc. is dedicated to serving the life-long needs of adults with significant learning disabilities within their residential communities. LIFE is committed to providing these men and women with the adult education and the opportunities to develop their personal and vocational/occupational skills to their maximum potential, and to supporting them appropriately in independent and group living.

4143 May Institute
41 Pacella Park Dr.
Randolph, MA 02368 800-778-7601
http://www.mayinstitute.org
info@mayinstitute.org
Lauren C. Solotar, Ph.D., President/CEO
Ralph B. Sperry, Chief Operating Officer
Kevin M. More, Chief Information Officer
The May Institute provides educational and rehabilitative services for individuals with autism, developmental disabilities, neurological disorders, and mental illness.

4144 Melmark New England
461 River Rd.
Andover, MA 01810 978-654-4300
http://www.melmarkne.org
admissions@melmarkne.org
Rita Gardner, President/CEO
Peter J. Troy, Vice President
Joseph M. Zakrzewski, VP/Chief Financial Officer
Serves children and adolescents within the autism spectrum disorders, and works to develop and enhance their abilities and confidence in a safe and nuturing environment.

4145 Riverbrook Residence
4 Ice Glen Rd.
P.O. Box 478
Stockbridge, MA 01262 413-298-4926
http://www.riverbrook.org
info@riverbrook.org
Rebecca Amuso Wendell, Executive Director
Lynn Ciccone, Clinical Program Director
Colleen Powers, Day Program Director
A residence in western Massachusetts, providing supported living to developmentally disabled women, with therapy and treatment focused on the arts.

4146 Riverview School
551 Route 6A
East Sandwhich, MA 02537 508-888-0489
Fax: 508-833-7001
http://www.riverviewschool.org
admissions@riverviewschool.org
Stewart Miller, Head of School
Riverview School is a co-educational residential school for adolescents and young adults with complex language, learning, and cognitive disabilities.

4147 Seven Hills Academy at Groton
Seven Hills Foundation
81 Hope Ave.
Worcester, MA 01603 508-755-2340
Fax: 508-849-3882
TTY: 508-890-5584
http://www.sevenhills.org
David A. Jordan, DHA, President
Kathleen M. Jordan, DHA, EVP/Chief Executive Officer
Joseph L. Tosches, DBA, EVP/Chief Operations Officer
Special education day programs for children and young adults with complex developmental and medical disabilities. Summer programs are also available.

4148 Son-Rise Program®
Autism Treatment Center of America
2080 S. Undermountain Rd.
Sheffield, MA 01257 413-229-2100
877-766-7473
http://www.autismtreatment.com
Barry Neil Kaufman, Co-Founder
Raun K. Kaufman, Group Facilitator
Samahria Lyte Kaufman, Co-Founder
Since 1983, the Autism Treatment Center of America has provided innovative training programs and workshops for parents and professionals caring for children challenged by Autism, Autism Spectrum Disorders, Pervasive Developmental Disorder (PDD), and other developmental difficulties.
1983

4149 Special Education School
The Protestant Guild for Human Services
521 Virginia Rd.
Concord, MA 01742 781-893-6000
Fax: 978-369-3602
http://www.guildhumanservices.org
admissions@guildhumanservices.org
Amy C. Sousa, Chief Executive Officer
Michael J. Clontz, Chief Operating Officer
Maureen Costello-Shea, Chief Program Officer
A private, 365-day community-based, educational program serving difficult to place students with a primary diagnosis of autism or other developmental disability. In addition, students may carry secondary diagnosis of hearing impairments and other communication disorders, traumatic brain injury, seizure disorders, Tourette's syndrome, and emotional and psychiatric disorders.

4150 The New England Center for Children
33 Turnpike Rd.
Southborough, MA 01772-2108 508-481-1015
Fax: 508-485-3421
http://www.necc.org
info@necc.org

Vincent Strully, Jr., President/CEO
Michael S. Downey, CPA, MBA, EVP/Chief Financial Officer
Jared Bouzan, MEd., Chief Development Officer
The New England Center for Children is a private, non-profit organization serving children with autism and other related disabilities.

4151 **The Perkins Day Treatment Program**
971 Main St.
Lancaster, MA 01523 978-365-7376
http://www.perkinsprograms.org
admissions@perkinschool.org
Michael W. Ames, President/CEO
Timothy R. Hammond, Chief Operating Officer
Lisa Harrington, Chief Financial Officer
The program offers comprehensive educational and clinical programs for children and adolescents with ADD, bi-polar disorder, depression, post traumatic stress disorder, asperger syndrome, and thought disorders. Some of the academic programs are speech and language therapy, math, reading, arts, music, and swimming.

4152 **Willow Hill School**
98 Haynes Rd.
Sudbury, MA 01776 978-443-2581
Fax: 978-443-0949
http://www.willowhillschool.org
Marilyn G. Reid, Head of School
Mark Hall, Director, Education
Tom Rimer, Director, Admissions
Willow Hill School provides supportive and individualized educational programs for middle and high school students in grades 6-12 who are capable of advancing along a strong academic curriculum, but have experienced frustration in earlier school settings.

Michigan

4153 **Eton Academy**
1755 Melton Rd.
Birmingham, MI 48009 248-642-1150
http://www.etonacademy.org
contact@etonacademy.org
Pete Pullen, Head of School
The Eton Academy is a co-educational private day school dedicated to educating students with learning differences. The mission is to educate students who will understand their learning styles and practice strategies that will prepare them for responsible independence, life-long learning and participation in school, family and in their community.

4154 **Lake Michigan Academy**
2428 Burton St., SE
Grand Rapids, MI 49546 616-464-3330
Fax: 616-285-1935
http://www.mylma.org
info@mylma.org
Robert Woodhouse, Jr., Chairman
Philip Wood, Vie Chairman
Bejamin Pitcher, Treasurer
Lake Michigan Academy is a state-certified, non-profit school for learning disabled children in grades 1 through 12 with average or above average intelligence. Lake Michigan Academy services students with varying learning disabilities such as dyslexia, dyscalculia, or dysgraphia.

4155 **Living & Learning Enrichment Center**
315 Griswold St.
Northville, MI 48167 248-308-3592
http://www.livingandlearningcenter.org
livingandlearningcenter@gmail.com
Rachelle Vartanian, President/Founder
Pamela Travis, Assistant Director
David Franco, Director, Business Development
A non-profit organization that teached social employment skills to children and teens with Autism Spectrum Disorders and other related challenges. The center also provides professional development skills training.

4156 **Reading Success Plus, Inc.**
4467 Cascade Rd., SE
Suite 4471
Grand Rapids, MI 49546 616-856-7262
http://readingsuccessplus.com
info@readingsuccessplus.com
Anne Kloth, Co-Founder
Lawrence G. Kloth, Jr., Co-Founder
An organization of specialists helping students with dyslexia by supporting them in the areas of reading, spelling, comprehension, fluency, handwriting, keyboarding, and math.

4157 **Specialized Language Development Center**
2650 Horizon Dr., SE
Suite 230
Grand Rapids, MI 49546 616-361-1182
http://www.sldcenter.org
info@sldcenter.org
Maura Race, Co-Executive Director
Carol McGlinn, Co-Executive Director
Evie Jefferies, Operations Coordinator
A community resource of West Michigan committed to bringing the power of reading, writing, and spelling to all individuals with dyslexia or other learning styles, enabling them to reach their full potential.

Minnesota

4158 **Groves Academy**
3200 Highway 100 South
Saint Louis Park, MN 55416 952-920-6377
Fax: 952-920-2068
http://www.grovesacademy.org
mainoffice@grovesacademy.org
Lawrence Graham, Director, Finance
John Alexander, Executive Director
Kim Peeples, Head of School
A day school for children who because of their learning disabilities have not been successful in a traditional school setting.

4159 **LDA Learning Center**
LDA Minnesota
6100 Golden Valley Rd
Golden Valley, MN 55422 952-582-6000
Fax: 952-582-6031
http://www.ldaminnesota.org
info@ldaminnesota.org
Jeff Fox, President
Sherry Holtz, Vice President
Jerry Golden, Treasurer
Maximizes the potential of children, youths, adults and families, especially those with learning disabilities and other learning difficulties so that they can lead more productive and fulfilled lives. Provides consultations, tutoring, assessments, parent workshops, training and outreach on sliding fee scale.

4160 **LearningRx Woodbury**
8425 Seasons Pkwy.
Suite 101
Woodbury, MN 55125 651-262-5900
http://www.learningrx.com/woodbury/
woodbury.mn@learningrx.net
Rich Frieder, Owner/Director
LearningRx helps children and adults with improving their cognitive skills relating to learning, reading, memory, and attention. LearningRx has helped people with ADD/ADHD, Dyslexia, Autism Specturm Disorders, and more.

4161 **The Reading Center/Dyslexia Institute of Minnesota**
847 5th St., NW.
Rochester, MN 55901 507-288-5271
Fax: 507-288-6424
http://www.thereadingcenter.org
read@TheReadingCenter.org
Cindy Russell, Executive Director
Sarah Carlson-Wallrath, Director, Development
Fay Can Vliet, Director, Programming
A non-profit organization that offers services for dyslexic students and their families. The Reading Center also provides training for teachers and parents.

Mississippi

4162 **The Learning Center of Rankin County School District**
200 School Rd.
Brandon, MS 39042 601-824-0334
Fax: 601-825-2988
http://www.rcsd.ms/learningcenter
George E. Jones, III, Head Principal
Monica Harris, Assistant Principal
Helps meet the educational needs of students who are unsuccessful in traditional school settings. The Learning Center equips students with the skills needed to return to a regular school environment.

Missouri

4163 **Churchill Center & School for Learning Disabilities**
1021 Municipal Center Dr.
Town & Country, MO 63131 314-997-4343
Fax: 314-997-2760
http://www.churchillstl.org
info@churchillstl.org
Sandra Gilligan, Director
Anne Evers, Director, Admissions
Deborah Warden, Assistant Director
The Churchill School is a private, not-for-profit, co-educational day school. It is designed to serve children between the ages of 8-16 with diagnosed learning disabilities. The goal is to help each child reach his or her full potential and prepare them for a successful return to a traditional classroom in as short a period of time as possible.

4164 **Cornerstones of Care**
300 E. 36th St.
Kansas City, MO 64111 816-508-1700
http://www.cornerstonesofcare.org
Denise Cross, President/CEO
Ryan Dowis, Chief Operating Officer
Eric Giovanni, Chief Financial Officer
Previously known as Gillis Center, Cornerstones of Care's mission is to help at-risk children and their families become contributing members of the community through education, counseling, and social services.

4165 **MPACT - Missouri Parents Act**
7421 Mexico Rd.
Suite 200
St. Peters, MO 63376 800-743-7634
http://www.missouriparentsact.org
info@missouriparentsact.org
Debby Loveall-Stewart, Executive Directorÿ
Amey McAllister, Operations Coordinator
Elizabeth Fox, Program Coordinatorÿ
MPACT assists parents to effectively advocate for their children's educational rights and services. MPACT is a statewide parent training and information center serving all disabilities. Their mission is to ensure that all children with special needs receive an education that allows them to achieve their personal goals.

4166 **Miriam School**
501 Bacon Ave.
St. Louis, MO 63119 314-968-5225
http://www.miriamschool.org
info@miriamschool.org
Mary Cognata, Head of School
Megan Gibson, Director, Admissions
Mary Bless, Director, Media Services
A non-profit day school for children between four and twelve years of age who are learning disabled and/or behaviorally disabled. Speech and language services and occupational therapy are integral components of the program. The focus of all the activities is to increase children's self-esteem and help them acquire the coping skills needed to successfully meet future challenges.

Montana

4167 **Parents, Let's Unite for Kids**
2345 King Ave. West
Suite B
Billings, MT 59102 406-255-0540
800-222-7585
Fax: 406-255-2523
http://www.mtpluk.org
info@mtpluk.org
PLUK is a private, non-profit organization formed in 1984 by parents and children with disabilities and chronic illnesses in the state of Montana for the purpose of information, support, training, and assistance to aid their children at home, school, and as adults.

4168 **Sage Learning Center**
2055 North 22nd Ave.
Suite 4
Bozeman, MT 59718 406-582-9570
http://www.sagelearningcenter.com
Carisa Fillback, Director
A private education center that helps students who have trouble with reading, writing, math, or paying attention in class. Sage Learning Center provides students with the skills needed to achieve learning success by using the Precision Teaching technique.

Nebraska

4169 **Nebraska Parents Training and Information Center**
PTI Nebraska
1941 S. 42nd St.
Suite 205
Omaha, NE 68105 402-346-0525
800-284-8520
Fax: 402-934-1479
http://www.pti-nebraska.org
reception@pti-nebraska.org
Lyris Peak, President
Seamus Kelly, Vice President
Mike Tufte, Executive Director
The Parent Training and Information Program views parents as full partners in the educational process and a significant source of support and assistance to each other. Funded by the Division of Personnel Preparation, Office of Special Education Programs, these programs provide training and information to parents to enable such individuals to participate more effectively with professionals in meeting the educational needs of disabled children.

New Hampshire

4170 **Becket Family of Services**
633 NH Route 10
Orford, NH 03777 603-353-9102
http://www.becket.org

Jay T. Wolter, Chief Executive Officer
Kerry Beck, Chief Operating Officer
Ladd Raine, Director, Human Resources
Becket guides and inspires adolescents having difficulties at home, in school or in the community.

4171 **Cedarcrest Center for Children with Disabilities**
91 Maple Ave.
Keene, NH 03431 603-358-3384
Fax: 603-358-6485
http://www.cedarcrest4kids.org
cgray@cedarcrest4kids.org
Cathy Gray, President/CEO
Thomas W. Connelly, Jr., Director, Nursing Services
Michael O'Hara, Director, Special Education
Provides long-term and short-term residential care, special education, and therapy services for children with complex medical and developmental needs.

4172 **Hampshire Country School**
28 Patey Circle
Rindge, NH 03461 603-899-3325
Fax: 603-899-6521
http://www.hampshirecountryschool.org
office@hampshirecountyschool.net
William Dickerman, Director, Admissions
Bernd Focking, Headmaster
Thomas Ciglar, Director, Operations
Hampshire Country School is a small boarding school for middle school students with Asperger's Syndrome, Nonverbal Learning Disabililties, and Attention Deficit Hyperactivity Disorder. Faculty to student ratio is 2:3.

4173 **Parent Information Center**
54 Old Suncook Rd.
Concord, NH 03301 603-224-7005
800-947-7005
Fax: 603-224-4365
TTY: 800-947-7005
http://www.parentinformationcenter.org
info@picnh.org
Michelle Lewis, PIC Executive Director
Marcia Bagley, Chair
Jocelyn Charles, Vice Chair
Parent Training and Information Program views parents as full partners in the educational process and a significant source of support and assistance to each other. Funded by the Division of Personnel Preparation, Office of Special Education Programs, these programs provide training and information to parents to enable such individuals to participate more effectively with professionals in meeting the educational needs of children with disabilities.

New Jersey

4174 **Bancroft**
1255 Caldwell Rd.
Cherry Hill, NJ 08034 856-348-1137
800-774-5516
http://www.bancroft.org
info@bancroft.org
Toni Pergolin, President/CEO
James P. Hartman, Chief Financial Officer
Dr. Scott Janney, Chief Development Officer
Non-profit organization offering educational/vocational programs, therapeutic support services, and a full range of community living opportunities for children and adults with brain injury in Maine, New Jersey, Delaware, and Louisiana. Residential options include community living supervised apartments, specialized supervised apartments, group homes, and supported living models.

4175 **ECLC of New Jersey**
Ho-Ho-Kus Campus
302 North Franklin Turnpike
Ho-Ho-Kus, NJ 07423 201-670-7880
http://www.eclcofnj.org
vlindorff@eclofnj.org
Vicki Lindorff, Principal
Bruce Litinger, Executive Director
Heather Alonge, Director, Development
A private school for individuals with disabilities between the ages of 5-21. Their mission is to help disabled students discover how they fit into the world and guide them towards becoming independent and employed adults.

4176 **Eden Autism Services**
2 Merwick Rd.
Princeton, NJ 08540 609-987-0099
Fax: 609-987-0243
http://edenautism.org
info@edenservices.org
Michael K. Decker, President/CEO
Jennifer Bizub, Chief Operating Officer
David Napoleon, Chief Financial Officer
Non-profit organization founded in 1975 to provide a comprehensive continuum of lifespan services for individuals with autism and their families.

4177 **Family Resource Associates, Inc.**
35 Haddon Ave
Shrewsbury, NJ 07702 732-747-5310
Fax: 732-747-1896
http://www.frainc.org
info@frainc.org
Nancy Phalanukorn, Executive Director
Christopher Curcia, President
Allan Proske, Vice President
A New Jersey nonprofit agency dedicated to helping individuals with disabilities and their families.

4178 **Forum School**
107 Wyckoff Ave.
Waldwick, NJ 07463 201-444-5882
http://www.theforumschool.com
info@theforumschool.com
Brian Detlefsen, Principal
Special education day school for developmentally disabled children. The Forum School offers a therapeutic education environment for children who cannot be accommodated in a public school setting.

4179 **Huntington Learning Centers, Inc.**
29 Nathaniel Pl.
Englewood, NJ 07631 201-871-2211
http://huntingtonhelps.com
Huntington Learning Center helps target your child's unique needs through diagnostic testing so they can better achieve their grades.

4180 **Matheny Medical and Educational Center**
65 Highland Ave.
P.O. Box 339
Peapack, NJ 07977 908-234-0011
http://www.matheny.org
info@matheny.org
Edana Desatnick, Co-Chair
Bruce Fisher, Co-Chair
William A. Krais, Esq., Vice Chair
Matheny School and Hospital is a special educational facility and hospital for children and adults with medically complex developmental disabilities. The school provides comprehensive educational programs and functional life skills for children and young adults ages 3-21.

4181 **Newgrange School**
526 South Olden Ave.
Hamilton, NJ 08629
609-688-1280
Fax: 609-430-3030
http://www.thenewgrange.org
info@thenewgrange.org
Tim Viands, Executive Director
Deardra Rosenberg, Director, Education
Ted Varias, Assistant Director
Newgrange is a non-profit organization established in 1977 to provide specialized educational programs for students with language based learning disabilities.

4182 **SEARCH Day Program**
73 Wickapecko Dr.
Ocean, NJ 07712
732-531-0454
http://www.searchdayprogram.com
info@searchdayprogram.com
Katherine Solana, Executive Director
SEARCH Day Program is a private, non-profit, New Jersey State certified agency serving children and adults with autism and their families.

4183 **Spectrum360**
414 Eagle Rock Ave.
Suite 200B
West Orange, NJ 07052
973-509-3050
Fax: 973-509-0185
http://spectrum360.org
Jonah Zimiles, Vice President
Michael J. Reimer, President
Kristen Olson, Vice President
Previously known as The Children's Institute, Spectrum360 is a private, non-profit school approved by the New Jersey State Board of Education, serving children facing learning, language, and social challenges. Programs include Academy360, FilmAcademy360, CulinaryAcademy360, and Independence360.

4184 **Statewide Parent Advocacy Network**
Central Office
35 Halsey St.
Fourth Fl.
Newark, NJ 07102
973-642-8100
800-654-7726
Fax: 973-642-8080
http://www.spanadvocacy.org
Diana Autin, Executive Co-Director
Debra Jennings, Executive Co-Director
A non-profit educational and advocacy center for parents of children from birth to 21 years of age. Assists families of infants, toddlers, children, and youth with and without disabilities. Serves as a vehicle for the exchange of ideas, promoting awareness of the abilities and needs of the children and youth and improves services for children and families in the state of NJ.

4185 **The Center School**
2 Riverview Dr.
Somerset, NJ 08873
908-253-3870
Fax: 732-764-8605
http://www.thecenterschool.com
Marcie Fiorentino, Executive Director
June Curau, Business Manager
Ron Rinaldi, Principal
A school designed for bright students in grades 1-12 with learning and behavioral difficulties. The Center School offers counseling, speech and language, and occupational therapy. The Center School is committed to helping each student become as self-sufficient and successful as possible.

4186 **The Craig School**
10 Tower Hill Rd.
Mountain Lakes, NJ 07046
973-334-1295
Fax: 973-334-1299
http://www.craigschool.org
info@craigschool.org
Grant L. Jacks, III, Head of School
Katie Burke, Director, Development
Karen Meisinger, Chief Financial Officer
The Craig School is an independent, non-profit school serving children who have difficulty succeeding in the traditional classroom environment. They specialize in a language-based curriculum for children of average or above average intelligence with such disorders as dyslexia, auditory processing, and attention deficit.

4187 **The Learning Connection (TLC)**
Georgian Court University
900 Lakewood Ave.
Lakewood, NJ 08701
732-987-2650
http://www.georgian.edu
admissions@georgian.edu
Robert E. Mulcahy III, Chair
Judith M. Persichilli, Vice Chair
Joseph R. Marbach, University President
The Learning Center is an assistance program designed to provide an environment for students with mild to moderate learning disabilities who desire a college education. The program is not one of remediation, but it is an individualized support program to assist candidates in becoming successful college students. Emphasis is placed on developing self-help strategies, study techniques, content tutoring, time management, organization skills, and social skills all taught by a certified professional.

4188 **The Lewis School and Clinic for Educational Therapy**
53 Bayard Ln.
Princeton, NJ 08540
609-924-8120
Fax: 609-924-5512
http://www.lewisschool.org
Marsha Lewis, Executive Director
The Clinic and School integrate teaching and diagnostic perspective of multisensory educational practices in the classrooms, and the perspective of clinical research into the brain's learning process.

4189 **The Midland School**
94 Readington Rd.
Branchburg, NJ 08876
908-722-8222
http://www.midlandschool.org
info@midlandschool.org
Kristen Zizelmann, Principal
A New Jersey approved non-profit school for children, ages 5-21 with developmental disabilities. Serving approx 210 students from public school districts throughout Northern and Central New Jersey. Midland provides a comprehensive special education program serving the individual social, emotional, academic, and career education needs of its students.

New Mexico

4190 **Abrazos Family Support Services**
412 Camino Don Tomas
P.O. Box 788
Bernalillo, NM 87004
505-867-3396
Fax: 505-867-3398
http://abrazosnm.org
info@abrazosnm.org
April Spaulding, Executive Director
Leonard Lopez, Financial Manager
Randi Malach, Program Manager
Abezos provides a variety of educational, health, developmental and parental support services.

4191 **Designs for Learning Differences Sycamore School**
8600 Academy Rd., NE
Albuquerque, NM 87111
505-822-0476
Fax: 505-858-4424
http://www.dldsycamoreschool.com
dldschool1@aol.com
Linda Murray, Principal

A private, non-profit school serving children and young adults in grades 1-12 with learning difficulties.

4192 Education for Parents of Indian Children with Special Needs (EPICS)
1600 San Pedro Dr., NE
Albuquerque, NM 87110 888-499-2070
http://www.epicsnm.org
Elizabeth Martin, Executive Director
Judy Wiley, Project Manager
Kelsey Woody, Project Coordinator
A community parent resource center for families with Native American children who have disabilities and/or developmental delays.

4193 Parents Reaching Out Network
1920 Columbia Dr., SE
Albuquerque, NM 87106 505-247-0192
800-524-5176
Fax: 505-247-1345
http://parentsreachingout.org/
info@parentsreachingout.org
Naomi Sandweiss, Executive Director
Ron Valek, Business Manager
Andrea Leon, Program Director
PRO views parents as full partners in the educational process and a significant source of support and assistance to each other. Programs provide training and information to parents to enable such individuals to participate more effectively with professionals in meeting the educational needs of disabled children.

New York

4194 Advocates for Children of New York
151 West 30th St.
5th Fl.
New York, NY 10001 212-947-9779
Fax: 212-947-9790
http://www.advocatesforchildren.org
info@advocatesforchildren.org
Kim Sweet, Executive Director
Matthew Lenaghan, Deputy Director
Melissa Atkinson, Administrative Assistant
Advocates for Children of New York, has worked in partnership with New York City's most impoverished and vulnerable families to secure quality and equal public education services. AFC works on behalf of children from infancy to age 21 who have disabilites, ethnic minorities, immigrants, homeless children, foster care children, limited English proficient children, and those living in poverty.

4195 Anderson Center for Autism
4885 Route 9
P.O. Box 367
Staatsburg, NY 12580 845-889-4034
Fax: 845-889-3104
http://www.andersoncenterforautism.org
Patrick Paul, Executive Director/CEO
Tina Covington, Chief Operating Officer
Tina M. Chirico, Chief Financial Officer
The Anderson Center for Autism provides the highest quality programs for children and adults with autism and other developmental disabilities.

4196 Andrus Children's Center
1156 N. Broadway
Yonkers, NY 10701 914-965-3700
800-647-2301
Fax: 914-965-3883
http://andruscc.org
Bryan R. Murphy, President/CEO
Jason R. Honecker, Vice President/COO
Tito Del Pilar, VP/Chief Administration Officer
For more than 75 years, Andrus has been a provider of programs and services for children and families with learning disabilities.

4197 Baker Victory Services
780 Ridge Rd.
Lackawanna, NY 14218 716-828-9500
888-287-1160
http://www.bakervictoryservices.org
Paul J.E. Burkard, President
BVS offers a wide range of services for individuals with physical, developmental, and/or behavorial challenges. In addition, they offer programming which supplies a lifetime of care; from infancy to late adulthood.

4198 Bridges to Adelphi Program
Adelphi University
1 South Ave
P.O. Box 701
Garden City, NY 11530-0701 516-877-4181
800-233-5744
Fax: 516-877-4552
http://bridges.adelphi.edu
bridges@adelphi.edu
Mitch Nagler, Director
Diana Damilatis, Associate Director
Stephanie Grindell, Academic Coordinator
A fee-for-service program designed to offer individualized comprehensive, academic, social, and vocational services to Adelphi University students who have autism spectrum disorder, another nonverbal learning disability, or problems with executive functioning/socialization, in order to make their college experience successful.

4199 Center for Spectrum Services
Special Education Program
4 Yankee Pl.
Ellenville, NY 12428 845-647-6464
Fax: 845-647-3456
http://www.centerforspectrumservices.org
info@centerforspectrumservices.org
Crystal C. Jacob, President
Brian Schug, Jr., Vice President
Samuel Kandel, Treasurer
Provides educational programs, diagnostic evaluations, and clinical services to children ages 2 to 12 with autism and Asperger Syndrome.

4200 EAC Network
50 Clinton St.
Suite 107
Hempstead, NY 11550 516-539-0150
Fax: 516-539-0160
http://eac-network.org
Glenn Stanis, Vice President, Finance
Lance W. Elder, President/CEO
Tania Peterson Chandler, Vice President, Operations
A social service agency whose mission is to empower, assist, and care for people in need across New York, including at-risk youth and people with disabilities.

4201 Eden II Programs
15 Beach St.
Staten Island, NY 10304 718-816-1422
Fax: 718-273-7106
http://www.eden2.org
Joanne Gerenser, Executive Director
Daniel Rauch, Chief Financial Officer
Eileen Hopkins, Deputy Executive Director
The mission of the Eden II/Genesis Programs is to provide people with autism specialized community-based programs and other opportunities, with the goal of enabling them to achieve the highest possible quality of living across life.

4202 Hallen School
97 Centre Ave.
New Rochelle, NY 10801 914-636-6600
Fax: 914-633-4294
http://www.thehallenschool.net
info@thehallenschool.net

Hallen School is a private, special education school that serves children who exhibit learning disabilities, speech and language impairments, emotional difficulties, autistic features, and mid-health impairments.

4203 **ICD Institute for Career Development**

123 William St.
5th Fl.
New York, NY 10038
212-585-6000
http://www.icdnyc.org

Dr. Richard Weber, Chair
Christopher Wu, Vice Chair
Susan Scheer, President/CEO

Serving children, adolescents, adults, and seniors with disabilities and other rehabilitative and developmental needs.

4204 **Just Kids: Early Childhood Learning Center**

35 Longwood Rd.
P.O. Box 12
Middle Island, NY 11953-0012
631-924-0008
Fax: 631-924-4602
http://justkidsschool.com

Steven Held, Executive Director
Cathy Cianfarano, Assistant Executive Director

Offers a developmentally appropriate curriculum to young children, ages birth to five years of age, who are disabled and non-disabled. Offers infant/toddler programs, pre-school education programs, mental health services, speech and language therapy, and physical and occupational therapy services.

4205 **Karafin School**

40-1 Radio Circle
P.O. Box 277
Mount Kisco, NY 10549-0277
914-666-9211
Fax: 914-666-9868
http://www.karafinschool.com

Bart A. Donow, PhD, Director

Private school serving students with disabilities in grades 9-12.

4206 **Kildonan School**

425 Morse Hill Rd.
Amenia, NY 12501
845-373-8111
Fax: 845-373-9793
http://www.kildonan.org
admissions@kildonan.org

C. Wilson Anderson, Jr., Chair
Richard S. Berg, Vice Chair
Bruce Karsk, Treasurer

Offers a fully accredited College Preparatory curriculum. The school is co-educational, enrolling boarding students in Grades 6-Postgraduate and day students in Grade 2-Postgraduate. Provides daily one-on-one Orton-Gillingham tutoring to build skills in reading, writing, and spelling. Daily independent reading and writing work reinforces skills and improves study habits. Interscholastic sports, horseback riding, clubs, and community service enhance self-confidence.

4207 **Maplebrook School**

5142 Route 22
Amenia, NY 12501
845-373-8191
Fax: 845-373-7029
http://www.maplebrookschool.org
admissions@maplebrookschool.org

Mark J. Metzger, Chairman
Robert S. Audia, Vice Chairman
George T. Whalen, Jr., Treasurer

A traditional boarding school enrolling students with learning differences and ADD. Offers strong academics and character development.

4208 **Mary McDowell Friends School**

20 Bergen St.
Brooklyn, NY 11201
718-625-3939
http://www.marymcdowell.org

Debbie Zlotowitz, Head of School
Beth Schneider, Associate Head of School
Horace Knight, Chief Financial Officer

An independent friends school for children with learning disabilities ages 5-12. There is also a middle and upper school for older children, also located in Brooklyn.

4209 **New Interdisciplinary School**

430 Sills Rd.
Yaphank, NY 11980
631-924-5583
Fax: 631-924-5687
http://www.niskids.org
info@niskids.org

Jay Silverstein, Ph.D., Executive Director
Susan Cali, Director, Development
Theresa Mahoney, Director, Special Education

Offers educational and therapeutic services to children with disabilities from birth to five years of age.

4210 **New York Institute for Special Education**

999 Pelham Pkwy., N.
Bronx, NY 10469
718-519-7000
http://www.nyise.org

Bernadette Kappen, Executive Director
Kim Benisatto, Operations Manager
Lisa Blasone, Human Resource Manager

Educational facility that provides quality programs for children who are blind or visually impaired, emotionally/learning disabled, or developmentally delayed. Students ages 3 to 21 attend NYISE. The school offers residential and day programs, physical programs, occupational and speech-language therapy, career guidance, and couseling.

4211 **Parent Network of WNY**

1000 Main St.
Buffalo, NY 14202
716-332-4170
Fax: 716-332-4171
http://www.parentnetworkwny.org
info@parentnetworkwny.org

Susan Barlow, Executive Director
Gary Pochatko, Business Manager
Peg Kovach, Administrative Coordinator

A non-profit agency with the mission of parents helping parents and professionals enabling individuals with disabilities to reach their own potential. Parent Network provides parents/caregivers of children with special needs the tools necessary to allow them to take an active role in their child's education. This is accomplished through information and referral services, workshops and conferences on various special education topics, and library and resource materials.

4212 **Pathways Program**

St. Thomas Aquinas College
125 Route 340
Sparkill, NY 10976
845-398-4230
http://www.stac.edu
pathways@stac.edu

Richard F. Heath, Director
Dustin Horvath, Assistant Director

Comprehensive support program for selected college students with learning disabilities and/or ADHD.

4213 **Responsibility Increases Self-Esteem (RISE) Program**

Maplebrook School
5142 Route 22
Amenia, NY 12501
845-373-8191
Fax: 845-373-7029
http://www.maplebrookschool.org
admissions@maplebrookschool.org

Mark J. Metzger, Chairman
Robert S. Audia, Vice Chairman
George T. Whalen, Jr., Treasurer

The RISE program provides the structure and support to awaken the learner in each student, promote responsibility and develop character, foster independence and growth, and enhances social development.

4214 **Robert Louis Stevenson School**
24 West 74th St.
New York, NY 10023 212-787-6400
http://www.stevenson-school.org
bcunningham@stevenson-school.org
Robert Cunningham, Head of School
Chris Ongaro, Associate Head of School
Lana Farina, Clinical Director
A college preparatory school that serves students who are functioning below their potential, whether because of adjustment difficulties, problems with peers, mild depression, or anxiety. Some have been diagnosed with a learning disability or ADD, but the program is for bright under-achievers.

4215 **Stephen Gaynor School**
148 West 90th St.
New York, NY 10024 212-787-7070
Fax: 212-787-3312
http://www.stephengaynor.org
jmay@stephengaynor.org
Scott Gaynor, Head of School
Grant Duers, Co-President
Ericka Leslie Horan, Co-President
The school offers a unique educational experience for children ages 5-14 with learning differences.

4216 **The Gow School**
2491 Emery Rd.
South Wales, NY 14139 716-652-3450
http://www.gow.org
admissions@gow.org
M. Bradley Rogers, Jr., Headmaster
A boarding school for boys, grades 7-12, with dyslexia and other language based learning disabilities.

4217 **The Norman Howard School**
275 Pinnacle Rd.
Rochester, NY 14623 585-334-8010
http://www.normanhoward.org
info@normanhoward.org
Joseph M. Martino, Executive Director
Julie Murray, Associate Director
Rosemary Hodges, Director, Education
Norman Howard School is an independent day school for students with disabilities in 5-12th grade.

4218 **Vocational Independence Program (VIP)**
New York Institute of Technology
Old Westbury, NY 11568 631-348-3114
Fax: 516-686-7414
http://www.nyit.edu/vip
vip@nyit.edu
Kevin D. Silva, Chair
Michael J. Merlo, Vice Chair
Peter J. Romano, Vice Chair
A 3-year certificate program that focuses on vocational, social, and independent living skills, with academics that support these areas. Also offers those that qualify the ability to take credit courses towards a degree.

4219 **Windward School**
13 Windward Ave.
White Plains, NY 10605 914-949-6968
http://www.thewindwardschool.org
Ellen Bowman, President
Timothy M. Jones, 1st Vice President
Susan C. Salice, 2nd Vice President
Independent school for language-based, learning disabled students in grades 1-9.

North Carolina

4220 **Exceptional Children's Assistance Center**
907 Barra Row
Suite 102-103
Davidson, NC 28036 704-892-1321
800-962-6817
Fax: 704-892-5028
http://www.ecac-parentcenter.org
ecac@ecacmail.org
Laura J. Weber, Executive Director
Grace Sisco, Business Manager
Denise Weir, Human Resources
A non-profit organization dedicated to helping children and adults with disabilities, as well as their parents and families. ECAC aims to empower families and improve the lives of children with disabilities from ages 0-26.

4221 **Hill Center**
3200 Pickett Rd.
Durham, NC 27705 919-489-7464
Fax: 919-489-7466
http://www.hillcenter.org
info@hillcenter.org
Beth Anderson, Executive Director
Bryan Brander, Head of School
Beth Hawkins, Director, Finance/Operations
Offers a unique half-day program to students in grades K-12 with diagnosed learning disabilities and attention deficit disorders. Also offers a comprehensive teacher training program.

4222 **Manus Academy**
6203 Carmel Rd.
Charlotte, NC 28226 704-542-6471
http://www.manusacademy.com
Rosanne Manus, Owner/Program Developer
Lesley Taylor, M.Ed., Head of School
Allison Osborn, Head of Instruction
Manus Academy works with students from grades 3-12 who experience learning disabilities, attention deficit disorder, and other neurological and developmental difficulties. Their services include an after-school tutoring services for K-12 students who attend other schools, testing, consultation, and parent and teacher training.

4223 **Piedmont School**
815 Old Mill Rd.
High Point, NC 27265 336-883-0992
http://www.thepiedmontschool.com
tmontgomery@thepiedmontschool.com
Tim Montgomery, Head of School
Pam Garner, Business Manager
Kori Mackall, Communications Director
Provides a unique, essential service to children with learning disabilites and/or an attention deficit disorder.

North Dakota

4224 **Anne Carlsen Center for Children**
701 3rd St., NW.
P.O. Box 8000
Jamestown, ND 58402 800-568-5175
http://annecarlsen.org
Tim Eissinger, Chief Executive Officer
Stephanie Nelson, Chief Operations Officer
Daniel Johnson, Chief Financial Officer
Offers education, therapy, medical care, and social and psychological services for children and young adults with special needs.

Ohio

4225 **Bellefaire Jewish Children's Bureau**
One Pollock Circle
22001 Fairmount Blvd.
Cleveland, OH 44118 216-932-2800
800-879-2522
Fax: 216-932-6704
http://www.bellefairejcb.org
info@bellefairejcb.org
Adam G. Jacobs, President
Jeffrey Lox, Executive Director
Tom Browne, Chief Financial Officer
Residential treatment center for adolescents, offering foster care, an adoption center, and Monarch School for Children with Autism.

4226 **Cincinnati Occupational Therapy Institute for Services and Study, Inc.**
4440 Carver Woods Dr.
Cincinnati, OH 45242-5545 513-791-5688
http://www.cintiotinstitute.com
Deborah Whitcomb, President/CEO
Linda Campbell, Executive Director
Rebecca Henderson, Programs Manager
Cincinnati Occupational Therapy Institute provides evaluation and treatment directly to children and adults with occupational therapy needs. COTI is owned and operated by therapists. The therapists are uniquely skilled at helping clients of all ages achieve or regain independence by offering creative adaptations and alternatives for carrying out daily activities, as well as remediating dysfunction through appropriate therapeutic modalities.

4227 **North Coast Education Services**
31300 Salon Rd.
Suite 1
Solon, OH 44139 440-914-0200
800-335-7984
http://www.northcoasted.com
info@northcoasted.com
Carole Richards, Executive Director/Founder
Kimberly Page, Director, Home Instruction
Nikki Claverie, VP, Education Services
Provides onsite education services to individual learners or groups. Uppermost in the delivery of these services is the development of self-esteem, expanding learner potential, and utilizing problem-solving to identify strengths and weaknesses. Specializing in working with at-risk learners which include learning disabled students.

4228 **Ohio Center for Autism and Low Incidence**
470 Glenmont Ave.
Columbus, OH 43214 614-410-0321
866-886-2254
Fax: 614-262-1070
http://www.ocali.org
ocali@ocali.org
Shawn Henry, Executive Director
Serves parents and educators of students with autism and low incidence disabilities including Autism Spectrum Disorders, deaf-blindness, deafness and hearing impairments, multiple disabilities, orthopedic impairments, other health impairments, traumatic brain injuries, and visual impairments.

4229 **Ohio Coalition for the Education of Children with Disabilities**
165 W. Center St.
Suite 302
Marion, OH 43302 740-382-5452
Fax: 740-383-6421
http://www.ocecd.org
ocecd@ocecd.org
Marcie Beers, Executive Director
Barbara Rice, Grants Manager/Bookkeeper
Non-profit parent training and information center serving Ohio families. Services are free.

4230 **Springer School and Center**
2121 Madison Rd.
Cincinnati, OH 45208 513-871-6080
http://www.springer-ld.org
Brett Marcoux, Executive Director
Kirstin Eismin, Development Director
Mark Priest, Business Director
Springer School and Center is the only organization in the Greater Cincinnati area whose program is devoted entirely to the education of children with learning disabilities.

4231 **The Children's Home Of Cincinnati**
5050 Madison Rd.
Cincinnati, OH 45227 513-272-2800
http://www.thechildrenshomecinti.org
John Banchy, President/CEO
Melanie L. Burden, VP, Human Resources
Heather Ellison, Chief Strategy Officer
Helps children with social, behavioral, and learning challenges by helping them build the skills and confidence that they need in life to succeed in school, home, and the community.

4232 **University Center for Excellence in Developmental Disabilities**
Division of Developmental & Behavioral Pediatrics
3333 Burnet Ave.
MLC 4002
Cincinnati, OH 45229 513-803-3627
http://www.ucucedd.org
ucucedd@cchmc.org
Ilka Riddle, Director
Kara Ayers, Associate Director
Rachel Miller, Communications Coordinator
UCEDD aims to help children and adults with disabilities through education, training, research, policy, and information sharing.

Oregon

4233 **Edison High School**
9020 S.W. Beaverton-Hillsdale Hwy.
Portland, OR 97225 503-297-2336
Fax: 503-297-2527
http://edisonhs.org/
Sean Preston, President
Jennifer Hogan, Development Director
Chris Cooper, Business Manager
A private high school in Oregon specifically designed to meet the needs of students with complex learning disabilities and attention deficit disorder issues. Edison High School empowers students with learning differences to experience academic success and personal growth, while preparing them for the future.

Pennsylvania

4234 **Barber National Institute**
100 Barber Pl.
Erie, PA 16507 814-453-7661
Fax: 814-455-1132
http://www.barberinstitute.org
BNIerie@barberinstitute.org
John Barber, President/CEO
Maureen Barber-Carey, Executive Vice President
Laurie Callaghan, Chief Information Officer
Offers a complete range of educational services and support to children and adults with disabilities.

4235 **Center for Alternative Learning**
6 East Eagle Rd.
Havertown, PA 19083 610-446-6126
800-869-8336
http://www.learningdifferences.com
rcooper-ldr@comcast.net

Dr. Richard Cooper, Ph.D., President
The Center for Alternative Learning was founded in 1987 to provide low cost and free educational services to individuals with learning differences, problems, and disabilities.

4236 **Center for Psychological Services**
125 Coulter Ave.
Ardmore, PA 19003
610-642-4873
Fax: 610-642-4886
http://www.centerpsych.com
CenterPsychServices@gmail.com
Moss A. Jackson, Director
Bruce V. Miller, Director
Individual, family, and group therapy, as well as psychoeducational evaluation and school consultation.

4237 **Devereux Center for Autism**
Devereux Pennsylvania
444 Devereux Dr.
Villanova, PA 19085
800-345-1292
http://www.devereux.org
Melanie Beidler, Vice President, Operations
Stephen Bruce, Vice President, Operations
Christopher Betts, Exec. Director, Adult Services
Addressing the particular needs of children, adolescents, and adults with Autism Spectrum Disorders, the center offers residential, educational, and vocational programs. All programs are geared to reaching these individuals, helping them overcome challenging behaviors, and teaching them crucial life skills.

4238 **Hill Top Preparatory School**
737 South Ithan Ave.
Rosemont, PA 19010
610-527-3230
Fax: 610-527-7683
http://www.hilltopprep.org
Tom Needham, Principal
Lex Nugent, Business Manager
Preparatory School for bright students in grades five through twelve with learning disabilities.

4239 **Hillside School**
2697 Brookside Rd.
Macungie, PA 18062
610-967-3701
http://www.hillsideschool.org
Donna Henry, Head of School
Darlene Stack, Business Manager
Jane Hottenstein, Administrative Assistant
A day school for children with learning differences in grades K-8. Scholarships are available.

4240 **KidsPeace Orchard Hills Campus**
4085 Independence Dr.
Schnecksville, PA 18078
800-257-3223
http://www.kidspeace.org
Will Isemann, President/CEO
Michael Slack, Chief Operating Officer
Michael Callan, Chief Financial Officer
Offers various programs including community residential care, specialized group homes, child and family guidance center, and student assistance programs.

4241 **Melmark**
2600 Wayland Rd.
Berwyn, PA 19312
610-325-2937
888-MEL-MARK
http://www.melmark.org
admissions@melmark.org
Rita M. Gardner, President/CEO
Peter J. Troy, Vice President
Karen Parenti, Executive Director
Provides residential, educational, therapeutic, and recreational services for children and adults with mild to severe developmental disabilities.

4242 **Pathway School**
162 Egypt Rd.
Jeffersonville, PA 19403
610-277-0660
http://www.pathwayschool.org
info@pathwayschool.org
William S. Harrigan, Chair
Edmond A. Watters III, Vice Chair
Brad Kerr, Treasurer
Provides day and residential programming for individuals ages 5-21, who have learning disabilities, neurological impairments, and neuropsychiatric disorders. Special education, counseling, speech and language therapy, reading therapy, and other specialized services are provided in a small, warm, and supportive atmosphere.

4243 **Stratford Friends School**
2 Bishop Hollow Rd.
Newtown Square, PA 19073
610-355-9580
Fax: 610-355-9585
http://www.stratfordfriends.org
info@stratfordfriends.org
Jill Dougherty, Head of School
Bethann Lynch, Director, Advancement
Corinne News, Associate Head of School
A Quaker elementary school for children with language-based learning differences who have had difficulty learning in a traditional classroom.

4244 **The Children's Institute**
1405 Shady Ave.
Pittsburgh, PA 15217-1350
412-420-2400
TTY: 412-420-2578
http://www.amazingkids.org
Wendy Pardee, President/CEO
Sharon Dorogy, Chief Information Officer
Tim Bittner, Vice President, Operations
Provides pediatric and adult rehabilitation services and programs.

4245 **Vanguard School**
1777 North Valley Rd.
Malvern, PA 19355
610-296-6700
Fax: 610-296-6530
http://www.vfes.net/vanguard
Dr. Grace Fornicola, Executive Director
Dr. Darren Levin, Director, Clinical Services
Lisa Wood, Director, Education
State licensed and approved private, non-profit, and non-sectarian day school serving children from four to twenty-one years of age who have been diagnosed with neurological disorders, emotional disturbances, or autism/PDD.

4246 **Woods Schools**
Woods Services
Route 413 & 213
P.O. Box 36
Langhorne, PA 19047-0036
215-750-4000
http://www.woods.org
communications@woods.org
Tina Hansen-Turton, President/CEO
Michael D. Haggerty, Senior VP, Operations
Tom Grant, Executive Vice President/CFO
Provides a full range of residential, special education, rehabilitation, recreation, and vocational training to children and adults with Autism Spectrum Disorder, developmental disabilities, neurological disorders, traumatic brain injuries, and emotional disturbances.

Rhode Island

4247 **Harmony Hill School**
63 Harmony Hill Rd.
Chepachet, RI 02814
401-949-0690
Fax: 401-949-4412
http://www.harmonyhillschool.org

Eric James, President/CEO
Cynthia McDermott, Education Director
Cheryl Raposa, Clinical Director
A private residential and day treatment center for behaviorally disordered and learning disabled boys, age eight through eighteen, who cannot be treated within their local educational system or community based mental health programs. Individual, group, and family psychotherapy and 24-hour crisis intervention are available. Other programs include: Extended Day, Sex Offender, Diagnostic Day, Transition Programming, Summer Day, Career Education Center, and a Formalized Life Skills Program.

4248 **Rhode Island Parent Information Network**
1210 Pontiac Ave.
Cranston, RI 02920 401-270-0101
Fax: 401-270-7049
http://www.ripin.org
info@ripin.org
Johnny Z. Luo, Chair
Jane Palmer, Vice Chair
Stephen Brunero, Executive Director
Rhode Island Parent Information Network is a statewide, non-profit organization that provides programs and services to families with children in RI, including families of children with special needs due to disabilities.

South Carolina

4249 **Parents Reaching Out to Parents of South Carolina**
652 Bush River Rd.
Suite 203
Columbia, SC 29210-7537 803-772-5688
Fax: 803-772-5341
http://www.proparents.org
Mary Eaddy, Executive Director
Private non-profit parent oriented organization providing information, individual assistance, and workshops to parents of children with disabilities ages birth-21. Services focus on enabling parents to have a better understanding of special education to participate more effectively with professionals in meeting the educational needs of disabled children. Funded by a grant from the US Department of Education and tax deductible contributions.

4250 **Trident Academy**
1455 Wakendaw Rd.
Mount Pleasant, SC 29464 843-884-7046
Fax: 843-881-8320
http://www.tridentacademy.com
admissions@tridentacademy.com
Mike Jeresaty, President
Chad Anderson, Vice President
Andrea Martin, Secretary
Trident Academy is for students with specific learning disabilities; offering an intensive, effective, multi-sensory program to remediate learning differences, tailored to each student's unique needs.

Tennessee

4251 **Bodine School**
2432 Yester Oaks Dr.
Germantown, TN 38139 901-754-1800
http://www.bodineschool.org
communications@bodineschool.org
John Murphy, Head of School
Loie Watkins, Director, Finance/Operations
Tom Hutton, Chair
The Bodine School has provided students with language based learning disabilities a nurturing environment and a challenging academic curriculum for the last 30 years. The Bodine School program is designed specifically for the dyslexic student and is based on current research findings on reading and reading disorders.

4252 **Genesis Learning Centers**
430 Allied Dr.
Nashville, TN 37211 615-832-4222
Fax: 615-832-4577
http://www.genesislearn.org
admin@genesislearn.org
Terance Adams, Executive Director/Co-Founder
Melissa Adams, Asst. Exec. Director/Co-Founder
Chuck Goon, Director, Human Resources
Genesis Learning Centers offer special educational services to children and youth with distinctive needs, including emotional and behavioral disorders, learning disabilities, developmental delays, and short-term severe illness, physical challenges, or misconduct.

Texas

4253 **Achievers' Center for Education**
University United Methodist Church
5084 DeZavala Rd.
San Antonio, TX 78249 210-690-7359
http://www.aceschool.org
annette@theu.org
Anne Zuber, Executive Director
Ida Ross, Director, Operations
Annette Griffin, Operations/Events Coordinator
Educational program for children and young adults in 5th through 8th grade who are behind academically due to dyslexia or other learning disabilities.

4254 **Bridges Academy**
4320 N. Stanton
El Paso, TX 79902 915-532-6647
Fax: 915-532-8767
http://www.bridgesacademy.org
bschool001@elp.rr.com
Irma Keys, Executive Director
Jesus Arreola, Assistant Director
Robert Brandmeyer, Chairman
Private School for students with learning disabilities.

4255 **Camelot Education**
7500 Rialto Blvd.
Building 1, Suite 260
Austin, TX 78735 512-858-9900
Fax: 512-858-9901
http://www.cameloteducation.org
info@cameloteducation.org
Andrew Morrison, Chief Executive Officer
Joseph Carter, Chief Operating Officer
Todd Bock, President
Accepts children ages 4-17 who have been referred by area school systems. The campus includes a horsebarn and pasture, in-ground swimming pool, playground areas, and pet therapy dogs.

4256 **Crisman School**
2455 N. Eastman Rd.
Longview, TX 75605 903-758-9741
Fax: 903-758-9767
http://www.crismanschool.org
Laura Lea Banks, Executive Director
A private school designed to meet the needs of students with learning differences, including dyslexia, Aspergers, sensory delays, ADD/ADHD, and language based delays.

4257 **Parish School**
11001 Hammerly Blvd.
Houston, TX 77043 713-467-4696
http://www.parishschool.org
info@parishschool.org
Nancy Bewley, Head of School
Mimi Branham, Clinic Director
Terry Clough, Director, Finance/Operations

Offers a multi-age, language-based, developmental curriculum for children ages 12-12. Children served have communication and learning differences, but average to above average learning potential. The Parish School utilizes a classroom based therapy program implemented by certified teachers and speech/language pathologists.

4258 **Partners Resource Network**
1090 Longfellow Dr.
Beaumont, TX 77706 409-898-4684
800-866-4726
Fax: 409-898-4869
http://prntexas.org
partnersresource@sbcglobal.net
Theresa Howell, Executive Director
Jon Howell, Co-Director
Statewide network of federally funded parent training and information centers. Provides services to parents of infants, toddlers, children, and youth ages birth to 26 with all types of disabilities.

4259 **Scottish Rite Dyslexia Center of Austin, Inc.**
12871 N. U.S. Highway 183
Suite 105
Austin, TX 78750 512-472-1231
Fax: 512-326-1877
http://www.scottishritelearningcenter.org
lmuse@scottishritedyslexiacenter.org
Lindsay Muse, Executive Director
Alice Marsel, Director, Education
Focuses on the evalation and treatment of dyslexia in children. The center also provides workshops, seminars, and resources for educators and parents.

4260 **Shelton School and Evaluation Center**
6001 Summerside Dr.
Suite 204
Dallas, TX 75252 972-774-1772
http://www.shelton.org
Suzanne Stell, Executive Director
Linda Kneese, Head of School
Gary Webb, Chairman
A co-educational day school serving 900 students in grades Pre-K-12. The school focuses on the development of learning disabled students of average to above average intelligence, enabling them to succeed in conventional classroom settings. Services include on-site Evaluation Center for diagnostic testing, a Speech, Language and Hearing Clinic, an Early Childhood Program, Out Reach Program, open summer school, and more.

4261 **Starpoint School**
Texas Christian University
TCU Box 297410
Fort Worth, TX 76109 817-257-7141
http://starpoint.tcu.edu
starpoint@tcu.edu
Dr. Marilyn Tolbert, Director
Kimberly Payne, Assistant Director
Provides individualized academic programs for children with learning disabilities.

4262 **The Winston School**
5707 Royal Ln.
Dallas, TX 75229 214-691-6950
http://www.winston-school.org
info@winston-school.org
Nancy W. Furney, Chair
Terri Anderson, Treasurer
Johnny M. Hea, Secretary
The environmment and curriculum of The Winston School are designed for bright students who learn differently. Through Winston's Testing and Evaluation Center, students are assessed and teachers are provided with the learning profiles, training, and resources needed to respond to the needs of each student.

Utah

4263 **Reid School**
2965 E. Evergreen Ave.
Salt Lake City, UT 84109 801-466-4214
Fax: 801-484-5938
http://www.reidschool.com
ereid@xmission.com
Dr. Ethna R. Reid, Principal
Mervin R. Reid, President
Reid School is a private, innovative center for students who need more attention with reading, writing, speaking, and language arts education.
1987Grade Range: K-9

4264 **Utah Parent Center**
230 West 200 South
Suite 1101
Salt Lake City, UT 84101 801-272-1051
800-468-1160
Fax: 801-272-8907
http://www.utahparentcenter.org
info@utahparentcenter.org
Helen Post, Executive Director
Gina Money, Associate Director
Jennie Dopp, Development Coordinator
Utah Parent Center offers free training, information, referral, and assistance to parents and professionals through the provision of information, referrals, individual assistance, workshops, presentations, and displays.

Vermont

4265 **Stern Center for Language and Learning**
183 Talcott Rd.
Suite 101
Williston, VT 05495 802-878-2332
Fax: 802-878-0230
http://www.sterncenter.org
learning@sterncenter.org
Blanche Podhajski, President
Jane Ashby, Senior Director, Education
Michael Shapiro, Chief Operating Officer
Founded in 1983, the center is a non-profit organization providing comprehensive services for children and adults with learning disabilities. The Center is also an educational resource serving all of Northern New England and Northern New York State. Programs include educational testing, individual instruction, psychotherapy, school consultation, professional training for educators, and a parent/professional resource library.

Virginia

4266 **Accotink Academy**
6215 Rolling Rd.
Springfield, VA 22003 703-451-5797
Fax: 703-451-0336
http://www.accotinkacademy.com
preschool@accotinkpreschool.com
Lexie Winsten, Educational Director
An early childhood program for children ages 2-6 that aims to recognize the unique educational needs of each child.

4267 **Behavioral Directions**
626 Grant St.
Suite I
Herndon, VA 20170 703-855-4032
http://www.BehavioralDirections.com
info@behavioraldirections.com
Jane Barbin, Ph.D, BCBA-D, Executive Director
A resource for applied behavior analysis and behavior disorders.

4268 **Blue Ridge Autism and Achievement Center (BRAAC)**
312 Whitwell Dr.
Roanoke, VA 24019
540-366-7399
Fax: 540-366-5523
http://braacroanoke.org
braac.roanoke@svhservices.org
Christina Giuliano, Executive Director
Lisa Hensley, Business Manager
Samantha McFarland, Clinical Director
A private day school offering many academic and educational programs for children with Autism and learning disabilities and their families.

4269 **Chesapeake Bay Academy**
821 Baker Rd.
Virginia Beach, VA 23462
757-497-6200
http://www.cba-va.org
Stanley F. Baldwin, Chair
Donald L. Glenum III, Vice Chair
Judy T. Jankowski, Ed.D., Head of School
Chesapeake Bay Academy is the only accredited independent school in Southeastern Virginia specifically dedicated to providing a strong academic program and individualized instruction for bright students with learning disabilities and ADHD. With a small student to teacher ratio, qualified professionals tailor their techniques to individual needs, allowing students who have difficulty learning in traditional settings to finally succeed.

4270 **Grafton School**
Grafton, Inc.
P.O. Box 2500
Winchester, VA 22604
888-955-5205
Fax: 540-542-1721
http://www.grafton.org
admissions@grafton.org
James H. Stewart, CEO/President
Kent Houchins, Chief Administrative Officer
Scott Zeiter, Chief Operating Officer
Grafton provides individualized educational and residential services and in-community supports for children, youth, and adults with severe emotional disturbances, learning disabilities, Autism Spectrum Disorders, behavioral disorders, and other complex challenges, including physical disabilities.

4271 **Learning Resource Center**
935 First Colonial Rd.
Virginia Beach, VA 23454
757-428-3367
Fax: 757-428-1630
http://www.learningresourcecenter.org
Nancy Harris-Kroll, Director/Owner
One-on-one remedial and tutorial sessions after school, during the school year, and all day and evening during the summer with specialists who have masters degrees. Advocacy services for parents of students with special needs. Psychoeducational testing is available. Special study skills and SAT courses given. Gifted, average, and learning disabled students attend.

4272 **Leary School Programs**
Lincolnia Educational Foundation
6349 Lincolnia Rd.
Alexandria, VA 22312
703-941-8150
http://www.learyschool.org
mail@learyschool.org
Ed Schultze, President/Executive Director
A private, day, co-educational, and special education facility that serves 130 students with emotional, learning, and behavioral problems. Along with individualized academic instruction, Leary School of Virginia offers a range of supportive and therapeutic services, including physical education, recreation therapy, group counseling, individual psychotherapy, and art therapy.

4273 **Little Keswick School**
P.O. Box 24
Keswick, VA 22947-0024
434-295-0457
Fax: 434-977-1892
http://www.littlekeswickschool.net
Marc J. Columbus, M.Ed., Headmaster
Terry Columbus, M.Ed., Director, Development
Jody Berkey, M.Ed., Assistant Head of School
Little Keswick School is a therapeutic boarding school for 33 learning disabled and/or emotionally disturbed boys between the ages of 10 to 15 at acceptance and served through 17. IQ range accepted is below average to superior. LKS provides a structured routine in a small, nurturing environment with services that include psychotherapy, occupational therapy, speech therapy, and art therapy. Five week summer session.

4274 **New Vistas School**
520 Eldon St.
Lynchburg, VA 24501
434-846-0301
Fax: 434-528-1004
http://www.newvistasschool.org
cmorgan@newvistasschool.org
Lisa J. DeJarnette, Head of School
Nancy Harrison, Assistant Head of School
Brooke Levens, Development Director
The New Vistas School provides individualized programs for students in grades 3-12 with Attention Deficit Disorder and learning disabilities.

4275 **Oakwood School**
7210 Braddock Rd.
Annandale, VA 22003
703-941-5788
Fax: 703-941-4186
http://www.oakwoodschool.com
oakwood@oakwoodschool.com
Robert McIntyre, Chairman of the Board
Oakwood School is a private, non-profit, co-educational day school for elementary and middle school students with mild to moderate learning disabilities. Students are of average to above average potential and exhibit a discrepancy between their potential and their current level of achievement.

4276 **Riverside School**
2110 McRae Rd.
North Chesterfield, VA 23235
804-320-3465
Fax: 804-320-6146
http://www.riversideschool.org
info@riversideschool.org
William J. Longan, Jr., President
Richard W. Fowlkes, Vice President
Juliette Sykes, Treasurer
Private school for children grages 1-8 with specific language based learning disabilities and Dyslexia.

4277 **The New Community School**
4211 Hermitage Rd
Richmond, VA 23227
804-266-2494
Fax: 804-264-3281
http://www.tncs.org
info@tncs.org
Nancy L. Foy, Head of School
The New Community School is an independent day school specializing in college preparatory instruction and intensive remediation for students in grades 5-12 with dyslexia and related learning differences.

Washington

4278 **Children's Institute for Learning Differences**
2640 Benson Rd. South
Renton, WA 98055
425-336-3260
866-492-4902
Fax: 425-277-7726
http://www.childnow.org
Carrie Fannin, Executive Director
Cathy DeLeon, Director, Clinical Services
Linda Foley, Director, Development

CHILD provides a therapeutic year-round day school, serving students who learn differently and who process information and life experiences in a unique way. Also provides on-site occupational and speech therapy, individual, group, and family counseling.

4279 Early Life Speech & Language
Scottish Rite Masons
1207 N. 152nd St.
Suite A
Shorline, WA 98133
206-324-6293
Fax: 203-365-0270
http://earlylifespeech.org
info@earlylifespeech.org
Angelique Leone, Executive Director
Jacqueline Brown, Director, Programs
Susie Beresford, Director, Development/Comm.
Provides diagnostic and therapeutic services to children whose primary disorder is a severe delay in language or speech development.

4280 Hamlin Robinson School
1701 20th Ave. South
Seattle, WA 98144
206-763-1167
Fax: 206-763-7149
http://www.hamlinrobinson.org
info@hamlinrobinson.org
Stacy Turner, Head of School
A non-profit, state approved elementary day school for children with specific language disabilities, providing a positive learning environment, and meeting individual needs to nurture the whole child. Small classes use the Slingerland multi-sensory classroom approach in reading, writing, spelling, and all instructional areas.

4281 STOMP Specialized Training of Military Parents
PAVE
6316 South 12th St.
Tacoma, WA 98465
253-565-2266
800-5-PARENT
Fax: 253-566-8052
http://wapave.org
pave@wapave.org
Tracy Kahlo, Executive Director
Elma Rounds, Chief Financial Officer
Nicol Walsh, Communications Specialist
STOMP (Specialized Training of Military Parents) is a federally funded center established to assist military families who have children with special education or health needs.

4282 St. Christopher Academy
4100 S.W. Genesee St.
Seattle, WA 98116
206-246-9751
http://www.stchristopheracademy.com
jevne@stchristopheracademy.com
Darlene Jevne, Founder/Executive Director
St. Christopher Academy is a private school for learning disabled, ADD, and/or academically at-risk students.

West Virginia

4283 West Virginia Parent Training and Information
99 Edmiston Way
Suite 101-102
Buckhannon, WV 26201
304-427-5697
800-281-1436
Fax: 304-472-3548
TDD: 304-624-1436
http://www.wvpti-inc.org
office@wvpti-inc.org
Brenda Lamkin, Executive Director
Provides information to parents and to professionals who work with children with disabilities.

Wisconsin

4284 Chileda Institute
1825 Victory St.
La Crosse, WI 54601
608-782-6480
http://www.chileda.org
Ruth Wiseman, President/CEO
Serves children and young adults ages 6-21 with learning disabilities. The Institute offers on-campus day school and residential programs, on/off campus summer school, after school and weekend respite programs, and individualized consulting and training programs for educators and families.

4285 Wisconsin FACETS
600 W. Virginia St.
Suite 501
Milwaukee, WI 53204
414-374-4645
877-374-0511
Fax: 414-374-4655
http://wifacets.org
Courtney Salzer, Executive Director
Cheryl Peterson, Accounting Director
Wisconsin Family Assistance Center for Education, Training & Support, also known as WI FACETS, is a non-profit organization that aims to help children and youth with special needs and their families by being an information center that connects them to much needed resources.

4286 Wisconsin Institute for Learning Disabilities/Dyslexia Inc.
6525 Grand Teton Plaza
Suite B
Madison, WI 53719
608-824-8980
Fax: 608-831-3840
http://wildd.org
madison@wildd.org
Ervin Carpenter, Co-Founder/Executive Director
Kim Campbell-Carpenter, Co-Founder/Director, Operations
Tim Mueller, Chairman
Through therapy, support, cummunity education, and advocacy the Wisconsin Institute for Learning Disabilities/Dyslexia helps children with learning disabilities achieve success in school and in their community.

Wyoming

4287 Parent Information Center of Wyoming
500 W. Lott St.
Suite A
Buffalo, WY 82834
307-684-2277
Fax: 888-389-6542
http://www.wpic.org
info@wpic.org
Terri Dawson, Executive Director
Juanita Bybee, Outreach Parent Liaison
Erin Swilling, PIC Director
Parent Training and Information Program views parents as full partners in the educational process and a significant source of support and assistance to each other. Funded by the Division of Personnel Preparation, Office of Special Education Programs, these programs provide training and information to parents to enable such individuals to participate more effectively with professionals in meeting the educational needs of disabled children.

Centers

4288 **American College Testing Program**
ACT Universal Testing
PO Box 168
Iowa City, IA 52243-168 319-337-1000
Fax: 319-339-3020
http://www.act.org
sandy.schlote@act.org

Jon Whitmore, CEO
Janet E. Godwin, Chief of Staff
Thomas J. Goedken, CFO/EVP
Helps individuals and organizations make informed decisions about education and work. We provide information for life's transitions.

4289 **Center for Child and Human Development**
Georgetown University
PO Box 571485
Washington, DC 20057-1485 202-687-5000
Fax: 202-687-1954
http://gucchd.georgetown.edu
gucchd@georgetown.edu

Phyllis Magrab, PhD, Executive Director
To improve the quality of life for all children and youth, especially those with, or at risk for, special needs and their families.

4290 **Diagnostic and Educational Resources**
115 Rowell Court
Suite 2
Falls Church, VA 22046-3126 703-534-5180
Fax: 703-534-5181
http://www.der-online.com
aspector@DER-online.com

Annette Spector, M.S. Ed., Executive Director
Elisabeth Wester, Course Coordinator
Focuses on what the child can do and builds self-esteem. Provides a full range of psychoeducational testing, parent advocacy, case management, and tutoring services. Diagnostic testing determines individual needs, which are addressed in one-on-one tutoring sessions in the child's home or school. Staff trained in LD/ADHD methodologies remediate learning disabilities and offer practical suggestions for home programs and for working with school systems.

4291 **Educational Diagnostic Center at Curry College**
Curry College
1071 Blue Hill Ave
Milton, MA 02186-2302 617-333-0500
Fax: 617-333-2114
http://www.curry.edu
curryadm@curry.edu

Jane Fidlery, Dean Of Admission
Keith Robichaud, Director Of Admission
Kenneth K. Quigley, Jr., President
A comprehensive evaluation and testing center specializing in the learning needs of adolescents and adults. The Diagnostic Center welcomes adolescents and adults in need of learning strategies, long term educational plans, and better understanding of their learning profiles.

4292 **Educational Testing Service**
660 Rosedale Road
Princeton, NJ 08541-0001 609-921-9000
Fax: 609-734-5410
TDD: 800-877-2540
http://www.ets.org
etsinfo@ets.org

Kurt M Landgraf, President
Our mission is to help advance quality and equity in education by providing fair and valid assessments, research and related services.

4293 **GED Testing Service**
American Council on Education
1 Dupont Cir NW
Washington, DC 20036-1193 202-939-9300
800-626-9433
Fax: 202-293-2223
http://www.gedtest.org
help@GEDtestingservice.com

Randy Trask, President and CEO
The American Council on Education, founded in 1918, is the nation's coordinating higher education association. ACE is dedicated to the belief that equal educational opportunity and a strong higher education system are essential cornerstones of a democratic society.

4294 **Huntington Learning Centers, Inc.**
496 Kinderkamack Rd
Oradell, NJ 07649 201-261-8400
800-226-7323
http://www.huntingtonlearning.com

Eileen Huntington, Founder
Helps students ages 5 to 17 achieve remarkable improvements in their grades, test scores and self esteem. Builds a personalized learning program for your child based on his or her individual strenths and needs, which is identified using their in-depth diagnostic evaluation. Helps child master a skill before moving on to more difficult tasks and mor advanced learning. Helps develop the skills to learn and solve problems independently.

4295 **Munroe-Meyer Institute for Genetics and Rehabilitation**
University of Nebraska Medical Center
985450 Nebraska Med Center
Omaha, NE 68198-5450 402-559-6430
800-656-3937
Fax: 402-559-5737
http://www.unmc.edu/mmi
munroemeyer@unmc.edu

J. Michael Leibowitz, Ph.D., Director, Munroe-Meyer Inst.
Diagnostic evaluation therapy, speech, physical, occupational, behavioral therapies, pediatrics, dentistry, nursing, psychology, social work, genetics, Media Resource Center, education, nutrition. Adult services for developmentally disabled, genetic evaluation and counseling, adaptive equipment, motion analysis laboratory, recreational therapy.

4296 **National Center for Fair & Open Testing FairTest**
P.O. Box 300204
Jamaica Plain, MA 02130 617-477-9792
Fax: 857-350-8209
http://www.fairtest.org
info@fairtest.org

Dr. Sophie Sa, Chair
Monty Neill, Ed.D, Executive Director
Robert Schaeffer, Public Education Director
Dedicated to ensuring that America's students and workers are assessed using fair, accurate, relevant and open tests.

4297 **Plano Child Development Center**
5401 S Wentworth Ave
Ste 14A
Chicago, IL 60609-6300 773-924-5297
Fax: 773-373-3548
http://www.planovision.org
pcdc59@yahoo.com

Dr. Henry R. Moore, Co-Founder
Albert Pritchett, Chairperson
Linda Ford, Vice Chairperson
A multi-disciplinary, not-for-profit optometric service organization that specializes in the identification, evaluation and treatment of individuals with learning related vision skills problems.

4298 **Providence Speech and Hearing Center**
1301 Providence Ave
Orange, CA 92868-3892
714-923-1521
855-901-7742
Fax: 714-639-2593
TTY: 714-532-4047
http://www.pshc.org
pshc@pshc.org

Raul Lopez, Founder
Linda Smith, CEO
Raul Lopez, COO/Director of Finance
Comprehensive services for testing and treatment of all speech, language and hearing problems. Individual and group therapy beginning with parent/infant programs.

4299 **Reading Assessment System**
Harcourt Achieve
222 Berkeley Street
Boston, MA 02116
617-351-5000
800-531-5015
Fax: 800-699-9459
http://www.steckvaughn.com
info@steckvaughn.com

Steck-Vaughn Staff, Author
Linda K. Zecher, President, CEO & Director
Eric Shuman, Chief Financial Officer
William Bayers, EVP/General Counsel
The Reading Assessment System provides an ongoing meaure of specific student's skills and offers detailed directions for individual instruction and remediation. Up to eight reports are available. This popular program generates individual scores, class scores, school scores, and district reports.

4300 **Rehabilitation Resource**
University Of Wisconsin - Stout
221 10th Avenue East
Room 101A
Menomonie, WI 54751
715-232-2470
800-447-8688
Fax: 715-232-5008
http://www3.uwstout.edu.com
luij@uwstout.edu

John W. Lui, Ph.D., Executive Director
Develops, publishes, and distributes a variety of rehabilitation related materials. Also makes referrals to other sources on rehabilitation.

4301 **Riley Child Development Center**
Indiana University School of Medicine
702 Barnhill Dr
Room 5837
Indianapolis, IN 46202-5225
317-944-8167
Fax: 317-944-9760
http://www.child-dev.com
info@child-dev.com

Dr. John Rau, M.D., Director
Provides an interdisciplinary evaluation for children with behanvior, learning and other developmental disabilities.

4302 **Rose F Kennedy Center**
Albert Einstein College of Medicine
1410 Pelham Pkwy S
Bronx, NY 10461-1116
718-430-8600
Fax: 718-892-2296
http://www.einsten.yu.edu.com

Steven U. Walkley, D.V.M., Ph.D., Director
John J. Foxe, Ph.D., Associate Director
Lisa L. Guillory, M.A., Administrator
Provides comprehensive diagnostic services and intervention services for children and adults with learning disabilities. The primary mission is to improve the quality of life of persons with developmental disabilites and their families.

4303 **Scholastic Testing Service**
480 Meyer Rd
Bensenville, IL 60106-1617
630-766-7150
800-642-6787
Fax: 630-766-8054
http://www.ststesting.com
sts@ststesting.com

John Kauffman, Marketing VP
Publisher of assessment materials from birth to adulthood, ability and achievement tests for kindergarten through grade twelve. Publishes the Torrance Tests of Creative Thinking, Thinking Creatively in Action and Movement, the STS High School Placement Test and Educational Development Series.

4304 **Services For Students with Disabilities**
PSAT/NMSQT Students With Disabilities
P.O. Box 8060
Mt. Vernon, IL 62864-0060
212-713-8333
Fax: 866-360-0114
TTY: 609-882-4118
http://www.collegeboard.com/ssd
ssd@info.collegeboard.org

Provides services and reasonable accommodations that are appropriate according to the type of disability and the purpose of the exam.

4305 **The Center for Learning Differences**
45 North Station Plaza
Great Neck, NY 11201
646-775-6646
http://www.centerforlearningdifferences.org
syellin@yellincenter.com

Susan Denberg Yellin J.D., Chairman/Executive Director
Stuart Rothman, PhD
Herman Davidovicz, PhD
A not-for-profit organization dedicated to providing information to families, physicians and other professionals in the New York metropolitan area about issues they face in dealing with children and parents of children who struggle in school with the hope that others can benefit from their experiences and the information they have learned. And by sharing your experinces with them, they hope to make them available to other families who are dealing with similar issues.

4306 **The Reading Group**
3011A Village Office Pl.
Champaign, IL 61822
217-351-9144
http://www.readinggroup.org
info@readinggroup.org

Winnie Crowder, Executive Director
Liz Miles, President
Penny Porter, Secretary
A non-profit learning center known for its work with students who have challenging learning difficulties/differences. Individualized one-on-one instruction is offered by educational specialists in reading, writing, early childhood development, giftedness, and English as a second language.

Behavior & Self Esteem

4307 **BASC Monitor for ADHD**
Pearson Assessments
4940 Pearl East Circle
Suite 200
Boulder, CO 80301
888-977-7900
800-328-5999
Fax: 888-556-2103
http://www.pearsonassessments.com
info@pearsonkt.com

Randy W Kamphaus, Author
Cecil R Reynolds, Co-Author
Doug Kubach, Group President & CEO
The BASC Monitor for ADHD is a powerful new tool to help evaluate the effectiveness of ADHD treatments using teacher and parent rating scales, and database software for tracking behavior changes.

4308 **Behavior Assessment System for Children**
Pearson Assessments
4940 Pearl East Circle
Suite 200
Boulder, CO 80301
888-977-7900
800-328-5999
Fax: 888-556-2103
http://www.pearsonassessments.com
info@pearsonkt.com

Randy W Kamphaus, Author
Cecil R Reynolds, Co-Author
Doug Kubach, Group President & CEO
A powerful assessment to evaluate child and adolescent behavior. Includes a self-report form for describing the behaviors and emotions of children and adolescents. Administration time: 10 - 20 minutes (TRS & PRS) 30 - 45 minutes for SRP.

4309 **Behavior Rating Profile**
Pro-Ed
8700 Shoal Creek Boulevard
Austin, TX 78757-6897
512-451-3246
800-897-3202
Fax: 512-451-8542
http://www.proedinc.com
general@proedinc.com

Donald D Hammill, Owner
Linda Brown, Author
A global measure of behavior providing student, parent, teacher and peer scales. It helps to identify behaviors that may cause a student's learning problems. *$211.00*

4310 **Child Behavior Checklist**
University of Vermont
1 S Prospect St
St. Joseph's Wing (3rd Floor, Room# 3207
Burlington, VT 05401-3456
802-656-5130
Fax: 802-656-5131
http://www.aseba.org
mail@aseba.org

Dr TM Achenbach, Director/Professor
Ramani Sunderaju, Operations Manager
Psychological assessments

4311 **Culture-Free Self-Esteem Inventories**
Pro-Ed
8700 Shoal Creek Boulevard
Austin, TX 78757-6897
512-451-3246
800-897-3202
Fax: 512-451-8542
http://www.proedinc.com
general@proedinc.com

Donald D Hammill, Owner
James Battle, Author
A series of self-report scales used to determine the level of self-esteem in children and adults. *$190.00*

4312 **Devereux Early Childhood Assessment Program Observation Journal**
Kaplan Early Learning Company
1310 Lewisville Clemmons Rd
Lewisville, NC 27023-9635
336-766-7374
800-334-2014
Fax: 800-452-7526
http://www.kaplanco.com
info@kaplanco.com

Hal Kaplan, President & CEO
Provides both sample and reproducible copies of suggested forms for early childhood programs to support appropriate observation and planning for individual children and the classroom. *$199.95*

4313 **Disruptive Behavior Rating Scale Kit**
Slosson Educational Publications, Inc.
538 Buffalo Road
East Aurora, NY 14052
716-652-0930
888-756-7766
Fax: 800-655-3840
http://www.slosson.com
slossonprep@gmail.com

Bradley T Erford, Author
Steven Slosson, President
John H Slosson, Vice President
Identifies common behavior problems such as attention deficit disorder, attention deficit hyperactivity disorder, oppositional disorders and anti-social conduct problems. *$186.25*

4314 **Draw a Person: Screening Procedure for Emotional Disturbance**
Pro-Ed
8700 Shoal Creek Boulevard
Austin, TX 78757-6897
512-451-3246
800-897-3202
Fax: 512-451-8542
http://www.proedinc.com
general@proedinc.com

Donald D Hammill, Owner
Jack A. Naglieri, Author
Timothy J. McNeish, Co-Author
A screening test that helps identify children and adolescents who have emotional problems and require further evaluation. *$145.00*

4315 **Fundamentals of Autism**
Slosson Educational Publications
538 Buffalo Road
East Aurora, NY 14052
716-652-0930
888-756-7766
Fax: 800-655-3840
http://www.slosson.com
slossonprep@gmail.com

Steven Slosson, President
Sue Larson, Author
Dr. Georgina Moynihan, Tech Support
The handbook and two accompanying checklists provide a quick, user-friendly approach to help in identifying and developing educationally related program objectives for the child diagnosed as Autistic. *$91.25*

4316 **Multidimensional Self Concept Scale**
Pro-Ed
8700 Shoal Creek Boulevard
Austin, TX 78757-6897
512-451-3246
800-897-3202
Fax: 512-451-8542
http://www.proedinc.com
general@proedinc.com

Donald D Hammill, Owner
Bruce Bracken, Author
A thoroughly researched, developed and standardized clinical instrument. It assesses global self-concept and six context-dependent self-concept domains that are functionally important in the social-emotional adjustment of youth and adolescents. *$114.00*

4317 **Revised Behavior Problem Checklist**
Psychological Assessment Resources
16204 N Florida Ave
Lutz, FL 33549-8119
813-449-4065
800-899-8378
Fax: 800-727-9329
http://www.parinc.com
chairman@parinc.com

Bob III, President/CEO
Kay Cunningham, Director
Cathy Smith, Vice President
Psychological test products and software designed by mental health professionals. *$195.00*

4318 **SSRS: Social Skills Rating System**
Pearson Assessments
4940 Pearl East Circle
Suite 200
Boulder, CO 80301
888-977-7900
800-328-5999
Fax: 888-556-2103
http://www.pearsonassessments.com
info@pearsonkt.com

Kevin Brueggman, President
Frank M Gresham, Author
Stephen N Elliot, Co-Author
A nationally standardized series of questionnaires that obtain information on the social behaviors of children and adolescents from teachers, parents and the students themselves. Administration time is 10-15 minutes per questionnaire.

4319 **Self-Esteem Index**
Pro-Ed
8700 Shoal Creek Boulevard
Austin, TX 78757-6897
512-451-3246
800-897-3202
Fax: 512-451-8542
http://www.proedinc.com
general@proedinc.com

Donald D Hammill, Owner
Linda Brown, Author
Jacquelyn Alexander, Co-Author
A new, multidimensional, norm-referenced measure of the way that individuals perceive and value themselves. *$132.00*

4320 **Social-Emotional Dimension Scale**
Pro-Ed
8700 Shoal Creek Boulevard
Austin, TX 78757-6897
512-451-3246
800-897-3202
Fax: 512-451-8542
http://www.proedinc.com
general@proedinc.com

Donald D Hammill, Owner
Jerry Hutton, Author
Timothy Roberts, Co-Author
A quick, well-standardized rating scale that can be used by teachers, counselors and psychologists to screen students who are at risk for conduct disorders or emotional disturbances. *$154.00*

4321 **Wings for Kids**
476 Meeting Street
Suite E
Charleston, SC 29403
843-442-2835
Fax: 866-562-8615
http://www.wingsforkids.org
hello@wingsforkids.org

Ginny Deerin, Founder
Suzan Zoukis, Chair
Alex Opoulos, Secretary
Wings for Kids is the only U.S. organization focused soley on social and emotional learning after school. Hot WINGS are social skill development activities that anyone can use to model, shape and reinforce the capabilities that equip a child to succeed. Through small lessons, you give kids the tools they need to navigate challenging situations and everyday problems. Activties include Positive Reinforcement, Cope with Anger and Stress, Express Emotions Constructively.

LD Screening

4322 **ADD-H Comprehensive Teacher's Rating Scale: 2nd Edition**
Slosson Educational Publications
538 Buffalo Road
East Aurora, NY 14052
716-652-0930
888-756-7766
Fax: 800-655-3840
http://www.slosson.com
slossonprep@gmail.com

Rina Ullmann, Robert Sprague, Author
Steven Slosson, President
John H Slosson, Vice President
Dr. Georgina Moynihan, Tech Support
This brief checklist assesses one of the most prevalent childhood behavior problems: attention-deficit disorder, with or without hyperactivity. Because this disorder manifests itself primarily in the classroom, it is best evaluated by teacher ratings. Also available in a Spanish translation; please indicate when ordering. *$62.00*

4323 **Attention-Deficit/Hyperactivity Disorder Test**
Slosson Educational Publications
538 Buffalo Road
East Aurora, NY 14052
716-652-0930
888-756-7766
Fax: 800-655-3840
http://www.slosson.com
slossonprep@gmail.com

James E Gilliam, Author
Steven Slosson, President
John H Slosson, Vice President
Dr. Georgina Moynihan, Tech Support
An effective instrument for identifying and evaluating ADHD. Contains 36 items that describe characteristic behaviors of persons with ADHD. These items comprise three subtests representing the core symptoms necessary for the diagnosis of ADHD: hyperactivity, impulsivity, and inattention. *$95.00*

4324 **BRIGANCE Screens: Early Preschool**
Curriculum Associates
153 Rangeway Road
North Billerica, MA 01862-901
978-667-8000
800-225-0248
Fax: 800-366-1158
http://www.curriculumassociates.com
info@CAinc.com

Frank E. Ferguson, Chairman
Albert Brigance, Author
Robert Waldron, Chief Executive Officer
An affordable, easy-to-administer, all-purpose solution. Accurately screen key developmental and early academic skills in just 10-15 minutes per child. Widely used in Early Head Start programs, it meets IDEA requirements and provides consistent results that support early childhood educator's observations and judgement. *$110.00*

4325 **BRIGANCE Screens: Infants and Toddler**
Curriculum Associates
153 Rangeway Road
North Billerica, MA 01862-901
978-667-8000
800-225-0248
Fax: 800-366-1158
http://www.curriculumassociates.com
info@CAinc.com

Frank E. Ferguson, Chairman
Albert Brigance, Author
Robert Waldron, Chief Executive Officer
An affordable, easy-to-administer, all-purpose solution. The Infant and Toddler Screen accurately assesses key developmental skills, and observes caregivers involvement and interactions. *$110.00*

4326 **BRIGANCE Screens: K and 1**
Curriculum Associates
153 Rangeway Road
North Billerica, MA 01862-901
978-667-8000
800-225-0248
Fax: 800-366-1158
http://www.curriculumassociates.com
info@CAinc.com

Frank E. Ferguson, Chairman
Albert Brigance, Author
Robert Waldron, Chief Executive Officer

The K and 1 Screen is an affordable, easy-to-administer, all-purpose solution. Accurately screen key developmental and early academic skills in just 10-15 mintues per child. School districts nationwide rely on BRIGANCE for screening children before entering kindergarten, grade 1, and grade 2. It meets IDEA requirements and provides consistant results that support early childhood educators observations and judgement. *$110.00*

4327 **Basic School Skills Inventory: Screen and Diagnostic**
Pro-Ed
8700 Shoal Creek Boulevard
Austin, TX 78757-6897
512-451-3246
800-897-3202
Fax: 512-451-8542
http://www.proedinc.com
general@proedinc.com
Lindy Jordaan, Marketing Coordinator
Donald D Hammill, Owner
Can be used to locate children who are high risk for school failure, who need more in-depth assessment and who should be referred for additional study. *$109.00*

4328 **DABERON Screening for School Readiness**
Pro-Ed
8700 Shoal Creek Boulevard
Austin, TX 78757-6897
512-451-3246
800-897-3202
Fax: 512-451-8542
http://www.proedinc.com
general@proedinc.com
Donald D Hammill, Owner
Virginia Danzer, Author
Theresa Lyons, Co-Author
Provides a standardized assessment of school readiness in children with learning or behavior problems. *$176.00*
Yearly

4329 **Developmental Assessment for Students with Severe Disabilities**
Pro-Ed
8700 Shoal Creek Boulevard
Austin, TX 78757-6897
512-451-3246
800-897-3202
Fax: 512-451-8542
http://www.proedinc.com
general@proedinc.com
Mary Kay Dykes & Jane Erin, Author
Donald D Hammill, Owner
Offers diagnostic and programming personnel concise information about individuals who are functioning between birth and 8 years of age developmentally. *$217.00*

4330 **Educational Developmental Series**
Scholastic Testing Service
480 Meyer Rd
Bensenville, IL 60106-1617
630-766-7150
800-642-6787
Fax: 630-766-8054
http://http://www.ststesting.com/
sts@ststesting.com
John Kauffman, Marketing VP
Scott Rich, J.D., Assessment Specialist
A standardized battery of ability and achievement tests. Administration time is approximately 2.5 - 5 hours, depending on grade level and subtests. The EDSERIES has the most comprehensive coverage of all the STS tests. It permits teachers, counselors and administrators to evaluate a student from the broadest possible perspective. A school may use the EDSERIES on a lease/score basis or it may purchase testing materials.

4331 **Fundamentals of Autism**
Slosson Educational Publications
538 Buffalo Road
East Aurora, NY 14052
716-652-0930
888-756-7766
Fax: 800-655-3840
http://www.slosson.com
slossonprep@gmail.com
Sue Larson, Author
Steven Slosson, President
John H Slosson, Vice President
Dr. Georgina Moynihan, Tech Support
Provides a quick, user-friendly, effective, and accurate approach to help in identifying and developing educationally related program objectives for children diagnosed as autistic.

4332 **Goodenough-Harris Drawing Test**
Pearson
19500 Bulverde Rd
San Antonio, TX 78259-3701
210-339-5000
800-627-7271
Fax: 800-232-1223
http://www.psychcorp.com
clinicalcustomersupport@pearson.com
Aurelio Prifitera, President
Florence Goodenough, Author
This test focuses on mental maturity without requiring verbal skills. The fifteen-minute examination provides standard scores for children ages 3-15. *$178.00*

4333 **Higher Education for Learning Problems (HELP)**
Marshall University
Myers Hall
520 18th St.
Huntington, WV 25755
304-696-6252
Fax: 304-696-3231
http://www.marshall.edu/help
help@marshall.edu
Debbie Painter, Director
Missi Fisher, Business Manager
Renna Moore, Administrative Assistant
The HELP program is committed to providing assistance through individual tutuoring, mentoring and support, as well as fair and legal access to educational opportunities for students diagnosed with learning disabilities and related disorders such as ADD/ADHD.

4334 **Kaufman Assessment Battery for Children**
Pearson
4940 Pearl East Circle
Suite 200
Boulder, CO 80301
888-977-7900
800-328-5999
Fax: 888-556-2103
http://www.pearsonassessments.com
info@pearsonkt.com
Alan Kaufman, Author
Nadeen Kaufman, Co-Author
Carol Watson, Publisher/Pres Clinical Asses
An individually administered measure of intelligence and achievement, using simultaneous and sequential mental processes.

4335 **Kaufman Brief Intelligence Test**
Pearson
4940 Pearl East Circle
Suite 200
Boulder, CO 80301
888-977-7900
800-328-5999
Fax: 888-556-2103
http://www.pearsonassessments.com
info@pearsonkt.com
Alan Kaufman, Author
Nadeen Kaufman, Co-Author
Doug Kubach, Group President & CEO
KBIT is a brief, individually administered test of verbal and non-verbal intelligence. Screens two cognitive functions quickly and easily.

4336 **Peabody Individual Achievement Test**
Pearson
4940 Pearl East Circle
Suite 200
Boulder, CO 80301
888-977-7900
800-328-5999
Fax: 888-556-2103
http://www.pearsonassessments.com
info@pearsonkt.com

Frederick Markwardt Jr, Author
Matt Keller, Marketing Manager
Doug Kubach, Group President & CEO
Efficient individual measure of academic achievement. Reading, mathematics and spelling are assessed in a simple nonthreatning format that requires only a revised pointing response for most items.

4337 **Peabody Test-Picture Vocabulary Test**
Pearson
4940 Pearl East Circle
Suite 200
Boulder, CO 80301
888-977-7900
800-328-5999
Fax: 888-556-2103
http://www.pearsonassessments.com
info@pearsonkt.com

Lloyd Dunn, Author
Leota Dunn, Co-Author
Doug Kubach, Group President & CEO
A measure of hearing vocabulary for Standard American English; administration time: 10-15 minutes.

4338 **Restless Minds, Restless Kids**
Slosson Educational Publications
538 Buffalo Road
East Aurora, NY 14052
716-652-0930
888-756-7766
Fax: 800-655-3840
http://www.slosson.com
slossonprep@gmail.com

Rick D'Alli, Author
Steven Slosson, President
John H Slosson, Vice President
Dr. Georgina Moynihan, Tech Support
Two leading specialists in the field of childhood behavioral disorders discuss the state-of-the-art approach to diagnosing and testing ADHD. They are joined by four mothers of ADHD children who share their experiences of the effects of this disorder on the family. *$67.00*

4339 **School Readiness Test**
Scholastic Testing Service
480 Meyer Rd
Bensenville, IL 60106-1617
630-766-7150
800-642-6787
Fax: 630-766-8054
http://www.ststesting.com
sts@ststesting.com

John Kauffman, Marketing VP
Scott Rich, J.D., Assessment Specialist
An effective tool for determining the readiness of each student for first grade. It allows a teacher to learn as much as possible about every entering student's abilities, and about any factors that might interfere with his or her learning.

4340 **Slosson Intelligence Test**
Pro-Ed
538 Buffalo Road
East Aurora, NY 14052
716-652-0930
888-756-7766
Fax: 800-655-3840
http://www.slosson.com
slossonprep@gmail.com

Steven Slosson, President
John H Slosson, Vice President
Richard.L Slosson, Author
A widely used individual screening test for those who need to evaulate the mental ability of individuals who are learning disabled, mentally retarded, blind, orthopedically disabled, normal, or gifted from ages 4 to adulthood. Revised by Charles Nicholson and Terry Hibpshman. *$147.00*

4341 **TOVA**
Universal Attention Disorders
3321 Cerritos Ave
Los Alamitos, CA 90720-2105
562-594-7700
800-729-2886
Fax: 562-594-7770
http://www.tovatest.com
support@tovatest.com

Tammy Dupuy, Medical Director
Karen Carlson, Marketing Director
The TOVA (Tests of Variables of Attention) is a computerized, objective measure of attention and impulsivity, used in the assessment and treatment of ADD/ADHD. It is standardized from 4 to 80 years of age. TOVA's report contains a full analysis and interpetation of data. Variables measured include omissions, commisions, response time and response time variability.

4342 **Test of Memory and Learning (TOMAL)**
Pro-Ed
8700 Shoal Creek Boulevard
Austin, TX 78757-6897
512-451-3246
800-897-3202
Fax: 512-451-8542
http://www.proedinc.com
general@proedinc.com

Donald D Hammill, Owner
Cecil Reynolds, Author
Judith K Voress, Co-Author
TOMAL provides ten subtests that evaluate general and specific memory functions. *$376.00*

4343 **Test of Nonverbal Intelligence (TONI-3)**
Pro-Ed
8700 Shoal Creek Boulevard
Austin, TX 78757-6897
512-451-3246
800-897-3202
Fax: 512-451-8542
http://www.proedinc.com
general@proedinc.com

Donald D Hammill, President
Linda Brown, Author
Susan Johnson, Co-Author
A language-free measure of reasoning and intelligence presents a variety of abstract problem solving tasks. *$285.00*

4344 **Vision, Perception and Cognition: Manual for Evaluation & Treatment**
Therapro
225 Arlington St
Framingham, MA 01702-8773
508-872-9494
800-257-5376
Fax: 508-875-2062
http://www.theraproducts.com
info@theraproducts.com

Karen Conrad, Owner
Barbara Zoltan, Author
Details methods for testing perceptual, visual and cognitive deficits, as well as procedure for evaluating test results in relation to cognitive loss. Clearly explains each deficit, provides step by step testing techniques and gives complete treatment guidelines. Also includes information on the use of computers in cognitive training. *$40.00*
232 pages

Math

4345 **3 Steps to Math Success**
Curriculum Associates
153 Rangeway Road
North Billerica, MA 01862-901 978-667-8000
800-225-0248
Fax: 800-366-1158
http://www.curriculumassociates.com
info@CAinc.com
Curriculum Associates, Author
Frank E. Ferguson, Chairman
Renee Foster, President and Publisher
Dave Caron, Chief Financial Officer
We developed an integrated approach to math that ensures academic success long after the final bell has rung. Together, these series create an easy-to-use system of targeted instruction designed to remedy math weakness and reinforce math strengths.

4346 **AfterMath Series**
Curriculum Associates
153 Rangeway Road
North Billerica, MA 01862-901 978-667-8000
800-225-0248
Fax: 800-366-1158
http://www.curriculumassociates.com
info@CAinc.com
Frank E. Ferguson, Chairman
Renee Foster, President and Publisher
Dave Caron, Chief Financial Officer
Galileo once said that mathematics is the alphabet in which the universe was created. This series helps students master that alphabet. As they puzzle their way through brainteasers and learn math magic, students build critical-thinking skills that are vital to comprehending and succeeding in today's world.

4347 **ENRIGHT Computation Series**
Curriculum Associates
153 Rangeway Road
North Billerica, MA 01862-901 978-667-8000
800-225-0248
Fax: 800-366-1158
http://www.curriculumassociates.com
info@CAinc.com
Frank E. Ferguson, Chairman
Renee Foster, President and Publisher
Dave Caron, Chief Financial Officer
Close the gap between expected and actual computation performance. The ENRIGHT Computation Series provides the practice necessary to master addition, subtraction, multiplication, and division of whole numbers, fractions, and decimals.

4348 **Figure It Out: Thinking Like a Math Problem Solver**
Curriculum Associates
153 Rangeway Road
North Billerica, MA 01862-901 978-667-8000
800-225-0248
Fax: 800-366-1158
http://www.curriculumassociates.com
info@CAinc.com
Frank E. Ferguson, Chairman
Renee Foster, President and Publisher
Dave Caron, Chief Financial Officer
Critical thinking is the key to unlocking the mystery of these nonroutine problems. Your students will eagerly accept the challenge! Students learn to apply eight strategies in each book including: draw a picture; use a pattern; work backwards; make a table; and guess and check.

4349 **Getting Ready for Algebra**
Curriculum Associates
153 Rangeway Road
North Billerica, MA 01862-901 978-667-8000
800-225-0248
Fax: 800-366-1158
http://www.curriculumassociates.com
info@CAinc.com
Frank E. Ferguson, Chairman
Renee Foster, President and Publisher
Dave Caron, Chief Financial Officer
NCTM encourages algebra instruction in the early grades to develop critical-thinking, communication, reasoning, and problem-solving skills. Getting Ready for Algebra exercises these skills in lessons that focus on key algebra concepts: adding and subtracting positive integers; patterns; set theory notation; open sentences; inequality and more.

4350 **Learning Disability Evaluation Scale: Renormed**
Hawthorne Educational Services
800 Gray Oak Dr
Columbia, MO 65201-3730 573-874-1710
800-542-1673
Fax: 800-442-9509
http://www.hawthorne-ed.com
info@hes-inc.com
Stephen McCarney, Author
Edina Laird, Director External Relations
Michele Jackson, Owner
The Learning Disability Evaluation Scale (LDES) is an initial screening and assessment instrument in the areas of listening, thinking, speaking, reading, writing, spelling, and mathematical calculations based on the federal definition (IDEA). The Learning Disability Intervention Manual (LDIM) is a companion to the LDES and contains goals, objectives, and intervention/instructional strategies for the learning problems identified by the LDES. *$152.00*
217 pages

4351 **QUIC Tests**
Scholastic Testing Service
480 Meyer Rd
Bensenville, IL 60106-1617 630-766-7150
800-642-6787
Fax: 630-766-8054
http://www.ststesting.com
sts@ststesting.com
John Kauffman, Marketing VP
Scott Rich, J.D., Assessment Specialist
The Quic Tests are used to determine the functional level of student comptetency in mathematics and/ or communicative arts for use in grades 2-12. Administration time is 30 minutes or less.

4352 **Skills Assessments**
Harcourt
222 Berkeley Street
Boston, MA 02116 617-351-5000
800-531-5015
Fax: 800-699-9459
http://www.hmhco.com/educators
international@harcourt.com
Linda K. Zecher, President, CEO & Director
Eric Shuman, Chief Financial Officer
William Bayers, EVP/General Counsel
This handy, all-in-one resource helps identify students strengths and weaknesses in order to determine appropriate instructional levels in each of five subjects areas: reading; language arts; math; science; and social studies. Assessments are identified by subtopics in each subject.

4353 **Test of Mathematical Abilities**
Pro-Ed
8700 Shoal Creek Boulevard
Austin, TX 78757-6897 512-451-3246
800-897-3202
Fax: 512-451-8542
http://www.proedinc.com
general@proedinc.com

Donald D Hammill, Owner
Virginia Brown, Author
Mary Cronin, Co-Author
Has been developed to provide standardized information about story problems and computation, attitude, vocabulary and general cultural application. *$95.00*

Professional Guides

4354 **Assessment Update**
Jossey-Bass
111 River St
Hoboken, NJ 07030-5774 201-748-6000
Fax: 201-748-6008
http://www.wiley.com
info@wiley.com
Stephen M. Smith, President/CEO
Ellis E. Cousens, EVP/COO
John Kritzmacher, EVP/CFO
Assessment Update is dedicated to covering the latest developments in the rapidly evolving area of higher education assessment. Assessment Update offers all academic leaders up-to-date information and practical advice on conducting assessments in a range of areas, including student learning and outcomes, factulty instruction, academic programs and curricula, student services, and overall institutional functioning.

4355 **Assessment of Students with Handicaps in Vocational Education**
Association for Career and Technical Education
1410 King St
Alexandria, VA 22314-2749 800-826-9972
Fax: 703-683-7424
http://www.acteonline.org
sheath@jeffco.k12.co.us
L Albright, Author
Sarah Heath, President
Katrina Plese, Finance Chair
Chuck Gallagher, Regional Representative
Includes teachers, supervisors, administrators and others interested in the development and improvement of career & technical and practical-arts education.

4356 **BRIGANCE Word Analysis: Strategies and Practice**
Curriculum Associates
153 Rangeway Road
North Billerica, MA 01862-901 978-667-8000
800-225-0248
Fax: 800-366-1158
http://www.curriculumassociates.com
info@CAinc.com
Albert Brigance, Author
Frank E. Ferguson, Chairman
Renee Foster, President and Publisher
Dave Caron, Chief Financial Officer
Our comprehensive, two-volume resource combines activities, strategies, and reference materials for teaching phonetic and structural word analysis. Two durable binders feature reproducible activity pages. Choose from more than 1,600 activities for corrective instruction or to reinforce your classroom reading program.

4357 **Career Planner's Portfolio: A School-to-Work Assessment Tool**
Curriculum Associates
153 Rangeway Road
North Billerica, MA 01862-901 978-667-8000
800-225-0248
Fax: 800-366-1158
http://www.curriculumassociates.com
info@CAinc.com
Robert G Forest, Author
Frank E. Ferguson, Chairman
Renee Foster, President and Publisher
Dave Caron, Chief Financial Officer
Students career plans develop and evolve over several school years. Our portfolio will help keep track of their progress.

4358 **Computer Scoring Systems for PRO-ED Tests**
Pro-Ed
8700 Shoal Creek Boulevard
Austin, TX 78757-6897 512-451-3246
800-897-3202
Fax: 512-451-8542
http://www.proedinc.com
general@proedinc.com
Donald D Hammill, Owner
Computer scoring systems have been developed to generate reports for many PRO-ED tests and to help examiners interpret test performance.

4359 **Goals and Objectives Writer Software**
Curriculum Associates
153 Rangeway Road
North Billerica, MA 01862-901 978-667-8000
800-225-0248
Fax: 800-366-1158
http://www.curriculumassociates.com
info@CAinc.com
Frank E. Ferguson, Chairman
Renee Foster, President and Publisher
Dave Caron, Chief Financial Officer
Using the Goals and Objectives program, you'll quickly and easily create, edit, and print IEPs. The CD allows you to install the program on your hard drive in order to save students data for future updates. You can easily export IEPs into any word processing program. CD-Rom for Windows and Macintosh.

4360 **Occupational Aptitude Survey and Interest Schedule**
Pro-Ed
8700 Shoal Creek Boulevard
Austin, TX 78757-6897 512-451-3246
800-897-3202
Fax: 512-451-8542
http://www.proedinc.com
general@proedinc.com
Donald D Hammill, Owner
Randall M Parker, Author
Consists of two related tests: the OASIS-2 Aptitude Survey and the OASIS-2 Interest Schedule. The tests were normed on the same national sample of 1,505 students from 13 states. The Aptitude Survey measures six broad aptitude factors that are directly related to skills and abilities required in over 20,000 jobs and the Interest Schedule measures 12 interest factors directly related to the occupations listed in Occupational Exploration.

4361 **Portfolio Assessment Teacher's Guide**
Harcourt
222 Berkeley Street
Boston, MA 02116 617-351-5000
800-531-5015
Fax: 800-699-9459
http://www.hmhco.com/educators
international@harcourt.com
Roger Farr, Author
Linda K. Zecher, President, CEO & Director
Eric Shuman, Chief Financial Officer
William Bayers, EVP/General Counsel
Start your portfolio systems with tips from the expert. Roger Farr outlines the basic steps for evaluating a portfolio, offers ideas for organizing portfolios and making the most of portfolio conferences, and provides reproducible evaluation forms for primary through intermediate grades and above. *$23.60*

4362 **Teaching Test Taking Skills**
Brookline Books
8 Trumbull Rd
Suite B-001
Northampton, MA 01060
603-669-7032
800-666-2665
Fax: 413-584-6184
http://www.brooklinebooks.com
brbooks@yahoo.com
Margo Mastropieri,Thomas Scruggs, Author
Mike Beattie, Manager
Test-wise individuals often score higher than others of equal ability who may not use test-taking skills effectively. This work teaches general concepts about the test format or other conditions of testing, not specific items on the test. *$21.95*
ISBN 0-914797-76-X

4363 **Tests, Measurement and Evaluation**
American Institutes for Research
1000 Thomas Jefferson St
Washington, DC 20007-3835
202-342-5000
Fax: 202-403-5001
TTY: 877-344-3499
http://www.air.org
inquiry@air.org
David Myers, President/CEO
Marijo Ahlgrimm, EVP/CFO
Sabrina Laine, SVP/Director, Education
Our goal is to provide governments and the private sector with responsive services of the highest quality by applying and advancing the knowledge, theories, methods, and standards of the behavioral and social services to solve significant societal problems and improve the quality of life of all people.

Reading

4364 **3 Steps to Reading Success: CARS, STARS, CARS II**
Curriculum Associates
153 Rangeway Road
North Billerica, MA 01862-901
978-667-8000
800-225-0248
Fax: 800-366-1158
http://www.curriculumassociates.com
info@CAinc.com
Frank E. Ferguson, Chairman
Renee Foster, President and Publisher
Dave Caron, Chief Financial Officer
Equipping your students with the skills and strategies they need to achieve lifelong success can be a challenge. That's why we developed an integrated approach to learning that ensures academic success long after the final bell has rung.

4365 **BRIGANCE Readiness: Strategies and Practice**
Curriculum Associates
153 Rangeway Road
North Billerica, MA 01862-901
978-667-8000
800-225-0248
Fax: 800-366-1158
http://www.curriculumassociates.com
info@CAinc.com
Frank E. Ferguson, Chairman
Albert Brigance, Author
Dave Caron, Chief Financial Officer
Attend to the needs and differences of the children in your program using Readiness: Strategies and Practice. Skills are introduced, taught, and reinforced using both age-appropriate and individual appropriate activties. *$174.00*

4366 **Capitalization and Punctuation**
Curriculum Associates
153 Rangeway Road
North Billerica, MA 01862-901
978-667-8000
800-225-0248
Fax: 800-366-1158
http://www.curriculumassociates.com
info@CAinc.com
Frank E. Ferguson, Chairman
Renee Foster, President and Publisher
Dave Caron, Chief Financial Officer
Capitalization and Punctuation features structured, easy to understand lessons that are organized sequentially. Students read the rules, study sample exercises, apply the skills in practice lessons, and review the skills in maintenance lessons.

4367 **Dyslexia/ADHD Institute**
148 Eastern Blvd
Suite 406
Glastonbury, CT 06033
860-633-2604
877-342-7323
http://www.diaread.com
info@diaread.com
Les Fredette, Co-Operator/Co-Owner
Susan Fredette, Co-Operator/Co-Owner
Testing, diagnosis, and 1-on-1 tutoring for all ages and levels of need

4368 **Extensions in Reading**
Curriculum Associates
153 Rangeway Road
North Billerica, MA 01862-901
978-667-8000
800-225-0248
Fax: 800-366-1158
http://www.curriculumassociates.com
info@CAinc.com
Frank E. Ferguson, Chairman
Renee Foster, President and Publisher
Dave Caron, Chief Financial Officer
A unique new program teaching reading strategies and more. Extensions offers rich experiences with nonfiction and fiction. Each lesson extends to include: researching and writing; use of graphic organizers; vocabulary development; and comprehension questions with test-prep format.

4369 **Gray Diagnostic Reading Tests**
Pro-Ed
8700 Shoal Creek Boulevard
Austin, TX 78757-6897
512-451-3246
800-897-3202
Fax: 512-451-8542
http://www.proedinc.com
general@proedinc.com
Donald D Hammill, Owner
Brian Bryant, Author
Diane Bryant, Co-Author
Uses two alternate, equivalent forms to assess students who have difficulty reading continuous print and who require an evaluation of specific abilities and weaknesses. Item # 10965. *$259.00*

4370 **Gray Oral Reading Tests**
Pro-Ed
8700 Shoal Creek Boulevard
Austin, TX 78757-6897
512-451-3246
800-897-3202
Fax: 512-451-8542
http://www.proedinc.com
general@proedinc.com
Donald D Hammill, Owner
J Lee Wiederholt, Author
Brian Bryant, Co-Author
The latest revision provides an objective measure of growth in oral reading and an aid in the diagnosis of oral reading difficulties. *$233.00*

4371 **Reading Assessment System**
Steck-Vaughn Company
222 Berkeley Street
Boston, MA 02116
617-351-5000
800-289-4490
Fax: 800-289-3994
http://www.hmhco.com/educators
Linda K. Zecher, President, CEO & Director
Eric Shuman, Chief Financial Officer
William Bayers, EVP/General Counsel

The Reading Assessment System provides an ongoing measure of specific student's skills and offers detailed directions for individual instruction and remediation. Up to eight reports are available. This popular program generates individual scores, class scores, school scores, and district reports.

4372 **Scholastic Abilities Test for Adults**
Pro-Ed
8700 Shoal Creek Boulevard
Austin, TX 78757-6897
512-451-3246
800-897-3202
Fax: 512-451-8542
http://www.proedinc.com
general@proedinc.com
Donald D Hammill, Owner
Brian Bryant, Author
James Patton, Co-Author
Measures scholastic competence, aptitude and academic achievement for persons with learning difficulties. *$186.00*

4373 **Skills Assessments**
Steck-Vaughn Company
222 Berkeley Street
Boston, MA 02116
617-351-5000
800-531-5015
Fax: 800-269-5232
http://www.hmhco.com/educators
info@steck-vaughn.com
Linda K. Zecher, President, CEO & Director
Eric Shuman, Chief Financial Officer
William Bayers, EVP/General Counsel
This handy, all-in-one resource helps identify students strengths and weaknesses in order to determine appropriate instructional levels in each of five subjects areas: reading; language arts; math; science; and social studies. Assessments are identified by subtopics in each subject. Each book is $13.99 each. *$69.95*

4374 **Standardized Reading Inventory**
Pro-Ed
8700 Shoal Creek Boulevard
Austin, TX 78757-6897
512-451-3246
800-897-3202
Fax: 512-451-8542
http://www.proedinc.com
general@proedinc.com
Donald D Hammill, Owner
Phyllis Newcomer, Author
An instrument for evaluating students' reading ability. *$277.00*

4375 **Test of Early Reading Ability**
Pro-Ed
8700 Shoal Creek Boulevard
Austin, TX 78757-6897
512-451-3246
800-897-3202
Fax: 512-451-8542
http://www.proedinc.com
general@proedinc.com
Donald D Hammill, Owner
D Kim Reid, Author
Wayne Hresko, Co-Author
Unique test in that it measures the actual reading ability of young children. Items measure knowledge of contextual meaning, alphabet and conventions. *$274.00*

4376 **Test of Reading Comprehension**
Pro-Ed
8700 Shoal Creek Boulevard
Austin, TX 78757-6897
512-451-3246
800-897-3202
Fax: 512-451-8542
http://www.proedinc.com
general@proedinc.com
Donald D Hammill, Owner/Author
Virginia Brown, Co-Author
J Lee Wiederholt, Co-Author
A multidimensional test of silent reading comprehension for students. The test reflects current psycholinguistic theories that consider reading comprehension to be a constructive process involving both language and cognition. *$ 196.00*

Speech & Language Arts

4377 **A Calendar of Home Activities**
Curriculum Associates
153 Rangeway Road
North Billerica, MA 01862-901
978-667-8000
800-225-0248
Fax: 800-366-1158
http://www.curriculumassociates.com
info@CAinc.com
Frank E. Ferguson, Chairman
Donald Johnson, Author
Elaine Johnson, Co-Author
An activity-a-day: 365 activities for parents and children to share at home in just 10-15 minutes each day. Parents support their children's educational experiences in a meaningful and enjoyable way, such as cooking, playing ball, and sculpting clay.

4378 **Adolescent Language Screening Test**
Pro-Ed
8700 Shoal Creek Boulevard
Austin, TX 78757-6897
512-451-3246
800-897-3202
Fax: 512-451-8542
http://www.proedinc.com
general@proedinc.com
Donald D Hammill, Owner
Denise Morgan, Author
Arthur Guilford, Co-Author
Provides speech/language pathologists and other interested professionals with a rapid thorough method for screening adolescents' speech and language. *$145.00*

4379 **Advanced Skills For School Success Series: Module 4**
Curriculum Associates
153 Rangeway Road
North Billerica, MA 01862-901
978-667-8000
800-225-0248
Fax: 800-366-1158
http://www.curriculumassociates.com
info@CAinc.com
Anita Archer, Mary Gleason, Author
Frank E. Ferguson, Chairman
Renee Foster, President and Publisher
Dave Caron, Chief Financial Officer
Develops oral and written language abilities. Students learn valuable strategies for note-taking, brainstorming, and effectively participating in class dicussions. *$19.90*

4380 **Aphasia Diagnostic Profiles**
Pro-Ed
8700 Shoal Creek Boulevard
Austin, TX 78757-6897
512-451-3246
800-897-3202
Fax: 512-451-8542
http://www.proedinc.com
general@proedinc.com
Donald D Hammill, Owner
Nancy Helm-Estrabrooks, Author
This is a quick, efficient, and systematic assessment of language and communication impairment associated with aphasia that should be administered individually. The test can be administered in 40-45 minutes. *$175.00*

4381 **BRIGANCE Assessment of Basic Skills**
Curriculum Associates
153 Rangeway Road
North Billerica, MA 01862-901
978-667-8000
800-225-0248
Fax: 800-366-1158
http://www.curriculumassociates.com
info@CAinc.com

Frank E. Ferguson, Chairman
Albert Brigance, Author
Dave Caron, Chief Financial Officer
Critiqued and field tested by Spanish linguists and educators nationwide, the Assessment of Basic Skills meets nondiscriminatory testing requirements for Limited English Proficient students.

4382 **BRIGANCE Comprehensive Inventory of Basic Skills**
Curriculum Associates
153 Rangeway Road
North Billerica, MA 01862-901 978-667-8000
800-225-0248
Fax: 800-366-1158
http://www.curriculumassociates.com
info@CAinc.com
Frank E. Ferguson, Chairman
Albert Brigance, Author
Dave Caron, Chief Financial Officer
Designed for use in elementary and middle schools, the CIBS-R is a valuable resource for programs emphasizing individualized instruction. The Inventory is especially helpful in programs serving students with special needs, and continues to be indispensable in IEP development and program planning.

4383 **BRIGANCE Employability Skills Inventory**
Curriculum Associates
153 Rangeway Road
North Billerica, MA 01862-901 978-667-8000
800-225-0248
Fax: 800-366-1158
http://www.curriculumassociates.com
info@CAinc.com
Frank E. Ferguson, Chairman
Albert Brigance, Author
Dave Caron, Chief Financial Officer
Extensive criterion-referenced tool assesses basic skills and employability skills in the context of job-seeking or employment situations: reading grade placement; rating scales; career awareness and self-understanding; reading skills; speaking and listening; job-seeking skills and knowledge; pre-employment writing; math and concepts.

4384 **BRIGANCE Life Skills Inventory**
Curriculum Associates
153 Rangeway Road
North Billerica, MA 01862-901 978-667-8000
800-225-0248
Fax: 800-366-1158
http://www.curriculumassociates.com
info@CAinc.com
Frank E. Ferguson, Chairman
Albert Brigance, Author
Dave Caron, Chief Financial Officer
Assesses listening, speaking, reading, writing, comprehending, and computing skills in nine life-skill sections: speaking and listening; money and finance; functional writing; food; words on common signs and warning labels; clothing; health; telephone; travel and transportation.

4385 **Bedside Evaluation and Screening Test**
Pro-Ed
8700 Shoal Creek Boulevard
Austin, TX 78757-6897 512-451-3246
800-897-3202
Fax: 512-451-8542
http://www.proedinc.com
general@proedinc.com
Donald D Hammill, Owner
Joyce West, Author
Elaine Sands, Co-Author
Access and quantify language disorders in adults resulting from aphasia. *$171.00*

4386 **Boone Voice Program for Adults**
Pro-Ed
8700 Shoal Creek Boulevard
Austin, TX 78757-6897 512-451-3246
800-897-3202
Fax: 512-451-8542
http://www.proedinc.com
general@proedinc.com
Donald D Hammill, Owner
Daniel Boone, Author
Kay Wiley, Co-Author
Provides for diagnosis and remediation of adult voice disorders. This program is based on the same philosophy and therapy as The Program for Children but is presented at an adult interest level. *$153.00*

4387 **Boone Voice Program for Children**
Pro-Ed
8700 Shoal Creek Boulevard
Austin, TX 78757-6897 512-451-3246
800-897-3202
Fax: 512-451-8542
http://www.proedinc.com
general@proedinc.com
Donald D Hammill, Owner
Daniel Boone, Author
Provides a cognitive approach to voice therapy and is designed to give useful step-by-step guidelines and materials for diagnosis and remediation of voice disorders in children. *$208.00*

4388 **Connecting Reading and Writing with Vocabulary**
Curriculum Associates
153 Rangeway Road
North Billerica, MA 01862-901 978-667-8000
800-225-0248
Fax: 800-366-1158
http://www.curriculumassociates.com
info@CAinc.com
Frank E. Ferguson, Chairman
Deborah P Adcock, Author
Dave Caron, Chief Financial Officer
This vocabulary enrichment series builds successful writers and speakers by implementing strategic word techniques. Students will add 120 writing words and other word forms to their word banks. Each lesson introduces ten vocabulary words in a variety of contexts: a letter, poem, story, journal entry, classified ad, etc.

4389 **Diamonds in the Rough**
Slosson Educational Publications
538 Buffalo Road
East Aurora, NY 14052 716-652-0930
888-756-7766
Fax: 800-655-3840
http://www.slosson.com
slossonprep@gmail.com
Steven Slosson, President
Peggy Strass Dras, Author
Dr. Georgina Moynihan, Tech Support
College reference/rehabilitation guide for people with attention deficit disorder and learning disabilities. *$36.00*

4390 **Easy Talker: A Fluency Workbook for School Age Children**
Pro-Ed
8700 Shoal Creek Boulevard
Austin, TX 78757-6897 512-451-3246
800-897-3202
Fax: 512-451-8542
http://www.proedinc.com
general@proedinc.com
Donald D Hammill, Owner
Barry Guitar, Author
Julie Reville, Co-Author
A diagnostic, criterion-referenced instrument to be used with children, to determine which stutterers would benefit from early intervention. Item #4855. *$45.00*

4391 Fluharty Preschool Speech & Language Screening Test-2
Speech Bin
PO Box 1579
Appleton, WI 54912-1579
888-388-3224
Fax: 800-845-1535
http://www.schoolspecialty.com
orders@schoolspecialty.com
Joseph M. Yorio, President & CEO
James R. Henderson, Chairman
Patrick T. Collins, EVP, Distribution
Carefully normed on 705 children, the Fluharty yields standard scores, percentiles, and age equivalents. The form features space for speech-language pathologists to note phonelogical processes, voice quality, and fluency; a Teacher Questionnaire is also provided. Item number P882. *$153.00*

4392 Help for the Learning Disabled Child
Slosson Educational Publications
538 Buffalo Road
East Aurora, NY 14052
716-652-0930
888-756-7766
Fax: 800-655-3840
http://www.slosson.com
slossonprep@gmail.com
Steven Slosson, President
John H Slosson, Vice President
Dr. Georgina Moynihan, Tech Support
Symptoms and solutions for learning disabled children. Features issues from a medical, psychological and educational basis and illustrates learning disabilities from emotional and mental impairment. *$48.75*

4393 Learning Disability Evaluation Scale
Hawthorne Educational Services
800 Gray Oak Dr
Columbia, MO 65201-3730
573-874-1710
800-542-1673
Fax: 800-442-9509
http://www.hawthorne-ed.com
info@hes-inc.com
Stephen B McCarney Ed-D, Author
Tamara J Arthaud PhD, Co-Author
The Learning Disability Evaluation Scale - Renormed Second Edition (LDES-R2) was developed to enable instructional personnel to document those performance behaviors most characteristic of learning disabilities in children and youth. The LDES-R2 avoids the nature of a testing situation by relying on the performance observations of the classroom teacher or other instructional personnel. *$189.00*

4394 Oral Speech Mechanism Screening Examination
Pro-Ed
8700 Shoal Creek Boulevard
Austin, TX 78757-6897
512-451-3246
800-897-3202
Fax: 512-451-8542
http://www.proedinc.com
general@proedinc.com
Donald D Hammill, Owner
Kenneth St Louis, Author
Dennis Ruscello, Co-Author
Provides an efficient, quick, and reliable method to examine the oral speech mechanism of all types of speech, language, and related disorders where oral structure and function are of concern. *$105.00*

4395 Peabody Picture Vocabulary Test
4940 Pearl East Circle
Suite 200
Boulder, CO 80301
888-977-7900
800-328-5999
Fax: 888-556-2103
http://www.pearsonassessments.com
info@pearsonkt.com
Lloyd M Dunn, Author
Leota M Dunn, Co-Author
Doug Kubach, Group President & CEO
A wide-range measure of receptive vocabulary for standard English, and a screening test of verbal ability.

4396 Peabody Picture Vocabulary Test: Fourth Edition
Pearson Assessments
4940 Pearl East Circle
Suite 200
Boulder, CO 80301
888-977-7900
800-328-5999
Fax: 888-556-2103
http://www.pearsonassessments.com
info@pearsonkt.com
Karen Dahlen, Associate Director
Matt Keller, Marketing Manager
Lisa Dunttam, Development Assistant
A wide range measure of receptive vocabulary for standard English and screen of verbal ability. *$379.99*

4397 Preschool Motor Speech Evaluation & Intervention
Speech Bin
PO Box 1579
Appleton, WI 54912-1579
888-388-3224
Fax: 800-845-1535
http://www.schoolspecialty.com
orders@schoolspecialty.com
Joseph M. Yorio, President & CEO
James R. Henderson, Chairman
Patrick T. Collins, EVP, Distribution
This comprehensive criterion-based assessment tool differentiates motor-based speech disorders from those of phonology and determines if speech difficulties of children 18 months to six years old are characteristic of: oral nonverbal apraxia; dysarthria; developmental verbal dyspraxia; hypersensitivity; differences in tone and hyposensitivity. Item number J322. *$59.00*

4398 Receptive One-Word Picture Vocabulary Test
Speech Bin
PO Box 1579
Appleton, WI 54912-1579
888-388-3224
Fax: 800-845-1535
http://www.schoolspecialty.com
orders@schoolspecialty.com
Rick Brownell, Author
Joseph M. Yorio, President & CEO
James R. Henderson, Chairman
Patrick T. Collins, EVP, Distribution
This administered, untimed measure assessess the vocabulary comprehension of 0-2 through 11-18 years. New full-color test pictures are easy to recognize; many new test items have been added. It is ideal for children unable or reluctant to speak because only a gestural response is required. *$140.00*

4399 Receptive-Expressive Emergent Language Tests
Pro-Ed
8700 Shoal Creek Boulevard
Austin, TX 78757-6897
512-451-3246
800-897-3202
Fax: 512-451-8542
http://www.proedinc.com
general@proedinc.com
Donald D Hammill, Owner
Kenneth Bzoch, Author
Richard League, Co-Author
Designed to use with at-risk infants and toddlers to provide a multidimensional analysis of emergency language skills. *$104.00*

4400 Say and Sign Language Program
Slosson Educational Publications
538 Buffalo Road
East Aurora, NY 14052
716-652-0930
888-756-7766
Fax: 800-655-3840
http://www.slosson.com
slossonprep@gmail.com
Roger Hoffmann, Author
John H Slosson, Vice President
Dr. Georgina Moynihan, Tech Support

Addresses articulation skills, speech production, basic sign language skills, and finger spelling. *$71.50*

4401 **Sequenced Inventory of Communication Development (SICD)**
Speech Bin
PO Box 1579
Appleton, WI 54912-1579 888-388-3224
Fax: 800-845-1535
http://www.schoolspecialty.com
orders@schoolspecialty.com
Joseph M. Yorio, President & CEO
James R. Henderson, Chairman
Patrick T. Collins, EVP, Distribution
SICD uses appealing toys to assess communication skills of children at all levels of ability, including those with impaired hearing or vision. SICD looks at child and environment, measuring receptive and expressive language. Item number W710. *$395.00*

4402 **Skills Assessments**
222 Berkeley Street
Boston, MA 02116 617-351-5000
800-531-5015
Fax: 800-269-5232
http://www.hmhco.com/educators
info@steck-vaughn.com
Linda K. Zecher, President, CEO & Director
Eric Shuman, Chief Financial Officer
William Bayers, EVP/General Counsel
This handy, all-in-one resource helps identify students strengths and weaknesses in order to determine appropriate instructional levels in each of five subjects areas: reading; language arts; math; science; and social studies. Assessments are identified by subtopics in each subject.

4403 **Slosson Intelligence Test**
Slosson Educational Publications, Inc.
538 Buffalo Road
East Aurora, NY 14052 716-652-0930
888-756-7766
Fax: 800-655-3840
http://www.slosson.com
slossonprep@gmail.com
Steven Slosson, President
John H Slosson, Vice President
Dr. Georgina Moynihan, Tech Support
A quick and reliable individual screening test of Crystallized Verbal Intelligence. Tests include SIT-R3: Slosson Intelligence Test, Rev. - Third Edition; SORT-R3: Slosson Oral Reading Test, Rev. - Third Edition; S-VMPT: Slosson Visual Motor Performance Test; EASYOT: Educational Assessment of School Youth for Occupational Therapists. *$147.00*

4404 **Slosson Intelligence Test Primary**
Slosson Educational Publications
538 Buffalo Road
East Aurora, NY 14052 716-652-0930
888-756-7766
Fax: 800-655-3840
http://www.slosson.com
slossonprep@gmail.com
Steven Slosson, President
Bradley Erford, Author
Gary Vitali, Co-Author
Designed to facilitate the screening identification of children at risk of educational failure. Provides a quick estimate of mental ability to identify children who may be appropriate candidates for deeper testing services. *$ 168.00*

4405 **Stuttering Severity Instrument for Children and Adults**
Pro-Ed
8700 Shoal Creek Boulevard
Austin, TX 78757-6897 512-451-3246
800-897-3202
Fax: 512-451-8542
http://www.proedinc.com
general@proedinc.com
Donald D Hammill, Owner
Glyndon Riley, Author
With these easily administered tools you can determine whether to schedule a child for therapy using the Stuttering Prediction Instrument or to evaluate the effects of treatment using the Stuttering Severity Instrument. *$114.00*

4406 **Test for Auditory Comprehension of Language: TACL-3**
Speech Bin
PO Box 1579
Appleton, WI 54912-1579 888-388-3224
Fax: 800-845-1535
http://www.schoolspecialty.com
orders@schoolspecialty.com
Joseph M. Yorio, President & CEO
James R. Henderson, Chairman
Patrick T. Collins, EVP, Distribution
The newly revised TACL-3 evaluates the 0-3 to 9-11-year old's understanding of spoken language in three subtests: Vocabulary, Grammatical Morphemes and Elaborated Phrases and Sentences. Each test item is a word or sentence read aloud by the examiner; the child responds by pointing to one of three pictures. Item number P792. *$261.00*

4407 **Test of Adolescent & Adult Language: TOAL-3**
Pro-Ed
8700 Shoal Creek Boulevard
Austin, TX 78757-6897 512-451-3246
800-897-3202
Fax: 512-451-8542
http://www.proedinc.com
general@proedinc.com
Donald D Hammill, Owner/Author
Virginia Brown, Co-Author
Stephen Larson, Co-Author
This test is a measure of receptive and expressive language skills. In this revision easier items were added to the subtests, making them more appropriate for testing disabled students. *$202.00*

4408 **Test of Auditory Reasoning & Processing Skills: TARPS**
Speech Bin
PO Box 1579
Appleton, WI 54912-1579 888-388-3224
Fax: 800-845-1535
http://www.schoolspecialty.com
orders@schoolspecialty.com
Morrison Gardner, Author
Joseph M. Yorio, President & CEO
James R. Henderson, Chairman
Patrick T. Collins, EVP, Distribution
TARPS assesses how 5-14 year old children understand, interpret, draw conclusions, and make inferences from auditorily presented stimuli. It tests their ability to think, understand, reason, and make sense of what they hear. Item number H787. *$64.00*

4409 **Test of Auditory-Perceptual Skills: Upper TAPS-UL**
Speech Bin
PO Box 1579
Appleton, WI 54912-1579 888-388-3224
Fax: 800-845-1535
http://www.schoolspecialty.com
orders@schoolspecialty.com
Wayne Hresko, Shelley Herron, Pamela Peak, Author
Joseph M. Yorio, President & CEO
James R. Henderson, Chairman
Patrick T. Collins, EVP, Distribution
This highly respected, well-normed test evaluates a 13-18 year old's ability to perceive auditory stimuli and helps you diagnose auditory disorders in just 15-20 minutes. TAPS: UL measures the auditory perceptual skills of processing, word and sequential memory, interpretation of oral directions, and discrimination. Item number H769. *$95.00*

4410 **Test of Early Language Development**
Pro-Ed, Inc.
8700 Shoal Creek Boulevard
Austin, TX 78757-6897
512-451-3246
800-897-3202
Fax: 512-451-8542
http://www.proedinc.com
general@proedinc.com
Wayne P Hresko, Author

4411 **Test of Early Language Development: TELD-3**
Pro-Ed, Inc.
8700 Shoal Creek Boulevard
Austin, TX 78757-6897
512-451-3246
800-897-3202
Fax: 512-451-8542
http://www.proedinc.com
general@proedinc.com
Donald D Hammill, President/Author
Wayne Hresko, Co-Author
Kim Reid, Co-Author
An individually administered test of spoken language abilities. This test fills the need for a well-constructed, standardized instrument, based on a current theory, that can be used to assess spoken language skills at early ages. Now including scores for receptive language and expressive language subtests. Administration Time: 20 minutes. *$295.00*

4412 **Test of Early Written Language**
Pro-Ed
8700 Shoal Creek Boulevard
Austin, TX 78757-6897
512-451-3246
800-897-3202
Fax: 512-451-8542
http://www.proedinc.com
general@proedinc.com
Donald D Hammill, Owner
Shelley Herron, Author
Wayne Hresko, Co-Author
Measures the merging written language skills of young children and is especially useful in identifying mildy disabled students. *$197.00*

4413 **Test of Written Language: TOWL-3**
Pro-Ed
8700 Shoal Creek Boulevard
Austin, TX 78757-6897
512-451-3246
800-897-3202
Fax: 512-451-8542
http://www.proedinc.com
general@proedinc.com
Donald D Hammill, Owner/Author
Stephen Larson, Co-Author
Offers a measure of written language skills to identify students who need help improving their writing skills. Administration Time: 65 minutes. *$217.00*

4414 **Test of Written Spelling**
Pro-Ed
8700 Shoal Creek Boulevard
Austin, TX 78757-6897
512-451-3246
800-897-3202
Fax: 512-451-8542
http://www.proedinc.com
general@proedinc.com
Donald D Hammill, Owner/Author
Stephen Larsen, Co-Author
Louisa Cook Moats, Co-Author
Assesses students' ability to spell words whose spellings are readily predictable in sound-letter patterns, words whose spellings are less predictable and both types of words considered together. *$88.00*

4415 **Testing & Remediating Auditory Processing (TRAP)**
Speech Bin
PO Box 1579
Appleton, WI 54912-1579
888-388-3224
Fax: 800-845-1535
http://www.schoolspecialty.com
orders@schoolspecialty.com
Lynn Baron Berk, Author
Joseph M. Yorio, President & CEO
James R. Henderson, Chairman
Patrick T. Collins, EVP, Distribution
TRAP gives you an easy-to-implement program to assess and treat school-age auditory processing problems. It gives you two major components: Screening Test of Auditoring Processing Skills that identifies children at risk due to auditory processing deficits; and Remediating Auditory Processing Skills that presents interactional stories, sequence pictures, and illustrated activities. Item number 1233. *$38.00*

4416 **Voice Assessment Protocol for Children and Adults**
Pro-Ed
8700 Shoal Creek Boulevard
Austin, TX 78757-6897
512-451-3246
800-897-3202
Fax: 512-451-8542
http://www.proedinc.com
general@proedinc.com
Donald D Hammill, Owner
Rebekah Pindzola, Author
Easily guides the speech pathologist through a systematic evaluation of vocal pitch, loudness, quality, breath features and rate/rhythm. *$78.00*

Visual & Motor Skills

4417 **BRIGANCE Inventory of Early Development-II**
Curriculum Associates
153 Rangeway Road
North Billerica, MA 01862-901
978-667-8000
800-225-0248
Fax: 800-366-1158
http://www.curriculumassociates.com
info@CAinc.com
Albert H Brigance, Author
Frank E. Ferguson, Chairman
Dave Caron, Chief Financial Officer
The Inventory of Early Development simplifies and combines the assessment, diagnostic, recordkeeping, and instructional planning process, and it encourages communication between teachers and parents.

4418 **Benton Visual Retention Test**
Pearson Assessments
4940 Pearl East Circle
Suite 200
Boulder, CO 80301
888-977-7900
800-328-5999
Fax: 888-556-2103
http://www.pearsonassessments.com
info@pearsonkt.com
Abigail Benton Sivan, Author
Matt Keller, Marketing Manager
Doug Kubach, Group President & CEO
Assess visual perception, memory, visoconstructive abilities. Test administration 15-20 minutes. *$199.00*

4419 **Boston Diagnostic Aphasia Exam**
Speech Bin
PO Box 1579
Appleton, WI 54912-1579
888-388-3224
Fax: 800-845-1535
http://www.schoolspecialty.com
orders@schoolspecialty.com

Harold Goodglass, Edith Kaplan, Barbara Barresi, Author
Joseph M. Yorio, President & CEO
James R. Henderson, Chairman
Patrick T. Collins, EVP, Distribution
BDAE-3 now gives you an instructive 90-minute video plus two separate forms of the test. Item number L235. *$150.00*

4420 **Developmental Test of Visual Perception (D TVP-2)**
Pro-Ed
8700 Shoal Creek Boulevard
Austin, TX 78757-6897
512-451-3246
800-897-3202
Fax: 512-451-8542
http://www.proedinc.com
general@proedinc.com
Donald D Hammill, Owner/Author
Nils Pearson, Co-Author
Judith Voress, Co-Author
A test that measures both visual perception and visual-motor integration skills, has eight subtests, is based on updated theories of visual perceptual development, and can be administered to individuals in 45 minutes. *$207.00*

4421 **Differential Test of Conduct and Emotional Problems**
Slosson Educational Publications
538 Buffalo Road
East Aurora, NY 14052
716-652-0930
888-756-7766
Fax: 800-655-3840
http://www.slosson.com
slossonprep@gmail.com
Steven Slosson, President
Edward Kelly, Author
Dr. Georgina Moynihan, Tech Support
Designed to address one of the most critical challenges in education and juvenile care. Administration of test is 15-20 minutes. *$120.75*

4422 **Educational Assessment of School Youth for Occupational Therapists**
Slosson Educational Publications
538 Buffalo Road
East Aurora, NY 14052
716-652-0930
888-756-7766
Fax: 800-655-3840
http://www.slosson.com
slossonprep@gmail.com
Sharon Kenmotsu, Author
Katy Tressler, Co-Author
Dr. Georgina Moynihan, Tech Support
The E.A.S.Y. is a school-based occupational therapy assessment tool developed by occuaptional therapists. *$280.00*

4423 **Khan-Lewis Phonological Analysis: KLPA-2**
Pro-Ed
8700 Shoal Creek Boulevard
Austin, TX 78757-6897
512-451-3246
800-897-3202
Fax: 512-451-8542
http://www.proedinc.com
general@proedinc.com
Donald D Hammill, President
Linda Klan, Author
Nancy Lewis, Co-Author
An in-depth measure of phonological processes for assessment and remediation planning. Administration Time: 10-30 minutes. *$144.00*

4424 **Peabody Developmental Motor Scales-2**
Speech Bin
PO Box 1579
Appleton, WI 54912-1579
888-388-3224
Fax: 800-845-1535
http://www.schoolspecialty.com
orders@schoolspecialty.com
Joseph M. Yorio, President & CEO
James R. Henderson, Chairman
Patrick T. Collins, EVP, Distribution
PDMS-2 gives you in-depth standardized assessment of motor skills in children birth to six years. Subtests include: fine motor object manipulation; grasping; gross motor; locomotion; reflexes; visual-motor integration and stationary. Item number P624. *$43.00*

4425 **Perceptual Motor Development Series**
Therapro
225 Arlington St
Framingham, MA 01702-8773
508-872-9494
800-257-5376
Fax: 508-875-2062
http://www.theraproducts.com
info@theraproducts.com
Karen Conrad, Owner
Jack Capon, Author
Use these classroom tested movement education activities to assess motor strengths and weaknesses in preschool and early elementary grades or special education classes. The sequence of easily given tests and tasks requires minimal instruction time and your kids will find the activities to be interesting, challenging, and fun! Each book has 25-54 pages and costs $9.99 each. *$49.95*

4426 **Phonic Reading Lessons**
Academic Therapy Publications
20 Commercial Blvd
Novato, CA 94949-6120
415-883-3314
800-422-7249
Fax: 888-287-9975
http://www.academictherapy.com
sales@academictherapy.com
Jim Arena, President
Joanne Urban, Manager
Samuel Kirk, Author
A step-by-step program for teaching reading to children who failed to learn by conventional methods. Consistent sound-symbol relationships are presented and reinforced using a grapho-vocal method. A two book set (Book 1: Skills; Book 2: Practice). *$140.00*
ISBN 1-571284-68-6

4427 **Preschool Motor Speech Evaluation & Intervention**
Speech Bin
PO Box 1579
Appleton, WI 54912-1579
888-388-3224
Fax: 800-845-1535
http://www.schoolspecialty.com
orders@schoolspecialty.com
Joseph M. Yorio, President & CEO
James R. Henderson, Chairman
Patrick T. Collins, EVP, Distribution
This comprehensive criterion-based assessment tool differentiates motor-based speech disorders from those of phonology and determines if speech difficulties of children 18 months to six years old are characteristic of: oral nonverbal apraxia; dysarthria; developmental verbal dyspraxia; hypersensitivity; differences in tone and hyposensitivity. Item number J322. *$59.00*

4428 **Slosson Full Range Intelligence Test Kit**
Slosson Educational Publications
538 Buffalo Road
East Aurora, NY 14052
716-652-0930
888-756-7766
Fax: 800-655-3840
http://www.slosson.com
slossonprep@gmail.com
Steven Slosson, President
H Robert Vance, Author
Bob Algozzine, Co-Author
Intended to supplement the use of more extensive cognitive assessment instruments. Administration of test 25-45 minutes. *$175.00*

4429 **Slosson Visual Motor Performance Test**
Slosson Educational Publications
538 Buffalo Road
East Aurora, NY 14052
716-652-0930
888-756-7766
Fax: 800-655-3840
http://www.slosson.com
slossonprep@gmail.com
Steven Slosson, President
Richard.L Slosson, Author
Dr. Georgina Moynihan, Tech Support
A test of visual motor integration in which individuals are asked to copy geometric figures increasing in complexity without the use of a ruler, compass or other aids. *$86.75*

4430 **Test of Gross Motor Development**
Pro-Ed
8700 Shoal Creek Boulevard
Austin, TX 78757-6897
512-451-3246
800-897-3202
Fax: 512-451-8542
http://www.proedinc.com
general@proedinc.com
Donald D Hammill, Owner
Dale Urlich, Author
Assists you in identifying children who are significantly behind their peers in gross motor skill development and who should be eligible for special education services in phyiscal education. *$109.00*

4431 **Test of Information Processing Skills**
Academic Therapy Publications
20 Commercial Blvd
Novato, CA 94949-6120
415-883-3314
800-422-7249
Fax: 888-287-9975
http://www.academictherapy.com
sales@academictherapy.com
Jim Arena, President
Joanne Urban, Manager
Raymond Webster, Author
The TIPS (formerly The Learning Efficiency Test) provides a quick and accurate measure of a child or adult's information processing abilities, sequential and nonsequential, in both visual and auditory modalities. Additional subtests include Delayed Recall and Semantic Fluency. *$140.00*
ISBN 1-571284-68-6

4432 **Visual Skills Appraisal**
Academic Therapy Publications
20 Commercial Blvd
Novato, CA 94949-6120
415-883-3314
800-422-7249
Fax: 888-287-9975
http://www.academictherapy.com
sales@academictherapy.com
Jim Arena, President
Regina Richards, Author
Gary Oppenheim, Co-Author
This test identifies visual problems in children ages 5-9. Can be administered by an experienced examiner. Set includes manual, stimulus cards and test forms, design completion forms, and red/green glasses. *$100.00*
ISBN 0-878794-53-0

National Programs

4433 **ACT Universal Testing**
ACT
500 ACT Drive
P.O. Box 168
Iowa City, IA 52243-0168
319-337-1332
Fax: 319-339-3021
TDD: 319-337-1701
http://www.act.org
sandy.schlote@act.org

Jon Whitmore, CEO
Janet E. Godwin, Chief of Staff
Thomas J. Goedken, CFO/EVP
To help individuals and organizations make informed decisions about education and work. We provide information for life's transitions.

4434 **American College Testing Program**
ACT Universal Testing
500 ACT Drive
P.O. Box 168
Iowa City, IA 52243-0168
319-337-1000
Fax: 319-339-3021
TDD: 319-337-1701
http://www.act.org
sandy.schlote@act.org

Jon Whitmore, CEO
Janet E. Godwin, Chief of Staff
Thomas J. Goedken, CFO/EVP
ACT provides a broad array of assessment, information, research and program management solutions pertaining to education and workforce development.

4435 **Center For Accessible Technology**
Alliance For Technology Access
3075 Adeline
Suite 220
Berkeley, CA 94703
510-841-3224
Fax: 510-841-7956
http://www.cforat.org
info@cforat.orgg

Guy Thomas, Board President
Sara Armstrong Ph.D., Board Treasurer
A national organization dedicated to providing access to technology for people with disabilities through its coalition of 39 community-based resource centers in 28 states and in the Virgin Islands. Each center provides information, awareness, and training for professionals and provides guided problem solving and technical assistance for individuals with disabilities and family members.

4436 **Division on Career Development**
Council for Exceptional Children
2900 Crystal Drive
Suite 1000
Arlington, VA 22202-3557
888-232-7733
Fax: 703-264-9494
TTY: 866-915-5000
http://www.cec.sped.org
service@ces.sped.org

Robin D. Brewer, President
James P. Heiden, President Elect
Joni L. Baldwin, Board Member
Focuses on the career development of individuals with disabilities and/or who are gifted and their transition from school to adult life. Members include professionals and others interested in career development and transition for individuals with any exception at any age. Members receive a journal twice yearly and newsletter three times per year.

4437 **Independent Living Research Utilization Program**
TIRR Memorial Hermann Research Center
1333 Moursund
Houston, TX 77030
713-520-0332
Fax: 713-520-5785
TTY: 713-520-0232
http://www.ilru.org
ilru@ilru.org

Lex Frieden, Director
Richard Petty, Co-Director
Darrell Jones, Program Director
A national resource center for information, training, research, and technical assistance in independent living; produces and disseminates materials, develops and conducts training, and publishes a monthly newsletter. Provides a listing of Statewide Independent Living Councils (SILCS) in each state.

4438 **Job Accommodation Network (JAN)**
West Virginia University
PO Box 6080
Morgantown, WV 26506-6080
800-526-7234
Fax: 304-293-5407
TDD: 877-781-9403
http://askjan.org
jan@jan.wvu.edu

Anne Hirsh, Co-Director
Louis Orslene, Co-Director
Melanie Whetzel, Senior Consultant
Source of free, expert, and confidential guidance on workplace accomodations and disability employment issues. Working toward practical solutions that benefit both employer and employee, helps people with disabilities enhance their employability and shows employers how to capitalize on the value and talent that people with disabilities add to the workplace.

4439 **National Federation of the Blind**
200 E. Wells St.
at Jernigan Place
Baltimore, MD 21230
410-659-9314
Fax: 410-685-5653
http://www.nfb.org
pmaurer@nfb.org

Mark A. Riccobono, President
Pam Allen, First VP/Board Chair
Ron Brown, Second Vice President
Provides education, information, literature, and publications to the public about blindness. The National Federation of the Blind also provides programs and jobs to blind individuals, which helps them build self-confidence and self-respect.

4440 **U.S. Department of Education: Office of Vocational & Adult Education**
400 Maryland Avenue, SW
Lyndon Baines Johnson, Dept Ed. Bldg.
Washington, DC 20202-0001
202-401-1576
800-872-5327
http://www2.ed.gov
ovae@ed.gov

Arne Duncan, Secretary of Education
Emma Vadehra, Chief of Staff
Massie Ritsch, Acting Assistant Secretary
These agencies can provide job training, counseling, financial assistance, and employment placement to individuals who meet eligibility criteria.

Publications

4441 **ADD on the Job**
Taylor Publishing
7211 Circle S Road
Austin, TX 78745
512-444-0571
800-225-3687
Fax: 512-440-2160
http://www.balfour.com
Yearbooks@balfour.com

Lynn Weiss PhD, Author
Practical, sensitive advice for the ADD employee, his boss, and his co-workers. The book suggests advantages that the ADD worker has, how to find the right job, and how to keep it. Employers and co-workers will learn what to expect from fellow workers with ADD and the most effective ways to work with them.
232 pages Paperback
ISBN 0-878339-17-5

4442 **Ability Magazine**
Ability Awareness
PO Box 10878
Costa Mesa, CA 10878
949-854-8700
Fax: 949-548-5966
http://www.abilitymagazine.com
editorial@abilitymagazine.com
Chet Cooper, President
Brings disabilities into mainstream America. By interviewing high profile personalities such as President Clinton, Elizabeth Taylor, Mary Tyler Moore, Richard Pryor, Jane Seymour and many more, Ability Magazine is able to bring articles to the public's attention that may in the past have gone unnoticed.
80+ pages Bimonthly

4443 **Building a Bridge from School to Adult Life**
State Education Resource Center
100 Roscommon Dr
Middletown, CT 06457-1520
860-632-1485
Fax: 860-632-8870
http://www.ctserc.org
info@ctserc.org
A guide for students and their families to help with the transition from high school to an independent adult life.
1909

4444 **Current Developments in Employment and Training**
National Governors Association
444 N Capitol St NW
Ste 267
Washington, DC 20001-1512
202-624-5300
Fax: 202-624-5313
http://www.nga.org
mjensen@nga.org
John Hickenlooper, Chair
Gary Herbert, Vice Chair
Dan Crippen, Executive Director
Highlights issues and areas of interest related to employment and training.
Bimonthly

4445 **Fundamentals of Job Placement**
RPM Press
737 N. Cental Avenue
Wood Dale, IL 60191
630-422-7393
888-810-1990
Fax: 630-422-7246
http://www.rpmpress.com
info@rpmpress.com
James Costello, Author
Paul McCray, President
Provides step-by-step guidance for educators, special counselors and vocational rehabilitation personnel on how to develop job placement opportunities for special needs students and adults.

4446 **Fundamentals of Vocational Assessment**
RPM Press
737 N. Cental Avenue
Wood Dale, IL 60191
630-422-7393
888-810-1990
Fax: 630-422-7246
http://www.rpmpress.com
info@rpmpress.com
Paul McCray, President
Provides step-by-step guidance for educators, counselors and vocational rehabilitation personnel on how to conduct professional vocational assessments of special needs students.

4447 **Handbook for Developing Community Based Employment**
RPM Press
737 N. Cental Avenue
Wood Dale, IL 60191
630-422-7393
888-810-1990
Fax: 630-422-7246
http://www.rpmpress.com
info@rpmpress.com
Paul McCray, President
Provides step-by-step guidance for educators and vocational rehabilitation personnel on how to develop community-based employment training programs for severely challenged workers.

4448 **JOBS V**
PESCO International
21 Paulding St
Pleasantville, NY 10570-3108
914-769-4266
800-431-2016
Fax: 914-769-2970
http://www.pesco.org
pesco@pesco.org
Joseph Kass, President
A software program matching people with jobs, training, employment and local employers. Provides job outlooks for the next five years.

4449 **Job Access**
Ability Awareness
PO Box 10878
Costa Mesa, CA 92627-4512
949-548-1986
Fax: 949-548-5966
TDD: 949-548-5966
http://www.jobaccess.org
custserv@jobtarget.com
Chet Cooper, President
Job Access, a program of ability awareness, is an internet driven system dedicated to employ qualified people with disabilities. Employers can list job postings and review our resume bank. People with disabilities seeking employment can also search for jobs.

4450 **Job Accommodation Handbook**
RPM Press
737 N. Cental Avenue
Wood Dale, IL 60191
630-422-7393
888-810-1990
Fax: 630-422-7246
http://www.rpmpress.com
info@rpmpress.com
Paul McCray, President
Provides how-to-do-it for counselors, job placement specialists, educators and others on how to modify jobs for special needs workers.

4451 **Life Centered Career Education: Assessment Batteries**
Council for Exceptional Children
2900 Crystal Drive
Suite 1000
Arlington, VA 22202-3557
703-620-3660
888-232-7733
Fax: 703-264-9494
TTY: 866-915-5000
http://www.cec.sped.org
service@ces.sped.org
Robin D. Brewer, President
James P. Heiden, President Elect
Joni L. Baldwin, Board Member

The LCCE Batteries are curriculum-based assessment instruments designed to measure the career education knowledge and skills of regular and special education students. There are two alternative forms of a Knowledge Battery and two forms of the Performance Batteries. These assessment tools can be combined with instruction to determine the instructional goals most appropriate for a particular student.
827 pages

4452 **National Governors Association Newsletter**
444 N Capitol St NW
Ste 267
Washington, DC 20001-1512 202-624-5300
Fax: 202-624-5313
http://www.nga.org
mjensen@nga.org
John Hickenlooper, Chair
Gary Herbert, Vice Chair
Dan Crippen, Executive Director
Highlights issues and areas of interest related to employment and training.
Bimonthly

4453 **PWI Profile**
Goodwill Industries of America
15810 Indianola Dr
Derwood, MD 20855-2674 301-530-6500
800-GOODWILL
http://www.goodwill.org
contactus@goodwill.org
David Hadani, Director
Rev. Edgar J Helms, Founder
Newsletter that deals with employment of persons with disabilities.

4454 **Self-Supervision: A Career Tool for Audiologists, Clinical Series 10**
American Speech-Language-Hearing Association
2200 Research Boulevard
Rockville, MD 20850-3289 301-897-5700
800-638-2255
Fax: 301-897-7358
TDD: 301-897-5700
http://www.asha.org
jjanota@asha.org
Elizabeth S. McCrea, President
Judith L. Page, President-Elect
Arlene A. Pietranton, Chief Executive Officer
Describes concepts of supervision, defines and presents strategies for self-supervision, discusses supervisory accountability and covers issues of self-supervision within supervisor format.

4455 **Succeeding in the Workplace**
4156 Library Road
Pittsburgh, PA 15234-1349 412-341-1515
Fax: 412-344-0224
http://ldaamerica.org
lathamlaw@gmail.com
Nancie Payne, President
Ed Schlitt, First Vice President
Beth McGaw, Secretary
Comprehensive review: understanding disabilities, how to find and get the right job, how to succeed on the job, strategies, job accommodations, legal rights and personal experiences.

4456 **Tales from the Workplace**
Ste 707
2700 Virginia Ave NW
Washington, DC 20037-1909 202-333-1713
Fax: 202-333-1735
lathamlaw@gmail.com
Peter S Latham JD, Director
Patricia Horan Latham JD, Director
Easy to read. Explores through stories: What is the right job match? Should I disclose my disability? What are the signs of job trouble?

4457 **Transition and Students with Learning Disabilities**
Pro-Ed
8700 Shoal Creek Boulevard
Austin, TX 78757-6897 512-451-3246
800-897-3202
Fax: 512-451-8542
http://www.proedinc.com
general@proedinc.com
Patton Blalock, Author
Donald D Hammill, Owner
Provides important information about academic, social and vocational planning for students with learning disabilities.

4458 **Vocational Training and Employment of Autistic Adolescents**
Charles C Thomas
2600 S 1st St
Springfield, IL 62704-4730 217-789-8980
800-258-8980
Fax: 217-789-9130
http://www.ccthomas.com
books@ccthomas.com
Michael P Thomas, President
Publisher of Education and Special Education books.

4459 **Workforce Investment Quarterly**
National Governor's Association (NGA)
444 N Capitol St NW
Ste 267
Washington, DC 20001-1512 202-624-5300
Fax: 202-624-5313
http://www.nga.org
info@nga.org
John Hickenlooper, Chair
Gary Herbert, Vice Chair
Dan Crippen, Executive Director
Highlights issues and area interests related to employment and training. Contact NGA for more information.

Alabama

4460 **Achievement Center**
Easter Seals Of East Central Alabama
510 W Thomason Cir
Opelika, AL 36801-5499 334-745-3501
866-239-2237
Fax: 334-749-5808
http://www.achievement-center.org
info@achievement-center.org
Jason Lazenby, Chairman
Kenneth Burton, Vice-Chairman
Phyllis Horace, Secretary
Provides vocational development and employment programs to developmentally and physically disabiled individuals. The programs help individuals build self-esteem, self-confidence and helps to maximize their independent living skills.

4461 **Easter Seals - Alabama**
5960 E Shirley Ln
Montgomery, AL 36117 334-395-4489
Fax: 334-395-4492
http://www.easterseals.com/alabama
info@al.easterseals.comÿ
John Ives, Chairman
Randy Thomas, Chairman Elect
Lynne Stokley, Chief Executive Officer
Job training and employment services, senior community service employment program.

4462 **Easter Seals - Camp ASCCA**
PO Box 21
Jacksons Gap, AL 36861-21 256-825-9226
800-843-2267
Fax: 256-825-8332
http://www.alabama.easter-seals.org
matt@campascca.org

Richard W. Davidson, Chairman
Sandra L. Bouwman, 1st Vice Chairman
Lynne Stokley, CEO
Camp respite for adults and children, camperships, canoeing, day camping for adults, day camping for children, therapeutic horseback riding.

4463 **Easter Seals - Disability Services**
2448 Gordon Smith Dr
Mobile, AL 36617-2319 251-471-1581
800-411-0068
Fax: 251-476-4303
TTY: 334-872-8421
http://www.alabama.easterseals.org
info@al.easterseals.comÿ
S.Lynne Stokley, CEO
Easter Seals has been helping individuals with disabilities and special needs, and their families, live better lives for more than 80 years. Whether helping someone improve physical mobility, return to work or simply gain greater independence for everyday living, Easter Seals offers a variety of services to help people with disabilities address life's challenges and achieve personal goals.

4464 **Easter Seals - Opportunity Center**
United Way
6300 McClellan Blvd
Anniston, AL 36206 256-820-9960
Fax: 256-820-9592
http://www.alabama.easter-seals.org
mikenancyoppcen@aol.com
Richard W. Davidson, Chairman
Sandra L. Bouwman, 1st Vice Chairman
Lynne Stokley, CEO
Job training and employment services, occupational skills training, job placement/competitive-supported employment, vocational evaluation/situation assessment, work adjustment.

4465 **Easter Seals - Rehabilitation Center, Northwest Alabama**
1450 E Avalon Ave
Muscle Shoals, AL 35661-3110 256-381-1110
Fax: 256-314-5105
http://www.alabama.easter-seals.org
info@al.easterseals.comÿ
Richard W. Davidson, Chairman
Sandra L. Bouwman, 1st Vice Chairman
Lynne Stokley, CEO
Job training and employment services, occupational skills training, job placement/competitive-supported employment, vocational evaluation/situation assessment, work services.

4466 **Easter Seals - West Alabama**
1140 James I Harrison, Jr. Pkwy E
Tuscaloosa, AL 35405 205-759-1211
800-726-1216
Fax: 205-349-1162
http://www.eswaweb.org
eswa@eswaweb.org
Kenneth Gaddy, Chair
Sandra Ray, Vice Chair
Ronny Johnston, Executive Director
Job training and employment services, occupational skills training, job placement/competitive-supported employment, vocational evaluation/situation assessment, work adjustment.

4467 **Good Will Easter Seals**
2448 Gordon Smith Dr
Mobile, AL 36617-2319 251-471-1581
800-411-0068
Fax: 251-476-4303
TTY: 800-411-0068
http://www.gesgc.org
bill@gesgc.org
Frank Harkins, President/CEO
John McCain, Chief Operating Officer
Terri Bolin, VP Program Services
Job training and employment services, occupational skills training, job placement/competitive-supported employment, vocational evaluation/situation assessment, work adjustment.

4468 **State Vocational Rehabilitation Agency**
Alabama Dept Of Rehabilitation Services
602 South Lawrence Street
Montgomery, AL 36104 334-293-7500
800-441-7607
Fax: 334-293-7383
TDD: 334-613-2249
http://www.rehab.state.al.us
sshivers@rehab.state.al.us
Steve Shivers, Director
State vocational rehabilitation agencies provide direct services to persons with disabilities, including persons with learning disabilities. The services may include evaluation and diagnosis; counseling, guidance, and referral services; vocational and other training services; transportation to rehabilitation services; and assistive devices.

4469 **Workforce Development Division**
Alabama Dept of Economic & Community Affairs
P.O.Box 5690
Montgomery, AL 36103-5690 334-242-5100
Fax: 334-242-5099
http://www.adeca.state.al.us
stevew@adeca.state.al.us
Tim Alford, Executive Director
Customer focused to help Americans access the tools they need to manage their careers through information and high quality services and to help US companies find skilled workers. Alabama's Career Center System is a network of one-stop centers designed to offer these services. These centers are co-located or electronically linked to provide streamlined services.

Alaska

4470 **AK Dept. of Labor and Workforce Dev.**
Division of Voc. Rehab.
801 W. 10th Street
Suite A
Juneau, AK 99801-1894 907-465-2814
800-478-2815
Fax: 907-465-2856
http://www.labor.state.ak.us/dvr
Cheryl Walsh, Director
Assists individuals with disabilities to obtain and maintain employment.

Arizona

4471 **Arizona Vocational Rehabilitation**
Arizona Department of Economic Security
1717 W. Jefferson
Room 119
Phoenix, AZ 85007 602-542-4791
Fax: 602-241-7158
TTY: 602-241-1048
http://www.azdes.gov
Michael Scione, Program Manager
Jon Ellerston, Assistant Program Manager
Programs provide a variety of specialized services for individuals with physical or mental disabilities that create barriers to employment or independent living. RSA offers three major service programs and several specialized programs/services.

4472 **Rehabilitation Services Administration**
Arizona Dept Of Economic Security
1717 W. Jefferson
Room 119
Phoenix, AZ 85007 602-542-4791
Fax: 602-241-7158
TTY: 602-241-1048
http://www.azdes.gov
Katharine Levandowsky, Director
The mission of the Rehabilitation Services Administration (RSA) is to work with individuals with disabilities to achieve increased independence and/or gainful employment through the provision of comprehensive rehabilitative and employment support services in a partnership with all stakeholders.

Arkansas

4473 **Arkansas Department of Career Education**
Luther Hardin Building
Three Capitol Mall
Little Rock, AR 72201-1005 501-682-1500
Fax: 501-682-1509
http://ace.arkansas.gov
Mike Beebe, Governor
William L. Walker, Jr., Director
James H. Smith, Jr., Deputy Director
Formerly the Dept. of Workforce Education, the Arkansas Dept. of Career Education (ACE) provides many resources to serve the educational needs of Arkansas individuals living with disabilities.

4474 **Arkansas Department of Health & Human Services: Division of Developmental Disabilities**
425 W. Capital Avenue
Suite 1620
Little Rock, AR 72201 501-324-8900
http://www.arkansas.gov
James Green PhD, Director
The mission of the Division of Developmental Disabilities Services is to provide a variety of supports to improve the quality of life for individuals with mental retardation, autism, epilepsy, cerebral palsy or other conditions that cause a person to function as if they had a mental impairment.

4475 **Arkansas Employment Security Department: Office of Employment & Training Services**
425 W. Capital Avenue
Suite 1620
Little Rock, AR 72201 501-324-8900
http://www.arkansas.gov
Artee Williams, Director
Employment related services that contribute to the economic stability of Arkansa and its citizens. These services are provided to employers, the workforce and the general public.

4476 **Arkansas Rehabilitation Services**
Three Capitol Mall
Little Rock, AR 72201 501-682-1500
Fax: 501-682-1509
TDD: 501-686-9686
http://ace.arkansas.gov
ssholt@ars.state.ar.us
Mike Beebe, Governor
William L. Walker, Jr., Director
James H. Smith, Jr., Deputy Director
For persons who are clients of Arkansas Rehabilitation Services, individual psychological/educational evaluations and college preparatory training are provided if approved by vocational rehabilitation counselor.

4477 **Department of Human Services: Division of Developmental Disabilities Services**
425 W. Capital Avenue
Suite 1620
Little Rock, AR 72201 501-324-8900
http://www.state.ar.us
Dr. Charlie Fleetwood, Chairman
Angela Harrison-King, Vice Chairman
Michael Stock, Treasurer
Offers a wide range of services and supports to Arkansans with developmental disabilities and their families.

4478 **Easter Seals - Adult Services Center**
Easter Seals Arkansas
3920 Woodland Heights Rd
Little Rock, AR 72212 501-367-1200
http://www.easterseals.com/arkansas
ctw@eastersealsar.com
Jay Heflin, Chair
Dr. James Hunt, Vice Chair
Elaine Eubank, President & CEO
An Easter Seals day program for adults with disabilities to interact with other members of the community, learn life skills and employment training.

4479 **Office For The Deaf And Hearing Impaired**
Arkansas Rehabilitation Services
Three Capitol Mall
Little Rock, AR 72201 501-682-1500
Fax: 501-682-1509
TDD: 501-686-9686
http://ace.arkansas.gov
Mike Beebe, Governor
William L. Walker, Jr., Director
James H. Smith, Jr., Deputy Director
Providing opportunities for individuals with hearing impairment to work and have productive and independent lives.

4480 **State Vocational Rehabilitation Agency of Arkansas**
ARS, Vocational & Technical Education Division
Three Capitol Mall
Little Rock, AR 72201 501-682-1500
Fax: 501-682-1509
TDD: 501-686-9686
http://ace.arkansas.gov
William L. Walker, Jr., Director
James H. Smith, Jr., Deputy Director
Provides direct services to persons with disabilities, including persons with learning disabilities. The services may include evaluation and diagnosis, counseling, guidance, and referral services, vocational and other training services, transportation to rehabilitation services, and assistive devices. Offering opportunities for individuals with disabilities to lead productive and independent lives.

4481 **Workforce Investment Board**
Arkansas State Employment Board
425 W. Capital Avenue
Suite 1620
Little Rock, AR 72201 501-324-8900
http://www.arkansas.gov
Cindy Verner, Division Chief
Operates workforce centers that offer locally developed and operated services linking employers and jobseekers through a statewide delivery system. Conveinient centers are designed to eliminate the need to visit different locations. The centers integrate multiple workforce development programs into a single system, making the resources much more accessible and user friendly to jobseekers as well as expanding services to employers.

California

4482 **Adult Education**
California Department of Education
Ste 400
1430 N St
Sacramento, CA 95814-5901 916-319-0800
Fax: 916-319-0100
http://www.cde.ca.gov
scheduler@cde.ca.gov
Jack O'Connell, Director
Elementary basic skills and tutor/literacy training are offered on or off site using language masters, audiocassettes, videos and computers with internet access. Workplace literacy training will also be provided, with groups of students physically coming into the Center or hooking up to the Center from their workplace by borrowing materials or going online. In the latter case, instructors will meet with students at the work site on a regular schedule for evaluation and consultation.

4483 **California Department of Education**
1430 N St
Sacramento, CA 95814-5901 916-319-0800
800-331-6316
TTY: 916-445-4556
http://www.cde.ca.gov
gedoffic@cde.ca.gov
Nancy Edmunds, Program Coordinator
Provides access to a general high school education by providing many local classes and testing services.

4484 **California Department of Rehabilitation**
California Health & Human Services Agency
721 Capitol Mall
P.O. Box 944222
Sacramento, CA 94244-2220 916-324-1313
Fax: 916-558-5807
http://www.dor.ca.gov
externalaffairs@dor.ca.gov
Catherine Campisi PhD, Executive Director
California Department of Rehabilitation works in partnership with consumers and other stakeholders to provide services and advocacy resulting in employment, independent living and equality for individuals with disabilities.

4485 **California Employment Development Department**
800 Capitol Mall
Sacramento, CA 95814-4807 916-654-8210
Fax: 916-657-5294
TTY: 800-815-9387
http://www.edd.ca.gov
phenning@edd.ca.gov
Patrick Henning, Director
The California Employment Development Department (EDD) offers a wide variety of services to millions of Californians under the Job Service, Unemployment Insurance, Disability Insurance, Workforce Investment, and Labor Market Information programs.

4486 **Easter Seals - Central California, Aptos**
9010 Soquel Dr
Ste 1
Aptos, CA 95003-4002 831-684-2166
Fax: 831-684-1018
TTY: 831-684-1054
http://www.easterseals.com/centralcal
Scott Webb, Executive Director
Twila Chaffee, Finance Manager
Jeff Terpstra, Chair
Create solutions that change lives of children and adults with disabilities or other special needs and their families.

4487 **Easter Seals - Pacoima**
Eastern Seals Southern California
12510 Van Nuys Blvd
Ste 103
Pacoima, CA 91331 818-996-9902
800-996-6302
Fax: 818-975-8299
http://www.easterseals.com
paula.pompa-craven@essc.org
Richard W. Davidson, Chairman
Sandra L. Bouwman, 1st Vice Chairman
Joseph G. Kern, 2nd Vice Chairman
Job training and employment services, occupational skills training, job placement/competitive-support employment, vocational evaluation/situational assessment and work adjustment.

4488 **Easter Seals - Redondo Beach**
Ste 201
700 N Pacific Coast Hwy
Redondo Beach, CA 90277-2147 310-376-3445
800-404-3445
Fax: 310-376-5567
http://www.easterseals.com
dee.prescott@cssc.org
Richard W. Davidson, Chairman
Sandra L. Bouwman, 1st Vice Chairman
Joseph G. Kern, 2nd Vice Chairman
Job training and employment services, occupational skills training, job placement/competitive-support employment, vocational evaluation/situational assessment and work adjustment.

4489 **Easter Seals - Southern California**
1063 McGaw Ave
Irvine, CA 92614 714-834-1111
http://www.easterseals.com/southerncal
Mark Whitley, Chief Executive Officer
Molly Pyott, Chair
Andre Bertrand, First Vice Chair
Provides exceptional services to ensure that all people with disabilities or other special needs and their families have equal opportunities to live, learn, work and play in their communities.

4490 **Easter Seals - Superior California**
3205 Hurley Way
Sacramento, CA 95864-3898 916-485-6711
888-887-3257
Fax: 916-485-2653
http://www.easterseals.com
info@easterseals-superiorca.org
Richard W. Davidson, Chairman
Sandra L. Bouwman, 1st Vice Chairman
Joseph G. Kern, 2nd Vice Chairman
Job training and employment services, occupational skills training, job placement/competitive-support employment, vocational evaluation/situational assessment and work adjustment.

4491 **WorkFirst**
Easter Seals Of Southern California
Ste C
11110 Artesia Blvd
Cerritos, CA 90703-2546 760-737-3990
877-855-2279
Fax: 562-860-1680
http://www.workfirst.us
dee.prescott@essc.org
Sandra Meredith, Executive Director
WorkFirst helps individuals with disabilities to find work and keep working in a job that is more suited to their talents. The program also helps those individuals who are looking to open a business of their own.

Colorado

4492 **Colorado Department of Human Services: Division for Developmental Disabilities**
1575 Sherman Street
Denver, CO 80203-3111 303-866-5700
Fax: 303-866-4047
TDD: 303-866-7471
http://www.cdhs.state.co.us
cdhs_communications@state.co.us.
Karen L. Beye, Executive Director
A state office that provides leadership for the direction, funding and operation of community based services to people with developmental disabilities within Colorado.

4493 **Easter Seals - Colorado**
5755 W Alameda Ave
Lakewood, CO 80226-3500 303-233-1666
Fax: 303-569-3857
http://www.co.easterseals.com
info@eastersealscolorado.org
Lynn Robinson, President/CEO
Nancy Hanson, VP, Human Resources
Job training and employment services, occupational skills training, job placement/competitive-support employment, vocational evaluation/situational assessment and work adjustment.

4494 **Human Services: Division of Vocational**
1575 Sherman St
4th Fl
Denver, CO 80203-1702 303-866-4150
866-870-4595
Fax: 303-866-4905
TDD: 303-866-4150
http://www.dvrcolorado.com
Voc.Rehab@state.co.us
Nancy Smith, Director
Assists individuals whose disabilities result in barriers to employment to succeed at work and live independently. Building partnerships to improve opportunities for safety, self-sufficiency and dignity for the people of Colorado.

Connecticut

4495 **Department of Social Services: Vocational Rehabilitation Program**
55 Farmington Avenue
Hartford, CT 06105 860-424-5241
800-842-1508
TDD: 800-842-4524
http://www.ct.gov
pgr.dss@ct.gov
John Galiette, Director
Brenda Moore, Executive Director
Provides services to people with most significant physical or mental disabilities to assist them in their effort to enter or maintain employment. The agency also oversees a statewide network of community based, consumer controlled, independent living centers that promote independence for people with disabilities.

4496 **Easter Seals - Connecticut**
85 Jones Street
PO Box 198
Hebron, CT 06248-0100 860-228-9496
800-874-7687
Fax: 860-228-2091
http://www.easterseals.com
Richard W. Davidson, Chairman
Sandra L. Bouwman, 1st Vice Chairman
Joseph G. Kern, 2nd Vice Chairman
Easter Seals Connecticut creates solutions that change the lives of children and adults with disabilities or special needs, their families and communities.

4497 **Easter Seals - Employment Industries**
Easter Seals Rehabilitation Center
122 Avenue of Industry
Waterbury, CT 06705-3901 203-236-0188
Fax: 203-236-0183
http://www.easterseals.com
eswct@eswct.com
Fran DeBlasio, CEO
Ron Bourque, Primary Contact
Job training, employment services, vocational evaluation/situational assessment and work services.

4498 **Easter Seals - Fulfillment Enterprises Easter Seals Connecticut**
24 Stott Ave
Norwich, CT 06360-1508 860-859-4148
Fax: 860-455-1372
http://www.easterseals.com
Richard W. Davidson, Chairman
Sandra L. Bouwman, 1st Vice Chairman
Joseph G. Kern, 2nd Vice Chairman
Job training, employment services, vocational evaluation/situational assessment and work services.

4499 **Easter Seals - Job Training And Placement Services**
Easter Seals Waterbury, Connecticut
22 Tompkins St
Waterbury, CT 06708-1496 203-754-5141
Fax: 203-757-1198
TTY: 203-754-5141
http://www.waterburyct.easterseals.com
Curtis Audibert, Chairman
David Segal, Vice Chairman
Francis DeBlasio, President
Offers a number of vocational rehabilitation services, application & interviewing support, individualized employment planning & supported employment, and on the job training.

Delaware

4500 **Division of Vocational Rehabilitation**
Delaware Department of Labor
4425 N Market St
PO Box 9969
Wilmington, DE 19809-0969 302-761-8085
Fax: 302-761-6601
TTY: 302-761-8275
http://www.delawareworks.com
cynthia.fairwell@state.de.us
Andrea Guest, Director
Mission is to provide information opportunities and resources to individuals with disabilities, leading to success in employment and independent living. Facebook: http://www.facebook.com/DE.DVR.1

4501 **Easter Seals - Dover Enterprise**
Easter Seals Delaware & Maryland's Eastern Shore
100 Enterprise Pl
Ste 1
Dover, DE 19904 302-324-4444
Fax: 302-324-4441
TDD: 302-324-4442
http://www.easterseals.com/de
mblankenship@esdel.org
Kenan Sklenar, Chief Executive Officer
Jeffrey Gosnear, Chair
Gary W Spitzer, Vice Chair
Easter Seals offers a variety of programs and activities for children and adults with disabililties.

4502 **Easter Seals Delaware & Maryland's Eastern Shore**
61 Corporate Cir
New Castle, DE 19720 302-324-4444
Fax: 302-324-4441
TDD: 302-324-4442
http://www.easterseals.com/de

Kenan Sklenar, Chief Executive Officer
Jeffrey Gosnear, Chair
Gary W Spitzer, Vice Chair
Provides exceptional services to ensure that all people with disabilities or special needs and their families have equal opportunities to live, learn, work and play in their communities.

District of Columbia

4503 **Department of Employment Services**
District of Columbia
4058 Minnesota Avenue, NE
Washington, DC 20019
202-724-7000
Fax: 202-673-6993
TTY: 202-698-4817
http://www.does.dc.gov
does@dc.gov
Gregory Irish, Director
Helps consider career decisions and offer vocational and placement assistance at several area training locations.

4504 **District of Columbia Department of Education: Vocational & Adult Education**
400 Maryland Ave SW
Washington, DC 20202
202-842-0973
800-872-5327
Fax: 202-205-8748
TTY: 800-437-0833
http://www2.ed.gov
ovae@ed.gov
Arne Duncan, Secretary of Education
Emma Vadehra, Chief of Staff
Massie Ritsch, Acting Assistant Secretary
To help all people achieve the knowledge and skills to be lifelong learners, to be successful in their chosen careers, and to be effective citizens.

4505 **The DC Center For Independent Living, Inc.**
1400 Florida Ave NE
Washington, DC 20002-5032
202-388-0033
Fax: 202-398-3018
TDD: 202-388-0277
TTY: 202-388-0277
http://www.dccil.org
info@dccil.org
Richard Simms, Executive Director
Kandra Hall, Coordinator
Promotes independent life styles for persons with significant disabilities. Programs offered include advocacy/legal/information and referral services, and independent living skills training.

Florida

4506 **Children's Therapy Services Center**
Easter Seals Of Southwest Florida
350 Braden Ave
Sarasota, FL 34243-2001
941-355-7637
800-807-7899
Fax: 941-358-3069
http://www.swfl.easterseals.com
Bill Lloyd, President
Job training, employment services, vocational evaluation/situational assessment and work services.

4507 **College Living Experience**
6555 Nova Drive
Suite 300
Davie, FL 33317-7404
954-370-5142
800-486-5058
Fax: 954-370-1895
http://www.experiencecle.com
secretary@cleinc.net
Stephanie Martin, President
Amy Radochonski, Vice President
Tiffany Prior, Assistant VP
A post-secondary program for students with Autism spectrum disorders, Dyslexia, Traumatic Brain Injury, ADD/ADHD, auditory/visual processing disorders and nonverbal learning disorders. The program offers students additional support with academic, social and living skills which helps them in adulthood.

4508 **Division of Vocational Rehabilitation**
Florida Department of Education
2002 Old Saint Augustine Road
Building A
Tallahassee, FL 32301-4862
850-245-3399
800-451-4327
Fax: 850-245-3316
TDD: 800-451-4327
http://www.rehabworks.org
Bill Palmer, Director
Statewide employment resource for businesses and people with disabilities. Our mission is to enable individuals with disabilities to obtain and keep employment.

4509 **Easter Seals - Florida**
6050 Babcock St SE
Ste 18
Palm Bay, FL 32909-3996
321-723-4474
Fax: 321-676-3843
http://www.fl.easterseals.org
scaporina@fl.easterseals.com
Gail Edwards, President
Offers vocational training to adults with disabilities and special needs, giving them the opportunity to receive job and life skills training so they gain greater independence.

4510 **Easter Seals - South Florida**
1475 NW 14th Ave
Miami, FL 33125-1616
305-325-0470
Fax: 305-325-0578
TTY: 305-326-7351
http://www.southflorida.easterseals.com
lwelch@sfl.easterseals.com
Luanne K Welch, Executive President/CEO
Malerie Sloshay, VP Operations
Job training, employment services, vocational evaluation/situational assessment and work services, adult day services, outpatient medical rehabilitation.

4511 **Florida Workforce Investment Act**
Department of Labor & Employment Security
1580 Waldo Palmer Lane
Suite 1
Tallahassee, FL 32308
850-921-1119
Fax: 850-921-1101
http://careersourceflorida.com
Kathleen McLeskey, Director
Provides job-training services for economically disadvantaged adults and youth, dislocated workers and others who face significant employment barriers.

4512 **TILES Project: Transition/Independent Living/Employment/Support**
Family Network on Disabilities, Inc.
2196 Main Street
Suite K
Dunedin, FL 34698-1610
727-523-1130
800-825-5736
Fax: 727-523-8687
http://www.fndfl.org
fnd@fndfl.org
Tracy Stewart, President/Parliamentarian
Jennifer Morgan-Byrd, Vice President
Molly Jacobson, Secretary

Provides training information to enable individuals with disabilities and the parents, family members, guardians, advocates, or other authorized representatives to participate more effectively with professionals in meeting the vocational, independent living and rehabilitation needs of people with disabilities in Florida.

Georgia

4513 **Easter Seals - East Georgia**
1500 Wrightsboro Rd
PO Box 2441
Augusta, GA 30903-4079
706-667-9695
866-667-9695
Fax: 706-667-8831
http://www.ga-ea.easterseals.com
shthomas@esega.org
Sheila Thomas, President/CEO
Job training for disabled individuals, employment services, vocational evaluation/situational assessment and work services.

4514 **Easter Seals - Middle Georgia**
604 Kellam Rd
PO Box 847
Dublin, GA 31040
478-275-8850
Fax: 478-275-8852
http://www.easterseals.com/middlega
Wayne Peebles, President
Job training, employment services, vocational evaluation/situational assessment and work services.

4515 **Easter Seals - Southern Georgia**
1906 Palmyra Rd
Albany, GA 31701
229-439-7061
Fax: 229-435-6278
http://www.easterseals.com/southerngeorgia
Beth English, Executive Director
Matt Hatcher, Chief Operating Officer
Kyle Nichols, Chairman
Helps individuals with disabilities and special needs by providing many services such as job training, employment services, vocational evaluation/situational assessment and work services.

4516 **Vocational Rehabilitation Services**
Georgia Department of Labor
10 Park Place South, SE
Suite 602
Atlanta, GA 30303-1732
404-657-2239
Fax: 404-657-4731
TTY: 404-657-2239
http://www.vocrehabga.org
rehab@dol.state.ga.us
Peggy Rosser, Director
Operates 5 integrated and interdependent programs that share a primary goal — to help people with disabilities to become fully productive members of society by achieving independence and meaningful employment.

Hawaii

4517 **Vocational Rehabilitation and Services For The Blind Division (VRSBD)**
State Of Hawaii, Department Of Human Services
1901 Bachelot Street
Honolulu, HI 96817-0339
808-586-5268
http://www.hawaii.gov
Lilian Poller, Director
State vocational rehabilitation agencies provide direct services to persons with disabilities, including persons with learning disabilities. The services may include evaluation and diagnosis, counseling, guidance, and referral services, vocational and other training services, transportation to rehabilitation services, and assistive devices.

Idaho

4518 **Idaho Department of Commerce & Labor**
State Of Idaho Department of Labor
317 W Main St
Boise, ID 83735-0001
208-332-3570
Fax: 208-334-6430
TDD: 800-377-1363
http://www.labor.idaho.gov
labor.idaho.gov
Roger Madsen, Director
Renee Bade, Project Coordinator
Alexis Neufeld, Administrative Assistant
Provides vocational training services for economically disadvantaged adults and youth, dislocated workers and others who face significant employment barriers.

4519 **Idaho Division of Vocational Rehabilitation Administration**
Idaho State Board of Education
650 W. State Street
Room 150
Boise, ID 83702-0001
208-334-3390
Fax: 208-334-5305
http://www.vr.idaho.gov
department.info@vr.idaho.gov
Michael Graham, Director
State vocational rehabilitation agencies provide direct services to persons with disabilities, including persons with learning disabilities. The services may include evaluation and diagnosis, counseling, guidance, and referral services, vocational and other training services, transportation to rehabilitation services, and assistive devices.

4520 **State Of Idaho Department Of Labor**
317 W Main St
Boise, ID 83735-0001
208-332-3570
Fax: 208-334-6430
TDD: 800-377-1363
http://www.labor.idaho.gov
labor.idaho.gov
Roger Madsen, Director
Renee Bade, Project Coordinator
Alexis Neufeld, Administrative Assistant
An equal opportunity employer/program with auxiliary aids and services available upon request to individuals with disabilities.

Illinois

4521 **State Vocational Rehabilitation Agency**
100 S Grand Ave
Springfield, IL 62762-0001
217-782-2094
800-843-6154
Fax: 217-558-4270
TDD: 217-557-2507
TTY: 888-440-8982
http://www.dhs.state.il.us
dhs.ors@illinois.gov
Rob Kilbury, Director
Assists people with physical, visual, and hearing disabilities in achieving their education, employment, and independent living goals, including preparing for and finding quality employment.

4522 **Timber Pointe Outdoor Center**
Easter Seals Of Illinois
507 East Armstrong Avenue
Peoria, IL 61603-3197
309-686-1177
http://www.easterseals-ci.org
info@easterseals-ci.org
Debbie England, President
Timber Pointe provides specialized camping and respite programs for individuals with disabilities or special needs and their families. For ages 7 and up. Children enjoy activities such as swimming, boating, fishing, sports, music and arts and crafts.

Indiana

4523 **Easter Seals - Arc of Northeast Indiana**
4919 Colwater Rd
Fort Wayne, IN 46825 260-456-4534
http://www.easterseals.com/neindiana
Donna K. Elbrecht, President & CEO
Sheri Ward, Director, Development
Misty Woltman, CFO/Controller
The Easter Seals Arc of Northeast Indiana covers 16 counties and offers many services and programs to children and adults with special needs or disabilities.

4524 **Easter Seals - Crossroads**
4740 Kingsway Dr
Indianapolis, IN 46205-1521 317-466-1000
Fax: 317-466-2000
TTY: 317-479-3232
http://www.eastersealscrossroads.org
J. Patrick Sandy, President / CEO
Susan Saunders, CFO/Security Officer
Bruce Schnaith, VP Workforce Dev Services
Works with children and adults with disabilities or special needs to promote growth, dignity and independence.

4525 **INdiana Camp R.O.C.K.S.**
Easter Seals Crossroads
4740 Kingsway Drive
Indianapolis, IN 46205 317-466-1000
Fax: 317-466-2000
TDD: 317-479-3232
http://www.eastersealscrossroads.org
Anne Shupe, Director
J. Patrick Sandy, President / CEO
Susan Saunders, CFO/Security Officer
Camp for chidlren and young adults ages 10-17 who have autism.

4526 **Vocational Rehabilitation Services**
1452 Vaxter Ave
Clarksville, IN 47129-7721 812-288-8261
877-228-1967
Fax: 812-282-7048
TDD: 812-288-8261
http://www.in.gov
Delbert Hayden, Director
Purpose is to assist the community by providing services which allow individuals to maximize their potential and to participate in work, family and the community. To do this we will provide rehabilitation, education and training.

Iowa

4527 **Division of Community Colleges and Workforce Preparation**
Iowa Department of Education
400 E 14th St
Des Moines, IA 50319-146 515-281-5294
Fax: 515-242-5988
http://educateiowa.gov
kathy.petosa@iowa.gov
Dr. Jason Glass, Director
Kathy Petosa, Administrative Assistant
The Iowa Department of Education (the Department) works with the Iowa State Board of Education (State Board) to provide oversight, supervision, and support for the state education system that includes public elementary and secondary schools, nonpublic schools that receive state accreditation, area education agencies (AEAs), community colleges, and teacher preparation programs.

4528 **Easter Seals - Iowa**
401 NE 66th Ave
Des Moines, IA 50313-1200 515-289-1933
866-533-9344
Fax: 515-289-1281
TDD: 515-274-8348
TTY: 515-289-4069
http://www.ia.easterseals.com
info@eastersealsia.org
Sherri Nielsen, President/CEO
Krable Mentzer, Chief Development Officer
Kevin Small, Chief Financial Officer
Offers many programs and services for children and adults with disabilities or special needs.

4529 **Easter Seals Center**
2920 30th St
Des Moines, IA 50310-5299 515-274-1529
866-533-9344
Fax: 515-274-6434
TDD: 515-274-8348
TTY: 515-274-8348
http://www.easterseals.com
info@eastersealsia.org
Richard W. Davidson, Chairman
Sandra L. Bouwman, 1st Vice Chairman
Joseph G. Kern, 2nd Vice Chairman
Job training, employment services, vocational evaluation/situational assessment and work services.

4530 **State Vocational Rehabilitation Agency**
Iowa Division of Vocational Rehabilitation Service
510 E 12th St
Des Moines, IA 50319-9025 515-281-4211
800-532-1486
Fax: 515-281-7645
TDD: 515-281-4211
TTY: 800-532-1486
http://www.ivrs.iowa.gov
Stephen Wooderson, Director
We work for and with individuals with disabilities to achieve their employment, independence and economic goals. Economic independence and more and better jobs are what we are about for Iowans with disabilities.

Kansas

4531 **Office of Vocational Rehabilitation**
Department of Vocational Rehabilitation
915 SW Harrison St
Topeka, KS 66612-1505 888-369-4777
TTY: 785-296-1491
http://www.srskansas.org
cmxa@srskansas.org
Clarissa Ashdown, Director
Partnering to connect Kansans with support and services to improve lives. Vocational and transitional training.

Kentucky

4532 **Easter Seals - West Kentucky**
801 N 29th St
Paducah, KY 42001-3067 270-442-9687
866-673-3565
Fax: 270-442-4933
http://www.easterseals.com/westkentucky
George Kennedy, President
Provides programs and services for children and adults with disabilities and/or special needs. Provides job training, employment services, vocational evaluation/situational assessment and work services.

4533 **Office of Vocational Rehabilitation**
275 E Main St
Mail Drop 2EK
Frankfort, KY 40621
502-564-4440
800-372-7172
Fax: 502-564-6745
TTY: 888-420-9874
http://www.kydor.state.ky.us
wfd.vocrehab@mail.state.ky.us
Beth Smith, Executive Director
Pam Jarboe, Program Services Director
Provides direct services to persons with disabilities, including persons with learning disabilities. The services may include evaluation and diagnosis; counseling, guidance, and referral services, vocational and other training services, transportation to rehabilitation services, and assistive devices.

Maine

4534 **State Vocational Rehabilitation Agency**
Maine Bureau of Rehabilitation Services
150 State House Station
Augusta, ME 04333-0150
207-623-6799
800-698-4440
Fax: 207-287-5292
http://www.maine.gov/rehab
Carolyn Lockwood, Executive Director
Betsy Hopkins, Director
Works to bring about full access to employment, independence and community integration for people with disabilities. Our three service provision units are Vocational Rehabilitation, Division for the Blind and Visually Impaired and Division of Deafness.

Maryland

4535 **Maryland Technology Assistance Program**
Maryland Department of Disabilities
217 E. Redwood Street
Suite 1300
Baltimore, MD 21202
410-767-3660
800-637-4113
http://www.mdod.maryland.gov
Beth Lash, Director
Offers information and referrals, reduced rate loan program for assistive technology, five regional display centers, presentations and training on request.

4536 **State Vocational Rehabilitation Agency**
Maryland State Dept Of Education/Div Rehab Svcs.
2301 Argonne Dr
Baltimore, MD 21218-1696
410-554-9442
888-554-0334
TTY: 410-554-9411
http://www.dors.state.md.us
Robert Burns, Director
Operates more than 20 statewide offices and also operates the Workforce and Technology Center, a comprehensive rehabilitation facility in Baltimore. Rehabilitation representatives also work in many Maryland One-Stop Career Centers.

Massachusettes

4537 **Easter Seals - Massachusetts**
484 Main St
Worcester, MA 01608-1817
800-244-2756
http://www.easterseals.com/ma
Paul Nedeiros, President & CEO
Kathy Kittle, Chair
David Hoffman, Vice Chair
Job training, employment services, vocational evaluation/situational assessment and work services. Camp programs, assistive technology and augmentative communication.

4538 **State Vocational Rehabilitation Agency**
Massachusetts Rehabilitation Commission
59 Temple Place
Suite 905
Boston, MA 02111-1619
617-357-8137
800-245-6543
Fax: 617-482-5576
TDD: 800-223-3212
TTY: 800-245-6543
http://www.mass.gov
Elmer Bartels, Director
Provides public vocational rehabilitation, independent living and disability determination services for residents with disabilities in Massachusetts.

Michigan

4539 **Easter Seal - Michigan**
2399 E Walton Blvd
Auburn Hills, MI 48326
248-475-6400
http://www.easterseals.com/michigan
Brent Wirth, President & CEO
Juliana Harper, Chief Program Officer/SVP
Ron Hocking, Chief Financial Officer/SVP
Job training, employment services, vocational evaluation/situational assessment and work services.

4540 **State Vocational Rehabilitation Agency**
Dept Of Labor & Economic Grwth-Rehabilitation Svcs
201 N. Washington Square, 4th Floor
P.O. Box 30010
Lansing, MI 48909-7510
517-373-4026
800-605-6722
Fax: 517-335-7277
TDD: 888-605-6722
TTY: 888-605-6722
http://www.michigan.gov
Jaye Balthazar, Director
State vocational rehabilitation agencies provide direct services to persons with disabilities, including persons with learning disabilities. The services may include evaluation and diagnosis; counseling, guidance, and referral services; vocational and other training services; transportation to rehabilitation services; and assistive devices.

Minnesota

4541 **Goodwill - Easter Seals Minnesota**
553 Fairview Ave N
Saint Paul, MN 55104-1708
651-379-5800
Fax: 651-379-5803
http://www.goodwilleasterseals.org
The Goodwill stores help individuals achieve their goals for employment, education, training and independence.

4542 **Minnesota Vocational Rehabilitation Agency: Rehabilitation Services Branch**
Department of Employment & Economic Development
1st National Bank Building
332 Minnesota Street, Suite E-200
Saint Paul, MN 55101-1351
651-259-7114
800-657-3858
Fax: 651-297-5159
TTY: 651-296-3900
http://www.deed.state.mn.us
DEED.CustomerService@state.mn.us
Katie Clark Sieben, Commissioner
Blake Chaffee, Deputy Commissioner /COO
Robin Sternberg, Deputy Commissioner Eco Dev
Provides basic vocational rehabilitation services to consumers including vocational counseling, planning, guidance and placement, as well as certain special services based on individual circumstances.

4543 **State Vocational Rehabilitation Agency: Minnesota Department of Economics Security**
Rehabilitation Service Branch
1st National Bank Building
332 Minnesota Street, Suite E-200
Saint Paul, MN 55101-1351 651-259-7114
800-657-3858
Fax: 651-296-3900
TTY: 651-296-3900
http://www.deed.state.mn.us
DEED.CustomerService@state.mn.us
Katie Clark Sieben, Commissioner
Blake Chaffee, Deputy Commissioner /COO
Robin Sternberg, Deputy Commissioner Eco Dev
State vocational rehabilitation agencies provide direct services to persons with disabilities, including persons with learning disabilities. The services may include evaluation and diagnosis, counseling, guidance, and referral services, vocational and other training services, transportation to rehabilitation services, and assistive devices.

Mississippi

4544 **Office Of Vocational Rehabilitation**
Mississippi Dept Of Rehabilitation Services
P.O.Box 1698
Jackson, MS 39215-1698 601-853-5100
800-443-1000
Fax: 601-853-5158
TDD: 601-351-1586
http://www.mdrs.ms.gov
Chris Howard, Deputy Executive Director???
Anita Naik, Office Director???
Billy Taylor, Special Assistant???
Helps individuals with physical or mental disabilities to find employment, retain employment and so they feel better about themselves and can live more independently.

Missouri

4545 **Rehabilitation Services for the Blind**
615 E 13th St
Ste 409
Kansas City, MO 64106-2829 816-889-2677
800-592-6004
Fax: 816-889-2504
http://www.dss.mo.gov/fsd/rsb/index.htm
Rachel.M.Labrado@dss.mo.gov
Rachel Labrado, District Supervisor
Provides services to people with varing degrees of visual impairment, ranging from those who cannot read regular print to those who are totally blind. Services may include: job training, job placement, vocational rehabilitation, assistive technology, independent living skills, personal and home management, meal preparation, communications assistance, independent travel instruction, counseling and guidance, leisure activities and client assistant program.

4546 **State Vocational Rehabilitation Agency Department of Elementary & Secondary Education**
205 Jefferson St.
Jefferson City, MO 65109-6188 573-751-4212
877-222-8963
Fax: 573-751-1441
TDD: 573-751-0881
http://www.dese.mo.gov
Jeanne Loyd, Director
State vocational rehabilitation agencies provide direct services to persons with disabilities, including persons with learning disabilities. The services may include evaluation and diagnosis, counseling, guidance, and referral services, vocational and other training services, transportation to rehabilitation services, and assistive devices.

Montana

4547 **Easter Seals - Goodwill Career Designs Mountain**
Regional Service Center
4400 Central Ave
Great Falls, MT 59405-1641 406-761-3680
800-771-2153
Fax: 406-761-5110
http://www.esg.easterseals.com
sharonod@esgw.org
Michelle Belknap, President
Job skill training programs for adults with developmental disabilities.

4548 **Easter Seals - Goodwill Store**
425 1st Ave N
Great Falls, MT 59405-1641 406-761-3680
800-771-2153
Fax: 406-761-5110
TDD: 800-253-4093
http://www.esgw-nrm.easterseals.com
gwbillings@mcn.net
Shalene Sparling, Director
Provides vocational training sites for individuals with emotional, developmental and physical disabilities. Employees develop and improve work skills while gaining work experience.

4549 **Easter Seals - Goodwill Working Partners, Great Falls**
425 1st Ave N
Great Falls, MT 59405-1641 406-761-3680
800-771-2153
Fax: 406-761-5110
TDD: 800-253-4093
http://www.esgw-nrm.easterseals.com
joelc@csgw.org
Michelle Belknap, President
Russell Plath, Board Chair
Scott Wilson, 1st Vice Chair and Treasurer
Job training, employment services, vocational evaluation/situational assessment and work services.

4550 **Goodwill Staffing Services**
Easter Seals Goodwill Northern Rocky Mountain
425 1st Ave. N.
Great Falls, MT 59401 406-761-3680
http://www.easterseals.com/esgw
Marcie Bailey, Director
Temporary staffing company which provides effective solutions to businesses in Idaho by customizing staffing solutions to fit individual needs, fill orders promptly, and monitors job performance to ensure customer satisfaction.

4551 **State Vocational Rehabilitation Agency**
Department of Public Health & Human Services
111 North Sanders
P.O. Box 4210
Helena, MT 59604-4210 406-444-2590
877-296-1197
Fax: 406-444-3632
http://www.dphhs.mt.gov
Robert Wynia, Executive Director
Joe Mathews, Director
State vocational rehabilitation agencies provide direct services to persons with disabilities, including persons with learning disabilities. The services may include evaluation and diagnosis, counseling, guidance, and referral services, vocational and other training services, transportation to rehabilitation services, and assistive devices.

4552 **Workforce Development Services**
Easter Seals-Goodwill Northern Rocky Mountains
425 1st Ave. N.
Great Falls, MT 59401 406-761-3680
http://www.easterseals.com/esgw
Kim Osadchuk, Director
Job training, employment services, vocational evaluation/situational assessment and work services.

Nebraska

4553 **Camp Kaleo**
Easter Seals Nebraska
12565 West Center Road
Suite 100
Omaha, NE 68144-8144
402-345-2200
800-471-6425
TTY: 402-462-4721
http://www.ne.easterseals.com
Karen Ginder, President
Job training, employment services, vocational evaluation/situational assessment and work services.

4554 **State Vocational Rehabilitation Agency: Nebraska**
Nebraska Dept Of Educ. Vocational Rehabilitation
PO Box 94987
Lincoln, NE 68509-4987
402-471-3644
877-637-3422
Fax: 402-471-0788
TTY: 402-471-3659
http://www.vocrehab.state.ne.us
vr_stateoffice@vocrehab.state.ne.us
Cherly Ferree, Director
We help people with disabilities make career plans, learn job skills, get and keep a job. Our goal is to prepare people for jobs where they can make a living wage and have access to medical insurance.

Nevada

4555 **Bureau of Services to the Blind & Visually Impaired**
Nevada Dept Of Employment,Training&Rehabilitation
2800 E. St. Louis Avenue
Las Vegas, NV 89104
702-486-5230
800-326-6868
Fax: 775-684-4186
TTY: 702-486-1018
http://www.detr.state.nv.us
InternetHelp@nvdetr.org
Dennis A. Perea, Deputy Director/Interim Director
Services to the Blind and Visually Impaired (BSBVI) provides a variety of services to eligible individuals, whose vision is not correctable by ordinary eye care. Adaptive training, independence skills, low vision exams and aids, mobility training and vocational rehabilitation are offered.

4556 **Nevada Governor's Council on Rehabilitation & Employment of People with Disabilities**
2800 E. St. Louis Avenue
Carson City, NV 89713
775-684-3849
Fax: 775-684-3850
TTY: 775-687-5353
http://www.detr.state.nv.us
InternetHelp@nvdetr.org
Dennis A. Perea, Deputy Director/Interim Director
To help insure vocational rehabilitation programs are consumer oriented, driven and result in employment outcomes for Nevadans with disabilities. Funding for innovation and expansion grants.

4557 **Rehabilitation Division Department of Employment, Training & Rehabilitation**
Bureau of Services to Blind and Visually Impaired
500 East Third Street
Carson City, NV 89713
775-684-4040
Fax: 775-684-4184
TDD: 775-684-8400
TTY: 800-326-6868
http://www.detr.state.nv.us
InternetHelp@nvdetr.org
Dennis A. Perea, Deputy Director/Interim Director
Providing options and choices for Nevadans with disabilities to work and live independently. Our mission will be accomplished through planning, implementing and coordinating assessment, employment, independent living and training.

New Hampshire

4558 **Camp Sno Mo**
Easter Seals New Hampshire
Hidden Valley Reservation
260 Griswold Ln.
Gilmanton Iron Works, NH 03837
603-364-5818
Fax: 603-364-0230
http://www.nh.easterseals.com
rkelly@eastersealsnh.org
Larry J. Gammon, President
Elin A. Treanor, Chief Financial Officer
Robert Kelly, Camp Director
The camp gives children and young adults ages 11-21 with disabililties or special needs the chance to explore new adventures which develop confidence, gain courage and build new friendships. Some of the activities include swimming, canoeing, hiking, archery, woodcarving, and arts & crafts. Camp is also its own Venture Crew Troop No. 1990 as of the 2018 season. Allowing campers to become scouts and earn merit badges and advancement.

4559 **Easter Seals - Keene**
20 Norway Ave
Keene, NH 03431-3825
603-209-5619
800-307-2737
Fax: 603-352-1879
http://www.easterseals.com
Larry J. Gammon, President
Diana Castor, Primary Contact
Job training, employment services, vocational evaluation/situational assessment and work services.

4560 **Easter Seals - Manchester**
555 Auburn St
Manchester, NH 03103
603-623-8863
800-870-8728
http://www.easterseals.com/nh/
Larry Gammon, President
Elin Treanor, Chief Financial Officer
Nancy Rollins, Chief Operating Officer
Job training, employment services, vocational evaluation/situational assessment and work services.

4561 **New Hampshire Department of Health & Human Services**
129 Pleasant Street
Concord, NH 03301-3852
603-271-6200
800-322-9191
TDD: 800-735-2964
http://www.dhhs.nh.gov
Nick Toumpas, Director
Programs for individuals with disabilities or special needs.

4562 **State Vocational Rehabilitation Agency**
Department of Education
101 Pleasant Street
Concord, NH 03301-3494
603-271-3494
800-299-1647
Fax: 603-271-7095
TDD: 603-271-3471
TTY: 603-271-3471
http://www.education.nh.gov
Paul K Leather, Executive Director
Assisting eligible New Hampshire citizens with disabilities secure suitable employment, financial and personal independence by providing rehabilitation services.

New Jersey

4563 **Assistive Technology Advocacy Center-ATAC**
New Jersey Protection and Advocacy
210 South Broad Street
3rd Floor
Trenton, NJ 08608-2407
609-292-9742
800-922-7233
Fax: 609-777-0187
TTY: 609-633-7106
http://www.njpanda.org
advocate@drnj.com
Ellen Catanese, Director
Assists individuals in overcoming barriers in the system and making assistive technology more accessible to individuals with disabilities throughout the state.

4564 **Division of Family Development: New Jersey Department of Human Services**
Quakerbridge Plaza, Building 6
P.O. Box 716
Trenton, NJ 08625-0716
609-588-2000
Fax: 609-588-3051
http://www.state.nj.us
Jeanette Page-Hawkins, Director
Offers programs to individuals with disabilities.

4565 **Eden Family of Services**
Eden Services
One Eden Way
Princeton, NJ 08540-5711
609-987-0099
Fax: 609-987-0243
http://www.edenservices.org
info@edenservices.org
Tom Mc Cool, President
David Holmes EdD, Executive Director
Provides year round educational services, early intervention, parent training, respite care, outreach services, community based residential services and employment opportunities for individuals with autism.

4566 **New Jersey Council on Developmental Disabilities**
P.O. Box 700
Trenton, NJ 08625-0700
609-292-3745
800-792-8858
Fax: 609-292-7114
TDD: 609-777-3238
http://www.njddc.org
njddc@njddc.org
Elaine Buschbaum, Chair
Dr Allison Lozano, Executive Director
Douglas McGruher, Deputy Director
Promotes systems change, coordinates advocacy and research for 1.2 million residents with developmental and other disabilities.

4567 **New Jersey State Department of Education**
P.O.Box 500
Trenton, NJ 08625-0500
609-292-4469
http://www.state.nj.us
Lucille E Davy, Commissioner
Assists the disabled student with changes from the school environment to the working world.

4568 **Programs for Children with Special Health Care Needs**
NJ Department of Health
P.O. Box 360
Trenton, NJ 08625-0360
609-292-7837
800-367-6543
Fax: 609-292-9288
http://www.nj.gov/health/fhs/sch
Gloria Rodriguez, President
Assists families caring for children with long-term medical and developmental disabilities. Programs include early intervention and case management units

New Mexico

4569 **New Mexico Department of Labor: Job Training Division**
Office of Workforce Training and Development
401 Broadway NE
Albuquerque, NM 87102-3960
505-841-4000
http://www.dws.state.nm.us
reese.fullerton@state.nm.us
Reese Fullerton, Executive Director
Veronica Moya, Office Assistant
Helps citizens of New Mexico from all walks of life find appropriate vocational trainings, and job placement.

4570 **State of New Mexico Division of Vocational Rehabilitation**
491 Old Santa Fe Trail
Santa Fe, NM 87501-2753
505-827-6328
877-696-1470
TTY: 505-476-0412
http://www.dvrgetsjobs.com
rsmith@state.nm.us
Jim Parker, Director
Commited to improving the quality of life of those with disabilities by addressing program accessibility and economic self-sufficiency.

New York

4571 **Commission for the Blind & Visually Handicapped**
NYS Office Of Children & Family Services
52 Washington Street
Rensselaer, NY 12144-2796
518-473-7793
Fax: 518-486-7550
TDD: 518-473-1698
http://ocfs.ny.gov/main
Professionals and paraprofessionals are available to help those with low vision or blindness with vocational rehabilitation services.

4572 **Office of Curriculum & Instructional Support**
New York State Education Department
89 Washington Ave
Albany, NY 12234-1000
518-474-8892
Fax: 518-474-0319
http://www.p12.nysed.gov
NYSEDP12@mail.nysed.gov
Jean Stevens, Director
Works with those seeking General Educational Development diplomas and technical training.

4573 **Office of Vocational and Educational Services for Individuals with Disabilities**
New York State Department of Education
1 Commerce Plaza
Room 1624e Plz
Albany, NY 12234-0001
518-436-0008
800-222-5627
TTY: 519-486-3773
http://www.p12.nysed.gov
NYSEDP12@mail.nysed.gov
Harvey Rosenthal, Executive Director
Nancy Lauria, Director
Promotes educational equality and excellence for students with disabilities while ensuring that they receive the rights and protection to which they are entitled, assure appropriate continuity between the child and adult services systems, and provide the highest quality vocational rehabilitation and independent living services to all eligible people.

North Dakota

4574 **North Dakota Department of Career and Technical Education**
State Capital, 15th Floor
600 E Boulevard Ave, Dept. 270
Bismarck, ND 58505-0610 701-328-3180
Fax: 701-328-1255
http://www.nd.gov/cte
cte@nd.gov
Wayne Kutzer, Director and Executive Officer
Dwight Crabtree, Assistant State Director
Brenda Schuler, Administrative Officer
The mission of the Board for Vocational and Technical Education is to work with others to provide all North Dakota citizens with the technical skills, knowledge, and attitudes necessary for successful performance in a globally competitive workplace.

4575 **North Dakota Workforce Development Council**
North Dakota Department of Commerce
1600 E. Century Ave.
Suite 2
Bismarck, ND 58503-2057 701-328-5000
Fax: 701-328-5320
TTY: 800-366-6888
http://www.workforce.nd.gov
NDWorkforce@nd.gov
James Hirsch, Director
The role of the North Dakota Workforce Development Council is to advise the Governor and the Public concerning the nature and extent of workforce development in the context of North Dakota's economic development needs, and how to meet these needs effectively while maximizing the efficient use of available resources and avoiding unnecessary duplication of effort.

4576 **Vocational Rehabilitation**
North Dakota Department of Human Services
1237 West Divide Avenue
Suite 1B
Bismarck, ND 58501-1208 701-328-8950
800-755-2745
Fax: 701-328-8969
TDD: 701-328-8968
TTY: 701-328-8802
http://www.nd.gov/dhs/dvr
dhsvr@nd.gov
Nancy Mc Kenzie, Director
Assists individuals with disabilities to achieve competitive employment and increased independence through rehabilitation services.

4577 **Workforce Investment Act**
Governor's Employment & Training Forum
1000 E Divide Ave
POBox 5507
Bismarck, ND 58506-5507 701-328-2836
Fax: 701-328-1612
TDD: 800-366-6888
http://www.jobnd.com
mdaley@nd.gov
Maren Daley, Executive Director
Job service North Dakota

Ohio

4578 **Office of Workforce Development**
Ohio Department of Job and Family Services
30 E. Broad Street 32nd Floor
Columbus, OH 43215-1618 888-296-7541
Fax: 614-728-8366
http://jfs.ohio.gov/owd
John Weber, Deputy Director
Operates several US department of labor-funded programs that focus on improving Ohio's workforce through career and job search realted services, assistance to employers, training and education.

4579 **State Vocational Rehabilitation Agency**
Ohio Dept Of Rehabilitation Services Commission
150 E. Campus View Blvd.
Columbus, OH 43235-4604 614-438-1200
800-282-4536
Fax: 614-438-1257
TDD: 614-438-1726
TTY: 614-438-1200
http://ood.ohio.gov
rsc_rir@vscnet.a1.state.oh.us
John M Connelly, Executive Director
Bill Bishilany, Assistant Executive Director
Erik Williamson, Deputy Director
State vocational rehabilitation agencies provide direct services to persons with disabilities, including persons with learning disabilities. The services may include evaluation and diagnosis, counseling, guidance, and referral services, vocational and other training services, transportation to rehabilitation services, and assistive devices.

Oklahoma

4580 **State Vocational Rehabilitation Agency: Oklahoma Department of Rehabilitation Services**
3535 NW. 58th St.
Suite 500
Oklahoma City, OK 73112 405-951-3400
800-845-8476
Fax: 405-951-3529
http://www.okrehab.org
info@okdrs.gov
Noel Tyler, Executive Director
Mark Kinnision, Administrator, Vocational Rehab.
Tracy Brigham, Visual Services Administrator
State vocational rehabilitation agency that provides direct services to persons with disabilities, including persons with learning disabilities. The services may include evaluation and diagnosis counseling, guidance, referral services, vocational and other training services, transportation to rehabilitation services, and assistive devices.

4581 **Workforce Investment Act**
Oklahoma Employment Security Commission
Will Rogers Memorial Office Bldg.
2401 N. Lincoln Blvd., P.O. Box 52003
Oklahoma City, OK 73152-2003 405-557-7100
Fax: 405-557-7256
TDD: 800-722-0353
http://www.ok.gov
John Brock, Executive Director
Partnership of local goverments offering resource conservation and development and workforce development.

Oregon

4582 **Oregon Employment Department**
875 Union St NE
Salem, OR 97311 503-947-1470
877-345-3484
TTY: 503-947-1472
http://www.employment.oregon.gov
Laurie Warner, Director
Tom Fuller, Communciations Manager
Craig Spivey, Backup Manager
Supports economic stability for Oregonians and communities during times of unemployment through the payment of unemployment benefits. Serves businesses by recruiting and referring the best qualified applicants to jobs, and provides resources to diverse job seekers in support of their employment needs.

4583 **Recruitment and Retention Special Education Jobs Clearinghouse**
Teaching Research Institute
Western Oregon University
345 Monmouth Ave
Monmouth, OR 97361 503-838-8391
Fax: 503-838-8150
TTY: 503-838-9623
http://teachingresearchinstitute.org
samplesb@wou.edu
John Killoran, Director
A free on-line jobs clearinghouse with access to position openings in Oregon in the area of Special Education and related services. A Job Seeker Listing and resumes also sent via e-mail to districts and agencies looking for qualified individuals.

Pennsylvania

4584 **State Vocational Rehabilitation Agency: Pennsylvania**
Department of Labor & Industry
1521 N 6th St
Harrisburg, PA 17102-1104 717-787-5244
800-442-6351
Fax: 717-783-5221
TTY: 717-787-5244
http://www.portal.state.pa.us
wgannon@dli.state.pa.us
William Gannon, Executive Director
Provides individualized services to assist people with disabilities to pursue, obtain, and maintain satisfactory employment. Counselors are available for training, planning and placement services.

Rhode Island

4585 **Rhode Island Vocational and Rehabilitation Agency**
Rhode Island Department of Human Services
40 Fountain St
Providence, RI 02903-1898 401-421-7005
Fax: 401-421-9259
TDD: 401-421-7016
http://www.ors.ri.gov
ronald.racine@dhs.ri.gov
Ronald Racine, Acting Associate Director
John Microulis, Administrator
Roberta Greene-Whittemore, Assistant Administrator of VR
Assists people with disabilities to become employed and to live independently in the community. In order to achieve this goal, we work in partnership with the State Rehabilitation Council, our customers, staff and community.

4586 **State Vocational Rehabilitation Agency: Rhode Island**
Rhode Island Department of Human Services
40 Fountain St
Providence, RI 02903-1830 401-421-7005
Fax: 401-421-9259
TDD: 401-421-7016
http://www.ors.ri.gov
ronald.racine@dhs.ri.gov
Ronald Racine, Acting Associate Director
John Microulis, Administrator
Roberta Greene-Whittemore, Assistant Administrator of VR
Assists people with disabilities to become employed and to live independently in the community. In order to achieve this goal, we work in partnership with the State Rehabilitation Council, our customers, staff and community.

South Carolina

4587 **Americans with Disabilities Act Assistance Line**
Employment Security Commission
1550 Gadsden Street
P.O. Box 995
Columbia, SC 29202-1406 803-737-9935
800-436-8190
Fax: 803-737-0140
http://www.sces.org
rratterree@sces.org
Regina Ratterree, Director
Provides information, technical assistance and training on the Americans with Disabilities Act.

4588 **South Carolina Vocational Rehabilitation Department**
PO Box 15
West Columbia, SC 29171-0015 803-896-6500
Fax: 803-896-6529
TTY: 803-896-6500
http://www.scvrd.net
info@scrvd.state.sc.us
Barbara G Hollis, Commissioner
Enabling eligible South Carolinians with disabilities to prepare for, achieve and maintain competitive employment.

South Dakota

4589 **South Dakota Department of Labor**
700 Governors Dr
Pierre, SD 57501-2291 605-773-3165
800-952-3216
Fax: 605-773-6184
TDD: 605-773-5017
TTY: 605-773-3101
http://www.dss.sd.gov
Mike Ryan, Director
Job training programs provide an important framework for developing public-private sector partnerships. We help prepare South Dakotans of all ages for entry or re-entry into the labor force.

4590 **South Dakota Department of Social Services**
700 Governors Dr
Pierre, SD 57501-2291 605-773-3165
Fax: 605-773-4855
http://www.dss.sd.gov
Deborah K Bowman, Director

4591 **South Dakota Rehabilitation Center forthe Blind**
Department of Human Services
Ste 101
2900 W 11th St
Sioux Falls, SD 57104-2594 605-334-4491
800-658-5441
Fax: 605-367-5263
TTY: 605-367-5260
http://www.dss.sd.gov
dawn.backer@state.sd.us
Gaye Mattke, Director
Helping people lead a full, productive life — regardless of how much one does or does not see. Upon completion of training, individuals usually return to their community and use these new skills in their home, school or job.

4592 **State Vocational Rehabilitation Agency**
Division of Rehabilitation Services
East Highway 34
Hillsview Plaza
Pierre, SD 57501-5070 605-773-3195
800-265-9684
Fax: 605-773-5483
TDD: 605-773-3195
http://www.dhs.sd.gov/drs
steve.stewart@state.sd.us
Grady Kickul, Executive Director

Assists individuals with disabilities to obtain employment, economic self-sufficiency, personal independence and full inclusion into society.

Tennessee

4593 State Vocational Rehabilitation Agency
Tennessee Department of Human Services
Citizens Plaza State Office Buildin
2nd Floor, 400 Deaderick Street
Nashville, TN 37243-1403
615-313-4891
866-311-4288
Fax: 615-741-6508
TTY: 615-313-5695
http://tennessee.gov/humanserv/rehab/vrs.html
car.w.brown@state.tn.us
Terry Smith, Director
State vocational rehabilitation agencies provide direct services to persons with disabilities, including persons with learning disabilities. The services may include evaluation and diagnosis counseling, guidance, and referral services, vocational and other training services, transportation to rehabilitation services and assistive devices.

4594 Tennessee Department of Education
Tennessee Department of Education
710 James Robertson Parkway
Nashville, TN 37243-0382
615-741-5158
800-531-1515
http://www.tn.gov/education/
education.comments@tn.gov
Kevin S. Huffman, Commissioner
Kathleen Airhart, Deputy Commissioner
Hanseul Kang, Chief of Staff
Mission is to take Tennessee to the top in education. Guides administration of the state's K-12 public schools.

4595 Tennessee Department of Labor & Workforce Development: Office of Adult Education
11th Fl
500 James Robertson Pkwy
Nashville, TN 37243-1204
615-741-7054
800-531-1515
Fax: 615-532-4899
TDD: 800-848-0299
http://www.tn.gov/labor-wfd/AE/
Phyllis.Pardue@tn.gov
Burns Phillips, Commissioner
Dustin Swayne, Deputy Commissioner
Marva Doremus, Administrator

4596 Tennessee Services for the Blind
Tennessee Department Of Human Services
400 Deaderick Street
2nd Floor
Nashville, TN 37243-1403
615-313-4700
800-628-7818
Fax: 615-313-6617
TDD: 615-313-6601
TTY: 615-313-6601
http://www.state.tn.us
Human-Services.Webmaster@state.tn.us
Terry Smith, Director
Offering training and services to help blind or low-vision citizens of Tennessee become more independent at home, in the community and at work.

Texas

4597 Department of Assistive & Rehabilitative Services
Texas Department of Health & Human Services
4800 N Lamar Blvd
Austin, TX 78756-3106
512-377-0500
800-628-5115
TTY: 866-581-9328
http://www.dars.state.tx.us
DARS.Inquiries@dars.state.tx.us
Veronda L. Durden, Commissioner
Glenn Neal, Deputy Commissioner
Karin Hill, Director of Internal Audit
Transitional and vocational programs aid independence in the home, community and at work for Texans who are blind, deaf, or have other impairments that would benefit from assistive technology.

4598 State Vocational Rehabilitation Agency
Texas State Rehabilitation Commission
4800 N Lamar Blvd
Austin, TX 78756-3106
512-424-4000
800-628-5115
Fax: 512-424-4337
TTY: 800-628-5115
http://www.dars.state.tx.us
DARS.Inquiries@dars.state.tx.us
Veronda L. Durden, Commissioner
Glenn Neal, Deputy Commissioner
Karin Hill, Director of Internal Audit
State vocational rehabilitation agencies provide direct services to persons with disabilities, including persons with learning disabilities. The services may include evaluation and diagnosis, counseling, guidance, and referral services, vocational and other training services, transportation to rehabilitation services and assistive devices.

4599 Texas Department of Assistive and Rehabilitative Services
4800 N Lamar Blvd
Austin, TX 78756-3106
512-377-0500
800-628-5115
Fax: 512-424-4730
TTY: 866-581-9328
http://www.dars.state.tx.us
DARS.Inquiries@dars.state.tx.us
Veronda L. Durden, Commissioner
Glenn Neal, Deputy Commissioner
Karin Hill, Director of Internal Audit
A place where people with disabilities and families with children who have developmental delays enjoys independent and productive lives. The mission is to wo

4600 Texas Workforce Commission
101 E 15th St
Austin, TX 78778-0001
512-463-2294
Fax: 512-475-2321
TDD: 800-735-2989
http://www.twc.state.tx.us
larry.temple@twc.state.tx.us
Larry Temple, Executive Director
Provides oversight, coordination, guidance, planning, technical assistance and implementation of employment and training activities with a focus on meeting the needs of employers throughout the state of Texas.

Utah

4601 Adult Education Services
Utah State Office of Education
250 East 500 South
Salt Lake City, UT 84114-4200
801-538-7500
Fax: 801-538-7882
http://www.schools.utah.gov
marty.kelly@schools.utah.gov
Marty Kelly, Director

Provides oversight of state and federally funded adult education programs. Offers adult basic education, adult high school completion, English as a second language, and general education development programs.

4602 **Utah State Office of Rehabilitation**
250 E 500 S
Salt Lake City, UT 84111-4200 801-538-7500
Fax: 801-538-7882
http://www.schools.utah.gov
Russell Thelin, Director
Assisting and empowering eligible individuals. Disabled, learning disabled, blind, low vision and deaf people can prepare for and obtain employment and increase their independence through job training and assistive technology.

Vermont

4603 **Adult Education & Literacy**
State Department of Education
120 State St
Montpelier, VT 05602-2703 802-828-3101
Fax: 802-828-3146
http://wwww.education.vermont.gov
edinfo@education.state.vt.us
Kay Charron, Director
Provides adults with educational opportunities to acquire the essential skills and knowledge to achieve career, post-secondary and life goals.

4604 **State of Vermont Department of Education: Adult Education and Literacy**
120 State Street
Montpelier, VT 05602 802-828-3101
Fax: 802-828-3146
http://www.vermont.gov
Kay Charron, Director
Adult Education and Literacy Programs provide adults with educational opportunities to acquire the essential skills and knowledge to achieve career, post-secondary and life goals. The Department of Education supports and administers a number of programs that focus on essential literacy and academic skills as well as workplace and introductory occupational skills.

4605 **Vermont Dept of Employment & Training**
5 Green Mountain Drive
P.O. Box 488
Montpelier, VT 05601-0488 802-828-4000
Fax: 802-828-4022
TDD: 802-825-4203
http://www.labor.vermont.gov
Mike Calcagni, Director
The Disability Program Navigator Initiative provides professionals who help individuals with disabilities to find jobs, gain access to jobs, or help in re-entering the job market.

4606 **Vermont Division of Vocational Rehabilitation**
VocRehab Of Vermont
103 South Main Street
Weeks 1A Building
Waterbury, VT 05671-2303 866-879-6757
TTY: 802-241-1455
http://www.vocrehab.vermont.gov
jana.sherman@ahs.state.vt.us
Diane Dalmasse, Director of VocRehab Division
VocRehab's mission is to assist Vermonters with disabilities, find and maintain meaningful employment in their communities. VocRehab Vermont works in close partnership with the Vermont Association of Business, Industry and Rehabilitation. Contact local VocRehab office for information about services.

4607 **Vermont Family Network**
600 Blair Park Road
Suite 240
Williston, VT 05495-7549 802-876-5315
800-800-4005
Fax: 802-876-6291
http://www.vermontfamilynetwork.org
info@vtfn.org
June Heston, President/CEO
Provides educational programs for children and young adults with special educational needs.

4608 **VocRehab Reach-Up Program**
VocRehab Of Vermont
103 South Main Street
Weeks 1A Building
Waterbury, VT 05671-2303 802-241-1455
866-879-6757
Fax: 802-241-2830
http://www.vocrehabvermont.org
jana.sherman@ahs.state.vt.us
Pamela Dalley, Director
The program helps individuals with disabilities find meaningful work at a level that is appropriate for them.

Virginia

4609 **Virginia Department of Rehabilitative Services**
8004 Franklin Farms Dr
Richmond, VA 23229-5019 804-662-7000
800-552-5019
Fax: 804-662-9532
TTY: 804-662-9040
http://www.vadrs.org
James.Rothrock@drs.virginia.gov
James Rothrock, Commissioner
In partnership with people with disabilities and their families, the Virginia Department of Rehabilitative Services collaborates with the public and private sectors to provide and advocate for the highest quality services that empower individuals with disabilities to maximize their employment, independence and engagement in the community.

Washington

4610 **State Vocational Rehabilitation Agency: Washington Division of Vocational Rehabilitation**
Department of Social Services & Health
P.O.Box 45340
Olympia, WA 98504-5340 360-725-3636
800-637-5627
Fax: 360-438-8007
TDD: 360-438-8000
TTY: 360-438-8000
http://www.dshs.wa.gov
obrien@dshs.wa.gov
Michael O'Brien, Director
State vocational rehabilitation agencies provide direct services to persons with disabilities, including persons with learning disabilities. The services may include evaluation and diagnosis, counseling, guidance, and referral services, vocational and other training services, transportation to rehabilitation services, and assistive devices.

4611 **State of Washington, Division of Vocational Rehabilitation**
P.O. Box 45340
Olympia, WA 98504-5340 360-725-3636
800-637-5627
Fax: 360-438-8007
http://www1.dshs.wa.gov
ruttllm@dshs.wa.gov
Lynnea Ruttledge, Director

Provides employment-related services to individuals with disabilities who want to work but need assistance. These individuals might experience difficulty getting or keeping a job due to a physical, sensory and/or mental disability. A DVR counselor works with each individual to develop a customized plan of services designed to help the individual achieve his or her job goal.

West Virginia

4612 **West Virginia Division of Rehabilitation Services**
West Virginia Department of Education & the Arts
107 Capitol St.
Charleston, WV 25301
304-356-2375
800-642-8207
http://www.wvdrs.org
Angela.r.walker@wv.gov

Marijane Waldron, Director
Susan Weinberger, Assistant Director
Angela Walker, Program Specialist, Trans./Ed.
A state agency responsible for the operation of the state and federal vocational rehabilitation program in West Virginia. Specializes in providing Pre-Employment Transition Services, as well as services to employers to facilitate transition to employment for individuals with disabilities.

Wisconsin

4613 **Wisconsin Division of Vocational Rehabilitation**
PO Box 7852
Madison, WI 53707-7852
608-261-0050
800-442-3477
Fax: 608-266-1133
TDD: 888-877-5939
http://dwd.wisconsin.gov/dvr
dwddvr@dwd.wisconsin.gov

Charlene Dwyer, Administrator
Federal and state program designed to obtain, maintain and improve employment for people with disabilities by working with vocational rehabilitation consumers, employers and other partners.

Wyoming

4614 **Wyoming Department of Workforce Services: State Vocational Rehabilitation Agency**
1510 E Pershing Blvd
Cheyenne, WY 82002-0001
307-777-3700
Fax: 307-777-5870
TTY: 307-777-7389
http://www.wyomingworkforce.org
jmcint@state.wy.us

Norma Whitney, Vocational Rehabilitation
Assists Wyoming citizens with disabilities to prepare for, enter into, and return to suitable employment. Individuals with a disability that prevents them from working may apply for these services as long as a physical or mental impairment which constitutes or results in a substantial impediment to employment exists, and they have the ability to benefit in terms of an employment outcome from vocational services.

A

B

C

D

E

F

G

H

I

J

K

L

M

O

P

Q

R

S

T

V

W

X

Y

Z

Alabama

Alaska

Arizona

Arkansas

California

Canada

Colorado

Connecticut

Delaware

District of Columbia

Florida

Georgia

Hawaii

Idaho

Illinois

Indiana

Iowa

Kansas

Kentucky

Louisiana

Maine

Maryland

Massachusetts

Michigan

Minnesota

Mississippi

Missouri

Montana

Nebraska

Nevada

New Hampshire

New Jersey

New Mexico

New York

North Carolina

North Dakota

Ohio

Oklahoma

Oregon

Pennsylvania

Rhode Island

South Carolina

South Dakota

Tennessee

Texas

Utah

Vermont

Virginia

Washington

West Virginia

Wisconsin

Wyoming

ADD/ADHD

Animation

Aphasia

Apraxia

Aptitude

Articulation

Arts

At-Risk

Autism

Behavioral Disorders

Bilingual Resources

Camps

Child Welfare

Civil Rights

Clearinghouses

Cognitive Disorders

College

Communication Disorders

Community Integration

Comprehension

Conceptual Skills

Conferences

Contemporary Education

Cooperative Learning Centers

Creative Expression

Crisis Intervention

Critical Thinking

Curriculum Guides

Daily Living

Databases

Developmental Disabilities

Directories

Discrimination

Dispute Resolution Dyslexia

Dyscalculia

Dyslexia

ESL

Economic Skills

Education

Elementary Education

Equality

Ethics

Evaluations

Eye/Hand Coordination

Family Involvement

Family Resources

Financial Resources

Fluency

Gameboards

Gifted Education

Graphing

Health Care

Hearing Impaired

Higher Education

History

Hotlines

Human Services

Inclusion

Infancy

Information Resources

Integration

International Associations

Intervention

Job/Vocational Resources

Keyboards

Kits

Language Skills

Leadership

Legal Issues

Libraries

Listening Skills

Literacy

Literature

Logic

Mainstreaming

Matching

Mathematics

Maturity

Memorization Skills

Motivation

Motor Development

Multicultural Education

Multisensory Education

Music

Neurological Disorders

Newsletters

Occupational Therapy

Pathology

Peer Programs

Perception Skills

Pets

Phonics

Physical Education

Play Therapy

Program Planning

Public Awareness & Interest

Publishers

Puzzles

Recognition Skills

Rehabilitation

Remediation

Research

Resource Centers

School Administration

Science

Secondary Education

Self-Advocacy

Self-Esteem

Sensory Integration

Siblings

Sign Language

Software

Sound Recognition

Special Education

Speech Skills

Spelling

Strategies

Student Workshops

Support Groups

Surveys

Switches

Synthesizers

Tape Recorders

Technology

Tourette Syndrome

Training

Transportation

Treatment

Visual Assistive Devices

Visual Discrimination

Vocabulary

Voice Output Devices

Volunteer

Workshop Training

Writing

2018 Title List

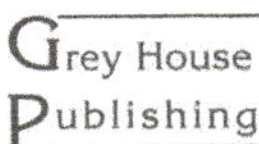

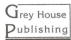

Visit www.GreyHouse.com for Product Information, Table of Contents, and Sample Pages

General Reference

America's College Museums
American Environmental Leaders: From Colonial Times to the Present
Encyclopedia of African-American Writing
Encyclopedia of Constitutional Amendments
Encyclopedia of Human Rights and the United States
Encyclopedia of Invasions & Conquests
Encyclopedia of Prisoners of War & Internment
Encyclopedia of Religion & Law in America
Encyclopedia of Rural America
Encyclopedia of the Continental Congress
Encyclopedia of the United States Cabinet, 1789-2010
Encyclopedia of War Journalism
Encyclopedia of Warrior Peoples & Fighting Groups
The Environmental Debate: A Documentary History
The Evolution Wars: A Guide to the Debates
From Suffrage to the Senate: America's Political Women
Gun Debate: An Encyclopedia of Gun Rights & Gun Control in the U.S.
Opinions throughout History: National Security vs. Civil and Privacy Rights
Opinions throughout History: Immigration
Opinions throughout History: Drug Abuse & Drug Epidemics
Political Corruption in America
Privacy Rights in the Digital Era
The Religious Right: A Reference Handbook
Speakers of the House of Representatives, 1789-2009
This is Who We Were: 1880-1900
This is Who We Were: A Companion to the 1940 Census
This is Who We Were: In the 1900s
This is Who We Were: In the 1910s
This is Who We Were: In the 1920s
This is Who We Were: In the 1940s
This is Who We Were: In the 1950s
This is Who We Were: In the 1960s
This is Who We Were: In the 1970s
This is Who We Were: In the 1980s
This is Who We Were: In the 1990s
This is Who We Were: In the 2000s
U.S. Land & Natural Resource Policy
The Value of a Dollar 1600-1865: Colonial Era to the Civil War
The Value of a Dollar: 1860-2014
Working Americans 1770-1869 Vol. IX: Revolutionary War to the Civil War
Working Americans 1880-1999 Vol. I: The Working Class
Working Americans 1880-1999 Vol. II: The Middle Class
Working Americans 1880-1999 Vol. III: The Upper Class
Working Americans 1880-1999 Vol. IV: Their Children
Working Americans 1880-2015 Vol. V: Americans At War
Working Americans 1880-2005 Vol. VI: Women at Work
Working Americans 1880-2006 Vol. VII: Social Movements
Working Americans 1880-2007 Vol. VIII: Immigrants
Working Americans 1880-2009 Vol. X: Sports & Recreation
Working Americans 1880-2010 Vol. XI: Inventors & Entrepreneurs
Working Americans 1880-2011 Vol. XII: Our History through Music
Working Americans 1880-2012 Vol. XIII: Education & Educators
Working Americans 1880-2016 Vol. XIV: Industry Through the Ages
Working Americans 1880-2017 Vol. XV: Politics & Politicians
World Cultural Leaders of the 20th & 21st Centuries

Education Information

Charter School Movement
Comparative Guide to American Elementary & Secondary Schools
Complete Learning Disabilities Directory
Educators Resource Handbook
Special Education: Policy and Curriculum Development

Health Information

Comparative Guide to American Hospitals
Complete Directory for Pediatric Disorders
Complete Directory for People with Chronic Illness
Complete Directory for People with Disabilities
Complete Mental Health Directory
Diabetes in America: Analysis of an Epidemic
Guide to Health Care Group Purchasing Organizations
Guide to U.S. HMO's & PPO's
Medical Device Market Place
Older Americans Information Directory

Business Information

Complete Television, Radio & Cable Industry Directory
Directory of Business Information Resources
Directory of Mail Order Catalogs
Directory of Venture Capital & Private Equity Firms
Environmental Resource Handbook
Financial Literacy Starter Kit
Food & Beverage Market Place
Grey House Homeland Security Directory
Grey House Performing Arts Directory
Grey House Safety & Security Directory
Hudson's Washington News Media Contacts Directory
New York State Directory
Sports Market Place Directory

Statistics & Demographics

American Tally
America's Top-Rated Cities
America's Top-Rated Smaller Cities
Ancestry & Ethnicity in America
The Asian Databook
Comparative Guide to American Suburbs
The Hispanic Databook
Profiles of America
"Profiles of" Series - State Handbooks
Weather America

Financial Ratings Series

Financial Literacy Basics
TheStreet Ratings' Guide to Bond & Money Market Mutual Funds
TheStreet Ratings' Guide to Common Stocks
TheStreet Ratings' Guide to Exchange-Traded Funds
TheStreet Ratings' Guide to Stock Mutual Funds
TheStreet Ratings' Ultimate Guided Tour of Stock Investing
Weiss Ratings' Consumer Guides
Weiss Ratings' Financial Literary Basic Guides
Weiss Ratings' Guide to Banks
Weiss Ratings' Guide to Credit Unions
Weiss Ratings' Guide to Health Insurers
Weiss Ratings' Guide to Life & Annuity Insurers
Weiss Ratings' Guide to Property & Casualty Insurers

Bowker's Books In Print® Titles

American Book Publishing Record® Annual
American Book Publishing Record® Monthly
Books In Print®
Books In Print® Supplement
Books Out Loud™
Bowker's Complete Video Directory™
Children's Books In Print®
El-Hi Textbooks & Serials In Print®
Forthcoming Books®
Law Books & Serials In Print™
Medical & Health Care Books In Print™
Publishers, Distributors & Wholesalers of the US™
Subject Guide to Books In Print®
Subject Guide to Children's Books In Print®

Canadian General Reference

Associations Canada
Canadian Almanac & Directory
Canadian Environmental Resource Guide
Canadian Parliamentary Guide
Canadian Venture Capital & Private Equity Firms
Canadian Who's Who
Financial Post Directory of Directors
Financial Services Canada
Governments Canada
Health Guide Canada
The History of Canada
Libraries Canada
Major Canadian Cities

SALEM PRESS SALEM PRESS

2018 Title List

Visit www.SalemPress.com for Product Information, Table of Contents, and Sample Pages

Science, Careers & Mathematics

Ancient Creatures
Applied Science
Applied Science: Engineering & Mathematics
Applied Science: Science & Medicine
Applied Science: Technology
Biomes and Ecosystems
Careers in the Arts: Fine, Performing & Visual
Careers in Building Construction
Careers in Business
Careers in Chemistry
Careers in Communications & Media
Careers in Environment & Conservation
Careers in Financial Services
Careers in Green Energy
Careers in Healthcare
Careers in Hospitality & Tourism
Careers in Human Services
Careers in Law, Criminal Justice & Emergency Services
Careers in Manufacturing
Careers in Outdoor Jobs
Careers in Overseas Jobs
Careers in Physics
Careers in Sales, Insurance & Real Estate
Careers in Science & Engineering
Careers in Sports & Fitness
Careers in Social Media
Careers in Sports Medicine & Training
Careers in Technology Services & Repair
Computer Technology Innovators
Contemporary Biographies in Business
Contemporary Biographies in Chemistry
Contemporary Biographies in Communications & Media
Contemporary Biographies in Environment & Conservation
Contemporary Biographies in Healthcare
Contemporary Biographies in Hospitality & Tourism
Contemporary Biographies in Law & Criminal Justice
Contemporary Biographies in Physics
Earth Science
Earth Science: Earth Materials & Resources
Earth Science: Earth's Surface and History
Earth Science: Physics & Chemistry of the Earth
Earth Science: Weather, Water & Atmosphere
Encyclopedia of Energy
Encyclopedia of Environmental Issues
Encyclopedia of Environmental Issues: Atmosphere and Air Pollution
Encyclopedia of Environmental Issues: Ecology and Ecosystems
Encyclopedia of Environmental Issues: Energy and Energy Use
Encyclopedia of Environmental Issues: Policy and Activism
Encyclopedia of Environmental Issues: Preservation/Wilderness Issues
Encyclopedia of Environmental Issues: Water and Water Pollution
Encyclopedia of Global Resources
Encyclopedia of Global Warming
Encyclopedia of Mathematics & Society
Encyclopedia of Mathematics & Society: Engineering, Tech, Medicine
Encyclopedia of Mathematics & Society: Great Mathematicians
Encyclopedia of Mathematics & Society: Math & Social Sciences
Encyclopedia of Mathematics & Society: Math Development/Concepts
Encyclopedia of Mathematics & Society: Math in Culture & Society
Encyclopedia of Mathematics & Society: Space, Science, Environment
Encyclopedia of the Ancient World
Forensic Science
Geography Basics
Internet Innovators
Inventions and Inventors
Magill's Encyclopedia of Science: Animal Life
Magill's Encyclopedia of Science: Plant life
Notable Natural Disasters
Principles of Artificial Intelligence & Robotics
Principles of Astronomy
Principles of Biology
Principles of Biotechnology
Principles of Chemistry
Principles of Climatology
Principles of Physical Science
Principles of Physics
Principles of Programming & Coding
Principles of Research Methods
Principles of Sustainability
Science and Scientists
Solar System
Solar System: Great Astronomers
Solar System: Study of the Universe
Solar System: The Inner Planets
Solar System: The Moon and Other Small Bodies
Solar System: The Outer Planets
Solar System: The Sun and Other Stars
World Geography

Literature

American Ethnic Writers
Classics of Science Fiction & Fantasy Literature
Critical Approaches: Feminist
Critical Approaches: Multicultural
Critical Approaches: Moral
Critical Approaches: Psychological
Critical Insights: Authors
Critical Insights: Film
Critical Insights: Literary Collection Bundles
Critical Insights: Themes
Critical Insights: Works
Critical Survey of American Literature
Critical Survey of Drama
Critical Survey of Graphic Novels: Heroes & Super Heroes
Critical Survey of Graphic Novels: History, Theme & Technique
Critical Survey of Graphic Novels: Independents/Underground Classics
Critical Survey of Graphic Novels: Manga
Critical Survey of Long Fiction
Critical Survey of Mystery & Detective Fiction
Critical Survey of Mythology and Folklore: Heroes and Heroines
Critical Survey of Mythology and Folklore: Love, Sexuality & Desire
Critical Survey of Mythology and Folklore: World Mythology
Critical Survey of Novels into Film
Critical Survey of Poetry
Critical Survey of Poetry: American Poets
Critical Survey of Poetry: British, Irish & Commonwealth Poets
Critical Survey of Poetry: Cumulative Index
Critical Survey of Poetry: European Poets
Critical Survey of Poetry: Topical Essays
Critical Survey of Poetry: World Poets
Critical Survey of Science Fiction & Fantasy
Critical Survey of Shakespeare's Plays
Critical Survey of Shakespeare's Sonnets
Critical Survey of Short Fiction
Critical Survey of Short Fiction: American Writers
Critical Survey of Short Fiction: British, Irish, Commonwealth Writers
Critical Survey of Short Fiction: Cumulative Index
Critical Survey of Short Fiction: European Writers
Critical Survey of Short Fiction: Topical Essays
Critical Survey of Short Fiction: World Writers
Critical Survey of World Literature
Critical Survey of Young Adult Literature
Cyclopedia of Literary Characters
Cyclopedia of Literary Places
Holocaust Literature
Introduction to Literary Context: American Poetry of the 20th Century
Introduction to Literary Context: American Post-Modernist Novels
Introduction to Literary Context: American Short Fiction
Introduction to Literary Context: English Literature
Introduction to Literary Context: Plays
Introduction to Literary Context: World Literature
Magill's Literary Annual 2018
Masterplots
Masterplots II: African American Literature
Masterplots II: American Fiction Series
Masterplots II: British & Commonwealth Fiction Series
Masterplots II: Christian Literature
Masterplots II: Drama Series
Masterplots II: Juvenile & Young Adult Literature, Supplement
Masterplots II: Nonfiction Series
Masterplots II: Poetry Series
Masterplots II: Short Story Series
Masterplots II: Women's Literature Series
Notable African American Writers
Notable American Novelists
Notable Playwrights
Notable Poets
Recommended Reading: 600 Classics Reviewed
Short Story Writers

SALEM PRESS

2018 Title List

Visit www.SalemPress.com for Product Information, Table of Contents, and Sample Pages

History and Social Science

The 2000s in America
50 States
African American History
Agriculture in History
American First Ladies
American Heroes
American Indian Culture
American Indian History
American Indian Tribes
American Presidents
American Villains
America's Historic Sites
Ancient Greece
The Bill of Rights
The Civil Rights Movement
The Cold War
Countries, Peoples & Cultures
Countries, Peoples & Cultures: Central & South America
Countries, Peoples & Cultures: Central, South & Southeast Asia
Countries, Peoples & Cultures: East & South Africa
Countries, Peoples & Cultures: East Asia & the Pacific
Countries, Peoples & Cultures: Eastern Europe
Countries, Peoples & Cultures: Middle East & North Africa
Countries, Peoples & Cultures: North America & the Caribbean
Countries, Peoples & Cultures: West & Central Africa
Countries, Peoples & Cultures: Western Europe
Defining Documents: American Revolution
Defining Documents: American West
Defining Documents: Ancient World
Defining Documents: Asia
Defining Documents: Civil Rights
Defining Documents: Civil War
Defining Documents: Court Cases
Defining Documents: Dissent & Protest
Defining Documents: Emergence of Modern America
Defining Documents: Exploration & Colonial America
Defining Documents: Immigration & Immigrant Communities
Defining Documents: LGBTQ
Defining Documents: Manifest Destiny
Defining Documents: Middle Ages
Defining Documents: Middle East
Defining Documents: Nationalism & Populism
Defining Documents: Native Americans
Defining Documents: Political Campaigns, Candidates & Discourse
Defining Documents: Postwar 1940s
Defining Documents: Reconstruction
Defining Documents: Renaissance & Early Modern Era
Defining Documents: Secrets, Leaks & Scandals
Defining Documents: 1920s
Defining Documents: 1930s
Defining Documents: 1950s
Defining Documents: 1960s
Defining Documents: 1970s
Defining Documents: The 17th Century
Defining Documents: The 18th Century
Defining Documents: The 19th Century
Defining Documents: The 20th Century: 1900-1950
Defining Documents: Vietnam War
Defining Documents: Women
Defining Documents: World War I
Defining Documents: World War II
Education Today
The Eighties in America
Encyclopedia of American Immigration
Encyclopedia of Flight
Encyclopedia of the Ancient World
Fashion Innovators
The Fifties in America
The Forties in America
Great Athletes
Great Athletes: Baseball
Great Athletes: Basketball
Great Athletes: Boxing & Soccer
Great Athletes: Cumulative Index
Great Athletes: Football
Great Athletes: Golf & Tennis
Great Athletes: Olympics
Great Athletes: Racing & Individual Sports
Great Contemporary Athletes
Great Events from History: 17th Century
Great Events from History: 18th Century
Great Events from History: 19th Century
Great Events from History: 20th Century (1901-1940)
Great Events from History: 20th Century (1941-1970)
Great Events from History: 20th Century (1971-2000)
Great Events from History: 21st Century (2000-2016)
Great Events from History: African American History
Great Events from History: Cumulative Indexes
Great Events from History: LGBTG
Great Events from History: Middle Ages
Great Events from History: Secrets, Leaks & Scandals
Great Events from History: Renaissance & Early Modern Era
Great Lives from History: 17th Century
Great Lives from History: 18th Century
Great Lives from History: 19th Century
Great Lives from History: 20th Century
Great Lives from History: 21st Century (2000-2017)
Great Lives from History: American Women
Great Lives from History: Ancient World
Great Lives from History: Asian & Pacific Islander Americans
Great Lives from History: Cumulative Indexes
Great Lives from History: Incredibly Wealthy
Great Lives from History: Inventors & Inventions
Great Lives from History: Jewish Americans
Great Lives from History: Latinos
Great Lives from History: Notorious Lives
Great Lives from History: Renaissance & Early Modern Era
Great Lives from History: Scientists & Science
Historical Encyclopedia of American Business
Issues in U.S. Immigration
Magill's Guide to Military History
Milestone Documents in African American History
Milestone Documents in American History
Milestone Documents in World History
Milestone Documents of American Leaders
Milestone Documents of World Religions
Music Innovators
Musicians & Composers 20th Century
The Nineties in America
The Seventies in America
The Sixties in America
Sociology Today
Survey of American Industry and Careers
The Thirties in America
The Twenties in America
United States at War
U.S. Court Cases
U.S. Government Leaders
U.S. Laws, Acts, and Treaties
U.S. Legal System
U.S. Supreme Court
Weapons and Warfare
World Conflicts: Asia and the Middle East

Health

Addictions & Substance Abuse
Adolescent Health & Wellness
Cancer
Complementary & Alternative Medicine
Community & Family Health
Genetics & Inherited Conditions
Health Issues
Infectious Diseases & Conditions
Magill's Medical Guide
Nutrition
Nursing
Psychology & Behavioral Health
Psychology Basics

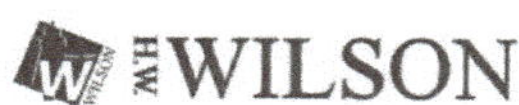

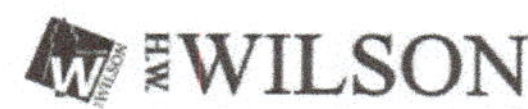

2018 Title List

Visit **www.HWWilsonInPrint.com** for Product Information, Table of Contents and Sample Pages

Current Biography

Current Biography Cumulative Index 1946-2013
Current Biography Monthly Magazine
Current Biography Yearbook: 2003
Current Biography Yearbook: 2004
Current Biography Yearbook: 2005
Current Biography Yearbook: 2006
Current Biography Yearbook: 2007
Current Biography Yearbook: 2008
Current Biography Yearbook: 2009
Current Biography Yearbook: 2010
Current Biography Yearbook: 2011
Current Biography Yearbook: 2012
Current Biography Yearbook: 2013
Current Biography Yearbook: 2014
Current Biography Yearbook: 2015
Current Biography Yearbook: 2016
Current Biography Yearbook: 2017

Core Collections

Children's Core Collection
Fiction Core Collection
Graphic Novels Core Collection
Middle & Junior High School Core
Public Library Core Collection: Nonfiction
Senior High Core Collection
Young Adult Fiction Core Collection

The Reference Shelf

Aging in America
Alternative Facts: Post Truth & the Information War
The American Dream
American Military Presence Overseas
The Arab Spring
Artificial Intelligence
The Brain
The Business of Food
Campaign Trends & Election Law
Conspiracy Theories
The Digital Age
Dinosaurs
Embracing New Paradigms in Education
Faith & Science
Families: Traditional and New Structures
The Future of U.S. Economic Relations: Mexico, Cuba, and Venezuela
Global Climate Change
Graphic Novels and Comic Books
Guns in America
Immigration
Immigration in the U.S.
Internet Abuses & Privacy Rights
Internet Safety
LGBTQ in the 21st Century
Marijuana Reform
The News and its Future
The Paranormal
Politics of the Ocean
Prescription Drug Abuse
Racial Tension in a "Postracial" Age
Reality Television
Representative American Speeches: 2008-2009
Representative American Speeches: 2009-2010
Representative American Speeches: 2010-2011
Representative American Speeches: 2011-2012
Representative American Speeches: 2012-2013
Representative American Speeches: 2013-2014
Representative American Speeches: 2014-2015
Representative American Speeches: 2015-2016
Representative American Speeches: 2016-2017
Representative American Speeches: 2017-2018
Rethinking Work
Revisiting Gender
Robotics
Russia
Social Networking
Social Services for the Poor
South China Seas Conflict
Space Exploration & Development
Sports in America
The Supreme Court
The Transformation of American Cities
U.S. Infrastructure
U.S. National Debate Topic: Educational Reform
U.S. National Debate Topic: Surveillance
U.S. National Debate Topic: The Ocean
U.S. National Debate Topic: Transportation Infrastructure
Whistleblowers

Readers' Guide

Abridged Readers' Guide to Periodical Literature
Readers' Guide to Periodical Literature

Indexes

Index to Legal Periodicals & Books
Short Story Index
Book Review Digest

Sears List

Sears List of Subject Headings
Sears: Lista de Encabezamientos de Materia

Facts About Series

Facts About American Immigration
Facts About China
Facts About the 20th Century
Facts About the Presidents
Facts About the World's Languages

Nobel Prize Winners

Nobel Prize Winners: 1901-1986
Nobel Prize Winners: 1987-1991
Nobel Prize Winners: 1992-1996
Nobel Prize Winners: 1997-2001

World Authors

World Authors: 1995-2000
World Authors: 2000-2005

Famous First Facts

Famous First Facts
Famous First Facts About American Politics
Famous First Facts About Sports
Famous First Facts About the Environment
Famous First Facts: International Edition

American Book of Days

The American Book of Days
The International Book of Days

Monographs

American Reformers
The Barnhart Dictionary of Etymology
Celebrate the World
Guide to the Ancient World
Indexing from A to Z
Nobel Prize Winners
The Poetry Break
Radical Change: Books for Youth in a Digital Age
Speeches of American Presidents

Wilson Chronology

Wilson Chronology of Asia and the Pacific
Wilson Chronology of Human Rights
Wilson Chronology of Ideas
Wilson Chronology of the Arts
Wilson Chronology of the World's Religions
Wilson Chronology of Women's Achievements